Contents

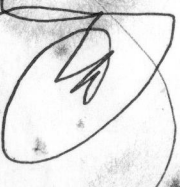

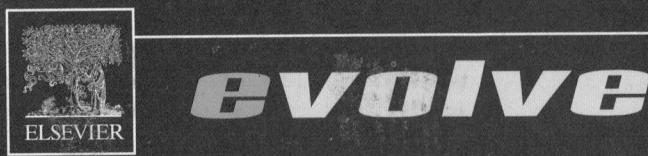

ELSEVIER

⁝• To access your Student Resources, visit the web address below:

http://evolve.elsevier.com/Sorrentino/NurseAsst/

Evolve® Student Resources for *Mosby's Textbook for Nursing Assistants,* **Seventh Edition,** offer the following features:

Student Resources

- **Video Clips**—Demonstrate important steps in procedures included in this textbook

- **Audio Glossary**—Provides definitions of all key terms in addition to audio pronunciations for selected key terms

- **Useful Spanish Vocabulary and Phrases**—Includes helpful translations of common healthcare terms and phrases

- **Skills Evaluation**—Reviews procedures that may be covered on certification reviews

- **Checklists**—Allow for instructor and self-evaluation

- **Body Spectrum**—Provides interactive review of Anatomy and Physiology content

Mosby's Textbook for Nursing Assistants

7th Edition

SHEILA A. SORRENTINO, PhD, RN

Curriculum and Health Care Consultant
Anthem, Arizona

With 752 Illustrations

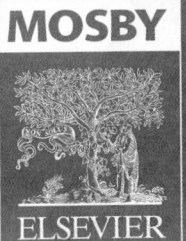

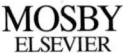

MOSBY
ELSEVIER

11830 Westline Industrial Drive
St. Louis, Missouri 63146

International Standard Book Number: 978-0-323-04994-8 (Softcover Edition)
978-0-323-04998-6 (Hardcover Edition)

Executive Editor: Susan R. Epstein
Senior Developmental Editor: Maria Broeker
Publishing Services Manager: John Rogers
Project Manager: Kathleen L. Teal
Text Designer: Teresa McBryan

Printed in Canada

Last digit is the print number: 9 8 7 6 5 4 3 2

To my nephew, Christopher Michael Bookhout,
Berklee College of Music Class of 2007,

I am so proud of you.
May you share your music and talents with the world.

With much love,
Aunt Sheila

About the Author

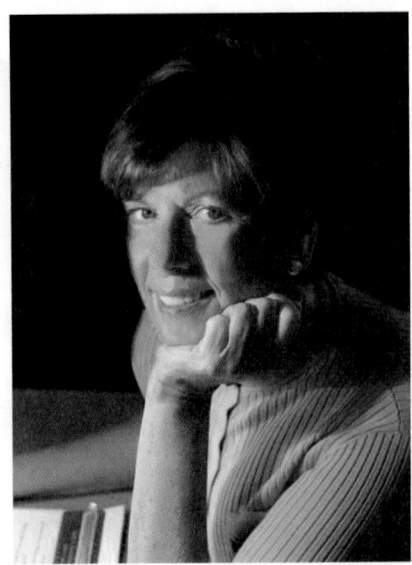

http://www.spindelvisions.com

Sheila A. Sorrentino is currently a curriculum and health care consultant focusing on effective delegation and partnering with nursing assistive personnel in hospitals, long-term care centers, and home care agencies.

Dr. Sorrentino was instrumental in the development and approval of CNA-PN-ADN programs in the Illinois Community College System and has taught in nursing assistant, practical nursing, associate degree, and baccalaureate and higher degree programs. Her career includes experiences as a nursing assistant, staff nurse, charge nurse, head nurse, nursing educator, assistant dean, dean, and consultant.

A Mosby author since 1982, Dr. Sorrentino is the author of several textbooks for nursing assistants and other nursing assistive personnel. She was also involved in the development of *Mosby's Nursing Assistant Skills Videos* and *Mosby's Nursing Skills Videos*, winner of the 2003 AJN Book of the Year Award (electronic media). An earlier version of nursing assistant skills videos won the 1992 International Medical Films Award on caregiving.

Dr. Sorrentino has a bachelor of science degree in nursing, a master of arts in education, a master of science degree in community nursing, and a PhD in higher education administration. She is a member of Sigma Theta Tau and former member and chair of the Central Illinois Higher Education Health Care Task Force. She also served on the Iowa-Illinois Safety Council Board of Directors and the Board of Directors of Our Lady of Victory Nursing Center in Bourbonnais, Ill. In 1998 she received an alumni achievement award from Lewis University for outstanding leadership and dedication in nursing education. In 2005 she was inducted into the Illinois State University College of Education Hall of Fame. Her presentations at national and state conferences focus on delegation and other issues relating to nursing assistive personnel.

Consultants and Reviewers

CONSULTANTS

Nancy J. Brent, RN, MS, JD
Nancy J. Brent, Attorney At Law
Wilmette, Illinois

Diann Muzyka, PhD, RN
Clinical Associate Professor
Arizona State University
College of Nursing and Healthcare Innovation
Phoenix, Arizona

REVIEWERS

Kathleen J. Bogucki, BSN, MA
Health Careers Instructor
Kent Career/Tech Center
Grand Rapids, Michigan

Ellen V. Gerlach, RN
Coordinator—CNA Programs
Southern Maine Community College
South Portland, Maine

Amy E. Green, RN, BSN
Registered Nurse
Edward Hospital and Health Services
Naperville, Illinois

Wendy Maleki, MS, RN
Associate Professor
Chaffey College
Rancho Cucamonga, California

Carla Wright, RN
Nursing Assistant Program Director
School of Health Sciences
College of Southern Nevada
Las Vegas, Nevada

Acknowledgments

Many individuals and agencies have contributed to this new, seventh edition of *Mosby's Textbook for Nursing Assistants* by providing information, insights, and resources. I am especially grateful and appreciative of the efforts by:

- The staff at Illinois Valley Community Hospital (IVCH) in Peru, Illinois, for graciously sharing policies and hosting the photo shoot. Jeanette Coughlin, MS, RN (Assistant Administrator of Patient Services), Mary Beth Sorrentino Herron (Benefits Coordinator–Human Resources), and Rose Mary Carrico, MS, RN (Nurse Manager) were especially helpful and accommodating. Maureen Rebholz, MS, RN (Director of Education) also contributed to the effort.
- The individuals who so graciously participated in the photo shoot: Linda Puchalski (a dear friend), Sophia Ferrari (family), and IVCH personnel: Rosemary Carrico (MS, RN), Dasia Barajas (CNA), Dave Fessler (RN), Kristina Martin (RN) and her son Travis, Karen Krysiak (RT), and Roger Tidaback (volunteer). Thank you all very, very much.
- Jane DeBlois, RN, Clinical Educator at OSF St. Joseph's Medical Center in Bloomington, Illinois, for being a valuable resource and always responding to information requests in a most timely manner.
- Tammy Taylor, RN, MSN, Associate Professor of Nursing at Heartland Community College in Normal, Illinois, and Julie White, RN, MSN, Dean of Allied Health at Wilbur Wright College (one of the City Colleges of Chicago) in Chicago, Illinois, for providing valuable insights and information and for serving as informal consultants.
- Diann Muzyka, PhD, RN, Clinical Associate Professor at Arizona State University College of Nursing and Healthcare Innovation in Phoenix, Arizona (formerly Coordinator of Health Programs and Community Education and Workforce Development at Columbus State Community College in Columbus, Ohio), for serving as a consultant, for her ideas and insights, and for writing the competency review section in the workbook. It is a valuable new workbook feature.
- Nancy Brent, JD, MS, RN (Willmette, Illinois), for researching legal cases to include in the "Focus on Ethics and Laws" boxes and for reviewing my work.
- Pamela K. Randolph, MSN, RN, Associate Director of Education and Evidenced Based Regulation and Joey Ridenour, MSN, RN, Executive Director at the Arizona State Board of Nursing (Phoenix, Arizona), for providing Board information and for sharing and reviewing cases for the "Focus on Ethics and Laws" boxes.
- Mary Beth Sorrentino Herron (family; IVCH in Peru, Illinois) for promptly accommodating countless requests for documents, deliveries, research, finding things in my office, facilitating the photo shoot, and many favors. What would I do without you?
- Ron Kurzejka, MD, Director of Emergency Medical Services at Provena St. Mary's Hospital in Kankakee, Illinois, for answering questions about emergency measures and procedures.
- The artists at Graphic World in St Louis, Missouri, for their talented work.
- Photographer Mike DeFilipo of St Louis, Missouri, for his great photos. He is very patient, cooperative, and flexible during photo shoots.
- Photographic artist David M. Spindel of Anthem, Arizona, for doing his very best to make me look good. And to his wife, Barbara, for assisting David and for helping me primp, straighten, and fluff!
- Kathleen J. Bogucki, BSN, MA, Ellen V. Gerlach, RN, Amy E. Green, BSN, RN, Wendy Maleki, MS, RN, and Carla Wright, RN for reviewing the manuscript and for their candor and suggestions. They have contributed to the thoroughness and accuracy of this book.
- Beth Welch (Columbus, Ohio) for serving as copy editor. It was a pleasure talking to her.
- Tina Kult, Tyson Sturgeon, Maria Broeker, and Kathy Teal—all of Elsevier/Mosby—for all their efforts in developing and producing the CD-ROM. It was a challenging but rewarding experience for all.
- And finally, to the talented and dedicated Elsevier/Mosby staff, especially:
  - Suzi Epstein (Executive Editor)—Suzi once again gave guidance and support and kept the project on track. She also stressed the importance of taking care of self and family. Suzi believes in me and supports me. Her vision, creativity, and resourcefulness are amazing. She is dedicated to her authors and titles and is a master at what she does.
  - Maria Broeker (Senior Developmental Editor)—Maria handled numerous details, manuscript needs, tasks, and issues. She always has an empathetic ear and time to listen to author wants, needs, and frustrations. I've said it many, many times, what would I do without Maria?
  - Mary Jo Adams (Editorial Assistant)—Mary Jo provided prompt clerical and secretarial assistance. She is simply pleasant and a delight to work with.
  - John Rogers (Publishing Services Manager) and members of his team—Kathy Teal (Senior Project Manager) and Beth Hayes (Senior Project Manager). With all the features and design elements of this book, Kathy again produced a user friendly and attractive layout.
  - Teresa McBryan (Senior Designer). Teresa took all of our ideas, some rather abstract, and created a unique and colorful book and cover design. As always, the book is distinctive from the rest.

And to all those who contributed to this effort in any way, I am sincerely grateful.

Sheila A. Sorrentino

Instructor Preface

As with previous editions of *Mosby's Textbook for Nursing Assistants*, the seventh edition serves to prepare students to function as nursing assistants in nursing centers, hospitals, and home care settings. This textbook serves the needs of students and instructors in community colleges, technical schools, high schools, nursing centers, hospitals, and other agencies. As students complete their education, the book is a valuable resource for the competency test review. And as part of one's personal library, the book is a reference for the nursing assistant who seeks to review or learn additional information for safe care.

The book emphasizes the needs of individuals across the life span. Patients and residents of all ages are presented as *persons* with dignity and value who have a past, a present, and a future. Caring, understanding, and protecting and respecting the person's rights, and respecting patients and residents as persons with dignity and value are attitudes conveyed throughout the book.

Nursing assistants of today and tomorrow must have a firm understanding of the legal principles affecting their role. Both federal and state laws directly and indirectly define their roles, range of functions, and limitations. Nursing assistant roles and functions also vary among states and agencies. Therefore emphasis is given to nursing assistant responsibilities, limitations, and professional boundaries—specifically in Chapters 2 and 3 which focus on the legal and ethical aspects of the role. To further stress the importance of ethics and laws, a new seventh edition feature is *Focus on Ethics and Laws* boxes. Court cases and discipline actions taken by state boards of nursing are presented to illustrate the consequences of negligent actions and unprofessional conduct.

Nursing assistant functions and role limits also depend on effective delegation. Building on the delegation principles presented in Chapter 2, *Delegation Guidelines* are presented as they relate to procedures. They empower the student to seek information from the nurse and the care plan about critical aspects of the procedure and the observations to report and record. Step 1 of most procedures refers the student to the appropriate *Delegation Guidelines* boxes.

Safety and comfort have been core values of *Mosby's Textbook for Nursing Assistants*. The Safety Alert feature in the sixth edition has been expanded to *Promoting Safety and Comfort*. Integrated throughout the book, these boxes focus the student's attention on the need to be safe and cautious and to promote comfort when giving care. Step 1 of most procedures refers the student to the appropriate *Promoting Safety and Comfort* boxes. "Safety" and "Comfort" subtitles are used.

Besides legal aspects, delegation, and safety and comfort, work ethics also affect how nursing assistants function. To foster a positive work ethic, Chapter 4 focuses on workplace behaviors and practices. The goal is for the nursing assistant to be a proud, professional member of the nursing and health teams.

Being a productive and efficient member of the nursing and health teams requires good communication, teamwork, and time management. And good communication skills are needed when interacting with patients and residents. According to *Nurse Aide Training* (a November 2002 report from the Department of Health and Human Services, Office of the Inspector General), nursing assistant education has not adequately prepared nursing assistants with communication, teamwork, and time management skills. Therefore, two new features are:
- *Focus on Communication* boxes that suggest what to say and questions to ask when interacting with patients and residents and the nursing team.
- *Teamwork and Time Management* boxes that suggest ways to efficiently work with and help other nursing team members.

Because some chapters in the sixth edition were long and were going to be longer because of new guidelines and content, some lengthy chapters are divided into shorter ones to facilitate the teaching/learning process. And some features are combined for more efficient use of space and to allow new features:
- *Focus on Long-Term Care* and *Focus on Home Care* boxes in the sixth edition are now *Focus on Long-Term Care and Home Care*. "Long-Term Care" and "Home Care" are subtitles within the boxes.
- *Focus on Children* and *Focus on Older Persons* boxes in the sixth edition are now *Focus on Children and Older Persons*. "Children" and "Older Persons" are subtitles within the boxes.
- *The Nursing Assistant* chapter was divided into two chapters—*The Nursing Assistant* and *Ethics and Laws*.
- Fall prevention content was moved from the *Safety* chapter to Chapter 12, *Preventing Falls*.
- Body mechanics, moving the person in bed, turning, and transferring content and procedures are in two chapters: Chapter 15, *Body Mechanics* and Chapter 16, *Safely Handling, Moving, and Transferring the Person*.
- Enteral nutrition and IV therapy, previously in the chapter on *Nutrition and Fluids*, are now in Chapter 24, *Nutritional Support and IV Therapy*.
- The chapter on *Oxygen Needs* was made into two chapters: *Oxygen Needs* and *Respiratory Support and Therapies*.

- The *Common Health Problems* chapter is now five chapters with expanded content:
  - *Cancer, Immune System, and Skin Disorders*
  - *Nervous System and Musculoskeletal System Disorders*
  - *Cardiovascular and Respiratory System Disorders*
  - *Digestive and Endocrine System Disorders*
  - *Urinary and Reproductive System Disorders*

A most exciting feature is the CD-ROM in this book! Using video clips and animations, key procedures are presented along with interactive exercises. The CD also includes an audio glossary and the *Body Spectrum* program.

ORGANIZATIONAL STRATEGIES

These concepts and principles—that the patient or resident is a person, ethical and legal aspects, delegation, safety and comfort, and work ethics—serve as the guiding framework for this book. Other organizational strategies and values include:

- Understanding the work setting and the individuals in that setting
- Respecting patients and residents as physical, social, psychological, and spiritual beings with basic needs and protected rights
- Respecting personal choice and the person's dignity
- Appreciating the role of cultural heritage and religion in health and illness practices
- Understanding that knowledge about body structure and function is needed to give safe care and to safely perform nursing skills
- Following the principle that learning proceeds from the simple to the complex
- Recognizing that certain concepts and functions are foundational—safety, body mechanics, and preventing infection are central to other procedures
- Embracing the nursing process as the basis for planning and delivering nursing care and the role that nursing assistants play in assisting with the process

CONTENT ISSUES

With every edition, revision and content decisions are made. When changes are made in laws or in guidelines and standards issued by government or accrediting agencies, the decisions are easy. Content decisions also are based on state curricula and competency testing services. For example, while many agencies use electronic thermometers, some testing services test the skill of measuring an oral temperature with a glass (non-mercury) thermometer. Every attempt is made to make the book as up-to-date as possible with changes sometimes made right before publication.

Other content issues are more difficult. The learning needs and abilities of the student, instructor desires, work-related issues, and course/program and book length are among the factors considered. With such issues in mind, new and expanded content includes:

Chapter 1: Introduction to Health Care Agencies
- FOCUS ON LONG-TERM CARE AND HOME CARE: Organization

Chapter 2: The Nursing Assistant
- TEAMWORK AND TIME MANAGEMENT: Other OBRA Requirements
- FOCUS ON COMMUNICATION: Job Description
- Certification
- Working in Another State
- Nursing Assistant Standards
- FOCUS ON COMMUNICATION: Refusing a Task

Chapter 3: Ethics and Laws
- Professional Boundaries
- Box 3-2 Rules for Maintaining Professional Boundaries
- Box 3-3 Boundary Signs
- FOCUS ON COMMUNICATION: Professional Boundaries
- FOCUS ON ETHICS AND LAWS: Unintentional Torts
- Vulnerable Adults
- FOCUS ON LONG-TERM CARE AND HOME CARE: Vulnerable Adults
- Self-Neglect
- Box 3-6 Prosecuted Cases of Elder Abuse
- FOCUS ON LONG-TERM CARE AND HOME CARE: Domestic Abuse

Chapter 4: Work Ethics
- TEAMWORK AND TIME MANAGEMENT: Attendance
- FOCUS ON COMMUNICATION: Confidentiality
- FOCUS ON ETHICS AND LAWS: Sexual Harassment
- Drug Testing
- FOCUS ON ETHICS AND LAWS: Drug Testing

Chapter 5: Communicating With the Health Team
- TEAMWORK AND TIME MANAGEMENT: Reporting
- FOCUS ON ETHICS AND LAWS: Recording
- TEAMWORK AND TIME MANAGEMENT: End-of-Shift Report
- PROMOTING SAFETY AND COMFORT: End-of-Shift Report
- Commons Terms and Phrases
- Box 5-4 Common Health Care Terms and Phrases
- FOCUS ON COMMUNICATION: Dealing With Conflict

Chapter 6: Assisting With the Nursing Process
- Box 6-2 Observations to Report at Once
- FOCUS ON COMMUNICATION: Planning
- TEAMWORK AND TIME MANAGEMENT: Assignment Sheets

Chapter 7: Understanding the Person

- Addressing the Person
- Optimal Level of Function
- Persons With Disabilities
- TEAMWORK AND TIME MANAGEMENT: Behavior Issues

Chapter 10: Care of the Older Person

- Box 10-1 Myths and Facts About Aging
- FOCUS ON COMMUNICATION: Social Changes
- FOCUS ON ETHICS AND LAWS: Freedom from Abuse, Mistreatment, and Neglect
- TEAMWORK AND TIME MANAGEMENT: Activities
- FOCUS ON COMMUNICATION: Activities

Chapter 11: Safety

- FOCUS ON LONG-TERM CARE AND HOME CARE: Safety
- TEAMWORK AND TIME MANAGEMENT: A Safe Setting
- Gun Safety
- PROMOTING SAFETY AND COMFORT: Identifying the Person
- Lead Poisoning
- Box 11-4 Lead Poisoning
- FOCUS ON ETHICS AND LAWS: Choking
- FOCUS ON COMMUNICATION: Fire and the Use of Oxygen
- PROMOTING SAFETY AND COMFORT: What to Do During a Fire

Chapter 12: Preventing Falls

- TEAMWORK AND TIME MANAGEMENT: Causes and Risk Factors for Falls
- FOCUS ON COMMUNICATION: Fall Prevention Programs
- PROMOTING SAFETY AND COMFORT: Fall Prevention Programs
- FOCUS ON ETHICS AND LAWS: Transfer/Gait Belts
- FOCUS ON CHILDREN AND OLDER PERSONS: The Falling Person

Chapter 13: Promoting a Restraint-Free Environment

- Centers for Medicare and Medicaid (CMS) Guidelines
- FOCUS ON COMMUNICATION: Legal Aspects
- FOCUS ON COMMUNICATION: Safety Guidelines
- TEAMWORK AND TIME MANAGEMENT: Safety Guidelines

Chapter 14: Preventing Infection

- FOCUS ON LONG-TERM CARE AND HOME CARE: Healthcare-Associated Infection
- FOCUS ON ETHICS AND LAWS: Hand Hygiene
- Guideline for Isolation Precautions: Preventing Transmission of Infectious Agents in Healthcare Settings 2007
- FOCUS ON ETHICS AND LAWS: Isolation Precautions
- TEAMWORK AND TIME MANAGEMENT: Isolation Precautions
- FOCUS ON LONG-TERM CARE AND HOME CARE: Isolation Precautions
- FOCUS ON LONG-TERM CARE AND HOME CARE: Transmission-Based Precautions
- PROMOTING SAFETY AND COMFORT: Protective Measures
- PROMOTING SAFETY AND COMFORT: Goggles and Face Shields
- FOCUS ON COMMUNICATION: Meeting Basic Needs

Chapter 15: Body Mechanics

- FOCUS ON ETHICS AND LAWS: Ergonomics

Chapter 16: Safely Handling, Moving, and Transferring the Person

- PROMOTING SAFETY AND COMFORT: Safely Handling, Moving, and Transferring the Person
- FOCUS ON COMMUNICATION: Safely Handling, Moving, and Transferring the Person
- TEAMWORK AND TIME MANAGEMENT: Safely Handling, Moving, and Transferring the Person
- Preventing Work-Related Injuries
- DELEGATION GUIDELINES: Preventing Work-Related Injuries
- TEAMWORK AND TIME MANAGEMENT: Preventing Work-Related Injuries
- FOCUS ON CHILDREN AND OLDER PERSONS: Preventing Work-Related Injuries
- FOCUS ON ETHICS AND LAWS: Preventing Work-Related Injuries
- PROMOTING SAFETY AND COMFORT: Moving the Person Up in Bed
- PROMOTING SAFETY AND COMFORT: Moving the Person Up in Bed With an Assist Device
- FOCUS ON ETHICS AND LAWS: Raising the Person's Head and Shoulders
- TEAMWORK AND TIME MANAGEMENT: Transferring Persons
- Slings
- PROMOTING SAFETY AND COMFORT: Transferring the Person To and From a Toilet

Chapter 17: The Person's Unit

- FOCUS ON CHILDREN AND OLDER PERSONS: Noise
- FOCUS ON CHILDREN AND OLDER PERSONS: Lighting

Chapter 40: Cardiovascular and Respiratory System Disorders

- FOCUS ON CHILDREN AND OLDER PERSONS: Cardiovascular Disorders

Chapter 41: Digestive and Endocrine System Disorders

- Gastroesopahgeal Reflux Disease
- Gallstones

Chapter 42: Urinary and Reproductive System Disorders

- Prostate Enlargement

Chapter 43: Mental Health Problems

- Post-Traumatic Stress Disorder
- Box 43-3 Signs and Symptoms of Post-Traumatic Stress Disorder
- FOCUS ON ETHICS AND LAWS: Substance Abuse and Addiction
- Alcoholism and Alcohol Abuse
- FOCUS ON CHILDREN AND OLDER PERSONS: Alcoholism and Alcohol Abuse
- Drug Abuse and Addiction
- Suicide
- FOCUS ON CHILDREN AND OLDER PERSONS: Suicide
- FOCUS ON LONG-TERM CARE AND HOME CARE: Suicide
- Suicide Contagion
- Box 43-7 Risk Factors for Suicide
- FOCUS ON ETHICS AND LAWS: Care and Treatment

Chapter 44: Confusion and Dementia

- Mild Cognitive Impairment
- FOCUS ON COMMUNICATION: Care of Persons With AD and Other Dementias
- TEAMWORK AND TIME MANAGEMENT: Care of Persons With AD and Other Dementias
- FOCUS ON ETHICS AND LAWS: Care of Persons With AD and Other Dementias

Chapter 45: Developmental Disabilities

- FOCUS ON COMMUNICATION: Intellectual Disabilities (Mental Retardation)

Chapter 46: Sexuality

- FOCUS ON COMMUNICATION: The Sexually Aggressive Person
- FOCUS ON ETHICS AND LAWS: Protecting the Person

Chapter 47: Caring for Mothers and Newborns

- FOCUS ON HOME CARE AND LONG-TERM CARE: Cleaning Baby Bottles
- PROMOTING COMFORT AND SAFETY: Care of the Umbilical Cord

Chapter 48: Assisted Living

- TEAMWORK AND TIME MANAGEMENT: Laundry
- FOCUS ON COMMUNICATION: Medication Assistance

Chapter 49: Basic Emergency Care

- TEAMWORK AND TIME MANAGEMENT: Emergency Care
- Defibrillation
- PROCEDURE: Adult CPR With AED—Two Rescuers
- PROCEDURE: Child CPR With AED—Two Rescuers
- PROCEDURE: Infant CPR—Two Rescuers
- Rescue Breathing
- Epilepsy

Chapter 50: The Dying Person

- TEAMWORK AND TIME MANAGEMENT: The Dying Person
- FOCUS ON COMMUNICATION: Psychological, Social, and Spiritual Needs

Features and Design

Besides content issues, attention also is given to improving the book's features and designs. To make the book readable and user friendly, new features and design elements are added while others are retained (see Student Preface, p. xvi).

- **Illustrations**—the book contains numerous full-color photographs and line art.
- **Objectives**—list the learning objectives for the chapter.
- **Procedures**—a list of the procedures in the chapter follows the objectives. A CD icon identifies the procedures in the chapter that are part of *Mosby's Nursing Assistant CD Companion* and a video icon alerts you to a video clip on the Evolve website. *New!*
- **Key Terms with definitions**—are at the beginning of each chapter.
- **Key Abbreviations**—for quick reference, the abbreviations used in the chapter are listed in the chapter opening section. *New!*
- **Key Terms in bold print**—are throughout the text. The definition is presented in narrative in the text. Unlike other books, students do not have to turn to the margin for the definition, return to the text, and then try to understand the context of the term.

- **Boxes and tables**—list principles, guidelines, signs and symptoms, nursing measures, and other information. They are an efficient way for instructors to highlight content. And they are useful study guides for students.
- **Procedure icons**—in section headings alert the student to an associated procedure. Procedure boxes contain the same icon.
- **Delegation Guidelines**—are associated with procedures. They focus on the information needed from the nurse and the care plan about critical aspects of the procedure and the observations to report and record. Step 1 of most procedures refers the student to the appropriate *Delegation Guidelines.*
- **Promoting Safety and Comfort**—focus the student's attention on the need to be safe and cautious and promote comfort when giving care. "Safety" and "Comfort" subtitles are used. Step 1 of most procedures refers the student to the appropriate *Promoting Safety and Comfort* boxes.
- **Procedure boxes divided into Quality of Life, Pre-Procedure, Procedure, and Post-Procedure steps**—Each procedure section has a subtitle. *Quality of Life*, *Pre-Procedure* and *Post-Procedure* steps are included to show the procedure as a whole and reinforce learning. The *Quality of Life* section in the procedure boxes reminds the student of six fundamental courtesies:
  - Knock before entering the room.
  - Address the person by name.
  - Introduce one's self by name and title.
  - Explain the procedure to the person before beginning and during the procedure.
  - Protect the person's rights during the procedure.
  - Handle the person gently during the procedure.
- **CD icon**—in the procedure title bar alerts the student to an associated procedure on *Mosby's Nursing Assistant CD Companion*. *New!*
- **Video icon**—in the procedure title bar alerts the student to a video clip on the EVOLVE website. *New!*
- **NNAAP™**—appears in the procedure box title bar for skills included in the National Nurse Aide Assessment Program (NNAAP™).

- **Caring About Culture boxes**—serve to sensitize the student to cultural diversity and how culture influences health and illness practices.
- **Focus on Children and Older Persons boxes**—provide age-specific information about needs, considerations, and special circumstances of children. The feature is useful in meeting age-specific training requirements of The Joint Commission. Subtitles—"Children" and "Older Persons"—are used. The "Older Persons" sections contain useful information about persons with Alzheimer's disease and other dementias.
- **Focus on Long-Term Care and Home Care boxes**—highlight information unique to long-term care settings and for safe functioning in home settings. "Long-Term Care" and "Home Care" subtitles are used. For long-term care, information is included about the requirements of the Omnibus Budget Reconciliation Act of 1987 (OBRA).
- **Teamwork and Time Management boxes**—suggest ways to efficiently work with and help other nursing team members. *New!*
- **Focus on Communication boxes**—suggest what to say and questions to ask when interacting with residents and the nursing team. *New!*
- **Focus on Ethics and Laws boxes**—present summaries of court cases and state cases involving nursing assistant discipline actions. The intent is to sensitize the student to the consequences of not acting in a safe or professional manner. *New!*
- **Review Questions**—are found at the end of each chapter. A page number is given for where to find the answers. The goal is to provide the student with a mechanism to review the chapter content. The questions are not intended to be test questions. They are structured to allow a thorough review of the content.

May this book serve you and your students well. My intent is to provide you and your students with the current information needed to teach and learn safe and effective care during this time of dynamic change in health care.

Sheila A. Sorrentino, BSN, MA, MSN, PhD, RN

Student Preface

This book was designed for you. It was designed to help you learn. The book is a useful resource as you gain experience and expand your knowledge.

This preface gives some study guidelines and helps you use the book. When given a reading assignment do you read from the first page to the last page without stopping? How much do you remember? You will learn more if you use a study system. A useful study system has these steps:

- Survey or preview
- Question
- Read and record
- Recite and review

PREVIEW

Before you start a reading assignment, preview or survey the assignment. This gives you an idea of what the assignment covers. It also helps you recall what you already know about the subject. Carefully look over the assignment. Preview the chapter title, headings, subheadings, and terms or ideas in bold print or italics. Also survey the objectives, key terms, boxes, and review questions at the end of the chapter. Previewing only takes a few minutes. Remember, previewing helps you become familiar with the material.

QUESTION

After previewing, you need to form questions to answer while you read. Questions should relate to what might be asked on a test or how the information applies to giving care. Use the title, headings, and subheadings to form questions. Avoid questions that have one word answers. Questions that begin with what, how, or why are helpful. While reading, you may find that a question does not help you study. If so, just change the question. Remember, questioning sets a purpose for reading. So changing a question only makes this step more useful.

READ AND RECORD

Reading is the next step. Reading is more productive after determining what you already know and what you need to learn. Read to find answers to your questions. The purpose of reading is to:

- Gain new information
- Connect new information to what you know already

Break the assignment into smaller parts. Then answer your questions as you read each part. Also, mark important information—underline, highlight, or make notes. Underlining and highlighting remind you of what you need to learn. Go back and review the marked parts later. Making notes results in more immediate learning. To make notes, write down important information in the margins or in a notebook. Use words and statements to jog your memory about the material.

You need to remember what you read. To do so, work with the information. Organize information into a study guide. Study guides have many forms. Diagrams or charts show relationships or steps in a process. Note taking in outline format is also very useful. The following is a sample outline.

1. Main heading
   a. Second level
   b. Second level
      i. Third level
      ii. Third level
2. Main heading

RECITE AND REVIEW

Finally, recite and review. Use your notes and study guides. Answer the questions you formed earlier. Also answer other questions that came up when reading and answering the *Review Questions* at the end of a chapter. Answer all questions out loud (recite).

Reviewing is more about when to study rather than what to study. You already determined what to study during the preview, question, and reading steps. The best times to review are right after the first study session, one week later, and before a quiz or test.

This book was also designed to help you study. Special design features are described on the next pages.

I hope you enjoy learning and your work. You and your work are important. You and the care you give make a difference in the person's life!

Sheila A. Sorrentino

Objectives tell what is presented in the chapter.

Procedures list identifies the procedures presented in the chapter. A CD icon precedes those procedures that are also on the CD-ROM in this book. A video icon alerts you to a video clip on the Evolve website.

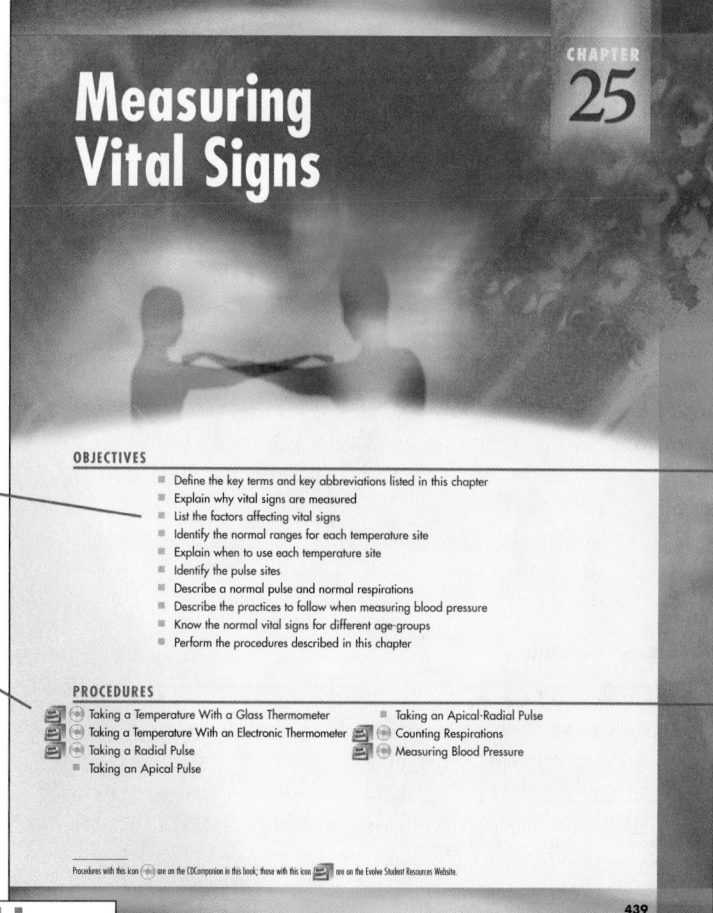

CHAPTER 25

Measuring Vital Signs

OBJECTIVES

- Define the key terms and key abbreviations listed in this chapter
- Explain why vital signs are measured
- List the factors affecting vital signs
- Identify the normal ranges for each temperature site
- Explain when to use each temperature site
- Identify the pulse sites
- Describe a normal pulse and normal respirations
- Describe the practices to follow when measuring blood pressure
- Know the normal vital signs for different age-groups
- Perform the procedures described in this chapter

PROCEDURES

- Taking a Temperature With a Glass Thermometer
- Taking a Temperature With an Electronic Thermometer
- Taking a Radial Pulse
- Taking an Apical Pulse
- Taking an Apical-Radial Pulse
- Counting Respirations
- Measuring Blood Pressure

Procedures with this icon are on the CDCompanion in this book; those with this icon are on the Evolve Student Resources Website.

439

---

440 MOSBY'S TEXTBOOK FOR NURSING ASSISTANTS

KEY TERMS

apical-radial pulse Taking the apical and radial pulses at the same time

blood pressure The amount of force exerted against the walls of an artery by the blood

body temperature The amount of heat in the body that is a balance between the amount of heat produced and the amount lost by the body

bradycardia A slow *(brady)* heart rate *(cardia)*; less than 60 beats per minute

diastole The period of heart muscle relaxation; the period when the heart is at rest

diastolic pressure The pressure in the arteries when the heart is at rest

fever Elevated body temperature

hypertension Blood pressure measurements that remain above *(hyper)* a systolic pressure of 140 mm Hg or a diastolic pressure of 90 mm Hg

hypotension When the systolic blood pressure is below *(hypo)* 90 mm Hg and the diastolic pressure is below 60 mm Hg

pulse The beat of the heart felt at an artery as a wave of blood passes through the artery

pulse deficit The difference between the apical and radial pulse rates

pulse rate The number of heartbeats or pulses felt in 1 minute

respiration Breathing air into *(inhalation)* and out of *(exhalation)* the lungs

sphygmomanometer A cuff and measuring device used to measure blood pressure

stethoscope An instrument used to listen to sounds produced by the heart, lungs, and other body organs

systole The period of heart muscle contraction; the period when the heart is pumping blood

systolic pressure The amount of force needed to pump blood out of the heart into the arterial circulation

tachycardia A rapid *(tachy)* heart rate *(cardia)*; more than 100 beats per minute

vital signs Temperature, pulse, respirations, and blood pressure

Key Terms are the important words and phrases in the chapter. Definitions are given for each term. The key terms introduce you to the chapter content. They are also a useful study guide.

KEY ABBREVIATIONS

A Axillary
Ap Apical
BP Blood pressure
C Centigrade; Celsius
CPR Cardiopulmonary resuscitation
F Fahrenheit

Hg Mercury
IV Intravenous
mm Millimeters
mm Hg Millimeters of mercury
R Rectal
TPR Temperature, pulse, and respirations

Key Abbreviations are a quick reference of the abbreviations used in the chapter. They are listed after the "Key Terms."

V ital signs reflect the function of three body processes essential for life: regulation of body temperature, breathing, and heart function. The four vital signs of body function are:

- Temperature
- Pulse
- Respirations
- Blood pressure

Vital signs are often called TPR (temperature, pulse, and respiration) and BP (blood pressure). Some agencies consider "pain" to be a vital sign. See Chapter 27 for how to assist the nurse with pain assessment.

MEASURING AND REPORTING VITAL SIGNS

A person's vital signs vary within certain limits. They are affected by sleep, activity, eating, weather, noise, exercise, drugs, anger, fear, anxiety, pain, and illness.

Vital signs are measured to detect changes in normal body function. They tell about responses to treatment. They often signal life-threatening events. Vital signs are part of the assessment step in the nursing process. Vital signs are measured:

- During physical exams
- When the person is admitted to a health care agency
- As often as required by the person's condition
- Before and after surgery
- Before and after complex procedures or diagnostic tests
- After some care measures, such as ambulation
- After a fall or other injury
- When drugs affect the respiratory or circulatory system
- When there are complaints of pain, dizziness, light-headedness, feeling faint, shortness of breath, a rapid heart rate, or not feeling well
- As stated on the care plan (usually daily or weekly in nursing centers)

Vital signs show even minor changes in the person's condition. Accuracy is essential when you measure, record, and report vital signs. If unsure of your measurements,

Safely Handling, Moving, and Transferring the Person   **Chapter 16**   **247**

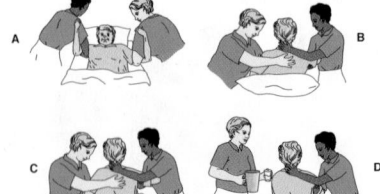

FIGURE 16-7 Raising the person's head and shoulders with a co-worker. **A,** Two nursing assistants lock arms with the person. **B,** The nursing assistants have their arms under the person's head and neck. **C,** The nursing assistants raise the person to a semi-sitting position. **D,** One nursing assistant supports the person in the semi-sitting position while the other gives care.

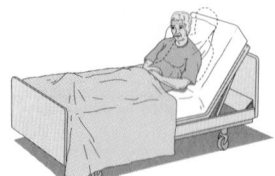

FIGURE 16-8 A person in poor alignment after sliding down in bed.

Moving the Person Up in Bed

When the head of the bed is raised, it is easy to slide down toward the middle and foot of the bed (Fig. 16-8). The person is moved up in bed for good alignment and comfort.

You can usually move small children up in bed alone. You can sometimes move lightweight adults up in bed alone if they can assist and use a trapeze. However, it is best to have help and to use an assist device—lift sheet, large incontinence product, slide sheet (p. 249). Two or more staff members are needed to move heavy, weak, and very old persons up in bed. Always protect the person and yourself from injury.

See *Promoting Safety and Comfort: Moving the Person Up in Bed.*

PROMOTING SAFETY AND COMFORT: Moving the Person Up in Bed

SAFETY
This procedure is best done with at least two staff members. Assist devices are used as directed by the nurse and the care plan.

Perform this procedure alone *only if:*
- The person is small in size.
- The person can follow directions.
- The person can assist with much of the moving.
- The person uses a trapeze.
- The person can push against the mattress with his or her feet.
- The nurse says it is safe to do so.
- You are comfortable doing so.

Follow the nurse's directions and the care plan. Ask any questions before you begin the procedure.

Measuring Vital Signs   **Chapter 25**   **441**

FOCUS ON CHILDREN AND OLDER PERSONS

Measuring and Reporting Vital Signs

OLDER PERSONS

Measuring vital signs on persons with dementia may be difficult. The person may move about, hit at you, and grab equipment. This is not safe for the person or for you. Two workers may be needed. One uses touch and a soothing voice to calm and distract the person. The other measures the vital signs.

You may need to try the procedure when the person is calmer. Or take the pulse and respirations at one time. Then take the temperature and blood pressure at another time.

Always approach the person calmly. Use a soothing voice. Tell the person what you are going to do. Do not rush the person. Follow the care plan. If you cannot measure vital signs, tell the nurse right away.

FOCUS ON COMMUNICATION

Measuring and Reporting Vital Signs

Patients and residents like to know their measurements. If agency policy allows, you can tell the person the measurements. Remember, this information is private and confidential. Roommates and visitors must not hear what you are saying.

A measurement may be abnormal. Or you may not be able to feel a pulse or hear a blood pressure. Do not alarm the person. You can say:
- "I'm not sure that I counted your pulse correctly. I want the nurse to take it too."
- "I'm not sure that I heard your blood pressure correctly. I'll ask the nurse to take it again."
- "Your pulse is a little slow (or fast). I'll ask the nurse to check it."
- "Your temperature is higher than normal. I'm going to check it with another thermometer. I'll also ask the nurse to check you."

BOX 25-1 Temperature Sites

ORAL SITE
Oral temperatures are *not* taken if the person:
- Is under 4 or 5 years of age
- Is unconscious
- Has had surgery or an injury to the face, neck, nose, or mouth
- Is receiving oxygen
- Breathes through the mouth
- Has a nasogastric tube
- Is delirious, restless, confused, or disoriented
- Is paralyzed on one side of the body
- Has a sore mouth
- Has a convulsive (seizure) disorder

RECTAL SITE
The rectal site is used for infants and children under 3 years old. Rectal temperatures are taken when the oral site cannot be used. Rectal temperatures are *not* taken if the person:
- Has diarrhea
- Has a rectal disorder or injury
- Has heart disease
- Had rectal surgery
- Is confused or agitated

TYMPANIC MEMBRANE SITE
The site has fewer microbes than the mouth or rectum. Therefore the risk of spreading infection is reduced. This site is *not* used if the person has:
- An ear disorder
- Ear drainage

TEMPORAL ARTERY SITE
Measures body temperature at the temporal artery in the forehead. The site is non-invasive.

AXILLARY SITE
Less reliable than the other sites. It is used when the other sites cannot be used.

---

promptly ask the nurse to take them again. Unless otherwise ordered, take vital signs with the person lying or sitting. The person is at rest when vital signs are measured. Report the following at once:
- Any vital sign that is changed from a prior measurement
- Vital signs above the normal range
- Vital signs below the normal range

Vital signs are recorded in the person's medical record. If they are measured often, a flow sheet is used. The doctor or nurse compares current and previous measurements.

See *Focus on Children and Older Persons: Measuring and Reporting Vital Signs.*

See *Focus on Communication: Measuring and Reporting Vital Signs.*

BODY TEMPERATURE

Body temperature is the amount of heat in the body. It is a balance between the amount of heat produced and the amount lost by the body. Heat is produced as cells use food for energy. It is lost through the skin, breathing, urine, and feces. Body temperature stays fairly stable. It is lower in the morning and higher in the afternoon and evening. Body temperature is affected by age, weather, exercise, emotions, stress, and illness. Pregnancy and the menstrual cycle are other factors.

Thermometers are used to measure temperature. It is measured using the Fahrenheit (F) and centigrade or Celsius (C) scales.

Temperature Sites

Temperature sites are the mouth, rectum, axilla (underarm), tympanic membrane (ear), and temporal artery (forehead) (Box 25-1). Each site has a normal range (Table 25-1, p. 442). Fever means an elevated body temperature. Always report temperatures that are above or below the normal range.

See *Focus on Children and Older Persons: Temperature Sites,* p. 442.

See *Promoting Safety and Comfort: Temperature Sites,* p. 442.

Color illustrations and photographs visually present key ideas, concepts, or procedure steps. They help you apply and remember the written material.

Boxes and tables contain important rules, principles, guidelines, signs and symptoms, nursing measures, and other information in a list format. They identify important information and are useful study guides.

Focus on Children and Older Persons provides age-specific information about needs, considerations, and special circumstances of children. Subtitles— "Children" and "Older Persons"—are used. The "Older Persons" sections contain useful information about persons with Alzheimer's disease and other dementias.

Focus on Communication suggests what to say and questions to ask when interacting with patients, residents, and the nursing team.

Bolded type is used to highlight the key terms in the text. You again see the key term and read its definition. This helps reinforce your learning.

Caring About Culture contains information to help you learn about the various practices of other cultures.

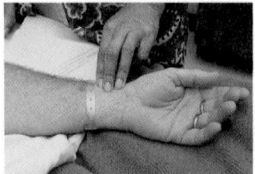

FIGURE 19-2 Structures of the skin.

Openings of sweat ducts
Hair shaft
Pigment layer
Sensory nerve ending for touch
Oil (sebaceous) gland
Hair follicle
Sweat gland
Epidermis
Dermis
Subcutaneous fatty tissue

FOCUS ON CHILDREN AND OLDER PERSONS

Personal Hygiene

OLDER PERSONS
Some older persons resist your efforts to assist with hygiene. Illness, disability, dementia, and personal choice are common reasons. Follow the care plan to meet the person's needs.
Older and disabled persons may have a hard time bending and reaching. Some have weak hand grips. They cannot hold onto soap or a washcloth. To maintain independence, the person may use an adaptive device for hygiene (Fig. 19-3). Remember, the person should do as much for himself or herself as safely possible.

CARING ABOUT CULTURE

Personal Hygiene

Personal hygiene is very important to *East Indian Hindus*. Their religion requires at least one bath a day. Some believe it is harmful to bathe after a meal. Another Hindu belief is that a cold bath prevents blood disease. Some believe that eye injuries can occur if a bath is too hot. Hot water can be added to cold water. However, cold water is not added to hot water. After bathing, the body is carefully dried with a towel.

From Giger JN, Davidhizar RE: *Transcultural nursing: assessment and intervention*, ed 4, St Louis, 2004, Mosby.

FOCUS ON COMMUNICATION

Personal Hygiene

During hygiene procedures, you must make sure that the person is warm enough. You can ask:
• "Is the water warm enough?" "Is it too hot?" "Is it too cold?"
• "Are you warm enough?"
• "Do you need another bath blanket?"
• "Is the water starting to cool?"
• "Is the room warm enough?"

Heading icons alert you to associated procedures. Procedure boxes contain the same icon.

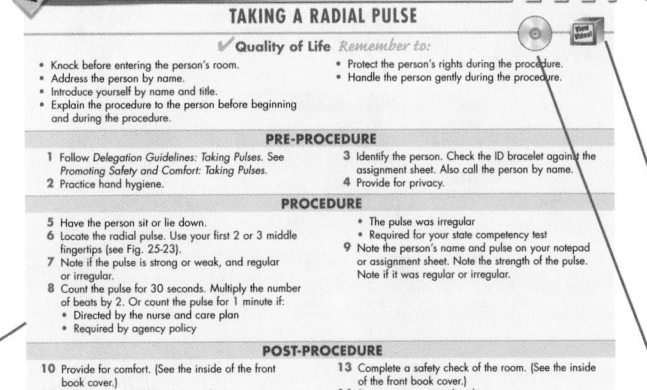

452 MOSBY'S TEXTBOOK FOR NURSING ASSISTANTS

PROMOTING SAFETY AND COMFORT: Taking Pulses

SAFETY
Do not use your thumb to take a pulse. The thumb has a pulse. You could mistake the pulse in your thumb for the person's pulse. Reporting and recording the wrong pulse rate can harm the person.

Taking a Radial Pulse
The radial pulse is used for routine vital signs. Place the first 2 or 3 fingertips of one hand against the radial artery. The radial artery is on the thumb side of the wrist (Fig. 25-23). Count the pulse for 30 seconds. Then multiply the number by 2. This gives the number of beats per minute. If the pulse is irregular, count it for 1 minute.
In some agencies, all radial pulses are taken for 1 minute. Follow agency policy.

FIGURE 25-23 The middle three fingertips are used to take the radial pulse.

NNAAP™ Skill

TAKING A RADIAL PULSE

✓ **Quality of Life** *Remember to:*

• Knock before entering the person's room.
• Address the person by name.
• Introduce yourself by name and title.
• Explain the procedure to the person before beginning and during the procedure.
• Protect the person's rights during the procedure.
• Handle the person gently during the procedure.

PRE-PROCEDURE

1 Follow *Delegation Guidelines: Taking Pulses.* See *Promoting Safety and Comfort: Taking Pulses.*
2 Practice hand hygiene.
3 Identify the person. Check the ID bracelet against the assignment sheet. Also call the person by name.
4 Provide for privacy.

PROCEDURE

5 Have the person sit or lie down.
6 Locate the radial pulse. Use your first 2 or 3 middle fingertips (see Fig. 25-23).
7 Note if the pulse is strong or weak, and regular or irregular.
8 Count the pulse for 30 seconds. Multiply the number of beats by 2. Or count the pulse for 1 minute if:
• Directed by the nurse and care plan
• Required by agency policy
• The pulse was irregular
• Required for your state competency test
9 Note the person's name and pulse on your notepad or assignment sheet. Note the strength of the pulse. Note if it was regular or irregular.

POST-PROCEDURE

10 Provide for comfort. (See the inside of the front book cover.)
11 Place the signal light within reach.
12 Unscreen the person.
13 Complete a safety check of the room. (See the inside of the front book cover.)
14 Decontaminate your hands.
15 Report and record pulse rate and your observations. Report an abnormal pulse at once.

Procedure icons in the title bar alert you to associated content areas. Heading icons and procedure icons are the same.

Procedures are written in a step-by-step format. They are divided into *Quality of Life, Pre-Procedure, Procedure,* and *Post-Procedure* sections for easy studying. The Quality of Life section lists six simple courtesies that show respect for the resident as a person.

NNAAP™ in the procedure title bar alerts you to those skills that are part of the National Nurse Aide Assessment Program (NNAAP™). Note: All states do not participate in NNAAP™. Ask your instructor for a list of the skills tested in your state.

Video icon in the *Procedures* list and the procedure box title bar alerts you to video clips on the EVOLVE website.

CD icon appears in the *Procedures* list and the procedure box title bar for the skills included on the

---

138 MOSBY'S TEXTBOOK FOR NURSING ASSISTANTS

closet, drawers, purse, or other space without the person's knowledge and consent. A nurse may ask you to inspect closets and drawers. Center policy should require that a co-worker and the person or legal representative be present. The co-worker is a witness to your activities. Follow center policy for reporting and recording the inspection.

Freedom From Abuse, Mistreatment, and Neglect

Residents have the right to be free from verbal, sexual, physical, or mental abuse (Chapter 3). They also have the right to be free from **involuntary seclusion:**

▶ Separating a person from others against his or her will
▶ Confining the person to a certain area
▶ Keeping the person away from his or her room without consent

No one can abuse, neglect, or mistreat a resident. This includes center staff, volunteers, and staff from other agencies or groups. It also includes other residents, family members, visitors, and legal representatives. Nursing centers must investigate suspected or reported cases of abuse. They cannot employ persons who were convicted of abusing, neglecting, or mistreating others.

See Focus on Ethics and Laws: Freedom From Abuse, Mistreatment, and Neglect.

Freedom From Restraint

Residents have the right not to have body movements restricted. Restraints and certain drugs can restrict body movements. Some drugs can restrain the person because they affect mood, behavior, and mental function. Sometimes residents are restrained to protect them from harming themselves or others. A doctor's order is needed for restraint use. Restraints are not used for staff convenience or to discipline a person. Restraints are discussed in Chapter 13.

Quality of Life

Nursing centers must care for residents in a manner that promotes dignity and self-esteem. Centers must also promote physical, psychological, and mental well-being. Protecting resident rights promotes quality of life. It shows respect for the person.

The person is spoken to in a polite and courteous manner (Chapter 7). Good, honest, and thoughtful care enhances the person's quality of life. Box 10-6 lists OBRA-required actions that promote dignity and privacy. Surveyors check for these actions in the person's care.

Activities

Nursing centers must provide activity programs that promote physical, intellectual, social, spiritual, and emotional well-being. The person is allowed to choose activities that appeal to his or her interests. Many centers provide religious servi[...]
and from a[...]
with activiti[...]

See Tea[...]
See Foc[...]

FOCUS ON ETHICS AND LAWS

Freedom from Abuse, Mistreatment, and Neglect

For about 3 months, a certified nursing assistant (CNA) worked at a nursing home in Texas. During that time, she received a warning for standing on a resident's bed to turn him onto his side. She was a "no call/no show before the last day of her resignation notice."

While working in an Arizona nursing home, the following were reported by the CNA's co-workers:

• Twice in one day the CNA was heard saying to a resident "You're full of xxxx."
• About 4 days later, the CNA told a resident "that if he grabbed her again, she would break his fingers." On the same day she was heard telling a resident that she "didn't want to hear the same xxxx she had already heard thirty times before."

The CNA's employment was terminated the next day.

On November 17, 2005, the Arizona State Board of Nursing found that the CNA's actions violated the state's Nurse Practice Act. The Board offered the CNA a stayed revocation agreement for 12 months with terms. The CNA failed to sign the agreement.

On March 20, 2006, the Arizona State Board of Nursing revoked the CNA's certificate. She could apply for re-instatement after a 5-year period.

(Arizona State Board of Nursing, March 20, 2006. NOTE: Names withheld by request of the Arizona State Board of Nursing.)

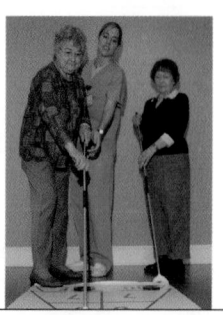

Focus on Ethics and Laws presents summaries of court cases and state cases involving nursing assistant discipline actions. The intent is to sensitize the student to the consequences of not acting in a safe or professional manner.

Admissions, Transfers, and Discharges **Chapter 28** **491**

Admission to a hospital or nursing center causes anxiety and fear in patients, residents, and families. They may worry about treatments and surgeries and their outcomes. They may fear serious health problems. The fear of pain is common.

Patients, residents, and their families are in new, strange settings. They may have concerns and fears about:

▶ Where to go, what to do, and what to expect
▶ Never returning home
▶ Who gives care, how care is given, and if the correct care is given
▶ Getting meals
▶ Finding the bathroom
▶ How to get help
▶ Being abused
▶ Strange sights and sounds
▶ Being apart from family and friends
▶ Making new friends
▶ Leaving homes and possessions behind

Discharge is usually a happy time. However, the person may need home care or long-term care.

Admission, transfer, and discharge are critical events. They involve:

▶ Privacy and confidentiality
▶ Reporting and recording
▶ Understanding and communicating with the person
▶ Communicating with the health team
▶ Respect for the person and the person's property
▶ Being kind, courteous, and respectful

See Focus on Long-Term Care and Home Care: Admissions, Transfers, and Discharges.

See Teamwork and Time Management: Admissions, Transfers, and Discharges.

See Delegation Guidelines: Admissions, Transfers, and Discharges.

See Promoting Safety and Comfort: Admissions, Transfers, and Discharges.

ADMISSIONS

The admission process usually starts in the admitting office. Admission is the official entry of a person into an agency. Admitting staff or a nurse obtains information for the admission record. This includes the person's:

▶ Full name
▶ Age and birth date
▶ Doctor's name
▶ Religion

The person is given an identification number and an ID bracelet (Chapter 11). Admitting papers and a general consent for treatment are signed at this time.

The admitting office tells the nursing unit when there is a new patient or resident. The person's room and bed number are given. In some agencies, the person can walk to the room if able. Most persons require transport by wheelchair or stretcher.

See Focus on Long-Term Care and Home Care: Admissions, p. 492.

FOCUS ON LONG-TERM CARE AND HOME CARE

Admissions, Transfers, and Discharges

LONG-TERM CARE

The Omnibus Budget Reconciliation Act of 1987 (OBRA) has standards for transfers and discharges. The person's rights must be protected. Therefore reasons for a transfer or discharge are part of the person's medical record. The person and family are told of the transfer or discharge plans. A procedure is followed if the person objects. An ombudsman makes sure the person's best interests are considered.

TEAMWORK AND TIME MANAGEMENT

Admissions, Transfers, and Discharges

Transfers and discharges are easier if a co-worker helps you. When asking for help, politely tell your co-worker:

• The procedure you need help with
• When you plan to do the procedure
• What you need the person to do
• How much time it will take

Remember to thank the person for helping you.

DELEGATION GUIDELINES: Admissions, Transfers, and Discharges

When admitting, transferring, or discharging a person, you need this information from the nurse:

• If you need to admit, transfer, or discharge the person
• The person's method of transportation to or from the agency—car, ambulance, or wheelchair van
• How the person will move about within the agency—walking, wheelchair, stretcher, or bed
• The person's room and bed number
• What special equipment and supplies are needed
• If the person can stay dressed or needs to wear a gown or sleepwear
• If the person stays in bed or can be in a chair
• When to report observations
• What specific patient or resident concerns to report at once

---

PROMOTING SAFETY AND COMFORT: Admissions, Transfers, and Discharges

SAFETY

The person may develop pain or become distressed during admission, a transfer, or discharge. If so, call for the nurse at once. Stay with the person. When the nurse arrives, assist as needed.

COMFORT

Admission, transfer, or discharge may be stressful for the person. Some persons are happy. Others are sad and fearful. Some anxiety is expected. To provide for the person's mental comfort:

• Explain what you are doing and why
• Do not rush the person
• Be sensitive to the person's needs and feelings

Focus on Long-Term Care and Home Care highlights information unique to long-term care settings for safe functioning in home settings. "Long-Term Care" and "Home Care" subtitles are used. For long-term care, information is included about the requirements of the Omnibus Budget Reconciliation Act of 1987 (OBRA).

Teamwork and Time Management boxes suggest ways to efficiently work with and help other nursing team members.

Delegation Guidelines describe what information you need from the nurse and care plan before performing a procedure. They also tell you what information to report and record.

Promoting Safety and Comfort boxes focus your attention on the need to be safe and cautious and promote comfort when giving care. "Safety" and "Comfort" subtitles are used.

Date	Time	Weight	T	P	R	BP			Signatures
10/19	0700	126	98.8	72	20	142/84			Mary Smith CNA
10/26	0715	125	98.6	72	18	140/89			Jane Doe CNA
11/2	0715	126	98.6	70	18	144/82			Mary Smith CNA

FIGURE 25-29 Charting sample.

Charting samples provide a guide for effective recording of care and observations.

Review Questions are useful study guides. They help you to review what you have learned. They can also be used when studying for a test or the competency evaluation. Answers are given at the back of the book beginning on p. 779.

REVIEW QUESTIONS

Circle the BEST answer.

1 Which statement is *false?*
   a The vital signs are temperature, pulse, respirations, and blood pressure.
   b Vital signs detect changes in body function.
   c Vital signs change only during illness.
   d Sleep, exercise, drugs, emotions, and noise affect vital signs.

2 Which should you report at once?
   a An oral temperature of 98.4° F
   b A rectal temperature of 101.6° F
   c An axillary temperature of 97.6° F
   d An oral temperature of 99.0° F

3 A rectal temperature is taken when the person
   a Is unconscious
   b Has heart disease
   c Is confused
   d Has diarrhea

4 Which gives the *least* accurate measurement of body temperature?
   a Oral site
   b Rectal site
   c Axillary site
   d Tympanic membrane site

5 Which site is used to take an infant's temperature?
   a Oral site
   b Rectal site
   c Axillary site
   d Tympanic membrane site

6 Which is usually used to take an adult's pulse?
   a The radial pulse
   b The apical pulse
   c The apical-radial pulse
   d The brachial pulse

7 Which is reported to the nurse at once?
   a An adult has a pulse of 120 beats per minute.
   b An infant has a pulse of 130 beats per minute.
   c An adult has a pulse of 80 beats per minute.
   d An adult has a pulse of 64 beats per minute.

8 Which statement about the apical-radial pulse is *true?*
   a The radial pulse can be greater than the apical pulse.
   b The apical pulse can be greater than the radial pulse.
   c The apical and radial pulses are always equal.
   d The pulse deficit is 0.

9 In an adult, normal respirations are
   a 10 to 18 per minute
   b 12 to 20 per minute
   c Less than 20 per minute
   d More than 20 per minute

10 Normal respirations
   a Are heard as the person inhales
   b Are heard as the person exhales
   c Are quiet
   d Sound like wheezing with inhalation and exhalation

11 Respirations are usually counted
   a After taking the temperature
   b After taking the pulse
   c Before taking the pulse
   d After taking the blood pressure

12 Which blood pressure is normal for an adult?
   a 88/54 mm Hg
   b 140/90 mm Hg
   c 100/60 mm Hg
   d 112/78 mm Hg

13 When measuring blood pressure, you should do the following except
   a Use the arm with an IV infusion
   b Apply the cuff to a bare upper arm
   c Turn off the TV
   d Locate the brachial artery

14 The systolic pressure is the point
   a Where the pulse is no longer felt
   b Where the first sound is heard
   c Where the last sound is heard
   d 30 mm Hg above where the pulse was felt

Answers for these questions are on p. 781.

Contents

Procedures

Procedures with this icon are also on the CD-ROM in this book.

Procedures with this icon are also on the Evolve website for this book.

Procedures—cont'd

Introduction to Health Care Agencies

OBJECTIVES

- Define the key terms and key abbreviations listed in this chapter
- Describe the types, purposes, and organization of health care agencies
- Describe members of the health team and nursing team
- Describe the nursing service department
- Describe four nursing care patterns
- Describe the programs that pay for health care
- Explain why standards are met

KEY TERMS

acute illness A sudden illness from which a person is expected to recover

assisted living residence Provides housing, personal care, support services, health care, and social activities in a home-like setting

case management A nursing care pattern; a case manager (an RN) coordinates a person's care from admission through discharge and into the home setting

chronic illness An ongoing illness, slow or gradual in onset; it has no known cure; the illness can be controlled and complications prevented with proper treatment

functional nursing A nursing care pattern focusing on tasks and jobs; each nursing team member has certain tasks and jobs to do

health team The many health care workers whose skills and knowledge focus on the person's total care; interdisciplinary health care team

hospice A health care agency or program for persons who are dying

licensed practical nurse (LPN) A nurse who has completed a 1-year nursing program and has passed a licensing test; called *licensed vocational nurse (LVN)* in some states

licensed vocational nurse (LVN) Licensed practical nurse

nursing assistant A person who has passed a nursing assistant training and competency evaluation program; performs delegated nursing tasks under the supervision of a licensed nurse

nursing team Those who provide nursing care—RNs, LPNs/LVNs, and nursing assistants

patient-focused care A nursing care pattern; services are moved from departments to the bedside

Continued

1

KEY TERMS—cont'd

primary nursing A nursing care pattern; an RN is responsible for the person's total care
registered nurse (RN) A nurse who has completed a 2-, 3-, or 4-year nursing program and has passed a licensing test

team nursing A nursing care pattern; a team of nursing staff is led by an RN who decides the amount and kind of care each person needs
terminal illness An illness or injury for which there is no reasonable expectation of recovery

KEY ABBREVIATIONS

CMG Case mix group
DON Director of nursing
DRG Diagnosis-related group
HHRG Home health resource group
HMO Health maintenance organization
LPN Licensed practical nurse
LVN Licensed vocational nurse

NATCEP Nursing assistant training and competency evaluation program
PPO Preferred provider organization
RN Registered nurse
RUG Resource utilization group
SNF Skilled nursing facility

Health care agencies offer services to persons needing health care (Box 1-1). Agencies vary in size, services, hours open, and staff. The *person* is always the focus of care.

Staff members have special talents, knowledge, and skills. All work to meet the person's needs.

AGENCY PURPOSES

Services range from simple to complex. Some agencies have one purpose and offer one service. Others have many purposes. They offer many services.

The purposes of health care are:

▶ *Health promotion.* This includes physical and mental health. The goal is to reduce the risk of illnesses. People receive teaching and counseling about healthy living. Diet and exercise are examples. People learn the warning signs and symptoms of illness. They learn how to manage and cope with health problems as needed.

▶ *Disease prevention.* Risk factors and early warning signs of disease are identified. Measures are taken to reduce risk factors and prevent disease. Immunizations prevent some infectious diseases. Polio, measles, mumps, smallpox, and hepatitis B are examples. Simple life-style changes can prevent health problems. For example, high blood pressure can lead to heart attacks and strokes. Diet and exercise can help lower blood pressure.

▶ *Detection and treatment of disease.* This involves diagnostic tests, physical exams, surgery, emergency care, and drugs. Often respiratory, physical, and occupational therapies are needed. The nursing team observes signs and symptoms, gives care, and carries out the doctor's orders.

▶ *Rehabilitation and restorative care.* The goal is to return persons to their highest possible level of physical and

mental functioning and to independence. *Independence* means not relying on or requiring care from others. The process starts when the person first seeks health care. The person learns or relearns skills needed to live, work, and enjoy life. Maintaining function is important. Help is given with making needed changes at home.

These purposes are all related. For example, Mr. Parsons has severe chest pain and problems breathing. He goes to a hospital emergency department. After an exam and tests, the doctor diagnoses a heart attack. Mr. Parsons is admitted to the hospital for treatment. He also receives teaching and counseling about heart attack risk factors and healthy living. The goals are to promote health and

---

BOX 1-1 Types of Health Care Agencies

- Hospitals
- Long-term care centers (nursing homes, nursing facilities, nursing centers)
- Home care agencies
- Adult day-care centers
- Assisted living residences
- Board and care homes
- Rehabilitation and subacute care facilities
- Hospices
- Doctors' offices
- Clinics
- Centers for persons with mental illnesses
- Centers for persons with developmental disabilities
- Drug and alcohol treatment centers
- Crisis centers for rape, abuse, suicide, and other emergencies

prevent another heart attack. A rehabilitation program is planned. Activity starts slowly and may progress from walking to jogging and swimming. Teaching and counseling focus on diet, drugs, life-style, activity, and how to cope with fears and concerns. Successful rehabilitation promotes health and may prevent another heart attack.

Student Learning

Many agencies are learning sites for students. (See "The Health Team," p. 4.) The students assist in the purposes of health care. They are involved with and provide care.

TYPES OF AGENCIES

Nursing assistants work in many settings. Some work in doctors' offices and clinics. Most work in the following agencies.

Hospitals

Hospital services include emergency care, surgery, nursing care, x-ray procedures and treatments, and laboratory testing. Services also include respiratory, physical, occupational, and speech therapies.

People of all ages need hospital care. They go to have babies, for physical and mental health problems, for surgery, to heal broken bones, or to die. They have acute, chronic, or terminal illnesses:

▶ **Acute illness** is a sudden illness from which the person is expected to recover.
▶ **Chronic illness** is an ongoing illness that is slow or gradual in onset. There is no known cure. The illness can be controlled and complications prevented with proper treatment.
▶ **Terminal illness** is an illness or injury for which there is no reasonable expectation of recovery. The person will die (Chapter 50).

Rehabilitation and Subacute Care Agencies

Hospital stays are usually short. This is because of insurance coverage. Some people do not need hospital care but are too sick to go home. However, medical and nursing care and rehabilitation are needed. Care needs fall between hospital care and long-term care. Complex equipment and care measures are needed. Common programs include:

▶ *Cardiac rehabilitation*—for heart disorders (Chapter 40)
▶ *Brain injury rehabilitation*—for nervous system disorders including traumatic brain injury (Chapter 39)
▶ *Spinal cord rehabilitation*—for spinal cord injuries (Chapter 39)
▶ *Stroke rehabilitation*—after a stroke (Chapter 39)
▶ *Respiratory rehabilitation*—for respiratory system disorders such as chronic obstructive pulmonary disease, after lung surgery, for respiratory complications from other health problems (Chapter 40), and for mechanical ventilation (Chapter 35)
▶ *Musculoskeletal rehabilitation*—for fractures, joint replacement surgery, and so on (Chapter 39)

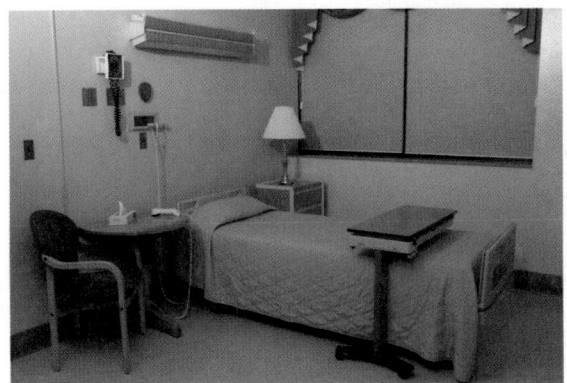

FIGURE 1-1 Room in a long-term care setting.

▶ *Rehabilitation for complex medical and surgical conditions*—for wound care (Chapter 32), diabetes (Chapter 41), burns (Chapter 49), and so on

Some hospitals and long-term care centers have rehabilitation and subacute care units. Some are separate agencies. Many persons fully recover. Others may need long-term care.

Long-Term Care Centers

Some persons cannot care for themselves at home. But they do not need hospital care. Long-term care centers (nursing homes, nursing facilities, nursing centers) can help them. Care needs range from simple to complex. Medical, nursing, dietary, recreational, rehabilitative, and social services are provided. So are housekeeping and laundry services.

Persons in long-term care centers are called *residents*. They are not *patients*. This is because the center is their temporary or permanent home.

Most residents are older. They have chronic diseases, poor nutrition, or poor health. Long-term care centers are designed to meet their needs (Fig. 1-1).

Not all residents are old. Some are disabled from birth defects, accidents, or diseases. People are often discharged from hospitals while still sick or still recovering from surgery. Home care is an option for some. Others need long-term care. Some recover and return home. Others need nursing care until death.

Skilled Nursing Facilities

Skilled nursing facilities (SNFs) provide more complex care than do nursing centers. They are part of hospitals or nursing centers. SNF residents need rehabilitation or time to recover from illness or surgery. Often they return home after a short stay. Others become permanent nursing center residents.

Assisted Living Residences

An **assisted living residence** provides housing, personal care, support services, health care, and social activities in a home-like setting (Chapter 48). Some are part of nursing centers or retirement communities (Chapter 10).

The person has a room or an apartment. Three meals a day are provided. So are housekeeping, laundry, and transportation services. Help is given with personal care and drugs. Social and recreational activities are provided. There is access to health and medical care.

Mental Health Centers

Mental health centers are for persons with mental illnesses. Some persons have problems dealing with life events. Others present dangers to themselves or others because of how they think and behave. Out-patient care is common. Some need short-term or life-long in-patient care.

Home Care Agencies

A wide range of services are provided to people where they live. Services are provided by nurses and nursing assistants and other health team members. Services range from health teaching and supervision to bedside nursing care. Physical therapy, rehabilitation, and food services are common. Hospitals, health care systems, public health departments, and private businesses offer home care services.

Some older persons need home health care. So do some persons who are dying.

Hospices

A **hospice** is a health care agency or program for persons who are dying. Such persons no longer respond to treatments aimed at cures. Usually they have less than 6 months to live.

The physical, emotional, social, and spiritual needs of the person and family are met. The focus is on comfort, not cure. Children and pets can visit. Family and friends can assist with care.

Hospice care is provided by hospitals, nursing centers, and home care agencies.

Health Care Systems

Agencies join together as one provider of care. A system usually has hospitals, nursing centers, home care agencies, hospice settings, and doctors' offices (Fig. 1-2). An

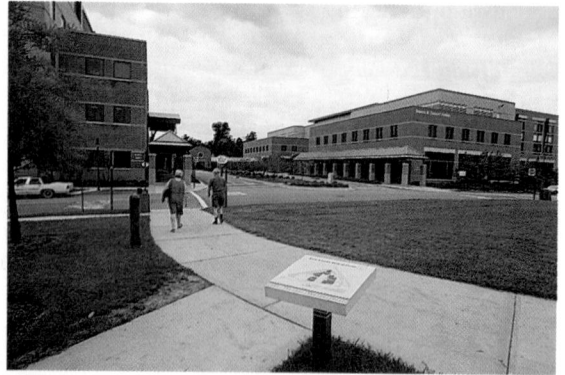

FIGURE 1-2 The hospital and doctors' offices are part of a health care system. (Courtesy Anne Arundel Health System, Inc., Annapolis, Md.)

BOX 1-2 Using a Health Care System

A health care system owns Mercy Hospital. Dr. Moore and Dr. Gills work there. The hospital has a rehabilitation unit and a home care service. LifeCare Ambulance Service and a medical supply store are part of the system. So is Lakeside Nursing Center.

June Adams is 78 years old. She sees Dr. Moore in his office. She complains of tightness in her chest, dizziness, and a "pounding heart." Dr. Moore admits her to the hospital. While in the hospital she has a heart attack. Dr. Gills, a heart specialist, takes over her care. A few days later she has a stroke. She cannot move her left side. She is given needed medical care. When stable, she is transferred to the rehabilitation unit.

Mrs. Adams spends 2 weeks on the rehabilitation unit. She needs home care if she returns home. Or she can go to a nursing center. She wants to go home. Her family wants to help care for her. They need a hospital bed, commode, bedpan, wheelchair, and other items. They rent some items and buy others at the medical supply store.

Mrs. Adams is transported home by LifeCare Ambulance Service. Mercy Hospital's home care agency provides home care services. A nursing assistant visits every day to help Mrs. Adams with hygiene and grooming needs. A nurse visits three times a week.

A month later Mrs. Adams has another stroke. She returns to Mercy Hospital by LifeCare Ambulance Service. After 8 days, she is transferred to the rehabilitation unit. The second stroke has caused more disabilities. Dr. Gills suggests nursing home care. Mrs. Adams and her family agree with him.

The nurse arranges for Mrs. Adams to be admitted to Lakeside Nursing Center. She is transferred there by LifeCare Ambulance Service.

---

ambulance service and medical supply store for home care are common. The system may serve a community or a large region.

The goal is to serve all health care needs. A person uses other system providers as needed (Box 1-2).

ORGANIZATION

An agency has a governing body called the *board of trustees* or *board of directors*. The board makes policies. It makes sure that safe care is given at the lowest possible cost. Local, state, and federal rules are followed.

An administrator manages the agency. He or she reports directly to the board. Directors or department heads manage certain areas (Fig. 1-3).

See *Focus on Long-Term Care and Home Care: Organization.*

The Health Team

The **health team** involves the many health care workers whose skills and knowledge focus on the person's total care (Table 1-1). (It is also called the *interdisciplinary health care team*.) The goal is to provide quality care. The person is the focus of their care (Fig. 1-4, p. 7).

Many health care workers are involved in the care of each person. Coordinated care is needed. An RN leads this team.

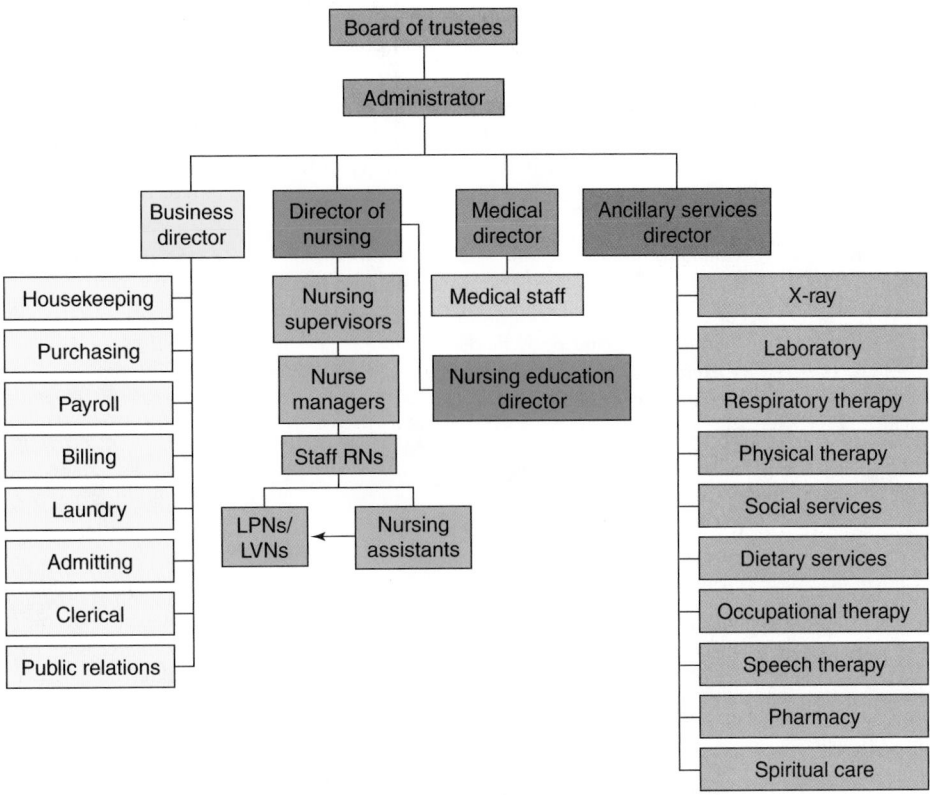

FIGURE 1-3 Organization of a health care agency.

FOCUS ON **LONG-TERM CARE** AND **HOME CARE**

Organization

LONG-TERM CARE

Nursing centers are usually owned by an individual or a corporation. Some are owned by county health departments.

Each center has an administrator. Department directors report to the administrator. Most nursing centers have nursing, therapy, and food service departments. They also have housekeeping, maintenance, and laundry departments. A human resources director handles personnel matters such as hiring staff. A finance director handles resident billing. A social services director meets the social needs of residents and families. An activities director plans resident activities.

By law, nursing centers must have a medical director. This person is a doctor. This doctor consults with the staff about medical problems not handled by a resident's doctor. Guidance is given about resident care policies and programs.

TABLE 1-1 **Health Team Members**

TITLE	DESCRIPTION	CREDENTIALS
Activities director	Assesses, plans, and implements recreational needs	Varies with state and/or employer; ranges from no training to bachelor's degree
Audiologist	Tests hearing; prescribes hearing aids; works with persons who are hard of hearing	Master's degree; 1 year of supervised employment; national test; license in some states
Cleric (clergyman; clergywoman)	Assists with spiritual needs	Priest, minister, rabbi, sister (nun), deacon, or other pastoral training
Clinical nurse specialist	Provides nursing care and consultation in a nursing specialty—geriatrics, critical care, diabetes, rehabilitation, and wound care are examples	RN with master's degree or doctorate as a clinical nurse specialist
Dental hygienist	Focuses on preventing dental disorders; supervised by a licensed dentist	Completion of an accredited dental hygiene program; state license
Dentist	Prevents and treats disorders and diseases of the teeth, gums, and oral structures	Doctor of dental science (DDS); state license

Continued

TABLE 1-1 Health Team Members—cont'd

TITLE	DESCRIPTION	CREDENTIALS
Dietitian	Assesses and plans for nutritional needs; teaches good nutrition, food selection, and preparation	Bachelor's degree; registered dietitian (RD) must pass a national registration test; license or certification in some states
Licensed practical/vocational nurse (LPN/LVN)	Provides direct nursing care, including giving drugs, under the direction of an RN	Certificate or diploma (usually 1 year in length); state license
Medical laboratory technician (MLT)	Collects samples and performs laboratory tests on blood, urine, and other body fluids, secretions, and excretions	Associate's degree; national certifying test; license in some states
Medical records and health information technician	Maintains medical records; transcribes medical reports, files records, completes required reports	Associate's degree; national test
Medical technologist (MT)	Performs complicated laboratory tests on blood, urine, and other body fluids, secretions, and excretions; organizes, supervises, and performs diagnostic analyses; supervises MLTs	Bachelor's degree; national certification test; license in some states
Medication assistant-certified (MA-C)	Gives medications as allowed by state law under the supervision of a licensed nurse	Certified nursing assistant with additional education and training as required by state law; state certification
Nurse practitioner	Works with the health team to plan and provide care; does physical exams, health assessments, and health education	RN with master's degree and clinical experience in an area of nursing; certification test may be required
Nursing assistant	Assists nurses and gives nursing care; supervised by a licensed nurse	Completion of a state-approved training and competency evaluation program to work in long-term care or in home care agencies receiving Medicare funds; state registry; state certification or license
Occupational therapist (OT)	Assists persons to learn or retain skills needed to perform activities of daily living; designs adaptive equipment for activities of daily living	Bachelor's degree; national certification; state license
Occupational therapy assistant	Performs tasks and services supervised by an OT	Associate's degree; national certification; license in some states
Pharmacist	Fills drug orders written by doctors; monitors and evaluates drug interactions; consults with doctors and nurses about drug actions and interactions	Degree from a college of pharmacy; state license
Physical therapist (PT)	Assists persons with musculoskeletal problems; focuses on restoring function and preventing disability	Bachelor's degree; state license
Physical therapy assistant	Performs selected physical therapy tasks and functions; supervised by a PT	Associate's degree; national certification or license in some states
Physician (doctor)	Diagnoses and treats diseases and injuries	Medical school graduation (MD), residency, and national board certification; state license
Physician's assistant	Assists doctors in diagnosis and treatment; performs many medical tasks; supervised by a doctor	Associate's, bachelor's, or master's degree; national certification or state license
Podiatrist	Prevents, diagnoses, and treats foot disorders	Doctor of podiatric medicine (DPM); state license
Radiographer/radiologic technologist	Takes x-rays and processes film for viewing	Certificate, associate's, or bachelor's degree; national registry test; license in some states
Registered nurse (RN)	Assesses, makes nursing diagnoses, plans, implements, and evaluates nursing care; supervises LPNs/LVNs and nursing assistants	Associate's degree, diploma, or bachelor's degree; state license
Respiratory therapist (RT)	Assists in treatment of lung and heart disorders; gives respiratory treatments and therapies	Associate's or bachelor's degree; national certification test; license in some states
Social worker	Deals with social, emotional, and environmental issues affecting illness and recovery; coordinates community agencies to assist patients, residents, and families	Bachelor's or master's degree in social work; license, certification, or registration
Speech-language pathologist	Evaluates speech and language and treats persons with speech, voice, hearing, communication, and swallowing disorders	Master's degree; 1 year supervised work experience; national test; license in some states

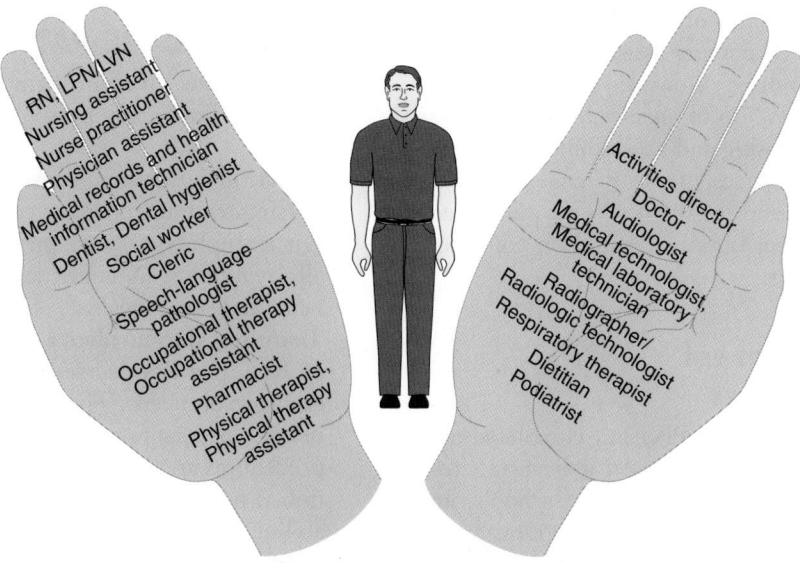

FIGURE 1-4 Members of the health team. The person is the focus of care.

Nursing Service

Nursing service is a large department. The director of nursing (DON) is an RN. (*Director of nursing services, vice president of nursing,* and *vice president of patient services* are some other titles used.) Usually a bachelor's or master's degree is required. The DON is responsible for the entire nursing staff. This includes giving safe care.

Nurse managers (usually RNs) assist the DON. They manage and carry out nursing department functions. Shift managers coordinate patient or resident care for a certain shift. Hospital nursing areas include surgical, medical, intensive care, pediatric, and mental health units. They also include operating and recovery areas, an emergency department, and a maternity department.

Other nurse managers are responsible for a nursing area or a certain function. Staff development, restorative nursing, infection control, and continuous quality improvement are examples. Nurse managers are responsible for all nursing care and the actions of nursing staff in their areas.

Nursing areas usually have charge nurses for each shift. They are usually RNs. In some states, LPNs/LVNs are charge nurses. The charge nurse is responsible for all patient or resident care and for the actions of nursing staff during that shift. Staff RNs report to the charge nurse. LPNs/LVNs report to staff RNs or to the charge nurse. You report to the nurse supervising your work.

Nursing education (staff development) is part of nursing service. Nursing education staff:

▶ Plan and present educational programs (in-service programs)
▶ Provide the nursing team with new and changing information
▶ Teach the nursing team how to use new equipment and supplies

▶ Review key policies and procedures on a regular basis
▶ Educate and train nursing assistants
▶ Conduct new employee orientation programs
▶ Provide programs that meet federal and state educational requirements

THE NURSING TEAM

The **nursing team** involves those who provide nursing care—RNs, LPNs/LVNs, and nursing assistants. Their roles and responsibilities differ. All focus on the physical, social, emotional, and spiritual needs of the person and family.

Registered Nurses

A **registered nurse (RN)** has completed a 2-, 3-, or 4-year nursing program and has passed a licensing test:

▶ Community college programs—2 years
▶ Hospital-based diploma programs—2 or 3 years
▶ College or university programs—4 years

Nursing and the biological, social, and physical sciences are studied. The graduate nurse takes a licensing test offered by a state board of nursing. The nurse receives a license and becomes *registered* when the test is passed. RNs must have a license recognized by the state in which they work.

RNs assess, make nursing diagnoses, plan, implement, and evaluate nursing care (Chapter 6). They develop care plans for each person, provide care, and make sure care plans are followed. They also delegate nursing care and tasks to the nursing team. They evaluate how the care plans and nursing care affect each person. RNs teach persons how to improve health and independence. They also teach the family.

RNs carry out the doctor's orders. They may delegate them to LPNs/LVNs or nursing assistants. RNs do not prescribe treatments or drugs. However, RNs can study to become *clinical nurse specialists* or *nurse practitioners*. These RNs have limited diagnosing and prescribing functions.

RNs work as staff nurses, nurse managers, DONs, agency administrators, and instructors. They have many other job options. Career options depend on education, abilities, and experiences.

Licensed Practical Nurses and Licensed Vocational Nurses

A **licensed practical nurse (LPN)** has completed a 1-year nursing program and has passed a licensing test. Hospitals, community colleges, vocational schools, and technical schools offer programs. Some programs are 10 months long; others take 18 months. Some high schools offer 2-year programs.

Graduates take a licensing test for practical nursing. After passing the test, the person receives a license to practice and the title of *licensed practical nurse*. **Licensed vocational nurse (LVN)** is used in some states. LPNs/LVNS must have a license required by the state in which they work.

LPNs/LVNs are supervised by RNs, licensed doctors, and licensed dentists. They have fewer responsibilities and functions than RNs do. They need little supervision when the person's condition is stable and care is simple. They assist RNs in caring for acutely ill persons and with complex procedures.

Nursing Assistants

A **nursing assistant** has completed a nursing assistant training and competency evaluation program (NATCEP). Nursing assistants perform delegated nursing tasks under the supervision of a licensed nurse. There are many titles for nursing assistants (Box 1-3). The title depends on the setting, roles, functions, and state laws.

Community colleges, technical schools, and high schools offer nursing assistant courses. So do hospitals and nursing centers. Nursing assistants are discussed in Chapter 2.

BOX 1-3 Nursing Assistant Titles

- Certified nursing assistant (CNA)
- Clinical technician
- Health care assistant
- Health care technician
- Licensed nursing assistant (LNA)
- Nurse extender
- Nurse's aide
- Nurse technician
- Nursing support technician
- Patient care assistant
- Patient care attendant
- Patient care monitor
- Patient care technician
- Patient care worker
- State tested nursing assistant
- Support partner
- Registered nurse aide (RNA)

NURSING CARE PATTERNS

Nursing care is given in many ways. The pattern used depends on how many persons need care, the staff, and the cost.

▶ **Functional nursing** focuses on tasks and jobs. Each nursing team member has certain tasks and jobs to do. For example, one nurse gives all drugs. Another gives all treatments. Nursing assistants give baths, make beds, and serve meals.

▶ **Team nursing** involves a team of nursing staff led by an RN. The RN decides the amount and kind of care each person needs. The team leader delegates the care of certain persons to other nurses. Nursing tasks and procedures are delegated to nursing assistants. Delegation is based on the person's needs and team member abilities. Team members report to the team leader about observations made and the care given.

▶ **Primary nursing** involves total care. The primary nurse (an RN) is responsible for the person's total care. The nursing team assists as needed. The RN gives nursing care and makes discharge plans. If needed, home care or long-term care is arranged. The RN teaches and counsels the person and family.

▶ **Case management** is like primary nursing. A case manager (an RN) coordinates a person's care from admission through discharge and into the home setting. He or she communicates with the person's doctor and the health team. There also is communication with the insurance company and community agencies as needed. The case manager also helps the health team work together. Some case managers work with certain doctors. Others deal with certain health problems. Heart diseases and cancer are examples.

▶ **Patient-focused care** is when services are moved from departments to the bedside. The nursing team performs basic skills usually done by other health team members. The number of people caring for each person is reduced. This reduces care costs.

PAYING FOR HEALTH CARE

Health care is a major focus in society. The goals are to provide health care to everyone and to reduce the high cost of care. Hospital and nursing center care is costly. So are doctor visits, drugs, medical supplies, and home care. Most people cannot afford these costs. Some avoid medical care because they cannot pay. Others pay doctor bills but go without food or drugs. Health care bills cause worry, fear, and emotional upset. If the person has insurance, some care costs are covered. Rarely is the total cost of long-term care covered.

These programs help pay for health care:
▶ *Private insurance* is bought by individuals and families. The insurance company pays for some or all health care costs.

▶ *Group insurance* is bought by groups or organizations for individuals. This is often an employee benefit.

▶ *Medicare* is a federal health insurance program for persons 65 years of age or older. Some younger people with certain disabilities are covered. Part A pays for some hospital, SNF, hospice, and home care costs. Part B helps pay for doctors' services, out-patient hospital care, physical and occupational therapists, some home care, and many other services. Part B is voluntary. The person pays a monthly premium.

▶ *Medicaid* is a health care payment program. Sponsored by the federal government, it is operated by the states. People with low incomes usually qualify. So do some older, blind, and disabled persons. There is no insurance premium. The amount paid for covered services is limited.

Prospective Payment Systems

Prospective payment systems limit the amount paid by insurers, Medicare, and Medicaid. Prospective means *before* care.

▶ *Diagnosis-related groups (DRGs)* are for hospital costs.
▶ *Resource utilization groups (RUGs)* are for SNF payments.
▶ *Case mix groups (CMGs)* are used for rehabilitation centers.
▶ *Home health resource groups (HHRGs)* are used for home health care.

Length of stay and treatment costs are determined for each group. If the treatment costs are less than the amount paid, the agency keeps the extra money. If costs are greater, the agency takes the loss.

Managed Care

Managed care deals with health care delivery and payment (Box 1-4). Insurers contract with doctors and hospitals for reduced rates or discounts. The insured person uses doctors and agencies providing the lower rates. If others are used, care is covered in part or not at all. The person pays for costs not covered by insurance.

Managed care limits the choice of where to go for health care. It also limits the care that doctors provide. Many states require managed care for Medicaid and Medicare coverage.

Managed Care as Pre-Approval for Services

Many insurers must approve the need for health care services. If the need is approved, the insurer pays for the services. If the need is not approved, the person pays for the costs. The pre-approval process depends on the insurer.

BOX 1-4 Types of Managed Care

Health Maintenance Organization (HMO)—provides health care services for a prepaid fee. For the fee, persons receive needed services offered by the HMO. Some have an annual physical exam. Others need hospital care. Whatever services are used, the cost is covered by the prepaid fee. HMOs focus on preventing disease and maintaining health. Keeping someone healthy costs far less than treating illness.

Preferred Provider Organization (PPO)—is a group of doctors and hospitals. They provide health care at reduced rates. Usually the agreement is between the PPO and an employer or an insurance company. Employees or those insured receive reduced rates for the services used. The person can choose any doctor or hospital in the PPO.

This pre-approval process is also called *managed care*. It includes monitoring care. The purpose is to reduce unneeded services and procedures. The insurer decides what to pay. With HMOs and PPOs, the insurer may decide where the person goes for services.

MEETING STANDARDS

Health care agencies must meet certain standards. Standards are set by the federal and state governments. They also are set by accrediting agencies. Standards relate to agency policies and procedures, budget and finances, and quality of care. An agency must meet standards for:

▶ *Licensure.* A license is issued by the state. An agency must have a license to operate and provide care.
▶ *Certification.* This is required to receive Medicare and Medicaid funds.
▶ *Accreditation.* This is voluntary. It signals quality and excellence.

The Survey Process

Surveys are done to see if the agency meets set standards. A survey team will:
▶ Review policies and procedures
▶ Review medical records
▶ Interview staff, patients and residents, and families
▶ Observe how care is given
▶ Observe if dignity and privacy are promoted
▶ Check for cleanliness and safety
▶ Review budgets and finances
▶ Make sure the staff meets state requirements (Are doctors and nurses licensed? Are nursing assistants on the state registry?)

The survey team decides if the agency meets the standards. If standards are met, the agency receives a license, certification, or accreditation.

Sometimes problems are found. A problem is called a *deficiency.* The agency is given time to correct it. Usually 60 days are given. Sometimes less time is given. The agency can be fined for uncorrected or serious deficiencies. Or it can lose its license, certification, or accreditation.

Your Role

You have an important role in meeting standards and in the survey process. You must:

▶ Provide quality care.
▶ Protect the person's rights.
▶ Provide for the person's and your own safety.
▶ Help keep the agency clean and safe.
▶ Conduct yourself in a professional manner.
▶ Have good work ethics.
▶ Follow agency policies and procedures.
▶ Answer questions honestly and completely.

REVIEW QUESTIONS

Circle the BEST answer.

1 Helping persons return to their highest physical and mental function is called
   a Maintaining independence
   b Promoting health
   c Preventing disease
   d Rehabilitation

2 Rehabilitation starts when the
   a Person is ready to leave the agency
   b Person first seeks health care
   c Doctor writes the order
   d Health team thinks the person is ready

3 A health care program for dying persons is a
   a Hospice
   b Board and care home
   c Skilled nursing facility
   d Home care agency

4 Who controls policy in a health care agency?
   a The survey team
   b The board of directors
   c The health team
   d Medicare and Medicaid

5 Who is responsible for the entire nursing staff and safe nursing care?
   a The case manager
   b The director of nursing
   c The charge nurse
   d The RN

6 You are member of
   a The health team and the nursing team
   b The health team and the medical team
   c The nursing team and the medical team
   d An HMO and a PPO

7 The nursing team does *not* include
   a Doctors
   b LPNs/LVNs
   c Nursing assistants
   d RNs

8 Nursing assistants are supervised by
   a Licensed nurses
   b Other nursing assistants
   c The health team
   d The medical director

9 The nursing assistant's role is to
   a Meet Medicare and Medicaid standards
   b Perform delegated nursing tasks
   c Carry out the doctor's orders
   d Manage care

10 Nursing tasks are delegated according to a person's needs and staff member abilities. This nursing care pattern is called
   a Team nursing
   b Functional nursing
   c Case management
   d Primary nursing

11 Medicare is for persons who
   a Are 65 years of age and older
   b Receive DRGs and RUGs
   c Have group insurance
   d Have low incomes

12 Which is required for an agency to operate and provide care?
   a A license
   b Certification
   c Accreditation
   d A survey

13 Which is voluntary for health care agencies?
   a Licensure
   b Certification
   c Accreditation
   d Surveys

14 A survey team is at your agency. A team member asks you some questions. You should
   a Refer all questions to the nurse
   b Answer as the DON tells you to
   c Give as little information as possible
   d Give honest and complete answers

Answers to these questions are on p. 779.

The Nursing Assistant

OBJECTIVES

- Define the key terms and key abbreviations listed in this chapter
- Explain the history and current trends affecting nursing assistants
- Explain the laws that affect nursing assistants
- List the reasons for denying, suspending, or revoking a nursing assistant's certification, license, or registration
- Describe the training and competency evaluation requirements for nursing assistants
- Identify the information in the nursing assistant registry
- Explain how to obtain certification, a license, or registration in another state
- Describe what nursing assistants can do and their role limits
- Describe the standards for nursing assistants developed by the National Council of State Boards of Nursing
- Explain why a job description is important
- Describe the delegation process
- Explain your role in the delegation process
- Explain how to accept or refuse a delegated task

KEY TERMS

accountable Being responsible for one's actions and the actions of others who performed the delegated tasks; answering questions about and explaining one's actions and the actions of others

delegate To authorize another person to perform a nursing task in a certain situation

job description A document that describes what the agency expects you to do

nursing task Nursing care or a nursing function, procedure, activity, or work that can be delegated to nursing assistants when it does not require an RN's professional knowledge or judgment

responsibility The duty or obligation to perform some act or function

KEY ABBREVIATIONS

CNA Certified nursing assistant, certified nurse aide

EMT Emergency medical technician

IV Intravenous infusion; intravenous

LNA Licensed nursing assistant

LPN Licensed practical nurse

LVN Licensed vocational nurse

MLT Medical laboratory technician

OBRA Omnibus Budget Reconciliation Act of 1987

NATCEP Nursing assistant training and competency evaluation program

NCSBN National Council of State Boards of Nursing

RN Registered nurse

RNA Registered nurse aide

Federal and state laws and agency policies combine to define the roles and functions of each health team member. Everyone must protect patients and residents from harm. To do so, you need to know:

▶ What you can and cannot do

▶ Your legal limits

Laws, job descriptions, and the person's condition shape your work. So does the amount of supervision you need.

HISTORY AND CURRENT TRENDS

For decades, nursing assistants have helped nurses with basic nursing care. Often called *nurse's aides*, they gave baths and made beds. They helped with grooming, elimination, and other needs. Their work was similar in hospitals and nursing homes. Until the 1980s, training was not required by law. RNs gave on-the-job training. Some hospitals, nursing homes, and schools offered nursing assistant courses.

Before the 1980s, team nursing was common. A registered nurse (RN) was the team leader. The RN assigned care to nurses and nursing assistants. Care was assigned according to each person's needs and condition. It also depended on the staff member's education and experiences.

Primary nursing was common in the 1980s. RNs planned and gave care. Many hospitals only hired RNs. Meanwhile, nursing homes relied on nursing assistants for resident care.

Home care increased during the 1980s. Prospective payment systems limit health care payments (Chapter 1). To reduce care costs, hospital stays also are limited. Therefore patients are discharged earlier than in the past. Often they are still quite ill and need home care.

Efforts to reduce health care costs include:

▶ *Hospital closings.* Many do not make enough money to stay open.

▶ *Hospital mergers.* Hospitals merge to share resources and to avoid the same costly services. For example, one hospital offers heart surgery. The other serves women and children.

▶ *Health care systems.* Agencies join together as one provider of care. A system often has hospitals, nursing centers, and home care agencies. It also has hospice settings, ambulance services, and doctors. For example, a hospital patient needs long-term care. The person transfers from the hospital to a system nursing center. The person is transported by the system-owned ambulance service. After rehabilitation, the person returns home. The system-owned home care agency provides needed services in the home setting. The person's care stays within the system from the hospital to the home setting.

▶ *Managed care.* Insurers have contracts with doctors, hospitals, and health care systems for reduced rates. See Chapter 1.

▶ *Staffing mix.* Hospitals hire RNs, licensed practical nurses/licensed vocational nurses (LPNs/LVNs), and nursing assistants. Most hospitals require a state-approved nursing assistant training and competency evaluation for employment. More training is given for tasks not in the training program.

▶ *Patient-focused care.* Services are moved from departments to the bedside. Staff members are cross-trained to perform basic skills performed by other health team members. For example, the doctor orders a blood test for Ms. Tyler. The nurse tells the unit secretary who calls the laboratory. The laboratory secretary tells a medical laboratory technician (MLT). The MLT sends a staff member to Ms. Tyler's room to draw the blood sample. Five people are involved so far. With patient-focused care and cross-training, Ms. Tyler's blood is drawn by a nursing team member when the order is given. Ms. Tyler does not wait for the MLT to arrive. She is served faster by fewer staff members. Fewer staff members reduce costs.

FEDERAL AND STATE LAWS

The U.S. Congress makes federal laws for all 50 states to follow. State legislatures make state laws. For example, the New York legislature makes state laws for New York. The Texas legislature for Texas. You must know the state and federal laws that affect your work. They provide direction for what you can do.

Nurse Practice Acts

Each state has a nurse practice act. It regulates nursing practice in that state. It does so to protect the public's welfare and safety. A nurse practice act:

▶ Defines RN and LPN/LVN. Some acts also define nursing assistant.
▶ Describes the scope of practice for RNs and LPNs/LVNs.
▶ Describes education and licensing requirements for RNs and LPNs/LVNs.
▶ Protects the public from persons practicing nursing without a license. Persons who do not meet the state's requirements cannot perform nursing functions.

The law allows for denying, revoking, or suspending a nursing license. The purpose for doing so is to protect the public from unsafe nurses. Reasons include:

▶ Being convicted of a crime in any state
▶ Selling or distributing drugs
▶ Using the person's drugs for oneself
▶ Placing a person in danger from the overuse of alcohol or drugs
▶ Demonstrating grossly negligent nursing practice
▶ Being convicted of abusing or neglecting children or older persons
▶ Violating a nurse practice act and its rules and regulations
▶ Demonstrating incompetent behaviors
▶ Aiding or assisting another person to violate a nurse practice act and its rules and regulations
▶ Making medical diagnoses
▶ Prescribing drugs and treatments

Nursing Assistants

A state's nurse practice act is used to decide what nursing assistants can do. Some nurse practice acts also regulate nursing assistant roles, functions, education, and certification requirements. In other states, there are separate laws for nursing assistants.

Legal and advisory opinions about nursing assistants are based on the state's nurse practice act. So are any state laws about their roles and functions. If you do something beyond the legal limits of your role, you could be practicing nursing without a license. This creates serious legal problems for you and the nurse supervising your work.

In most states, nursing assistants are certified after passing the state's education and competency evaluation program (p. 14). They have the title of certified nursing assistant (CNA). Some states license nursing assistants or register nurse aides. They are LNAs or RNAs.

Nursing assistants must be able to function with reasonable skill and safety. Like nurses, nursing assistants can have their certification, license, or registration denied, revoked, or suspended (Fig. 2-1). The National Council

CNA VIOLATIONS 2000-2005
ARIZONA STATE BOARD OF NURSING

Category	Total	2000	2001	2002	2003	2004	2005
Criminal conviction	2196	205	415	500	496	288	292
Drug related	907	90	212	207	146	108	144
Misconduct	824	67	126	182	157	141	151
Fraud deceit	526	82	119	84	101	84	56
Unprofessional conduct	492	23	90	72	125	85	97
Failure to cooperate	486		4	48	183	131	120
Violating board order	179		20	28	43	46	42
Sexual misconduct	98	7	31	17	14	8	21
Other	50		10	21	6		13
Practicing without certificate	24		2	1	11	10	
Violating State/Federal statutes/rules	21		14	7			
Inability to practice safely	11	2	3	2	2	1	1
Action in another jurisdiction	7	1	1	2	3		
Adjudication	7		5			1	1
Failure to renew	6				3	3	
Failure to report violations	3	1		2			

A

TRH, 1/26/2006

FIGURE 2-1 A, Types of nursing assistant violations in Arizona from 2000 through 2005. (Courtesy Arizona State Board of Nursing, 2006, Phoenix, Ariz.)

Continued

**CNA DISCIPLINARY ACTIONS TAKEN 2000-2005
ARIZONA STATE BOARD OF NURSING**

B

Discipline	Total	2000	2001	2002	2003	2004	2005
Certificate denied	957	80	166	221	228	119	143
Civil penalty	493	10	66	110	109	117	81
Revocation	708	80	117	165	127	114	105
Stayed revocation	20					5	15
Stayed suspension	69			1	19	31	18
Suspension	130	9	13	17	34	33	25
Voluntary surrender	110	10	23	13	6	21	37

TRH, 1/26/2006

FIGURE 2-1, cont'd B, Nursing assistant disciplinary actions taken in Arizona from 2000 through 2005. (Courtesy Arizona State Board of Nursing, 2006, Phoenix, Ariz.)

of State Boards of Nursing (NCSBN) lists these reasons for doing so:

▶ Substance abuse or dependency
▶ Abandoning a patient or resident
▶ Abusing a patient or resident
▶ Fraud or deceit; examples include:
  ▶ Filing false personal information
  ▶ Providing false information when applying for initial certification
  ▶ Providing false information when applying to have certification re-instated
  ▶ Providing false information when applying for certification renewal
▶ Neglecting a patient or resident
▶ Violating professional boundaries (Chapter 3)
▶ Giving unsafe care
▶ Performing acts beyond the nursing assistant role
▶ Misappropriation (stealing, theft) or misusing property
▶ Obtaining money or property from a patient or resident; the nursing assistant did so through fraud, falsely representing oneself, or through force
▶ Having been convicted of a crime; examples include murder, assault, kidnapping, rape or sexual assault, robbery, sexual crimes involving children, criminal mistreatment of children or a vulnerable adult (Chapter 3), drug trafficking, embezzlement (to take a person's property for one's own use), theft, and arson (starting fires)
▶ Failing to conform to the standards of nursing assistants (p. 17)
▶ Putting patients and residents at risk for harm
▶ Violating the privacy of a patient or resident
▶ Failing to maintain the confidentiality of patient or resident information

The Omnibus Budget Reconciliation Act of 1987

The Omnibus Budget Reconciliation Act of 1987 (OBRA) is a federal law. Therefore it applies to all 50 states. Its purpose is to improve the quality of life of nursing center residents.

This law sets minimum training and competency evaluation requirements for nursing assistants. Each state must have a nursing assistant training and competency

evaluation program (NATCEP). It must be successfully completed by nursing assistants working in nursing centers, hospital long-term care units, and home care agencies receiving Medicare funds.

The Training Program

OBRA requires at least 75 hours of instruction. Some states require more hours. There must be at least 16 hours of supervised practical training. Such training occurs in a laboratory or clinical setting (Fig. 2-2). Students perform nursing care and procedures on another person. A nurse supervises this practical training (clinical practicum or clinical experience).

The training program includes the knowledge and skills needed to give basic nursing care. Areas of study include:

▶ Communication
▶ Infection control
▶ Safety and emergency procedures
▶ Residents' rights
▶ Basic nursing skills
▶ Personal care skills
▶ Feeding methods
▶ Elimination procedures
▶ Skin care
▶ Transferring, positioning, and turning methods
▶ Dressing
▶ Helping the person walk
▶ Range-of-motion exercises
▶ Signs and symptoms of common diseases
▶ How to care for cognitively impaired persons (those who have problems with thinking and memory)

Competency Evaluation

The competency evaluation has a written test and a skills test (Appendix A, p. 783). The written test has multiple-choice questions. Each has 4 choices. Only 1 answer is correct. The number of questions varies from state to state.

The skills test involves performing nursing skills. You will perform certain skills learned in your training program.

You take the competency evaluation after your training

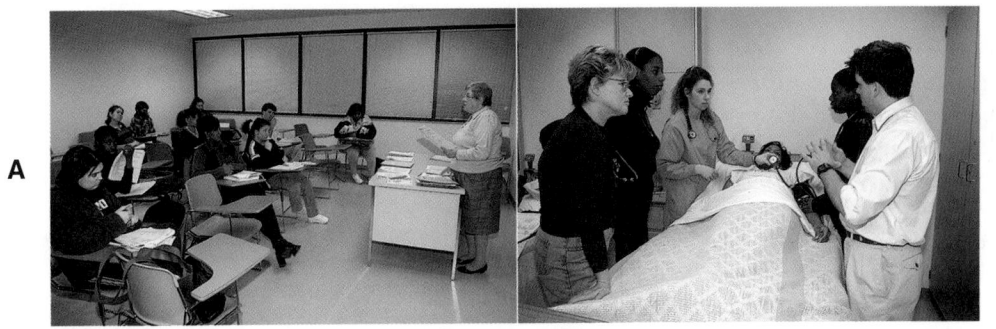

FIGURE 2-2 Nursing assistant training program. **A,** Students study in a classroom setting. **B,** Students practice nursing in a laboratory setting.

program. Your instructor tells you when and where the tests are given. He or she helps you complete the application. There is a fee for the evaluation. If you work in a nursing center, the employer pays this fee. You are told the place and time of the tests after your application is processed. Some states give a choice of test dates and sites.

Your training prepares you for the competency evaluation. If you listen, study hard, and practice safe care, you should do well. If the first attempt was not successful, you can retest. OBRA allows at least 3 attempts to successfully complete the evaluation.

Nursing Assistant Registry

OBRA requires a nursing assistant registry in each state. It is an official record or listing of persons who have successfully completed that state's state-approved NATCEP. The registry has information about each nursing assistant:

- Full name, including maiden name and any married names
- Last known home address
- Registration number and the date it expires
- Date of birth
- Last known employer, date hired, and date employment ended
- Date the competency evaluation was passed
- Information about findings of abuse, neglect, or dishonest use of property. It includes the nature of the offense and supporting evidence. If a hearing was held, the date and its outcome are included. The person has the right to include a statement disputing the finding. All information stays in the registry for at least 5 years.

Any agency can access registry information. You also receive a copy of your registry information. The copy is provided when the first entry is made and when information is changed or added. You can correct wrong information.

Other OBRA Requirements

Retraining and a new competency evaluation program are required for nursing assistants who have not worked for 24 months. It does not matter how long you worked as a

---

TEAMWORK AND TIME MANAGEMENT

Other OBRA Requirements

Required educational programs are commonly called in-service programs or in-service training. Some programs are required; others are optional. Program announcements and schedules are posted on bulletin boards on nursing units, in staff locker rooms and lounges, and by the time clock. Some are included with your paycheck. Know where your agency posts in-service information. Check those areas often.

Such training is scheduled before your shift begins, during your shift, or after your shift. If scheduled before work, plan to arrive early. If scheduled after work, plan to stay late. Arrange for transportation and childcare as needed (Chapter 4).

If the program is during your shift, you need to plan with your co-workers. Some staff stay on the unit while others attend the program. Staff on the unit tend to all patients and residents. A person may have special care needs while you are off the unit. Share this information with the staff who will provide such care. When you return to the unit, thank your co-workers for helping you. Help your co-workers when they leave the unit to attend in-service programs.

---

nursing assistant. What matters is how long you did *not* work. States can require:

- A new competency evaluation
- Both retraining and a new competency evaluation

Agencies covered under OBRA must provide 12 hours of educational programs to nursing assistants every year. Performance reviews also are required. That is, the nursing assistant's work is evaluated. These requirements help ensure that nursing assistants have current knowledge and skills to give safe, effective care.

See *Teamwork and Time Management: Other OBRA Requirements.*

Certification

Each state NATCEP must meet OBRA requirements. Some states require more training hours. And each state has its own competency evaluation. After successfully completing your state's NATCEP, you have the title used in your state:

- Certified nursing assistant (CNA) or certified nurse aide (CNA) (CNA is used in most states.)
- Licensed nursing assistant (LNA)
- Registered nurse aide (RNA)

Working in Another State

If you want to work in another state, you must meet that state's registry requirements. To do so, contact the state agency responsible for NATCEPs and the nursing assistant registry. To find that agency, do one of the following:

▶ Contact your current nursing assistant registry.
▶ Go to the National Council of State Boards of Nursing website. Find the link to the state agency.

You need to apply to the state agency to be a CNA (LNA, RNA). The state will use one of the following terms: *endorsement*, *reciprocity*, or *equivalency*. The terms essentially mean that:

▶ Your application for CNA (LNA, RNA) is reviewed to see if you meet the state's requirements.
  ▶ Your certification (license, registration) is current and in good standing.
  ▶ You meet that state's education, work, and legal requirements.
▶ Certification, a license, or registration is granted if the requirements are met.

Follow the application instructions. Expect to:

▶ Complete the required forms.
▶ Provide proof of successfully completing a NATCEP. You may need to send a copy of the certificate of completion from your NATCEP. Do not send the original.
▶ Request written registry verification from the state in which you are currently certified (licensed, registered). Pay the required fee.
▶ Provide fingerprints.
▶ Pay the required application fee.

A criminal background check is a common requirement. Registry information is checked. Expect an investigation if the check shows a criminal history. Or if the registry check shows findings of abuse, neglect, dishonest use of property, or other actions against you.

You must be truthful. False or misleading information may result in:

▶ Denial of certification (a license, registration)
▶ Disciplinary action
▶ A fine

The review results in one more of the following:

▶ Being granted or denied certification, a license, or registration
▶ Having to take a competency test; this may be the written test, the skills test, or both
▶ Having to take a NATCEP in that state

ROLES AND RESPONSIBILITIES

Nurse practice acts, OBRA, state laws, and legal and advisory opinions direct what you can do. To protect persons from harm, you must understand what you can do, what you cannot do, and the legal limits of your role. In some states, this is called *scope of practice*. The NCSBN calls it *range of functions*.

BOX 2-1 Rules for Nursing Assistants

- You are an assistant to the nurse.
- A nurse assigns and supervises your work.
- You report observations about the person's physical and mental status to the nurse. Report changes in the person's condition or behavior at once.
- The nurse decides what should be done for a person. The nurse decides what should not be done for a person. You do not make these decisions.
- Review directions and the care plan with the nurse before going to the person.
- Perform no nursing task that you are not trained to do.
- Perform no nursing task that you are not comfortable doing without a nurse's supervision.
- Perform only the nursing tasks that your state and job description allow.

Licensed nurses supervise your work. You assist them in giving care. You also perform nursing tasks related to the person's care. A **nursing task** is the nursing care or a nursing function, procedure, activity, or work that can be delegated to nursing assistants when it does not require an RN's professional knowledge or judgment. Often you function without a nurse in the room. At other times you help nurses give care. In some agencies, you assist doctors with procedures. The rules in Box 2-1 will help you understand your role.

Nursing assistant functions and responsibilities vary among states and agencies. Before you perform a nursing task make sure that:

▶ Your state allows nursing assistants to do so
▶ It is in your job description
▶ You have the necessary education and training
▶ A nurse is available to answer questions and to supervise you

You perform nursing tasks to meet the person's hygiene, safety, comfort, nutrition, exercise, and elimination needs. You also handle and move persons, make observations, and collect specimens. You assist with admitting and discharging patients and residents. You also measure temperatures, pulses, respirations, and blood pressures. And you have a role in the person's mental comfort.

Box 2-2 describes the limits of your role. These are the nursing tasks that you should never do. State laws differ. You must know what you can do in the state in which you are working. For example, you move from Vermont to Maine. You must learn the laws and rules in Maine. Or you might work in two states. For example, you work in agencies in Illinois and Iowa. You must know the laws and rules of both states.

Some nursing assistants are also emergency medical technicians (EMTs). EMTs give emergency care outside of health care settings. These settings are called "in the field." EMTs work under the direction of doctors in hospital emergency departments. State laws and rules for EMTs and nursing assistants differ. For example, Joan

BOX 2-2 Role Limits for Nursing Assistants

- **Never give drugs.** This includes drugs given orally, rectally, vaginally, and by injection. It also includes drugs given by application to the skin, eyes, ears, and nose. Nor do you give drugs directly into the bloodstream or through an intravenous (IV) line. Nurses give drugs. Many states allow nursing assistants to give drugs under certain conditions. To do so, you must complete a state-approved medication assistant training program. The function must be in your job description. And you must have the necessary supervision.
- **Never insert tubes or objects into body openings. Do not remove them from the body.** You must not insert tubes into a person's bladder, esophagus, trachea, nose, ears, bloodstream, or surgically created body openings. Exceptions to this rule are those procedures described in this textbook (giving enemas is an example). You may study and practice these procedures during your training. To perform them, they must be in your job description. And you must have the necessary supervision.
- **Never take oral or phone orders from doctors.** Politely give your name and title, and ask the doctor to wait for a nurse. Promptly find a nurse to speak with the doctor.
- **Never perform procedures that require sterile technique.** With sterile technique, all objects in contact with the person are free of microorganisms (Chapter 14). Sterile technique and procedures require skills, knowledge, and judgment beyond your training. You can assist a nurse with a sterile procedure. However, you will not perform the procedure yourself.
- **Never tell the person or family the person's diagnosis or medical or surgical treatment plans.** This is the doctor's responsibility. Nurses may clarify what the doctor has said.
- **Never diagnose or prescribe treatments or drugs for anyone.** Doctors diagnose and prescribe.
- **Never supervise others including other nursing assistants.** This is a nurse's legal responsibility. You will not be trained to supervise others. Supervising others can have serious legal problems.
- **Never ignore an order or request to do something.** This includes nursing tasks that you can do, those you cannot do, and those that are beyond your legal limits. Promptly and politely explain to the nurse why you cannot carry out the order or request. The nurse assumes you are doing what you were told to do unless you explain otherwise. You cannot neglect the person's care.

Woods is an EMT for a fire department. When off duty, she is a nursing assistant at Deer Valley Hospital. Her state allows EMTs to start intravenous infusions (IVs) in the field. However, nursing assistants do not start IVs. Ms. Woods cannot start IVs when working at the hospital as a nursing assistant.

The situation is similar for persons who were medics or corpsmen in military service. They can suture wounds. Nursing assistants cannot do so. When working as nursing assistants, medics and corpsmen must follow their state's laws and rules for nursing assistants. As with EMTs, the ability to do something does not give the right to do so in all settings.

FOCUS ON LONG-TERM CARE AND HOME CARE

Roles and Responsibilities

HOME CARE

You provide personal care and home services. Home services depend on the needs of the person and family. They may include:
- Doing laundry. Clothing and linens are washed, ironed or folded, and mended. This may include family laundry.
- Shopping for groceries and household items.
- Preparing and serving meals. You plan menus, follow diets, and feed the person if necessary.
- Doing light housekeeping. You do not do heavy housekeeping. This includes moving heavy furniture, waxing floors, shampooing carpets, washing windows, and cleaning rugs or drapes. You do not carry firewood, coal, or ash containers.

State laws and rules limit nursing assistant functions. Your job description reflects those laws and rules. An agency can further limit what you can do. So can a nurse based on the person's needs. However, no agency or nurse can expand your range of functions beyond what is allowed by your state's laws and rules.

See *Focus on Long-Term Care and Home Care: Roles and Responsibilities.*

BOX 2-3 Nursing Assistant Standards

The nursing assistant:
- Performs nursing tasks within the range of functions allowed by the state's nurse practice act and its rules.
- Is honest and shows integrity in performing nursing tasks. (*Integrity* involves following a code of ethics [Chapter 3].)
- Bases nursing tasks on his or her education and training. Also bases them on the nurse's directions.
- Is accountable for his or her behavior and actions while assisting the nurse and helping patients and residents.
- Performs delegated aspects of the person's nursing care.
- Assists the nurse in observing patients and residents. Also assists in identifying their needs.
- Communicates:
  - Progress toward completing delegated nursing tasks
  - Problems in completing delegated nursing tasks
  - Changes in the person's status
- Asks the nurse to clarify what is expected when unsure.
- Uses educational and training opportunities as available.
- Practices safety measures to protect the person, others, and self.
- Respects the person's rights, concerns, decisions, and dignity.
- Functions as a member of the health team. Helps implement the care plan (Chapter 6).
- Respects the person's property and the property of others. Protects confidential information unless required by law to share the information.

Modified from National Council of State Boards of Nursing: *Draft model language: nursing assistive personnel,* Chicago, Ill, 2005.

Nursing Assistant Standards

OBRA defines the basic range of functions for nursing assistants. All NATCEPs include those functions (p. 14). Some states allow other functions. NATCEPs also prepare nursing assistants to meet the standards listed in Box 2-3, p. 17.

Job Description

The **job description** is a document that describes what the agency expects you to do (Fig. 2-3). It also states educational requirements.

Always obtain a written job description when you apply for a job. Ask questions about it during your job interview. Before accepting a job, tell the employer about functions you did not learn. Also advise the employer of functions you cannot do for moral or religious reasons. Clearly understand what is expected before taking a job. Do not take a job that requires you to:

▶ Act beyond the legal limits of your role
▶ Function beyond your training limits
▶ Perform acts that are against your morals or religion

No one can force you to do something beyond the legal limits of your role. Sometimes jobs are threatened for refusing to follow a nurse's orders. Often staff obey out of fear. That is why you must understand your roles and responsibilities. You also need to know what you can safely do, the things you should never do, and your job description. Understanding the ethical and legal aspects of your role is equally important (Chapter 3).

See *Focus on Communication: Job Description.*

See *Focus on Communication: Job Description.*

FOCUS ON COMMUNICATION

Job Description

Your training prepares you to perform certain nursing tasks. The agency may not let you do everything you learned. Other agencies may want you to do things that you did not learn. Use your job description if you need to discuss these issues with your supervisor.

For example, Mr. Wey is in the bathroom when the nurse brings a drug to him. The nurse tells you to give him the drug when he comes out of the bathroom. If you give the drug, you are performing a task and responsibility beyond the limits of your role. With respect, you must firmly refuse to follow the nurse's direction. You can say: "I'm sorry, but I cannot give Mr. Wey that drug. I was not trained to give drugs, and that task is not in my job description. I'll let you know when Mr. Wey comes out of the bathroom."

JOB DESCRIPTION

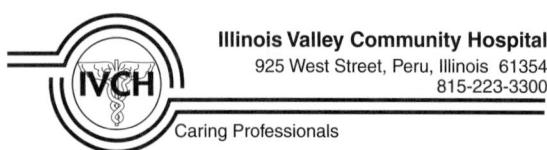

Illinois Valley Community Hospital
925 West Street, Peru, Illinois 61354
815-223-3300
Caring Professionals

CRITERIA: NURSE ASSISTANT   NAME: _____   UNIT: _____

The following criteria are to be considered as an integral part of this job description and are used in the evaluation process.

ASSISTING WITH NURSING CARE	Met	Not Met
ASSISTS WITH ASSESSING Recognizes abnormal vital signs and reports them to the nurse in charge immediately.		
Observes patients and reports problems (e.g., bleeding, drainage, voiding, machine functions, IV drip, safety situations) immediately and/or current status to the nurse in charge.		
Checks on patients regularly, making frequent rounds.		
ASSISTS WITH PLANNING/ORGANIZING Consistently organizes and appropriately executes personal work assignments in an effort to achieve maximum productivity and efficiency during the assigned shift.		
Demonstrates a time-conscious awareness and consistently strives to use time effectively, completing assigned procedures during scheduled shift.		
Responds to changes in the unit workload, patient census, and staffing levels; plans patient care accordingly.		
Demonstrates an ability to recognize and deal with priorities promptly.		

FIGURE 2-3 Nursing assistant job description. Note that the job description is also a performance evaluation tool. (Modified from Illinois Valley Community Hospital, Peru, Ill.)

Continued

ASSISTING WITH NURSING CARE (CONT'D)	Met	Not Met
ASSISTS WITH IMPLEMENTING Administers patient care based on the plan of care.		
Effectively implements nursing orders after consulting appropriate sources regarding unfamiliar or questionable orders.		
Responds to patient's condition/needs and acts in a timely and appropriate manner.		
Demonstrates a reliable and dependable ability to follow through with designated responsibilities in collecting, labeling, and transporting specimens to the proper area at the appropriate time: always correctly labels type of specimen collected, including patient's name and room number.		
Assists the nurse with complicated treatment procedures.		
Completes work left from previous shifts and reports all incomplete assignments to ensure continuity of care.		
As required, provides for patient comfort (by positioning, extra bathing, straightening linens, putting personal articles within reach) with courtesy and responsiveness.		
Routinely assists patients with elimination (bedpan, bathroom) as required.		
Regularly ambulates patients as assigned; demonstrates proper techniques.		
Consistently demonstrates competence in providing morning, evening, and general care routines in accordance with established nursing care procedures to ensure patients' comfort and safety.		
Regularly prepares patients for meals, sets up each patient and patient's tray, assists in feeding patients (if necessary), positions patients to avoid choking and for ease in eating, and distributes water and other nourishments according to patients' needs; regularly provides patients with fresh water.		
Always follows the nursing care plan; observes established policies and procedures for proper patient treatment and care.		
Promptly answers patient signal lights, whether that of assigned patient or not.		
ASSISTS WITH EVALUATING Checks physical environment of unit to determine what needs to be done in terms of smooth operation.		
Evaluates need for linen changes.		
Reviews basic care provided to patients and reports if changes are needed.		
ASSISTS WITH TEACHING/LEARNING Regularly provides patient information on admission in regard to: correct storage of patients' valuables, eyeglasses, and dentures; use of equipment, bed controls, nurse/patient communication system; location of bathroom and emergency call signals; and specimen collection.		
Serves as a resource person for new employees during orientation.		
Demonstrates the knowledge and skills necessary to provide care appropriate to pediatric, adolescent, adult, and geriatric patients. (Attends two age-specific in-services.)		
Demonstrates the knowledge of the principles of growth and development over the life span. (Score at least 80% on post-test.)		
Recognizes own inadequacies, and seeks assistance appropriately.		
COMMUNICATING		
Communicates to appropriate members of the health care team specific observations or changes in patient's condition.		
Explains information to patients, visitors, and co-workers in a clear and thorough manner; leaves no questions unanswered and follows up on information not readily available.		
Consistently communicates appropriately with patients: speaks respectfully, addresses patients by name, responds to patients' needs or requests for assistance.		

FIGURE 2-3, cont'd Nursing assistant job description. Note that the job description is also a performance evaluation tool. (Modified from Illinois Valley Community Hospital, Peru, Ill.)
Continued

	Met	Not Met
JUDGMENT/LEADERSHIP		
Promotes teamwork among staff.		
Reports all patient care or management problems as appropriate, using chain of command.		
Functions in a calm manner during emergency and crisis situations.		
MAINTAINING SAFETY/INFECTION CONTROL/PATIENT RIGHTS		
Always demonstrates knowledge of and rationale for safe use of equipment; reports any equipment malfunctions and orders service, as necessary.		
Ensures patient safety by maintaining bed in a low position and signal light within reach at all times. Identifies patients before performing procedures. Follows the care plan for bed rail use.		
Uses proper techniques of body mechanics.		
Assists in maintaining a clean, safe, and attractive environment in all areas of the patient unit.		
Practices hand hygiene before and after each patient contact; uses aseptic technique during procedures and treatments.		
Uses principles of Standard and Transmission-Based Precautions. Follows the Bloodborne Pathogen Standard.		
Adheres to *The Patient Care Partnership: Understanding Expectations, Rights, and Responsibilities,* and respects the patient's right to privacy, dignity, and confidentiality.		
Handles all patients' clothing, dentures, eyeglasses, and other valuables with care.		
RELATIONSHIP WITH OTHERS		
Demonstrates a high level of mental and emotional tolerance and even temperament when dealing with ill people; uses tact, sensitivity, sound judgment, and a professional attitude when relating with patients, families, co-workers, and physicians.		
Greets all patients in a courteous manner by introducing self and calling the patient by name.		
Displays an unhurried, caring manner in all personal contact; demonstrates the ability to remain friendly and cooperative during all work situations.		
Consistently responds to others in a helpful manner, especially in times of increased patient activities or short staffing situations.		
Promotes an atmosphere of acceptance for new staff members on the unit.		
ATTENDANCE AND RELIABILITY		
Consistently is on time and ready to work at the start of the shift; requires no start-up time.		
Willingly accepts reassignments to other units when necessary.		
Consistently returns promptly from errands, coffee breaks, and meals.		
Complies with Absenteeism Policy.		

FIGURE 2-3, cont'd Nursing assistant job description. Note that the job description is also a performance evaluation tool. (Modified from Illinois Valley Community Hospital, Peru, Ill.)

	Met	Not Met
COOPERATION/SUPPORT		
Attends and actively participates in unit meetings (75% of the time).		
Accepts additional assignments willingly.		
Consistently promotes good public relations for the unit, nursing department, and hospital.		
Supports hospital philosophy, policies and procedures, and management decisions.		
INITIATIVE		
Takes initiative in recognition and resolution of problems.		
Reports to the nurse manager or appropriate supervisor any suggestions or recommendations for positive changes within the departmental policies and procedures.		
Ensures that supplies are maintained according to established guidelines, and notifies appropriate person to restock.		
PROFESSIONAL GROWTH/APPEARANCE		
Always appears well-groomed and observes the hospital dress code; wears identification badge while on duty; maintains a professional appearance at all times; is clean and well-groomed.		
Maintains professional code of ethics.		
Attends all mandatory programs including those on safety, infection control, and CPR.		
Attends a minimum of 5 other programs throughout the year.		
Identifies own self-development needs, and writes goals for same. Strives to achieve those goals.		
Demonstrates ability to perform unit-specific competencies.		
PARTICIPATES IN PROFESSIONAL/COMMUNITY ORGANIZATIONS/ACTIVITIES OR HOSPITAL-RELATED COMMUNITY ACTIVITIES. **LIST:** **BONUS**		
DEMONSTRATES PROFESSIONAL GROWTH BY ACQUIRING COLLEGE CREDIT, CEUs, OR CERTIFICATION. **BONUS**		
REGULARLY CONTRIBUTES TO NURSING AND HOSPITAL FUNCTIONS THROUGH ACTIVE PARTICIPATION ON COMMITTEES. **BONUS**		
WORKS EXTRA WEEKENDS/HOLIDAYS TO ASSIST IN PROVIDING ADEQUATE STAFFING. **BONUS**		
ROTATES SHIFTS AND WORKS EXTRA HOURS TO ASSIST IN PROVIDING ADEQUATE STAFFING. **BONUS**		

FIGURE 2-3, cont'd Nursing assistant job description. Note that the job description is also a performance evaluation tool. (Modified from Illinois Valley Community Hospital, Peru, Ill.)

DELEGATION

Nurse practice acts give nurses certain responsibilities. They also give them the legal authority to perform nursing actions. A **responsibility** is the duty or obligation to perform some act or function. For example, RNs are responsible for supervising LPNs/LVNs and nursing assistants. Only RNs can carry out this responsibility.

Delegate means to authorize another person to perform a nursing task in a certain situation. The person must be competent to perform a task in a given situation. For example, you know how to give a bed bath. However, Mr. Jones is a new resident. The RN wants to spend time with him and assess his nursing needs. You do not assess. Therefore the RN gives the bath.

Who Can Delegate

RNs can delegate nursing tasks to LPNs/LVNs and nursing assistants. In some states, LPNs/LVNs can delegate tasks to nursing assistants. RNs and LPNs/LVNs can only delegate tasks within their scope of practice. And they can only delegate tasks that are in the nursing assistant's job description.

Delegation decisions must protect the person's health and safety. The delegating nurse is legally accountable for the nursing task. **Accountable** means to be responsible for one's actions and the actions of others who performed the delegated tasks. It also involves answering questions about the task and explaining one's actions and the actions of others.

The delegating nurse must make sure that the task was completed safely and correctly. If the RN delegates, the RN is responsible for the delegated task. If the LPN/LVN delegates, the LPN/LVN is responsible for the delegated task. The RN also supervises LPNs/LVNs. Therefore the RN is legally accountable for the tasks that LPNs/LVNs delegate to nursing assistants. The RN is accountable for all nursing care.

Nursing assistants cannot delegate. You cannot delegate any task to other nursing assistants or to any other worker. You can ask someone to help you. But you cannot ask or tell someone to do your work.

Delegation Process

To make delegation decisions, the nurse follows a process. The person's needs, the nursing task, and the staff member doing the task must fit. The nurse can decide to delegate the task to you. Or the nurse can decide not to delegate the task. The person's needs and the task may require a nurse's knowledge, judgment, and skill. You may be asked to assist.

Do not get offended or angry if you cannot perform a task that is usually delegated to you. The nurse decides what is best for the person at the time. That decision is also best for you at that time. You should not do something that requires a nurse's judgment. For example, you always care for Mrs. Mills. Now she is weak and not eating well. The nurse wants to observe and evaluate the changes in her condition. The nurse decides to give needed care. At this time Mrs. Mills needs the nurse's judgment and knowledge.

The person's circumstances are central factors in delegation decisions. Delegation decisions must result in the best care for the person. A nurse risks a person's health and safety with poor delegation decisions. Also, the nurse may face serious legal problems. If you perform a task that places the person at risk, you can also face serious legal problems.

The NCSBN describes the delegation process in four steps.

Step 1—Assess and Plan

Step 1 is done by the nurse. To safely delegate, the nurse needs to understand the person's needs. And the nurse needs to know your knowledge, skills, and job description.

When assessing the person's needs, the nurse answers these questions.

- What is the nature of the person's needs? How complex are the needs? How can they vary? How urgent are the care needs?
- What are the most important long-term needs? What are the most important short-term needs?
- How much judgment is needed to meet the person's needs and give care?
- How predictable is the person's health status? How does the person respond to health care?
- What kind of problems might arise from the nursing task? How severe might the problems be?
- What actions are needed if a problem arises? How complex are those actions?
- What kind of emergencies or incidents might arise? How likely might they occur?
- How involved is the person in health care decisions? How involved is the family?
- How will delegating the nursing task help the person? What are the risks to the person?

To assess your knowledge and skills, the nurse answers these questions.

- What knowledge and skills are needed to safely perform the nursing task?
- What is your role in the agency? What is in your job description?
- What are the conditions under which the nursing task will be performed?
- What is expected after the nursing task is performed?
- What problems can arise from the nursing task? What problems might the person develop during the nursing task?

The nurse then decides if it is safe to delegate the nursing task. It must be safe for the person and safe for you. If unsafe, the nurse stops the delegation process. If it is safe for the person and you, the nurse moves to step 2.

Step 2—Communication

This step involves the nurse and you. The nurse must provide clear and complete directions about:

- How to perform and complete the task
- What observations to report and record
- When to report observations
- What specific patient and resident concerns to report at once
- Priorities for nursing tasks
- What to do if the person's needs or condition changes

The nurse needs to make sure that you understand the directions. The nurse asks you questions to make sure you understand. He or she may ask you to explain what you are going to do. Do not be insulted by the nurse's questions. The nurse must make sure that safe care is given. This protects the person and you.

Before performing a delegated nursing task, you must have the opportunity to discuss the task with the nurse. Make sure that you:

- Ask questions about the delegated task.
- Ask questions about what you are expected to do.
- Tell the nurse if you have not done the task before. Also tell the nurse if you have not done it often.
- Ask for needed training or supervision.
- Restate what is expected of you.
- Restate what specific patient or resident concerns to report to the nurse.
- Explain how and when you will report your progress in completing the task.
- Know how to contact the nurse if there is an emergency.
- Know what the nurse wants you to do if there is an emergency.

After completing a delegated task, you must report and record the care given. You also report and record your observations. See "Reporting and Recording" in Chapter 5.

Step 3—Surveillance and Supervision

Surveillance means to keep a close watch over someone or something. *Supervise* means to oversee, direct, or manage. In this step, the nurse observes the care you give. The nurse has to make sure that you complete the task correctly. The nurse also observes the person's condition and response to your care. How often the nurse makes observations depends on:

- The person's health status and needs
- If the person's condition is stable or unstable
- If the nurse can predict the person's responses and risk to care
- The setting where the nursing task occurs
- The resources and support available
- If the nursing task is simple or complex

The nurse must follow up on any problems or concerns. For example, the nurse must take action if you did not complete the nursing task in a timely manner. The nurse also must take action if the nursing task did not meet expectations. An unexpected change in the person's condition is also cause for the nurse to act.

The nurse must be alert for signs and symptoms that signal a possible change in the person's condition. This way the nurse, with your help, can take action before the person's condition changes in a major way.

Sometimes problems arise in completing a nursing task. By supervising you, the nurse can detect and solve problems early. This helps you complete the task safely and on time.

After you complete the task, the nurse may review and discuss what happened with you. This helps you learn. If a similar situation happens in the future, you have ideas about how to adjust.

Step 4—Evaluation and Feedback

This step is done by the nurse. *Evaluate* means to judge. The nurse decides if the delegation was successful. The nurse answers these questions:

- Was the nursing task done correctly?
- Did the person respond to the nursing task as expected?
- Was the outcome (the result) as desired? Was it satisfactory or not satisfactory?
- Was communication between you and the nurse timely and effective?
- What went well? What were the problems?
- Does the care plan need to change (Chapter 6)? Or can the plan stay the same?
- Did the nursing task present ways for the nurse or you to learn?
- Did the nurse give you the right feedback? *Feedback* means to respond. The nurse tells you what you did correctly. If you did something wrong, the nurse tells you that too. Feedback is another way in which you can learn and improve the care you give.
- Did the nurse thank you for completing the nursing task?

See *Focus on Long-Term Care and Home Care: Communication.*

FOCUS ON LONG-TERM CARE AND HOME CARE

Communication

HOME CARE

The delegating nurse is not with you when you give home care. The nurse may be at the agency or at another person's home. The nurse and you must decide on the best way to communicate with each other. You must know how to get help at once if you need it. Work out a communication plan with the nurse before you leave the agency.

The Five Rights of Delegation

The NCSBN's *Five Rights of Delegation* is another way to view the delegation process. In using the "five rights," the nurse answers the questions listed in the four steps described above. The *Five Rights of Delegation* are:

▶ *The right task.* Can the task be delegated? Is the nurse allowed to delegate the task? Is the task in your job description?
▶ *The right circumstances.* What are the person's physical, mental, emotional, and spiritual needs at this time?
▶ *The right person.* Do you have the training and experience to safely perform the task for this person?
▶ *The right directions and communication.* The nurse must give clear directions. The nurse tells you what to do and when to do it. The nurse tells you what observations to make and when to report back. The nurse allows questions and helps you set priorities.
▶ *The right supervision.* The nurse guides, directs, and evaluates the care you give. The nurse demonstrates tasks as necessary and is available to answer questions. The less experience you have with a task, the more supervision you need. Complex tasks require more supervision than do basic tasks. Also, the person's circumstances affect how much supervision you need. The nurse assesses how the task affected the person and how well you performed the task. The nurse tells you what you did well and how to improve your work. This helps you learn and give better care.

Your Role in Delegation

You perform delegated nursing tasks for or on *a person.* You must protect the person from harm. You have two choices when a task is delegated to you. You either *agree* or *refuse* to do the task. Use the *Five Rights of Delegation* in Box 2-4.

Accepting a Task

When you agree to perform a task, you are responsible for your own actions. What you do or fail to do can harm the person. *You must complete the task safely.* Ask for help when you are unsure or have questions about a task. Report to the nurse what you did and the observations you made.

BOX 2-4 The Five Rights of Delegation for Nursing Assistants

THE RIGHT TASK
- Does your state allow you to perform the task?
- Were you trained to do the task?
- Do you have experience performing the task?
- Is the task in your job description?

THE RIGHT CIRCUMSTANCES
- Do you have experience performing the task given the person's condition and needs?
- Do you understand the purposes of the task for the person?
- Can you perform the task safely under the current circumstances?
- Do you have the equipment and supplies to safely complete the task?
- Do you know how to use the equipment and supplies?

THE RIGHT PERSON
- Are you comfortable performing the task?
- Do you have concerns about performing the task?

THE RIGHT DIRECTIONS AND COMMUNICATION
- Did the nurse give clear directions and instructions?
- Did you review the task with the nurse?
- Do you understand what the nurse expects?

THE RIGHT SUPERVISION
- Is a nurse available to answer questions?
- Is a nurse available if the person's condition changes or if problems occur?

Modified from National Council of State Boards of Nursing: *The Five Rights of Delegation,* 1997, Chicago.

Refusing a Task

You have the right to say "no." Sometimes refusing to follow the nurse's directions is your right and duty. You should refuse to perform a task when:

▶ The task is beyond the legal limits of your role.
▶ The task is not in your job description.
▶ You were not prepared to perform the task.
▶ The task could harm the person.
▶ The person's condition has changed.
▶ You do not know how to use the supplies or equipment.
▶ Directions are not ethical or legal.
▶ Directions are against agency policies.
▶ Directions are unclear or incomplete.
▶ A nurse is not available for supervision.

Use common sense. This protects you and the person. Ask yourself if what you are doing is safe for the person.

Never ignore an order or a request to do something. Tell the nurse about your concerns. If the task is within the legal limits of your role and in your job description, the nurse can help increase your comfort with the task. The nurse can:

- Answer your questions
- Demonstrate the task
- Show you how to use supplies and equipment
- Help you as needed
- Observe you performing the task
- Check on you often
- Arrange for needed training

Do not refuse a task because you do not like it or do not want to do it. You must have sound reasons. Otherwise, you place the person at risk for harm. You also could lose your job.

See *Focus on Communication: Refusing a Task*.

FOCUS ON COMMUNICATION

Refusing a Task

A nurse may delegate a task that you did not learn in your training program. The task is in your job description. You can say: "I know this task is in my job description. But I did not learn that in school. Can you show me what to do and then observe me doing it? That would really help me."

REVIEW QUESTIONS

Circle the BEST answer.

1 Nursing practice is regulated by
   a The National Council of State Boards of Nursing
   b Nurse practice acts
   c Medicare
   d Medicaid

2 What state law affects what nursing assistants can do?
   a Standards for nursing assistants
   b OBRA
   c Nurse practice act
   d Medicaid

3 Your nursing assistant certification can be revoked for
   a Refusing a nursing task
   b Asking the nurse questions
   c Performing acts beyond your role
   d Keeping the person's information confidential

4 Which requires a training and competency evaluation program for nursing assistants?
   a Medicare   c NCSBN
   b Medicaid   d OBRA

5 As a nursing assistant, you
   a Must perform all nursing tasks as directed by the nurse
   b Make decisions about a person's care
   c Should have a written job description before employment
   d Should give a drug when a nurse tells you to

6 As a nursing assistant, you
   a Can take verbal or telephone orders from doctors
   b Are responsible for your own actions
   c Can remove tubes from the person's body
   d Should ignore a nursing task if it is not in your job description

7 Which statement is *false*?
   a You are accountable for your actions.
   b You must be honest when performing nursing tasks.
   c You can use the person's property for your own needs.
   d A law can require you to share the person's confidential information.

Continued

8 Who assigns and supervises your work?
 a Other nursing assistants
 b The health team
 c Nurses
 d Doctors

9 You are responsible for
 a Supervising other nursing assistants
 b Delegation decisions
 c Completing delegated tasks safely
 d Adding information to the nursing assistant registry

10 You perform a task not allowed by your state. Which is *true*?
 a If a nurse delegated the task, there is no legal problem.
 b You could be practicing nursing without a license.
 c You can perform the task if it is in your job description.
 d If you complete the task safely, there is no legal problem.

11 These statements are about delegation. Which is *false*?
 a Nurses can delegate their responsibilities to you.
 b A delegated task must be safe for the person.
 c The delegated task must be in your job description.
 d The delegating nurse is responsible for the safe completion of the task.

12 A task is in your job description. Which is *false*?
 a The nurse must delegate the task to you.
 b The nurse can delegate the task if the person's circumstances are right.
 c You must have the necessary education and training to complete the task.
 d You must have clear directions before you perform the task.

13 A nurse delegates a task to you. You must
 a Complete the task
 b Decide to accept or refuse the task
 c Delegate the task if you are busy
 d Ignore the request if you do not know what to do

14 You can refuse to perform a task for these reasons *except*
 a The task is beyond the legal limits of your role
 b The task is not in your job description
 c You do not like the task
 d A nurse is not available to supervise you

15 You decide to refuse a task. What should you do?
 a Delegate the task to a nursing assistant.
 b Communicate your concerns to the nurse.
 c Ignore the request.
 d Talk to the director of nursing.

Answers to these questions are on p. 779.

Ethics and Laws

OBJECTIVES

■ Define the key terms and key abbreviations used in this chapter
■ Describe ethical conduct
■ Describe the rules of conduct for nursing assistants
■ Explain how to maintain professional boundaries
■ Explain how to prevent negligent acts
■ Give examples of false imprisonment, defamation, assault, battery, and fraud
■ Describe how to protect the right to privacy
■ Explain the purpose of informed consent
■ Explain your role in relation to wills
■ Describe elder, child, and domestic abuse

KEY TERMS

abuse The intentional mistreatment or harm of another person

assault Intentionally attempting or threatening to touch a person's body without the person's consent

battery Touching a person's body without his or her consent

boundary crossing A brief act or behavior outside of the helpful zone

boundary sign An act, behavior, or thought that warns of a boundary crossing or violation

boundary violation An act or behavior that meets your needs, not the person's needs

civil law Laws concerned with relationships between people

crime An act that violates a criminal law

criminal law Laws concerned with offenses against the public and society in general

defamation Injuring a person's name and reputation by making false statements to a third person

ethics Knowledge of what is right conduct and wrong conduct

false imprisonment Unlawful restraint or restriction of a person's freedom of movement

fraud Saying or doing something to trick, fool, or deceive a person

invasion of privacy Violating a person's right not to have his or her name, photo, or private affairs exposed or made public without giving consent

Continued

KEY TERMS—cont'd

law A rule of conduct made by a government body

libel Making false statements in print, writing, or through pictures or drawings

malpractice Negligence by a professional person

neglect Failure to provide the person with the goods or services needed to avoid physical harm, mental anguish, or mental illness

negligence An unintentional wrong in which a person did not act in a reasonable and careful manner and a person or the person's property was harmed

professional boundary That which separates helpful behaviors from behaviors that are not helpful

professional sexual misconduct An act, behavior, or comment that is sexual in nature

protected health information Identifying information and information about the person's health care that is maintained or sent in any form (paper, electronic, oral)

self-neglect A person's behaviors that put him or her at high risk for harm; health and safety are threatened

slander Making false statements orally

standard of care The skills, care, and judgments required by a health team member under similar conditions

tort A wrong committed against a person or the person's property

vulnerable adult A person 18 years old or older who has a disability or condition that makes him or her at risk to be wounded, attacked, or damaged

will A legal document of how a person wants property distributed after death

KEY ABBREVIATIONS

ANA American Nurses Association

HIPAA Health Insurance Portability and Accountability Act of 1996

LNA Licensed nursing assistant

LPN Licensed practical nurse

LVN Licensed vocational nurse

NFLPN National Federation of Licensed Practical Nurses

OBRA Omnibus Budget Reconciliation Act of 1987

RN Registered nurse

Nurse practice acts, your training and job description, and safe delegation serve to protect patients and residents from harm (Chapter 2). Protecting them from harm also involves a complex set of rules and standards of conduct. They form the ethical and legal aspects of care.

ETHICAL ASPECTS

Ethics is knowledge of what is right conduct and wrong conduct. Morals are involved. It also deals with choices or judgments about what should or should not be done. An ethical person behaves and acts in the right way. He or she does not cause a person harm.

Ethical behavior also involves not being *prejudiced* or *biased*. To be prejudiced or biased means to make judgments and have views before knowing the facts. Judgments and views usually are based on one's values and standards. They are based on the person's culture, religion, education, and experiences. The person's situation may be very different from your own. For example:

▶ Children want their mother to have nursing home care. In your culture, children care for older parents at home.

▶ A person has many tattoos and body piercings. You do not like tattoos or body piercings.

▶ An 80-year-old man does not want life-saving measures. You believe that everything should be done to save life.

Do not judge the person by your values and standards. Do not avoid persons whose standards and values differ from your own.

Ethical problems involve making choices. You must decide what is the right thing to do. For example:

▶ You find a co-worker in an empty room drinking from a cup. You smell alcohol on her breath. She asks you not to tell anyone.

▶ A resident has bruises all over her body. She told the nurse that she fell. She tells you that her son is very mean to her. She asks you not to tell the nurse.

Professional groups have codes of ethics. The code has rules, or standards of conduct, for group members to follow. The American Nurses Association (ANA) has a code of ethics for registered nurses (RNs). The National Federation of Licensed Practical Nurses (NFLPN) has one for licensed practical nurses/licensed vocational nurses (LPNs/LVNs.) The rules of conduct in Box 3-1 can guide your thinking and behavior. See Chapter 4 for ethics in the workplace.

Boundaries

A *boundary* limits or separates something. For example, a fence forms a boundary. It tells you to stay within or on the side of the fenced area. As a nursing assistant, you help patients, residents, and families. Therefore you enter into a helping relationship with them. The helping relationship has professional boundaries.

Professional boundaries separate helpful behaviors from behaviors that are not helpful (Fig. 3-1). The boundaries create a helpful zone. If your behaviors are outside of the helpful zone, you are over-involved with the person or under-involved. Boundary crossings,

BOX 3-1 Code of Conduct for Nursing Assistants

- Respect each person as an individual.
- Know the limits of your role and knowledge.
- Perform only those tasks that are within the legal limits of your role.
- Perform only those tasks that you have been prepared to do.
- Perform no act that will cause the person harm.
- Take no drug without the prescription and supervision of a doctor.
- Carry out the directions and instructions of the nurse to your best possible ability.
- Follow the agency's policies and procedures.
- Complete each task safely.
- Be loyal to your employer and co-workers.
- Act as a responsible citizen at all times.
- Keep the person's information confidential.
- Protect the person's privacy.
- Protect the person's property.
- Consider the person's needs to be more important than your own.
- Report errors and incidents at once.
- Be accountable for your actions.

PROFESSIONAL BOUNDARIES

Under-involved	Helpful zone	Over-involved

FIGURE 3-1 Professional boundaries. (Redrawn from the National Council of State Boards of Nursing: *Professional boundaries: a nurse's guide to the importance of appropriate professional boundaries,* Chicago, Ill, 1996.)

boundary violations, or professional sexual misconduct can occur.

▶ A **boundary crossing** is a brief act or behavior outside of the helpful zone. The act or behavior may be thoughtless or something you did not mean to do. Or it could be on purpose if it meets the person's needs. For example, you give a crying patient a hug. The hug meets the person's needs at that time. If you give the hug to meet your needs, the act is wrong. Also, it is wrong to hug the person every time you see him or her.

▶ A **boundary violation** is an act or behavior that meets your needs, not the person's needs. The act or behavior is unethical. It violates the code of conduct in Box 3-1. The person could be harmed. Boundary violations include:
  ▶ Abuse (p. 32)
  ▶ Giving a lot of personal information about yourself (You tell a person about your personal relationships or problems.)
  ▶ Keeping secrets with the person

Professional Boundaries

Some patients, residents, and families want to thank the staff for the care given. Sometimes they send thank you cards and letters. Sometimes they offer gifts—candy, cookies, money, gift certificates, flowers, and so on. Accepting gifts is a boundary violation. When offered a gift, you can say:

- "Thank you so much for thinking of me. It's very kind of you. However, it is against center policy to accept gifts of any kind. I do appreciate your offer."
- "Thank you for wanting me to have the flowers your friend sent. They are lovely. However, staff cannot receive gifts because it is against hospital policy. Let me help you find a way to take them home."

▶ **Professional sexual misconduct** is an act, behavior, or comment that is sexual in nature. It is sexual misconduct even if the person consents or makes the first move.

Some boundary violations and some professional sexual misconduct also are crimes. To maintain professional boundaries, follow the rules in Box 3-2 (p. 30). Be alert to boundary signs. **Boundary signs** are acts, behaviors, or thoughts that warn of a boundary crossing or violation (Box 3-3, p. 30).

See *Focus on Communication: Professional Boundaries.*

LEGAL ASPECTS

Ethics is concerned with what you *should or should not do.* Laws tell you want you *can and cannot do.* A **law** is a rule of conduct made by a government body. The U.S. Congress and state legislatures make laws. Enforced by the government, laws protect the public welfare.

Criminal laws are concerned with offenses against the public and society in general. An act that violates a criminal law is called a **crime.** A person found guilty of a crime is fined or sent to prison. Murder, robbery, rape, kidnapping, and abuse (p. 32) are crimes.

Civil laws are concerned with relationships between people. Examples of civil laws are those that involve contracts and nursing practice. A person found guilty of breaking a civil law usually has to pay a sum of money to the injured person.

Torts

Tort comes from the French word meaning wrong. Torts are part of civil law. A **tort** is a wrong committed against a person or the person's property. Torts may be unintentional. Harm was not intended. Some torts are intentional. Harm was intended.

Unintentional Torts

Negligence is an unintentional wrong. The negligent person did not act in a reasonable and careful manner. As a result, a person or the person's property was harmed. The person causing the harm did not intend or mean to

---

BOX 3-2 Rules for Maintaining Professional Boundaries

- Follow the code of conduct listed in Box 3-1.
- Talk to the nurse if you sense a boundary sign, crossing, or violation.
- Avoid caring for family, friends, and people with whom you do business. This may be hard to do in a small community. Always tell the nurse if you know the person. The nurse may need to change your assignment.
- Do not date, flirt with, kiss, or have a sexual relationship with current patients or residents. The same applies to family members of current patients or residents.
- Do not make sexual comments or jokes.
- Do not use offensive language.
- Do not discuss your sexual relationships with patients, residents, or their families.
- Do not say or write things that could suggest a romantic or sexual relationship with a patient, resident, or family member.
- Use touch correctly (Chapter 7). Do not touch or handle sexual and genital areas unless when necessary to give care. Such areas include the breasts, nipples, perineum, buttocks, and anus.
- Do not accept gifts, loans, money, credit cards, or other valuables from a patient, resident, or family member.
- Do not give gifts, loans, money, credit cards, or other valuables to a patient, resident, or family member.
- Do not borrow from a patient, resident, or family member. This includes money, personal items, and transportation.
- Maintain a professional relationship at all times. Do not develop any personal relationship or friendship with the person or family member.
- Do not visit or spend extra time with a person that is not part of your assignment.
- Do not share personal or financial information with a person or family member.
- Do not help a person or family member with his or her finances.
- Do not take a person home with you. This includes for holidays or other events.
- Ask these questions before you date or marry a person whom you cared for. Be aware of the risk for sexual misconduct.
  - How long ago did you assist with the person's care?
  - Was the person's care short-term or long-term?
  - What kind and how much information do you have about the person? How will that information affect your relationship with the person?
  - Will the person need more care in the future?
  - Does dating or marrying the person place the person at risk for harm?

BOX 3-3 Boundary Signs

- You think about the person when you are not at work.
- You organize your work and provide other care around the person's needs.
- You spend free time with the person. You visit with the person during breaks, mealtimes, when off duty, and so on.
- You trade assignments with other nursing assistants so you can provide the person's care.
- You give more care or attention to the person at the expense of other patients and residents.
- You believe that you are the only person who understands the person and his or her needs.
- The person gives you gifts or money.
- You give the person gifts or money.
- You share information about yourself with the person.
- You talk about your work situation with the person.
- You flirt with the person.
- You make comments that have a sexual message.
- You tell the person "off-color" jokes.
- You notice more touch between you and the person.
- You use foul, vulgar, or offensive language when talking to the person.
- You and the person have secrets.
- You choose the person's side when he or she disagrees with other staff or the family.
- You select what you report and record. You do not give complete information.
- You do not like questions about the care you give or your relationship with the person.
- You change how you dress or your appearance when you will work with the person.
- You receive gifts from the person after he or she leaves the agency.
- You have contact with the person after he or she leaves the agency.

---

cause harm. The person failed to do what a reasonable and careful person would have done. Or he or she did what a reasonable and careful person would not have done. The negligent person may have to pay damages (a sum of money) to the one injured.

Malpractice is negligence by a professional person. A person has professional status because of training and the service provided. Nurses, doctors, dentists, and pharmacists are examples.

What you do or do not do can lead to a lawsuit if harm results to the person or property of another. **Standard of care** refers to skills, care, and judgments required by a health team member under similar conditions. Standards of care come from:

▶ Laws, including nurse practice acts
▶ Textbooks
▶ Agency policy and procedure manuals (Fig. 3-2) (These explain how to perform certain procedures.)
▶ Manufacturer instructions for equipment and supplies
▶ Job descriptions
▶ Approval and accrediting agency standards
▶ Standards and guidelines issued by government agencies

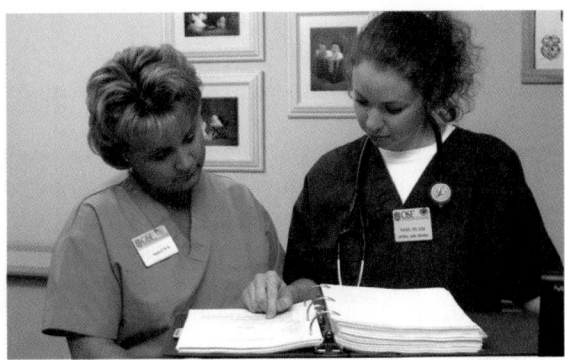

FIGURE 3-2 A nurse and nursing assistant review the policy and procedure manual. It is kept at the nurse's station.

The following actions could lead to charges of negligence:

▶ A nurse asks you to apply a hot soak. You fail to test water temperature. The water is too hot. The person is burned.

▶ Mrs. Parks needs help getting to the bathroom. You do not answer her signal light promptly. She gets up without help. She falls and breaks a leg.

▶ A mechanical lift is used to transfer Mr. Brown from bed to a chair. You do not follow the manufacturer's instructions for using the lift. Mr. Brown slips out of the lift and falls to the floor. He fractures a hip.

▶ Mrs. Clark complains of chest pain. You do not tell the nurse. Mrs. Clark has a heart attack and dies.

▶ Two residents have the same last name. You do not identify the person before a procedure. You perform the procedure on the wrong person. Both residents are harmed. One had a procedure that was not ordered. The other did not have a needed procedure.

You are legally responsible *(liable)* for your own actions. The nurse is liable as your supervisor. However, you are not relieved of personal liability. Remember, sometimes refusing to follow the nurse's directions is your right and duty (Chapter 2).

Intentional Torts

Intentional torts are acts meant to be harmful. The act is done knowingly.

Defamation is injuring a person's name and reputation by making false statements to a third person. **Libel** is making false statements in print, writing, or through pictures or drawings. **Slander** is making false statements orally. Never make false statements about a patient, resident, co-worker, or any other person. Examples of defamation include:

▶ Implying or suggesting that a person uses drugs
▶ Saying that a person is insane or mentally ill
▶ Implying or suggesting that a person steals money from the staff

False imprisonment is the unlawful restraint or restriction of a person's freedom of movement. It involves:

▶ Threatening to restrain a person
▶ Restraining a person
▶ Preventing a person from leaving the agency

Invasion of privacy is violating a person's right not to have his or her name, photo, or private affairs exposed or made public without giving consent. You must treat the person with respect and ensure privacy. Only staff involved in the person's care should see, handle, or examine his or her body. See Box 3-4 for measures to protect privacy.

The Health Insurance Portability and Accountability Act of 1996 (HIPAA) protects the privacy and security of a person's health information. **Protected health information** refers to identifying information and information about the person's health care that is maintained or sent in any form (paper, electronic, oral). Failure to comply with HIPAA rules can result in fines, penalties, and criminal action including jail time. You must follow agency policies and procedures. Direct any questions about the person or the person's care to the nurse. Also follow the rules for using computers and other electronic devices (Chapter 5).

Fraud is saying or doing something to trick, fool, or deceive a person. The act is fraud if it does or could cause harm to a person or the person's property. Telling a person or family that you are a nurse is fraud. So is giving wrong or incomplete information on a job application.

Assault and battery may result in both civil and criminal charges. **Assault** is intentionally attempting or threatening to touch a person's body without the person's consent. The person fears bodily harm. Threatening to "tie down" a person is an example of assault. **Battery** is touching a person's body without his or her consent. Consent is the important factor in assault and battery. The person must consent to any procedure, treatment, or other act that involves touching the body. The person has the right to withdraw consent at any time.

Protect yourself from being accused of assault and battery. Explain to the person what is to be done and get the person's consent. Consent may be verbal—"yes" or "okay." Or it can be a gesture—a nod, turning over for a back rub, or holding out an arm so you can take a pulse.

See *Focus on Ethics and Laws: Intentional Torts*, p. 32.

BOX 3-4 Protecting the Right to Privacy

- Keep all information about the person confidential.
- Cover the person when he or she is being moved in hallways.
- Screen the person. Close the privacy curtain as in Figure 3-3, p. 32. Close the door when giving care. Also close window coverings.
- Expose only the body part involved in care or a procedure.
- Do not discuss the person or the person's treatment with anyone except the nurse supervising your work. "Shop talk" is a common cause of invasion of privacy.
- Ask visitors to leave the room when care is given.
- Do not open the person's mail.
- Allow the person to visit with others in private.
- Allow the person to use the phone in private.
- Follow agency policy and procedures required to protect privacy.

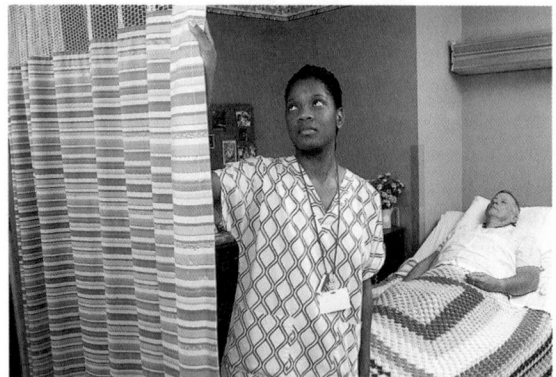

FIGURE 3-3 Pulling the privacy curtain around the bed helps protect the person's privacy.

Informed Consent

A person has the right to decide what will be done to his or her body and who can touch his or her body. The doctor is responsible for informing the person about all aspects of treatment. Consent is informed when the person clearly understands:
- The reason for a treatment, procedure, or care measure
- What will be done
- How it will be done
- Who will do it
- The expected outcomes
- Other treatment, procedure, or care options
- The effects of not having the treatment, procedure, or care measure

Persons under legal age (usually 18 years of age) cannot give consent. Nor can mentally incompetent persons. Such persons are unconscious, sedated, or confused. Or they have certain mental health problems. Informed consent is given by a responsible party—a wife, husband, daughter, son, or a legal representative.

Consent is given when the person enters the agency. A form is signed giving general consent to treatment. Special consent forms are required for surgery and other complex procedures. In nursing centers, consent is needed before admission to a secured Alzheimer's unit. The doctor informs the person about all aspects of the procedure. The nurse may be given this responsibility.

You are never responsible for obtaining written consent. In some agencies, you can witness the signing of a consent. To be a witness, you must be present when the person signs the consent.

Wills

A **will** is a legal document of how a person wants property distributed after death. You can ethically and legally witness the signing of a will. You can also refuse to do so without fear of legal action.

A person may ask you to prepare a will. You must politely refuse. Explain that you do not have the legal knowledge or ability to prepare a will. Report the request to the nurse. The nurse will speak to the person or family member about contacting a lawyer.

Do not witness the signing of a will if you are named in the will. To do so prevents you from receiving what was left to you. As a witness, be prepared to testify that:
- The person was of sound mind when the will was signed
- The person stated that the document was his or her last will

Many agencies do not let employees witness wills. Know your agency's policy before you agree to witness a will. If you have questions, ask the nurse. If you witness a will, tell the nurse.

REPORTING ABUSE

Abuse is the intentional mistreatment or harm of another person. Abuse is a crime. It can occur at home or in a health care agency. Abuse has one or more of these elements:
- Willful causing of injury
- Unreasonable confinement
- Intimidation (to make afraid with threats of force or violence)
- Punishment
- Depriving the person of the goods or services needed for physical, mental, or psychosocial well-being

Abuse causes physical harm, pain, or mental anguish. Protection against abuse extends to persons in a coma.

The abuser is usually a family member or caregiver—spouse, partner, adult child, and others. The abuser can be a friend, neighbor, landlord, or other person. Both men and women are abusers. Both men and women are abused.

Many states, accrediting agencies, and the Omnibus Budget Reconciliation Act of 1987 (OBRA) do not allow agencies to employ persons who were convicted of abuse, neglect, or mistreatment. Before hiring, the agency must thoroughly check the applicant's work history. All references are checked. Efforts must be made to find out about any criminal records.

The agency also checks the nursing assistant registry for findings of abuse, neglect, or mistreatment. It also is checked for misusing or stealing a person's property.

Vulnerable Adults

Vulnerable comes from the Latin word *vulnerare*, which means *to wound*. **Vulnerable adults** are persons 18 years old or older who have disabilities or conditions that make them at risk to be wounded, attacked, or damaged. They have problems caring for or protecting themselves due to:

▶ A mental, emotional, physical, or developmental disability (see Chapter 45)
▶ Brain damage
▶ Changes from aging

Patients and residents, regardless of age, are considered vulnerable. Older persons and children are at risk for abuse.

See *Focus on Long-Term Care and Home Care: Vulnerable Adults.*

FOCUS ON **LONG-TERM CARE** AND **HOME CARE**

Vulnerable Adults

HOME CARE

Some persons have behaviors that put themselves at high risk for harm. Health and safety are threatened. This is called **self-neglect.** Causes include declining health and chronic disease. Other causes are disorders that impair judgment or memory—Alzheimer's disease, dementia, depression, and drug or alcohol abuse. Some persons refuse care.

The person has the right to personal choice, to make decisions for oneself, and to be independent. However, there are warning signs of self-neglect. Report the following to the nurse:

• Hoarding. The persons saves, hides, or stores things. For example, people may save newspapers, magazines, food containers, shopping bags, and so on. The hoarding can present fire, pest (mice, rats, insects), and other safety hazards.
• Absence of food, water, heat, and other necessities.
• Failing to take needed drugs.
• Refusing to seek medical treatment for serious illnesses.
• Dehydration—poor urinary output, dry skin, dry mouth, confusion.
• Leaving a stove or oven unattended.
• Poor hygiene.
• Not wearing the correct clothing for the weather.
• Confusion.
• Not attending to or not being able to attend to housekeeping.
• Safety hazards in the home (Chapter 11).

Elder Abuse

Elder abuse is any knowing, intentional, or negligent act by a caregiver or any other person to an older adult. The act causes harm or serious risk of harm. Elder abuse can take these forms:

▶ *Physical abuse.* This involves inflicting, or threatening to inflict, physical pain or injury. Grabbing, hitting, slapping, kicking, pinching, hair-pulling, or beating are examples. It also includes *corporal punishment*—punishment inflicted directly on the body. Beatings, lashings, and whippings are examples. Depriving the person of a basic need also is physical abuse.
▶ *Neglect.* Failure to provide the person with the goods or services needed to avoid physical harm, mental anguish, or mental illness is called **neglect.** This includes failure to provide health care or treatment, food, clothing, hygiene, shelter, or other needs. In health care, neglect includes but is not limited to:
  ▶ Leaving persons lying or sitting in urine or feces
  ▶ Keeping persons alone in their rooms or other areas
  ▶ Failing to answer signal lights
▶ *Verbal abuse.* Using oral or written words or statements that speak badly of, sneer at, criticize, or condemn the person is called verbal abuse. It includes unkind gestures.
▶ *Involuntary seclusion.* This involves confining the person to a certain area. People have been locked in closets, basements, attics, bathrooms, and other spaces.
▶ *Financial exploitation or misappropriation.* To *exploit* means to use unjustly. *Misappropriate* means to dishonestly, unfairly, or wrongly take for one's own use. The older person's resources (money, property, assets) are misused by another person. Or the resources are used for the other person's profit or benefit. The person's money is stolen or used by another person. It is also misusing a person's property.
▶ *Emotional abuse.* This involves inflicting mental pain, anguish, or distress through verbal or nonverbal acts. Humiliation, harassment, ridicule, and threats of punishment are examples. It includes being deprived of needs such as food, clothing, care, a home, or a place to sleep.
▶ *Sexual abuse.* The person is harassed about sex or is attacked sexually. The person may be forced to perform sexual acts out of fear of punishment or physical harm.
▶ *Abandonment. Abandon* means to leave or desert someone. The person is deserted by someone who is responsible for his or her care.

There are many signs of elder abuse. The abused person may show only some of the signs in Box 3-5, p. 34.

Federal and state laws require the reporting of elder abuse. If abuse is suspected, it must be reported. Where and how to report abuse vary among states. You may suspect abuse. If so, discuss the matter and your observations with the nurse. Give as many details as possible. The nurse contacts health team members as needed.

BOX 3-5 Signs of Elder Abuse

- Living conditions are unsafe, unclean, or inadequate.
- Personal hygiene is lacking. The person is not clean. Clothes are dirty.
- Weight loss—there are signs of poor nutrition and inadequate fluid intake.
- Assistive devices are missing or broken—eyeglasses, hearing aids, dentures, cane, walker, and so on.
- Medical needs are not met.
- Frequent injuries—conditions behind the injuries are strange or seem impossible.
- Old and new injuries—bruises, pressure marks, welts, scars, fractures, punctures, and so on.
- Complaints of pain or itching in the genital area.
- Bleeding and bruising around the breasts or in the genital area.
- Burns on the feet, hands, buttocks, or other parts of the body. Cigarettes and cigars cause small circle-like burns.
- Pressure ulcers (Chapter 32) or contractures (Chapter 26).
- The person seems very quiet or withdrawn.
- Unexplained withdrawal from normal activities.
- The person seems fearful, anxious, or agitated.
- Sudden change in alertness.
- Depression.
- Sudden changes in finances.
- The person does not seem to want to talk or answer questions.
- The person is restrained. Or the person is locked in a certain area for long periods.
- The person cannot reach toilet facilities, food, water, and other needed items.
- Private conversations are not allowed. The caregiver is present during all conversations.
- Strained or tense relationships with a caregiver.
- Frequent arguments with a caregiver.
- The person seems anxious to please the caregiver.
- Drugs are not taken properly. Drugs are not bought. Or too much or too little of the drug is taken.
- Visits to the emergency room may be frequent.
- The person may change doctors often. Some people do not have a doctor.

BOX 3-6 Prosecuted Cases of Elder Abuse

- A resident was complaining of pain while he was being cleaned. To stop him from complaining, a nursing assistant stuck a rag down his throat.
- A patient was screaming. To stop the patient from screaming, a nurse poured water down her throat.
- A nursing assistant beat and kicked a 92-year-old man who was lying on the floor.
- A nursing assistant stepped on a resident's face.
- A person was visiting his grandmother. While in the agency, he sexually abused a patient with head injuries.
- A female patient in a wheelchair was dragged into a room by a nursing assistant. The nursing assistant forced the patient to have sex with him.
- A nursing assistant teased and taunted a resident with dementia.
- A health care worker repeatedly insulted an older woman because her son was gay.
- A nursing assistant forced a person to urinate in bed. Then the nursing assistant made fun of the person.
- Two older women lived in a board and care home. Both had Alzheimer's disease. The operator of the home left the women in a room with blood splattered on the walls. The carpet was caked with feces, vomitus, and urine. The women were partially dressed. One woman was tied to the bed with a sheet.
- A nursing assistant failed to feed a resident who could not feed herself. A video camera caught the nursing assistant dumping the resident's food into trash cans.
- A resident could not talk. She was totally dependent on the staff for care. She did not have a bowel movement for 26 days. She was given a laxative every 3 days. No other treatment was given for her constipation.
- Caregivers willfully neglected to give drugs to residents.

From *Elder abuse and neglect: prosecution and prevention,* San Francisco, American Society on Aging.

The nurse also contacts community agencies that investigate elder abuse. They act at once if the problem is life-threatening. Sometimes the help of police or the courts is necessary.

Helping abused older persons is not always easy or possible. Some abuse is not reported or recognized. Or the investigating agency cannot gain access to the person. Sometimes older persons are abused by a spouse or adult child. A victim may want to protect the spouse or child. Some victims are embarrassed or believe abuse is deserved. A victim may fear what will happen. He or she may think that the present situation is better than no care at all. Some people fear not being believed if they report the abuse themselves.

Box 3-6 lists some severe cases of elder abuse. The abusers were convicted of crimes. The examples that follow are more common. However, such abuse is still wrong. It will be investigated. You can lose your job. Your state nursing assistant registry will be notified. Nursing assistants have lost their certification, license, or registration because of elder abuse.

- A person constantly crying out for help is taken to his room. He is left alone with the door closed.
- A nursing assistant tells a person to be nice. Otherwise care will not be given.
- A person cannot control her bowels. She is called "dirty" and "disgusting."
- A person is turned in a rough and hurried manner.
- The nurse uses the person's phone to call a friend.
- A person lies in a wet and soiled bed all night.
- Money is taken from a person's wallet.
- A person uses the signal light a lot. It is taken away from the person.
- A person's mouth is forced open. Food is forced into the person's mouth.

See *Focus on Long-Term Care and Home Care: Elder Abuse.*

Child Abuse and Neglect

Child abuse and neglect involve the following:

- A child 18 years old or younger
- Any recent act or failure to act on the part of a parent or caregiver
- The act or failure to act results in death, serious physical or emotional harm, sexual abuse, or exploitation
- The act or failure to act presents a likely or immediate risk for harm

Child abuse and neglect occur at every social level. They occur in low-, middle-, and high-income families. The abuser may have little education or be highly educated. The abuser usually is a household member—parent, a parent's partner, brother or sister, nanny. Usually an abuser is someone the family knows. Risk factors for child abuse include:

- Stress
- Family crisis (divorce, unemployment, moving, poverty, crowded living conditions)
- Drug or alcohol abuse
- Abuser history of being abused as a child
- Discipline beliefs that include physical punishment
- Lack of emotional attachment to the child
- A child with birth defects or chronic illness
- A child with personality or behaviors that the abuser considers "different" or not acceptable
- Unrealistic expectations for the child's behavior or performance
- Families that move often and do not have family or friends nearby

Types of Child Abuse and Neglect

Child abuse and neglect can take different forms. Often more than one type is present.

- *Physical abuse* is injuring the child on purpose. It can cause death. Forms of physical abuse include striking, kicking, burning, or biting the child. Any action that causes physical impairment of the child is physical abuse.
- *Neglect* can be physical or emotional. *Physical neglect* means to deprive the child of food, clothing, shelter, and medical care. *Emotional neglect* is not meeting the child's need for affection and attention.
- *Sexual abuse* is using, persuading, or forcing a child to engage in sexual conduct. It can take many forms:
  - *Rape or sexual assault*—forced sexual acts with a person against his or her will.
  - *Molestation*—sexual advances toward a child. It includes kissing, touching, or fondling sexual areas. The abuser may kiss, touch, or fondle the child. Or the child is forced to kiss, touch, or fondle the abuser.
  - *Incest*—sexual activity between family members. The abuser may be a parent, step-parent, brother or sister, step-brother or step-sister, aunt or uncle, cousin, or grandparent.
  - *Child pornography*—taking pictures or videotaping a child involved in sexual acts or poses.
  - *Child prostitution*—forcing a child to engage in sexual activity for money. Usually the child is forced to have many sexual partners.
- *Emotional abuse* is injuring the child mentally. The child has changes in behavior, emotional responses, thinking, reasoning, learning, and so on. The child may show anxiety, depression, withdrawal, or aggressive behaviors.
- *Substance abuse* is part of child abuse and neglect in some states. A *controlled substance* is a drug or chemical substance whose possession and use are controlled by law. Substance abuse involves:
  - Making a controlled substance in the presence of a child
  - Making a controlled substance on the premises occupied by a child
  - Allowing a child to be present where there are chemicals or equipment used to make or store a controlled substance
  - Selling, distributing, or giving drugs or alcohol to a child
  - Using a controlled substance (a caregiver) that impairs the caregiver's ability to adequately care for the child
  - Exposing the child to equipment and supplies for using, selling, or distributing drugs
  - Exposing the child to other drug-related activities
- *Abandonment* is when a parent's identity or whereabouts are unknown. The child was left by the parent in circumstances where the child suffers serious harm. Or the parent fails to maintain contact with the child or provide support for the child.

BOX 3-7 Signs and Symptoms of Child Abuse and Neglect

PHYSICAL ABUSE
- Bruises on the face (eyes, lips, mouth, cheeks), back, buttocks, abdomen, chest, and inner thighs
- Welts on the face (lips, mouth, cheeks), back, buttocks, abdomen, chest, and inner thighs
  - The shape of the object causing the welt may be seen. The shape may be of a belt, belt buckle, wooden spoon, chain, clothes hanger, rope, or other object.
- Burns and scalds on the feet, hands, back, buttocks, or other body parts
  - Intentional burns leave a pattern from the item causing the burn: cigarettes, irons, curling irons, ropes, stove burners, and radiators are examples.
  - In scalds, the area put in hot liquid is clearly marked. For example, a scald to the hand looks like a glove. A scald to the foot looks like a sock.
- Fractures of the nose, skull, arms, or legs
- Bite marks

NEGLECT
- Fails to gain weight
- Shows great affection to others
- Wants to eat large amounts of food
- Steals food
- Is dirty or has a severe body odor
- Lacks the correct clothing for the weather
- Abuses alcohol or drugs
- States that no one is home

SEXUAL ABUSE
- Bleeding, cuts, and bruises of the genitalia, anus, breasts, or mouth
- Stains or blood on underclothing
- Painful urination
- Signs and symptoms of urinary tract infection (Chapter 42)
- Vaginal discharge
- Genital odor
- Genital pain
- Difficulty walking or sitting
- Pregnancy
- Fearful behaviors—nightmares, depression, unusual fears, attempts to run away
- Sexual behavior that does not fit with one's age

EMOTIONAL ABUSE
- Sudden changes in self-confidence
- Headaches
- Stomach aches
- Abnormal fears
- Nightmares
- Attempts to run away

Box 3-7 lists the signs of child abuse and neglect. You must be alert for any unexplained changes in the child's body or behavior. Child and parent behaviors may signal that something is wrong. The child may be quiet and withdrawn. He or she may fear adults. Sometimes children are afraid to go home. Sudden behavior changes are common in sexual abuse. Bed-wetting, thumb-sucking, loss of appetite, poor grades, and running away from home are examples. Some children attempt suicide.

Parents give different stories about what happened. Injuries are blamed on play accidents or other children. Frequent emergency room visits are common.

Child abuse is complex. Many more behaviors, signs, and symptoms are present than discussed here. The health team must be alert for signs and symptoms of child abuse. All states require the reporting of suspected child abuse. However, someone should not be falsely accused.

If you suspect child abuse, share your concerns with the nurse. Give as much detail as you can. The nurse contacts health team members and child protection agencies as needed.

Domestic Abuse

Domestic abuse—also called domestic violence, intimate partner abuse, partner abuse, and spousal abuse—occurs in relationships. One partner has power and control over the other through abuse. Fear and harm occur. Abuse may be physical, sexual, verbal, economic, or social. Usually more than one type of abuse is present.
- *Physical abuse*—unwanted punching, slapping, grabbing, choking, poking, biting, pulling hair, twisting arms, or kicking. It may involve burns and weapons. Physical injuries occur. Death is a constant threat.
- *Sexual abuse*—unwanted sexual contact.
- *Verbal abuse*—unkind and hurtful remarks. They make the person feel unwhole, unattractive, and without value.
- *Economic abuse*—controlling money. Having or not having a job is controlled by the abuser. So are paychecks, money gifts from family and friends, and money for household expenses (food, clothing).
- *Social abuse*—controlling friendships and other relationships. The abuser controls phone calls, car use, leaving the home, and visits with family and friends.

Patients and residents can suffer from domestic abuse. For example, a husband slaps his wife during a visit. Or a wife uses her husband's money for her own benefit rather than buying her husband's drugs.

Domestic abuse is a safety issue. Like child and elder abuse, domestic abuse is complex. The victim often hides the abuse. He or she may protect the abusive partner. State laws vary about reporting domestic abuse. However, the health team has an ethical duty to give information about safety and community resources. If you suspect domestic abuse, share your concerns with the nurse. The nurse gathers information to help the person.

See *Focus on Long-Term Care and Home Care: Domestic Abuse.*

FOCUS ON LONG-TERM CARE AND HOME CARE

Domestic Abuse

LONG-TERM CARE
Under OBRA, the resident has the right to be free from abuse, mistreatment, or neglect. If a resident is abused by anyone, the abuse must be reported. This includes abuse by a partner.

Circle the BEST answer.

1 Ethics is
a Making judgments before you have the facts
b Knowledge of what is right and wrong conduct
c A behavior that meets your needs, not the person's
d Skills, care, and judgments required of a health team member

2 Which of the following is ethical behavior?
a Sharing information about a patient with your family
b Accepting gifts from a resident's family
c Reporting errors
d Calling your family before answering a signal light

3 On your days off, you call the agency to check on a patient. This is a
a Professional boundary
b Boundary crossing
c Boundary violation
d Boundary sign

4 To maintain professional boundaries, your behaviors must
a Help the person
b Meet your needs
c Be biased
d Show that you care

5 A patient asks you out to dinner. You accept. This is a
a Professional boundary
b Boundary crossing
c Boundary violation
d Boundary sign

6 A friend is admitted to the hospital. You helped with the person's care. This is a
a Professional boundary
b Boundary crossing
c Boundary violation
d Boundary sign

7 Which is *not* a crime?
a Abuse
b Murder
c Negligence
d Robbery

8 These statements are about negligence. Which is *false*?
a It is an unintentional tort.
b The negligent person did not act in a reasonable manner.
c Harm was caused to a person or a person's property.
d A prison term is likely.

9 Threatening to touch the person's body without the person's consent is
a Assault
b Battery
c Defamation
d False imprisonment

10 Restraining a person's freedom of movement is
a Assault
b Battery
c Defamation
d False imprisonment

11 Photos of Mr. Blue are shown to others without his consent. This is
a Battery
b Fraud
c Invasion of privacy
d Malpractice

12 A person asks if you are a nurse. You answer "yes." This is
a Negligence
b Fraud
c Libel
d Slander

13 Informed consent is when the person
a Fully understands all aspects of his or her treatment
b Signs a consent form
c Is admitted to the agency
d Decides how to distribute property after his or her death

14 Who is at risk for being wounded, attacked, or damaged?
a Children
b Older adults
c Persons with disabilities
d All patients and residents

15 Self-neglect is when
a A caregiver harms a person
b The person's behaviors put him or her at risk for harm
c A person is deprived of food, clothing, hygiene, and shelter
d The person does not receive attention or affection

16 You scold an older person for not eating lunch. This is
a Physical abuse
b Neglect
c Emotional abuse
d Verbal abuse

17 You leave a home care patient before the next caregiver arrives. This is abuse by
a Abandonment
b Neglect
c Involuntary seclusion
d Financial exploitation

18 Which is *not* a sign of elder abuse?
a Stiff joints and joint pain
b Old and new bruises
c Poor personal hygiene
d Frequent injuries

19 A child is deprived of food, clothing, and shelter. This is
a Physical abuse
b Neglect
c Abandonment
d Emotional abuse

Continued

20 A child has a black eye, bruises on her face, and bite marks on her arms. These are signs of
  a Physical abuse
  b Sexual abuse
  c Neglect
  d Substance abuse

21 A child is dirty and has a body odor. These are signs of
  a Physical abuse
  b Sexual abuse
  c Neglect
  d Substance abuse

22 You find blood stains on a child's underpants. This is a sign of
  a Physical abuse
  b Sexual abuse
  c Neglect
  d Substance abuse

23 These statements are about domestic abuse. Which is *true*?
  a It always involves physical harm.
  b It always involves violence.
  c One partner has control over the other partner.
  d Only one type of abuse is usually present.

24 You suspect a person was abused. What should you do?
  a Tell the family.
  b Call the police.
  c Tell the nurse.
  d Ask the person about the abuse.

Answers to these questions are on p. 779.

Work Ethics

OBJECTIVES

- Define the key terms and key abbreviations listed in this chapter
- Identify good health and hygiene practices
- Describe how to look professional
- Describe the qualities and traits of a successful nursing assistant
- Explain how to get a job
- Explain how to plan for childcare and transportation
- Describe ethical behavior on the job
- Explain how to manage stress
- Explain the aspects of harassment
- Explain how to resign from a job
- Identify the common reasons for losing a job
- Explain the reasons for drug testing

KEY TERMS

confidentiality Trusting others with personal and private information

courtesy A polite, considerate, or helpful comment or act

gossip To spread rumors or talk about the private matters of others

harassment To trouble, torment, offend, or worry a person by one's behavior or comments

preceptor A staff member who guides another staff member

professionalism Following laws, being ethical, having good work ethics, and having the skills to do your work

stress The response or change in the body caused by any emotional, physical, social, or economic factor

stressor The event or factor that causes stress

work ethics Behavior in the workplace

KEY ABBREVIATIONS

CNA Certified nursing assistant
CEU Continuing education unit
GED General equivalency diploma

NATCEP Nursing assistant training and competency evaluation program
OBRA Omnibus Budget Reconciliation Act of 1987

A s a nursing assistant, you must act and function in a professional manner. **Professionalism** involves following laws, being ethical, having good work ethics, and having the skills to do your work. Laws and ethics are discussed in Chapter 3. Laws are rules of conduct made by government bodies. Ethics deal with right and wrong conduct. Ethics involve choices and judgments about what to do or what not to do. An ethical person does the right thing. In the workplace, certain behaviors (conduct), choices, and judgments are expected. **Work ethics** deal with behavior in the workplace. Your conduct reflects your choices and judgments. Work ethics involve:

▶ How you look
▶ What you say
▶ How you behave
▶ How you treat others
▶ How you work with others

To get and keep a job, you must conduct yourself in the right way.

HEALTH, HYGIENE, AND APPEARANCE

Patients, residents, families, and visitors expect the health team to look and act healthy. For example, a person is told to stop smoking. Yet he or she sees health team members smoking. If you are not clean, people wonder if you give good care. You are a member of the health team. Your health, appearance, and hygiene need careful attention.

Your Health

You must give safe and effective care. To do so, you must be physically and mentally healthy. Otherwise you cannot function at your best.

▶ *Diet.* You need a balanced diet (Chapter 23). Start your day with a good breakfast. To maintain your weight, balance the calories you take in with your energy needs. To lose weight, take in fewer calories than your energy needs. Avoid foods high in fat, oil, and sugar. Also avoid salty foods and crash diets.
▶ *Sleep and rest.* Sleep and rest are needed for health and to do your job well. Most adults need about 7 hours of sleep daily. Fatigue, lack of energy, and irritability mean you need more rest and sleep.
▶ *Body mechanics.* You will bend, carry heavy objects, and handle, move, and turn persons. These tasks place stress and strain on your body. You need to use your muscles correctly (Chapter 15).

▶ *Exercise.* Exercise is needed for muscle tone, circulation, and weight loss. Walking, running, swimming, and biking are good forms of exercise. Regular exercise helps you feel better physically and mentally. Consult your doctor before starting a vigorous exercise program.
▶ *Your eyes.* You will read instructions and take measurements. Wrong readings can cause the person harm. Have your eyes checked. Wear needed eyeglasses or contact lenses. Provide enough light for reading and fine work.
▶ *Smoking.* Smoking causes lung, heart, and circulatory disorders. Smoke odors stay on your breath, hands, clothing, and hair. Hand washing and good personal hygiene are needed.
▶ *Drugs.* Some drugs affect thinking, feeling, behavior, and function. Working under the influence of drugs affects the person's safety. Take only those drugs ordered by a doctor. Take them in the prescribed way.
▶ *Alcohol.* Alcohol is a drug that depresses the brain. It affects thinking, balance, coordination, and mental alertness. Never report to work under the influence of alcohol. Do not drink alcohol while working. Like other drugs, alcohol affects the person's safety.

Your Hygiene

Personal hygiene needs careful attention. Bathe daily. Use a deodorant or antiperspirant to prevent body odors. Brush your teeth often—upon awakening, before and after meals, and at bedtime. Use a mouthwash to prevent breath odors. Shampoo often. Style hair in a simple, attractive way. Keep fingernails clean, short, and neatly shaped.

Menstrual hygiene is important. Change tampons or sanitary pads often, especially if flow is heavy. Wash your genital area with soap and water at least twice a day. Also practice good hand washing.

Foot care prevents odors and infection. Wash your feet daily. Dry thoroughly between the toes. Cut toenails straight across after bathing or soaking them.

Your Appearance

Good health and hygiene practices help you look and feel well. Follow the practices in Box 4-1. They help you look clean, neat, and professional (Fig. 4-1).

BOX 4-1 Practices for a Professional Appearance

- Practice good hygiene.
- Wear uniforms that fit well. They are modest in length and style. Follow the agency's dress code.
- Keep uniforms clean, pressed, and mended. Sew on buttons. Repair zippers, tears, and hems.
- Wear a clean uniform daily.
- Wear your name badge or photo ID at all times when on duty. Wear it according to agency policy.
- Wear undergarments that are clean and fit properly. Change them daily.
- Do not wear colored (red, pink, blue, and so on) undergarments. They can be seen through white and light-colored uniforms. Undergarments should not be visible. They should be the correct color for your skin tone.
- Cover tattoos. They may offend others.
- Follow the agency's dress code for jewelry. Wedding and engagement rings may be allowed. Rings and bracelets can scratch a person. Confused or combative persons can easily pull on jewelry (necklaces, dangling earrings). So can young children.
- Do not wear jewelry in pierced eyebrows, nose, lips, or tongue while on duty.
- Follow the agency's dress code for earrings. Usually small, simple earrings are allowed. For multiple ear piercings, usually only one set of earrings is allowed.
- Wear a wristwatch with a second hand.
- Wear clean stockings and socks that fit well. Change them daily.
- Wear shoes that fit properly, are comfortable, give needed support, and have non-skid soles. Do not wear sandals or open-toed shoes.
- Clean and polish shoes often. Wash and replace laces as needed.
- Keep fingernails clean, short, and neatly shaped. Long nails can scratch a person. Nails must be natural.
- Do not wear nail polish. Chipped nail polish may provide a place for microbes to grow.
- Have a simple, attractive hairstyle. Hair is off your collar and away from your face. Use simple pins, combs, barrettes, and bands to keep long hair up and in place.
- Keep beards and mustaches clean and trimmed.
- Use makeup that is modest in amount and moderate in color. Avoid a painted and severe look.
- Do not wear perfume, cologne, or after-shave lotion. The scents may offend, nauseate, or cause breathing problems in patients and residents.

GETTING A JOB

There are easy ways to find out about jobs:
- Newspaper ads
- Local state employment services
- Agencies where you would like to work
- Phone book yellow pages
- People you know—your instructor, family, and friends
- The Internet
- Job placement counselors at your school or college
- Your clinical experience site

Your clinical experience site is an important source. The staff always look at students as future employees. They look for good work ethics. They watch how students treat patients, residents, and co-workers. They look for the qualities and traits described in Box 4-2, p. 42. If that agency is not hiring, the staff may suggest other places to apply.

What Employers Look For

If you had your own business, who would you want to hire? Your answer helps you better understand the employer's point of view. Employers want to hire people who:
- Are dependable
- Are well-groomed
- Have needed job skills and training
- Have values and attitudes that fit with the agency

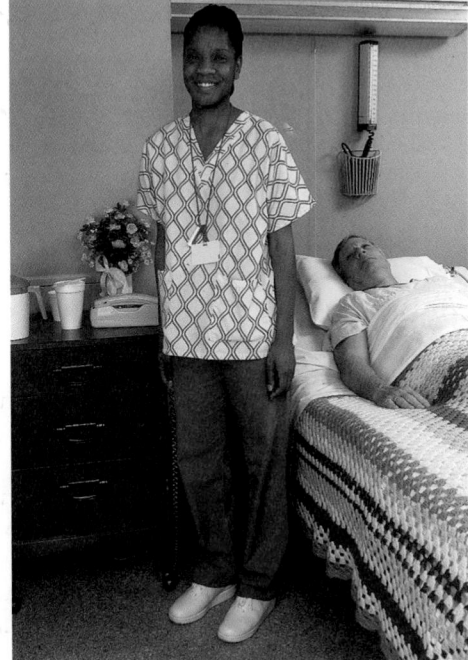

FIGURE 4-1 This nursing assistant is well-groomed. Her uniform and shoes are clean. Her hair has a simple style. It is away from her face and off of her collar. She does not wear jewelry.

Good work ethics involve the qualities and traits described in Box 4-2, p. 42. They are necessary for you to function well (Fig. 4-2, p. 42).

Applicants who look good communicate many things to the employer. You have one chance to make a good first

BOX 4-2 Qualities and Traits for Good Work Ethics

- **Caring.** Have concern for the person. Help make the person's life happier, easier, or less painful.
- **Dependable.** Report to work on time and when scheduled. Perform delegated tasks. Keep obligations and promises.
- **Considerate.** Respect the person's physical and emotional feelings. Be gentle and kind toward patients, residents, families, and co-workers.
- **Cheerful.** Greet and talk to people in a pleasant manner. Do not be moody, bad-tempered, or unhappy while at work.
- **Empathetic.** Empathy is seeing things from the person's point of view—putting yourself in the person's place. How would you feel if you had the person's problems?
- **Trustworthy.** Patients, residents, and staff have confidence in you. They believe you will keep information confidential. They trust you not to gossip about patients, residents, or the health team.
- **Respectful.** Patients and residents have rights, values, beliefs, and feelings. They may differ from yours. Do not judge or condemn the person. Treat the person with respect and dignity at all times. Also show respect for the health team.
- **Courteous.** Be polite and courteous to patients, residents, families, visitors, and co-workers. See p. 50 for common courtesies in the workplace.
- **Conscientious.** Be careful, alert, and exact in following instructions. Give thorough care. Do not lose or damage the person's property.
- **Honest.** Accurately report the care given, your observations, and any errors.
- **Cooperative.** Willingly help and work with others. Also take that "extra step" during busy and stressful times.
- **Enthusiastic.** Be eager, interested, and excited about your work. Your work is important.
- **Self-aware.** Know your feelings, strengths, and weaknesses. You need to understand yourself before you can understand patients and residents.

FOCUS ON **LONG-TERM CARE** AND **HOME CARE**

What Employers Look for

HOME CARE

Besides the qualities and traits listed in Box 4-2, working in home care requires:

- *The ability to work alone.* The nurse makes some home visits. Usually a nurse is not with you in the home or at the bedside. If problems occur, you can reach the nurse by phone. You must provide skillful and safe care.
- *Self-discipline.* You must arrive at homes on time. Plan activities so personal care needs and housekeeping tasks get done. Avoid temptations. This includes watching TV, talking on the phone, visiting, and stopping for a cup of coffee.
- *Honesty.* You might need to shop for the person. Be honest and thrifty with the person's money. Accurately report to the person or family what you bought, the cost with receipts, amount spent, and amount of money returned.
- *Respect for the person's property.* You will handle valuables and personal property in health care settings. Access to the person's property is greater in the home. You use home furnishings, appliances, linens, and household items to give care and for housekeeping. Treat personal and family property with respect. Prevent damage. Read the manufacturer's instructions before using any appliance. Clean the appliance after use.

impression. A well-groomed person is likely to get the job. A sloppy person with wrinkled or dirty clothes is not likely to get the job. Nor is someone with body or breath odors. See p. 43 for how to dress for an interview.

Being dependable is important. You must be at work on time and when scheduled. Undependable people cause everyone problems. Other staff take on extra work. Fewer people give care. Quality of care suffers. Supervisors spend time trying to find out if the person is coming to work. They also have to find someone to cover for the absent employee. You want co-workers to work when scheduled. Otherwise, you have extra work. You have less time to spend with patients and residents. Likewise, co-workers also expect you to work when scheduled.

See *Focus on Long-Term Care and Home Care: What Employers Look For.*

Job Skills and Training

Employers need to know that you can do the required job skills. The employer checks the nursing assistant registry and requests proof of training:

▶ A certificate of course completion
▶ A high school, college, or technical school transcript
▶ An official grade report (report card)

Give the employer only a *copy* of your certificate, transcript, or grade report. Never give the original to the employer. Keep it for future use. The employer may want a transcript sent directly from the school or college.

See *Focus on Long-Term Care and Home Care: Job Skills and Training.*

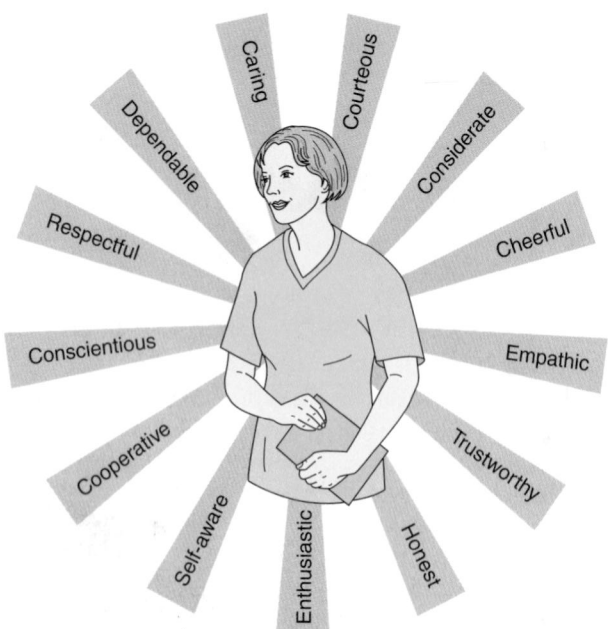

FIGURE 4-2 Good work ethics involve these qualities and traits.

Job Skills and Training

LONG-TERM CARE

To work in long-term care, you must complete a state-approved nursing assistant training and competency evaluation program (NATCEP). This is an OBRA requirement. The employer requests proof of training. The nursing assistant registry is checked. Nursing centers cannot hire persons convicted of abuse, neglect, or mistreatment. This also is an OBRA requirement.

HOME CARE

Home care agencies receiving Medicare funds must meet OBRA requirements. You must complete a NATCEP outlined by OBRA. Some states have additional training requirements for working in home care.

Job Applications

You get a job application from the *personnel office* or *human resources* office (Fig. 4-3, p. 44). You can complete the application there. Or you can take it home, and return it by mail or in person. You must be well-groomed and behave pleasantly when seeking or returning a job application. It may be your first chance to make a good impression.

To complete a job application, follow the guidelines in Box 4-3, p. 46. How you fill out the application may mean getting or not getting the job. Often the application is your first chance to impress the employer. A neat, readable, and complete application gives a good image. A sloppy or incomplete one does not.

Some agencies provide job applications on-line. Follow the agency's instructions for completing and sending an on-line application.

A job application is easier to complete if you have a file of your education and work history. The file should contain:

▶ A copy of your high school diploma or general equivalency diploma (GED)
▶ A copy of any grade reports, degrees, certificates, or military training
▶ A copy of your NATCEP certificate of completion
▶ Nursing assistant registry information (Include information for each state in which you are registered.)
▶ Copies of communications involving your state board of nursing or nursing assistant registry agency
▶ Copies of court records for criminal convictions
▶ A copy of your Social Security card
▶ Names, addresses, and phone numbers of references
▶ Names, addresses, and phone numbers of current and past employers. Include:
  ▶ Your job title
  ▶ The dates that employment started and ended
  ▶ Your supervisor's name
  ▶ Hourly salary
▶ Proof of in-services attended and continuing education units (CEUs)

The Job Interview

A job interview is the employer's chance to get to know and evaluate you. You also find out more about the agency.

The interview may be when you complete the job application. Some agencies schedule interviews after reviewing applications. Write down the interviewer's name and the interview date and time. If you need directions to the agency, ask for them at this time.

Box 4-4, p. 47 lists common interview questions. Prepare your answers before the interview. Also type a list of your skills. Give the list to the interviewer.

You must present a good image. You need to be neat, clean, and well-groomed. How you dress is important. Follow the guidelines in Box 4-5, p. 47.

Be on time. It shows you are dependable. Go to the agency some day before your interview. Note how long it takes to get there and where to park. Also find the personnel office. A *dry run* (practice run) gives an idea of how long it takes to get from your home to the personnel office.

When you arrive for the interview, turn off your wireless phone or pager. Tell the receptionist your name and why you are there. Also give the interviewer's name. Then sit quietly in the waiting area. Do not smoke or chew gum. Use the time to review your answers to the common interview questions. Waiting may be part of the interview. The interviewer may ask the receptionist about how you acted while waiting. Smile, and be polite and friendly.

Greet the interviewer in a polite manner. A firm handshake is correct for men and women. Address the interviewer as Miss, Mrs., Ms., Mr., or Doctor. Stand until asked to take a seat. When sitting, use good posture. Sit in a professional manner. If offered a beverage, it is correct to accept. Be sure to thank the person.

Good eye contact is needed. Look directly at the interviewer when answering or asking questions. Poor eye contact sends negative information—being shy, insecure, dishonest, or lacking interest.

Watch your body language (Chapter 7). Body language involves facial expressions, gestures, posture, and body movements. What you say is important. However, how you use and move your body also tells a great deal. Avoid distracting habits—biting nails; playing with jewelry, clothing, or your hair; crossing your arms; and swinging legs back and forth. Keep your mind on the interview. Do not touch or read things on the person's desk.

The interview lasts 15 to 45 minutes. Give complete and honest answers. Speak clearly and with confidence. Avoid short and long answers. "Yes" and "no" answers give little information. Briefly explain "yes" and "no" responses (Chapter 7).

The interviewer will ask about your skills. Share your skills list. He or she may ask about a skill not on your list. Explain that you are willing to learn the skill if your state allows nursing assistants to perform the task.

Text continued on p. 46

(Please Print in Ink)

In considering your application for employment, the facility may conduct a detailed and thorough investigation which may include but is not limited to a criminal record check, interviews or inquiries of prior employers, coworkers, acquaintances, relatives or friends.

PERSONAL

LAST NAME	FIRST	MIDDLE

HOME TELEPHONE NO.

PRESENT ADDRESS	CITY	STATE	ZIP CODE

CONTACT TELEPHONE NO.

PERMANENT ADDRESS	CITY	STATE	ZIP CODE

E-MAIL ADDRESS (optional)

ANY PREVIOUS NAME(S)? YES ☐ NO ☐ IF YES, IDENTIFY ALL OTHER NAMES INCLUDING MAIDEN NAME:

BEST TIME TO CONTACT YOU: | DATE AVAILABLE FOR WORK:

POSITION APPLIED FOR: SALARY DESIRED:

CHECK ALL YOU WOULD CONSIDER WORKING:
FULL TIME / REGULAR ☐
FULL TIME / TEMPORARY ☐
PART TIME / REGULAR ☐
PART TIME / TEMPORARY ☐

HOW DID YOU LEARN ABOUT THIS POSITION? (NEWSPAPER, INTERNET, FRIEND, IF OTHER – PLEASE LIST)

RELATIVES OR FRIENDS EMPLOYED IN THIS FACILITY? YES ☐ NO ☐
NAME: DEPT: RELATIONSHIP:

WOULD YOU CONSIDER WORKING:
WEEKENDS & HOLIDAYS YES ☐ NO ☐
ROTATING SHIFTS YES ☐ NO ☐
ON CALL YES ☐ NO ☐
ANY SHIFT YES ☐ NO ☐

HAVE YOU EVER BEEN EMPLOYED BY THIS FACILITY?
YES ☐ NO ☐ WHEN?

ARE YOU 18 YRS OF AGE OR OLDER?
YES ☐ NO ☐

ARE YOU A U.S. CITIZEN OR AN ALIEN LEGALLY AUTHORIZED TO WORK IN THE UNITED STATES?
YES ☐ NO ☐

SHIFT AVAILABILITY (check all that apply):
DAYS ☐ EVENINGS ☐ NIGHTS ☐

LONG RANGE OCCUPATIONAL GOALS:

HAVE YOU EVER BEEN CONVICTED OF, OR PLEAD GUILTY TO, A CRIME OTHER THAN **A MISDEMEANOR TRAFFIC VIOLATION?** YES ☐ NO ☐
IF YES, WHICH STATE(S), AND EXPLAIN: (You are not required to disclose any SEALED or EXPUNGED criminal records.)

HAVE YOU EVER BEEN INVOLVED IN THE SUBSTANTIATED ABUSE OR NEGLECT OF CHILDREN OR ADULTS UNDER THE LAWS OF THIS OR ANY OTHER STATE OF THE UNITED STATES? YES ☐ NO ☐ IF YES, WHICH STATE(S), AND EXPLAIN:

HAVE YOU BEEN SANCTIONED, CITED, REPORTED, OR EXCLUDED FROM PARTICIPATION IN MEDICARE, MEDICAID, OR ANY OTHER HEALTHCARE RELATED LAW OR REGULATION? YES ☐ NO ☐ IF YES, EXPLAIN:

If your answer is "yes" to any of the above, you will not be automatically disqualified from employment consideration, except as required by state or federal law.

EDUCATION / SKILLS

SCHOOL	NAME AND ADDRESS OF SCHOOL	COURSE OF STUDY	CHECK LAST YEAR COMPLETED				DID YOU GRADUATE?	LIST DIPLOMA OR DEGREE
HIGH			1	2	3	4	☐ YES ☐ NO	
COLLEGE			1	2	3	4	☐ YES ☐ NO	
COLLEGE			1	2	3	4	☐ YES ☐ NO	

OTHER Business College or Special Courses: (Include Special Military Training, Post Graduate and Nursing)

AREA(S) OF SPECIALIZATION OR MAJOR INTEREST: | LIST OFFICE SKILLS INCLUDING COMPUTER/SOFTWARE EXPERIENCE:

LIST HEALTH CARE, BUSINESS, OR INDUSTRIAL EQUIPMENT OPERATED: | WORD PROCESSING: (Approx. WPM)

PROFESSIONAL LICENSES

☐ CURRENTLY LICENSED ☐ ELIGIBLE FOR LICENSE
☐ CURRENTLY REGISTERED ☐ ELIGIBLE FOR REGISTRATION
LICENSE OR REGISTRATION **EVER** SUSPENDED, REVOKED OR ON PROBATION? ☐ YES ☐ NO IF YES, EXPLAIN:
TYPE:
NO: STATE: DATE:

PROFESSIONAL CERTIFICATIONS

☐ CURRENTLY CERTIFIED
☐ ELIGIBLE FOR CERTIFICATION
TYPE:
STATE: DATE:

☐ CURRENTLY LICENSED ☐ ELIGIBLE FOR LICENSE
☐ CURRENTLY REGISTERED ☐ ELIGIBLE FOR REGISTRATION
LICENSE OR REGISTRATION **EVER** SUSPENDED, REVOKED OR ON PROBATION? ☐ YES ☐ NO IF YES, EXPLAIN:
TYPE:
NO: STATE: DATE:

☐ CURRENTLY CERTIFIED
☐ ELIGIBLE FOR CERTIFICATION
TYPE:
STATE: DATE:

FIGURE 4-3 A sample job application. (Courtesy Association Management Resources, Naperville, Ill, ©2006.)

Briefly describe duties and skills acquired through military or volunteer service: (include dates)

_____

_____

_____

_____

PREVIOUS EXPERIENCE

PROVIDE INFORMATION REGARDING PREVIOUS EMPLOYMENT BEGINNING WITH MOST RECENT EMPLOYER.

	FROM: (MO/YR)	TO: (MO/YR)	SUPERVISOR'S NAME:	SALARY: (Hr/ Mo/Yr)

JOB TITLE: _____

EMPLOYER NAME:_____PHONE: _____

ADDRESS: _____

DUTIES:_____

_____

REASON FOR LEAVING: _____

MAY WE CONTACT YOUR CURRENT EMPLOYER?   YES ❏   NO ❏

	FROM: (MO/YR)	TO: (MO/YR)	SUPERVISOR'S NAME:	SALARY: (Hr/ Mo/Yr)

JOB TITLE: _____

EMPLOYER NAME:_____PHONE: _____

ADDRESS: _____

DUTIES:_____

_____

REASON FOR LEAVING: _____

	FROM: (MO/YR)	TO: (MO/YR)	SUPERVISOR'S NAME:	SALARY: (Hr/ Mo/Yr)

JOB TITLE: _____

EMPLOYER NAME:_____PHONE: _____

ADDRESS: _____

DUTIES:_____

_____

REASON FOR LEAVING: _____

	FROM: (MO/YR)	TO: (MO/YR)	SUPERVISOR'S NAME:	SALARY: (Hr/ Mo/Yr)

JOB TITLE: _____

EMPLOYER NAME:_____PHONE: _____

ADDRESS: _____

DUTIES:_____

_____

REASON FOR LEAVING: _____

PLEASE IDENTIFY AND EXPLAIN ANY GAPS IN EMPLOYMENT LONGER THAN THREE (3) MONTHS:

_____

FIGURE 4-3, cont'd   A sample job application. (Courtesy Association Management Resources, Naperville, Ill, ©2006.)

LANGUAGE

LANGUAGE SKILLS - DO NOT COMPLETE UNLESS REQUESTED

LANGUAGE	DO YOU?	☐ SPEAK	☐ FAIR ☐ GOOD ☐ FLUENT	☐ READ	☐ FAIR ☐ GOOD ☐ FLUENT	☐ WRITE	☐ FAIR ☐ GOOD ☐ FLUENT
LANGUAGE	DO YOU?	☐ SPEAK	☐ FAIR ☐ GOOD ☐ FLUENT	☐ READ	☐ FAIR ☐ GOOD ☐ FLUENT	☐ WRITE	☐ FAIR ☐ GOOD ☐ FLUENT

REFERENCES

LIST AT LEAST THREE (3) PROFESSIONAL / WORK / SCHOOL REFERENCES WHO ARE NOT RELATIVES OR PERSONAL ACQUAINTANCES:

NAME AND RELATIONSHIP	TITLE	COMPANY NAME AND ADDRESS	TELEPHONE

SIGNATURE

CAREFULLY READ THIS SECTION PRIOR TO PROVIDING SIGNATURE BELOW

I hereby affirm that the information provided on this application (and accompanying resume, if any) is true and complete. I understand that any false or misleading representations or omissions made on the application or during the hiring process may disqualify me from further consideration for employment and may result in discharge even if discovered at a later date.

I understand that employment may be conditioned upon successfully passing a medical examination and that I may be required to satisfactorily complete a drug screening as a condition of employment.

I hereby authorize persons, schools, my current employer (if applicable) and previous employers and other organizations to provide this facility and its affiliates with any requested information regarding my application or suitability for employment, and I completely release all such persons or entities from any and all liability related to the providing or use of such information.

I understand that my employment is at-will which means that I may terminate the employment relationship at any time and for any reason with or without notice, and that the facility has the same right. I understand that no one has the authority to enter into any agreement contrary to the preceding sentence, except for a written agreement signed by an administrative representative of this facility and notarized.

Date _____ Signature _____

FIGURE 4-3, cont'd   A sample job application. (Courtesy Association Management Resources, Naperville, Ill, ©2006.)

BOX 4-3 Guidelines for Completing a Job Application

- Read and follow the directions. They may ask you to print using black ink. Following directions is needed on the job. Employers look at job applications to see if you can follow directions.
- Write neatly. Your writing must be readable. A messy application gives a bad image. Readable writing gives the correct information. The agency cannot contact you if unable to read your phone number. You may miss getting the job.
- Complete the entire form. Something may not apply to you. If so, write "non-applicable" or "N/A" for non-applicable. Or draw a line through the space. This tells the employer that you read the section. It also shows that you did not skip the item on purpose.
- Report any felony arrests or convictions as directed. Write "no" or "none" as appropriate. Criminal background and fingerprint checks are common requirements.
- Give information about employment gaps. If you did not work for a time, the employer wonders why. Provide this information to give a good impression about your honesty. Some of the reasons are going to school, raising your children, caring for an ill or older family member, or your own illness.
- Tell why you left a job, if asked. Be brief, but honest. People leave jobs for one that pays better. Some leave for career advancement. Other reasons include those given for employment gaps. If you were fired from a job, give an honest but positive response. Do not talk badly about a former employer.
- Provide references. Be prepared to give names, titles, addresses, and phone numbers of at least four references who are not relatives or personal acquaintances. You should have this information written down before completing an application. (Always ask references if an employer can contact them.) You may get the job faster or over another applicant if the employer can quickly check references. If they are missing or not complete, the employer waits for all of the information. This wastes your time and the employer's time. Also, the employer wonders if you are hiding something with incomplete reference information.
- Be prepared to provide the following:
  - Social Security number
  - Proof of citizenship or legal residency
  - Proof of required training and competency evaluation
  - Identification—driver's license or government-issued ID card
- Give honest responses. Lying on an application is fraud. It is grounds for being fired.
- Keep a file of your education and work history.

You want to find the right job for you. An employer wants to hire someone who will be happy in the job and at the agency. You can ask questions at the end of the interview. Box 4-6 lists some questions to ask. The person's answers will help you decide if the job is right for you.

Review the job description with the interviewer. If you have questions, ask them at this time. Advise the interviewer of functions you cannot perform because of training, legal, ethical, or religious reasons. Honesty now prevents problems later.

BOX 4-4 Common Interview Questions

- Tell me about yourself.
- Tell me about your career goals.
- What are you doing to reach these goals?
- Describe your idea of *professional* behavior.
- Tell me about your last job. Why did you leave?
- What did you like the most about your last job? What did you like the least?
- What would your supervisor and co-workers tell me about you? Your dependability? Your skills? Your flexibility?
- Which functions are the hardest for you? How do you handle this difficulty?
- How do you set your priorities?
- How have your experiences prepared you for this job?
- What would you like to change about your last job?
- How do you handle problems with patients, residents, and co-workers?
- Why do you want to work here?
- Why should this agency hire you?

BOX 4-5 Grooming and Dressing for an Interview

- Bathe and brush your teeth. Wash your hair.
- Use deodorant or antiperspirant.
- Make sure your hands and fingernails are clean.
- Apply makeup in a simple, attractive manner.
- Style your hair in a neat and attractive way. Wear it as you would for work.
- Do not wear jeans, shorts, tank tops, halter tops, or other casual clothing.
- Iron clothing. Sew on loose buttons and mend garments as needed.
- Wear a simple dress, skirt and blouse, or suit (women). Men should wear a suit or dark slacks and a shirt and tie. A jacket is optional. A long-sleeved white or light blue shirt is best. (See Figure 4-4).
- Wear socks (men and women) or hose (women). Hose should be free of runs and snags.
- Make sure shoes are clean and in good repair.
- Avoid heavy perfumes, colognes, and after-shave lotions. A lightly scented fragrance is acceptable.
- Wear only simple jewelry that complements your clothes. Avoid adornments in body piercings. If you have multiple ear piercings, wear only one set of earrings.
- Stop in the restroom when you arrive for the interview. Check your hair, makeup, and clothes.

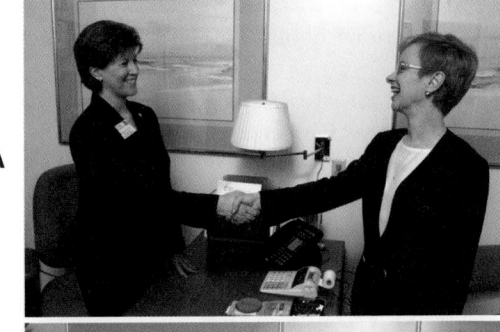

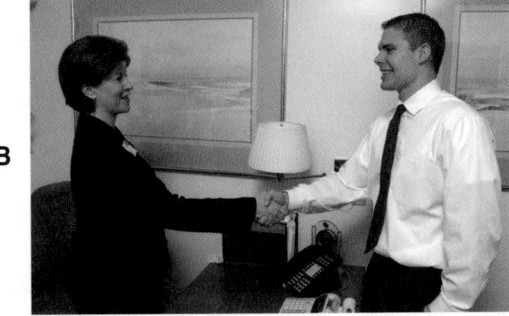

FIGURE 4-4 A, A simple suit is worn for a job interview. **B,** This man wears slacks and a shirt and tie for his interview.

BOX 4-6 Questions to Ask the Interviewer

- Which job functions do you think are the most important?
- What employee qualities and traits are the most important to you?
- What nursing care pattern is used here (Chapter 1)?
- Who will I work with?
- When are performance evaluations done? Who does them? How are they done?
- What performance factors are evaluated?
- How does the supervisor handle problems?
- What are the most common reasons that nursing assistants lose their jobs here?
- What are the most common reasons that nursing assistants resign from their jobs here?
- How do you see this job in the next year? In the next 5 years?
- What is the greatest reward from this job?
- What is the greatest challenge from this job?
- What do you like the most about nursing assistants who work here?
- What do you like the least about nursing assistants who work here?
- Why should I work here rather than in another agency?
- Why are you interested in hiring me?
- May I have a tour of the agency and the unit I will work on? Will you introduce me to the nurse manager and unit staff?
- Can I have a few minutes to talk to the nurse manager?

Also ask questions about:

▶ Pay rate
▶ Work hours
▶ Benefits—health and disability insurance, vacation, and continuing education
▶ Tuition reimbursement and scholarship programs for educational and career advancement
▶ Uniform requirements
▶ The new employee orientation program

The interviewer signals when the interview is over. You may be offered a job at this time. Or you are told when to expect a call or letter. Follow-up is acceptable. Ask when you can check on your application. Before leaving, thank the interviewer. Say that you look forward to hearing from him or her. Shake the person's hand before you leave.

A thank-you letter or note is advised (Fig. 4-5, p. 48). Write this within 24 hours of the interview. Your writing must be neat and readable. Use a computer or typewriter

December 12

Dear Ms. O'Neal,

Thank you for the interview yesterday. I enjoyed meeting you and learning more about the nursing center. I was impressed by the friendliness of the staff and would enjoy working in that environment.

Again, thank you. I look forward to hearing from you soon.

Sincerely,
Alison M. Teal

FIGURE 4-5 Sample thank-you note written after a job interview.

FOCUS ON LONG-TERM CARE AND HOME CARE

The Job Interview

HOME CARE

You need to ask more questions when interviewing with a home care agency:

- What part of the community does the agency serve?
- What neighborhoods will you go to?
- How far will you have to travel between homes?
- Do you use your own car or is an agency car provided?
- If you use your own car, how are you paid for mileage?
- Will you use public transportation? If yes, who pays for bus or train fares? If the agency pays, are you given fare money beforehand or repaid later?

---

if your writing is hard to read. The thank-you note should include:

- The date
- The interviewer's formal name using Miss, Mrs., Ms., Mr., or Dr.
- A statement thanking the person for the interview
- Comments about the interview, the agency, and your eagerness to hear about the job
- Your signature using your first and last names

See *Focus on Long-Term Care and Home Care: The Job Interview.*

Accepting a Job

Accept the job that is best for you. You can apply several places and have many interviews. Think about all offers before accepting one. You might have more questions about an agency. Ask them before accepting the job. Discussing the offer with a family member, friend, co-worker, or your instructor might help you decide what to do.

When you accept a job, agree on a starting date, pay rate, and work hours. Find out where to report on your first day. Ask for such information in writing. That way you and the agency have the same understanding of the job offer. You can use the written offer later if questions arise. Also ask for the employee handbook and other agency information. Read everything before you start working.

New Employee Orientation

Agencies have orientation programs for new employees. The agency's policy and procedure manual is reviewed. Your skills are checked. That is, the agency has you perform procedures in your job description. This is to make sure that you do them safely and correctly. Also, you are shown how to use the agency's supplies and equipment.

Many agencies have preceptor programs. A **preceptor** is a staff member who guides another staff member. In a preceptor program, a nurse or nursing assistant:

- Helps you learn the agency's layout so you can find what you need

---

- Introduces you to patients, residents, and staff
- Helps you organize your work
- Helps you feel comfortable as a part of the nursing team
- Answers questions about the policy and procedure manual

A nursing assistant preceptor is not your supervisor. Only nurses can supervise. A preceptor program usually lasts 2 to 4 weeks. Its purpose is to help you succeed in your role. It also helps ensure quality care. After the preceptor program, you should feel comfortable with the setting and your role. If not, ask for more orientation time.

PREPARING FOR WORK

Having a job is a privilege. It is not a right. It is not something owed to you. You obtained the necessary education and training. You succeeded in a job interview. To keep your job, you must function well and work well with others. You must:

- Work when scheduled
- Get to work on time
- Stay the entire shift

Absences and tardiness (being late) are common reasons for losing a job. Childcare and transportation issues often interfere with getting to work. Plan for them in advance.

Childcare

Someone needs to care for your children when you leave for work, while you are at work, and before you get home from work. Also plan for emergencies:

- Your childcare provider is ill or cannot care for your children that day.
- A child becomes ill while you are at work.
- You will be late getting home from work.

Transportation

Plan for how you get to and from work. If you drive, keep your car in good working order. Keep plenty of gas in the car. Or leave early to get enough gas.

Carpooling is an option. Carpool members depend on

each other. If the driver is late leaving, everyone is late for work. If one person is not ready when the driver arrives, everyone is late for work. Carpool with persons you trust to be ready and on time. When you drive, leave and pick up others on time. As a passenger, be ready to be picked up on time.

Know your bus or train schedule. Know what other bus or train to take if delays occur. Always carry enough money for fares to and from work.

Always have a back-up plan for getting to work. Your car may not start, the carpool driver may not go to work, or public transportation may not operate.

TEAMWORK ON THE JOB

How you look, how you behave, and what you say affect everyone in the agency. Practice good work ethics:

▶ Work when scheduled.
▶ Be cheerful and friendly.
▶ Perform delegated tasks.
▶ Be available to help others. Help them willingly.
▶ Be kind to others.

The *Employee Handbook* of OSF Saint Francis Medical Center (Peoria, Ill.) says it best:

You are what people see when they arrive here; yours are the eyes they look into when they're frightened and lonely. Yours are the voices people hear when they ride the elevators, when they try to sleep, and when they try to forget their problems. You are what they hear on their way to appointments which could affect their destinies, and what they hear after they leave those appointments. Yours are the comments people hear when you think they can't.

Yours is the intelligence and caring that people hope they'll find here. If you're noisy, so is the medical center. If you're rude, so is the medical center. And if you're wonderful, so is the medical center.

You are an important member of the health team. Quality care is affected by how you work with others and how you feel about your job.

Attendance

Report to work when scheduled and on time. The entire unit is affected when just one person is late. Call the agency if you will be late or cannot go to work. Follow the agency's attendance policy. It is explained in your employee handbook. Poor attendance can cause you to lose your job.

Be *ready to work* when your shift starts. Store your coat, purse, backpack, and other items before your shift starts. Use the restroom when you arrive at the agency. Arrive on your nursing unit a few minutes early. This gives you time to greet others and settle yourself.

Attendance also means staying the entire shift. You must prepare for childcare emergencies. Watching the clock for when your shift ends gives a bad image. You may need to work overtime. You need to prepare to stay longer if necessary. When it is time to leave, report off-duty to the nurse.

TEAMWORK AND TIME MANAGEMENT

Attendance

Sometimes your nursing unit may not have enough staff. Someone is late for work. Or someone does not show up for work. Until a replacement arrives, you and other staff members will have extra work. Patient and resident care cannot suffer.

You need to promote teamwork and manage your time. To do so:

• Ask the nurse how you can help.
• Do not complain about not having enough staff.
• Ask the nurse to list the most important tasks and care measures.

FOCUS ON LONG-TERM CARE AND HOME CARE

Attendance

HOME CARE
You must complete home care assignments. Never leave in the middle of an assignment. Nor should you leave before someone from the next shift arrives. Leaving before you complete an assignment is abandonment (Chapter 3).

Sometimes conflicts or problems occur. Make every effort to finish the assignment. Explain the problem to your supervisor. He or she will try to make needed changes. Do not walk out on the person. That would leave the person in an unsafe situation. Walking out is very unethical behavior. It also is abuse and a boundary violation (Chapter 3).

See *Teamwork and Time Management: Attendance.*
See *Focus on Long-Term Care and Home Care: Attendance.*

Your Attitude

A good attitude is needed (see Box 4-2). Show that you enjoy your work. Listen to others. Be willing to learn. Stay busy, and use your time well.

Your work is very important. Nurses, patients, residents, and families rely on you to give good care. They expect you to be pleasant and respectful. You must believe that you and your work have value.

Always think before you speak. These statements signal a bad attitude:

▶ "That's not my resident (patient)."
▶ "I can't. I'm too busy."
▶ "I didn't do it."
▶ "I don't feel like it."
▶ "It's not my fault."
▶ "Don't blame me."
▶ "It's not my turn. I did it yesterday."
▶ "Nobody told me."
▶ "That's not my job."
▶ "You didn't say that you needed it right away."
▶ "I work harder than anyone else."
▶ "No one appreciates what I do."
▶ "I'm tired of this place."
▶ "Is it time to leave yet?"

Gossip

To **gossip** means to spread rumors or talk about the private matters of others. Gossiping is unprofessional and hurtful. To avoid being a part of gossip:

► Remove yourself from a group or situation where gossip is occurring.
► Do not make or repeat any comment that can hurt a person, family member, visitor, co-worker, or the agency.
► Do not make or repeat any comment that you do not know to be true. Making or writing false statements about another person is defamation (Chapter 3).
► Do not talk about patients, residents, family members, visitors, co-workers, or the agency at home or in social settings.

Confidentiality

The person's information is private and personal. **Confidentiality** means trusting others with personal and private information. The person's information is shared only among health team members involved in his or her care. The person has the right to privacy and confidentiality. Agency and co-worker information also is confidential.

Avoid talking about patients, residents, the agency, or co-workers when others are present. Share information only with the nurse. Do not talk about patients, residents, the agency, or co-workers in hallways, elevators, dining areas, or outside the agency. Others may overhear you. Patients, residents, and visitors are very alert to comments. They think you are talking about them or their loved ones. This leads to wrong information and wrong impressions about the person's condition. You can easily upset the person or family. Be very careful about what, how, when, and where you say things.

Avoid eavesdropping. To eavesdrop means to listen in or overhear what others are saying. It invades a person's privacy.

Many agencies have intercom systems. They allow for communication between the beside and the nurses' station (Chapter 17). The person uses the intercom to signal when help is needed. Someone at the nurses' station answers the intercom. The nursing team also uses the intercom to communicate with each other. Be careful what you say over the intercom. It is like a loud speaker. Others nearby can hear what you are saying.

See *Focus on Communication: Confidentiality.*

Hygiene and Appearance

How you look affects the way people think about you and the agency. If staff members are clean and neat, people think the agency is clean and neat. They think the agency is unclean if staff members are messy and unkempt. People also wonder about the quality of care given.

Home and social attire is often improper at work. You cannot wear jeans, halter tops, tank tops, or short skirts. Clothing must not be tight, revealing, or sexual. Females cannot show cleavage, the tops of breasts, or upper thighs.

FOCUS ON COMMUNICATION

Confidentiality

Your family members and friends may ask you about people they know in the agency. They may ask about patients, residents, or employees. For example, your mother says: "Mrs. Drew goes to our church. I heard that she's in your nursing home. What's wrong with her?"

You must not share any information with your family and friends. To do so violates the person's right to privacy and confidentiality (Chapter 3). You can say: "I'm sorry, but I can't tell you about any person in the center. It is unprofessional and against center policies. And it violates the person's right to privacy and confidentiality. Please don't ask me about anyone in the center."

Males must avoid tight pants and exposing their chests. Only the top shirt button is open. Follow the practices in Box 4-1.

Speech and Language

Your speech and language must be professional. Speech and language used in home and social settings may be improper at work. Words used with family and friends may offend patients, residents, families, visitors, and co-workers. Remember the following:

► Do not swear or use foul, vulgar, or abusive language.
► Do not use slang.
► Control the volume and tone of your voice. Speak softly and gently.
► Speak clearly. The person may have a hearing problem (Chapter 37).
► Do not shout or yell.
► Do not fight or argue with a person, family member, visitor, or co-worker.

Courtesies

A **courtesy** is a polite, considerate, or helpful comment or act. Courtesies are easy. They require little time or energy. And they mean so much to people. Even the smallest kind act can brighten someone's day:

► Address others by Miss, Mrs., Ms., Mr., or Doctor. Use a first name only if the person asks you to do so.
► Say "please." Begin or end each request with "please."
► Say "thank you" whenever someone does something for you.
► Apologize. Say "I'm sorry" when you make a mistake or hurt someone. Even little things—like bumping into someone in the hallway—need an apology.
► Be thoughtful. Compliment others. Wish others a happy birthday, a happy day or weekend off, or a happy holiday.
► Wish the person and family well when they leave the agency. "Stay well" or "stay healthy" are good phrases to use.

- Hold doors open for others. If you are at the door first, open the door and let others pass through. In business, men and women hold doors open for each other.
- Hold elevator doors open for others coming down the hallway.
- Let patients, residents, families, and visitors enter elevators first.
- Stand to greet visitors and families.
- Help others willingly when asked.
- Give praise. If you see a co-worker do or say something that impresses you, tell that person. Also tell your co-workers.
- Do not take credit for another person's deeds. Give the person credit for the action.

Personal Matters

You were hired to do a job. Personal matters cannot interfere with the job. Otherwise care is neglected. You could lose your job for tending to personal matters while at work. To keep personal matters out of the workplace:

- Make personal phone calls during meals and breaks. Use a pay phone or your wireless phone.
- Do not let family and friends visit you on the unit. If they must see you, have them meet you during a meal or break.
- Make appointments (doctor, dentist, lawyer, and others) for your days off.
- Do not use the agency's computers, printers, fax machines, copiers, or other equipment for your personal use.
- Do not take agency supplies (pens, paper, and others) for your personal use.
- Do not discuss personal problems at work.
- Control your emotions. If you need to cry or express anger, do so in a private place. Get yourself together quickly and return to your work.
- Do not borrow money from or lend it to co-workers. This includes meal money and bus or train fares. Borrowing and lending can lead to problems with co-workers.
- Do not sell things or engage in fund-raising at work. Do not sell your child's candy or raffle tickets to co-workers.
- Do not have personal pagers or wireless phones turned on while at work.

Meals and Breaks

Meal breaks are usually for 30 minutes. Other breaks are usually for 15 minutes. Meals and breaks are scheduled so that some staff are always on the unit. Staff remaining on the unit cover for the staff on break.

Staff members depend on each other. Leave for and return from breaks on time. That way other staff can have their turn. Do not take longer than allowed. Tell the nurse when you leave and return to the unit.

Job Safety

You must protect patients, residents, families, visitors, co-workers, and yourself from harm. Everyone is responsible for safety. Negligent behavior affects the safety of others (Chapter 3). Safety practices are presented throughout this book. These guidelines apply to everything you do:

- Understand the roles, functions, and responsibilities in your job description.
- Know the contents and policies in the employee handbook and policy and procedure manuals.
- Know what is right and wrong.
- Know what you can and cannot do.
- Develop the qualities and traits in Box 4-1.
- Follow the nurse's directions and instructions.
- Question unclear directions and things you do not understand.
- Help others willingly when asked.
- Follow agency rules.
- Ask for any training that you might need.
- Report measurements, observations, the care given, the person's complaints, and any errors accurately (Chapter 5).
- Accept responsibility for your actions. Admit when you are wrong or make mistakes. Do not blame others. Do not make excuses for your actions. Learn what you did wrong and why. Try to learn from your mistakes.
- Handle the person's property carefully and prevent damage.

Planning Your Work

You will give care and perform routine tasks on the nursing unit. You must complete some things by certain times. Others are done by the end of the shift. Plan your work to give safe, thorough care and to make good use of your time (Box 4-7, p. 52).

MANAGING STRESS

Stress is the response or change in the body caused by any emotional, physical, social, or economic factor. Stress is normal. It occurs every minute of every day. It occurs in everything you do.

A **stressor** is the event or factor that causes stress. Many stressors are pleasant—watching a child play, planning a party, laughing with family and friends, enjoying a nice day. Some are not pleasant—illness, injury, family problems, death of loved ones, divorce, money concerns. Many parts of your job are stressful.

No matter the cause, stress affects the whole person:

- *Physically*—sweating, increased heart rate, faster and deeper breathing, increased blood pressure, dry mouth, and so on.
- *Mentally*—anxiety, fear, anger, dread, depression, and using defense mechanisms (Chapter 43).
- *Socially*—changes in relationships, avoiding others, needing others, blaming others, and so on.
- *Spiritually*—changes in beliefs and values and strengthening or questioning one's belief in God or a higher power.

BOX 4-7 Planning Your Work

- Discuss priorities with the nurse.
- Know the routine of your shift and nursing unit.
- Follow unit policies for shift reports.
- List care or procedures that are on a schedule. For example, some persons are turned or offered the bedpan every 2 hours.
- Judge how much time you need for each person, procedure, and task.
- Identify which tasks and procedures can be done while patients or residents are eating, visiting, or involved with activities or therapies.
- Plan care around mealtimes, visiting hours, and therapies. If working in a nursing center, also consider recreation and social activities.
- Identify when you will need help from a co-worker. Ask a co-worker to help you. Give the time when you will need help and for how long.
- Schedule equipment or rooms for the person's use. Some agencies have only one shower or bathtub to a nursing unit.
- Review delegated tasks. Gather needed supplies beforehand.
- Do not waste time. Stay focused on your work.
- Do not leave a messy work area. Make sure rooms are neat and orderly. Also clean utility areas.
- Be a self-starter. Have initiative. Ask others if they need help. Follow unit routines, stock supply areas, and clean utility rooms. Stay busy.

Prolonged or frequent stress can threaten your health. Physical and mental problems can occur. Some problems are minor—headaches, sleep problems, muscle tension, and so on. Others are life-threatening—high blood pressure, heart attack, stroke, ulcers, and so on.

Dealing with stress is important. If your job causes stress, it affects your family and friends. If you have stress in your personal life, it affects your work. Stress affects you, the care you give, the person's quality of life, and how you relate to co-workers. These guidelines can help you reduce or cope with stress:

- Exercise regularly. It has physical and mental benefits—cardiovascular health, weight control, tension release, emotional well-being, and relaxation.
- Get enough rest and sleep.
- Eat healthy.
- Plan personal and quiet time for you. Read, take a hot bath, go for a walk, meditate, or listen to music. Do what makes you feel good.
- Use common sense about what you can do. Do not try to do everything that family and friends ask you to do. Consider the amount of time and energy that you have.
- Do one thing at a time. The demands on you may seem overwhelming. List each thing that you have to do. Set priorities.
- Do not judge yourself harshly. Do not try to be perfect or expect too much from yourself.

- Give yourself praise. You do good and wonderful things every day.
- Have a sense of humor. Laugh at yourself. Laugh with others. Spend time with those who make you laugh.
- Talk to the nurse if your work or a person is causing too much stress. The nurse can help you deal with the matter.

HARASSMENT

Harassment means to trouble, torment, offend, or worry a person by one's behavior or comments. Harassment can be sexual. Or it can involve age, race, ethnic background, religion, or disability. You must respect others. Do not offend others by your gestures, remarks, or use of touch. Do not offend others with jokes, photos, or other pictures (drawings, cartoons, and so on). Harassment is not legal in the workplace.

Sexual Harassment

Sexual harassment involves unwanted sexual behaviors by another. The behavior may be a sexual advance. Or it may be a request for a sexual favor. Some remarks, comments, and touching are sexual. The behavior affects the person's work and comfort. In extreme cases, the person's job is threatened if sexual favors are not granted.

Victims of sexual harassment may be men or women. Men harass women or men. Women harass men or women. You might feel that you are being harassed. If so, report the matter to your supervisor and the human resource officer.

Be careful about what you say or do. Even innocent remarks and behaviors can be viewed as harassment. Employee orientation programs address harassment. You might not be sure about your own or another person's remarks or behaviors. If so, discuss the matter with the nurse. You cannot be too careful.

See *Focus on Ethics and Laws: Sexual Harassment.*

RESIGNING FROM A JOB

A job closer to home, better pay, or new opportunities may prompt you to leave your job. School, childcare, and illness are other reasons. Whatever the reason, you need to tell your employer. Give a written notice. Write a resignation letter. Or complete a form in the human resource

FOCUS ON ETHICS AND LAWS

Sexual Harassment

A female hospital employee sued a hospital in federal court for sexual harassment. She claimed sexual harassment because of a co-worker's sexually suggestive poster. She claimed that her rights were violated because:
- Of her co-worker's conduct
- The hospital failed to correct the situation
  The hospital asked the court to dismiss the lawsuit. However, the court found enough facts to allow the lawsuit to continue.

(*Cotton v South Suburban Hospital*, United States District Court, Northern District, Ill, 2002.)

office. Giving 2-weeks notice is a good practice. Do not leave a job without notice. Doing so can affect patient and resident care. Include the following in your notice:

▶ Reason for leaving
▶ The last date you will work
▶ Comments thanking the employer for the opportunity to work in the agency

An exit interview is common practice. You and the employer talk before you leave the agency. Usually the employer asks what you liked about the agency and your job. Often employees are asked how the agency can improve.

LOSING A JOB

A job is a privilege. You must perform your job well and protect patients and residents from harm. No pay raise or losing your job results from poor performance. Failure to follow agency policy is often grounds for termination. So is failure to get along with others. Box 4-8 lists the many reasons why you can lose your job. To protect your job, function at your best. Always practice good work ethics.

DRUG TESTING

Drug and alcohol use affects patient, resident, and staff safety. Quality of care suffers. Those who use drugs or alcohol are late to work or absent more often than staff members who do not use such substances. Therefore some agencies have drug testing policies. Review your agency's policy for when and how you might be tested.

See *Focus on Ethics and Laws: Drug Testing*.

BOX 4-8 Common Reasons For Losing a Job

- Poor attendance—not showing up for work or excessive tardiness (being late)
- Abandonment—leaving the job during your shift
- Falsifying a record—job application or a person's record
- Violent behavior in the workplace
- Having weapons in the work setting—guns, knives, explosives, or other dangerous items
- Having, using, or distributing alcohol in the work setting
- Having, using, or distributing drugs in the work setting (this excludes taking drugs ordered by a doctor)
- Taking a person's drugs for your own use or giving it to others
- Harassment
- Using offensive speech and language
- Stealing the agency's or a person's property
- Destroying the agency's or a person's property
- Showing disrespect to patients, residents, families, visitors, co-workers, or supervisors
- Abusing or neglecting a person
- Invading a person's privacy
- Failing to maintain patient, resident, agency, or co-worker confidentiality (includes access to computer and other electronic information)
- Using the agency's supplies and equipment for your own use
- Defamation—see Chapter 3 and "Gossip," p. 50
- Abusing meal breaks and break periods
- Sleeping on the job
- Violating the agency's dress code
- Violating any agency policy
- Failing to follow agency procedures for providing care
- Tending to personal matters while on duty

FOCUS ON ETHICS AND LAWS

Drug Testing

A certified nursing assistant (CNA) started working at an Arizona hospital in April 1999. While employed, she received Employee Corrective Action reports for:
- Poor communication with co-workers
- Arguing with an RN who gave her instructions
- Not being able to work in a team environment
- Excess time off the nursing unit for breaks
- Not taking the initiative in answering signal lights, collecting needed equipment, or transferring patients' belongings
- Excess socializing with staff in other departments
- Not meeting standards relating to customer service relations
  She was terminated from the hospital in January 2000.

In April 2003 she applied for a job at another Arizona hospital. A pre-employment urine drug screen was positive for benzodiazepine. The CNA reported the drug test to the Arizona State Board of Nursing. The CNA reported that she had a headache the night before her interview at the hospital. She admitted taking a Valium (benzodiazepine) that was prescribed for her mother. The CNA explained that "she knew this was wrong, that this was a one time occurrence and that it would not happen again."

In June 2003 the Board requested that the CNA submit to a urine drug screen. It was positive for benzodiazepine. The CNA did not have a prescription for that drug.

The Board revoked the CNA's certificate for unprofessional conduct. The Arizona State Board of Nursing found that the CNA's actions violated these aspects of the state's Nurse Practice Act:
- Conduct or practice that is or might be harmful or dangerous to the health of a patient or the public
- Committing an act that deceives, defrauds, or harms the public
- Obtaining, possessing, using, or selling any narcotic, controlled substance, or illegal drug in violation of any federal or state criminal law, or in violation of the policy of any employer
- Using violent or abusive behavior in any work setting
- Failing to cooperate with the Board during an investigation
- Practicing in any other manner that gives the Board reasonable cause to believe that the health of a client or the public may be harmed
  She can apply for re-instatement of her certificate after a 5-year period.

(Arizona State Board of Nursing, November 16, 2005. NOTE: Names withheld by request of the Arizona State Board of Nursing.)

REVIEW QUESTIONS

Circle T if the statement is true or F if the statement is false.

1 (T) F You wear needed eyeglasses. This helps protect the person's safety.

2 (T) F Childcare requires planning before you go to work.

3 (T) (F) Being on time for work means arriving at the agency when your shift begins.

4 (T) F You share information about a person with a friend. This is grounds for losing your job.

5 (T) F You must be careful what you say over the intercom system.

6 (T) F You do not follow the agency's dress code. You could lose your job.

7 T (F) You can use the agency's computer for your homework.

8 T (F) You can keep your wireless phone turned on while at work.

9 (T) F You should know your agency's attendance policy.

10 T (F) Harassment is legal in the workplace.

Circle the BEST answer.

11 Which will *not* help you do your job well?
a Enough rest and sleep
(c) Using drugs and alcohol
b Regular exercise
d Good nutrition

12 Which is *not* a good hygiene practice?
a Bathing daily
b Using a deodorant
c Brushing teeth after meals
(d) Having long and polished fingernails

13 You are getting ready for work. Which is *not* a good practice?
(a) Wearing jewelry
b Ironing your uniform
c Wearing your name badge
d Styling hair up and off your collar

14 When should you ask questions about your job description?
a After completing the job application
b Before completing the job application
c When your interview is scheduled
(d) During the interview

15 Lying on a job application is
a Negligence
c Libel
(b) Fraud
d Defamation

16 You are completing a job application. You should do the following *except*
a Write neatly and clearly
b Provide references
c Give information about employment gaps
(d) Leave spaces blank that do not apply to you

17 Which of the following do employers look for the *most*?
a Cooperation
(c) Dependability
b Courtesy
d Empathy

18 What should you wear to a job interview?
a A uniform
(c) A simple dress or suit
b Party clothes
d What is most comfortable

19 Which is a poor behavior during a job interview?
a Good eye contact with the interviewer
b Shaking hands with the interviewer
c Asking the interviewer questions
(d) Crossing your arms and legs

20 Which is the best response to an interview question?
a "Yes" or "no"
(c) Brief explanations
b Long answers
d A written response

21 Which statement reflects a good work attitude?
a "It's not my fault."
c "That's not my job."
(b) "I'm sorry. I didn't know."
d "I did it yesterday. It's your turn."

22 A co-worker says that a doctor and nurse are dating. This is
(a) Gossip
c Confidential information
b Eavesdropping
d Sexual harassment

23 Which is professional speech and language?
(a) Speaking clearly
c Shouting
b Using vulgar words
d Arguing

24 Which is *not* a courteous act?
a Saying "please" and "thank you"
(b) Wanting others to open doors for you
c Saying "I'm sorry"
d Complimenting others

25 You are on a meal break. Which is *false*?
a You can make personal phone calls.
b Family members can meet you.
(c) You can take a few extra minutes if needed.
d The nurse needs to know that you are off the unit.

26 You are planning your work. You should do the following *except*
a Discuss priorities with the nurse
b Ask others if they need help
c Stay busy
(d) Plan care so that you can watch the person's TV

27 These statements are about stress. Which is *false*?
a Stress affects the whole person.
b A stressor is an event that causes stress.
(c) All stress is unpleasant.
d Stress is normal.

28 Which is *not* harassment?
(a) Using touch to comfort a person
b Joking about a person's religion
c Asking for a sexual favor
d Acting like a disabled person

29 A resignation letter should *not* include
a Your reasons for leaving
b The last day you will work
c A thank-you to the employer
(d) Problems you had during your work

30 Which is *not* a reason for losing your job?
a Leaving the job during your shift
b Using alcohol in the work setting
c Sleeping on the job
(d) Taking a meal break

Answers to these questions are on p. 779.

Communicating With the Health Team

OBJECTIVES

- Define the key terms and key abbreviations listed in this chapter
- Explain why health team members need to communicate
- Describe the rules for good communication
- Explain the purpose, parts, and information found in the medical record
- Describe the legal and ethical aspects of medical records
- Describe the purpose of the Kardex
- List the information you need to report to the nurse
- List the rules for recording
- Use the 24-hour clock, medical terminology, and medical abbreviations
- Explain how computers and other electronic devices are used in health care
- Explain how to protect the right to privacy when using computers
- Describe the rules for answering phones
- Explain how to problem solve and deal with conflict

KEY TERMS

abbreviation A shortened form of a word or phrase

anterior At or toward the front of the body or body part; ventral

chart The medical record; clinical record

communication The exchange of information—a message sent is received and correctly interpreted by the intended person

conflict A clash between opposing interests or ideas

distal The part farthest from the center or from the point of attachment

dorsal Posterior

Kardex A type of card file that summarizes information found in the medical record—drugs, treatments, diagnoses, routine care measures, equipment, and special needs

lateral Away from the midline; at the side of the body or body part

medial At or near the middle or midline of the body or body part

medical record A written or electronic account of a person's condition and response to treatment and care; chart or clinical record

posterior At or toward the back of the body or body part; dorsal

prefix A word element placed before a root; it changes the meaning of the word

proximal The part nearest to the center or to the point of origin

recording The written account of care and observations; charting

reporting The oral account of care and observations

root A word element containing the basic meaning of the word

suffix A word element placed after a root; it changes the meaning of the word

ventral Anterior

word element A part of a word

KEY ABBREVIATIONS

ADL Activities of daily living

EPHI; ePHI Electronic protected health information

ID Identification

IV Intravenous

LNA Licensed nursing assistant

OBRA Omnibus Budget Reconciliation Act of 1987

PDA Personal digital assistant

PHI Protected health information

Health team members communicate with each other to give coordinated and effective care. They share information about:

▶ What was done for the person
▶ What needs to be done for the person
▶ The person's response to treatment

For example, the doctor ordered a blood test for Mrs. Lund. Food and fluids affect the test results. Mrs. Lund must fast from midnight until the blood is drawn. A nurse tells the dietary department that Mrs. Lund will have breakfast later. She explains the breakfast delay to you and Mrs. Lund. A technician tells the nurse the blood sample was drawn. The nurse orders the meal. A dietary worker brings the tray to the nursing unit. You serve Mrs. Lund's tray. After she is done eating, you remove the tray and observe what she ate. You report your observations to the nurse. You or the nurse record them in Mrs. Lund's medical record.

Team members communicated with each other and Mrs. Lund. Her care was coordinated and effective. She knew that she was not neglected or forgotten.

You need to understand the rules of communication. Then you can learn how to communicate information to the nursing and health teams.

COMMUNICATION

Communication is the exchange of information—a message sent is received and correctly interpreted by the intended person. For good communication:

▶ Use words that mean the same thing to you and the receiver of the message. "Small," "moderate," and "large" mean different things to different people. Is small the size of a dime? Or is it the size of a quarter? In health care, different meanings can cause serious problems. Avoid words with more than one meaning.

▶ Use familiar words. You will learn medical terminology. If do not know what a term means, ask the nurse. Or use a medical dictionary. You must understand the message. Otherwise communication does not occur. Likewise, do not use terms unfamiliar to the person and family.

▶ Be brief and concise. Do not add unrelated or unnecessary information. Stay on the subject. Avoid wandering in thought. Do not get wordy.

▶ Give information in a logical and orderly manner. Organize your thoughts. Present them step-by-step.

▶ Give facts and be specific. The receiver should have a clear picture of what you are saying. You report a pulse rate of 110. It is more specific and factual than saying the "pulse is fast."

THE MEDICAL RECORD

The **medical record (chart)** is a written or electronic account of a person's condition and response to treatment and care. (The Omnibus Budget Reconciliation Act of 1987 [OBRA] calls the medical record the *clinical record*.) It is a way for the health team to share information about the person. The record is permanent. It can be used years later if the person's health history is needed. The record is a legal document. It can be used as evidence in a court of law of the person's problems, treatment, and care.

The record has many forms. They are organized into sections for easy use. Each page has the person's name, room and bed number, and other identifying information. This helps prevent errors and improper placement of records. The record includes the person's:

▶ Admission sheet
▶ Health history
▶ Physical examination results
▶ Doctor's orders
▶ Doctor's progress note
▶ Progress notes (nursing team and health team)
▶ Graphic sheet
▶ Flow sheets
▶ Laboratory results
▶ X-ray reports
▶ IV (Intravenous) therapy record
▶ Respiratory therapy record
▶ Consultation reports
▶ Surgery and anesthesia reports
▶ Assessments and reports from social services, dietary services, and physical, occupational, speech, and recreational therapies
▶ Special consents

Health team members record information on the forms for their departments. Other health team members read the information. It tells the care provided and the person's response (Fig. 5-1).

Agencies have policies about medical records and who can see them. Policies address:

▶ Who records
▶ When to record
▶ Abbreviations
▶ Correcting errors
▶ Ink color
▶ Signing entries

Some agencies allow nursing assistants to record observations and care. Others do not. You must know your agency's policies.

Professional staff involved in a person's care can review the chart. Cooks, laundry, housekeeping, and office staff have no need to read charts. Some agencies let nursing assistants read charts. If not, the nurse shares information as needed.

You have an ethical and legal duty to keep the person's information confidential. You may know someone in the agency. If you do not give care to that person, you have no right to review the person's chart. To do so is an invasion of privacy.

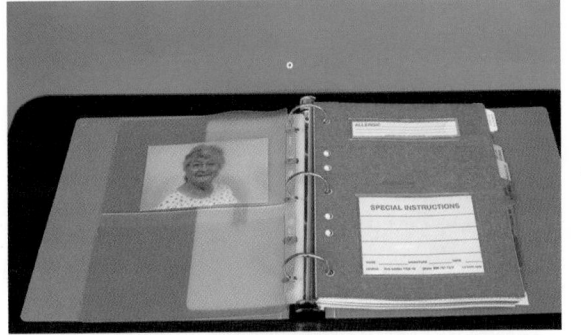

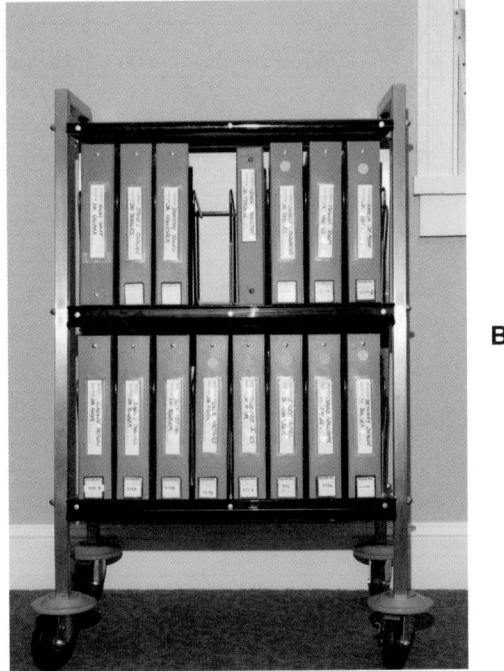

FIGURE 5-1 A, A medical record. **B,** Medical records are kept in chart rack.

Patients and residents have the right to the information in their medical records. The person or the person's legal representative may ask you for the chart. Report the request to the nurse. The nurse deals with the request.

The following parts of the medical record relate to your work.

The Admission Sheet

The admission sheet is completed when the person is admitted to the agency. It contains the person's identifying information—legal name, birth date, age, gender (male or female), current address, and marital status. The names of the person's nearest relative and legal representative also are included. Other information includes known allergies, diagnoses, date and time of admission, and doctor's name. Religion, place of worship, occupation, and employer are often included.

Each person receives an identification (ID) number. It is on the admission sheet. So is information about advance directives. An *advance directive* is a document stating a

Med-Forms, Inc.
FORM #MF37079 (Rev 9/95)

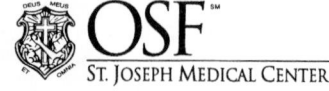

OSF
ST. JOSEPH MEDICAL CENTER
Bloomington, Illinois 61701

DAILY SUMMARY AND GRAPHIC

TEMPERATURE
Write in 105° or over

DATE																									
HOSPITAL DAY																									
POST OP DAY																									
HOUR	2400	0400	0800	1200	1600	2000	2400	0400	0800	1200	1600	2000	2400	0400	0800	1200	1600	2000	2400	0400	0800	1200	1600	2000
B/P																									

TEMPERATURE

104 40
102.2 39
100.4 38
98.6 37 •
96.6 36

PULSE				
RESPIRATION				
WEIGHT				
DR. VISIT				

INTAKE	2300-0700	0700-1500	1500-2300	TOTAL	2300-0700	0700-1500	1500-2300	TOTAL	2300-0700	0700-1500	1500-2300	TOTAL	2300-0700	0700-1500	1500-2300	TOTAL
Oral																
IV																
Tube Feedings																
PPN/TPN/Lipids																
Blood/Blood Products																
IV Meds																
Chemotherapy																
Unreturned irr. sol.																
TOTAL INTAKE																
OUTPUT	2300-0700	0700-1500	1500-2300	TOTAL	2300-0700	0700-1500	1500-2300	TOTAL	2300-0700	0700-1500	1500-2300	TOTAL	2300-0700	0700-1500	1500-2300	TOTAL
Urine																
GI																
Emesis																
Drains																
TOTAL OUTPUT																
Feces																

FIGURE 5-2 Graphic sheet. (Courtesy OSF St Joseph Medical Center, Bloomington, Ill.)

person's wishes about life support measures (Chapter 50).

Use the admission sheet to fill out other forms that require the same information. That way the person does not have to answer the same question many times.

Health History

The health history is completed when the person is admitted. In some agencies it is called the *nursing history*. The nurse interviews the person. You can use the form to learn about the person's background and health history. It contains information about:

▶ The person's chief complaint—why the person sought health care
▶ History of the current illness—sudden or gradual in onset, when it started, signs and symptoms, and so on
▶ Past health problems, surgeries, and injuries
▶ Childhood illnesses
▶ Allergies
▶ Current drugs
▶ Family health history
▶ Life-style—habits, diet, sleep, hobbies, and so on
▶ If the person wears dentures, eyeglasses, or hearing aids
▶ Problems with activities of daily living
▶ Education and occupation

The Graphic Sheet

The graphic sheet is used to record measurements and observations made daily, every shift, or 3 to 4 times a day (Fig. 5-2). Information includes vital signs—blood pressure, temperature, pulse, respirations. It also includes weight, intake and output, bowel movements (feces), and doctor's visits.

Progress Notes

The progress note describes the care given and the person's response and progress (Fig. 5-3). The nurse records:

▶ The person's signs and symptoms
▶ Information about treatments and drugs
▶ Information about patient or resident teaching and counseling
▶ Procedures performed by the doctor
▶ Visits by other health team members
See *Focus on Long-Term Care and Home Care: Progress Notes.*

FOCUS ON LONG-TERM CARE AND HOME CARE

Progress Notes

LONG-TERM CARE

The nurse writes progress notes when there is an unusual event, a problem, or a change in the person's condition. OBRA requires that summaries of care be written at least every 3 months. They reflect the person's progress toward the goals set in the care plan (Chapter 6). They also reflect the person's response to care. Some centers require summaries more often.

Date	Time	Nursing Margin / Other Depts Margin
3-19	1700	Out with family for dinner. Jane Doe, LPN
	1930	Returned from outing accompanied by her son. States she had a pleasant time. Mary Smith, CNA
3-20	0900	In bed. Complains of headache. T 98.4 orally, radial pulse 72 and regular, respirations 18 and unlabored. BP 134/84 left arm lying down. Alice Jones, RN notified of resident complaint and vital signs. Ann Adams, CNA
	0910	In bed resting. States she has had a headache for about 1/2 hour. Denies nausea and dizziness. No other complaints. PRN Tylenol given. Instructed resident to use signal light if headache worsens or other symptoms occur. Alice Jones, RN
	0945	Resting quietly. Denies headache at this time. T 98.4 orally, radial pulse 70 and regular, respirations 18 and unlabored. BP 132/84 left arm lying down. Alice Jones, RN

FIGURE 5-3 Progress notes. Note that other members of the health team also can record on this form.

Activities of Daily Living Flow Sheet

JAN FEB (MAR) APR MAY JUN JUL AUG SEP OCT NOV DEC

ORDER/INSTRUCTION	TIME	1	2	3	4	5	6	7	8	9	10	11	12	13	14	15	16	17	18	19	20	21	22	23	24	25	26	27	28	29	30	31
Bowel Movements L = Large M = Medium S = Small IC = Incontinent	11-7	M																														
	7-3			L																												
	3-11																															
Bladder Elimination I = Independent IC = Incontinent FC = Foley catheter	11-7	I	I	I	I																											
	7-3	I	I	I	I																											
	3-11	I	IC	I	I																											
Weight Bearing Status TT = Toe touch AT = As tol. P = Partial F = Full NWB = No weight bearing	11-7	AT	AT	AT	AT																											
	7-3	AT	AT	AT	AT																											
	3-11	AT	AT	AT	AT																											
Transfer Status ML = Mech lift SBA = Stand by assist; Assist of 1 or 2	11-7	SBA	SBA	SBA	SBA																											
	7-3	SBA	SBA	SBA	SBA																											
	3-11	SBA	SBA	SBA	A-1																											
Activity A = Ambulate GC = Gerichair T = Turn every 2 hrs. W/C = Wheelchair	11-7	T	T	T	T																											
	7-3	A	A	A	A																											
	3-11	A	A	A	A																											
Safety LT = Lap tray BR = Bed rails BA = Bed alarm SB = Seat belt	11-7																															
	7-3																															
	3-11																															
Feeding Status I = Independent S = Set up F = Staff feed SP = Swallow precautions TL = Thickened liquids	Breakfast	S	S	S	S																											
	Lunch	S	S	S	S																											
	Supper	S	S	S	S																											
Amount of food taken in %	Breakfast	75	100	100	75																											
	Lunch	75	75	100	75																											
	Supper	50	50	50	75																											
Bath and Shampoo every *Monday* & *Thursday* on *7-3* shift T = Tub S = Shower B = Bed bath	11-7																															
	7-3		T																													
	3-11																															
Oral Care Own/(Dentures)/No teeth I = Independent S = Set up A = Assist	11-7	S	S	S	S																											
	7-3	S	S	S	S																											
	3-11	S	S	S	S																											
Dressing I = Independent S = Set up A = Assist T = Total care	11-7	A	A	S	S																											
	7-3																															
	3-11	A	A	A	A																											
Grooming: Washing Face and Hands Combing Hair I = Independent S = Set up A = Assist T = Total care	11-7	A	A	A	A																											
	7-3	A	A	A	A																											
	3-11	A	A	A	A																											
Trim Fingernails weekly *Thursday*	11-7																															
	7-3		✓																													
	3-11																															
Lotion Arms and Legs twice daily	11-7																															
	7-3	✓	✓	✓	✓																											
	3-11	✓	✓	✓	✓																											
Shave Men daily Shave (Women) every *Monday* & *Thursday* on *7-3* shift	11-7																															
	7-3		✓																													
	3-11																															
Amount Between-Meal Nourishment taken in %	AM	100	75	100	50																											
	PM	100	100	75	75																											
	HS	50	75	75	75																											
Intake and Output	11-7																															
	7-3																															
	3-11																															
Vital Signs Every *Thursday*	11-7																															
	7-3		✓																													
	3-11																															
Weight Every *Thursday*	11-7		✓																													
	7-3																															
	3-11																															

FIGURE 5-4 Some items on an activities of daily living flow sheet.

Flow Sheets

LONG-TERM CARE

An activities of daily living (ADL) flow sheet is used to record a person's ability to perform ADL (Fig. 5-4). This flow sheet addresses hygiene, food and fluids, elimination, rest and sleep, activities, and social interactions.

HOME CARE

Flow sheets are used in home care. For example, a weekly record has boxes for each day of the week and for care activities. You check the box for the day care was given. There are boxes for vital signs and weight. You record the measurements on the day they were done.

Flow Sheets

Flow sheets are used to record frequent measurements or observations. For example, a person's vital signs are measured every 30 minutes. The graphic sheet does not have room for frequent measurements. A vital signs flow sheet does. The bedside intake and output record is another flow sheet (Chapter 23).

See *Focus on Long-Term Care and Home Care: Flow Sheets.*

THE KARDEX

The **Kardex** is a type of card file. It summarizes information found in the medical record—drugs, treatments, diagnoses, routine care measures, equipment, and special needs. The Kardex is a quick, easy source of information about the person (Fig. 5-5, p. 62).

REPORTING AND RECORDING

The health team communicates by reporting and recording. **Reporting** is the oral account of care and observations. **Recording** (*charting*) is the written account of care and observations.

Reporting

You report care and observations to the nurse. Report to the nurse:

▶ Whenever there is a change in the person's condition
▶ When the nurse asks you to do so
▶ When you leave the unit for meals, breaks, or for other reasons
▶ Before the end-of-shift-report
  Follow these rules:
▶ Be prompt, thorough, and accurate.
▶ Give the person's name and room and bed number.
▶ Give the time your observations were made or the care was given.
▶ Report only what you observed or did yourself.
▶ Report care measures that you expect the person to need. For example, you expect that the person will need the bedpan during your meal break. Explain why you expect the need.

▶ Report expected changes in the person's condition. For example, you are going off duty. The person has not voided since returning from surgery.
▶ Give reports as often as the person's condition requires. Or give them when the nurse asks you to.
▶ Report any changes from normal or changes in the person's condition. Report these changes at once. See Chapter 6.
▶ Use your written notes to give a specific, concise, and clear report (Fig. 5-6).
  See *Teamwork and Time Management: Reporting.*

End-of-Shift Report

The nurse gives a report at the end of the shift. This is called the *end-of-shift report* or the *change-of-shift report*. It is given to the nursing team of the on-coming shift. The nurse reports the following information about:

▶ The care given
▶ The care that must be given during other shifts
▶ The person's current condition
▶ Likely changes in the person's condition

In some agencies, the entire nursing team hears the end-of-shift report as they come on duty. In other agencies, only nurses hear the report. After the report, they share important information with nursing assistants.

See *Teamwork and Time Management: End-of-Shift Report*, p. 63.

See *Promoting Safety and Comfort: End-of-Shift Report*, p. 63.

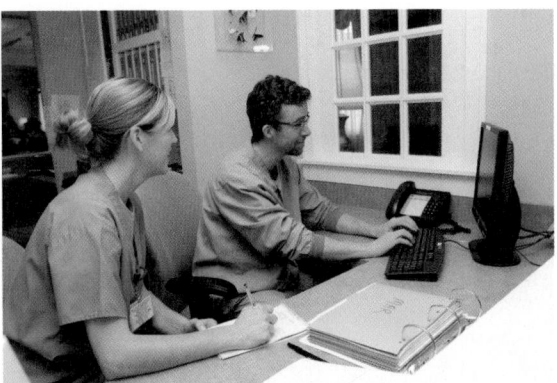

FIGURE 5-6 The nursing assistant uses notes to report to the nurse.

Reporting

You must give the nurse your full attention when reporting. If distracted, you could omit or forget to give important information.

Nurses need to give their full attention when receiving reports. If someone is reporting to a nurse, do not interrupt that process unless the matter is urgent. You must not distract the nurse.

DIET	NOURISHMENT/SPECIAL FEEDING	INTAKE/OUTPUT
Regular	*Health shake at Bedtime*	Encourage/**Restrict** Fluids *2000* mL/24 Hr.
Hold:		7-3 *1000* 3-11 *800* 11-7 *200*

FUNCTIONAL STATUS

	SELF	ASSIST	TOTAL	OTHER	SPECIFY
Feeding	☐	☒	☐	☐	
Bathing	☐	☒	☐	☐	
Toileting	☐	☒	☐	☐	
Oral Care	☐	☒	☐	☐	
Positioning	☒	☐	☐	☐	
Transferring	☒	☐	☐	☐	
Wheeling	☐	☐	☐	☐	
Walking	☒	☐	☐	☐	
	☐	☐	☐	☐	

ACTIVITIES

Bedrest & BRP	
Bedside Commode	
Up ad Lib	*X*
Chair	
Ambulatory	*X*
Ambulate & Assist	
Turn	
Dangle	
Mode of Travel	

ELIMINATION

Bladder - Cont. (**Incont.**)	
Catheter	
Date Changed	
Irrigations	
Bowel - (**Cont.**) / Incont.	
Ostomy	
Irrigations	

VITALS

Temp.	*4 times a day*
Pulse	*4 times a day*
Resp.	*4 times a day*
BP	*4 times a day*
Weight	*daily*
Other:	*Pulse OX daily*

COMMUNICATION DEFICITS   ☐ None

Hearing *Hard-of-hearing*
Vision *Impaired*
Speech
Language *Impaired*

PROSTHESIS   ☐ None

Glasses *X*   Dentures *X*
Contacts _____   Limb _____
Hearing Aid *L ear*

SPECIAL CONDITIONS (Paralysis, Pressure Ulcers, Etc.)

SAFETY/SUPPORTIVE MEASURES

Bed rails: ☐ Nights Only   ☐ Constant   ☐ No Need
Restraints: ☐ PRN   ☐ Constant

Support Devices: ☐ PRN   ☐ Constant

RESPIRATORY THERAPY

Aerosol
IPPB
Ultrasonic

Rx Med _____

OXYGEN

_____ *2* _____ Liter/Minute
☒ PRN   ☐ Constant

___ Tent   ___ Catheter
___ Mask   *X* Cannula

SPECIAL EQUIPMENT/PROCEDURES/ANCILLARY SERVICES/ETC.

Speech therapy 3 times/wk.

DATE	TREATMENTS/MISCELLANEOUS

ORDERED	SCHEDULED	COMPLETED	X-RAY AND SPECIAL DIAGNOSTIC EXAMS
10-20	*10-20*	*10-20*	*Chest x-ray*

START DATE	SCHEDULED MEDICATIONS	STOP DATE	RENEW	START DATE	STOP OR RENEW	SITE	IV FLUID & RATE	DATE & TIME CHANGED TUBING	DRESS.	SITE
10-19	*Lasix 40 mg daily*									
10-19	*Lanoxin 0.25 mg daily*									

DATE	ONE TIME ORDERS

DATE	DAILY/REPEATING ORDERS
10-20	*Serum potassium daily*

DATE	TIME	PRN MEDICATIONS
10-19	*2100*	*Ativan 0.25 mg*

MISCELLANEOUS

ALLERGIES:
☒ None Known

NURSING ALERTS:

EMERGENCY CONTACT:
Telephone No.
Name: *Parker, Marie*   Home: *555-1212*
Relationship: *Wife*   Bus:

ROOM	NAME	PHYSICIAN	ADMITTING DIAGNOSIS/PROBLEM	HOSP. NO.
310	*Parker, Edwin*	*Dr. S Epstein*	1. *CHF* 2. *Dementia*	*1035B*

FIGURE 5-5 A sample Kardex. (Modified from Briggs Corporation, Des Moines, Iowa.)

TEAMWORK AND TIME MANAGEMENT

End-of-Shift Report

Two staffs are present at the end of a shift—the staff going off duty and the staff coming on duty. The entire on-coming shift may attend the end-of-shift report. If so, staff members going off duty answer all signal lights, provide care, and tend to routine tasks. If only nurses attend the end-of-shift report, nursing assistants of the on-coming shift also answer signal lights, provide care, and tend to routine tasks.

The end-of-shift is a time for good teamwork. Continue to do your job. Your attitude is important. If going off duty, avoid saying or thinking the following:

- "I'm ready to go home. Let them do it."
- "It's their turn. I've been here all day (evening or night)."
- "No one helped us when we came on duty."

Some agencies have clear duties for the two shifts. For example, those going off duty continue to answer signal lights. They know about changes in the person's condition and care plan and about new orders. They also know about the care needs of new patients or residents. The on-coming shift has yet to learn this information. The on-coming shift uses this time to perform routine tasks for the shift and to collect needed supplies and equipment.

Recording

When recording on the person's chart, you must communicate clearly and thoroughly. Follow the rules in Box 5-1. The charting sample in Figure 5-7 (p. 64) shows how the rules apply.

Anyone who reads your charting should know:

▶ What you observed
▶ What you did
▶ The person's response

See *Focus on Ethics and Laws: Recording*, p. 64.

Recording Time

The 24-hour clock (military time or international time) has four digits (Fig. 5-8, p. 64). The first two digits are for the hours: 0100 = 1:00 AM; 1300 = 1:00 PM. The last two digits are for minutes: 0110 = 1:10 AM. The AM and PM abbreviations are not used.

As Box 5-2 (p. 64) shows, the hour is the same for morning times, but AM is not used. For PM times add 12 to the clock time. If it is 2:00 PM, add 12 and 2 for 1400. For 8:35 PM, add 12 and 835 for 2035.

Communication is better with the 24-hour clock. You must use AM and PM with conventional clock time. Someone may forget to use AM or PM. Or writing may be unclear. This means that the correct time is not communicated. Harm to the person could result.

PROMOTING SAFETY AND COMFORT: End-of-Shift Report

SAFETY

You may not hear the end-of-shift report as you come on duty. Yet you need to answer signal lights and give care before the nurse shares new information with you. To give safe care:

- Check the care plan and Kardex before granting a request. The person's condition or care plan may have changed since you last worked. There may be new orders from the doctor.
- Ask a nurse about the care needs of new patients or residents. If necessary, politely interrupt the end-of-shift report to ask your questions.
- Do not take directions or orders from another nursing assistant. Remember, nursing assistants cannot supervise or delegate to other nursing assistants.

BOX 5-1 Rules for Recording

- Always use ink. Use the ink color required by the agency.
- Include the date and time for every recording. Use conventional time (AM or PM) or 24-hour clock time according to agency policy.
- Make sure writing is readable and neat.
- Use only agency-approved medical abbreviations (p. 65).
- Use correct spelling, grammar, and punctuation.
- Do not use ditto marks.
- Never erase or use correction fluid. Draw a line through the incorrect part. Date and initial the line. Write "mistaken entry" over it if this is agency policy. Then rewrite the part. Follow agency policy for correcting errors.
- Sign all entries with your name and title as required by agency policy.
- Do not skip lines. Draw a line through the blank space of a partially completed line or to the end of the page. This prevents others from recording in a space with your signature.
- Make sure each form has the person's name and other identifying information.
- Record only what you observed and did yourself. Do not record for another person.
- Never chart a procedure, treatment, measurement, or care measure until after it is completed.
- Chart a procedure, treatment, measurement, or care measure after completing it. If not recorded, the action is considered not done.
- Be accurate, concise, and factual. Do not record judgments or interpretations.
- Record in a logical and sequential manner.
- Be descriptive. Avoid terms with more than one meaning.
- Use the person's exact words whenever possible. Use quotation marks to show that the statement is a direct quote.
- Chart any changes from normal or changes in the person's condition. Also chart that you informed the nurse (include the nurse's name), what you told the nurse, and the time you made the report.
- Do not omit information.
- Record safety measures. Examples include placing the signal light within reach, assisting a person when up, or reminding a person not to get out of bed.

Date	Time	Nursing Margin	Other Depts Margin
7/18	1045	Requested assistance to lie down. States. "I don't feel well. I have a little upset stomach."	
		Denies pain. VS taken. T-99(O). P-76 regular rate and rhythm. R-18 unlabored.	
		BP 134/84 L arm lying down. Signal light within reach. Paula Jones, RN notified at 1040	
		of resident's complaint and VS. Mary Jensen, CNA ————	
	1100	Asleep in bed. Appears to be resting comfortably. Color good. No signs of	
		discomfort or distress noted at this time. Paula Jones, RN ————	
	1145	Refused to go to the dining room for lunch. Complains of nausea.	
		Denies abdominal pain. Has not had an emesis. Abdomen soft to	
		palpation. Good bowel sounds. VS taken. T-98.2 99.2. P-76 regular *(Mistaken entry 4-10, PJ)*	
		rate and rhythm. R-18 unlabored. BP-134/84. States she will try to	
		eat something. Full liquid room tray ordered. Paula Jones, RN ————	

FIGURE 5-7 Charting sample.

FOCUS ON ETHICS AND LAWS

Recording

A licensed nursing assistant (LNA) worked at a home health and hospice agency. On November 9, 2001, she recorded on a time sheet that she was in a patient's home for about 30 minutes. However, the patient was in the hospital from November 8 through November 14, 2001.

The LNA admitted to unprofessional conduct. Her conduct violated Administrative Rules of the Board of Nursing for:

- Making inaccurate or misleading entries
- Failing to comply with federal or state laws or rules

The LNA was given a reprimand by the Board.

(Author note: A reprimand means that the Board considered her conduct to be improper. However, the Board did not limit her right to work as an LNA.)

(State of Vermont Board of Nursing in regard to T. Brigham, 2003.)

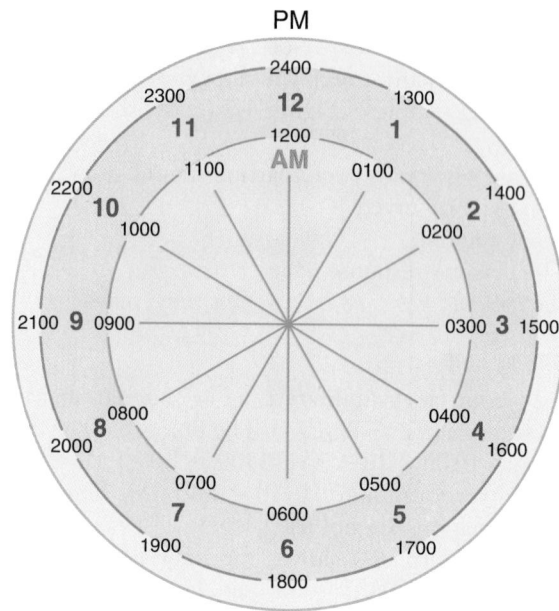

FIGURE 5-8 The 24-hour clock.

BOX 5-2 24-Hour Clock

Conventional Time	24-Hour Clock	Conventional Time	24-Hour Clock	Conventional Time	24-Hour Clock	Conventional Time	24-Hour Clock
1:00 AM	0100	7:00 AM	0700	1:00 PM	1300	7:00 PM	1900
2:00 AM	0200	8:00 AM	0800	2:00 PM	1400	8:00 PM	2000
3:00 AM	0300	9:00 AM	0900	3:00 PM	1500	9:00 PM	2100
4:00 AM	0400	10:00 AM	1000	4:00 PM	1600	10:00 PM	2200
5:00 AM	0500	11:00 AM	1100	5:00 PM	1700	11:00 PM	2300
6:00 AM	0600	12:00 NOON	1200	6:00 PM	1800	12:00 MIDNIGHT	2400 or 0000

MEDICAL TERMINOLOGY AND ABBREVIATIONS

Medical terminology and abbreviations are used in health care. Someone may use a term or phrase that you do not understand. If so, ask a nurse or use a medical dictionary. If you do not understand the term or phrase, communication does not occur. You may want to buy a medical dictionary so you can learn new words.

Like all words, medical terms are made up of parts or **word elements**—prefixes, roots, and suffixes (Box 5-3). Most are from Greek or Latin. They are combined to form medical terms. A term is translated by separating the word into its elements.

Prefixes, Roots, and Suffixes

A **prefix** is a word element placed before a root. It changes the meaning of the word. The prefix *olig* (scant, small amount) is placed before the root *uria* (urine) to make *oliguria*. It means a scant amount of urine. Prefixes are always combined with other word elements. They are never used alone.

The **root** is the word element that contains the basic meaning of the word. It is combined with another root, with prefixes, and suffixes. A vowel (an *o* or an *i*) is added when two roots are combined or when a suffix is added to a root. The vowel makes the word easier to pronounce.

A **suffix** is a word element placed after a root. It changes the meaning of the word. Suffixes are not used alone. When translating medical terms, begin with the suffix. For example, *nephritis* means inflammation of the kidney. It was formed by combining *nephro* (kidney) and *itis* (inflammation).

Medical terms are formed by combining word elements. Remember, prefixes always come before roots. Suffixes always come after roots. A root can be combined with prefixes, roots, and suffixes. The prefix *dys* (difficult) is combined with the root *pnea* (breathing). This forms *dyspnea*. It means difficulty breathing.

Roots can be combined with suffixes. The root *mast* (breast) combined with the suffix *ectomy* (excision or removal) forms *mastectomy*. It means the removal of a breast.

Combining a prefix, root, and suffix is another way to form medical terms. *Endocarditis* has the prefix *endo* (inner), the root *card* (heart), and the suffix *itis* (inflammation). *Endocarditis* means inflammation of the inner part of the heart.

BOX 5-3 Medical Terminology

PREFIX	MEANING	PREFIX	MEANING
a-, an-	without, not, lack of	mono-	one, single
ab-	away from	neo-	new
ad-	to, toward, near	non-	not
ante-	before, forward, in front of	olig-	small, scant
anti-	against	para-	beside, beyond, after
auto-	self	per-	by, through
bi-	double, two, twice	peri-	around
brady-	slow	poly-	many, much
circum-	around	post-	after, behind
contra-	against, opposite	pre-	before, in front of, prior to
de-	down, from	pro-	before, in front of
dia-	across, through, apart	re-	again, backward
dis-	apart, free from	retro-	backward, behind
dys-	bad, difficult, abnormal	semi-	half
ecto-	outer, outside	sub-	under, beneath
en-	in, into, within	super-	above, over, excess
endo-	inner, inside	supra-	above, over
epi-	over, on, upon	tachy-	fast, rapid
eryth-	red	trans-	across
eu-	normal, good, well, healthy	uni-	one
ex-	out, out of, from, away from	**ROOT (COMBINING VOWEL)**	**MEANING**
hemi-	half	abdomin (o)	abdomen
hyper-	excessive, too much, high	aden (o)	gland
hypo-	under, decreased, less than normal	adren (o)	adrenal gland
in-	in, into, within, not	angi (o)	vessel
inter-	between	arterio	artery
intra-	within	athr (o)	joint
intro-	into, within	broncho	bronchus, bronchi
leuk-	white	card, cardi (o)	heart
macro-	large	cephal (o)	head
mal-	bad, illness, disease	chole, chol (o)	bile
meg-	large	chondr (o)	cartilage
micro-	small		

Continued

BOX 5-3 Medical Terminology—cont'd

ROOT (COMBINING VOWEL)	MEANING
colo	colon, large intestine
cost (o)	rib
crani (o)	skull
cyan (o)	blue
cyst (o)	bladder, cyst
cyt (o)	cell
dent (o)	tooth
derma	skin
duoden (o)	duodenum
encephal (o)	brain
enter (o)	intestines
fibr (o)	fiber, fibrous
gastr (o)	stomach
gloss (o)	tongue
gluc (o)	sweetness, glucose
glyc (o)	sugar
gyn, gyne, gyneco	woman
hem, hema, hemo, hemat (o)	blood
hepat (o)	liver
hydr (o)	water
hyster (o)	uterus
ile (o), ili (o)	ileum
laparo	abdomen, loin, flank
laryng (o)	larynx
lith (o)	stone
mamm (o)	breast, mammary gland
mast (o)	mammary gland, breast
meno	menstruation
my (o)	muscle
myel (o)	spinal cord, bone marrow
necro	death
nephr (o)	kidney
neur (o)	nerve
ocul (o)	eye
oophor (o)	ovary
ophthalm (o)	eye
orth (o)	straight, normal, correct
oste (o)	bone
ot (o)	ear
ped (o)	child, foot
pharyng (o)	pharynx
phleb (o)	vein
pnea	breathing, respiration
pneum (o)	lung, air, gas
proct (o)	rectum
psych (o)	mind
pulmo	lung
py (o)	pus
rect (o)	rectum
rhin (o)	nose
salping (o)	eustachian tube, uterine tube
splen (o)	spleen
sten (o)	narrow, constriction
stern (o)	sternum
stomat (o)	mouth

ROOT (COMBINING VOWEL)	MEANING
therm (o)	heat
thoraco	chest
thromb (o)	clot, thrombus
thyr (o)	thyroid
toxic (o)	poison, poisonous
toxo	poison
trache (o)	trachea
urethr (o)	urethra
urin (o)	urine
uro	urine, urinary tract, urination
uter (o)	uterus
vas (o)	blood vessel, vas deferens
ven (o)	vein
vertebr (o)	spine, vertebrae

SUFFIX	MEANING
-algia	pain
-asis	condition, usually abnormal
-cele	hernia, herniation, pouching
-centesis	puncture and aspiration of
-cyte	cell
-ectasis	dilation, stretching
-ectomy	excision, removal of
-emia	blood condition
-genesis	development, production, creation
-genic	producing, causing
-gram	record
-graph	a diagram, a recording instrument
-graphy	making a recording
-iasis	condition of
-ism	a condition
-itis	inflammation
-logy	the study of
-lysis	destruction of, decomposition
-megaly	enlargement
-meter	measuring instrument
-oma	tumor
-osis	condition
-pathy	disease
-penia	lack, deficiency
-phagia	to eat or consume, swallowing
-phasia	speaking
-phobia	an exaggerated fear
-plasty	surgical repair or reshaping
-plegia	paralysis
-ptosis	falling, sagging, dropping down
-rrhage, -rrhagia	excessive flow
-rrhaphy	stitching, suturing
-rrhea	profuse flow, discharge
-scope	examination instrument
-scopy	examination using a scope
-stasis	maintenance, maintaining a constant level
-stomy, -ostomy	creation of an opening
-tomy, -otomy	incision, cutting into
-uria	condition of the urine

Abdominal Regions

The abdomen is divided into regions (Fig. 5-9). They are used to describe the location of body structures, pain, or discomfort. The regions are:

▶ Right upper quadrant (RUQ)
▶ Left upper quadrant (LUQ)
▶ Right lower quadrant (RLQ)
▶ Left lower quadrant (LLQ)

Directional Terms

Certain terms describe the position of one body part in relation to another. These terms give the direction of the body part when a person is standing and facing forward (Fig. 5-10):

▶ **Anterior (ventral)**—at or toward the front of the body or body part
▶ **Distal**—the part farthest from the center or from the point of attachment
▶ **Lateral**—away from the midline; at the side of the body or body part
▶ **Medial**—at or near the middle or midline of the body or body part
▶ **Posterior (dorsal)**—at or toward the back of the body or body part
▶ **Proximal**—the part nearest to the center or to the point of origin

Medical Abbreviations

Abbreviations are shortened forms of words or phrases. They save time and space when recording. Each agency has a list of accepted medical abbreviations. Obtain the list when you are hired. Use only those accepted by the agency. If not sure that an abbreviation is acceptable, write the term out in full. This promotes accurate communication.

Common abbreviations are on the inside of the back book cover for easy use.

Common Terms and Phrases

Some terms and phrases apply to basic care and safety. Because they are used throughout this book, they are presented in Box 5-4, p. 68. Some are presented as key terms in other chapters.

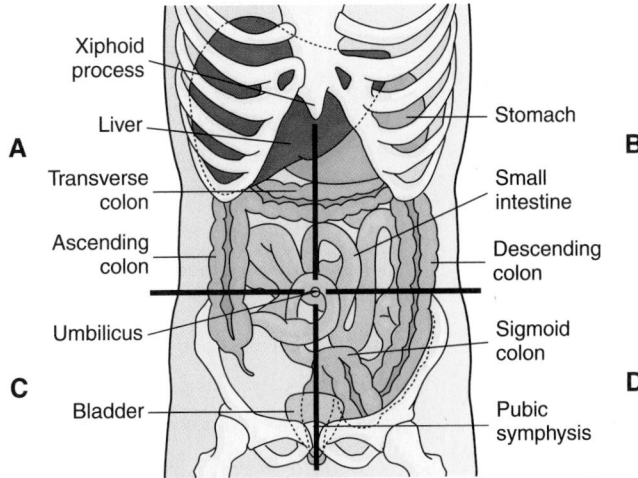

FIGURE 5-9 The four abdominal regions. **A,** Right upper quadrant. **B,** Left upper quadrant. **C,** Right lower quadrant. **D,** Left lower quadrant.

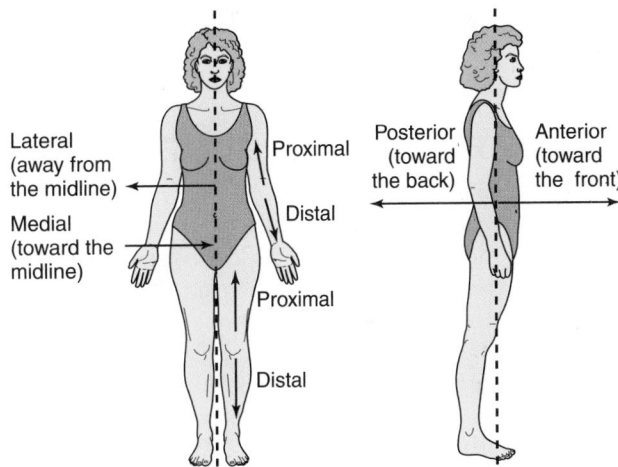

FIGURE 5-10 Directional terms describe the position of one body part in relation to another.

BOX 5-4 Common Health Care Terms and Phrases

activities of daily living (ADL)	The activities usually done during a normal day in a person's life
care plan	A written guide about the person's care
cognitive function	Involves memory, thinking, reasoning, ability to understand, judgment, and behavior
contracture	The lack of joint mobility caused by abnormal shortening of a muscle
dementia	The loss of cognitive and social function caused by changes in the brain; the loss of cognitive function that interferes with routine personal, social, and occupational activities
dysphagia	Difficulty (dys) swallowing (phagia)
dyspnea	Difficult, labored, or painful (dys) breathing (pnea)
feces	The semi-solid mass of waste products in the colon that are expelled through the anus
fever	Elevated body temperature
Fowler's position	A semi-sitting position; the head of the bed is raised between 45 and 60 degrees
incontinence	Not being able to control urination (urinary incontinence) or defecation (fecal incontinence)
pressure ulcer	A localized injury to the skin and/or underlying tissue, usually over a bony prominence
prone	Lying on the abdomen with the head turned to one side
semi-Fowler's position	The head of the bed is raised 30 degrees; or the head of the bed is raised 30 degrees and the knee portion is raised 15 degrees
signal light	Part of the call system that allows the person to signal the nurses' station for help
supine	The back-lying or dorsal recumbent position
vital signs	Temperature, pulse, respirations, and blood pressure (and pain)
voiding	Urinating

COMPUTERS AND OTHER ELECTRONIC DEVICES

Computer systems collect, send, record, and store information. So do some personal digital assistants (PDAs). Many agencies store charts and care plans (Chapter 6) on computers. Entering data on a computer is easier and faster than charting.

The health team uses computers, PDAs, and faxes to send messages and reports to the nursing unit. This reduces clerical work and phone calls. And information is sent with greater speed and accuracy.

Computers are used for measurements such as blood pressures, temperatures, and heart rates. The computer senses normal and abnormal measurements. When the abnormal is sensed, an alarm alerts the nursing staff. Life-threatening events are detected early. Computer monitoring is common in hospitals and in skilled nursing units.

Computers and other electronic devices save time. Quality care and safety are increased. Fewer errors are made in recording. Records are more complete (Fig. 5-11). Staff are more efficient.

Each staff member using computers and other electronic devices is issued a "unique user identification" and a password. They are used to access, send, receive, or store protected health information (PHI).

You must follow the agency's policies when using computers and other electronic devices. You must maintain the confidentiality of PHI and electronic protected health information (ePHI; EPHI). To do so follow the rules in Box 5-5 and the ethical and legal rules about privacy, confidentiality, and defamation (Chapter 2).

PHONE COMMUNICATIONS

You will answer phones at the nurse's station or in the person's room. Good communication skills are needed. The caller cannot see you. But you give much information by your tone of voice, how clearly you speak, and your attitude. Behave as if you are speaking to someone face-to-face. Be professional and courteous. Also practice good work ethics. Follow the agency's policy and the guidelines in Box 5-6, p. 570.

See *Focus on Long-Term Care and Home Care: Phone Communications.*

FOCUS ON LONG-TERM CARE AND HOME CARE

Phone Communications

HOME CARE

When answering phones in patients' homes, simply answer with "hello." This is for everyone's safety—the person, family, and you. The caller has too much information when you give the person's name ("Price residence") or your name and title.

People call homes for many reasons. Some make sales calls or want to obtain donations. Others have criminal intent. They want to know who is there. Saying that you are a home health assistant tells that an ill, older, or disabled person is in the home. These people have difficulty protecting and defending themselves. They are easy prey for criminals.

Do not give your name or the person's name until you know who is calling and why. Make sure that it is someone you want to talk to—the person's family or friend, your supervisor, or a caller expected by the person.

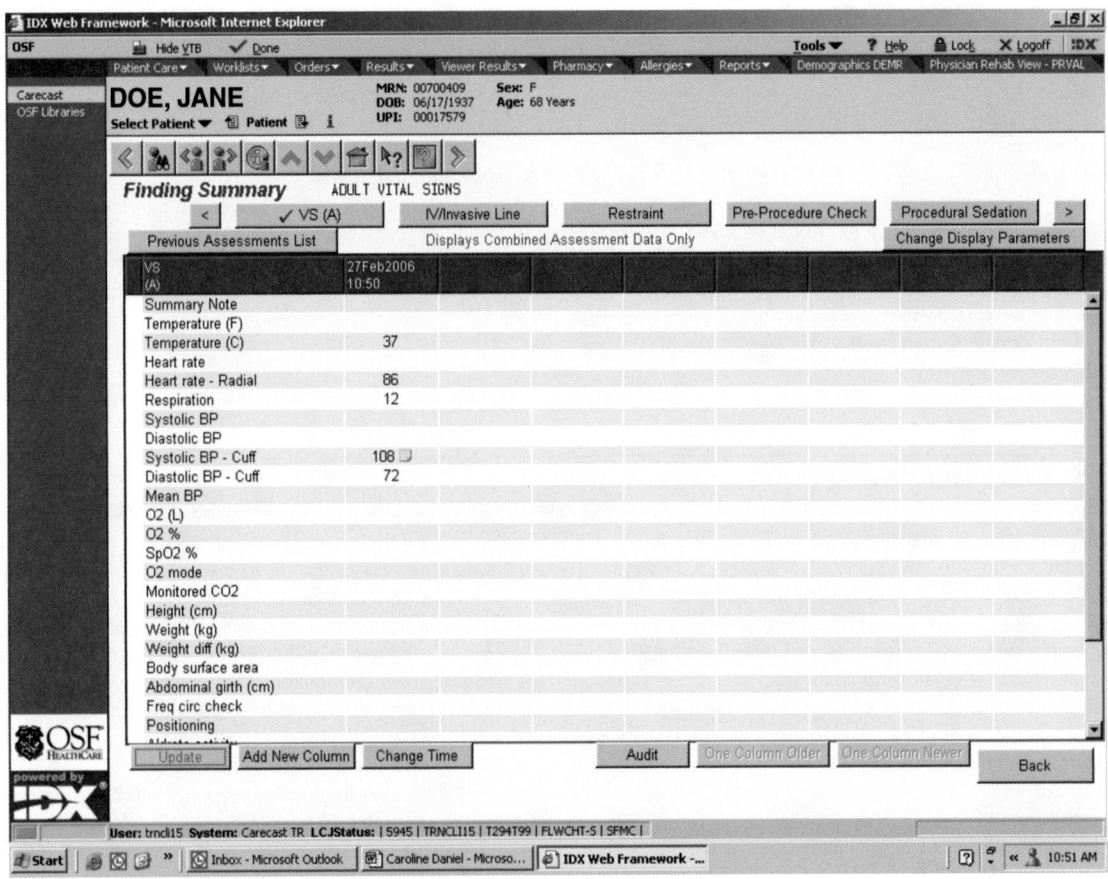

FIGURE 5-11 Computer charting. (Courtesy OSF St Joseph Medical Center, Bloomington, Ill.)

BOX 5-5 Using the Agency's Computer and Other Electronic Devices

COMPUTERS AND PDAs

- Do not tell anyone your "unique user identification" identification. If someone has your information, he or she can access, record, send, receive, or store PHI under your name. It will be hard to prove that someone else did so and not you.
- Do not write down, post, or expose your "unique user identification" or password in a manner that is not secure. For example, do not write them on a notepad or post them at your work station.
- Change your password often. Follow agency policy.
- Do not use another person's "unique user identification" or password.
- Follow the rules for recording (see Box 5-1).
- Enter data carefully. Double-check your entries.
- Prevent others from seeing what is on the screen:
  - Position the monitor or PDA so the screen cannot be seen in the hallway or by others.
  - Be aware of anyone standing behind you.
  - Stand or sit with your back to the wall if recording on a mobile computer unit.
  - Do not leave the computer or PDA unattended.
- Log off after making an entry.
- Do not leave printouts where others can read them or pick them up.
- Shred or destroy computer-printed documents or worksheets. Follow agency policy.
- Send e-mail and messages only to those needing the information.

- Do not use e-mail for information or messages that require immediate reporting. Give the report in person. (The person may not read the e-mail in a timely manner.)
- Do not use e-mail or messages to report confidential information. This includes addresses, phone numbers, and Social Security numbers. The computer system may not be secure.
- Do not use the agency's computer or PDA to:
  - Send personal e-mail messages
  - Send or receive e-mail or messages that are offensive, not legal, or sexual
  - Send or receive e-mail or messages for illegal activities, jokes, politics, gambling (including football and other pools), chain letters, or other non-work activities
  - Post information, opinions, or comments on Internet message boards
  - Take part in Internet discussion groups
  - Upload, download, or send materials containing a copyright, trademark, or patent
- Remember that any communication can be read or heard by someone other than the intended person.
- Remember that deleted communications can be retrieved by authorized staff.
- Remember that the agency has the right to monitor your use of computers, PDAs, and other electronic devices. This includes Internet use.
- Do not open another person's e-mail or messages.
- Follow agency policy for misdirected e-mails.

Continued

BOX 5-5 Using the Agency's Computer and Other Electronic Devices—cont'd

FAXES
- Use the agency's approved "cover sheet." The sheet has instructions about:
  - The confidentiality of PHI
  - The receiver's responsibilities concerning PHI
  - The receiver's responsibilities if the fax is received in error (misdirected fax)
- Complete the "cover sheet" according to agency policy. Usually the following information is required:
  - Name of the person to receive the PHI
  - Receiver's fax number

- Date
- Name of the person sending the fax
- Number of pages being faxed
- Department name
- Name and phone number of the employee sending the fax
- Follow agency policy for a misdirected fax.
- Do not leave sent or received faxes unattended in the fax machine or lying around.

BOX 5-6 Guidelines for Answering Phones

- Answer the call after the first ring if possible. Be sure to answer by the fourth ring.
- Do not answer the phone in a rushed or hasty manner.
- Give a courteous greeting. Identify the nursing unit, and give your name and title. For example: "Good morning. Three center. Mark Wills, nursing assistant."
- Write the following information when taking a message:
  - The caller's name and phone number (include area code and extension number)
  - The date and time
  - The message
- Repeat the message and phone number back to the caller.
- Ask the caller to "Please hold" if necessary. First find out who is calling. Then ask if the caller can hold. Do not put callers with an emergency on hold.

- Do not lay the phone down or cover the receiver with your hand when not speaking to the caller. The caller may overhear confidential conversations.
- Return to a caller on hold within 30 seconds. Ask if the caller can wait longer or if the call can be returned.
- Do not give confidential information to any caller. Patient, resident, and employee information is confidential. Refer such calls to a nurse.
- Transfer the call if appropriate:
  - Tell the caller that you are going to transfer the call.
  - Give the name of the department if appropriate.
  - Give the caller the phone number in case the call gets disconnected or the line is busy.
- End the conversation politely. Thank the person for calling, and say good-bye.
- Give the message to the appropriate person.

DEALING WITH CONFLICT

People bring their values, attitudes, opinions, experiences, and expectations to the work setting. Differences often lead to conflict. **Conflict** is a clash between opposing interests or ideas. People disagree and argue. There are misunderstandings and unrest.

Conflicts arise over issues or events. Work schedules, absences, and the amount and quality of work performed are examples. The problems must be worked out. Otherwise, unkind words or actions may occur. The work setting becomes unpleasant. Care is affected.

To resolve conflict, identify the real problem. This is part of *problem solving*. The problem solving process involves these steps:
- *Step 1:* Define the problem. *A nurse ignores me.*
- *Step 2:* Collect information. The information must be about the problem. Do not include unrelated information. *The nurse does not look at me. The nurse does not talk to me. The nurse does not respond when I call her by name. The nurse does not ask me to help with tasks that require two people. The nurse talks to other staff members.*
- *Step 3:* Identify possible solutions. *Ignore the nurse. Talk to my supervisor. Talk to co-workers about the problem. Change jobs.*
- *Step 4:* Select the best solution. *Talk to my supervisor.*
- *Step 5:* Carry out the solution. *See below.*
- *Step 6:* Evaluate the results. *See below.*

Communication and good work ethics help prevent and resolve conflicts. Identify and solve problems before they become major issues. These guidelines can help you deal with conflict:
- Ask your supervisor for some time to talk privately. Explain the problem. Give facts and specific examples. Ask for advice in solving the problem.
- Approach the person with whom you have the conflict. Ask to talk privately. Be polite and professional.
- Agree on a time and place to talk.
- Talk in a private setting. No one should hear you or the other person.
- Explain the problem and what is bothering you. Give facts and specific behaviors. Focus on the problem. Do not focus on the person.
- Listen to the person. Do not interrupt.
- Identify ways to solve the problem. Offer your thoughts. Ask for the co-worker's ideas.
- Set a date and time to review the matter.
- Thank the person for meeting with you.
- Carry out the solution.
- Review the matter as scheduled.
  See *Focus on Communication: Dealing With Conflict.*

FOCUS ON COMMUNICATION

Dealing With Conflict

You may find it hard to talk to someone with whom you have a conflict. Doing so is hard for many people. However, letting the problem or issue continue only makes the matter worse. The following may help you to start talking to the person:

- "You say 'no' when I ask you to help me. I help you when you ask me to. This really bothers me. Can we talk privately for a few minutes?"

- "I heard you tell John that you saw me sitting in Mr. Gordon's room. You seemed angry when you said it. Can we talk privately? I want to explain why I was sitting and find out why that bothers you."
- "The new schedule shows me working every weekend this month. Please tell me why. The employee handbook says that we work every other weekend."

REVIEW QUESTIONS

Circle the BEST answer.

1 To communicate, you should do the following *except*
  a Use terms with many meanings
  b Be brief and concise
  c Present information logically and in sequence
  d Give facts and be specific

2 When a person is discharged from the agency the medical record is
  a Destroyed
  b Sent home with the person
  c Permanent
  d Stored on a computer

3 These statements are about medical records. Which is *false?*
  a They are used to communicate information about patients and residents.
  b They are a written or electronic account of illness and response to treatment.
  c They can be used as evidence of the care given.
  d Anyone working in the agency can read them.

4 A person is weighed daily. The measurement is recorded on the
  a Admission sheet   c Flow sheet
  b Graphic sheet   d Progress notes

5 Where does the nurse describe the nursing care given?
  a Admission sheet   c Progress notes
  b Health history   d Graphic sheet

6 When recording, you do the following *except*
  a Use ink
  b Include the date and time
  c Erase errors
  d Sign all entries with your name and title

7 These statements are about recording. Which is *false?*
  a Use the person's exact words when possible.
  b Record only what you did and observed.
  c Sign your initials to a mistaken entry.
  d Chart a procedure before completing it.

8 In the evening the clock shows 9:26. In 24-hour clock time this is
  a 9:26 PM   c 0926
  b 926   d 2126

9 A suffix is
  a Placed at the beginning of a word
  b Placed after a root
  c A shortened form of a word or phrase
  d The main meaning of the word

10 These statements are about computers in health care. Which is *false?*
  a Computers are used to collect, send, record, and store information.
  b The person's privacy must be protected.
  c All employees have the same password.
  d Computers link one department to another.

11 You have access to the agency's computer. Which is *true?*
  a E-mail and messages are sent only to those needing the information.
  b E-mail is used for reports the nurse needs at once.
  c You can open another person's e-mail.
  d You can use the computer for your personal needs.

12 You answer a person's phone. How should you answer?
  a "Good morning. Mrs. Park's room."
  b "Good morning. Third floor."
  c "Hello."
  d "Good morning. Tammy Brown, nursing assistant, speaking."

13 Which term relates to the side of the body?
  a Anterior   c Posterior
  b Lateral   d Proximal

14 A co-worker is often late for work. This means extra work for you. To resolve the conflict you should do the following *except*
  a Explain the problem to your supervisor
  b Discuss the matter during the end-of-shift report
  c Give facts and specific behaviors
  d Suggest ways to solve the problem

Answers to these questions on p. 779.

Assisting With the Nursing Process

OBJECTIVES

- Define the key terms and key abbreviations listed in this chapter
- Explain the purpose of the nursing process
- Describe the steps of the nursing process
- Explain your role in each step of the nursing process
- Explain the difference between objective data and subjective data
- Identify the observations that you need to report to the nurse
- Explain the purpose of care conferences

KEY TERMS

assessment Collecting information about the person; a step in the nursing process

evaluation To measure if goals in the planning step were met; a step in the nursing process

goal That which is desired in or by the person as a result of nursing care

implementation To perform or carry out nursing measures in the care plan; a step in the nursing process

medical diagnosis The identification of a disease or condition by a doctor

nursing care plan A written guide about the person's care; care plan

nursing diagnosis Describes a health problem that can be treated by nursing measures; a step in the nursing process

nursing intervention An action or measure taken by the nursing team to help the person reach a goal

nursing process The method nurses use to plan and deliver nursing care; its five steps are assessment, nursing diagnosis, planning, implementation, and evaluation

objective data Information that is seen, heard, felt, or smelled; signs

observation Using the senses of sight, hearing, touch, and smell to collect information

planning Setting priorities and goals; a step in the nursing process

signs Objective data

subjective data Things a person tells you about that you cannot observe through your senses; symptoms

symptoms Subjective data

KEY ABBREVIATIONS

ADL Activities of daily living
IDCP Interdisciplinary care planning
MDS Minimum Data Set
NANDA North American Nursing Diagnosis Association
OBRA Omnibus Budget Reconciliation Act of 1987

OASIS Outcome and Assessment Information Set
PDA Personal digital assistant
RAPs Resident assessment protocols
RN Registered nurse

N urses communicate with each other about the person's strengths, problems, needs, and care. This information is shared through the nursing process. The **nursing process** is the method nurses use to plan and deliver nursing care. It has five steps:

▶ Assessment
▶ Nursing diagnosis
▶ Planning
▶ Implementation
▶ Evaluation

The nursing process focuses on the person's nursing needs. Good communication is needed between the person and the nursing team.

Each step is important. If done in order with good communication, nursing care is organized and has purpose. All nursing team members do the same things for the person. They have the same goals. The person feels safe and secure with consistent care.

The nursing process is used in all health care settings. It is used for all age-groups. The nursing process is ongoing. New information is gathered and the person's needs may change. However, the steps remain the same. You will see the continuous nature of the nursing process as each step is explained.

ASSESSMENT

Assessment involves collecting information about the person. Nurses use many sources. A health history is taken. This tells about current and past health problems. The family's history also is important. Many diseases are genetic. That is, the risk for certain diseases is inherited from parents. For example, a mother had breast cancer. Her daughters are at risk. Information from the doctor is reviewed. So are test results and past medical records.

An RN assesses the person's body systems and mental status. You play a key role in assessment. You make many observations as you give care and talk to the person.

Observation is using the senses of sight, hearing, touch, and smell to collect information:

▶ You *see* how the person lies, sits, or walks. You see flushed or pale skin. You see red and swollen body areas.
▶ You *listen* to the person breathe, talk, and cough. You use a stethoscope to listen to the heartbeat and to measure blood pressure.
▶ Through *touch*, you feel if the skin is hot or cold, or moist or dry. You use touch to take the person's pulse.

▶ *Smell* is used to detect body, wound, and breath odors. You also smell odors from urine and bowel movements.

Objective data (signs) are seen heard, felt, or smelled. You can feel a pulse. You can see the color of urine. **Subjective data (symptoms)** are things a person tells you about that you cannot observe through your senses. You cannot feel or see the person's pain, fear, or nausea.

Box 6-1, p. 74 lists the basic observations you need to make and report to the nurse. Box 6-2, p. 75 lists the observations that you must report at once. Make notes of your observations. Use them when reporting and recording observations. Carry a note pad and pen in your pocket. That way you can note observations as you make them. Your agency may provide personal data assistants (PDAs) for this purpose (Fig. 6-1, p. 75).

The assessment step never ends. New information is collected with every patient or resident contact. New observations are made. The person shares more information. Often the family adds more information.

See *Focus on Long-Term Care and Home Care: Assessment.*

FOCUS ON **LONG-TERM CARE** AND **HOME CARE**

Assessment

LONG-TERM CARE

The Omnibus Budget Reconciliation Act of 1987 (OBRA) requires the Minimum Data Set (MDS) for nursing center residents (Appendix B, p. 784). The MDS is an assessment and screening tool. The form is completed when the person is admitted to the center. It provides extensive information about the person. Examples include memory, communication, hearing and vision, physical function, and activities.

The nurse uses your observations to complete the MDS. The RN responsible for the person's care makes sure the MDS is complete. The MDS is updated before each care conference. A new MDS is completed once a year and whenever a significant change occurs in the person's health status. An RN signs the MDS. A signed MDS means that it is complete and accurate.

HOME CARE

Medicare-certified home health care agencies use the Outcome and Assessment Information Set (OASIS). It is used for adult home care patients. Besides assessment, OASIS is used for planning care.

BOX 6-1 Basic Observations

ABILITY TO RESPOND
- Is the person easy or hard to wake up?
- Can the person give his or her name, the time, and location when asked?
- Does the person identify others correctly?
- Does the person answer questions correctly?
- Does the person speak clearly?
- Are instructions followed correctly?
- Is the person calm, restless, or excited?
- Is the person conversing, quiet, or talking a lot?

MOVEMENT
- Can the person squeeze your fingers with each hand?
- Can the person move arms and legs?
- Are the person's movements shaky or jerky?
- Does the person complain of stiff or painful joints?

PAIN OR DISCOMFORT
- Where is the pain located? (Ask the person to point to the pain.)
- Does the pain go anywhere else?
- How does the person rate the severity of pain? Mild, moderate, severe?
- How does the person rate the pain on a scale of 0 to 10 (Chapter 27)?
- When did the pain begin?
- What was the person doing when the pain began?
- How long does the pain last?
- How does the person describe the pain?
  - Sharp
  - Severe
  - Knife-like
  - Dull
  - Burning
  - Aching
  - Comes and goes
  - Depends on position
- Was a pain-relief drug given?
- Did the pain-relief drug relieve the pain? Is the pain still present?
- Is the person able to sleep and rest?
- What is the position of comfort?

SKIN
- Is the skin pale or flushed?
- Is the skin cool, warm, or hot?
- Is the skin moist or dry?
- What color are the lips and nail beds?
- Is the skin intact? Are there broken areas? If so, where?
- Are sores or reddened areas present?
- Are bruises present? Where are they located?
- Does the person complain of itching? If yes, where?

EYES, EARS, NOSE, AND MOUTH
- Is there drainage from the eyes? What color is the drainage?
- Are the eyelids closed? Do they stay open?
- Are the eyes reddened?
- Does the person complain of spots, flashes, or blurring?
- Is the person sensitive to bright lights?
- Is there drainage from the ears? What color is the drainage?
- Can the person hear? Is repeating necessary? Are questions answered appropriately?
- Is there drainage from the nose? What color is the drainage?
- Can the person breathe through the nose?
- Is there breath odor?
- Does the person complain of a bad taste in the mouth?
- Does the person complain of painful gums or teeth?

RESPIRATIONS
- Do both sides of the person's chest rise and fall with respirations?
- Is breathing noisy?
- Does the person complain of pain or difficulty breathing?
- What is the amount and color of sputum?
- What is the frequency of the person's cough? Is it dry or productive?

BOWELS AND BLADDER
- Is the abdomen firm or soft?
- Does the person complain of gas?
- What are the amount, color, and consistency of bowel movements?
- What is the frequency of bowel movements?
- Can the person control bowel movements?
- Does the person have pain or difficulty urinating?
- What is the amount of urine?
- What is the color of urine?
- Is urine clear? Are there particles in the urine?
- Does the urine have a foul smell?
- Can the person control the passage of urine?
- What is the frequency of urination?

APPETITE
- Does the person like the food served?
- How much of the meal is eaten?
- What foods does the person like?
- Can the person chew food?
- What is the amount of fluid taken?
- What fluids does the person like?
- How often does the person drink fluids?
- Can the person swallow food and fluids?
- Does the person complain of nausea?
- What is the amount and color of material vomited?
- Does the person have hiccups?
- Is the person belching?
- Does the person cough when swallowing?

ACTIVITIES OF DAILY LIVING
- Can the person perform personal care without help?
  - Bathing?
  - Brushing teeth?
  - Combing and brushing hair?
  - Shaving?
- Which does the person use: toilet, commode, bedpan, or urinal?
- Does the person feed himself or herself?
- Can the person walk?
- What amount and kind of help is needed?

OTHER
- Is the person bleeding from any body part? If yes, where and how much?

BOX 6-2 **Observations to Report at Once**

- A change in the person's ability to respond
  - A responsive person is no longer responding.
  - A non-responsive person is now responding.
- A change in the person's mobility
  - The person cannot move a body part.
  - The person is now able to move a body part.
- Complaints of sudden, severe pain
- A sore or reddened area on the person's skin
- Complaints of a sudden change in vision
- Complaints of pain or difficulty breathing
- Abnormal respirations
- Complaints of or signs of difficulty swallowing
- Vomiting
- Bleeding
- Vital signs outside their normal ranges

NURSING DIAGNOSIS

The RN uses assessment information to make a nursing diagnosis. A **nursing diagnosis** describes a health problem that can be treated by nursing measures (Box 6-3). The problem may exist or develop.

Nursing diagnoses and medical diagnoses are not the same. A **medical diagnosis** is the identification of a disease or condition by a doctor. Cancer, stroke, heart attack, infection, and diabetes are examples. Doctors order drugs, therapies, and surgery to cure or heal.

A person can have many nursing diagnoses. They deal with the total person—physical, emotional, social, and spiritual needs. They may change as assessment information changes. Or new nursing diagnoses are added. For example, "Acute pain" is added after surgery.

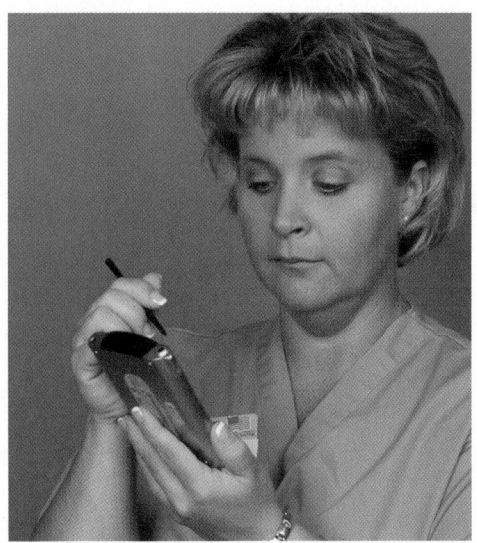

FIGURE 6-1 The nursing assistant uses a PDA to note observations.

BOX 6-3 **Nursing Diagnoses Approved by the North American Nursing Diagnosis Association International (NANDA-I)**

- Activity Intolerance
- Activity Intolerance, Risk for
- Airway Clearance, Ineffective
- Anxiety
- Aspiration, Risk for
- Bathing/Hygiene Self-Care Deficit
- Body Image, Disturbed
- Body Temperature, Risk for Imbalanced
- Breastfeeding, Effective
- Breastfeeding, Ineffective
- Breastfeeding, Interrupted
- Breathing Pattern, Ineffective
- Cardiac Output, Decreased
- Caregiver Role Strain
- Caregiver Role Strain, Risk for

- Comfort, Readiness for Enhanced
- Communication, Impaired Verbal
- Communication, Readiness for Enhanced
- Community Coping, Ineffective
- Community Coping, Readiness for Enhanced
- Confusion, Acute
- Confusion, Chronic
- Confusion, Risk for Acute
- Constipation
- Constipation, Perceived
- Constipation, Risk for
- Contamination
- Contamination, Risk for
- Coping, Defensive
- Coping, Ineffective

Modified from NANDA International: *Nursing diagnosis: definitions and classification 2007-2008*, Philadelphia, 2007, NANDA-I.   *Continued*

BOX 6-3 Nursing Diagnoses Approved by the North American Nursing Diagnosis Association International (NANDA-I) — cont'd

- Coping, Readiness for Enhanced
- Death Anxiety
- Decisional Conflict
- Decision Making, Readiness for Enhanced
- Denial, Ineffective
- Dentition, Impaired
- Development, Risk for Delayed
- Diarrhea
- Dignity, Human, Risk for Compromised
- Disuse Syndrome, Risk for
- Diversional Activity, Deficient
- Dressing/Grooming Self-Care Deficit
- Dysreflexia, Autonomic
- Dysreflexia, Autonomic, Risk for
- Energy Field, Disturbed
- Environmental Interpretation Syndrome, Impaired
- Failure to Thrive, Adult
- Falls, Risk for
- Family Coping, Compromised
- Family Coping, Disabled
- Family Coping, Readiness for Enhanced
- Family Processes, Dysfunctional: Alcoholism
- Family Processes, Interrupted
- Family Processes, Readiness for Enhanced
- Fatigue
- Fear
- Feeding Self-Care Deficit
- Fluid Balance, Readiness for Enhanced
- Fluid Volume, Deficient
- Fluid Volume, Excess
- Fluid Volume, Risk for Deficient
- Fluid Volume, Risk for Imbalanced
- Gas Exchange, Impaired
- Glucose Level, Blood, Risk for Unstable
- Grieving
- Grieving, Complicated
- Grieving, Risk for Complicated
- Growth and Development, Delayed
- Growth, Risk for Disproportionate
- Health Behavior, Risk-Prone
- Health Maintenance, Ineffective
- Health-Seeking Behaviors
- Home Maintenance, Impaired
- Hope, Readiness for Enhanced
- Hopelessness
- Hyperthermia
- Hypothermia
- Immunization Status, Readiness for Enhanced
- Incontinence, Bowel
- Incontinence, Urinary, Functional
- Incontinence, Urinary, Overflow
- Incontinence, Urinary, Reflex
- Incontinence, Urinary, Stress
- Incontinence, Urinary, Total
- Incontinence, Urinary, Urge
- Incontinence, Urinary, Urge, Risk for
- Infant Behavior, Disorganized
- Infant Behavior, Risk for Disorganized
- Infant Behavior, Organized, Readiness for Enhanced
- Infant Feeding Pattern, Ineffective
- Infection, Risk for
- Injury, Risk for

- Insomnia
- Intracranial Adaptive Capacity, Decreased
- Knowledge, Deficient (Specify)
- Knowledge, Readiness for Enhanced
- Latex Allergy Response
- Latex Allergy Response, Risk for
- Lifestyle, Sedentary
- Liver Function, Risk for Impaired
- Loneliness, Risk for
- Memory, Impaired
- Mobility, Impaired Bed
- Mobility, Impaired Physical
- Mobility, Impaired Wheelchair
- Moral Distress
- Nausea
- Neglect, Unilateral
- Noncompliance
- Nutrition, Imbalanced: Less Than Body Requirements
- Nutrition, Imbalanced: More Than Body Requirements
- Nutrition, Imbalanced: More Than Body Requirements, Risk for
- Nutrition, Readiness for Enhanced
- Oral Mucous Membrane, Impaired
- Pain, Acute
- Pain, Chronic
- Parent/Child Attachment, Risk for Impaired
- Parental Role Conflict
- Parenting, Impaired
- Parenting, Readiness for Enhanced
- Parenting, Risk for Impaired
- Perioperative-Positioning Injury, Risk for
- Peripheral Neurovascular Dysfunction, Risk for
- Personal Identity, Disturbed
- Poisoning, Risk for
- Post-Trauma Syndrome
- Post-Trauma Syndrome, Risk for
- Powerlessness
- Powerlessness, Risk for
- Power, Readiness for Enhanced
- Protection, Ineffective
- Rape-Trauma Syndrome
- Rape-Trauma Syndrome: Compound Reaction
- Rape-Trauma Syndrome: Silent Reaction
- Religiosity, Impaired
- Religiosity, Readiness for Enhanced
- Religiosity, Risk for Impaired
- Relocation Stress Syndrome
- Relocation Stress Syndrome, Risk for
- Role Performance, Ineffective
- Self-Care, Readiness for Enhanced
- Self-Concept, Readiness for Enhanced
- Self-Esteem, Chronic Low
- Self-Esteem, Situational Low
- Self-Esteem, Situational Low, Risk for
- Self-Mutilation
- Self-Mutilation, Risk for
- Sensory Perception, Disturbed (Specify type: visual, auditory, kinesthetic, gustatory, tactile, olfactory)
- Sexual Dysfunction
- Sexuality Pattern, Ineffective
- Skin Integrity, Impaired

Modified from NANDA International: *Nursing diagnosis: definitions and classification 2007-2008,* Philadelphia, 2007, NANDA-I.

BOX 6-3 Nursing Diagnoses Approved by the North American Nursing Diagnosis Association International (NANDA-I)—cont'd

- Skin Integrity, Risk for Impaired
- Sleep Deprivation
- Sleep, Readiness for Enhanced
- Social Interaction, Impaired
- Social Isolation
- Sorrow, Chronic
- Spiritual Distress
- Spiritual Distress, Risk for
- Spiritual Well-Being, Readiness for Enhanced
- Stress, Overload
- Sudden Infant Death Syndrome, Risk for
- Suffocation, Risk for
- Suicide, Risk for
- Surgical Recovery, Delayed
- Swallowing, Impaired
- Therapeutic Regimen Management, Effective
- Therapeutic Regimen Management, Ineffective
- Therapeutic Regimen Management, Ineffective Community
- Therapeutic Regimen Management, Ineffective Family

- Therapeutic Regimen Management, Readiness for Enhanced
- Thermoregulation, Ineffective
- Thought Processes, Disturbed
- Tissue Integrity, Impaired
- Tissue Perfusion, Ineffective (Specify type: renal, cerebral, cardiopulmonary, gastrointestinal, peripheral)
- Toileting Self-Care Deficit
- Transfer Ability, Impaired
- Trauma, Risk for
- Urinary Elimination, Impaired
- Urinary Elimination, Readiness for Enhanced
- Urinary Retention
- Ventilation, Impaired Spontaneous
- Ventilatory Weaning Response, Dysfunctional
- Violence, Risk for Other-Directed
- Violence, Risk for Self-Directed
- Walking, Impaired
- Wandering

PLANNING

Planning involves setting priorities and goals. Nursing measures or actions are chosen to help the person meet the goals. The person, family, and health team help the RN plan care.

Priorities relate to what is most important for the person. Maslow's theory of basic needs is useful for setting priorities (Chapter 7). The needs are arranged in order of importance. Some needs are required for life and survival (oxygen, water, and food). They must be met before all other needs. They have priority and must be done first.

Goals are then set. A **goal** is that which is desired in or by a person as a result of nursing care. Goals are aimed at the person's highest level of well-being and function—physical, emotional, social, spiritual. Goals promote health and prevent health problems. They also promote rehabilitation.

Nursing interventions are chosen after goals are set. An *intervention* is an action or measure. A **nursing intervention** is an action or measure taken by the nursing team to help the person reach a goal. *Nursing intervention*, *nursing action*, and *nursing measure* mean the same thing. A nursing intervention does not need a doctor's order. However, some nursing measures come from a doctor's order. For example, a doctor orders that Mrs. Lange walk 50 yards 2 times a day. The nurse includes this order in the care plan.

The **nursing care plan** (care plan) is a written guide about the person's care. It has the person's nursing diagnoses and goals. It also has the measures or actions for each goal. The care plan is a communication tool. Nursing staff use it to see what care to give. The care plan helps ensure that the nursing team members give the same care.

Each agency has a care plan form. It is found in the medical record, on the Kardex, or on a computer (Fig. 6-2, p. 78).

The RN may conduct a care conference to share information and ideas about the person's care. The purpose is to develop or revise the person's nursing care plan. Effective care is the goal. Nursing assistants usually take part in the conference.

The plan is carried out. It may change as the person's nursing diagnoses change.

See *Focus on Communication: Planning.*

See *Focus on Long-Term Care and Home Care: Planning,* p. 78.

FOCUS ON COMMUNICATION

Planning

You spend a lot of time with the patients and residents. You see what they like and do not like. You see what they can do and what they cannot do. Patients and residents talk to you. They tell you about their families and interests. You make observations every time you are with them. Share this information during care conferences. Also share your ideas about the person's care. Your sharing can improve the person's quality of life. For example, you can say:

- "Mr. Antonio never eats his squash. He says that he misses the fresh green beans and broccoli from his garden. Can he have those more often?"
- "Mrs. Clark can use her feet to propel her wheelchair. Why do we have to push her wheelchair?"
- "Miss Walsh never talks when her family visits. She just sits there. Yet she talks to her roommate all the time."

Nursing Diagnosis	Goal	Intervention
Constipation related to lack of privacy as evidenced by no BM for 5 days.	Patient will have regular bowel movements by 6/30.	Ask patient to use signal light when urge to have bowel movement is felt. Answer signal light promptly. Assist patient to bathroom. Close bathroom door for privacy. Leave the room if the patient can be alone; tell the patient you are leaving and that you will return when he turns on the signal light.
Insomnia related to noisy environment as evidenced by patient complaints of noise and lack of sleep.	Patient will report a restful sleep by 6/29.	Perform any necessary care measures before bedtime. Close the door to the patient's room. Turn off television or radio or keep volume low if patient prefers. Ask staff to avoid unnecessary talking outside the patient's room. Ask staff to speak in low voices. Turn off unneeded equipment.

FIGURE 6-2 Nursing care plan. Each nursing diagnosis has a goal. There are nursing interventions for each goal.

FOCUS ON LONG-TERM CARE AND HOME CARE

Planning

LONG-TERM CARE

OBRA requires two types of resident care conferences:
- *Interdisciplinary care planning (IDCP) conference.* This is held regularly to review and update care plans. It also is held to develop care plans for new residents. The RN, doctor, and other health team members attend.
- *Problem-focused conference.* This is held when one problem affects a person's care. Only staff directly involved with the problem attend.

The person has the right to take part in these planning conferences. Sometimes the family is involved. The person may refuse actions suggested by the health team.

The problems identified on the MDS give *triggers* (clues) for the Resident Assessment Protocols (RAPs). RAPs are guidelines used to develop the person's care plan (Appendix B, p. 784).

OBRA requires a *comprehensive care plan.* Like the nursing care plan, it is a written guide about the care a person should

receive. The health team develops it. The resident and family may give input. The care plan includes nursing diagnoses and goals. It has the person's problems, goals for care, and actions to take to help the person solve health problems.

For example, Mr. Smith is weak from illness and lack of exercise. The MDS shows that he cannot do activities of daily living (ADL). This triggers the RAPs. They provide guidelines to solve the problem. The goal is for Mr. Smith to perform his own ADL. Staff from occupational therapy, physical therapy, and nursing work to solve the problem. The actions to help Mr. Smith reach the goal are:
- Occupational therapy to work with Mr. Smith on ADL daily
- Physical therapy to work with Mr. Smith on exercises daily
- Nursing staff member to walk Mr. Smith 20 yards twice daily

The care plan also states the person's strengths. For example, Mr. Smith can feed himself. This strength increases his independence. The health team helps Mr. Smith continue to feed himself.

IMPLEMENTATION

To *implement* means to perform or carry out. The **implementation** step is performing or carrying out nursing measures in the care plan. Care is given in this step.

Nursing care ranges from simple to complex. The nurse delegates nursing tasks that are within your legal limits and job description. The nurse may ask you to assist with complex measures.

You report the care given to the nurse. In some agencies, you record the care given. Reporting and recording are done *after* giving care, not before. Also report and record your observations. Observing is part of assessment. New observations may change the nursing diagnoses. If so, care plan changes are made. To give correct care, you need to know about any changes in the care plan.

Assignment Sheets

The nurse communicates delegated measures and tasks to you. An assignment sheet is used for this purpose (Fig. 6-3). The assignment sheet tells you about:

▶ Each person's care
▶ What measures and tasks need to be done
▶ Which nursing unit tasks to do (cleaning kitchenettes and utility rooms and stocking tub and shower rooms are examples)

Talk to the nurse about any assignment that is unclear. You can also check the care plan and Kardex if you need more information.

See *Teamwork and Time Management: Assignment Sheets.*

TEAMWORK AND TIME MANAGEMENT

Assignment Sheets

Use your assignment sheet to organize your work and to set priorities:
• What do you need to do first?
• What can be done while the person is having breakfast, lunch, or dinner?
• What can you do while the person is at a therapy or an activity?
• Do you need to reserve the use of rooms (shower room, tub room) or equipment (portable tub, shower chair)?
• What do you need help with?
• How many co-workers are needed to complete nursing tasks such as turning and transferring a person?
• Ask a co-worker to help you. Tell the person what you need help with, when you need the help, and how long the task will take.
• Check off tasks as you complete them.

Assignment Sheet

Date: 9–10   Shift: Day   Nursing assistant: John Reed   Supervisor: Mary Adams, RN

Breaks: 1000   1400   Lunch: 1230   Unit Tasks: Pass ice water at 0900   Clean utility room at 1430

Check the care plan for other care measures and information

Room # 501A   Name: Mrs. Ann Lopez
ID Number: S1514491530   Date of birth: 11/04/1925
VS: Daily at 0700
T ___ P ___ R ___ BP ___
Wt: Weekly (Monday at 0700)
Intake ___ BM ___
Bath: Portable tub
Shampoo   Bed rails

Functional status/other care measures and procedures
Total assist with ADL
Stand-pivot transfers
Uses w/c
Incontinent of bowel and bladder – uses briefs
Bilateral passive ROM exercises to extremities twice daily
Turn and reposition q2h when in bed
Wears eyeglasses and dentures
Diet: High fiber (Total Assist)

Room # 510B   Name: Mr. Mark Monroe
ID Number: D4468947762   Date of birth: 12/29/1926
VS: 2 times daily, at 0700 and 1500
0700: T ___ P ___ R ___ BP ___
1500: T ___ P ___ R ___ BP ___
Wt: Daily at 0700
Intake ___ Output ___ BM ___
Bath: Shower

Functional status/other care measures and procedures
Independent with ADL
Independent with ambulation
Attends exercise group every morning
Continent of bowel and bladder – q4h bathroom schedule to maintain continence
Wears eyeglasses
Coughing and deep breathing exercises q4h
Diet: Sodium-controlled (Independent)

FIGURE 6-3 Sample assignment sheet. *NOTE:* This assignment sheet is a computer printout.

EVALUATION

Evaluation means to measure. The **evaluation** step involves measuring if the goals in the planning step were met. Progress is evaluated. Goals may be met totally, in part, or not at all. Assessment information is used for this step. Changes in nursing diagnoses, goals, and the care plan may result.

The nursing process never ends. Nurses constantly collect information about the person. Nursing diagnoses, goals, and the care plan may change as the person's needs change.

YOUR ROLE

You have a key role in the nursing process. The nurse uses your observations for nursing diagnoses and planning. You may help develop the care plan. In the implementation step, you perform nursing actions and measures in the care plan. Your assignment sheet tells you what to do. Your observations are used for the evaluation step.

REVIEW QUESTIONS

Circle the BEST answer.

1 Which is *not* a step in the nursing process?
  a Observation
  b Assessment
  c Planning
  d Implementation

2 The nursing process
  a Involves guidelines for care plans
  b Is a care conference
  c Involves triggers
  d Is the method nurses use to plan and deliver nursing care

3 What happens during assessment?
  a Goals are set.
  b Information is collected.
  c Nursing measures are carried out.
  d Progress is evaluated.

4 Which is a symptom?
  a Redness
  b Vomiting
  c Pain
  d Pulse rate of 78

5 Which is a sign?
  a Nausea
  b Headache
  c Dizziness
  d Dry skin

6 Which should you report at once?
  a The person had a bowel movement.
  b The person complains of sudden, severe pain.
  c The person does not like the food served for lunch.
  d The person complains of stiff, painful joints.

7 Which should you report at once?
  a The person can no longer move a body part.
  b The person answers questions correctly.
  c The person has a breath odor.
  d The person walked to the dining room.

8 Measures in the nursing care plan are carried out. This is
  a A nursing diagnosis
  b Planning
  c Implementation
  d Evaluation

9 Which statement about the nursing process is *true*?
  a It is done without the person's input.
  b You are responsible for it.
  c It is used to communicate the person's care.
  d Steps can be done in any order.

10 The nursing care plan is
  a Written by the doctor
  b The measures to help the person
  c The same for all persons
  d Also called the Kardex

11 What is used to communicate the nursing tasks delegated to you?
  a The care plan
  b The Kardex
  c An assignment sheet
  d Care conferences

12 Which is a nursing diagnosis?
  a Cancer
  b Heart attack
  c Kidney failure
  d Pain

Answers to these questions are on p. 779.

Understanding the Person

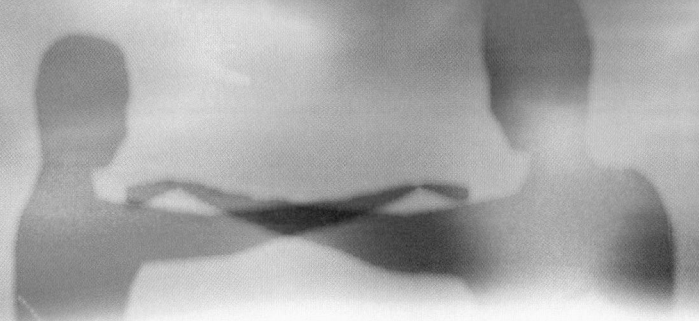

OBJECTIVES

- Define the key terms and key abbreviations listed in this chapter
- Identify the parts that make up the whole person
- Explain Abraham Maslow's theory of basic needs
- Explain how culture and religion influence health and illness
- Identify the emotional and social effects of illness
- Describe persons cared for in health care agencies
- Explain the American Hospital Association's *The Patient Care Partnership: Understanding Expectations, Rights, and Responsibilities*
- Identify the elements needed for good communication
- Describe how to use verbal and nonverbal communication
- Explain the methods and barriers to good communication
- Explain how to communicate with persons who have behavior problems
- Explain how to communicate with persons who have disabilities or who are comatose
- Explain why family and visitors are important to the person
- Identify the courtesies given to the person, family, and friends

KEY TERMS

body language Messages sent through facial expressions, gestures, posture, hand and body movements, gait, eye contact, and appearance

comatose Being unable to respond to verbal stimuli

culture The characteristics of a group of people—language, values, beliefs, habits, likes, dislikes, customs—passed from one generation to the next

disability Any lost, absent, or impaired physical or mental function

esteem The worth, value, or opinion one has of a person

geriatrics The branch of medicine concerned with the problems and diseases of old age and older persons

Continued

KEY TERMS — cont'd

holism A concept that considers the whole person; the whole person has physical, social, psychological, and spiritual parts that are woven together and cannot be separated

need Something necessary or desired for maintaining life and mental well-being

nonverbal communication Communication that does not use words

obstetrics The branch of medicine concerned with the care of women during pregnancy, labor, and childbirth and for the 6 to 8 weeks after birth

optimal level of function A person's highest potential for mental and physical performance

paraphrasing Restating the person's message in your own words

pediatrics The branch of medicine concerned with the growth, development, and care of children: they range in age from newborns to teenagers

psychiatry The branch of medicine concerned with mental health problems

religion Spiritual beliefs, needs, and practices

self-actualization Experiencing one's potential

self-esteem Thinking well of oneself and seeing oneself as useful and having value

verbal communication Communication that uses written or spoken words

KEY ABBREVIATIONS

ADL Activities of daily living
AHA American Hospital Association
OBRA Omnibus Budget Reconciliation Act of 1987

The patient or resident is the most important person in the agency. Age, religion, and nationality make each person unique. So do culture, education, occupation, and life-style. Each person is important and special. Each has value. Each has needs, fears, and rights. The person is treated as someone who thinks, acts, feels, and makes decisions.

CARING FOR THE PERSON

For effective care, you must consider the whole person. Holism means *whole*. **Holism** is a concept that considers the whole person. The whole person has physical, social, psychological, and spiritual parts. These parts are woven together and cannot be separated (Fig. 7-1).

Each part relates to and depends on the others. As a social being, a person speaks and communicates with others. Physically, the brain, mouth, tongue, lips, and throat structures must function for speech. Communication is also psychological. It involves thinking and reasoning.

To consider only the physical part is to ignore the person's ability to think, make decisions, and interact with others. It also ignores the person's experiences, life-style, culture, religion, joys, sorrows, and needs.

Disability and illness affect the whole person. For example, Mrs. Butler had a stroke. She needs help with her physical needs. She had to leave her home. Relationships with her husband and children are changed. She is angry with God for letting this happen to her. The health team plans care to help her deal with her problems.

Addressing the Person

You must know and respect the whole person to provide effective, quality care. Too often a person is referred to as a room number. For example: "12A needs the bedpan," rather than "Mrs. Brown in 12A needs the bedpan." This strips the person of his or her identity. It reduces the person to a thing.

Patients and residents are not things. They are not your relatives or children. They are complex human beings. Follow these rules to address them with dignity and respect:
- Call patients and residents by their titles—Mrs. Jones, Mr. Smith, Miss Turner, or Dr. Gonzalez.
- Do not call patients and residents by their first names unless they ask you to.
- Do not call patients and residents by any other name unless they ask you to.
- Do not call patients and residents Grandma, Papa, Sweetheart, Honey, or other names.

BASIC NEEDS

A **need** is something necessary or desired for maintaining life and mental well-being. According to Abraham Maslow, a famous psychologist, basic needs must be met for a person to survive and function. According to this theory, the needs are arranged in order of importance (Fig. 7-2). Lower-level needs must be met before the higher-level

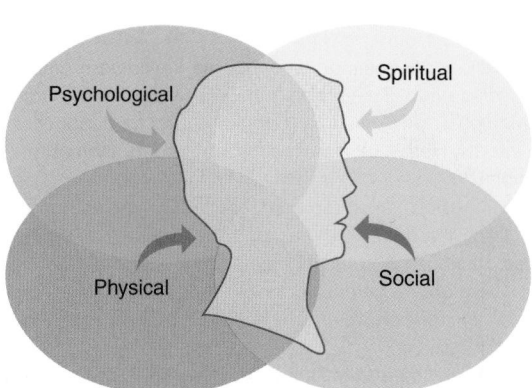

FIGURE 7-1 A person is a physical, psychological, social, and spiritual being. The parts overlap and cannot be separated.

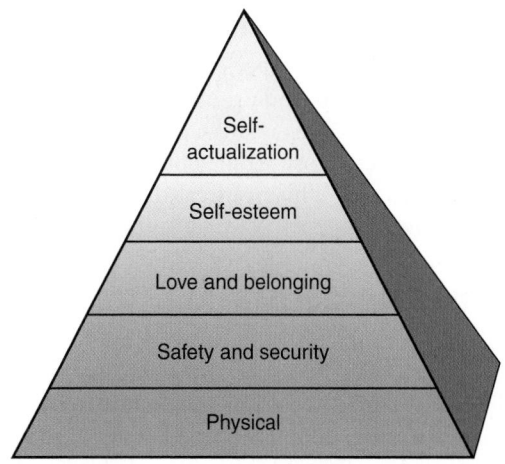

FIGURE 7-2 Basic needs for life as described by Maslow. (From Maslow AH: *Motivation and personality*, ed 3. Reprinted by permission of Pearson Education, Inc., Upper Saddle River, NJ.)

needs. Basic needs, from the lowest level to the highest level, are:

▶ Physical needs
▶ Safety and security needs
▶ Love and belonging needs
▶ Self-esteem needs
▶ The need for self-actualization

People normally meet their own needs. When they cannot, it is usually because of disease, illness, injury, or advanced age. Those who are ill or injured usually seek health care.

Physical Needs

Oxygen, food, water, elimination, rest, and shelter are needed for life. They are needed to survive. A person dies within minutes without oxygen. Without food or water, a person feels weak and ill within a few hours. The kidneys and intestines must function. Otherwise poisonous wastes build up in the blood. This can cause death. Without enough rest and sleep, a person becomes very tired. Without shelter, the person is exposed to extremes of heat and cold.

Safety and Security Needs

Safety and security needs relate to feeling safe from harm, danger, and fear. Many people are afraid of health care agencies. Some care involves strange equipment or entering the body. Some care causes pain or discomfort. People feel safer and more secure if they know what will happen. For every nursing task, even a simple bath, the person should know:

▶ Why it is needed
▶ Who will do it
▶ How it will be done
▶ What sensations or feelings to expect

See *Focus on Long-Term Care and Home Care: Safety and Security Needs*.

Love and Belonging Needs

Love and belonging needs relate to love, closeness, and affection. They also involve meaningful relationships with

---

FOCUS ON LONG-TERM CARE AND HOME CARE

Safety and Security Needs

LONG-TERM CARE

Many persons do not feel safe and secure when admitted to a nursing center. They are not in their usual, secure home settings. They are in a strange place with strange routines. Strangers care for them. Some become scared and confused.

Be kind and understanding. Show them the new setting. Listen to their concerns. Explain all routines and procedures. You may have to repeat information many times. Sometimes the information may need repeating for many days or weeks until the person feels safe and secure. Be patient.

---

others. There are many cases in which people became weaker or died because they lacked love and belonging. This is seen in children and in older persons who have outlived family and friends. Family, friends, and the health team can meet love and belonging needs.

Self-Esteem Needs

Esteem is the worth, value, or opinion one has of a person. **Self-esteem** means to think well of oneself and to see oneself as useful and having value. People often lack self-esteem when ill, injured, older, or disabled. For example:

▶ An older man once built his own home and worked a farm. He supported and raised a family. Now he cannot dress or feed himself.
▶ Cancer treatments caused a woman to lose her hair. She does not feel attractive or whole.
▶ A person has a slow, crippling disease.
▶ A person had a leg amputated.

You must treat all persons with respect. Although it takes more time, encourage them to do as much for themselves as possible. This helps increase self-esteem.

The Need for Self-Actualization

Self-actualization means experiencing one's potential. It involves learning, understanding, and creating to the limit of a person's capacity. This is the highest need. Rarely, if ever, is it totally met. Most people constantly try to learn and understand more. This need can be postponed, and life will continue.

CULTURE AND RELIGION

Culture is the characteristics of a group of people—language, values, beliefs, habits, likes, dislikes, and customs. They are passed from one generation to the next. The person's culture influences health beliefs and practices. Culture also affects thinking and behavior during illness and when in a hospital or nursing center.

People come from many cultures, races, and nationalities. Their family practices and food choices may differ from yours. So might their hygiene habits and clothing styles. Some speak a foreign language. Some cultures have beliefs about what causes and cures illness. (See *Caring About Culture: Health Care Beliefs.*) They may perform rituals to rid the body of disease. (See *Caring About Culture: Sick Care Practices.*) Many have beliefs and rituals about dying and death (Chapter 50). Culture also is a factor in communication.

Religion relates to spiritual beliefs, needs, and practices. A person's religion influences health and illness practices. Religions may have beliefs and practices about daily living, behaviors, relationships with others, diet, healing, days of worship, birth and birth control, drugs, and death.

Many people find comfort and strength from religion during illness. They may want to pray and observe religious practices. Hospitals and nursing centers offer religious services. Many have chapels or meditation areas for prayer. Assist the person to attend services as needed (Fig. 7-3). Some residents leave nursing centers to worship.

A person may want to see a spiritual leader or advisor. Report this to the nurse. Make sure the room is neat and orderly. Have a chair ready for the cleric. Provide privacy during the visit.

CARING ABOUT CULTURE

Health Care Beliefs

Some *Mexican Americans* believe that illness is caused by hot or cold. If hot causes illness, cold is used for the cure. Likewise, hot is used to cure illnesses caused by cold. Hot and cold are found in body organs, medicines (drugs), and food. For example, an earache may occur from cold air entering the body. Hot remedies are used to cure the earache.

The hot-cold balance is also a belief of some *Vietnamese Americans*. Illnesses, food, drugs, and herbs are either hot or cold. Hot is given to balance cold illnesses. Cold is given for hot illnesses.

(Modified from Giger JN, Davidhizar RE: *Transcultural nursing: assessment and intervention,* ed 4, St Louis, 2004, Mosby.)

CARING ABOUT CULTURE

Sick Care Practices

Folk practices are common among some *Vietnamese Americans.* They include *cao gio*—rubbing the skin with a coin to treat the common cold. Skin pinching *(bat gio)* is used for headaches and sore throats. Herbs, oils, and soups are used for many signs and symptoms.

Some *Russian Americans* practice folk medicine. Herbs are taken through drinks or enemas. For headaches, an ointment is placed behind the ears and temples and at the back of the neck. There are treatments for backaches. One involves making a dough of dark rye flour and honey. The dough is placed on the spinal column.

Folk healers are used by some *Mexican Americans.* Folk healers may be family members skilled in healing practices. Some folk healers are from outside the family. A *yerbero* uses herbs and spices to prevent or cure disease. A *curandero* (*curandera* if female) deals with serious physical and mental illnesses. Witches use magic. A male witch is called a *brujos.* A female witch is called a *brujas.*

(Modified from Giger JN, Davidhizar RE: *Transcultural nursing: assessment and intervention,* ed 4, St Louis, 2004, Mosby.)

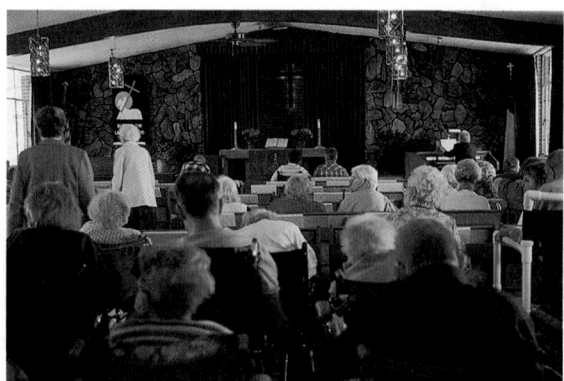

FIGURE 7-3 Residents attend a religious service at a nursing center.

The nursing process reflects the person's culture and religion. The care plan includes the person's cultural and religious practices.

You must respect and accept the person's culture and religion. You will meet people from other cultures and religions. Learn about their beliefs and practices. This helps you understand the person and give better care.

A person may not follow all beliefs and practices of his or her religion. Some people do not practice a religion. Each person is unique. Do not judge the person by your standards. And do not force your ideas on the person.

See *Focus on Long-Term Care and Home Care: Culture and Religion.*

EFFECTS OF ILLNESS AND DISABILITY

People do not choose sickness or injury. Physical, psychological, and social effects occur. Some result in disabilities. A **disability** is any lost, absent, or impaired physical or mental function. It may be temporary or permanent.

Normal activities—work, driving, fixing meals, yard work, hobbies—may be hard or impossible. Daily activities bring pleasure, worth, and contact with others. People often feel angry, upset, and useless when unable to perform them. These feelings may increase if others must help with routine functions.

Sick people fear death, disability, chronic illness, and loss of function. Some explain why they are afraid. Others do not share feelings. Some fear being laughed at for being afraid. A person with a broken leg may fear having a limp or not walking again. Persons having surgery may fear cancer. These feelings are normal and expected. You need to understand the effects of illness and disability. How would you feel and react if you had the person's problems?

Sick people are expected to behave in a certain way. They need to see a doctor, rest, and have others provide care and comfort. Sometimes recovery is delayed or does not occur. Then the psychological and social effects of illness or disability become greater.

Anger is a common response to illness and disability. Persons who need hospital or nursing center care are often angry. The person may direct anger at you. However, the person is usually angry at the situation. You might have problems dealing with the person's anger. If so, ask the nurse for help (p. 94).

You can help the person feel safe, secure, and loved. Take an extra minute to "visit," to hold a hand, or to give a hug. (Remember to maintain professional boundaries. See Chapter 3.) Treat each person with respect and dignity.

Optimal Level of Function

Sometimes the health team cannot prevent increasing loss of function. However, patients and residents are helped to maintain their **optimal level of function.** This is the person's highest potential for mental and physical performance. Encourage the person to be as independent as possible. Always focus on the person's abilities. Do not focus on disabilities.

Hospital patients are often treated as sick, dependent people. Promoting this "sick role" in a nursing center reduces quality of life. The health team focuses on improving the person's quality of life. You must help each person regain or maintain as much physical and mental function as possible.

PERSONS YOU WILL CARE FOR

People are grouped in health care agencies by their problems, needs, and age. Doctors and nurses have special knowledge and skills to care for these groups.

▶ *Mothers and newborns.* **Obstetrics** is the branch of medicine concerned with the care of women during pregnancy, labor, and childbirth and for the 6 to 8 weeks after birth. They are seen in clinics or doctors' offices during pregnancy. When labor begins, mothers usually go to a hospital. They are admitted to the obstetric (maternity) department. Pregnancy, labor, and childbirth are normal and natural events. However, problems can occur during and after pregnancy and childbirth.

▶ *Children.* **Pediatrics** is the branch of medicine concerned with the growth, development, and care of children. They range in age from newborns to teenagers (usually to age 16). Pediatric units are designed and equipped to meet the needs of children and parents. The nursing staff meets the child's physical, safety, and emotional needs (Fig. 7-4, p. 86).

▶ *Adults with medical problems.* Medical problems are illnesses, diseases, and injuries that do not need surgery. There are acute, chronic, and terminal illnesses. Examples are infections, strokes, and heart attacks.

▶ *Persons having surgery.* Surgical patients need care before and after surgery. Surgeries range from simple to very complex. Removal of the appendix (appendectomy) is a simple surgery. Heart and brain surgeries are complex. Before surgery, the person is prepared for the surgery and for what happens after it. This includes addressing the person's fears and concerns. Needs after surgery relate to relieving pain, preventing complications, and adjusting to body changes.

▶ *Persons with mental health problems.* **Psychiatry** is the branch of medicine concerned with mental health problems. Problems vary from mild to severe mental and emotional disorders (Chapter 43). Some persons need help making decisions or coping with life stresses. Others are severely disturbed. They cannot do simple things—eat, bathe, or get dressed. Some persons present dangers to themselves or others. They need special care and treatment.

▶ *Persons in special care units.* Some people are seriously ill or injured. Special care units are designed and equipped to treat and prevent life-threatening problems. They include emergency departments, and intensive care, coronary care, burn, and kidney dialysis units (Fig. 7-5, p. 86).

▶ *Persons needing subacute care or rehabilitation.* Some persons need more time to recover than hospital care allows. Others need rehabilitation (Chapter 36). They need to regain functions lost from surgery, illness, or accidents. Persons with birth defects learn skills using existing abilities.

▶ *Older persons.* **Geriatrics** is the branch of medicine concerned with the problems and diseases of old age and older persons. Aging is a normal process (Chapter 10). It is not an illness or disease. Many older people enjoy good health. Others have acute or chronic illnesses. Some have diseases common in older persons. Body changes normally occur with aging. Social and psychological changes also occur. (See *Focus on Long-Term Care and Home Care: Persons you will Care For.*)

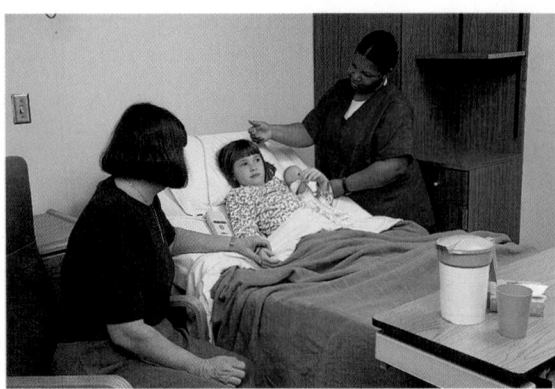

FIGURE 7-4 The nursing assistant gives care to a sick child.

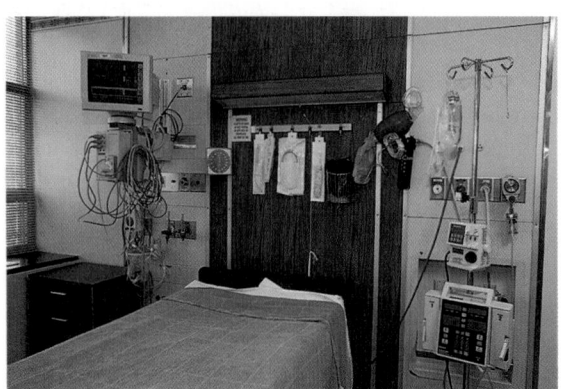

FIGURE 7-5 A room in an intensive care unit.

THE PERSON'S RIGHTS

People want information about their health problems and treatment. They also want better care at lower costs. They want to understand and be involved in treatment decisions. They do not accept the doctor's advice without question.

In April 2003, the American Hospital Association (AHA) adopted *The Patient Care Partnership: Understanding Expectations, Rights, and Responsibilities* (Box 7-1). The document explains the person's rights and expectations during hospital stays. The relationship between the doctor, the health team, and the patient is stressed.

See *Focus on Long-Term Care and Home Care: The Person's Rights.*

FOCUS ON LONG-TERM CARE AND HOME CARE

Persons You Will Care For

LONG-TERM CARE

Most nursing center residents are older. Their problems and care needs vary.

- *Alert, oriented persons.* They know who they are and where they are. They have physical problems. Some are paralyzed from a stroke, injury, or birth defect. Others are disabled from arthritis or multiple sclerosis. Still others have chronic heart, liver, kidney, or respiratory diseases. The amount of care required depends on the degree of disability.
- *Confused and disoriented persons.* These persons are mildly to severely confused and disoriented. Sometimes the problem is temporary. This is especially true for new residents. Some persons have Alzheimer's disease and other dementias. Confusion and disorientation are permanent and become worse (Chapter 44).
- *Persons needing complete care.* They are very disabled, confused, or disoriented. They need total assistance with all activities of daily living (ADL). They cannot meet any of their own needs. Some cannot say what they need or want.
- *Short-term residents.* These persons need to recover from acute illness, surgery, fractures, and other injuries. Often they are younger than most residents. They usually return home after subacute care or rehabilitation.
- *Persons needing respite care.* Some people are cared for at home. They are admitted to nursing centers for short stays. This is *respite care.* Respite means rest or relief. The caregiver can take a vacation, tend to business, or simply rest. Respite care may last from a few days to several weeks.
- *Life-long residents.* Some disabilities occur before 22 years of age. Called developmental disabilities (Chapter 45) they are caused by birth defects and childhood diseases and injuries. Impairments may be physical, intellectual, or both. The person needs life-long assistance, support, and special devices.
- *Mentally ill persons.* Behavior and function are affected. In severe cases, self-care and independent living are impaired. Some persons have physical and mental illnesses.
- *Terminally ill persons.* Terminally ill persons are dying (Chapter 50). The goal is a peaceful, dignified death.

FOCUS ON LONG-TERM CARE AND HOME CARE

The Person's Rights

LONG-TERM CARE

Residents have rights as United States citizens. They also have rights under the Omnibus Budget Reconciliation Act of 1987 (OBRA) (Chapter 10). They relate to everyday life and care in nursing centers.

Centers must protect and promote residents' rights. Residents must be free to exercise their rights without interference. Some residents are incompetent (not able). They cannot exercise their rights. Legal representatives do so for them.

Residents are informed of their rights orally and in writing. This occurs before or during admission to the center. It is given in the language the person uses and understands.

BOX 7-1 The Patient Care Partnership: Understanding Expectations, Rights, and Responsibilities

When you need hospital care, your doctor and the nurses and other professionals at our hospital are committed to working with you and your family to meet your health care needs. Our dedicated doctors and staff serve the community in all its ethnic, religious, and economic diversity. Our goal is for you and your family to have the same care and attention we would want for our families and ourselves.

The sections below explain some of the basics about how you can expect to be treated during your hospital stay. They also cover what we will need from you to care for you better. If you have questions at any time, please ask them. Unasked or unanswered questions can add to the stress of being in the hospital. Your comfort and confidence in your care are very important to us.

WHAT TO EXPECT DURING YOUR HOSPITAL STAY

- **High quality hospital care.** Our first priority is to provide you the care you need, when you need it, with skill, compassion, and respect. Tell your caregivers if you have concerns about your care or if you have pain. You have the right to know the identity of doctors, nurses, and others involved in your care, and you have the right to know when they are students, residents, or other trainees.
- **A clean and safe environment.** Our hospital works hard to keep you safe. We use special policies and procedures to avoid mistakes in your care and keep you free from abuse or neglect. If anything unexpected and significant happens during your hospital stay, you will be told what happened, and any resulting changes in your care will be discussed with you.
- **Involvement in your care.** You and your doctor often make decisions about your care before you go to the hospital. Other times, especially in emergencies, those decisions are made during your hospital stay. When decision-making takes place, it should include:
  - Discussing your medical condition and information about medically appropriate treatment choices. To make informed decisions with your doctor, you need to understand:
    - The benefits and risks of each treatment.
    - Whether your treatment is experimental or part of a research study.
    - What you can reasonably expect from your treatment and any long-term effects it might have on your quality of life.
    - What you and your family will need to do after you leave the hospital.
    - The financial consequences of using uncovered services or out of network providers.
      Please tell your caregivers if you need more information about treatment choices.
  - *Discussing your treatment plan.* When you enter the hospital, you sign a general consent to treatment. In some cases, such as surgery or experimental treatment, you may be asked to confirm in writing that you understand what is planned and agree to it. This process protects your right to consent to or refuse a treatment. Your doctor will explain the medical consequences of refusing recommended treatment. It also protects your right to decide if you want to participate in a research study.
  - *Getting information from you.* Your caregivers need complete and correct information about your health and coverage so that they can make good decisions about your care. That includes:
    - Past illnesses, surgeries, or hospital stays.
    - Past allergic reactions.

- Any medicines or dietary supplements (such as vitamins and herbs) that you are taking.
- Any network or admission requirements under your health plan.
- *Understanding your health care goals and values.* You may have health care goals and values or spiritual beliefs that are important to your well-being. They will be taken into account as much as possible throughout your hospital stay. Make sure your doctor, your family, and your care team know your wishes.
- Understanding who should make decisions when you cannot. If you have signed a health care power of attorney stating who should speak for you if you become unable to make health care decisions for yourself, or a "living will" or "advance directive" that states your wishes about end-of-life care, give copies to your doctor, your family, and your care team. If you or your family need help making difficult decisions, counselors, chaplains, and others are available to help.
- **Protection of your privacy.** We respect the confidentiality of your relationship with your doctor and other caregivers and the sensitive information about your health and health care that are part of that relationship. State and federal laws and hospital operating policies protect the privacy of your medical information. You will receive a Notice of Privacy Practices that describes the ways that we use, disclose, and safeguard patient information and that explains how you can obtain a copy of information from our records about your care.
- **Preparing you and your family for when you leave the hospital.** Your doctor works with hospital staff and professionals in your community. You and your family also play an important role in your care. The success of your treatment often depends on your efforts to follow medication, diet, and therapy plans. Your family may need to help care for you at home. You can expect us to help you identify sources of follow-up care and let you know if our hospital has a financial interest in any referrals. As long as you agree we can share information about your care with them, we will coordinate our activities with your caregivers outside the hospital. You can also expect to receive information and, where possible, training about the self-care you will need when you go home.
- **Help with your bill and filing insurance claims.** Our staff will file claims for you with health care insurers or other programs such as Medicare and Medicaid. They also will help your doctor with needed documentation. Hospital bills and insurance coverage are often confusing. If you have questions about your bill, contact our business office. If you need help understanding your insurance coverage or health plan, start with your insurance company or health benefits manager. If you do not have health coverage, we will try to help you and your family find financial help or make other arrangements. We need your help with collecting needed information and other requirements to obtain coverage or assistance.

While you are here, you will receive more detailed notices about some of the rights you have as a hospital patient and how to exercise them. We are always interested in improving. If you have questions, comments, or concerns, please contact

_____ .

COMMUNICATING WITH THE PERSON

You communicate with patients and residents every time you give care. You give information to the person. The person gives information to you. Your body sends messages all the time—at the bedside, in hallways, at the nurses' station, in the dining room, and elsewhere. The person and family are aware of what you say and what you do. Good work ethics and understanding the person are needed for good communication. What you say and do also are important.

Effective Communication

For effective communication between you and the person, you must:
▸ Follow the rules of communication (Chapter 5):
  ▸ Use words that have the same meaning for you and the person.
  ▸ Avoid medical terms and words not familiar to the person.
  ▸ Communicate in a logical and orderly manner. Do not wander in thought.
  ▸ Give facts and be specific.
  ▸ Be brief and concise.
▸ Understand and respect the patient or resident as a person.
▸ View the person as a physical, psychological, social, and spiritual human being.
▸ Appreciate the person's problems and frustrations.
▸ Respect the person's rights.
▸ Respect the person's religion and culture.
▸ Give the person time to process (understand) the information that you give.
▸ Repeat information as often as needed. Repeat exactly what you said. Use the exact same words. Do not give the person a new message to process. This is very important for persons with hearing problems.
▸ Ask questions to see if the person understood you.

▸ Be patient. People with memory problems may ask the same question many times. Do not say that you are repeating information. Accept the memory loss as a disability.
▸ Include the person in conversations when others are present. This includes when a co-worker is assisting you with care.

Verbal Communication

Words are used in **verbal communication**. Words are spoken or written. You talk to the person. You find out how the person is feeling and share information. Most verbal communication involves the spoken word. Follow these rules:
▸ Face the person. Look directly at the person.
▸ Position yourself at the person's eye level. You may have to sit or squat by the person.
▸ Control the loudness and tone of your voice.
▸ Speak clearly, slowly, and distinctly.
▸ Do not use slang or vulgar words.
▸ Repeat information as needed.
▸ Ask one question at a time. Wait for an answer.
▸ Do not shout, whisper, or mumble.
▸ Be kind, courteous, and friendly.

The written word is used when the person cannot speak or hear but can read. The nurse and care plan tell you how to communicate with the person. The devices shown in Figure 7-6 are often used. The person also may have poor vision. When writing messages:
▸ Keep them brief and concise.
▸ Use a black felt pen on white paper.
▸ Print in large letters.

Some persons cannot speak or read. Ask questions that have "yes" or "no" answers. The person can nod, blink, or use other gestures for "yes" and "no." Follow the care plan. A picture board may be helpful (Fig. 7-7, p. 90).

Persons who are deaf may use sign language. See Chapter 37.

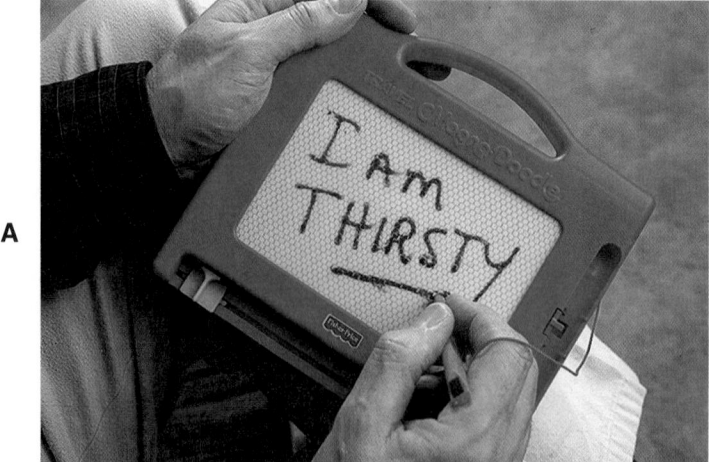

A

FIGURE 7-6 Communication aids. **A,** Magic Slate.

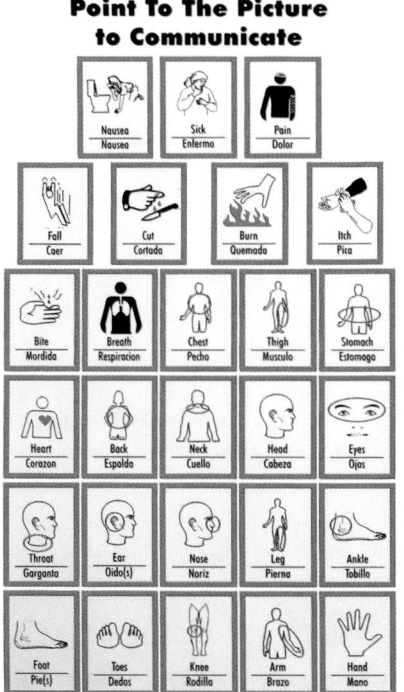

Point To The Picture to Communicate

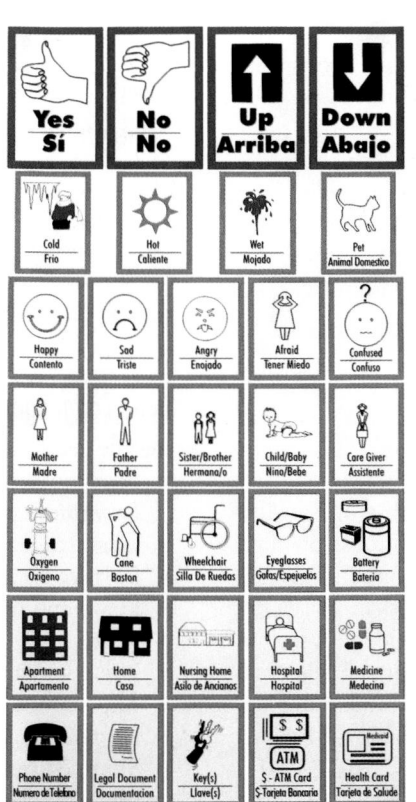

Indique A La Imágen Que Usted Quiere Comunicar

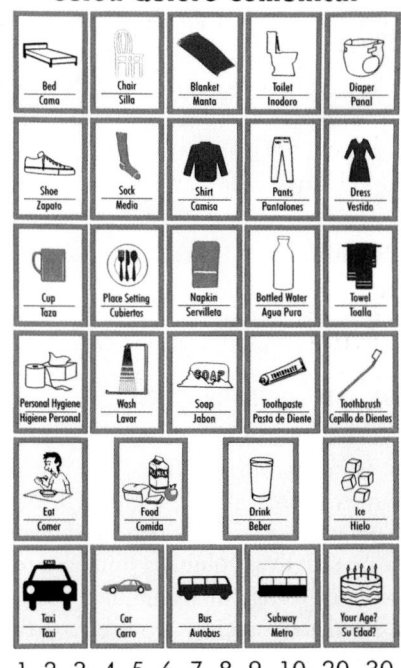

B

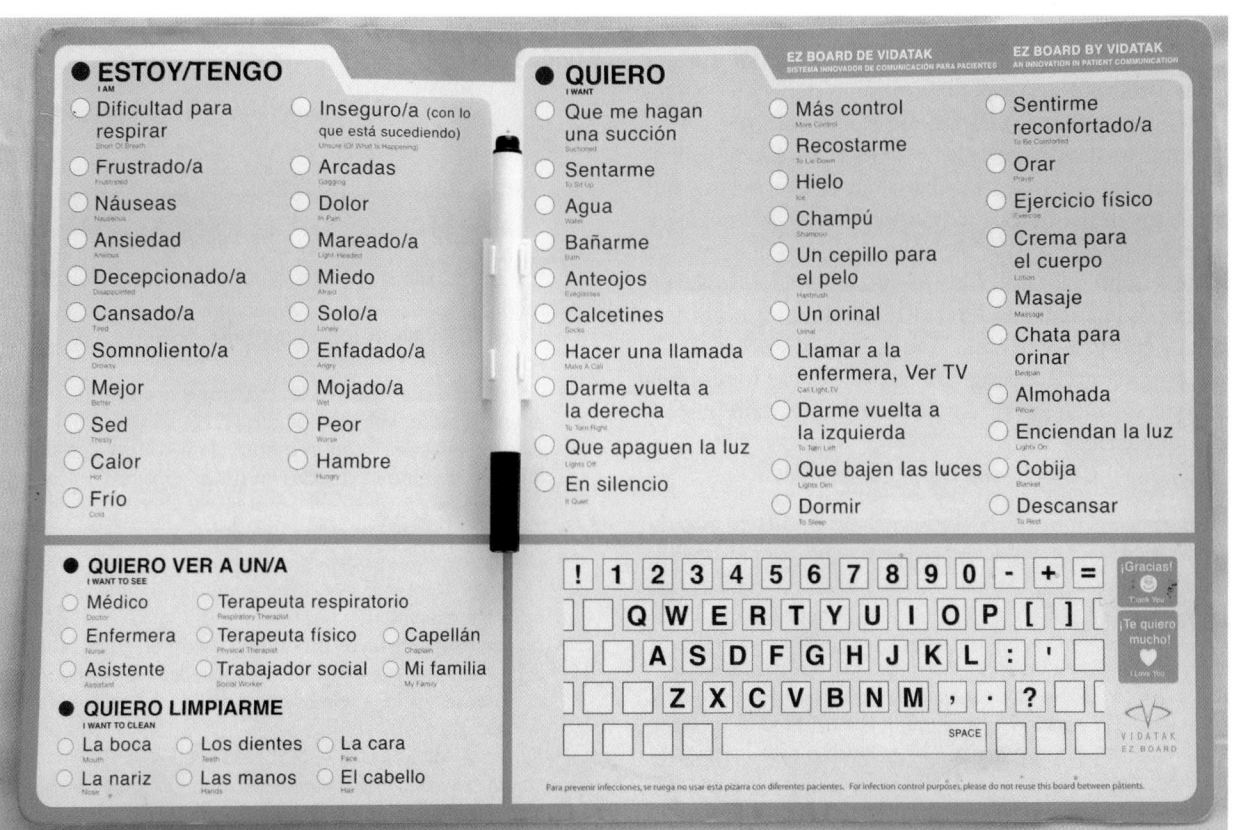

C

FIGURE 7-6, cont'd B, Picture board in English and Spanish. **C,** Communication board in Spanish.

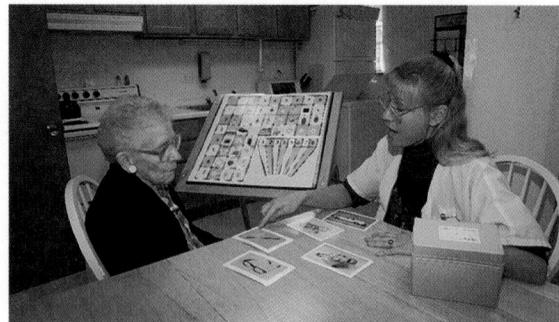

FIGURE 7-7 A resident uses a picture board and picture cards to communicate.

Nonverbal Communication

Nonverbal communication does not use words. Messages are sent with gestures, facial expressions, posture, body movements, touch, and smell. Nonverbal messages more accurately reflect a person's feelings than words do. They are usually involuntary and hard to control. A person may say one thing but act another way. Watch the person's eyes, hand movements, gestures, posture, and other actions. Sometimes they can tell you more than words.

Touch

Touch is a very important form of nonverbal communication. It conveys comfort, caring, love, affection, interest, trust, concern, and reassurance. Touch means different things to different people. The meaning depends on age, gender (male or female), experiences, and culture.

Cultural groups have rules or practices about touch. They relate to who can touch, when it can occur, and where to touch the body. (See *Caring About Culture: Touch Practices.*)

Some people do not like to be touched. However, touch can show caring and warmth. Stroking or holding a hand can comfort a person. Touch should be gentle. It should not be hurried, rough, or sexual. To use touch, follow the person's care plan. Remember to maintain professional boundaries.

See *Focus on Children and Older Persons: Touch.*

CARING ABOUT CULTURE

Touch Practices

Touch practices vary among cultural groups. Touch is used often in *Mexico*. Some people believe that using touch while complimenting a person is important. It is thought to neutralize the power of the evil eye *(mal de ojo)*. Touch also is important in the *Philippine* culture.

Persons from the *United Kingdom* tend not to use touch. Touch is socially acceptable in *Poland*.

In *India*, men shake hands with other men. Men do not shake hands with women. Similar practices occur in *Vietnam*.

People from *China* do not like being touched by strangers. A nod or slight bow is given during introductions.

(Modified from D'Avanzo CE, Geissler EM: *Pocket guide to cultural health assessment,* ed 3, St Louis, 2003, Mosby.)

FOCUS ON CHILDREN AND OLDER PERSONS

Touch

CHILDREN

Infants and young children respond to touch. It soothes and comforts them. They like to be held, stroked, rocked, and patted. They also like cuddling. Older children and teenagers like to give and receive hugs.

Contact must be professional, casual, and with consent. It should not be sexual or involve sexual areas.

Body Language

People send messages through their **body language**:
► Facial expressions (See *Caring About Culture: Facial Expressions.*)
► Gestures
► Posture
► Hand and body movements
► Gait
► Eye contact
► Appearance (dress, hygiene, jewelry, perfume, cosmetics, tattoos, body piercings, and so on)

Slumped posture may mean the person is not happy or feeling well. A person may deny pain. However, he or she protects the affected body part by standing, lying, or sitting in a certain way. Many messages are sent through body language.

CARING ABOUT CULTURE

Facial Expressions

Through facial expressions, *Americans* communicate:
• *Coldness*—there is a constant stare. Face muscles do not move.
• *Fear*—eyes are open wide. Eyebrows are raised. The mouth is tense with the lips drawn back.
• *Anger*—eyes are fixed in a hard stare. Upper lids are lowered. Eyebrows are drawn down. Lips are tightly compressed.
• *Tiredness*—eyes are rolled upward.
• *Disapproval*—eyes are rolled upward.
• *Disgust*—narrowed eyes. The upper lip is curled. There are nose movements.
• *Embarrassment*—eyes are turned away or down. The face is flushed. The person pretends to smile. He or she rubs the eyes, nose, or face. He or she twitches the hair, beard, or mustache.
• *Surprise*—direct gaze with raised eyebrows.
Italian, Jewish, African-American, and *Hispanic* persons smile readily. They use many facial expressions and gestures for happiness, pain, or displeasure. *Irish, English,* and *Northern European* persons tend to have less facial expression.

In some cultures, facial expressions mean the opposite of what the person is feeling. For example, *Asians* may conceal negative emotions with a smile.

(Modified from Giger JN, Davidhizar RE: *Transcultural nursing: assessment and intervention,* ed 4, St Louis, 2004, Mosby.)

Your actions, movements, and facial expressions send messages. So do how you stand, sit, walk, and look at the person. Your body language should show interest and enthusiasm. It should show caring and respect for the person. Often you will need to control your body language. Control reactions to odors from body fluids, secretions, excretions, or the person's body. Many odors are beyond the person's control. Embarrassment and humiliation increase if you react to odors.

Communication Methods

Certain methods help you communicate with others. They result in better relationships. More information is gained for the nursing process.

Listening

Listening means to focus on verbal and nonverbal communication. You use sight, hearing, touch, and smell. You focus on what the person is saying. You observe nonverbal clues. They can support what the person says. Or they can show other feelings. For example, Mr. Hart says, "I want to stay here. That way my daughter won't have to care for me." You see tears, and he looks away from you. His verbal says *happy*. His nonverbal shows *sadness*.

Listening requires that you care and have interest. Follow these guidelines:

▶ Face the person.
▶ Have good eye contact with the person. See *Caring About Culture: Eye Contact Practices*.
▶ Lean toward the person (Fig. 7-8). Do not sit back with your arms crossed.
▶ Respond to the person. Nod your head. Say "uh huh," "mmm," and "I see." Repeat what the person says. Ask questions.
▶ Avoid the communication barriers (p. 92).

Paraphrasing

Paraphrasing is restating the person's message in your own words. You use fewer words than the person did. Paraphrasing:

▶ Shows you are listening.
▶ Lets the person see if you understand the message.
▶ Promotes further communication.

The person usually responds to your statement. For example:

Mr. Hart: My wife was crying after she spoke with the doctor. I don't know what they talked about.
You: You don't know why your wife was crying.
Mr. Hart: He must have told her that I have a tumor.

Direct Questions

Direct questions focus on certain information. You ask the person something you need to know. Some direct questions have "yes" or "no" answers. Others require more information. For example:

You: Mr. Hart, do you want to shave this morning?
Mr. Hart: Yes.
You: Mr. Hart, when would you like to do that?

CARING ABOUT CULTURE

Eye Contact Practices

In the *American* culture, eye contact signals a good self-concept. It also shows openness, interest in others, attention, honesty, and warmth. Lack of eye contact can mean:

• Shyness
• Lack of interest
• Humility
• Guilt
• Embarrassment
• Low self-esteem
• Rudeness
• Dishonesty

For some *Asian* and *American Indian* cultures, eye contact is impolite. It is an invasion of privacy. In certain *Indian* cultures, eye contact is avoided with persons of higher or lower socioeconomic class. It is also given a special sexual meaning.

Direct eye contact is practiced in *Poland* and *Russia*. However, direct eye contact is rude in *Mexican* and *Vietnamese* cultures. In the *United Kingdom*, staring is a part of good listening.

Blinking has meaning. In *Vietnam*, it means that a message is received. It shows understanding in the *United Kingdom*.

(Modified from Giger JN, Davidhizar RE: *Transcultural nursing: assessment and intervention*, ed 4, St Louis, 2004, Mosby. Modified from D'Avanzo CE, Geissler EM: *Pocket guide to cultural health assessment*, ed 3, St Louis, 2003, Mosby.)

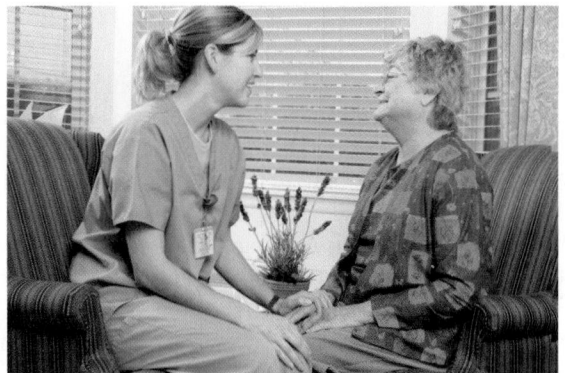

FIGURE 7-8 Listen by facing the person. Have good eye contact. Lean toward the person.

Mr. Hart: Could we start in 15 minutes? I'd like to call my son first.
You: Yes, we can start in 15 minutes. Did you have a bowel movement today?
Mr. Hart: No.
You: You said you didn't eat well this morning. Can you tell me what you ate?
Mr. Hart: I only had toast and coffee. I just don't feel like eating this morning.

Open-Ended Questions

Open-ended questions lead or invite the person to share thoughts, feelings, or ideas. The person chooses what to talk about. He or she controls the topic and the information given. Answers require more than a "yes" or "no." For example:

▶ "What do you like about living with your daughter?"
▶ "Tell me about your grandson."
▶ "What was your wife like?"
▶ "What do you like about being retired?"

The person chooses how to answer. Responses to open-ended questions are longer. They give more information than do responses to direct questions.

Clarifying

Clarifying lets you make sure that you understand the message. You can ask the person to repeat the message, say you do not understand, or restate the message. For example:

▶ "Could you say that again?"
▶ "I'm sorry, Mr. Hart. I don't understand what you mean."
▶ "Are you saying that you want to go home?"

Focusing

Focusing is dealing with a certain topic. It is useful when a person rambles or wanders in thought. For example, Mr. Hart talks at length about food and places to eat. You need to know why he did not each much breakfast. To focus on breakfast you say: "Let's talk about breakfast. You said you don't feel like eating."

Silence

Silence is a very powerful way to communicate. Sometimes you do not need to say anything. This is true during sad times. Just being there shows you care. At other times, silence gives time to think, organize thoughts, or choose words. Silence is useful when making decisions. It also helps when the person is upset and needs to gain control. Silence on your part shows caring and respect for the person's situation and feelings.

Sometimes pauses or long silences are uncomfortable. You do not need to talk when the person is silent. The person may need silence. Dealing with silence gets easier as you gain experience in your role. See *Caring About Culture: The Meaning of Silence.*

Communication Barriers

Communication barriers prevent the sending and the receiving of messages. Communication fails. You must avoid these barriers:

▶ *Using unfamiliar language.* You and the person must use and understand the same language. If not, messages are not accurately interpreted. See Appendix C, p. 795, for useful Spanish words and phrases.
▶ *Cultural differences.* The person may attach different meanings to verbal and nonverbal communication. See *Caring About Culture: Communicating With Persons From Other Cultures.*
▶ *Changing the subject.* Someone changes the subject when the topic is uncomfortable. Avoid changing the subject whenever possible.

CARING ABOUT CULTURE

The Meaning of Silence

In the *English* and *Arabic* cultures, silence is used for privacy. Among *Russian, French,* and *Spanish* cultures, silence means agreement between parties. In some *Asian* cultures, silence is a sign of respect, particularly to an older person.

(Modified from Giger JN, Davidhizar RE: *Transcultural nursing: assessment and intervention,* ed 4, St Louis, 2004, Mosby.)

CARING ABOUT CULTURE

Communicating With Persons From Other Cultures

• Ask the nurse about the beliefs and values of the person's culture. Learn as much as you can about the person's culture.
• Do not judge the person by your own attitudes, values, beliefs, and ideas.
• Follow the person's care plan. It includes the person's cultural beliefs and customs.
• Do the following when communicating with foreign speaking persons:
  • Convey comfort by your tone of voice and body language.
  • Do not speak loudly or shout. It will not help the person understand English.
  • Speak slowly and distinctly.
  • Keep messages short and simple.
  • Be alert for words the person seems to understand.
  • Use gestures and pictures.
  • Repeat the message in other ways.
  • Avoid using medical terms and abbreviations.
  • Be alert for signs the person is pretending to understand. Nodding and answering "yes" to all questions are signs that the person does not understand what you are saying.

(Modified from Geissler EM: *Pocket guide to cultural assessment,* ed 2, St Louis, 1998, Mosby.)

▶ *Giving your opinion.* Opinions involve judging values, behaviors, or feelings. Let others express feelings and concerns without adding your opinion. Do not make judgments or jump to conclusions.
▶ *Talking a lot when others are silent.* Talking too much is usually because of nervousness and discomfort with silence. Silences have meaning. They show acceptance, rejection, and fear. They also show the need for quiet and time to think.
▶ *Failure to listen.* Do not pretend to listen. It shows lack of interest and caring. This causes poor responses. You miss complaints of pain, discomfort, or other symptoms that you must report to the nurse.
▶ *Pat answers.* "Don't worry." "Everything will be okay." "Your doctor knows best." These make the person feel that you do not care about his or her concerns, feelings, and fears.
▶ *Illness and disability.* Some illnesses, injuries, and birth defects affect speech, hearing, vision, cognitive function, and body movements. Verbal and nonverbal communication are affected.
▶ *Age.* Values and communication styles vary among age-groups.

PERSONS WITH DISABILITIES

A person may acquire a disability any time from birth through old age. Disease and injury are common causes. For example, children can develop hearing problems from ear infections. Head injuries from accidents can impair cognitive function. Spinal cord injuries can affect movements. And loud noise (music, machinery) is linked to hearing loss. The cause of disability or the age of onset does not matter. The person does not choose to have a disability.

The person has to adjust to the disability. For many people, this can be long and hard (Chapter 36).

You will care for many people with disabilities. Your attitude is important for effective communication. People with disabilities have the same basic needs as you and everyone else. They feel joy, sorrow, happiness, sadness, and other emotions just like you and everyone else. They laugh and cry, have families, go to school, work, get married, and pay bills just like you and everyone else. And they have the right to dignity and respect just like you and everyone else.

To communicate with persons who have certain disabilities see persons:

▶ Who have speech impairments—Chapter 37
▶ Who are hard of hearing—Chapter 37
▶ Who are blind—Chapter 37
▶ Who are confused—Chapter 44
▶ With Alzheimer's disease and other dementias—Chapter 44

Common courtesies and manners (*etiquette*) apply to any person with a disability. See Box 7-2 for disability etiquette. The guidelines are from Easter Seals, an organization that helps persons with disabilities and their families.

BOX 7-2 Disability Etiquette

- Extend the same courtesies to the person as you would to anyone else.
- Allow the person privacy.
- Do not hang on or lean on a person's wheelchair.
- Treat adults as adults. Do not use the person's first name unless he or she asks you to do so.
- Do not pat a person in a wheelchair on the head.
- Speak directly to the person. Do not address questions intended for the person to his or her companion.
- Do not be embarrassed if you use words that relate to a disability. For example, you say "Did you see that?" to a person with a vision problem.
- Sit or squat to talk to a person in a wheelchair or chair. This puts you and the person at eye level.
- Ask the person if he or she needs help before acting. If the person says "no," respect the person's wishes. If the person wants help, ask the person what to do and how to do it.
- Think before giving directions to a person in a wheelchair. Think about distance, weather conditions, stairs, curbs, steep hills, and other obstacles.
- Allow the person extra time to say or do things. Let the person set the pace in walking, talking, or other activities.

Modified from *Disability Etiquette*, Easter Seals, 2005.

The Person Who Is Comatose

Comatose means being unable to respond to verbal stimuli. The person who is comatose is unconscious. The person cannot respond to others. Often the person can hear and can feel touch and pain. Often pain is shown by grimacing or groaning. Assume that the person hears and understands you. Use touch and give care gently. Practice these measures:

▶ Knock before entering the person's room.
▶ Tell the person your name, the time, and the place every time you enter the room.
▶ Give care on the same schedule every day.
▶ Explain what you are going to do. Explain care measures step-by-step as you do them.
▶ Tell the person when you are finishing care.
▶ Use touch to communicate care, concern, and comfort (p. 90).
▶ Tell the person what time you will be back to check on him or her.
▶ Tell the person when you are leaving the room.

FAMILY AND FRIENDS

Family and friends help meet safety and security, love and belonging, and self-esteem needs. They offer support and comfort. They lessen loneliness. Some also help with the person's care. This helps both the person and the family. The family knows they are doing something to help the person. And the person's physical and emotional needs are met. The presence or absence of family or friends affects the person's quality of life.

The person has the right to visit with family and friends in private and without unnecessary interruptions. You may need to give care when visitors are there. Protect the right to privacy. Do not expose the person's body in front of them. Politely ask them to leave the room. Show them where to wait. Promptly tell them when they can return. A partner or family member may want to help you. If the patient or resident consents, you may allow the person to stay.

Treat family and friends with courtesy and respect. They have concerns about the person's condition and care. They need support and understanding. However, do not discuss the person's condition with them. Refer their questions to the nurse.

Visiting rules depend on agency policy and the person's condition. Parents can visit children as often and as long as they want. Usually only short visits are allowed in special care units. Dying persons usually can have family members present all the time. This is policy for hospice units. Know your agency's visiting policies and what is allowed for the person.

Visitors may have questions about the chapel, gift shop, lounge, dining room, or business office. Know the location, special rules, and hours of these areas.

A visitor may upset or tire a person. Report your observations to the nurse. The nurse will speak with the visitor about the person's needs.

See *Caring About Culture: Family Roles in Sick Care.*

See *Focus on Children and Older Persons: Family and Friends.*

See *Focus on Long-Term Care and Home Care: Family and Visitors.*

CARING ABOUT CULTURE

Family Roles in Sick Care

In *Vietnam,* all family members are involved in the person's care. A similar practice is common in *China.* Family members bathe, feed, and comfort the person. However, women in *Mexico* cannot give care at home if it involves touching the genitals of adult men.

(Modified from D'Avanzo CE, Geissler EM: *Pocket guide to cultural health assessment,* ed 3, St Louis, 2003, Mosby.)

FOCUS ON CHILDREN AND OLDER PERSONS

Family and Friends

OLDER PERSONS

Sometimes older brothers, sisters, and cousins live together. They provide companionship and share living expenses. They care for each other during illness or disability.

Some older people live with their children. The older parent may be healthy, need some supervision, or be ill or disabled. The older parent moves in with the child. Or the child moves into the parent's home. Living with a child can help the older person feel safe and secure. Often the adult child gives care to an ill or disabled parent.

Adult children often need to work even though the parent cannot be left alone. Adult day-care centers provide meals, supervision, and supervised activities for older persons. Cards, board games, movies, crafts, dancing, walks, and lectures are common. Some provide bowling and swimming. Help is given as needed. Some provide transportation from home to the center.

Living with an adult child is a social change. The parent, child, and the child's family need to adjust. The child's family needs time alone. Other family members may help give care. Respite care provides a break for the family. The parent enters a nursing center for a few days or weeks. Caregivers can rest, go on vacation, or take a break from caregiving stresses. Church and community groups may have volunteers who help with care.

FOCUS ON LONG-TERM CARE AND HOME CARE

Family and Visitors

HOME CARE

Family personalities and attitudes affect the mood in the home. Many families are happy and supportive. Others have poor relationships. Mental or physical illness, drug or alcohol abuse, unemployment, and delinquency may affect the family. Some families have problems coping with or accepting the person's illness or disability.

Your supervisor explains family problems to you. Do not get involved. Be professional and have empathy. Do not give advice, take sides, or make judgments about family conflicts. Maintain professional boundaries at all times.

BEHAVIOR ISSUES

Many people accept illness, injury, and disability. Others do not adjust well. They have some of the following behaviors. These behaviors are new for some people. For others, they are life-long. They are part of one's personality.

► *Anger.* Anger is a common emotion. Causes include fear, pain, and dying and death. Loss of function and loss of control over health and life are causes. So are long waits for care or to see the doctor. Anger is a symptom of some diseases that affect thinking and behavior. Some people are generally angry. Anger is communicated verbally and nonverbally. Verbal outbursts, shouting, raised voices, and rapid speech are common. Some people are silent. Others are uncooperative. They may refuse to answer questions. Nonverbal signs include rapid movements, pacing, clenched fists, and a red face. Glaring and getting close to you when speaking are other signs. Violent behaviors can occur.

► *Demanding behavior.* Nothing seems to please the person. The person is critical of others. He or she wants care given at a certain time and in a certain way. Loss of independence, loss of health, and loss of control of life are causes. So are unmet needs. See *Teamwork and Time Management: Behavior Issues.*

► *Self-centered behavior.* The person cares only about his or her own needs. The needs of others are ignored. The person demands the time and attention of others. The person becomes impatient if needs are not met.

► *Aggressive behavior.* The person may swear, bite, hit, pinch, scratch, or kick. Fear, anger, pain, and dementia (Chapter 44) are causes. Protect the person, others, and yourself from harm (Chapter 11).

▶ *Withdrawal.* The person has little or no contact with family, friends, and staff. He or she spends time alone and does not take part in social or group events. This may signal physical illness or depression. Some people are generally not social. They prefer to be alone.

▶ *Inappropriate sexual behavior.* Some people make inappropriate sexual remarks. Or they touch others in the wrong way. Some disrobe or masturbate in public. These behaviors may be on purpose. Or they are caused by disease, confusion, dementia, or drug side effects.

A person's behavior may be unpleasant. You cannot avoid the person or lose control. Good communication is needed. Behaviors are addressed in the care plan. The care plan may include some of the guidelines in Box 7-3.

TEAMWORK AND TIME MANAGEMENT

Behavior Issues

Persons who are demanding can take a lot of time. A simple task such as filling a water pitcher can take several minutes. The pitcher may be too full or not full enough. The water may be too warm or too cold. Or the person may have a list of other care needs.

This may happen to you or to co-workers. Learn to recognize these situations. Offer to help co-workers with the person or other tasks. Hopefully they also will help you.

BOX 7-3 Dealing With Behavior Issues

- Recognize frustrating and frightening situations. Put yourself in the person's situation. How would you feel? How would you want to be treated?
- Treat the person with dignity and respect.
- Answer questions clearly and thoroughly. Ask the nurse to answer questions you cannot answer.
- Keep the person informed. Tell the person what you are going to do and when.
- Do not keep the person waiting. Answer signal lights promptly. If you tell the person that you will do something for him or her, do it promptly.
- Explain the reason for long waits. Ask if you can get or do something to increase the person's comfort.
- Stay calm and professional, especially if the person is angry or hostile. Often the person is not angry at you. He or she is angry at another person or situation.
- Do not argue with the person.
- Listen and use silence (p. 92). The person may feel better if able to express his or her feelings.
- Protect yourself from violent behaviors (Chapter 11).
- Report the person's behavior to the nurse. Discuss how you should deal with the person.

REVIEW QUESTIONS

Circle the BEST answer.

1 You work in a health care agency. You focus on
   a The person's care plan
   b The person's physical, safety and security, and self-esteem needs
   c The person as a physical, psychological, social, and spiritual being
   d The person's cultural and spiritual needs

2 Which basic need is the *most* essential?
   a Self-actualization
   b Self-esteem
   c Love and belonging
   d Safety and security

3 Based on Maslow's theory of basic needs, which person's needs must be met *first*?
   a The person who wants another blanket
   b The person who wants mail opened
   c The person who asks for more water
   d The person who is crying

4 A person says, "What are they doing to me?" Which basic needs are *not* being met?
   a Physical needs
   b Safety and security needs
   c Love and belonging needs
   d Self-esteem needs

5 A person has a garden behind the nursing center. This relates to
   a Self-actualization
   b Self-esteem
   c Love and belonging
   d Safety and security

6 Which is *false*?
   a Culture influences health and illness practices.
   b Culture and religion influence food practices.
   c Cultural and religious practices are allowed in health care agencies.
   d A person must follow all beliefs and practices of his or her culture or religion.

Continued

7 Which is *true?*
  a Mental health problems are the focus of psychiatry.
  b Sick children are the focus of pediatrics.
  c The diseases of aging are the focus of geriatrics.
  d Childbirth is the focus of obstetrics.

8 A hospital patient has the right to the following *except*
  a Compassionate and respectful care
  b Treatment information
  c Refuse treatment
  d Free care

9 These are statements about illness and disability. Which is *false?*
  a They are matters of personal choice.
  b They affect normal activities.
  c Anger is a common response.
  d A goal is for the person to maintain optimal level of function.

10 Alert and oriented residents need nursing center care because they
  a Are very disabled and confused
  b Have trouble remembering things
  c Have physical problems
  d Are dying

11 Which is *false?*
  a Verbal communication uses the written or spoken word.
  b Verbal communication is the truest reflection of a person's feelings.
  c Messages are sent by facial expressions, gestures, posture, and body movements.
  d Touch means different things to different people.

12 To communicate with a person, you should
  a Use medical words and phrases
  b Change the subject often
  c Give your opinions
  d Be quiet when the person is silent

13 Which might mean that you are *not* listening?
  a You sit facing the person.
  b You have good eye contact with the person.
  c You sit with your arms crossed.
  d You ask questions.

14 Which is a direct question?
  a "Do you feel better now?"
  b "What are your plans for home?"
  c "What will you do at home?"
  d "You said that you can't sleep."

15 A person wants to take a shower. You say, "You would like to take shower." This is
  a Focusing
  b Clarifying
  c Paraphrasing
  d An open-ended question

16 Focusing is useful when
  a A person is rambling
  b You want to make sure you understand the message
  c You want the person to share thoughts and feelings
  d You need certain information

17 Which promotes communication?
  a "Don't worry."
  b "Everything will be just fine."
  c "This is a good nursing center."
  d "Why are you crying?"

18 Which is *not* a barrier to communication?
  a Using silence
  b Giving your opinions
  c Changing the subject
  d Illness

19 A person uses a wheelchair. For effective communication, you should
  a Lean on the wheelchair
  b Pat the person on the head
  c Direct questions to the companion
  d Sit or squat next to the person

20 A person is comatose. Which action is *not correct?*
  a Assume that the person can hear and can feel touch.
  b Explain what you are going to do.
  c Use listening and silence to communicate.
  d Tell the person when you are leaving the room.

21 A person has many visitors. Which is *false?*
  a They can help meet basic needs.
  b Privacy should be allowed.
  c The nurse answers their questions about the person's care.
  d Visitors can stay in the room when care is given.

22 A visitor seems to tire a person. What should you do?
  a Ask the person to leave.
  b Tell the nurse.
  c Stay in the room to observe the person and visitor.
  d Find out the visitor's relationship to the person.

23 A person wants care given at a certain time and in a certain way. Nothing seems to please the person. The person is most likely demonstrating
  a Angry behavior
  b Demanding behavior
  c Withdrawn behavior
  d Aggressive behavior

24 A person is demonstrating problem behavior. You should do the following *except*
  a Put yourself in the person's situation
  b Tell the person what you are going to do and when
  c Ask the person to be nicer
  d Listen and use silence

Answers for these questions are on p. 779.

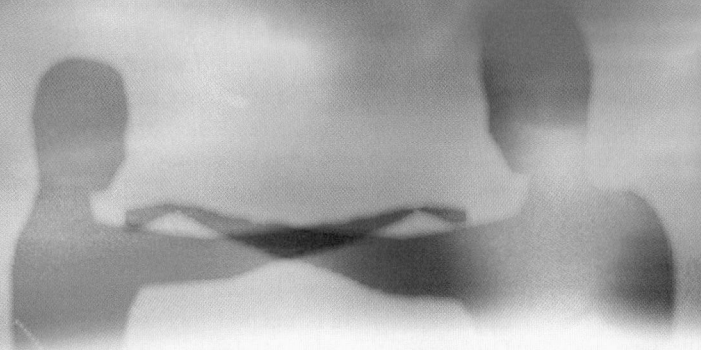

Body Structure and Function

CHAPTER

8

OBJECTIVES

- Define the key terms and key abbreviations listed in this chapter
- Identify the basic structures of the cell
- Explain how cells divide
- Describe four types of tissue
- Identify the structures of each body system
- Identify the functions of each body system
- Explain how to promote quality of life

KEY TERMS

artery A blood vessel that carries blood away from the heart

capillary A tiny blood vessel; food, oxygen, and other substances pass from the capillaries to the cells

cell The basic unit of body structure

digestion The process of physically and chemically breaking down food so that it can be absorbed for use by the cells

hemoglobin The substance in red blood cells that carries oxygen and gives blood its color

hormone A chemical substance secreted by the endocrine glands into the bloodstream

immunity Protection against a disease or condition; the person will not get or be affected by the disease

menstruation The process in which the lining of the uterus breaks up and is discharged from the body through the vagina

metabolism The burning of food for heat and energy by the cells

organ Groups of tissues with the same function

peristalsis Involuntary muscle contractions in the digestive system that move food down the esophagus through the alimentary canal

respiration The process of supplying the cells with oxygen and removing carbon dioxide from them

system Organs that work together to perform special functions

tissue A group of cells with similar functions

vein A blood vessel that returns blood back to the heart

97

KEY ABBREVIATIONS

ACTH Adrenocorticotropic hormone
ADH Antidiuretic hormone
CNS Central nervous system
GH Growth hormone
GI Gastrointestinal

mL Milliliter
RBC Red blood cell
TH Thyroid hormone; thyroxine
TSH Thyroid-stimulating hormone
WBC White blood cell

You help patients and residents meet basic needs. Their bodies do not work at peak levels because of illness, disease, or injury. Your care promotes comfort, healing, and recovery. You need to know the body's normal structure and function. It will help you understand signs, symptoms, and the reasons for care and procedures. You will give safe and more efficient care.

See Chapter 10 for changes in body structure and function that occur with aging.

CELLS, TISSUES, AND ORGANS

The basic unit of body structure is the **cell**. Cells have the same basic structure. Function, size, and shape may differ. Cells are very small. You need a microscope to see them. Cells need food, water, and oxygen to live and function.

Figure 8-1 shows the cell and its structures. The *cell membrane* is the outer covering. It encloses the cell and helps it hold its shape. The *nucleus* is the control center of the cell. It directs the cell's activities. The nucleus is in the center of the cell. The *cytoplasm* surrounds the nucleus.

Cytoplasm contains smaller structures that perform cell functions. *Protoplasm* means "living substance." It refers to all structures, substances, and water within the cell. Protoplasm is a semi-liquid substance much like an egg white.

Chromosomes are thread-like structures in the nucleus. Each cell has 46 chromosomes. Chromosomes contain *genes*. Genes control the traits children inherit from their parents. Height, eye color, and skin color are examples.

The nucleus controls cell reproduction. Cells reproduce by dividing in half. The process of cell division is called *mitosis*. It is needed for tissue growth and repair. During mitosis, the 46 chromosomes arrange themselves in 23 pairs. As the cell divides, the 23 pairs are pulled in half. The two new cells are identical. Each has 46 chromosomes (Fig. 8-2).

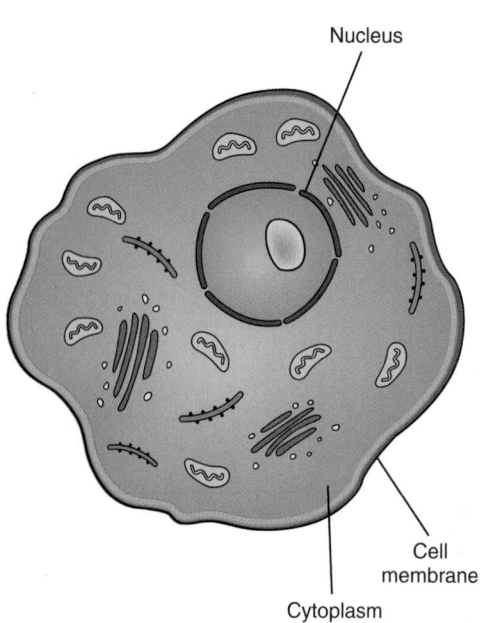

FIGURE 8-1 Parts of a cell.

Nucleus

Cell membrane

Cytoplasm

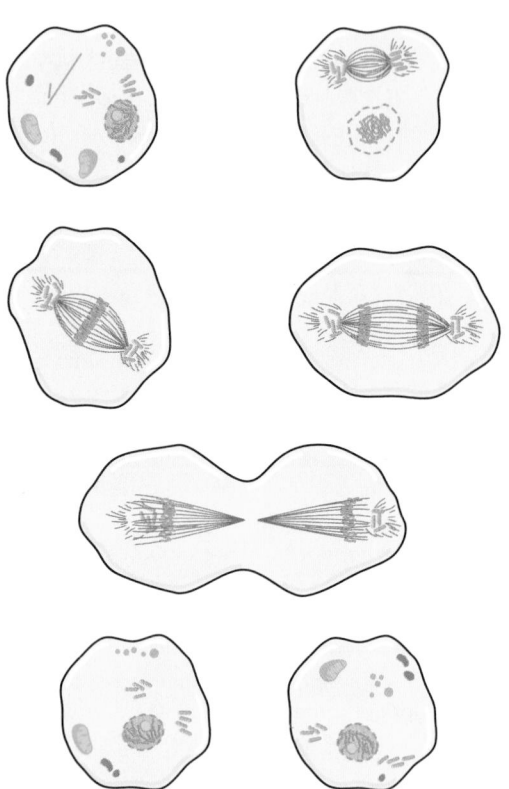

FIGURE 8-2 Cell division.

Cells are the body's building blocks. Groups of cells with similar functions combine to form **tissues:**

▶ *Epithelial tissue* covers internal and external body surfaces. Tissue lining the nose, mouth, respiratory tract, stomach, and intestines is epithelial tissue. So are the skin, hair, nails, and glands.

▶ *Connective tissue* anchors, connects, and supports other tissues. It is in every part of the body. Bones, tendons, ligaments, and cartilage are connective tissue. Blood is a form of connective tissue.

▶ *Muscle tissue* stretches and contracts to let the body move.

▶ *Nerve tissue* receives and carries impulses to the brain and back to body parts.

Groups of tissue with the same function form **organs.** An organ has one or more functions. Examples of organs are the heart, brain, liver, lungs, and kidneys. **Systems** are formed by organs that work together to perform special functions (Fig. 8-3).

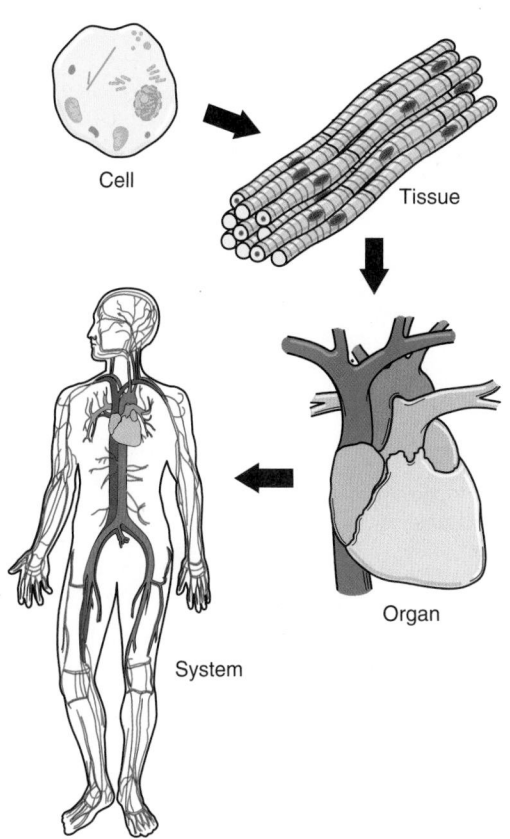

FIGURE 8-3 Organization of the body.

THE INTEGUMENTARY SYSTEM

The *integumentary system*, or *skin*, is the largest system. *Integument* means covering. The skin covers the body. It has epithelial, connective, and nerve tissue. It also has oil glands and sweat glands. There are two skin layers (Fig. 8-4):

▶ The *epidermis* is the outer layer. It has living cells and dead cells. The dead cells were once deeper in the epidermis. They were pushed upward as the cells divided. Dead cells constantly flake off. They are replaced by living cells. Living cells also die and flake off. Living cells of the epidermis contain *pigment*. Pigment gives skin its color. The epidermis has no blood vessels and few nerve endings.

▶ The *dermis* is the inner layer. It is made up of connective tissue. Blood vessels, nerves, sweat glands, and oil glands are found in the dermis. So are hair roots.

The epidermis and dermis are supported by *subcutaneous tissue.* The subcutaneous tissue is a thick layer of fat and connective tissue.

Oil glands and *sweat glands, hair,* and *nails* are skin appendages:

▶ Hair—covers the entire body, except the palms of the hands and the soles of the feet. Hair in the nose and ears and around the eyes protects these organs from dust, insects, and other foreign objects.

▶ Nails—protect the tips of the fingers and toes. Nails help fingers pick up and handle small objects.

▶ Sweat glands—help the body regulate temperature. Sweat consists of water, salt, and a small amount of wastes. Sweat is secreted through pores in the skin. The body is cooled as sweat evaporates.

▶ Oil glands—lie near the hair shafts. They secrete an oily substance into the space near the hair shaft. Oil travels to the skin surface. This helps keep the hair and skin soft and shiny.

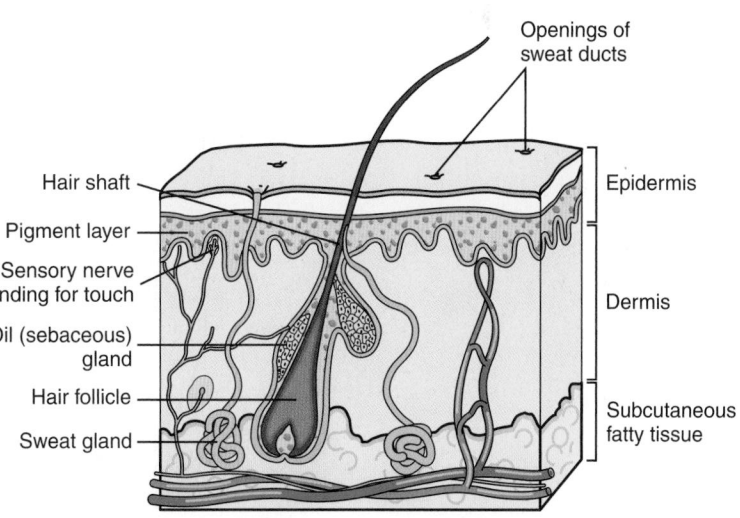

FIGURE 8-4 Layers of the skin.

The skin has many functions:
► It is the body's protective covering.
► It prevents microorganisms and other substances from entering the body.
► It prevents excess amounts of water from leaving the body.
► It protects organs from injury.
► Nerve endings in the skin sense both pleasant and unpleasant stimulation. Nerve endings are over the entire body. They sense cold, pain, touch, and pressure to protect the body from injury.
► It helps regulate body temperature. Blood vessels dilate (widen) when temperature outside the body is high. More blood is brought to the body surface for cooling during evaporation. When blood vessels constrict (narrow), the body retains heat. This is because less blood reaches the skin.

THE MUSCULOSKELETAL SYSTEM

The musculoskeletal system provides the framework for the body. It lets the body move. This system also protects and gives the body shape.

Bones

The human body has *206 bones* (Fig. 8-5). There are four types of bones:
► *Long bones* bear the body's weight. Leg bones are long bones.
► *Short bones* allow skill and ease in movement. Bones in the wrists, fingers, ankles, and toes are short bones.
► *Flat bones* protect the organs. They include the ribs, skull, pelvic bones, and shoulder blades.
► *Irregular bones* are the vertebrae in the spinal column. They allow various degrees of movement and flexibility.

Bones are hard, rigid structures. They are made up of living cells. They are covered by a membrane called *periosteum*. Periosteum contains blood vessels that supply bone cells with oxygen and food. Inside the hollow centers of the bones is a substance called *bone marrow*. Blood cells are formed in the bone marrow.

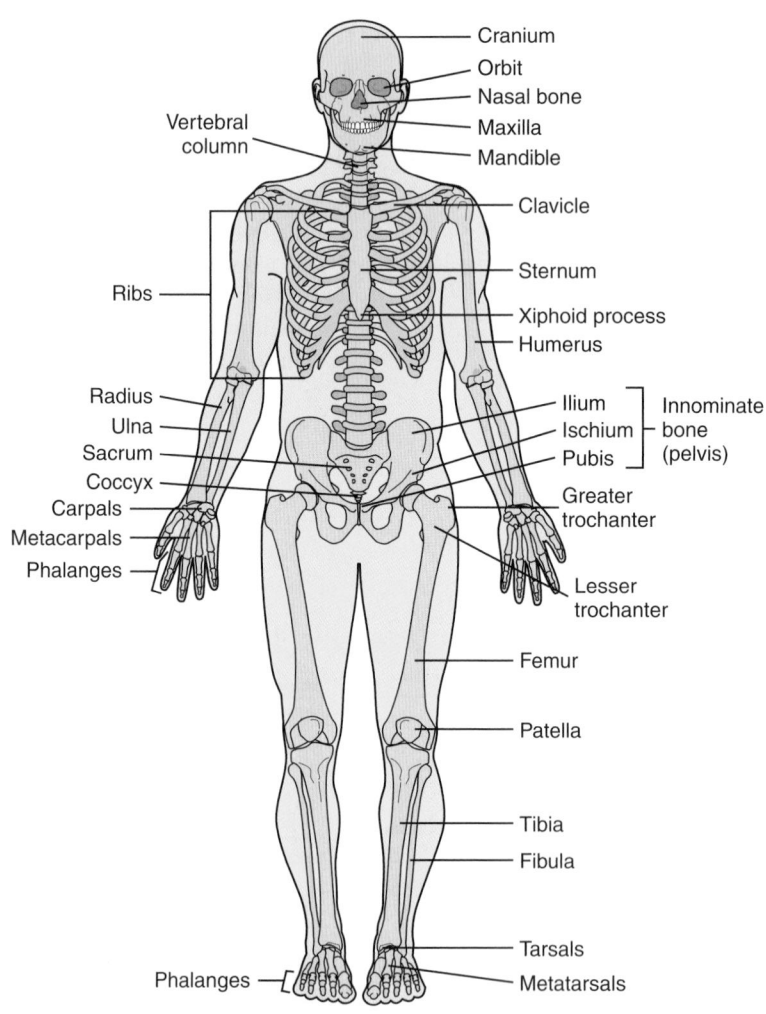

FIGURE 8-5 Bones of the body.

Joints

A *joint* is the point at which two or more bones meet. Joints allow movement (Chapter 26). *Cartilage* is the connective tissue at the end of the long bones. It cushions the joint so that the bone ends do not rub together. The *synovial membrane* lines the joints. It secretes *synovial fluid*. Synovial fluid acts as a lubricant so the joint can move smoothly. Bones are held together at the joint by strong bands of connective tissue called *ligaments*.

There are three major types of joints (Fig. 8-6):

▶ *Ball-and-socket joint* allows movement in all directions. It is made up of the rounded end of one bone and the hollow end of another bone. The rounded end of one fits into the hollow end of the other. The joints of the hips and shoulders are ball-and-socket joints.

▶ *Hinge joint* allows movement in one direction. The elbow is a hinge joint.

▶ *Pivot joint* allows turning from side to side. A pivot joint connects the skull to the spine.

Muscles

The human body has more than 500 *muscles* (Figs. 8-7 and 8-8). Some are voluntary. Others are involuntary.

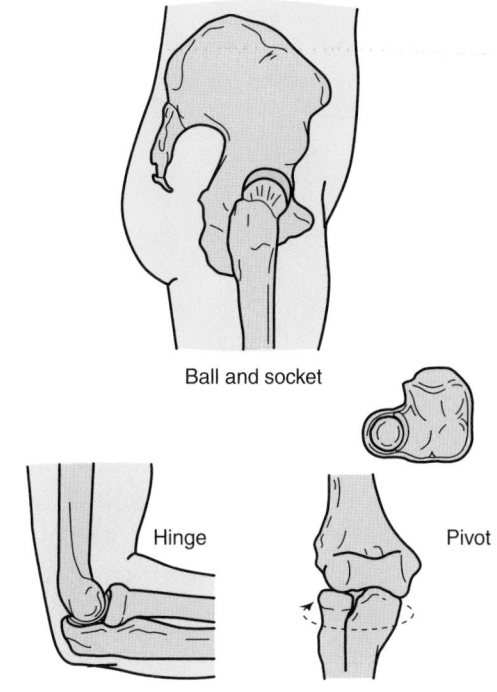

FIGURE 8-6 Types of joints.

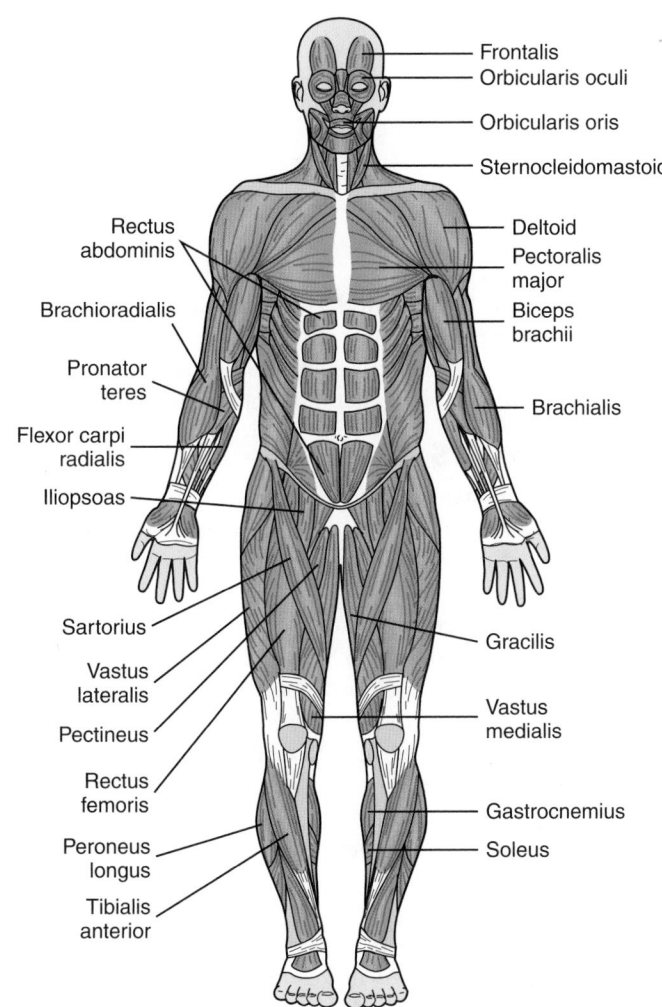

FIGURE 8-7 Anterior view of the muscles of the body.

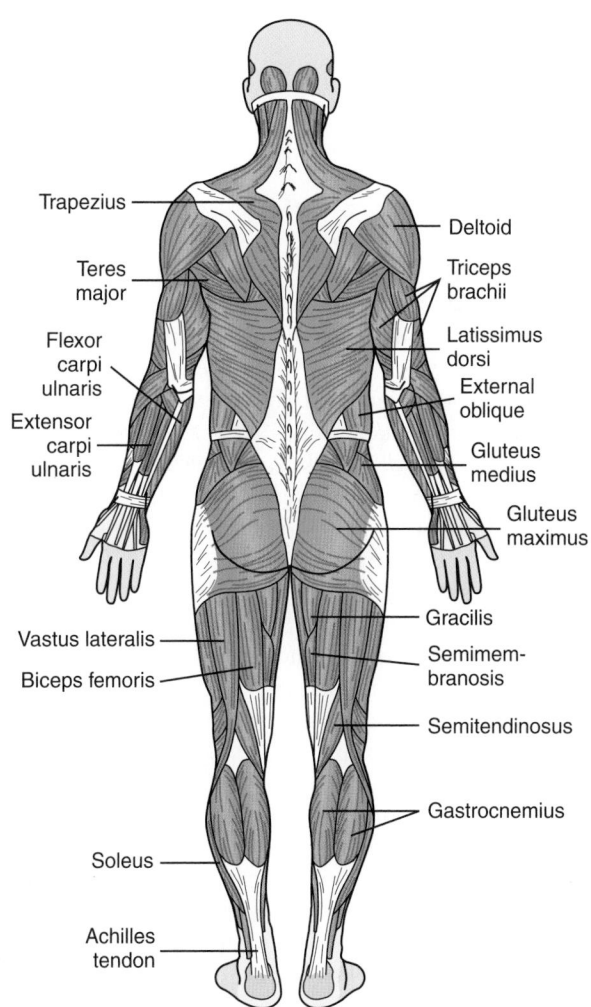

FIGURE 8-8 Posterior view of the muscles of the body.

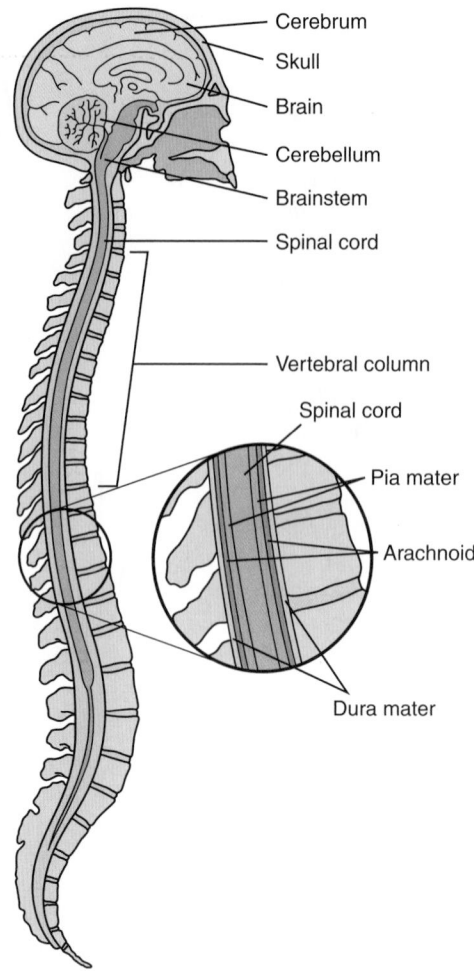

FIGURE 8-9 Central nervous system.

Voluntary muscles can be consciously controlled. Muscles attached to bones *(skeletal muscles)* are voluntary. Arm muscles do not work unless you move your arm; likewise for leg muscles. Skeletal muscles are *striated.* That is, they look striped or streaked.

Involuntary muscles work automatically. You cannot control them. They control the action of the stomach, intestines, blood vessels, and other body organs. Involuntary muscles also are called *smooth muscles.* They look smooth, not streaked or striped.

Cardiac muscle is in the heart. It is an involuntary muscle. However, it appears striated like skeletal muscle.

Muscles have three functions:
▶ Movement of body parts
▶ Maintenance of posture
▶ Production of body heat

Strong, tough connective tissues called *tendons* connect muscles to bones. When muscles contract (shorten), tendons at each end of the muscle cause the bone to move. The body has many tendons. See the Achilles tendon in Figure 8-8. Some muscles constantly contract to maintain the body's posture. When muscles contract, they burn food for energy. Heat is produced. The more muscle activity, the greater the amount of heat produced. Shivering is how the body produces heat when exposed to cold. Shivering is from rapid, general muscle contractions.

THE NERVOUS SYSTEM

The nervous system controls, directs, and coordinates body functions. Its two main divisions are:
▶ The *central nervous system* (CNS). It consists of the brain and spinal cord (Fig. 8-9).
▶ The *peripheral nervous system.* It involves the *nerves* throughout the body (Fig. 8-10).

Nerves carry messages or impulses to and from the brain. Nerves connect to the spinal cord. They are easily damaged and take a long time to heal. Some nerve fibers have a protective covering called a *myelin sheath.* The myelin sheath also insulates the nerve fiber. Nerve fibers covered with myelin conduct impulses faster than those fibers without it.

The Central Nervous System

The *brain* and *spinal cord* make up the central nervous system. The brain is covered by the skull. The three main

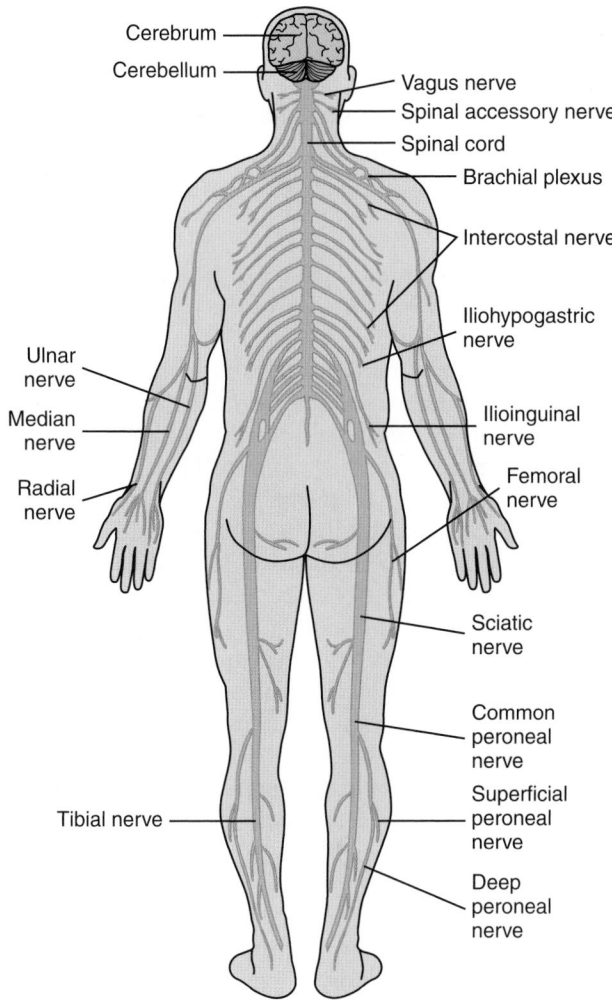

FIGURE 8-10 Peripheral nervous system.

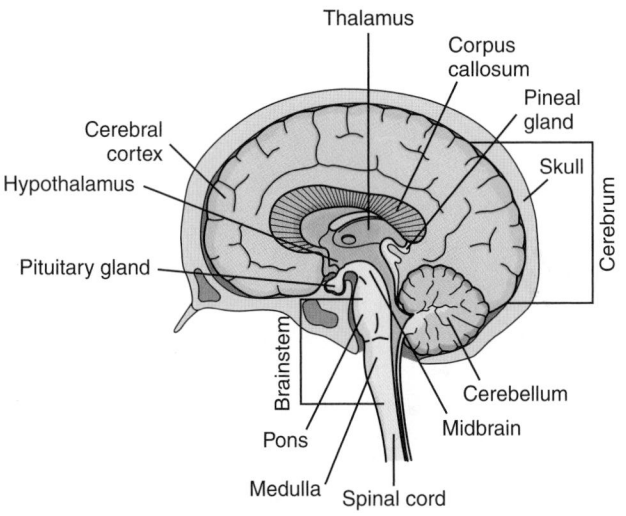

FIGURE 8-11 The brain.

parts of the brain are the *cerebrum*, the *cerebellum*, and the *brainstem* (Fig. 8-11).

The cerebrum is the largest part of the brain. It is the center of thought and intelligence. The cerebrum is

divided into two halves called the *right* and *left hemispheres*. The right hemisphere controls movement and activities on the body's left side. The left hemisphere controls the right side.

The outside of the cerebrum is called the *cerebral cortex*. It controls the highest functions of the brain. These include reasoning, memory, consciousness, speech, voluntary muscle movement, vision, hearing, sensation, and other activities.

The cerebellum regulates and coordinates body movements. It controls balance and the smooth movements of voluntary muscles. Injury to the cerebellum results in jerky movements, loss of coordination, and muscle weakness.

The brainstem connects the cerebrum to the spinal cord. The brainstem contains the *midbrain, pons*, and *medulla*. The midbrain and pons relay messages between the medulla and the cerebrum. The medulla is below the pons. The medulla controls heart rate, breathing, blood vessel size, swallowing, coughing, and vomiting. The brain connects to the spinal cord at the lower end of the medulla.

The spinal cord lies within the spinal column. The cord is 17 to 18 inches long. It contains pathways that conduct messages to and from the brain.

The brain and spinal cord are covered and protected by three layers of connective tissue called meninges:

▶ The outer layer lies next to the skull. It is a tough covering called the *dura mater*.
▶ The middle layer is the *arachnoid*.
▶ The inner layer is the *pia mater*.

The space between the middle layer (arachnoid) and inner layer (pia mater) is the *arachnoid space*. The space is filled with *cerebrospinal fluid*. It circulates around the brain and spinal cord. Cerebrospinal fluid protects the central nervous system. It cushions shocks that could easily injure brain and spinal cord structures.

The Peripheral Nervous System

The peripheral nervous system has 12 pairs of *cranial nerves* and 31 pairs of *spinal nerves*. Cranial nerves conduct impulses between the brain and the head, neck, chest, and abdomen. They conduct impulses for smell, vision, hearing, pain, touch, temperature, and pressure. They also conduct impulses for voluntary and involuntary muscles. Spinal nerves carry impulses from the skin, extremities, and the internal structures not supplied by cranial nerves.

Some peripheral nerves form the *autonomic nervous system*. This system controls involuntary muscles and certain body functions. The functions include the heartbeat, blood pressure, intestinal contractions, and glandular secretions. These functions occur automatically.

The autonomic nervous system is divided into the *sympathetic nervous system* and the *parasympathetic nervous system*. They balance each other. The sympathetic nervous system speeds up functions. The parasympathetic nervous system slows functions. When you are angry, scared, excited, or exercising, the sympathetic nervous system is stimulated. The parasympathetic system is activated when you relax or when the sympathetic system is stimulated for too long.

The Sense Organs

The five senses are *sight*, *hearing*, *taste*, *smell*, and *touch*. Receptors for taste are in the tongue. They are called *taste buds*. Receptors for smell are in the nose. Touch receptors are in the dermis, especially in the toes and fingertips.

The Eye

Receptors for vision are in the *eyes* (Fig. 8-12). The eye is easily injured. Bones of the skull, eyelids and eyelashes, and tears protect the eyes from injury. The eye has three layers:

▶ The *sclera*, the white of the eye, is the outer layer. It is made of tough connective tissue.
▶ The *choroid* is the second layer. Blood vessels, the *ciliary muscle*, and the *iris* make up the choroid. The iris gives the eye its color. The opening in the middle of the iris is the *pupil*. Pupil size varies with the amount of light entering the eye. The pupil constricts (narrows) in bright light. It dilates (widens) in dim or dark places.
▶ The *retina* is the inner layer. It has receptors for vision and the nerve fibers of the *optic nerve*.

Light enters the eye through the *cornea*. It is the transparent part of the outer layer that lies over the eye. Light rays pass to the *lens*, which lies behind the pupil. The light is then reflected to the retina. Light is carried to the brain by the optic nerve.

The *aqueous chamber* separates the cornea from the lens. The chamber is filled with a fluid called *aqueous humor*. The fluid helps the cornea keep its shape and position. The *vitreous humor* is behind the lens. It is a gelatin-like substance that supports the retina and maintains the eye's shape.

The Ear

The *ear* is a sense organ (Fig. 8-13). It functions in hearing and balance. It has three parts: the *external ear*, *middle ear*, and *inner ear*.

The external ear (outer part) is called the *pinna* or *auricle*. Sound waves are guided through the external ear into the *auditory canal*. Glands in the auditory canal secrete a waxy substance called *cerumen*. The auditory canal extends about 1 inch to the *eardrum*. The eardrum *(tympanic membrane)* separates the external and middle ear.

The middle ear is a small space. It contains the *eustachian tube* and three small bones called *ossicles*. The eustachian tube connects the middle ear and the throat. Air enters the eustachian tube so that there is equal pressure on both sides of the eardrum. The ossicles amplify sound received from the eardrum and transmit the sound to the inner ear. The three ossicles are:

▶ The *malleus*. It looks like a hammer.
▶ The *incus*. It looks like an anvil.
▶ The *stapes*. It is shaped like a stirrup.

The inner ear consists of *semicircular canals* and the *cochlea*. The cochlea looks like a snail shell. It contains fluid. The fluid carries sound waves from the middle ear to the *auditory nerve*. The auditory nerve then carries the message to the brain.

The three semicircular canals are involved with balance. They sense the head's position and changes in position. They send messages to the brain.

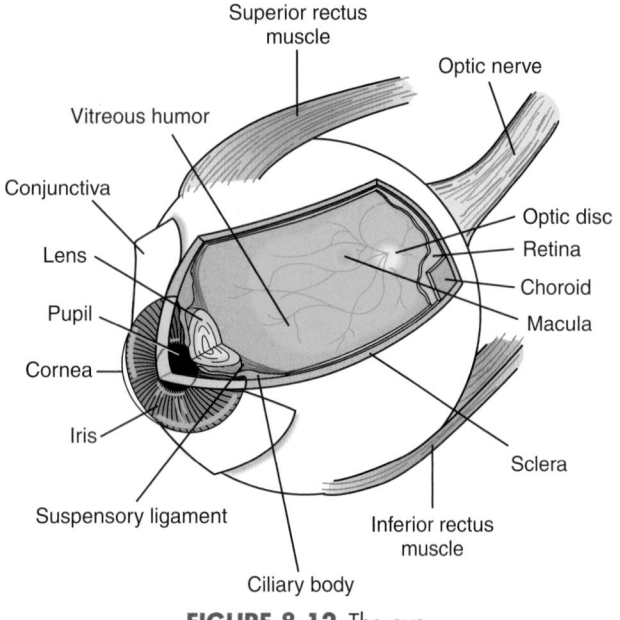

FIGURE 8-12 The eye.

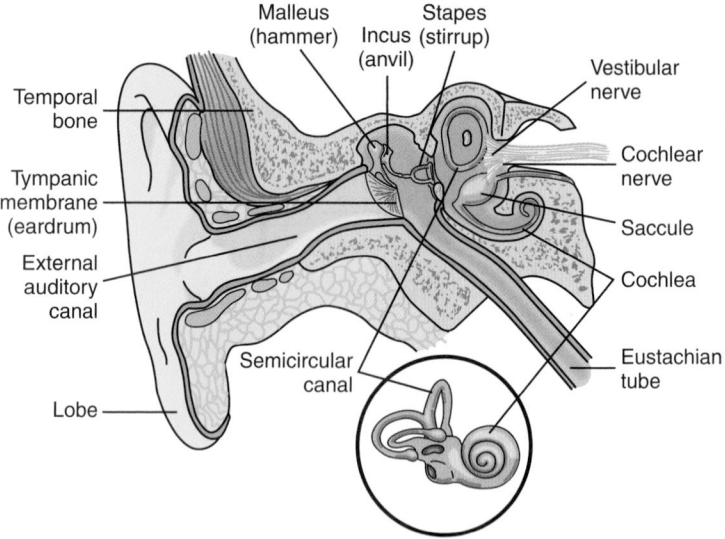

FIGURE 8-13 The ear.

THE CIRCULATORY SYSTEM

The circulatory system is made up of the *blood, heart,* and *blood vessels.* The heart pumps blood through the blood vessels. The circulatory system has many functions:

▶ Blood carries food, oxygen, and other substances to the cells.

▶ Blood removes waste products from cells.

▶ Blood and blood vessels help regulate body temperature. The blood carries heat from muscle activity to other body parts. Blood vessels in the skin dilate to cool the body. They constrict to retain heat.

▶ The system produces and carries cells that defend the body from microbes that cause disease.

The Blood

The blood consists of blood cells and *plasma.* Plasma is mostly water. It carries blood cells to other body cells. Plasma also carries substances that cells need to function. This includes food (proteins, fats, and carbohydrates), hormones (p. 110), and chemicals.

Red blood cells (RBCs) are called *erythrocytes.* They give blood its red color because of a substance in the cell called **hemoglobin.** As RBCs circulate through the lungs, hemoglobin picks up oxygen. Hemoglobin carries oxygen to the cells. When blood is bright red, hemoglobin in the RBCs is saturated (filled) with oxygen. As blood circulates through the body, oxygen is given to the cells. Cells release carbon dioxide (a waste product). It is picked up by the hemoglobin. RBCs saturated with carbon dioxide make the blood look dark red.

The body has about 25 trillion (25,000,000,000,000) RBCs. About 4½ to 5 million cells are in a cubic millimeter of blood (the size of a tiny drop). RBCs live for 3 or 4 months. They are destroyed by the liver and spleen as they wear out. New RBCs are formed in the bone marrow. About 1 million RBCs are produced every second.

White blood cells (WBCs) are called *leukocytes.* They have no color. They protect the body against infection. There are about 5,000 to 10,000 WBCs in a cubic millimeter of blood. At the first sign of infection, WBCs rush to the infection site. There they multiply rapidly. The number of WBCs increases when there is an infection. WBCs are formed by the bone marrow. They live about 9 days.

Platelets (thrombocytes) are needed for blood clotting. They are formed by the bone marrow. There are about 200,000 to 400,000 platelets in a cubic millimeter of blood. A platelet lives about 4 days.

The Heart

The heart is a muscle. It pumps blood through the blood vessels to the tissues and cells. The heart lies in the middle to lower part of the chest cavity toward the left side (Fig. 8-14). The heart is hollow and has three layers (Fig. 8-15):

▶ The *pericardium* is the outer layer. It is a thin sac covering the heart.

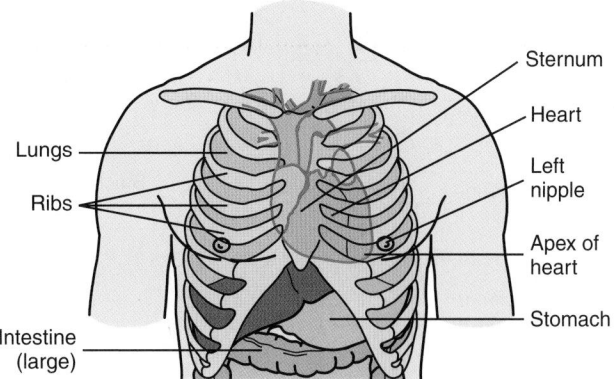

FIGURE 8-14 Location of the heart in the chest cavity.

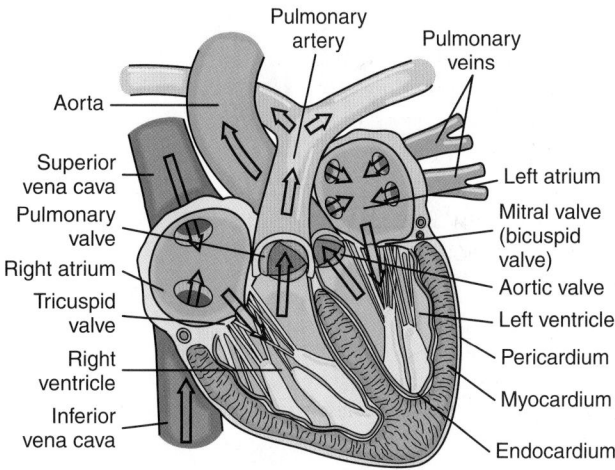

FIGURE 8-15 Structures of the heart.

▶ The *myocardium* is the second layer. It is the thick, muscular part of the heart.

▶ The *endocardium* is the inner layer. A membrane, it lines the inner surface of the heart.

The heart has four chambers (see Fig. 8-15). Upper chambers receive blood and are called *atria.* The *right atrium* receives blood from body tissues. The *left atrium* receives blood from the lungs. Lower chambers are called *ventricles.* Ventricles pump blood. The *right ventricle* pumps blood to the lungs for oxygen. The *left ventricle* pumps blood to all parts of the body.

Valves are between the atria and ventricles. The valves allow blood flow in one direction. They prevent blood from flowing back into the atria from the ventricles. The *tricuspid valve* is between the right atrium and the right ventricle. The *mitral valve (bicuspid valve)* is between the left atrium and left ventricle.

Heart action has two phases:

▶ *Diastole.* It is the resting phase. Heart chambers fill with blood.

▶ *Systole.* It is the working phase. The heart contracts. Blood is pumped through the blood vessels when the heart contracts.

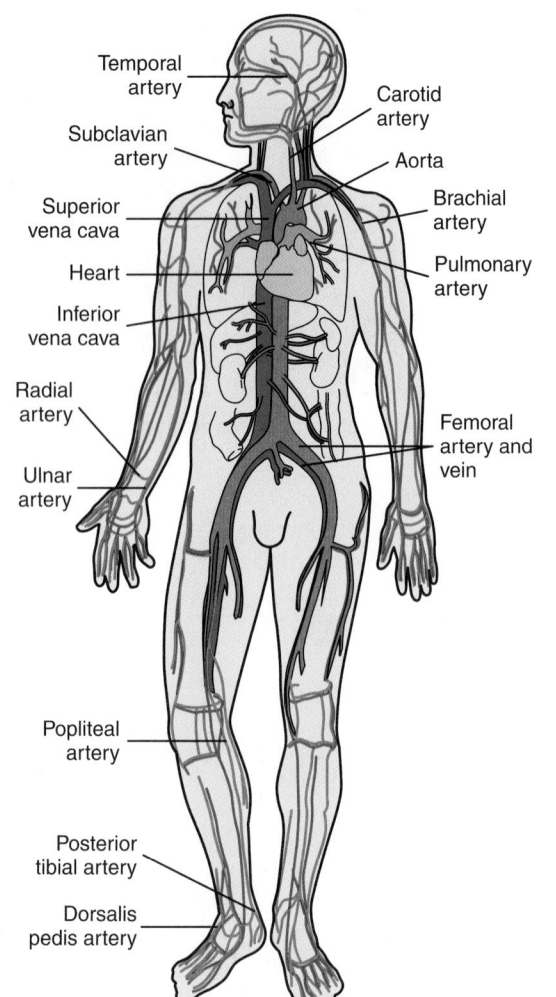

FIGURE 8-16 Arterial and venous systems. Arterial system is red. Venous system is blue.

The Blood Vessels

Blood flows to body tissues and cells through the blood vessels. There are three groups of blood vessels: arteries, capillaries, and veins.

Arteries carry blood away from the heart. Arterial blood is rich in oxygen. The *aorta* is the largest artery. It receives blood directly from the left ventricle. The aorta branches into other arteries that carry blood to all parts of the body (Fig. 8-16). These arteries branch into smaller parts within the tissues. The smallest branch of an artery is an *arteriole*.

Arterioles connect to **capillaries.** Capillaries are very tiny blood vessels. Food, oxygen, and other substances pass from capillaries into the cells. The capillaries pick up waste products (including carbon dioxide) from the cells. Veins carry waste products back to the heart.

Veins return blood to the heart. They connect to the capillaries by *venules.* Venules are small veins. Venules branch together to form veins. The many veins also branch together as they near the heart to form two main veins (see Fig. 8-16). The two main veins are the *inferior vena cava* and the *superior vena cava.* Both empty into the

right atrium. The inferior vena cava carries blood from the legs and trunk. The superior vena cava carries blood from the head and arms. Venous blood is dark red. It has little oxygen and a lot of carbon dioxide.

Blood flow through the circulatory system is shown in Fig. 8-15. The path of blood flow is as follows:

▶ Venous blood, poor in oxygen, empties into the right atrium.
▶ Blood flows through the tricuspid valve into the right ventricle.
▶ The right ventricle pumps blood into the lungs to pick up oxygen.
▶ Oxygen-rich blood from the lungs enters the left atrium.
▶ Blood from the left atrium passes through the mitral valve into the left ventricle.
▶ The left ventricle pumps the blood to the aorta. It branches off to form other arteries.
▶ Arterial blood is carried to the tissues by arterioles and to the cells by capillaries.
▶ Cells and capillaries exchange oxygen and nutrients for carbon dioxide and waste products.
▶ Capillaries connect with venules.
▶ Venules carry blood that has carbon dioxide and waste products.
▶ Venules form veins.
▶ Veins return blood to the heart.

THE RESPIRATORY SYSTEM

Oxygen is needed to live. Every cell needs oxygen. Air contains about 21% oxygen. This meets the body's needs under normal conditions. The respiratory system (Fig. 8-17) brings oxygen into the lungs and removes carbon dioxide. **Respiration** is the process of supplying the cells with oxygen and removing carbon dioxide from them. Respiration involves *inhalation* (breathing in) and *exhalation* (breathing out). The terms *inspiration* (breathing in) and *expiration* (breathing out) also are used.

Air enters the body through the *nose.* The air then passes into the *pharynx* (throat). It is a tube-shaped passageway for air and food. Air passes from the pharynx into the *larynx* (voice box). A piece of cartilage, the *epiglottis*, acts like a lid over the larynx. The epiglottis prevents food from entering the airway during swallowing. During inhalation the epiglottis lifts up to let air pass over the larynx. Air passes from the larynx into the *trachea* (windpipe).

The trachea divides at its lower end into the *right bronchus* and the *left bronchus.* Each bronchus enters a lung. Upon entering the lungs, the bronchi divide many times into smaller branches. The smaller branches are called *bronchioles.* Eventually the bronchioles subdivide. They end up in tiny, one-celled air sacs called *alveoli.*

Alveoli look like small clusters of grapes. They are supplied by capillaries. Oxygen and carbon dioxide are exchanged between the alveoli and capillaries. Blood in the capillaries picks up oxygen from the alveoli. Then the blood is returned to the left side of the heart and pumped

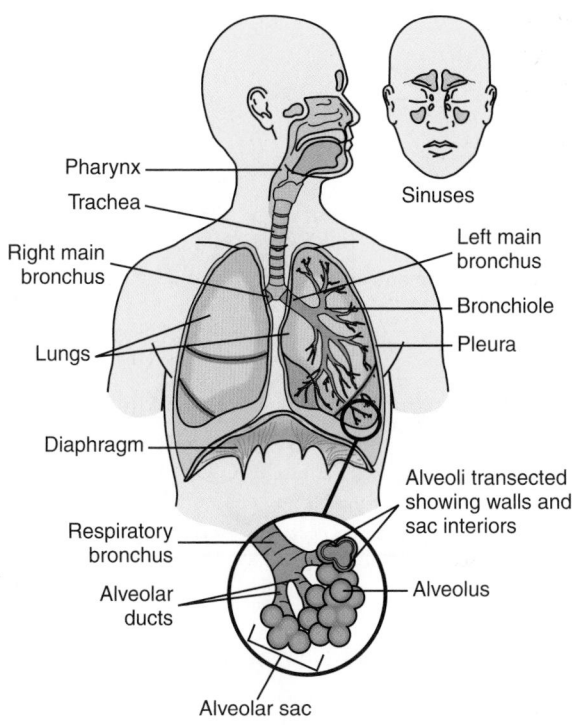

FIGURE 8-17 Respiratory system.

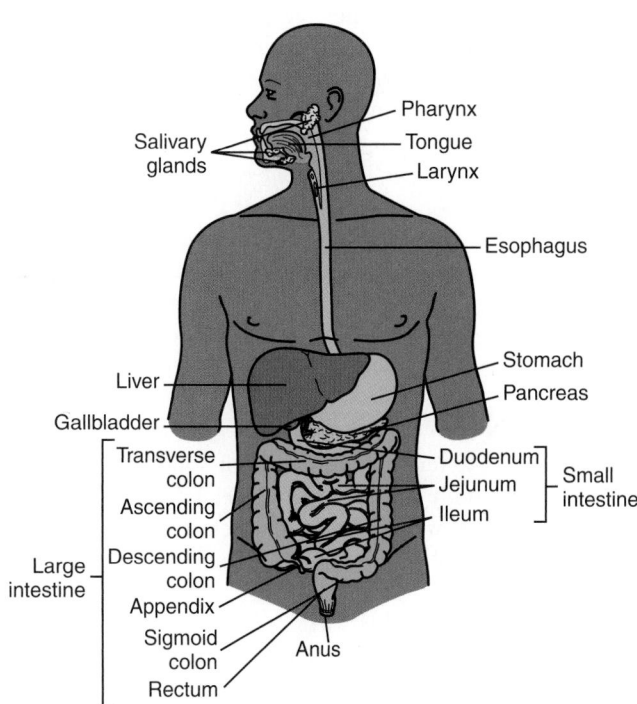

FIGURE 8-18 Digestive system.

to the rest of the body. Alveoli pick up carbon dioxide from the capillaries for exhalation.

The lungs are spongy tissues. They are filled with alveoli, blood vessels, and nerves. Each lung is divided into lobes. The right lung has three lobes; the left lung has two. The lungs are separated from the abdominal cavity by a muscle called the *diaphragm*.

Each lung is covered by a two-layered sac called the *pleura*. One layer is attached to the lung and the other to the chest wall. The pleura secretes a very thin fluid that fills the space between the layers. The fluid prevents the layers from rubbing together during inhalation and exhalation. A bony framework made up of the ribs, sternum, and vertebrae protects the lungs.

THE DIGESTIVE SYSTEM

The digestive system breaks down food physically and chemically so it can be absorbed for use by the cells. This process is called **digestion.** The digestive system is also called the *gastrointestinal (GI) system*. The system also removes solid wastes from the body.

The digestive system involves the *alimentary canal (GI tract)* and the accessory organs of digestion (Fig. 8-18). The alimentary canal is a long tube. It extends from the mouth to the anus. Its major parts are the mouth, pharynx, esophagus, stomach, small intestine, and large intestine. Accessory organs are the teeth, tongue, salivary glands, liver, gallbladder, and pancreas.

Digestion begins in the *mouth*. The mouth also is called the *oral cavity*. It receives food and prepares it for digestion. Using chewing motions, the *teeth* cut, chop,

and grind food into small particles for digestion and swallowing. The *tongue* aids in chewing and swallowing. Taste buds on the tongue's surface contain nerve endings. Taste buds allow sweet, sour, bitter, and salty tastes to be sensed. *Salivary glands* in the mouth secrete *saliva*. Saliva moistens food particles to ease swallowing and begin digestion. During swallowing, the tongue pushes food into the *pharynx*.

The pharynx (throat) is a muscular tube. Swallowing continues as the pharynx contracts. Contraction of the pharynx pushes food into the *esophagus*. The esophagus is a muscular tube about 10 inches long. It extends from the pharynx to the *stomach*. Involuntary muscle contractions called **peristalsis** move food down the esophagus through the alimentary canal.

The stomach is a muscular, pouch-like sac. It is in the upper left part of the abdominal cavity. Strong stomach muscles stir and churn food to break it up into even smaller particles. A mucous membrane lines the stomach. It contains glands that secrete *gastric juices*. Food is mixed and churned with the gastric juices to form a semi-liquid substance called *chyme*. Through peristalsis, the chyme is pushed from the stomach into the small intestine.

The *small intestine* is about 20 feet long. It has three parts. The first part is the *duodenum*. There more digestive juices are added to the chyme. One is called *bile*. Bile is a greenish liquid made in the *liver*. Bile is stored in the *gallbladder*. Juices from the *pancreas* and small intestine are added to the chyme. Digestive juices chemically break down food so it can be absorbed.

Peristalsis moves the chyme through the two other

parts of the small intestine: the *jejunum* and the *ileum*. Tiny projections called *villi* line the small intestine. Villi absorb the digested food into the capillaries. Most food absorption takes place in the jejunum and the ileum.

Some chyme is not digested. Undigested chyme passes from the small intestine into the *large intestine (large bowel* or *colon)*. The colon absorbs most of the water from the chyme. The remaining semi-solid material is called *feces*. Feces contain a small amount of water, solid wastes, and some mucus and germs. These are the waste products of digestion. Feces pass through the colon into the *rectum* by peristalsis. Feces pass out of the body through the *anus*.

THE URINARY SYSTEM

The digestive system rids the body of solid wastes. The lungs rid the body of carbon dioxide. Water and other substances are in sweat. There are other waste products in the blood from cells burning food for energy. The urinary system (Fig. 8-19):

▶ Removes waste products from the blood
▶ Maintains water balance within the body

The *kidneys* are two bean-shaped organs in the upper abdomen. They lie against the back muscles on each side of the spine. They are protected by the lower edge of the rib cage.

Each kidney has over a million tiny *nephrons* (Fig. 8-20). Each nephron is the basic working unit of the kidney. Each nephron has a *convoluted tubule*, which is a tiny coiled tubule. Each convoluted tubule has a *Bowman's capsule* at one end. The capsule partly surrounds a cluster

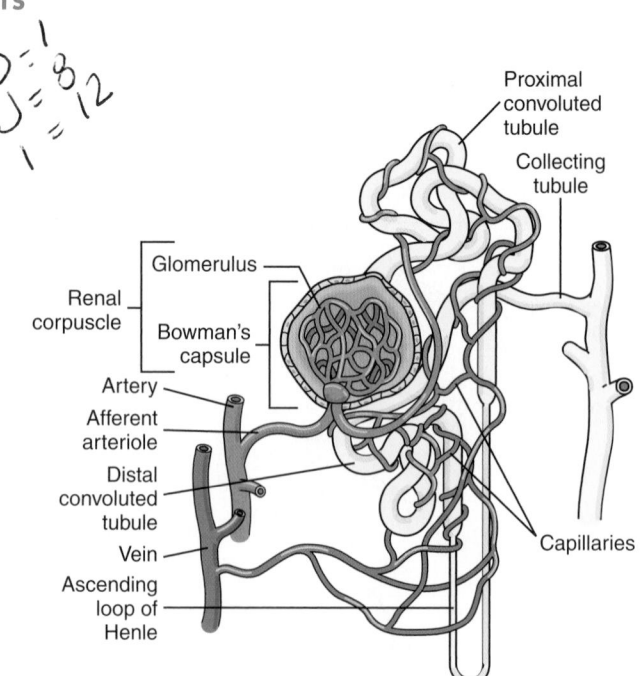

FIGURE 8-20 A nephron.

of capillaries called a *glomerulus*. Blood passes through the glomerulus and is filtered by the capillaries. The fluid part of the blood is squeezed into the Bowman's capsule. The fluid then passes into the tubule. Most of the water and other needed substances are reabsorbed by the blood. The rest of the fluid and the waste products form *urine* in the tubule. Urine flows through the tubule to a *collecting tubule*. All collecting tubules drain into the *renal pelvis* in the kidney.

A tube, called the *ureter*, is attached to the renal pelvis of the kidney. Each ureter is about 10 to 12 inches long. The ureters carry urine from the kidneys to the *bladder*. The bladder is a hollow, muscular sac. It lies toward the front in the lower part of the abdominal cavity.

Urine is stored in the bladder until the need to urinate is felt. This usually occurs when there is about a half pint (250 mL) of urine in the bladder. Urine passes from the bladder through the *urethra*. The opening at the end of the urethra is the *meatus*. Urine passes from the body through the meatus. Urine is a clear, yellowish fluid.

THE REPRODUCTIVE SYSTEM

Human reproduction results from the union of a male sex cell and a female sex cell. The male and female reproductive systems are different. This allows for the process of reproduction.

The Male Reproductive System

The male reproductive system is shown in Figure 8-21. The *testes (testicles)* are the male sex glands. Sex glands also are called *gonads*. The two testes are oval or almond-shaped glands. Male sex cells are produced in the testes. Male sex cells are called *sperm* cells.

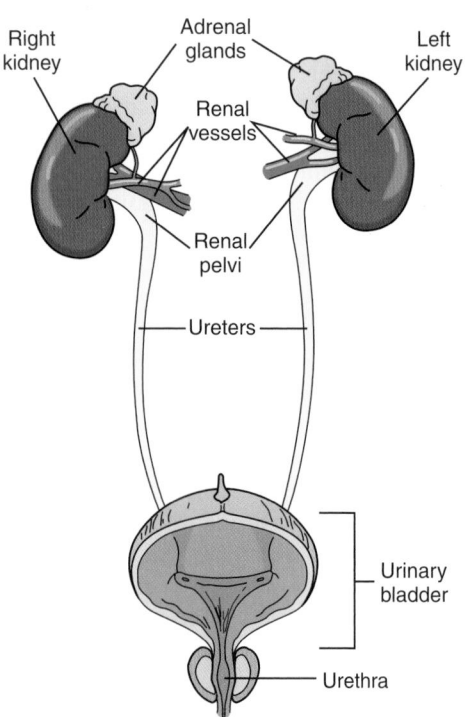

FIGURE 8-19 Urinary system.

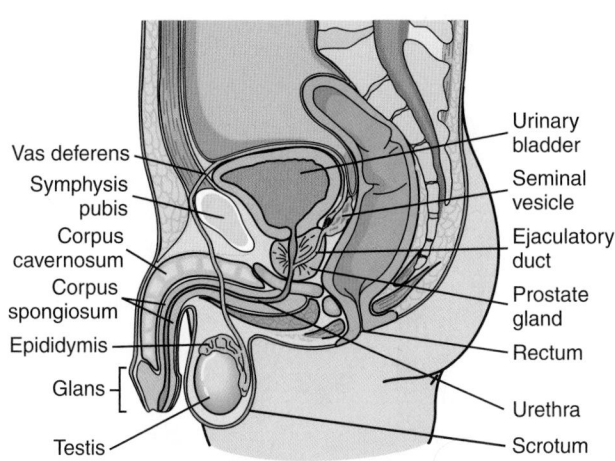

FIGURE 8-21 Male reproductive system.

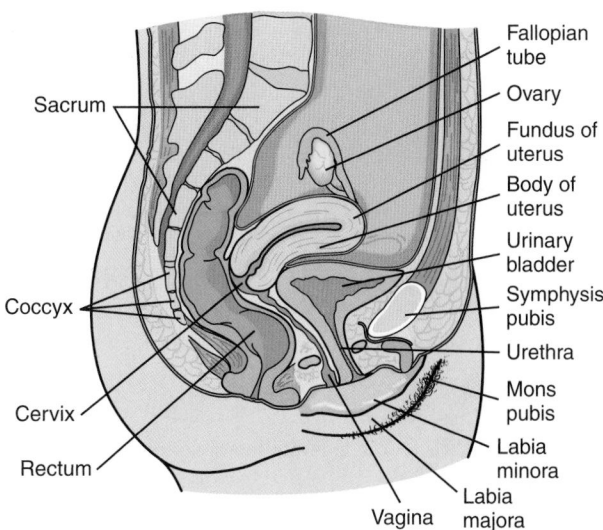

FIGURE 8-22 Female reproductive system.

Testosterone, the male hormone, is produced in the testes. This hormone is needed for reproductive organ function. It also is needed for the development of the male secondary sex characteristics. There is facial hair; pubic and axillary (underarm) hair; and hair on the arms, chest, and legs. Neck and shoulder sizes increase.

The testes are suspended between the thighs in a sac called the *scrotum*. The scrotum is made of skin and muscle.

Sperm travel from the testis to the *epididymis*. The epididymis is a coiled tube on top and to the side of the testis. From the epididymis, sperm travel through a tube called the *vas deferens*. Each vas deferens joins a seminal vesicle. The two seminal vesicles store sperm and produce *semen*. Semen is a fluid that carries sperm from the male reproductive tract. The ducts of the seminal vesicles unite to form the *ejaculatory duct*. It passes through the *prostate gland.*

The prostate gland lies just below the bladder. It is shaped like a donut. The gland secretes fluid into the semen. As the ejaculatory ducts leave the prostate, they join the *urethra*. The urethra runs through the prostate gland. The urethra is the outlet for urine and semen. The urethra is contained within the *penis*.

The penis is outside of the body and has *erectile* tissue. When a man is sexually excited, blood fills the erectile tissue. The penis enlarges and becomes hard and erect. The erect penis can enter a female's vagina. The semen, which contains sperm, is released into the vagina.

The Female Reproductive System

Figure 8-22 shows the female reproductive system. The female gonads are two almond-shaped glands called *ovaries*. An ovary is on each side of the uterus in the abdominal cavity.

The ovaries contain *ova* or eggs. Ova are the female sex cells. One ovum (egg) is released monthly during the woman's reproductive years. Release of an ovum is called *ovulation.*

The ovaries secrete the female hormones *estrogen* and *progesterone*. These hormones are needed for reproductive system function. They also are needed for the development of secondary sex characteristics in the female. These include increased breast size, pubic and axillary (underarm) hair, slight deepening of the voice, and widening and rounding of the hips.

When an ovum is released from an ovary, it travels through a *fallopian tube*. There are two fallopian tubes, one on each side. The tubes are attached at one end to the uterus. The ovum travels through the fallopian tube to the *uterus.*

The *uterus* is a hollow, muscular organ shaped like a pear. It is in the center of the pelvic cavity behind the bladder and in front of the rectum. The main part of the uterus is the *fundus*. The neck or narrow section of the uterus is the *cervix*. Tissue lining the uterus is called the *endometrium*. The endometrium has many blood vessels. If sex cells from the male and female unite into one cell, that cell implants into the endometrium. There the cell grows into a baby. The uterus serves as a place for the *fetus* (unborn baby) to grow and receive nourishment.

The cervix of the uterus projects into a muscular canal called the *vagina*. The vagina opens to the outside of the body. It is just behind the urethra. The vagina receives the penis during intercourse. It also is part of the birth canal. Glands in the vaginal wall keep it moistened with secretions. In young girls, the external vaginal opening is partially closed by a membrane called the *hymen*. The hymen ruptures when the female has intercourse for the first time.

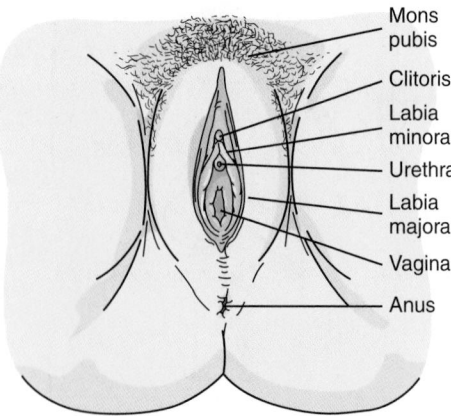

FIGURE 8-23 External female genitalia.

The external female genitalia are called the *vulva* (Fig. 8-23):
▶ The *mons pubis* is a rounded, fatty pad over a bone called the *symphysis pubis*. The mons pubis is covered with hair in the adult female.
▶ The *labia majora* and *labia minora* are two folds of tissue on each side of the vaginal opening.
▶ The *clitoris* is a small organ composed of erectile tissue. It becomes hard when sexually stimulated.

The *mammary glands (breasts)* secrete milk after childbirth. The glands are on the outside of the chest. They are made up of glandular tissue and fat (Fig. 8-24). The milk drains into ducts that open onto the *nipple*.

Menstruation

The endometrium is rich in blood to nourish the cell that grows into a fetus. If pregnancy does not occur, the endometrium breaks up. It is discharged from the body through the vagina. This process is called **menstruation**. Menstruation occurs about every 28 days. Therefore it is called the *menstrual cycle*.

The first day of the menstrual cycle begins with menstruation. Blood flows from the uterus through the vaginal opening. Menstrual flow usually lasts 3 to 7 days. Ovulation occurs during the next phase. An ovum matures in an ovary and is released. Ovulation usually occurs on or about day 14 of the cycle.

Meanwhile, estrogen and progesterone (the female hormones) are secreted by the ovaries. These hormones cause the endometrium to thicken for pregnancy. If pregnancy does not occur, the hormones decrease in amount. This causes the blood supply to the endometrium to decrease. The endometrium breaks up. It is discharged through the vagina. Another menstrual cycle begins.

Fertilization

To reproduce, a male sex cell (sperm) must unite with a female sex cell (ovum). The uniting of the sperm and ovum into one cell is called *fertilization*. A sperm has 23 chromosomes. An ovum has 23 chromosomes. When the two cells unite, the fertilized cell has 46 chromosomes.

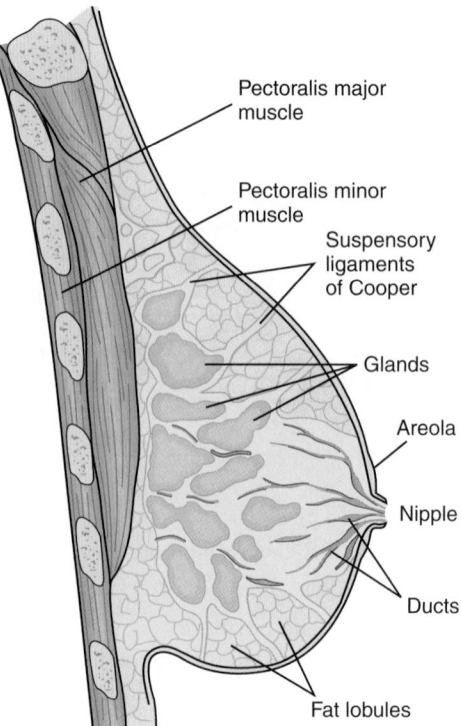

FIGURE 8-24 The female breast.

During intercourse, millions of sperm are deposited into the vagina. Sperm travel up the cervix, through the uterus, and into the fallopian tubes. If a sperm and an ovum unite in a fallopian tube, fertilization results. Pregnancy occurs. The fertilized cell travels down the fallopian tube to the uterus. After a short time, the fertilized cell implants in the thick endometrium and grows during pregnancy.

THE ENDOCRINE SYSTEM

The endocrine system is made up of glands called the *endocrine glands* (Fig. 8-25). The endocrine glands secrete chemical substances called **hormones** into the bloodstream. Hormones regulate the activities of other organs and glands in the body.

The *pituitary gland* is called the *master gland*. About the size of a cherry, it is at the base of the brain behind the eyes. The pituitary gland is divided into the *anterior pituitary lobe* and the *posterior pituitary lobe*. The anterior pituitary lobe secretes:
▶ *Growth hormone (GH)*—needed for growth of muscles, bones, and other organs. It is needed throughout life to maintain normal-size bones and muscles. Growth is stunted if a baby is born with deficient amounts of growth hormone. Too much of the hormone causes excessive growth.
▶ *Thyroid-stimulating hormone (TSH)*—needed for thyroid gland function.
▶ *Adrenocorticotropic hormone (ACTH)*—stimulates the adrenal gland.

The anterior lobe also secretes hormones that regulate growth, development, and function of the male and female reproductive systems.

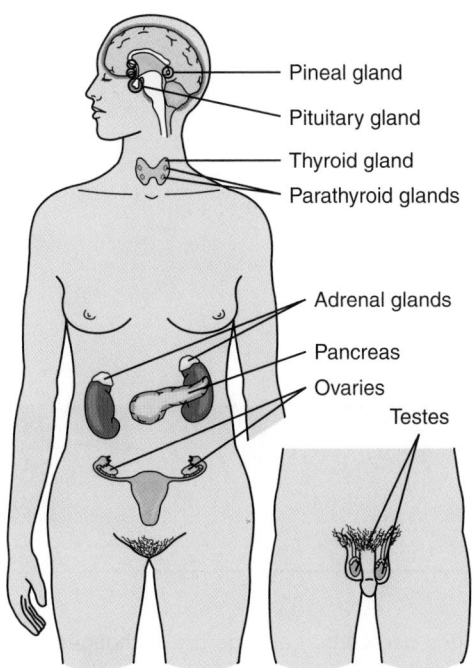

FIGURE 8-25 Endocrine system.

- Pineal gland
- Pituitary gland
- Thyroid gland
- Parathyroid glands
- Adrenal glands
- Pancreas
- Ovaries
- Testes

The posterior pituitary lobe secretes *antidiuretic hormone (ADH)* and *oxytocin.* ADH prevents the kidneys from excreting excessive amounts of water. Oxytocin causes uterine muscles to contract during childbirth.

The *thyroid gland,* shaped like a butterfly, is in the neck in front of the larynx. *Thyroid hormone (TH, thyroxine)* is secreted by the thyroid gland. It regulates **metabolism.** Metabolism is the burning of food for heat and energy by the cells. Too little TH results in slowed body processes, slowed movements, and weight gain. Too much TH causes increased metabolism, excess energy, and weight loss. Some babies are born with deficient amounts of TH. Their physical growth and mental growth are stunted.

The four *parathyroid glands* secrete *parathormone.* Two lie on each side of the thyroid gland. Parathormone regulates calcium use. Calcium is needed for nerve and muscle function. Insufficient amounts of calcium cause *tetany.* Tetany is a state of severe muscle contraction and spasm. If untreated, tetany can cause death.

There are two *adrenal glands.* An adrenal gland is on the top of each kidney. The adrenal gland has two parts: the *adrenal medulla* and the *adrenal cortex.* The adrenal medulla secretes *epinephrine* and *norepinephrine.* These hormones stimulate the body to quickly produce energy during emergencies. Heart rate, blood pressure, muscle power, and energy all increase.

The adrenal cortex secretes three groups of hormones needed for life:

- *Glucocorticoids*—regulate the metabolism of carbohydrates. They also control the body's response to stress and inflammation.
- *Mineralocorticoids*—regulate the amount of salt and water that is absorbed and lost by the kidneys.
- Small amounts of male and female sex hormones— p. 108.

The *pancreas* secretes *insulin.* Insulin regulates the amount of sugar in the blood available for use by the cells. Insulin is needed for sugar to enter the cells. If there is too little insulin, sugar cannot enter the cells. If sugar cannot enter the cells, excess amounts of sugar build up in the blood. This condition is called *diabetes.*

The *gonads* are the glands of human reproduction. Male sex glands (testes) secrete *testosterone.* Female sex glands (ovaries) secrete *estrogen* and *progesterone.*

THE IMMUNE SYSTEM

The immune system protects the body from disease and infection. Abnormal body cells can grow into tumors. Sometimes the body produces substances that cause the body to attack itself. Microorganisms (bacteria, viruses, and other germs) can cause an infection. The immune system defends against threats inside and outside the body.

The immune system gives the body **immunity.** Immunity means that a person has protection against a disease or condition. The person will not get or be affected by the disease:

- *Specific immunity* is the body's reaction to a certain threat.
- *Nonspecific immunity* is the body's reaction to anything it does not recognize as a normal body substance.

Special cells and substances function to produce immunity:

- *Antibodies*—normal body substances that recognize abnormal or unwanted substances. They attack and destroy such substances.
- *Antigens*—abnormal or unwanted substances. An antigen causes the body to produce antibodies. The antibodies attack and destroy the antigens.
- *Phagocytes*—white blood cells that digest and destroy microorganisms and other unwanted substances (Fig. 8-26, p. 112).
- *Lymphocytes*—white blood cells that produce antibodies. Lymphocyte production increases as the body responds to an infection.
- *B lymphocytes (B cells)*—cause the production of antibodies that circulate in the plasma. The antibodies react to specific antigens.
- *T lymphocytes (T cells)*—cells that destroy invading cells. *Killer T cells* produce poisons near the invading cells. Some T cells attract other cells. The other cells destroy the invaders.

When the body senses an antigen (an unwanted substance), the immune system acts. Phagocyte and lymphocyte production increases. Phagocytes destroy the invaders through digestion. The lymphocytes produce antibodies that attack and destroy the unwanted substances.

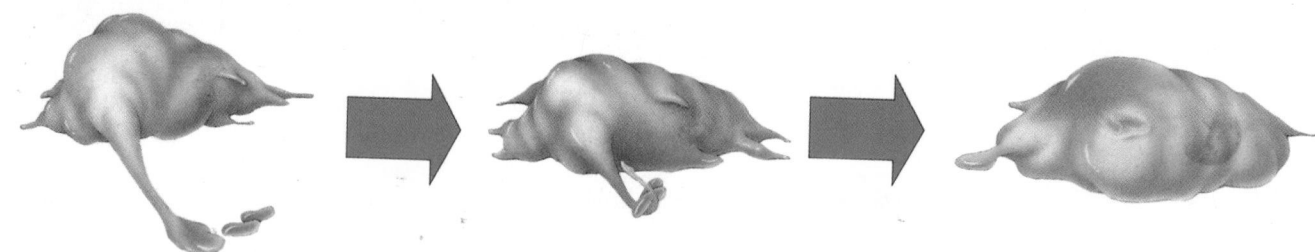

FIGURE 8-26 A phagocyte digests and destroys a microorganism. (From Thibodeau GA, Patton KT: *Structure and function of the body*, ed 11, St Louis, 2000, Mosby.)

REVIEW QUESTIONS

Circle the BEST answer.

1 The basic unit of body structure is the
   (a) Cell
   b Neuron
   c Nephron
   d Ovum

2 The outer layer of the skin is called the
   a Dermis
   (b) Epidermis
   c Integument
   d Myelin

3 Which is *not* a function of the skin?
   a Provides the protective covering for the body
   b Regulates body temperature
   c Senses cold, pain, touch, and pressure
   (d) Provides the shape and framework for the body

4 Which allows movement?
   a Bone marrow
   b Synovial membrane
   (c) Joints
   d Ligaments

5 Skeletal muscles
   a Are under involuntary control
   b Appear smooth
   (c) Are under voluntary control
   d Appear striped and smooth

6 The highest functions in the brain take place in the
   (a) Cerebral cortex
   b Medulla
   c Brainstem
   d Spinal nerves

7 The ear is involved with
   a Regulating body movements
   (b) Balance
   c Smoothness of body movements
   d Controlling involuntary muscles

8 The liquid part of the blood is the
   a Hemoglobin
   b Red blood cell
   (c) Plasma
   d White blood cell

9 Which part of the heart pumps blood to the body?
   a Right atrium
   b Left atrium
   c Right ventricle
   (d) Left ventricle

10 Which carry blood away from the heart?
   a Capillaries
   b Veins
   c Venules
   (d) Arteries

11 Oxygen and carbon dioxide are exchanged
   a In the bronchi
   (b) Between the alveoli and capillaries
   c Between the lungs and pleura
   d In the trachea

12 Digestion begins in the
   (a) Mouth
   b Stomach
   c Small intestine
   d Colon

13 Most food absorption takes place in the
   a Stomach
   (b) Small intestine
   c Colon
   d Large intestine

14 Urine is formed by the
   a Jejunum
   (b) Kidneys
   c Bladder
   d Liver

15 Urine passes from the body through the
   a Ureters
   (b) Urethra
   c Anus
   d Nephrons

16 The male sex gland is called the
   a Penis
   b Semen
   (c) Testis
   d Scrotum

17 The male sex cell is the
   a Semen
   b Ovum
   c Gonad
   (d) Sperm

18 The female sex gland is the
   (a) Ovary
   b Cervix
   c Uterus
   d Vagina

19 The discharge of the lining of the uterus is called
   a The endometrium
   b Ovulation
   c Fertilization
   (d) Menstruation

20 The endocrine glands secrete
   (a) Hormones
   b Mucus
   c Semen
   d Insulin

21 The immune system protects the body from
   a Low blood sugar
   (b) Disease and infection
   c Loss of fluid
   d Stunted growth

Answers for these questions are on p. 779.

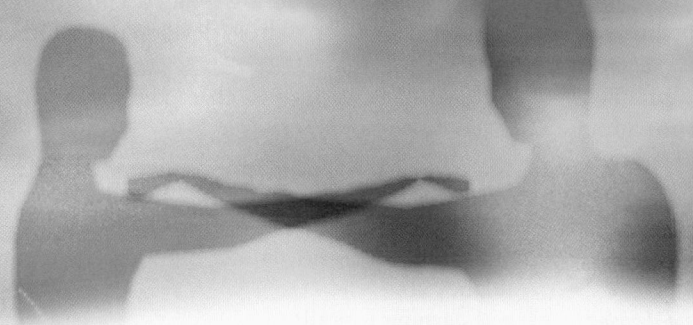

Growth and Development

OBJECTIVES

- Define the key terms listed in this chapter
- Explain the principles of growth and development
- Identify the stages of growth and development
- Identify the developmental tasks for each age-group
- Describe the normal growth and development for each age-group

KEY TERMS

adolescence The time between puberty and adulthood; a time of rapid growth and physical, sexual, emotional, and social changes

development Changes in mental, emotional, and social function

developmental task A skill that must be completed during a stage of development

ejaculation The release of semen

growth The physical changes that are measured and that occur in a steady, orderly manner

infancy The first year of life

menarche The first menstruation and the start of menstrual cycles

menopause The time when menstruation stops and menstrual cycles end

peer Persons of the same age-group and background

primary caregiver The person mainly responsible for providing or assisting with the child's basic needs

puberty The period when reproductive organs begin to function and secondary sex characteristics appear

reflex An involuntary movement

sexual orientation Sexual arousal or romantic attraction to persons of the other gender (heterosexual), the same gender (homosexual), or both genders (bisexual)

Y ou care for people of all ages. They are in different stages of growth and development. An understanding of growth and development helps you give better care. The person's needs are easier to understand. This chapter presents the basic changes that occur in normal, healthy persons from birth until death.

Growth and development are presented in stages. Age ranges and normal characteristics are given for each stage. The stages overlap. It is hard to see the start and end of each stage. Also, the rate of growth and development varies with each person.

Growth and development theories usually involve the two-parent family. However, single-parent households are common. A relative may care for children while the parent works or is in school. In this chapter *primary caregiver* is used in place of *mother* or *father*. The **primary caregiver** is the person mainly responsible for providing or assisting with the child's basic needs. A mother, father, grandparent, aunt, uncle, or court-appointed guardian may have this role. *Parent* and *parents* are sometimes used here. However, another primary caregiver may have the parent role.

Age ranges for each stage vary among growth and development experts. The groupings and content in this chapter are broad and general.

PRINCIPLES

Growth is the physical changes that are measured and that occur in a steady and orderly manner. Growth is measured in weight and height. Changes in appearance and body functions also measure growth.

Development relates to changes in mental, emotional, and social function. A person behaves and thinks in certain ways in each stage of development. A 2-year-old thinks in simple terms. A primary caregiver is needed for basic needs. A 40-year-old thinks in complex ways. Most basic needs are met without help.

The entire person is affected. Although they differ, growth and development:

- Overlap
- Depend on each other
- Occur at the same time

For example, an infant cannot coo or babble (development) until the physical structures for speech are strong enough (growth). Basic principles of growth and development are:

- The process starts at fertilization and continues until death.
- The process proceeds from the simple to the complex. A baby sits before standing, stands before walking, and walks before running.

- The process occurs in certain directions:
  - From head to foot. Babies hold up their heads before they sit; they sit before they stand.
  - From the center of the body outward. Babies control shoulder movements before they control hand movements.
- The process occurs in a sequence, order, and pattern. Certain skills must be completed during each stage. A **developmental task** is a skill that must be completed during a stage of development. A stage cannot be skipped. Each stage is the basis for the next stage.
- The rate of the process is uneven. It is not at a set pace. Growth is rapid during infancy. Children have growth spurts. Some children develop fast. Others develop slowly.
- Each stage has its own characteristics and developmental tasks.

INFANCY (BIRTH TO 1 YEAR)

Infancy is the first year of life. Growth and development are rapid during this time. The developmental tasks of infancy are:

- Learning to walk
- Learning to eat solid foods
- Beginning to talk and communicate with others
- Learning to trust
- Beginning to have emotional relationships with parents, brothers, and sisters
- Developing stable sleep and feeding patterns

The Newborn (Birth to 1 Month)

The neonatal period of infancy is from birth to 1 month. A baby is called a neonate or newborn at this time.

The average newborn weighs 6 to 9 pounds. Birth weight doubles by 5 to 6 months of age. At 6 months, the baby weighs an average of 16 pounds. Birth weight triples by 1 year of age. The average weight of a 1-year-old is 21½ pounds.

The average newborn is 19 to 21 inches long. Length increases in spurts. At 6 months, the average length is 25½ inches. The average 1-year-old is 29 inches.

The newborn's head is large compared with the rest of the body. The trunk is long. The abdomen is large, round, and soft. The newborn has fat, pudgy cheeks, a flat nose and a receding chin (Fig. 9-1).

The skin is smooth. It is bright red at birth in light-skinned babies but turns to pink a few days later. Dark-skinned newborns may appear pinkish to yellowish brown. The skin turns to its natural color in a few days. Eyes are a deep blue in light-skinned babies. Dark-skinned babies have brown eyes.

The central nervous system is not well developed in newborns. Movements are uncoordinated and lack purpose. Newborns can see clearly up to about 8 inches. They see in color. They prefer yellow, green, and pink

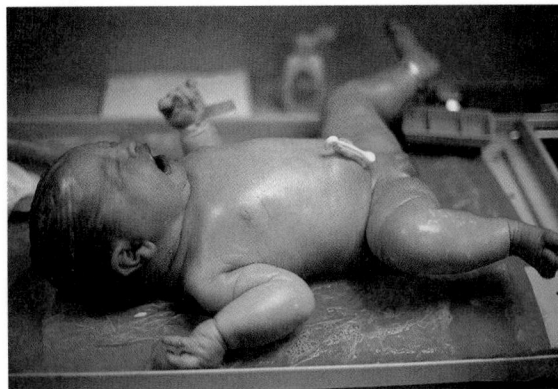

FIGURE 9-1 A newborn.

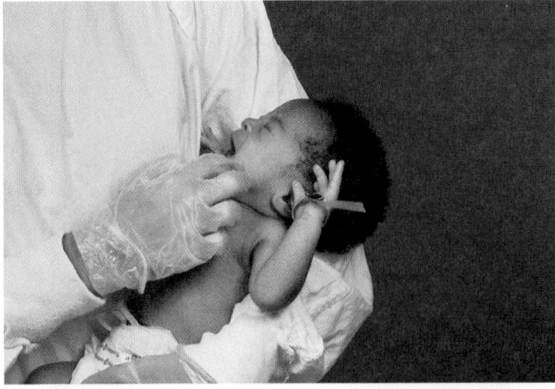

FIGURE 9-3 Rooting reflex. (From Seidel HM and others: *Mosby's guide to physical examination*, ed 3, St Louis, 1995, Mosby.)

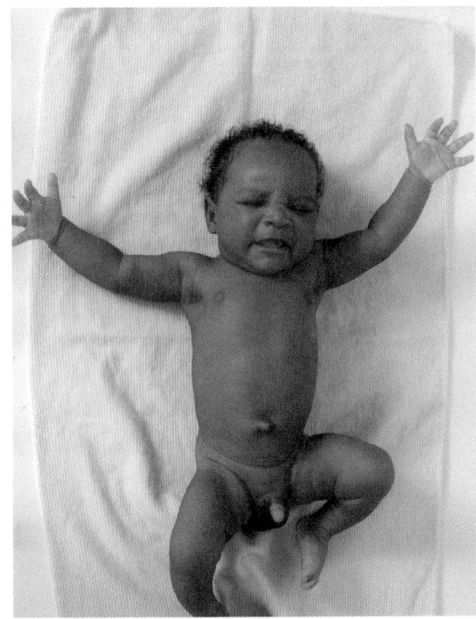

FIGURE 9-2 Moro reflex. (Courtesy Paul Vincent Kuntz, Texas Children's Hospital, as found in Hockenberry MJ and Wilson D: *Wong's nursing care of infants and children*, ed 8, St Louis, 2007, Mosby.)

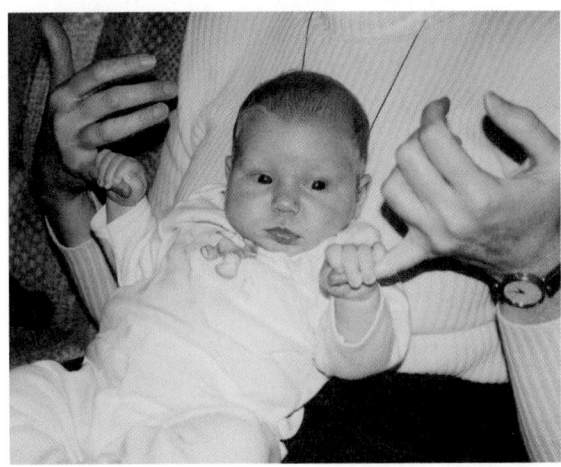

FIGURE 9-4 The grasp reflex.

colors. Newborns hear well. Loud sounds startle them. Soft sounds soothe them. They know the mother's voice. They react to touch and pain. They can taste and smell.

Newborns have certain **reflexes** (involuntary movements). These reflexes decline and then disappear as the central nervous system develops.

▶ *Moro reflex (startle reflex)*—occurs when a baby is startled by a loud noise, a sudden movement, or the head falling back. The arms are thrown apart. The legs extend and then flex. A brief cry is common. See Figure 9-2.

▶ *Rooting reflex*—occurs when the cheek is touched near the mouth. The mouth opens, and the head turns toward the touch. The rooting reflex is necessary for feeding. It guides the baby's mouth to the nipple. See Figure 9-3.

▶ *Sucking reflex*—occurs when the lips are touched.

▶ *Grasp (palmar) reflex*—occurs when the palm is stroked. The fingers close firmly around the object (Fig. 9-4).

▶ *Step (dance) reflex*—occurs when the baby is held upright and the feet touch a surface. The feet move up and down and in stepping motions (Fig. 9-5, p. 116).

Specific, voluntary, and coordinated movements occur as the nervous and muscular systems develop. Newborns cannot hold their heads up. They turn their heads from side to side.

Newborns sleep 16 to 18 hours a day. They awaken when hungry and fall asleep right after a feeding. Bottle-fed infants feed every 2½ to 4 hours. Breast-fed infants are hungry more often—every 2 to 3 hours. The time between feedings lengthens as infants grow and develop. They also stay awake more and sleep less.

Infants (1 Month to 1 Year)

When lying on their stomachs, 1-month-old infants can lift their heads up briefly (Fig. 9-6, p. 116). They also can turn their heads. They smile.

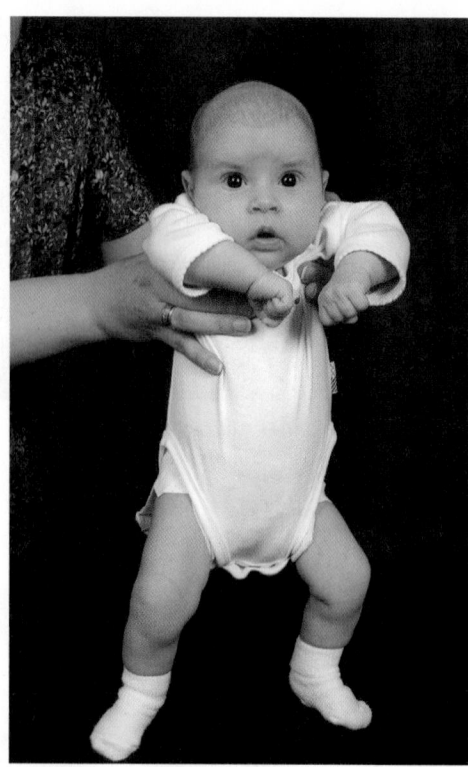

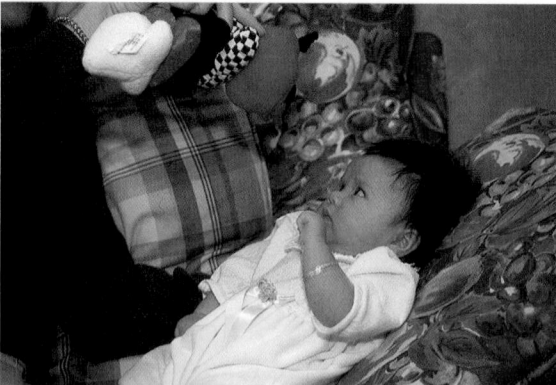

FIGURE 9-7 A 2-month-old child follows an object with her eyes.

FIGURE 9-5 Step (dance) reflex. (Courtesy Paul Vincent Kuntz, Texas Children's Hospital, as found in Hockenberry MJ and Wilson D: *Wong's nursing care of infants and children*, ed 8, St Louis, 2007, Mosby.)

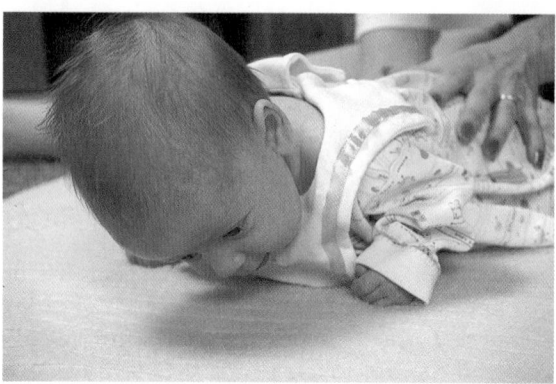

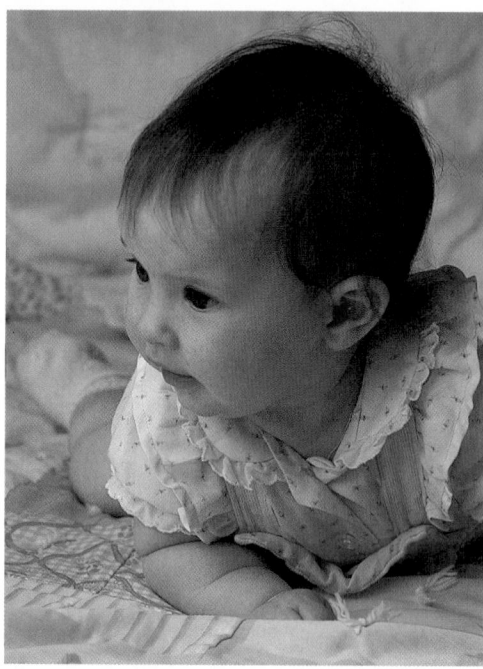

FIGURE 9-8 The 3-month-old child can raise the head and shoulders.

FIGURE 9-6 The 1-month-old can briefly lift her head when lying on her stomach.

Two-month-old infants can hold their heads up when held upright. When on their stomachs, they can turn their heads from side to side. They need support to sit in an angled position. They have tears and can follow objects with their eyes (Fig. 9-7). They smile when responding to others.

Infants 3 to 4 months of age can hold their heads up (Fig. 9-8). They reach for objects. Pleasure causes squealing. They babble, coo, gurgle, and laugh out loud. The Moro, rooting, and grasp reflexes disappear.

By 4 to 5 months, infants can roll from front to back. They roll from back to front by 5 to 6 months. They also can sit by leaning forward on their hands (Fig. 9-9). Teething may begin with the bottom front teeth. They sleep all night. They can play "peak-a-boo."

Solid foods are given at 4 to 6 months. Rice cereal mixed with milk is given first. It is given with an infant spoon. Fruits, vegetables, and meats are introduced slowly. These foods are thin in consistency at first. Thicker and chunkier foods are given as more teeth erupt and chewing and swallowing skills increase.

Infants have more skills at 6 months. They can bear weight when pulled up into a standing position. They sit with support and move around by rolling. Some start to drink from a cup. They smile at themselves in a mirror. They respond to their names.

Some infants start to crawl at 7 months. They can stand while holding on for support. They make sounds in response to caregivers.

Eight-month-old infants can sit for long periods. They also can change from lying to sitting and from sitting to lying positions. The pincer grasp develops—they can hold

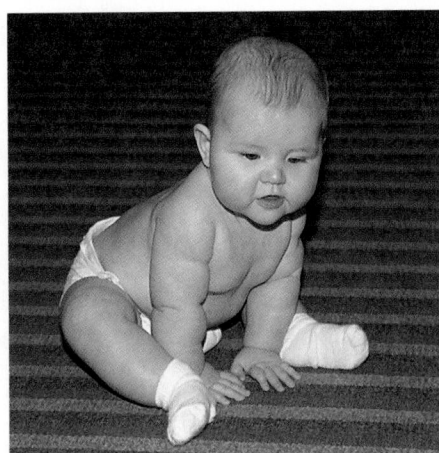

FIGURE 9-9 A 6-month-old sits forward leaning on the hands. (From James SR, Ashwill JW, Droske SC: *Nursing care of children: principles and practices,* ed 3, St Louis, 2007, Mosby.)

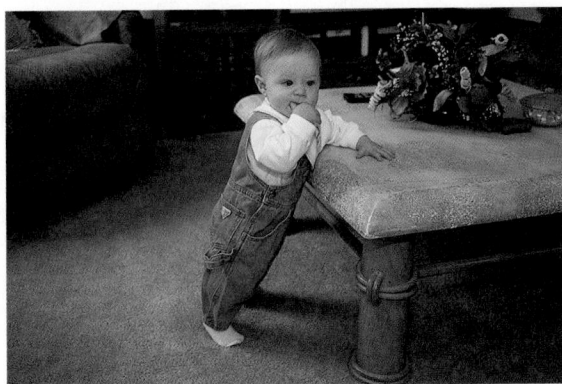

FIGURE 9-10 A 10-month-old infant can walk while holding onto furniture.

small objects with the thumb and index finger. They can pick up small finger foods. They learn to drink from a cup with handles. Language skills increase. They can say "mama" and "dada."

When holding onto something, 9-month-olds can pull up into a standing position. They can hold a bottle, play "pat-a-cake," and drink from a cup or glass. They understand their names and "no." They point and use gestures to communicate.

At 10 months, infants can stand alone. They may walk with help or while holding onto something (Fig. 9-10). They also may climb up and down stairs. At 11 months, they may walk alone and use push toys.

At 12 months, walking skills increase. They can climb onto furniture. They can turn book pages and put objects into a container. They can say a few words. Bottle weaning may begin.

The infant must develop a sense of trust. If successful, the infant trusts himself or herself and others. Trust develops when care is consistent. The infant's physical and safety needs are met—feeding, comfort, warmth, touch, stimulation, and caring.

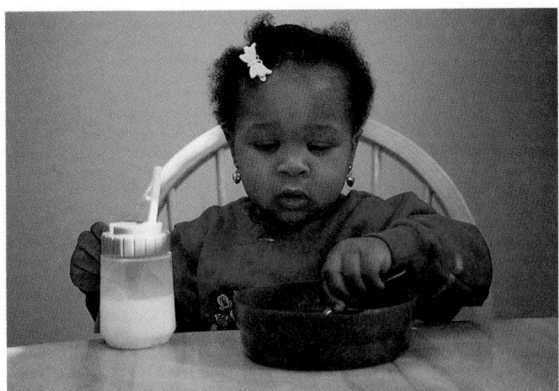

FIGURE 9-11 A toddler uses a spoon.

TODDLERHOOD (1 TO 3 YEARS)

Growth rate is slower than during infancy. Developmental tasks during this period are:

▶ Tolerating separation from the primary caregiver
▶ Gaining control of bowel and bladder function
▶ Using words to communicate
▶ Becoming less dependent on the primary caregiver

Toddlers need to assert independence. Therefore this time is called the "terrible twos." Toddlers learn to walk well. They are curious. They get into everything and anything. They touch, smell, and taste everything within reach. They climb on tables, chairs, counters, and other high places. With these new skills, toddlers can explore their environments. They venture farther away from primary caregivers. They learn to do some things without a primary caregiver. By the age of 3, they can run, jump, climb, ride a tricycle, and walk up and down stairs.

Hand coordination increases. They learn to feed themselves. They progress from eating with fingers to using a spoon (Fig. 9-11). Toddlers can drink from cups. They can scribble, build towers with blocks, and string beads. Right- or left-handedness is seen during the second year.

Toilet training is a major task for toddlers. Bowel and bladder control is related to central nervous system development. Children must be mentally and physically ready for toilet training. Some children are ready at age 2 years. Others are ready at 2½ to 3 years of age. The process starts with bowel control. Bladder control during the day occurs before bladder control at night.

Speech and language skills increase. Speech is clearer. Toddlers learn words by imitating others. They understand more words than they say. An 18-month-old knows 6 to 18 words. By age 2 years, the child knows about 300 words. "Me" and "mine" are used often.

Play skills increase. The child plays alongside other children but not with them. Toddlers do not share toys. They are very possessive and do not understand sharing.

Temper tantrums and saying "no" are common during this stage. Toddlers express anger and frustration by kicking and screaming. That is how they object to having independence challenged. Using "no" can frustrate primary caregivers. Almost every request may be answered "no," even if the child is following the request.

Another task is tolerating separation from the primary caregiver. As toddlers start to explore, they move away from the primary caregiver. With discomfort, frustration, or injury, they quickly return to primary caregivers or cry for their attention. If primary caregivers are consistently present when needed, children learn to feel secure. They learn to tolerate brief periods of separation.

PRESCHOOL (3 TO 6 YEARS)

The preschool years are from the ages of 3 to 6 years. Children grow 2 to 3 inches per year. They gain about 5 pounds per year. Preschoolers are thinner, more coordinated, and more graceful than toddlers.

Developmental tasks of the preschool years include:

▶ Increasing the ability to communicate and understand others
▶ Performing self-care
▶ Learning gender differences and developing sexual modesty
▶ Learning right from wrong and good from bad
▶ Learning to play with others
▶ Developing family relationships

The 3-Year-Old

Three-year-olds become more coordinated. They can walk on tiptoe, balance on one foot for a few seconds, and run, jump, kick a ball, and climb with ease.

Personal care skills increase. They can put on clothes and shoes, manage buttons, wash their hands, and brush their teeth (Fig. 9-12). They can feed themselves, pour from a bottle, and help set the table without breaking dishes. Hand skills also include drawing circles and crosses.

Language skills increase. Three-year-olds know about 900 words. They talk and ask questions ("how" and "why") constantly. They can name body parts, family members, and friends. They like talking toys and musical toys.

Play is important. They play with 2 or 3 other children and can share. They play simple games and learn simple rules. Imaginary friends and imitating adults are common. They enjoy crayons, cutting paper, pasting, painting, and

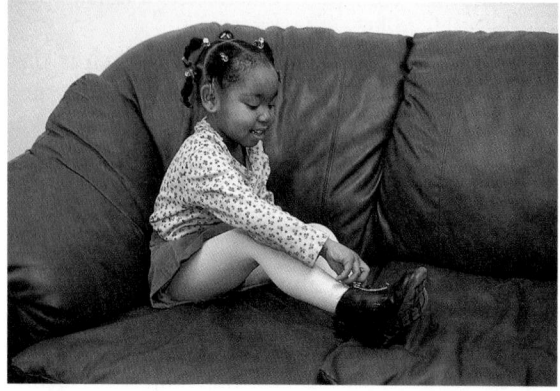

FIGURE 9-12 A 3-year-old has increased coordination.

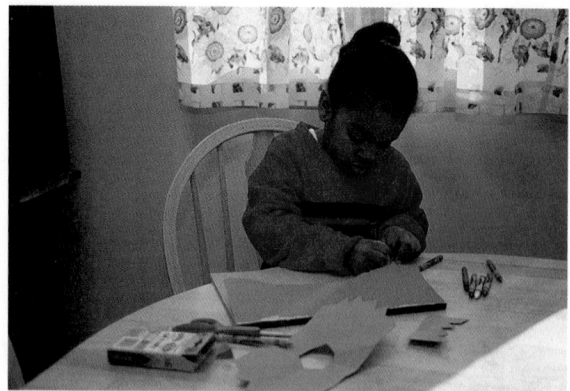

FIGURE 9-13 This 3-year-old enjoys cutting paper.

playing "house" and "dress-up" (Fig. 9-13). They also like wagons, tricycles, and other riding toys.

Three-year-olds know that there are two sexes. They know that male and female bodies differ. They also know their own sex. Little girls may wonder how the penis works and why they do not have one. Little boys may wonder how girls can urinate without a penis.

The concept of time develops. Three-year-olds may speak of the past, present, and future. "Yesterday" and "tomorrow" are confusing. Children may fear the dark and need night-lights in bedrooms. Nightmares are common.

Three-year-olds are less fearful of strangers. They can be away from primary caregivers for short periods. They are less jealous than toddlers of a new baby. They try to please primary caregivers.

The 4-Year-Old

Four-year-olds can hop, skip, and throw and catch a ball. They can lace shoes, draw faces, and copy a square. They try to print letters. With help, they can bathe and tend to toileting needs.

They know about 1500 words. They continue to ask many questions and tend to exaggerate stories. They can sing simple songs, repeat four numbers, count to five, and name a few colors.

Four-year-olds tend to tease, tattle, and tell fibs. When bad, they may blame an imaginary friend. Bragging, telling tales about family members, and showing off are common. They can play with other children. They are proud of accomplishments but have mood swings.

These children enjoy playing "dress-up," wearing costumes, and telling and hearing stories. They like to draw and make things. Imagination, drama, and imitating adults are part of play. They play in groups of two or three and tend to be bossy. Playing "doctor and nurse" is common as curiosity about the other sex continues (Fig. 9-14).

Four-year-olds prefer the primary caregiver of the other sex. Rivalries with brothers and sisters are seen, especially when a younger child takes the 4-year-old's things. Rivalries also occur when older children have more and different privileges. The family is often the focus of the child's frustrations and aggressive behavior. A 4-year-old may try to run away from home.

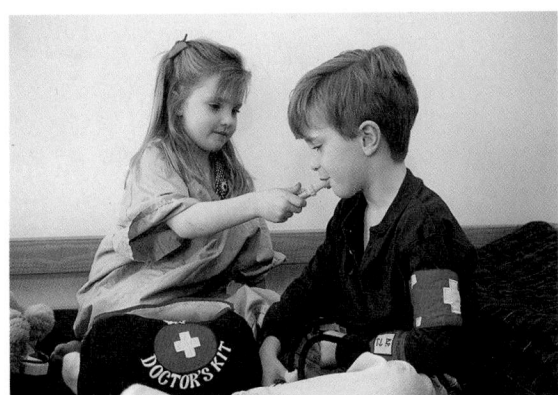

FIGURE 9-14 Four-year-olds play "doctor and nurse."

The 5-Year-Old

Coordination increases. Five-year-olds can jump rope, skate, tie shoelaces, dress, and bathe. They can use a pencil well and copy diamond and triangle shapes. They can print a few letters, numbers, and their first names. Drawings of people include body parts.

Communication skills increase. They speak in full sentences. Questions are fewer than before but have more meaning. They want words defined and take part in conversations. They can name colors, coins, days, and the months. They specify and describe drawings.

Five-year-olds are more responsible and truthful. They quarrel less than before. They are more aware of rules and are eager to do things correctly. They have manners, are independent, and can be trusted within limits. Fears are fewer, but nightmares and dreams are common. They are proud of accomplishments.

These children like books about animals and other children. They like board games and try to follow rules. They imitate adults during play and are interested in TV.

They also enjoy doing things with the primary caregiver of the same sex (Fig. 9-15). These include cooking, housekeeping, shopping, yard work, and sports.

Younger children are considered a nuisance. However, 5-year-olds usually protect them. They tolerate brothers and sisters well.

SCHOOL AGE (6 TO 9 OR 10 YEARS)

School-age children enter the world of peer groups, games, and learning. They grow 2 to 3 inches a year. They gain 4½ to 6½ pounds a year. Their developmental tasks are:

- Developing the social and physical skills needed for playing games
- Learning to get along with children of the same age and background (peers)
- Learning gender-appropriate behaviors and attitudes
- Learning basic reading, writing, and arithmetic skills
- Developing a conscience and morals
- Developing a good feeling and attitude about oneself

Baby teeth are lost. This starts at around age 6 years. Permanent teeth erupt.

Children are very active. They can run, jump, skip, hop, and ride a two-wheeled bike. They can swim, skate, dance, and jump rope. These children can take part in team sports. Soccer, T-ball, baseball, football, and volleyball are examples (Fig. 9-16, p. 120). Children learn to play in groups. They learn teamwork and sportsmanship and follow rules. Quiet play involves collections, board games, computer games, and crafts.

Language skills increase rapidly. Reading, writing, grammar, and math skills develop. They learn to print first. Printing is followed by cursive writing. Sentences are longer and more complex. As reading skills increase, so do language skills. Children like to read and be read to.

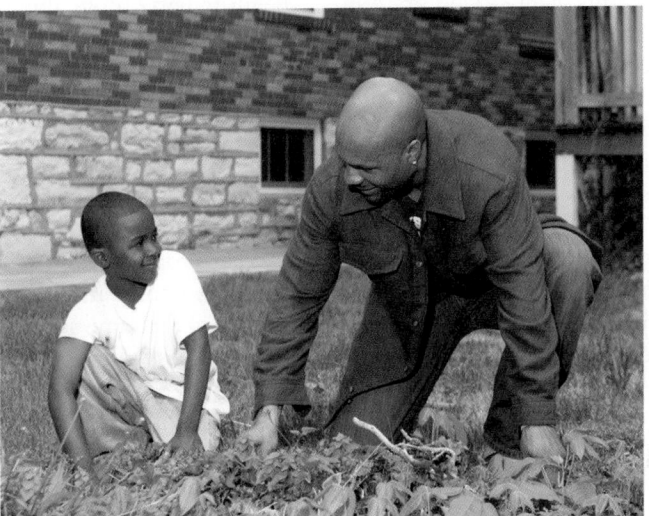

FIGURE 9-15 This 5-year-old does yard work with his father.

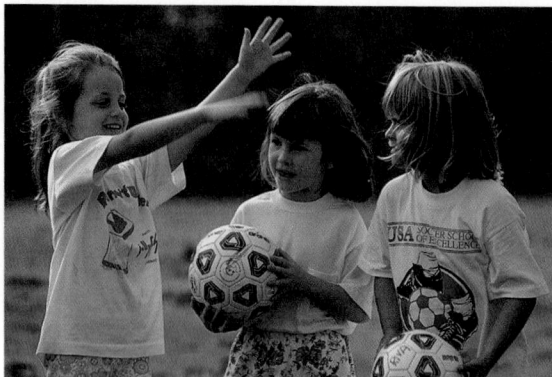

FIGURE 9-16 These 6-year-old girls enjoy soccer.

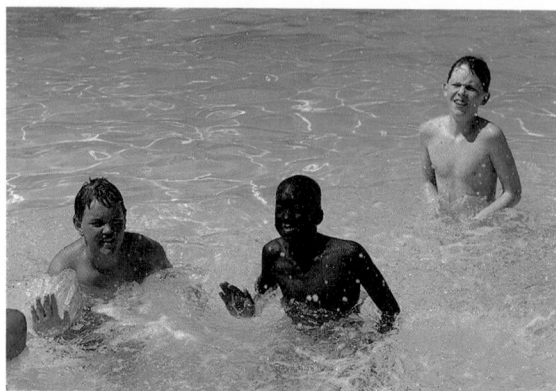

FIGURE 9-17 Belonging to a peer group is important to school-age children.

Play activities have purpose and involve "work." Children in this age-group like household tasks (cleaning, cooking, yard work). They also like crafts, building things, and scout groups. Rewards are important—good grades, trophies, payment for chores, scouting badges.

At about age 7, boys prefer playing with boys. Girls prefer playing with girls. From 8 to 9 years, they continue to play with children of their own sex. There is some play that involves boys and girls. Interest in boy-girl relationships starts at about 8 to 9 years. However, children may deny such interest.

School-age children are concerned about being well liked. A peer group is important for love, belonging, and self-esteem needs. These children get along well with and need adults. However, they prefer peer group fads, opinions, and activities (Fig. 9-17).

LATE CHILDHOOD (9 TO 10 or 12 YEARS)

Late childhood (pre-adolescence) is the time between childhood and adolescence. Developmental tasks are like

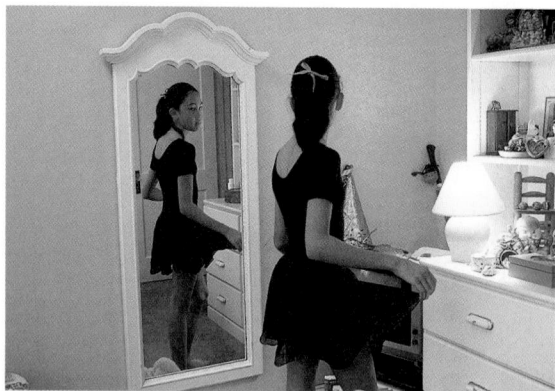

FIGURE 9-18 Movements are smooth and graceful in late childhood.

those for school-age children. Pre-adolescents are expected to show more refinement and maturity in achieving these tasks:

- Becoming independent of adults and learning to depend on oneself
- Developing and keeping friendships with peers
- Understanding the physical, psychological, and social roles of one's sex
- Developing moral and ethical behavior
- Developing greater muscular strength, coordination, and balance
- Learning how to study

Many permanent teeth erupt. Girls have a growth spurt. By age 12 years, they are taller and heavier than boys. Both boys and girls have more graceful and coordinated body movements (Fig. 9-18). Muscle strength and physical skills increase. Skill in team sports is important.

Math and language skills increase. These children read to find information and for pleasure. They read the news. They enjoy books and stories about romance, mystery, adventure, and science fiction.

The onset of puberty nears. **Puberty** is the period when reproductive organs begin to function and secondary sex characteristics appear. In girls, the hips widen and breast buds appear; some 9-, 10-, and 11-year-old girls begin puberty. Boys show fewer signs of maturing sexually. Genital organs begin to grow.

These children need factual sex education. Friends share information about sex. It is often not complete and not accurate. Parents and children may be uncomfortable discussing sex with each other. They may avoid the subject. When children ask questions, answers must be honest and complete and in terms that children understand.

Peer groups are the center of activities. The group affects the child's attitudes and behavior. Children prefer friends of the same sex. Friends are loyal and share problems. A "best friend" is common. Interest in the opposite sex begins.

These children are aware of the mistakes and faults of adults. They do not accept adult standards and rules without question. It is common to rebel against adults and test limits. Parents and children disagree. However, parents are needed for the child's development.

ADOLESCENCE (12 TO 18 YEARS)

Adolescence is the time between puberty and adulthood. It is a time of rapid growth and physical, sexual, emotional, and social changes. The stage begins with puberty. Girls reach puberty between the ages of 9 and 16 years. Boys reach puberty between the ages of 13 and 15 years.

The developmental tasks of adolescence include:

▶ Accepting changes in the body and appearance
▶ Developing appropriate relationships with males and females of the same age
▶ Accepting the male or female role appropriate for one's age
▶ Becoming independent from parents and adults
▶ Preparing for marriage and family life
▶ Preparing for a career
▶ Developing morals, attitudes, and values needed to function in society

Both boys and girls have a growth spurt. Both gain height and weight. They need about 9½ hours of sleep a night because of such rapid growth. Girls usually complete physical development by age 17. Boys usually stop growing between the ages of 18 and 21 years.

Oil glands are more active, leading to acne. Sweat glands are more active. Good hygiene is important. Deodorants or antiperspirants are needed to prevent body odors.

Menarche marks the onset of puberty in girls. **Menarche** is the first menstruation and the start of menstrual cycles (Chapter 8). *Pregnancy can occur with the onset of menarche.* Secondary sex characteristics appear. These include:

▶ Increase in breast size
▶ Pubic, axillary (underarm), and leg hair
▶ Slight deepening of the voice
▶ Widening and rounding of the hips

Ejaculation (the release of semen) signals the onset of puberty in boys. *Nocturnal emissions* ("wet dreams") occur. During sleep *(nocturnal)* the penis becomes erect. Semen is released *(emission)*. *The male can father children.* Other secondary sex characteristics include:

▶ Facial hair
▶ Pubic and axillary (underarm) hair
▶ Hair on the chest, arms, and legs
▶ Deepening of the voice
▶ Increases in neck and shoulder sizes

Movements often seem awkward and clumsy. Muscle and bone growth is uneven. Coordination and graceful movements develop as muscle and bone growth even out.

Acceptance of body changes and appearance occurs over time. Girls are concerned about weight gain. Breast development can embarrass girls, especially if breasts are very large or small. Some do not like to wear a bra. Others wear clothes that show off the breasts. Boys may worry about genital size. Height is a problem for both genders. Being small limits play in some sports. Boys do not like

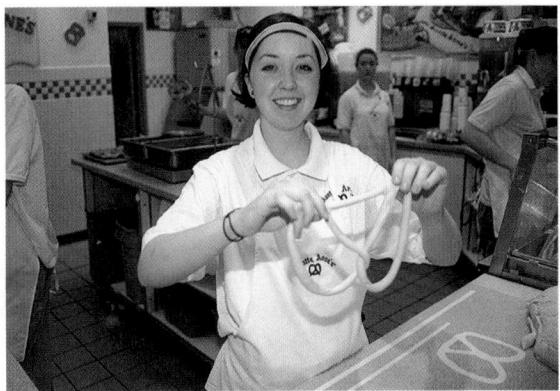

FIGURE 9-19 This teenager has a part-time job.

being shorter than their peers. Tall girls may feel embarrassed about being taller than other girls and boys.

Adolescents have mood swings. Emotional reactions vary from high to low. They can be happy one moment and sad the next. It is hard to predict their reaction to a comment or event. They control emotions better later in this stage. Fourteen- to 18-year-olds are sometimes sad and depressed. However, they have more control over the time and place of emotional reactions.

Adolescents need to become independent of adults, especially parents. They must learn to function, make decisions, and act responsibly without adult supervision. Many teenagers have part-time jobs or baby-sit (Fig. 9-19). They go to dances and parties, shop without an adult, and stay home alone. Many take part in school clubs and organizations.

Judgment and reasoning are not always sound. They still need guidance, discipline, and emotional and financial support from parents. The child and parents often disagree about behavior and activity restrictions and limits. Teenagers prefer being with peers than doing things with their families. They tend to confide in and seek advice from adults other than their parents.

Interests and activities also reflect the need to develop intimate relationships to act like males or females. Adolescents may begin to feel or show a sexual orientation (Chapter 46). **Sexual orientation** is sexual arousal or romantic attraction to persons of the other gender (heterosexual), the same gender (homosexual), or both genders (bisexual).

Both sexes like parties, dances, and other social events. Appearance is important (clothing, hairstyles). Teenagers spend time experimenting with makeup and hairstyles. They spend time talking to friends on the phone, listening to music, and reading teen magazines.

The age when dating begins varies. At first, dating is related to school events, such as a dance or football game. Group dating is common. The same group of girls just happens to be with the same group of boys. Pairing off and dating as a couple replace group dating. Couples may be sexual partners.

Many difficult choices and conflicts result as teens

mature physically, mentally, emotionally, and socially. Parents and teens often disagree about dating. Parents worry about sexual activities, pregnancy, and sexually transmitted diseases. Teen usually do not understand or appreciate these concerns. "Going steady" helps meet security, love and belonging, and self-esteem needs. Teens may have problems controlling sexual urges and considering the consequences of sexual activity.

Adolescents begin to think about careers and what to do after high school. Interests, skills, talents, and finances are some factors that influence the choice of college or getting a job.

Teens also need to develop morals, values, and attitudes for living in society. They need to develop a sense about good and bad, right and wrong, and the important and unimportant. Parents, peers, culture, religion, the media, and school are some influencing factors. Substance abuse, unwanted pregnancy, criminal acts, and suicide are risks for troubled teens.

YOUNG ADULTHOOD (18 TO 40 YEARS)

Mental and social development continues during young adulthood. There is little physical growth. Adult height has been reached. Body systems are fully developed. Developmental tasks of young adulthood include:

▶ Choosing education and a career
▶ Selecting a partner
▶ Learning to live with a partner
▶ Becoming a parent and raising children
▶ Developing a satisfactory sex life

Education and career are closely related. Most jobs require certain knowledge and skills. The education needed depends on career choice. Education usually increases job choices. Employment is needed for economic independence and to support a family.

Most adults marry at least once. Others choose to remain single. They may live alone or with friends of the same or opposite gender. Gay and lesbian persons may commit to a partner.

People marry for many reasons. They include love, emotional security, wanting a family, and sex. Some want to leave an unhappy home life. Some marry for social status, money, and companionship. Some marry to feel wanted, needed, and desirable.

Many factors affect the selection of a partner. They include age, religion, interests, education, race, personality, and love. Some marriages or partnerships are happy and successful. Others are not. There are no guarantees that a relationship will work. Therefore partners must work together to build a relationship based on trust, respect, caring, and friendship.

Partners must learn to live together. Habits, routines, meals, and pastimes are changed or adjusted to "fit" the other person's needs. They must learn to solve problems and make decisions together. They need to work toward

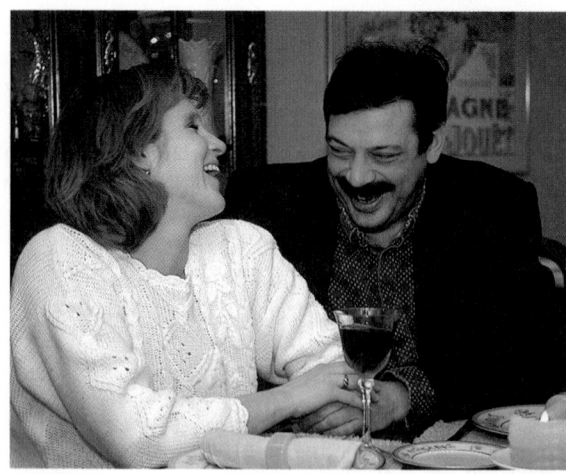

FIGURE 9-20 Communication is needed for a successful relationship.

the same goals. Open and honest communication is needed for a successful partnership (Fig. 9-20).

Adults need to develop a satisfactory sex life. Sexual frequency, desires, practices, and preferences vary. For a satisfying and intimate relationship, a partner must understand and accept the other's needs.

With modern birth control methods, couples can plan when to have children and how many to have. Some pregnancies are not planned. Some couples decide not to have children. The man or woman may have physical problems that interfere or prevent pregnancy.

Most couples have a child early in their marriage. Some wait several years to start a family. Parents must agree on child-rearing practices and discipline methods. They need to adjust to the child and to the child's needs for parental time, energy, and attention.

MIDDLE ADULTHOOD (40 TO 65 YEARS)

This stage is more stable and comfortable. Children are usually grown and have moved away. Partners have time to spend together. Worries about children and money are fewer. Developmental tasks relate to:

▶ Adjusting to physical changes
▶ Having grown children
▶ Developing leisure-time activities
▶ Adjusting to aging parents

Several physical changes occur. Many are gradual and are not noticed. Others are seen early. Energy and endurance begin to slow down. So do metabolism and physical activities. Therefore weight control becomes a problem. Facial wrinkles and gray hair appear. It is common to need eyeglasses. Hearing loss may begin. Menstruation stops, and menstrual cycles end. This is called **menopause.** It occurs between the ages of 45 and 55 years. Ovaries stop secreting hormones. The woman cannot have children.

Many diseases and illnesses can develop. The disorders become chronic and threaten life.

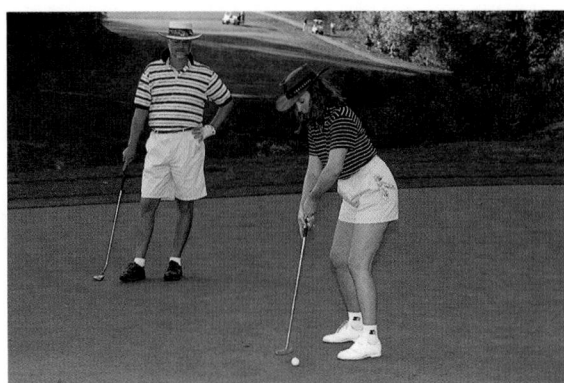

FIGURE 9-21 Middle-age adults usually have more time for leisure activities.

Children leave home for college, marry, move to their own homes, and start families. Adults have to cope with letting children go and being in-laws and grandparents. Parents must let children lead their own lives. However, they provide emotional support when needed.

These adults often have spare time as the demands of parenthood decrease. Hobbies and pastimes bring pleasure. They include gardening, fishing, painting, golfing, volunteer work, and being part of clubs and organizations (Fig. 9-21). These activities are even more important after retirement and during late adulthood.

Some middle-age adults have parents who are aging and in poor health. Responsibility for aging parents may begin during this stage. Many middle-age adults deal with the death of parents.

LATE ADULTHOOD (65 YEARS AND OLDER)

Chapter 10 describes the many changes that occur in older persons. Developmental tasks of this stage are:
▶ Adjusting to decreased strength and loss of health
▶ Adjusting to retirement and reduced income
▶ Coping with a partner's death
▶ Developing new friends and relationships
▶ Preparing for one's own death

REVIEW QUESTIONS

Circle the BEST answer.

1 Changes in mental, emotional, and social function are called
   a Growth
   b Development
   c A reflex
   d A stage

2 Which is *false*?
   a Growth and development occur from the simple to the complex.
   b Growth and development occur in an orderly pattern.
   c Growth and development occur at a set pace.
   d Each stage has its own characteristics.

3 Which reflexes does the infant need for feeding?
   a The Moro and startle reflexes
   b The rooting and sucking reflexes
   c The grasping and Moro reflexes
   d The rooting and grasping reflexes

4 Which occurs first in infants?
   a Holding the head up
   b Rolling from front to back
   c Rolling from back to front
   d The pincer grasp

5 An infant can stand alone at about
   a 9 months
   b 10 months
   c 11 months
   d 12 months

6 Infants point and use gestures to communicate at around
   a 5 months
   b 7 months
   c 9 months
   d 11 months

7 Toilet training begins
   a During infancy
   b During the toddler years
   c When the primary caregiver is ready
   d At the age of 3 years

8 The toddler can
   a Use a spoon and cup
   b Ride a bike
   c Help set the table
   d Name parts of the body

9 Playing with other children begins during
   a Infancy
   b The toddler years
   c The preschool years
   d Middle childhood

Continued

10 Loss of baby teeth usually begins at the age of
    a 4 years   **c** 6 years
    b 5 years   **d** 7 years

11 Peer groups become important to
    a Toddlers
    b Preschool children
    c School-age children
    d Adolescents

12 Reproductive organs being to function. Secondary sex characteristics appear. This is called
    a Late childhood
    b Adolescence
    c Puberty
    d Adulthood

13 Which is *false*?
    a Boys reach puberty earlier than girls.
    b Girls reach puberty between the ages of 9 and 16 years.
    c Menarche marks the onset of puberty in girls.
    d A growth spurt occurs during adolescence.

14 Dating usually begins
    a During late childhood
    b With group dating
    c With "pairing off"
    d During late adolescence

15 Adolescence is a time when parents and children
    a Talk openly about sex
    b Express love and affection
    c Disagree
    d Do things as a family

16 Which is *not* a developmental task of young adulthood?
    a Adjusting to changes in the body and appearance
    b Selecting a partner
    c Choosing a career
    d Becoming a parent

17 Middle adulthood is from about
    a 25 to 35 years
    b 30 to 40 years
    c 40 to 60 years
    d 40 to 65 years

18 Middle adulthood is a time when
    a Families are started
    b Physical energy and free time increase
    c Children are grown and leave home
    d People need to prepare for death

Answers to these questions are on p. 779.

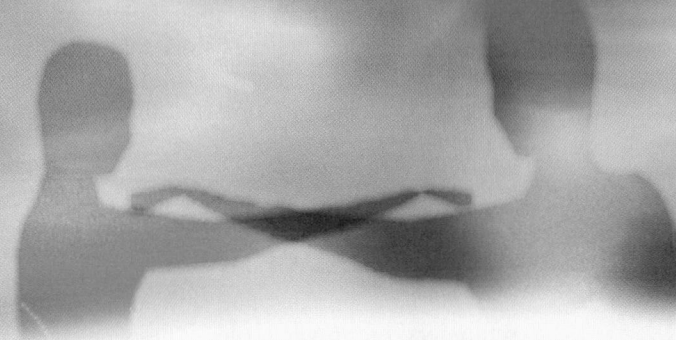

Care of the Older Person

OBJECTIVES

- Define the key terms and key abbreviations listed in this chapter
- Identify the psychological and social changes common in older adulthood
- Describe the physical changes from aging and the care required
- Describe housing options for older persons
- Describe resident rights

KEY TERMS

geriatrics The care of aging people

gerontology The study of the aging process

involuntary seclusion Separating a person from others against his or her will; keeping the person confined to a certain area or away from his or her room without consent

old Persons between 75 and 84 years of age

old-old Persons 85 years of age and older

ombudsman Someone who supports or promotes the needs and interests of another person

young-old Persons between 65 and 74 years of age

KEY ABBREVIATIONS

CCRC Continuing care retirement community

CNA Certified nursing assistant

ECHO Elder Cottage Housing Opportunity

OBRA Omnibus Budget Reconciliation Act of 1987

TRS Telecommunications Relay Services

TTD Telecommunications Devices for the Deaf

TTY Teletypewriter

People live longer than ever before. They are healthier and more active. U.S. Government reports show the following for the United States:

▶ In 2006 there were nearly 37,300,000 people age 65 and older.

▶ In 2005 there were 15,400,000 men age 65 and older. There were 21,400,000 women age 65 and older.

▶ In 2005 there were more older men who were married than older women. Widow-hood is more common in older women than in older men.

▶ In 2000 there were 4,200,000 people age 85 and older. In 2010 the number of older people is expected to increase to 6,100,000.

Chronic illness is common in older persons. Disability often results. Most older persons have at least one disability. Disabilities increase and become more severe with aging. They can interfere with:

▶ Self-care—bathing, dressing, eating, elimination

▶ Mobility and getting around one's home setting

▶ Fixing meals

▶ Shopping

▶ Managing money

▶ Using a phone

▶ Doing housework

▶ Taking drugs

▶ Leisure and recreational activities

Still, most older people live in a family setting. They live with a partner, children, brothers or sisters, or other family. Some live alone or with friends. Still others live in nursing centers. The need for nursing center care increases with aging.

Late adulthood involves these age ranges:

▶ **Young-old**—between 65 and 74 years of age

▶ **Old**—between 75 and 84 years of age

▶ **Old-old**—85 years of age and older

Gerontology is the study of the aging process. **Geriatrics** is the care of aging people. Aging is normal. It is not a disease. Normal changes occur in body structure and function. They increase the risk for illness, injury, and disability. Psychological and social changes also occur. Often changes are slow. Most people adjust well to these changes. They lead happy, meaningful lives.

As stated in Chapter 9, the developmental tasks of late adulthood are:

▶ Adjusting to decreased strength and loss of health

▶ Adjusting to retirement and reduced income

▶ Coping with a partner's death

▶ Developing new friendships and relationships

▶ Preparing for one's own death

There are many myths about aging and older persons. A *myth* is a widely believed story that is not true. To provide good care, you need to know the facts about older persons and aging. See Box 10-1 for some common myths and facts.

PSYCHOLOGICAL AND SOCIAL CHANGES

Graying hair, wrinkles, and slow movements are physical reminders of growing old. These changes affect self-esteem. They threaten self-image and feelings of self-worth. They also threaten independence.

Social roles also change. A parent may depend on an adult child for care. Retirees need activities to replace the work role. Adjusting to the death of a partner, family members, and friends is common. The person faces his or her own death.

People cope with aging in their own way. How they cope depends on:

▶ Health status

▶ Life experiences

▶ Finances

▶ Education

▶ Social support systems

BOX 10-1 Myths and Facts About Aging

Myth	Fact
All old people are the same.	Each person is unique. People age in different ways. Culture, religion, education, income, and life experiences affect aging. People develop throughout life.
Aging means illness and disability.	Older persons are at risk for health problems and disabilities. However, most are healthy. Not smoking, good nutrition, and exercise can reverse or slow many changes blamed on aging.
Older persons lose interest in sex.	Aging does not mean that sexual activity and expression must end. Many older people enjoy a fulfilling sex life. Sexuality is important throughout life. Intimacy, love, and companionship are needed.
Older people are lonely and isolated.	Most older people have frequent contact with their children. Older parents commonly live within 10 miles of their children. Most see a child at least once a week and take part in family activities. Regular contact with sisters and brothers is common. They can provide support and companionship. Many older persons have jobs, do volunteer work, and enjoy hobbies.
Mental function declines with age.	Older persons may receive and process information more slowly than younger people. However, people learn until very late in life. Many 90-year-olds have high levels of mental function.
Most older persons live in nursing centers.	In 2000 only 1,560,000 (4.5%) of the people 65 years and older lived in nursing centers.

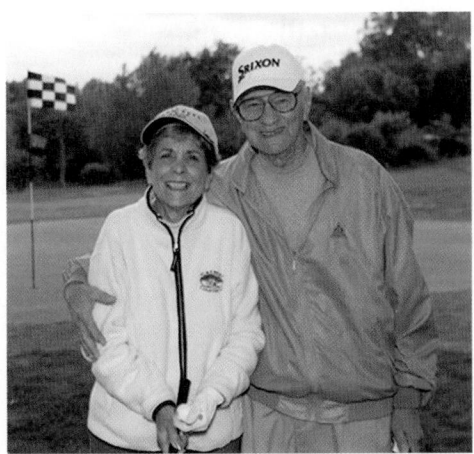

FIGURE 10-1 A retired couple enjoys golf as a leisure time activity.

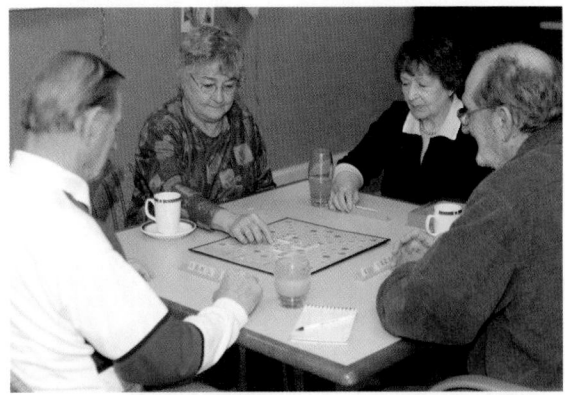

FIGURE 10-3 Older people enjoy being with others of their own age.

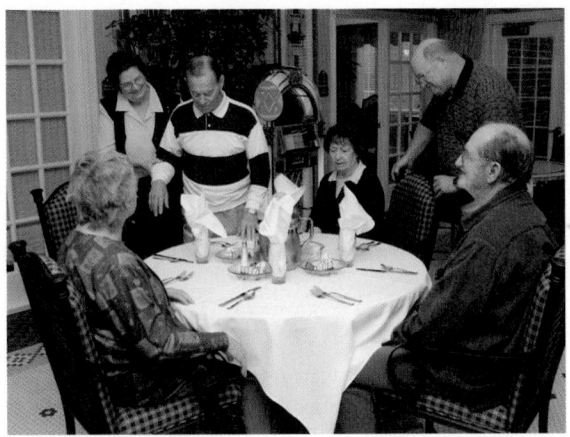

FIGURE 10-2 These older persons are nursing center volunteers.

Retirement

Age 65 is the usual retirement age. Some retire earlier. Others work into their 70s. Retirement is a reward for a life-time of work. The person can relax and enjoy life (Fig. 10-1). Travel, leisure, and doing what one desires are retirement "benefits." Many people enjoy retirement. Others are not so lucky. They are ill or disabled. Poor health and medical bills can make retirement very hard.

Work helps meet love, belonging, and self-esteem needs. The person feels fulfilled and useful. Friendships form. Co-workers share daily events. Leisure time, recreation, and companionship often involve co-workers. Some retired people want to work. They have part-time jobs or do volunteer work (Fig. 10-2).

Reduced Income

Retirement usually means reduced income. Social Security may provide the only income.

The retired person still has expenses. Rent or house payments continue. Food, clothing, utility bills, and taxes are other expenses. Car expenses, home repairs, drugs, and health care are other costs. So are entertainment and gifts.

Reduced income may force life-style changes. Examples include:

▶ Limiting social and leisure events
▶ Buying cheaper food, clothes, and household items
▶ Moving to cheaper housing
▶ Living with children or other family
▶ Avoiding health care or needed drugs
▶ Relying on children or other family for money or needed items

Severe money problems can result. Some people plan for retirement. They have savings, investments, retirement plans, and insurance. They are financially comfortable during retirement.

Social Relationships

Social relationships change throughout life. (See *Caring About Culture: Foreign-Born Persons*, p. 128.) Children grow up and leave home. They have their own families. Some live far away from parents. Older family members and friends die, move away, or are disabled. Yet most older people have regular contact with children, grandchildren, family, and friends. Others are lonely. Separation from children is a common cause. So is lack of companionship with people their own age (Fig. 10-3).

Many older people adjust to these changes. Hobbies, religious and community events, and new friends help prevent loneliness. Some community groups sponsor bus trips to ball games, shopping, plays, and concerts.

Grandchildren can bring great love and joy (Fig. 10-4, p. 128). Family times help prevent loneliness. They help the older person feel useful and wanted (Fig. 10-5, p. 128).

See *Focus on Communication: Social Changes*, p. 128.

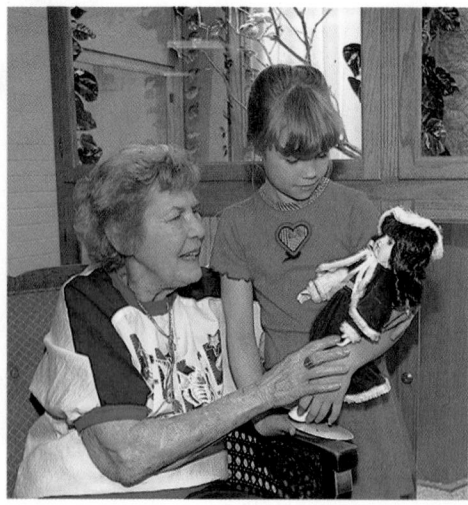

FIGURE 10-4 An older woman plays with her grandchild.

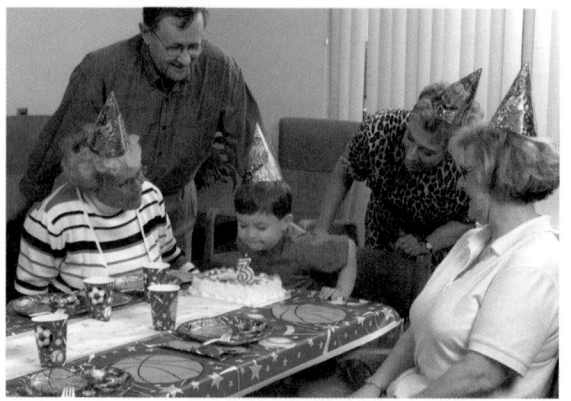

FIGURE 10-5 An older couple takes part in family activities.

FOCUS ON COMMUNICATION

Social Changes

The social changes of aging can cause loneliness. If nursing center care is needed, the loneliness can seem even greater. The person may be in the same building with other people. However, those people do not replace relationships with family and friends. To help the person feel less lonely, you can:
- Suggest that the person call a family member or friend. Offer to assist with finding phone numbers and dialing.
- Keep the phone within the person's reach. This helps him or her place or answer calls with ease.
- Suggest that the person read cards and letters. Offer to assist.
- Visit with the person a few times during your shift.
- Introduce new residents to other residents and staff.

CARING ABOUT CULTURE

Foreign-Born Persons

Some older persons speak and understand a foreign language. Communication occurs with family and friends who speak the same language. They also share cultural values and practices. These relatives and friends may move away or die. The person may not have anyone to talk to. He or she may not be understood by others. The person feels greater loneliness and isolation.

Children as Caregivers

Some children care for older parents. Parents and children change roles. The child cares for the parent. This helps some older persons feel more secure. Others feel unwanted, in the way, and useless. Some lose dignity and self-respect. Tensions may occur among the child, parent, and other household members. Lack of privacy is a cause. So are disagreements and criticisms about housekeeping, raising children, cooking, and friends.

Death of a Partner

As couples age, the chances increase that a partner will die. Women usually live longer than men. Therefore many women become widows.

A person may try to prepare for a partner's death. When death occurs, the loss is crushing. No amount of preparation is ever enough for the emptiness and changes that result. The person loses a lover, friend, companion, and confidant. Grief may be very great. The person's life will likely change. Serious physical and mental health problems result. Some lose the will to live. Some attempt suicide.

PHYSICAL CHANGES

Physical changes occur with aging. They happen to everyone (Box 10-2). Body processes slow down. Energy level and body efficiency decline. The rate and degree of change vary with each person. Influencing factors include diet, health, exercise, stress, environment, and heredity. The changes are slow. They occur over many years. Often they are not seen for a long time.

Normal aging does not mean loss of health. Quality of life does not have to decline. The person can adjust to many of the changes.

The Integumentary System

The skin loses its elasticity, strength, and fatty tissue layer. The skin thins and sags. Folds, lines, and wrinkles appear. Secretions from oil and sweat glands decrease. Dry skin occurs. The skin is fragile and easily injured. Skin breakdown, skin tears, and pressure ulcers are risks (Chapter 32). So are bruising and delayed healing. This is because blood vessels decrease in number.

Brown spots appear on the skin. They are called "age spots" or "liver spots." They are common on the wrists and hands.

Loss of the skin's fatty tissue layer also makes the person more sensitive to cold. Protect the person from drafts and cold. Sweaters, lap blankets, socks, and extra blankets are helpful. So are higher thermostat settings.

Dry skin causes itching. It is easily damaged. A shower or bath twice a week is enough for hygiene. Partial baths

---

BOX 10-2 **Common Physical Changes During the Aging Process**

INTEGUMENTARY SYSTEM
- Skin becomes less elastic
- Skin loses strength
- Brown spots ("age spots" or "liver spots") on the wrists and hands
- Fewer nerve endings
- Fewer blood vessels
- Fatty tissue layer is lost
- Skin thins and sags
- Skin is fragile and easily injured
- Folds, lines, and wrinkles appear
- Decreased secretion of oil and sweat glands
- Dry skin
- Itching
- Increased sensitivity to heat and cold
- Decreased sensitivity to pain
- Nails become thick and tough
- Whitening or graying hair
- Facial hair in some women
- Loss or thinning of hair
- Drier hair

MUSCULOSKELETAL SYSTEM
- Muscles atrophy
- Strength decreases
- Bone mass decreases
- Bones become brittle; can break easily
- Vertebrae shorten
- Joints become stiff and painful
- Hip and knee joints become flexed
- Gradual loss of height
- Decreased mobility

NERVOUS SYSTEM
- Fewer nerve cells
- Slower nerve conduction
- Reflexes slow
- Reduced blood flow to the brain
- Changes in brain cells
- Shorter memory
- Forgetfulness
- Slower ability to respond
- Confusion
- Dizziness
- Sleep patterns change
- Reduced sensitivity to touch
- Reduced sensitivity to pain
- Smell and taste decrease
- Eyelids thin and wrinkle
- Less tear secretion
- Pupils less responsive to light
- Decreased vision at night or in dark rooms
- Problems seeing green and blue colors
- Poor vision
- Changes in auditory nerve

- Eardrums atrophy
- High-pitched sounds are not heard
- Decreased earwax secretion
- Hearing loss

CIRCULATORY SYSTEM
- Heart pumps with less force
- Arteries narrow and are less elastic
- Less blood flows through narrowed arteries
- Weakened heart works harder to pump blood through narrowed vessels

RESPIRATORY SYSTEM
- Respiratory muscles weaken
- Lung tissue becomes less elastic
- Difficulty breathing (dyspnea)
- Decreased strength for coughing

DIGESTIVE SYSTEM
- Decreased saliva production
- Difficulty swallowing (dysphagia)
- Decreased appetite
- Decreased secretion of digestive juices
- Difficulty digesting fried and fatty foods
- Indigestion
- Loss of teeth
- Decreased peristalsis causing flatulence and constipation

URINARY SYSTEM
- Kidney function decreases
- Reduced blood supply to kidneys
- Kidneys atrophy
- Urine becomes concentrated
- Bladder muscles weaken
- Urinary frequency
- Urinary urgency may occur
- Urinary incontinence may occur
- Night-time urination may occur

REPRODUCTIVE SYSTEM
- Men
  - Testosterone decreases
  - Erections take longer
  - Longer phase between erection and orgasm
  - Less forceful orgasms
  - Erections lost quickly
  - Longer time between erections
- Women
  - Menopause
  - Estrogen and progesterone decrease
  - Uterus, vagina, and genitalia shrink (atrophy)
  - Thinning of vaginal walls
  - Vaginal dryness
  - Arousal takes longer
  - Less intense orgasms
  - Quicker return to pre-excitement state

---

are taken at other times. Mild soaps or soap substitutes are used to clean the underarms, genitals, and under the breasts. Often soap is not used on the arms, legs, back, chest, and abdomen. Lotions, oils, and creams prevent drying and itching. Deodorants may not be needed because sweat gland secretion is decreased. See Chapter 19 for hygiene.

Nails become thick and tough. Feet usually have poor circulation. A nick or cut can lead to a serious infection. See Chapter 20 for nail and foot care.

The skin has fewer nerve endings. This affects the ability to sense heat, cold, and pain. Burns are great risks. Fragile skin, poor circulation, and decreased ability to sense heat and cold increase the risk of burns. Older persons often complain of cold feet. Socks provide warmth. Hot water bottles and heating pads are not used because of the risk for burns.

White or gray hair is common. Hair loss occurs in men. Hair thins on men and women. Thinning occurs on the head, in the pubic area, and under the arms. Women and men may choose to wear wigs. Some color hair to cover graying. Facial hair (lip and chin) may occur in women.

Hair is drier from decreases in scalp oils. Brushing promotes circulation and oil production. Shampoo frequency depends on personal choice. Usually it decreases with age. It is done as needed for hygiene and comfort.

Skin disorders increase with age. They rarely cause death if treated early. The risk of skin cancers increases with age. Prolonged sun exposure is a cause.

Skin changes can be seen. Gray hair, hair loss, brown spots, and sagging skin are some examples. These changes can affect self-esteem and body image.

The Musculoskeletal System

Muscle cells decrease in number. Muscles atrophy (shrink). They decrease in strength. Bones lose minerals, especially calcium. Bones lose strength. They become brittle and break easily. Sometimes just turning in bed can cause fractures (broken bones).

Vertebrae shorten. Joints become stiff and painful. Hip and knee joints flex (bend) slightly. These changes cause gradual loss of height and strength. Mobility also decreases.

Older persons need to stay active. Activity, exercise, and diet help prevent bone loss and loss of muscle strength. Walking is good exercise. Exercise groups and range-of-motion exercises are helpful (Chapter 26). A diet high in protein, calcium, and vitamins is needed.

Bones can break easily. Protect the person from injury and prevent falls (Chapters 11 and 12). Turn and move the person gently and carefully (Chapter 16). Some persons need help and support getting out of bed. Some need help walking.

The Nervous System

Nerve cells are lost. Nerve conduction and reflexes slow. Responses are slower. For example, an older person slips. The message telling the brain of the slip travels slowly. The message from the brain to prevent the fall also travels slowly. The person falls.

Blood flow to the brain is reduced. Dizziness may occur. It increases the risk for falls. Practice measures to prevent falls (Chapter 12). Remind the person to get up slowly from a bed or a chair. This helps prevent dizziness (Chapter 26).

Changes occur in brain cells. This affects personality and mental function. So does reduced blood flow to the brain. Memory is shorter. Forgetfulness increases. Responses slow. Confusion, dizziness, and fatigue may occur. Older persons often remember events from long ago better than recent ones. Many older people are mentally active and involved in current events. They show fewer personality and mental changes. (See Chapter 44: Confusion and Dementia.)

Sleep patterns change. Older persons have a harder time falling asleep. Sleep periods are shorter. They wake often during the night, and have less deep sleep. Less sleep is needed. Loss of energy and decreased blood flow may cause fatigue. They may rest or nap during the day. They may go to bed early and get up early.

The Senses

Aging affects touch, smell, taste, sight, and hearing.

Touch. Touch and sensitivity to pain and pressure are reduced. So is sensing heat and cold. These changes increase the risk for injury. The person may not notice painful injuries or diseases. Or the person feels minor pain. You need to:
- Protect older persons from injury (Chapters 11 and 12)
- Follow safety measures for heat and cold (Chapter 33)
- Check for signs of skin breakdown (Chapters 19 and 32)
- Give good skin care (Chapter 19)
- Prevent pressure ulcers (Chapter 32)

Taste and smell. Taste and smell dull. Appetite decreases. Taste buds decrease in number. The tongue senses sweet, salty, bitter, and sour tastes. Sweet and salty tastes are lost first. Older people often complain that food has no taste. They like more salt and sugar on food.

The eye. Eyelids thin and wrinkle. Tear secretion is less. Therefore dust and pollutants can irritate the eyes.

The pupil becomes smaller and responds less to light. Vision is poor at night or in dark rooms. The eye takes longer to adjust to lighting changes. Vision problems occur when going from a dark to a bright room. They also occur when going from a bright to a dark room.

Clear vision is reduced. Eyeglasses are needed. The lens of the eye yellows. Therefore greens and blues are harder to see.

Older persons become more farsighted. This is called *presbyopia*. (*Presbly* relates to aging. *Opia* means eye.) The lens becomes more rigid with age. It is harder for the eye to shift from far to near vision and from near to far vision. These changes increase the risk of falls and accidents. The risk is greater on stairs and where lighting is poor. Eyeglasses are worn as needed. Keep rooms well-lit. Night-lights help at night.

The ear. Changes occur in the auditory nerve. Eardrums atrophy (shrink). High-pitched sounds are hard to hear. Severe hearing loss occurs if these changes progress. A hearing aid may be needed. It must be clean and correctly placed in the ear.

Wax secretion decreases. Wax becomes harder and thicker. It is easily impacted (wedged in the ear). This can cause hearing loss. A doctor or nurse removes the wax.

The Circulatory System

The heart muscle weakens. It pumps blood with less force. Problems may not occur at rest. Activity, exercise, excitement, and illness increase the body's need for oxygen and nutrients. A damaged or weak heart cannot meet these needs.

Arteries narrow and are less elastic. Less blood flows through them. Poor circulation occurs in many body parts. A weak heart must work harder to pump blood through narrowed vessels.

Exercise helps maintain health and well-being. Many older persons exercise daily. They walk, jog, golf, and bicycle. They also hike, ski, play tennis, swim, and play other sports. Older persons need to be as active as possible.

Sometimes circulatory changes are severe. Rest is needed during the day. Over-exertion is avoided. The person should not walk far, climb many stairs, or carry heavy things. Personal care items, TV, phone, and other needed items are kept nearby. Some exercise helps circulation. It also prevents blood clots in leg veins. Some persons need to stay in bed. They need range-of-motion exercises (Chapter 26). Doctors may order certain exercises and activity limits.

The Respiratory System

Respiratory muscles weaken. Lung tissue becomes less elastic. Often lung changes are not noted at rest. Difficult, labored, or painful breathing *(dypsnea)* may occur with activity. (*Dys* means difficult. *Pnea* means breathing.) The person may lack strength to cough and clear the airway of secretions. Respiratory infections and diseases may develop. These can threaten the older person's life.

Normal breathing is promoted. Avoid heavy bed linens over the chest. They prevent normal chest expansion. Turning, repositioning, and deep breathing are important. They help prevent respiratory complications from bedrest. Breathing usually is easier in semi-Fowler's position (Chapter 15). The person should be as active as possible.

The Digestive System

Salivary glands produce less saliva. This can cause difficulty swallowing *(dysphagia)*. (*Dys* means difficult. *Phagia* means swallowing.) Dry foods may be hard to swallow. Taste and smell dull. This decreases appetite.

Secretion of digestive juices decreases. As a result, fried and fatty foods are hard to digest. They may cause indigestion.

Loss of teeth and ill-fitting dentures cause chewing problems. This causes digestion problems. Hard-to-chew foods are avoided. Ground or chopped meat is easier to chew and swallow.

Peristalsis decreases. The stomach and colon empty slower. Flatulence and constipation can occur (Chapter 22).

Dry, fried, and fatty foods are avoided. This helps swallowing and digestion problems. Oral hygiene and denture care improve taste. Some people do not have teeth or dentures. Their food is pureed or ground.

High-fiber foods help prevent constipation. However, they are hard to chew and can irritate the intestines. They include apricots, celery, and fruits and vegetables with skins and seeds. Persons with chewing problems or constipation often need foods that provide soft bulk. They include whole-grain cereals and cooked fruits and vegetables.

Fewer calories are needed. Energy and activity levels decline. More fluids are needed for chewing, swallowing, digestion, and kidney function. Foods are needed to prevent constipation and bone changes. High-protein foods are needed for tissue growth and repair. However, some older persons lack protein in their diets. High-protein foods (meat and fish) are costly.

The Urinary System

Kidney function decreases. The kidneys shrink (atrophy). Blood flow to the kidneys is reduced. Waste removal is less efficient. Urine is more concentrated.

The ureters, bladder, and urethra lose tone and elasticity. Bladder muscles weaken. Bladder size decreases. Therefore the bladder stores less urine. Urinary frequency or urgency may occur. Many older persons have to urinate during the night. Urinary incontinence (inability to control the passage of urine from the bladder) may occur (Chapter 21).

In men, the prostate gland enlarges. This puts pressure on the urethra. Difficulty urinating or frequent urination occurs.

Urinary tract infections are risks. Adequate fluids are needed. The person needs water, juices, milk, and gelatin. Provide fluids according to the care plan. Remind the person to drink. Offer fluids often to those who need help. Most fluids should be taken before 1700 (5:00 PM). This reduces the need to urinate during the night.

Persons with incontinence may need bladder training programs. Sometimes catheters are needed. See Chapter 21.

The Reproductive System

Reproductive organs change with aging. For the effects of aging on sexuality, see Chapter 46.

▶ *Men.* The hormone *testosterone* decreases. It affects strength, sperm production, and reproductive tissues. These changes affect sexual activity. An erection takes longer. The phase between erection and orgasm also is longer. Orgasm is less forceful than when younger. Erections are lost quickly. The time between erections also is longer. Older men may need the penis stimulated for arousal. Fatigue, overeating, and drinking too much alcohol affect erections. Some men fear performance problems. They may avoid closeness.

▶ *Women. Menopause* is when menstruation stops. The woman can no longer have children. This occurs between 45 and 55 years of age. Female hormones *(estrogen* and *progesterone)* decrease. The uterus, vagina, and genitalia shrink (atrophy). Vaginal walls thin. There is vaginal dryness. These make intercourse uncomfortable or painful. Arousal takes longer. Orgasm is less intense. The pre-excitement state returns more quickly.

HOUSING OPTIONS

A person's home is more than a place to live. A home has family memories. It is a link to neighbors and the community. It brings pride and self-esteem. Aging can lead to changes in a person's home setting.

Most older people live in their own homes. Many function without help. Others need help from family or community agencies. In-home and community-based services assist older persons with activities of daily living (Box 10-3). Bathing, dressing, meals, housekeeping, shopping, and transportation are examples. Many services also provide social contact.

Some choose smaller homes when children are gone. Some retire to warmer climates. Others move closer to children and family. Still others have to give up their homes. Reduced income, taxes, home repairs, and yard work are factors. Some people cannot care for themselves.

Leaving a home is often very hard. Family, memories, gardens, neighbors, friends, churches, parks, and shopping provide close ties to one's home and neighborhood. Moving, whether a short or long distance, brings many losses.

Many housing options meet the needs of older people. A new home setting could maintain or improve the person's quality of life.

See *Focus on Long-Term Care and Home Care: Housing Options.*

Living With Family

Sometimes older brothers, sisters, and cousins live together. They:
▶ Provide companionship
▶ Share living expenses
▶ Provide care during illness or disability

Living with children is an option. The older parent (or parents) moves in with the child. Or the child moves to the parent's home. The parent may be healthy, may need some help, or may be ill or disabled. Some adult children give care to avoid nursing center care. A nursing center is an option if they cannot give needed care.

Living with an adult child is a social change. Everyone in the home must adjust. Sleeping plans may change if there is no spare bedroom. The parent may need a hospital bed. It can go in a family or living room, dining room, den, or bedroom.

The adult child's family needs time alone. Other family members may help give care. Respite care (Chapter 1) is an option for weekends and vacations. Many community and church groups have volunteers who help give care.

BOX 10-3 In-Home and Community Based Services

- *Adult day services.* Provide supervised group settings for those who cannot be alone during the day.
- *Case management.* A case manager assesses the needs of the older person and family. Needed services are arranged.
- *Meal programs.* Meals are provided in-home or in a senior center. Home delivery programs are often called *Meals on Wheels.*
- *Financial counseling.* Help is given with checking accounts, paying bills, income taxes, and insurance forms and claims.
- *Companionship services.* A volunteer visits the older person at home. Supervision and support services are provided as needed.
- *Home health care.* Nursing and physical, occupational, and speech therapies are provided. So are housekeeping and medical equipment services.
- *Homemaker services.* Help is given with household tasks. Cleaning, laundry, shopping, and preparing meals are examples. Some people need help with personal care.
- *Hospice care.* See Chapter 1. Nursing, comfort, and homemaker services are provided.
- *Personal care.* Help is given with eating, bathing, oral care, grooming, and dressing.
- *Rehabilitation.* Therapies are given to assist the person to regain or maintain his or her highest level of functioning.
- *Senior centers.* These centers offer many social and recreational activities. Classes, day trips, travel groups, performing arts, and nature activities are examples. Services also include meals, counseling, legal help, health screenings, and transportation.
- *Telephone reassurance.* Regular phone contact is provided. The person is called at various times. If the person does not answer, someone is sent to the person's home. Also, the older person can call the service when help is needed.
- *Transportation.* Older persons are given rides to and from doctor visits, appointments, shopping, religious services, and other places.
- *Wellness programs.* Blood pressure, blood sugar, and other tests are done to promote health. Sessions are held about fitness, nutrition, and other health topics.

Adult Day Care Centers

Many children need to work even though the parent cannot stay alone. Adult day care centers provide meals, supervision, and activities. Some provide rides to and from the center. Some serve persons with dementia (Chapter 44).

Requirements vary. Some require that the person be able to walk. A cane or walker is used as needed. Others allow wheelchairs. Most require that the person perform some self-care.

Many activities are offered. Cards, board games, movies, crafts, dancing, walks, exercise groups, and lectures are common (Fig. 10-7, p. 134). Some provide bowling and swimming. All activities are supervised. Needed help is given.

Some areas have intergenerational day care centers. Children and older persons are in the same center. They work together on some activities. They eat and play together. Young children bring much joy to older persons. They give older persons purpose, love, and affection. In turn, children learn about aging. They also receive love and affection from the older persons.

Housing Options

HOME CARE

Simple changes can make a home safe and easy to use. The nurse discusses needed changes with the patient and family.

The Bathroom
- Non-slick flooring
- Grab bars by showers, tubs, and toilets
- Non-skid surfaces in showers and tubs (bathmat, non-skid bath decals)
- Rugs with non-slip backing outside the tub and shower and in front of the toilet
- Hand-held shower nozzle or adjustable showerhead
- Shower chair for shower or bathtub
- Transfer bench
- Lever faucet handles
- Water controls close to the shower or tub entrance
- Anti-scald devices on faucets and showerheads
- Towel bars or hooks raised or lowered for the person's reach
- Raised toilet seat or a toilet seat riser
- Chair placed in front of the sink so the person can sit

The Bedroom
- Closet rods that adjust for height
- Lower shelves or pull-down shelves
- Pull-out drawers, bins, and baskets in closets
- A commode chair near the bed for night time use (Chapter 21)

The Kitchen
- Appliances within reach—side-by-side refrigerator/freezer, cook-top range, wall-mounted oven, dishwasher raised off the floor
- Stove controls on the front of the stove
- Stove controls easily marked and easy to see
- Lowered shelves or pull-down shelves
- Pull-out drawers, bins, and baskets
- Height of sink and countertops adjusted to meet the person's needs (lowered for the person who uses a wheelchair; raised for the person who cannot bend easily)
- Anti-scald devices on faucets
- Spray attachment to the sink—the person can fill pots after placing them on the stove

Other
- Lever door handles on all doors
- Easy-to-grasp cabinet and drawer handles
- Hand rails on stairways and outside steps
- Keyless locking system
- Security system
- Shelves near outside doors—the person can set items down to open the door
- Automatic garage door opener
- Rocker light switches that turn on and off with a push
- Electrical outlets 27 inches above the floor
- Peepholes or view panels in doors at the correct height for the person
- Washer and dryer on the main floor
- Wall-mounted, fold down ironing board
- Stair or platform lifts
- No scatter or throw rugs
- Thick carpeting replaced with low pile carpeting
- Furniture arranged to allow wheelchair use
- Phones in all rooms including the bathroom
- Cordless phone
- More chairs throughout the home so the person can sit when tired, weak, dizzy, and so on
- For poor eyesight:
  - Water controls that are color-coded or have large words
  - Light bulbs with increased wattage
  - Lights in closets and stairways
  - Outside lights by sidewalks, stairs, and doors
  - Task lighting under cabinets and over counters
  - Night-lights in bedrooms, bathrooms, and hallways
  - Phones with large keypads
- For hearing loss:
  - Phone volume increased
  - Smoke detectors with strobe lights
  - Teletypewriters (TTY) or Telecommunications Devices for the Deaf (TTD) (Fig. 10-6)
  - Amplified phone handset—increases sound and makes the caller's voice louder
  - Extension bells that make the phone ring louder
  - Doorbells that can be heard throughout the house

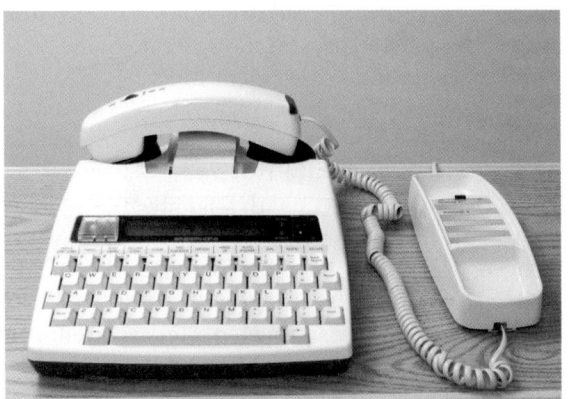

FIGURE 10-6 The Americans With Disabilities Act of 1990 requires that every state provide access to Telecommunications Relay Services (TRS). A communications assistant relays messages between the caller and the person with hearing loss. Messages are typed by the person with hearing loss. They are relayed orally to the caller. The communications assistant must relay everything that is said and maintain the confidentiality of all conversations.

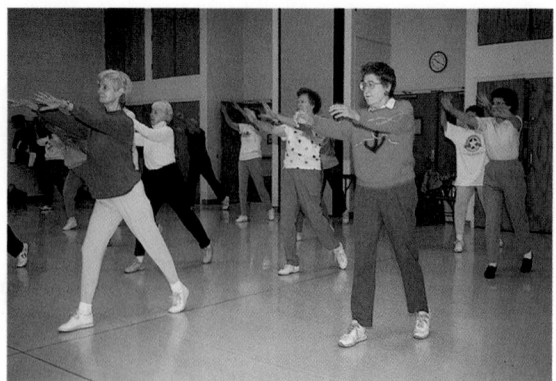

FIGURE 10-7 An adult day care center.

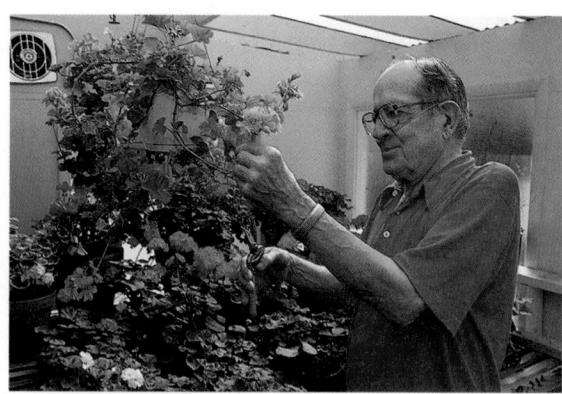

FIGURE 10-8 This man enjoys gardening.

Elder Cottage Housing Opportunity

Elder Cottage Housing Opportunity (ECHO) homes are small homes designed for older and disabled persons. The portable home is placed in the yard of a single-family home. The older person lives independently but near family or friends.

Apartments

Some older persons live in apartments. They pay rent and utility bills. The owner provides maintenance, yard work, snow removal, and appliance repair. Older persons remain independent. They can keep personal items. Many older persons like to garden or do yard work (Fig. 10-8). Apartment living usually does not provide such activities.

An *accessory apartment* is a separate living area in a home. It has a kitchen, bedroom, and bathroom. Some have a small living room. The older person lives independently near other people. Some children have these apartments for older parents. Or the older person's home may have an apartment. Renting other living space gives the older person more income.

Residential Hotels

Some cities have residential hotels. Private rooms or small apartments are rented. Food services may include a dining room, cafeteria, or room service. Some provide recreational activities and emergency medical services. Most hotels are close to shopping, places of worship, and other civic services.

Congregate Housing

Congregate means a group, gathering, or a cluster. In congregate housing, apartments are for older people. Buildings have wheelchair access, hand rails, elevators, and other safety features. The apartments are designed to meet the needs of older persons. Some are furnished.

There are many services. A doctor or nurse is on call. Someone checks on the person daily. A dining room is common. Rides are provided to places of worship, the doctor, or shopping areas. Tenants pay monthly rent.

Senior Citizen Housing

In many areas, state and federal funds support apartment complexes for older and disabled persons. Monthly rents are lower. The rent depends on the person's monthly income.

Homesharing

Two or more people share a house or apartment. Each person has a bedroom. They share other living space—kitchen, bathroom, living room. They share household chores and expenses. Or cooking, cleaning, and yard work are exchanged for rent.

Shared housing is a way to avoid living alone. It provides companionship. Some people feel safer when living with another person.

Assisted Living Residences

Assisted living residences are for persons who need help with daily living (Chapters 1 and 48). The person has social contact with others in a home-like setting. Health care and 24-hour oversight are provided. Nursing care is not provided.

Board and Care Homes

Board and care homes provide a room, meals, laundry, and supervision. Some homes are for older persons. Others are for people with certain problems. Dementia, mental health problems, and developmental disabilities are examples.

Homes vary in size—from housing 4 to 30 people or more. The care provided and rules vary from state to state. The person pays monthly rent. Some board and care homes receive government funds.

Adult Foster Care

Adult foster care can take two forms:
- An older person lives with a family.
- A single family home serves 4 to 5 persons with special needs. They may be older, disabled, or mentally ill.

The person receives help with daily living. A room, meals, and laundry are provided. Help is given with shopping and transportation. The person receives needed health care.

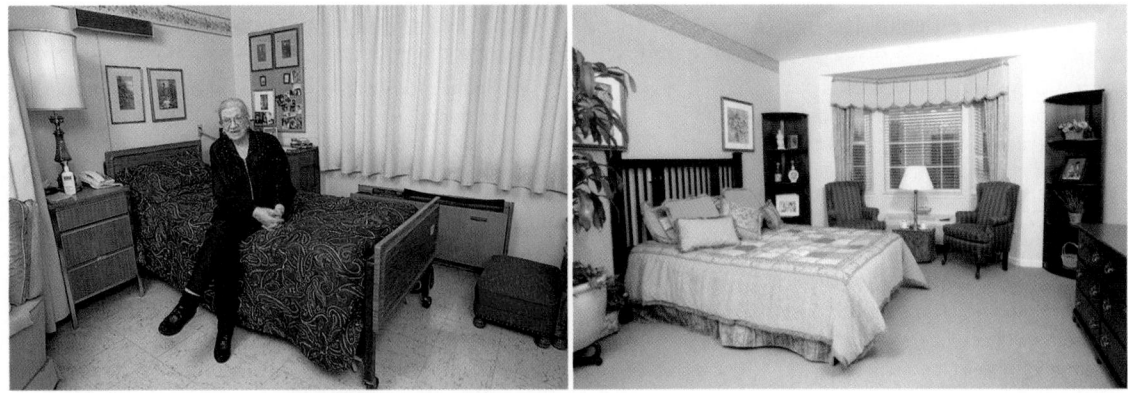

FIGURE 10-9 A nursing center is as home-like as possible.

Continuing Care Retirement Communities

Continuing care retirement communities (CCRCs) offer many services. They range from independent living units to 24-hour nursing care. A CCRC has housing, activity, and health care services. It meets the changing needs of older persons living alone or with a partner. CCRCs usually provide:

▶ Nursing care and other health care services
▶ Meals (including special diets)
▶ Housekeeping
▶ Transportation
▶ Personal assistance
▶ Recreational and educational activities

Independent living units are small apartments. Residents perform self-care and take their own drugs. Food service is provided. Help is nearby if needed. Many people have their own cars. They travel or drive about as desired. Rides are provided for those who need them.

Services are added as the person's needs change. Over time, some persons need nursing center care. They move into the nursing center within the CCRC. Many older couples find comfort in this plan. One partner needs nursing care. The other is close by and can visit often.

The person signs a contract with the CCRC. The contract is for a certain time or for the person's life-time. The contract lists services provided and the required fees.

Nursing Centers

Some older persons cannot care for themselves. Nursing centers are options for them (Chapter 1). Some people stay in nursing centers until death. Others stay until they can return home. The nursing center is the person's temporary or permanent home. The setting is as home-like as possible (Fig. 10-9).

The person needing nursing center care may suffer some or all of these losses:

▶ Loss of identity as a productive member of a family and community
▶ Loss of possessions—home, household items, car, and so on

▶ Loss of independence
▶ Loss of real-world experiences—shopping, traveling, cooking, driving, hobbies, and so on
▶ Loss of health and mobility

The person may feel useless, powerless, and hopeless. The health team helps the person cope with loss and improve quality of life. Treat the person with dignity and respect. Also practice good communication skills. Follow the care plan.

Nursing centers serve to meet the needs of older and disabled persons. Physical changes of aging are considered in the center's design. So are safety needs. Programs and services meet the person's basic needs. Box 10-4, p. 136 lists the features of a quality nursing center.

Some center designs, programs, and services follow the *Eden Alternative*™. Animals, plants, and children play a key role in giving residents dignity and purpose. The goal is to prevent residents from feeling lonely, helpless, and bored.

Most nursing centers receive Medicare or Medicaid funds. They must meet requirements of the Omnibus Budget Reconciliation Act of 1987 (OBRA). OBRA protects the person's rights. It also promotes quality of life. Funding is lost if requirements are not met (Box 10-5, p. 136). Surveys are conducted to determine if nursing centers are meeting OBRA requirements. These surveys are not announced.

Hospital Long-Term Care Units

Many hospitals have long-term care units. They are for persons who still need skilled care but not at the level once required. In time, some go home. Others transfer to nursing centers.

RESIDENT RIGHTS

OBRA is a federal law. It applies to all 50 states. Nursing centers must provide care in a manner and in a setting that maintains or improves each person's quality of life, health, and safety. Resident rights are a major part of OBRA.

BOX 10-4 Features of a Quality Nursing Center

- The center has a current state license.
- The administrator has a current state license.
- The center is Medicare- and Medicaid-certified.
- The location suits the resident. Family and friends can visit easily.
- There are safety features (Chapters 11 and 12). For example, hallways have hand rails. Bathrooms and showers have grab bars.
- Exits are clearly marked. They are not obstructed.
- State and/or federal fire codes are met.
- Residents' rooms open to the hallway.
- Residents' rooms have windows.
- A doctor is available for emergencies.
- No heavy odors are present. Scented sprays are not used to mask odors.
- Hallways are wide enough for 2 wheelchairs to pass with ease.
- Wheelchair ramps provide easy access into and out of the center.
- The kitchen has separate areas for food preparation, garbage, and dishwashing.
- There is enough refrigerator space for food.
- Toilet facilities allow wheelchair use.
- Dining rooms are attractive.
- Food looks, smells, and tastes good.
- Residents receive needed help with eating if required.
- Residents look clean.
- Residents are dressed properly for a full day of activity and social interaction inside or outside the center.
- There are attractive gardens and landscaping.
- There is an activity area for resident use.
- Staff is friendly and available to residents and visitors.
- There is a volunteer program.
- There is an active resident council.
- There is a residents' stated policy that identifies residents' individual rights.

Used with permission from the American Association of Homes and Services for the Aging.

BOX 10-5 OBRA Environment Requirements

- Dining areas are large enough and comfortable for the residents.
- Dining areas allow the use of wheelchairs, walkers, and other walking aids.
- Dining areas are equipped to meet the physical and social needs of residents.
- Recreation, program, and activity areas are large enough and comfortable for the residents.
  - There is enough space to store supplies and projects.
- Furnishings are sound and functional.
  - Chairs vary in size to meet residents' needs.
  - Wheelchairs can fit under dining room tables.
- Non-smoking areas are identified by signs.
- The space is well-ventilated.
- There is good air movement.
- Temperature, humidity, and odor levels are acceptable.
- Hand rails are secured to the walls in hallways.
- The area is free of pests (roaches, ants, flies, mice, rats, and so on).
- Toilet facilities are in or near each resident room.
- Resident rooms and toilet and bathing facilities are equipped with a call system. The call system functions properly.
- Lighting levels are adequate and comfortable.

Residents have rights as United States citizens. They also have rights relating to their everyday lives and care in a nursing center. These rights are protected by federal and state laws. Nursing centers must protect and promote such rights. The center cannot interfere with a resident's rights. Some residents are incompetent (not able). They cannot exercise their rights. A responsible party (partner, adult child) or legal representative does so for them.

Nursing centers must inform residents of their rights. This is done orally and in writing. Such information is given before or during admission to the center. It is given in the language the person uses and understands. Resident rights also are posted throughout the center.

Information

The right to information means access to all records about the person. They include the medical record, contracts, incident reports, and financial records. The request can be oral or written.

The person has the right to be fully informed of his or her health condition. Information is given in a language and in words the person can understand. Interpreters are used as needed. Sign language or other aids are used for those with hearing losses.

The person must also have information about his or her doctor. This includes the doctor's name, specialty, and how to contact the doctor.

Report any request for information to the nurse. *You do not give the information described above to the person or family (Chapter 2).*

Refusing Treatment

The person has the right to refuse treatment or to take part in research. Treatment means the care provided to relieve symptoms, improve function, or maintain or restore health. A person who does not give consent or refuses treatment cannot be given the treatment. The center must find out what the person is refusing and why.

Advance directives are part of the right to refuse treatment (Chapter 50). They include living wills and instructions about life support.

Report any treatment refusal to the nurse. The nurse may need to change the person's care plan.

Privacy and Confidentiality

Residents have the right to personal privacy. The person's body is not exposed unnecessarily. Only staff directly involved in care and treatments are present. The person must give consent for others to be present. For example, a student wants to observe a treatment. The person's consent is needed for the student to observe.

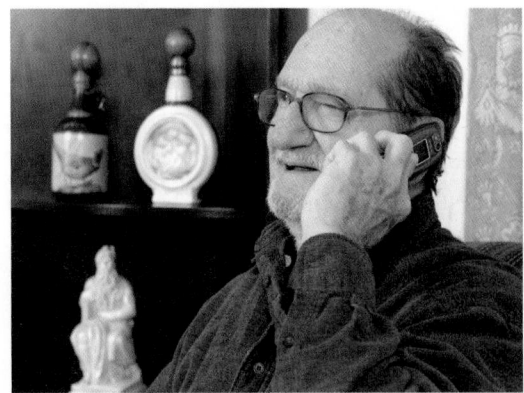

FIGURE 10-10 Resident talking privately on a phone.

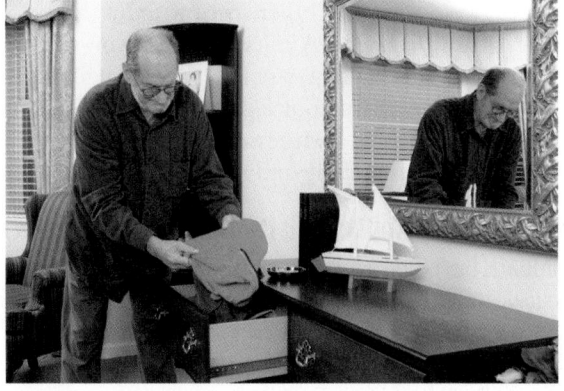

FIGURE 10-11 Resident choosing what clothing to wear.

A person has the right to use the bathroom in private. Privacy is maintained for all personal care measures. Bathing and dressing are examples.

Residents have the right to visit with others in private—in areas where others cannot see or hear them. This includes phone calls (Fig. 10-10). If requested, the center must provide private space. Offices, chapels, dining rooms, and meeting rooms are used as needed.

The right to privacy also involves mail. The person has the right to send and receive mail without others interfering. No one can open mail the person sends or receives without his or her consent. Mail is given to the person within 24 hours of delivery to the center.

Information about the person's care, treatment, and condition is kept confidential. So are medical and financial records. Consent is needed to release them to other agencies or persons.

You must provide privacy and protect confidentiality. Doing so shows respect for the person. It also protects the person's dignity. Privacy and confidentiality are discussed in Chapters 3 and 4.

Personal Choice

Residents can choose their own doctors. They also have the right to take part in planning and deciding about their care and treatment. They can choose activities, schedules, and care based on their preferences. They can choose when to get up and go to bed, what to wear, how to spend time, and what to eat (Fig. 10-11). They can choose friends and visitors inside and outside the center.

Personal choice promotes quality of life, dignity, and self-respect. You must allow personal choice whenever safely possible.

Disputes and Grievances

Residents have the right to voice concerns, questions, and complaints about treatment or care. The problem may involve another person. It may be about how care was given or not given. The center must promptly try to correct the matter. No one can punish the person in any way for voicing the grievance.

Work

The person does not work for care, care items, or other things or privileges. The person is not required to perform services for the center.

However, the person *can* work or perform services if he or she wants to. Some people like to garden, repair or build things, sew, mend, or cook. Other persons need work for rehabilitation or activity reasons. The desire or need for work is part of the person's care plan. The care plan states:

▸ The reason for the work—desire or need
▸ What work will be done
▸ If services are paid or voluntary

Taking Part in Resident and Family Groups

The person has the right to form and take part in resident and family groups. Families have the right to meet with other families. These groups can discuss concerns and suggest center improvements. They also can plan activities. They can provide support and comfort to group members.

Residents have the right to take part in social, cultural, religious, and community events. They have the right to help in getting to and from events of their choice.

Care and Security of Personal Items

Residents have the right to keep and use personal items. This includes clothing and some furnishings. The type and amount of personal items allowed depend on space needs and the health and safety of others.

Treat the person's property with care and respect. The items may not have value to you. However, they having meaning to the person. They also relate to personal choice, dignity, and quality of life.

The person's property is protected. Items are labeled with the person's name. The center must investigate reports of lost, stolen, or damaged items. Police help is sometimes needed. The person and family are advised not to keep jewelry and other costly items in the center.

Protect yourself and the center from being accused of stealing a person's property. Do not go through a person's closet, drawers, purse, or other space without the person's knowledge and consent. A nurse may ask you to inspect closets and drawers. Center policy should require that a co-worker and the person or legal representative be present. The co-worker is a witness to your activities. Follow center policy for reporting and recording the inspection.

Freedom From Abuse, Mistreatment, and Neglect

Residents have the right to be free from verbal, sexual, physical, or mental abuse (Chapter 3). They also have the right to be free from **involuntary seclusion:**

▶ Separating a person from others against his or her will
▶ Confining the person to a certain area
▶ Keeping the person away from his or her room without consent

No one can abuse, neglect, or mistreat a resident. This includes center staff, volunteers, and staff from other agencies or groups. It also includes other residents, family members, visitors, and legal representatives. Nursing centers must investigate suspected or reported cases of abuse. They cannot employ persons who were convicted of abusing, neglecting, or mistreating others.

See *Focus on Ethics and Laws: Freedom From Abuse, Mistreatment, and Neglect.*

Freedom From Restraint

Residents have the right not to have body movements restricted. Restraints and certain drugs can restrict body movements. Some drugs can restrain the person because they affect mood, behavior, and mental function. Sometimes residents are restrained to protect them from harming themselves or others. A doctor's order is needed for restraint use. Restraints are not used for staff convenience or to discipline a person. Restraints are discussed in Chapter 13.

Quality of Life

Nursing centers must care for residents in a manner that promotes dignity and self-esteem. Centers must also promote physical, psychological, and mental well-being. Protecting resident rights promotes quality of life. It shows respect for the person.

The person is spoken to in a polite and courteous manner (Chapter 7). Good, honest, and thoughtful care enhances the person's quality of life. Box 10-6 lists OBRA-required actions that promote dignity and privacy. Surveyors check for these actions in the person's care.

Activities

Nursing centers must provide activity programs that promote physical, intellectual, social, spiritual, and emotional well-being. The person is allowed to choose activities that appeal to his or her interests. Many centers provide religious services for spiritual health. You assist residents to and from activity programs. You may need to help them with activities.

See *Teamwork and Time Management: Activities.*
See *Focus on Communication: Activities.*

FOCUS ON ETHICS AND LAWS
Freedom from Abuse, Mistreatment, and Neglect

For about 3 months, a certified nursing assistant (CNA) worked at a nursing home in Texas. During that time, she received a warning for standing on a resident's bed to turn him onto his side. She was a "no call/no show before the last day of her resignation notice."

While working in an Arizona nursing home, the following were reported by the CNA's co-workers:
• Twice in one day the CNA was heard saying to a resident "You're full of xxxx."
• About 4 days later, the CNA told a resident "that if he grabbed her again, she would break his fingers." On the same day she was heard telling a resident that she "didn't want to hear the same xxxx she had already heard thirty times before."

The CNA's employment was terminated the next day.

On November 17, 2005, the Arizona State Board of Nursing found that the CNA's actions violated the state's Nurse Practice Act. The Board offered the CNA a stayed revocation agreement for 12 months with terms. The CNA failed to sign the agreement.

On March 20, 2006, the Arizona State Board of Nursing revoked the CNA's certificate. She could apply for re-instatement after a 5-year period.

(Arizona State Board of Nursing, March 20, 2006. NOTE: Names withheld by request of the Arizona State Board of Nursing.)

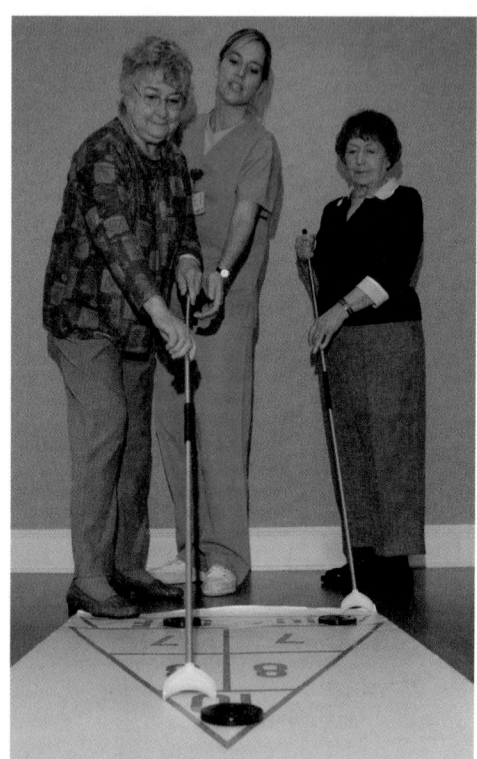

FIGURE 10-12 The nursing assistant is helping a resident with an activity.

BOX 10-6 OBRA-Required Actions to Promote Dignity and Privacy

COURTEOUS AND DIGNIFIED INTERACTIONS
- Use the right tone of voice.
- Use good eye contact.
- Stand or sit close enough as needed.
- Use the person's proper name and title. For example: "Mrs. Crane."
- Gain the person's attention before interacting with him or her.
- Use touch if the person approves.
- Respect the person's social status.
- Listen with interest to what the person is saying.
- Do not yell, scold, or embarrass the person.

COURTEOUS AND DIGNIFIED CARE
- Groom hair, beards, and nails as the person wishes.
- Assist with dressing in the right clothing for time of day and personal choice.
- Promote independence and dignity in dining.
- Respect private space and property.
- Assist with walking and transfers. Do not interfere with independence.
- Assist with bathing and hygiene preferences. Do not interfere with independence.
  - Appearance is neat and clean.
  - Person is clean shaven or has groomed beard and mustache.
  - Nails are trimmed and clean.

- Dentures, hearing aids, eyeglasses, and other devices are used correctly.
- Clothing is clean.
- Clothing is properly fitted and fastened.
- Shoes, hose, and socks are properly applied and fastened.
- Extra clothing for warmth is available as needed (sweaters and lap blanket are examples).

PRIVACY AND SELF-DETERMINATION
- Drape properly during care and procedures to avoid exposure and embarrassment.
- Drape properly in chair.
- Use privacy curtains or screens during care and procedures.
- Close the room door during care and procedures as the person desires. Also close window coverings.
- Knock on the door before entering. Wait to be asked in.
- Close the bathroom door when the person uses the bathroom.

MAINTAIN PERSONAL CHOICE AND INDEPENDENCE
- Person smokes in allowed areas.
- Person takes part in activities according to his or her interests.
- Person takes part in scheduling activities and care.
- Person gives input into the care plan about preferences and independence.
- Person is involved in room or roommate change.

TEAMWORK AND TIME MANAGEMENT

Activities

Residents may need help getting to and from activity programs. Know when an activity begins and ends. Do the following before assisting residents to activity areas:
- Assist with elimination needs and hand washing.
- Assist with grooming measures such as brushing and combing hair. A person may want to apply some perfume or makeup.
- Make sure the person wears the correct clothing and footwear for the activity.
- Make sure the person has needed assistive devices. Eyeglasses, hearing aids, canes, and walkers are examples. Allow 15 to 20 minutes to assist residents to and from the activity area. Help your co-workers as needed.

You may have to help residents with activities (Fig. 10-12). If not, use the activity time wisely. Provide needed care and visit residents who cannot leave their rooms. You can also clean and straighten rooms, bathrooms, shower rooms, and utility rooms.

FOCUS ON COMMUNICATION

Activities

You may need help assisting residents to and from activity programs. Politely ask a co-worker to help you. Share this information with your co-worker:
- What time you need the help.
- How much of the co-worker's time you need.
- The residents you need help with.
- If the person walks or uses a wheelchair.
- What assistive devices are used. Eyeglasses, hearing aids, canes, and walkers are examples.

Be sure to say "please" when asking for help. And thank the person for helping you. For example: "Jane, can you please help me assist two residents to the concert? It starts at 1300 so I'll need your help at 1245. Mr. Harris needs his glasses and hearing aid. He'll use a walker. Mrs. Janz uses a wheelchair. She needs her glasses and a blanket for her lap. The blanket is in her wheelchair. The concert is over at 1400. Please help me then, too. Thank you so much for helping me."

Environment

The center's environment must promote quality of life. It must be clean, safe, comfortable, and as home-like as possible (Chapters 11, 12, and 17). Letting the person have personal items enhances quality of life. They allow personal choice and promote a home-like setting.

OMBUDSMAN PROGRAM

The Older Americans Act is a federal law. It requires a long-term care ombudsman program in every state. An **ombudsman** is someone who supports or promotes the needs and interests of another person. Long-term care ombudsmen are employed by a state agency. Some are volunteers. They are not nursing center employees. They act on behalf of nursing center and assisted living residents.

Ombudsmen protect the health, safety, welfare, and rights of residents. They:

▶ Investigate and resolve complaints
▶ Provide services to assist residents
▶ Provide information about long-term care services
▶ Monitor nursing center care
▶ Monitor nursing center conditions
▶ Provide support to resident and family groups
▶ Help the resident and family resolve conflicts within the family
▶ Help the center manage difficult problems
▶ Educate residents, families, and the public about long-term care issues and concerns
▶ Represent residents' interests before local, state, and federal governments

Residents have the right to voice grievances and disputes. They also have the right to communicate privately with anyone of their choice. They can share concerns with anyone outside the center. Nursing centers must post the names, addresses, and phone numbers of local and state ombudsmen. This information must be posted where residents can easily see it.

A resident or family may share a concern with you. You must know state and center policies and procedures for contacting an ombudsman. Ombudsman services are useful when:

▶ There is concern about a person's care or treatment.
▶ Someone interferes with a person's rights, health, safety, or welfare.

REVIEW QUESTIONS

Circle the BEST answer.

1 People between the ages of 75 and 84 are
  a The young-old
  b Old
  c The old-old
  d Elderly

2 The study of the aging process is called
  a Geriatrics
  b Dysphagia
  c Gerontology
  d Dypsnea

3 Retirement usually means
  a Lowered income
  b Changes from aging
  c Less free time
  d Financial security

4 Which does *not* cause loneliness in older persons?
  a Children moving away
  b The death of family and friends
  c Problems communicating with others
  d Contact with other older persons

5 Older persons living with their children often feel
  a Independent
  b Wanted and a part of things
  c Useless
  d Dignified

6 These statements are about a partner's death. Which is *false*?
  a The person loses a lover, friend, companion, and confidant.
  b Preparing for the event lessens grief.
  c The survivor may develop health problems.
  d The survivor's life will likely change.

7 Skin changes occur with aging. Care should include the following *except*
  a Providing for warmth
  b Applying lotion
  c A daily bath with soap
  d Providing good skin care

8 An older person complains of cold feet. You should
  a Provide socks
  b Apply a hot water bottle
  c Soak the feet in hot water
  d Apply a heating pad

9 Aging causes changes in the musculoskeletal system. Which is *false*?
  a Bones become brittle. They can break easily.
  b Bedrest is needed for loss of strength.
  c Joints become stiff and painful.
  d Exercise slows musculoskeletal changes.

10 Changes occur in the nervous system. Which is *true*?
  a Less sleep is needed than when younger.
  b The person forgets events from long ago.
  c Sensitivity to pain increases.
  d Confusion occurs in all older persons.

11 Changes occur in the eye. Which is *false*?
  a Night vision decreases.
  b Blue and green colors are easy to see.
  c Eyelids thin and wrinkle.
  d The eye is easily irritated by dust.

12 Which is *not* a common cause of hearing loss in older persons?
  a Changes in the auditory nerve
  b Atrophy of the eardrums
  c Impacted earwax
  d Ear infections

13 Arteries narrow and lose their elasticity. These changes result in
  a A slower heart rate
  b Lower blood pressure
  c Poor circulation to many body parts
  d Less blood in the body

14 An older person has cardiovascular changes. Care includes the following *except*
  a Placing needed items nearby
  b A moderate amount of daily exercise
  c Avoiding exertion
  d Long walks

15 Respiratory changes occur with aging. Which is *false*?
  a Heavy bed linens are avoided.
  b The person is turned often if on bedrest.
  c The side-lying position is best for breathing.
  d The person should be as active as possible.

16 Older persons should avoid dry foods because of
  a Decreases in saliva
  b Loss of teeth or ill-fitting dentures
  c Decreased amounts of digestive juices
  d Decreased peristalsis

17 Changes occur in the digestive system. Older persons should eat
  a Fruits and vegetables with skins and seeds
  b Dry and fatty foods
  c Raw apricots and celery
  d Protein foods

18 Changes occur in the urinary system. Which is *true*?
  a Kidneys increase in size.
  b Fluids are needed for kidney function.
  c The bladder becomes larger.
  d Blood flow to the kidneys increases.

19 The doctor orders increased fluid intake for an older person. You should
  a Give most of the fluid before 1700 (5:00 PM)
  b Provide mostly water
  c Start a bladder training program
  d Insert a catheter

20 Most older people live
  a In nursing centers
  b In their own homes
  c With children
  d In senior citizen housing

21 These statements are about adult day care centers. Which is *false*?
  a They provide meals, supervision, and activities.
  b Usually the person must do some self-care.
  c All activities are supervised.
  d Personal care is provided.

22 Which housing option provides lodging, meals, and some help with personal care?
  a Apartments
  b Senior citizen housing
  c Board and care homes
  d Residential hotels

23 A continuing care retirement community provides the following *except*
  a Independent living units
  b A nursing center
  c Adult foster care
  d Meals, transportation, and recreational activities

24 A quality nursing center does the following *except*
  a Provides safety features
  b Uses scented sprays
  c Has dining rooms that allow wheelchair use
  d Has an activity area

25 As a nursing assistant, you must
  a Open the person's mail
  b Choose what the person wears
  c Provide for the person's privacy
  d Search the person's closet and drawers

26 Who decides how to style a person's hair?
  a The person
  b The nurse
  c You
  d The ombudsman

27 Residents do *not* have a right to
  a Free care
  b Refuse treatment
  c Contact an ombudsman
  d Make personal choices

28 A long-term care ombudsman
  a Is employed by the nursing center
  b Investigates resident complaints
  c Grants a nursing center a license or certification
  d Can prevent a resident from leaving the center

29 Which action does *not* promote a person's dignity?
  a Restraining the person
  b Providing privacy during personal care
  c Making sure the person has needed assistive devices
  d Listening to the person

30 Which is the correct way to address a person?
  a "Hello sweetie."
  b "Hello Mrs. Smith."
  c "Hello Jim."
  d "Hello Grandpa."

Answers to these questions are on p. 779.

Safety

OBJECTIVES

- Define the key terms and key abbreviations listed in this chapter
- Describe accident risk factors
- Identify safety measures for infants and children
- Explain why you identify a person before giving care
- Explain how to correctly identify a person
- Describe the safety measures to prevent burns, poisoning, and suffocation
- Identify the signs and causes of choking
- Explain how to prevent equipment accidents
- Explain how to handle hazardous substances
- Describe safety measures for fire prevention and oxygen use
- Explain what to do during a fire
- Give examples of natural and human-made disasters
- Explain how to report accidents and errors
- Explain how to protect yourself from workplace violence
- Describe your role in risk management
- Perform the procedures described in this chapter

PROCEDURES

- Relieving Choking—The Responsive Adult or Child (Over 1 Year of Age)
- Relieving Choking in the Infant
- Using A Fire Extinguisher

KEY TERMS

coma A state of being unaware of one's surroundings and being unable to react or respond to people, places, or things

disaster A sudden catastrophic event in which people are injured and killed and property is destroyed

electrical shock When electrical current passes through the body

ground That which carries leaking electricity to the earth and away from an electrical item

hazardous substance Any chemical in the workplace that can cause harm

hemiplegia Paralysis on one side of the body

incident Any event that has harmed or could harm a patient, resident, visitor, or staff member

paralysis Loss of muscle function, loss of sensation, or loss of both muscle function and sensation

paraplegia Paralysis in the legs and lower trunk

quadriplegia Paralysis in the arms, legs, and trunk

suffocation When breathing stops from the lack of oxygen

workplace violence Violent acts (including assault and threat of assault) directed toward persons at work or while on duty

KEY ABBREVIATIONS

AED Automated external defibrillator

CPR Cardiopulmonary resuscitation

EMS Emergency Medical Services

FBAO Foreign-body airway obstruction

ID Identification

MSDS Material safety data sheet

OBRA Omnibus Budget Reconciliation Act of 1987

OSHA Occupational Safety and Health Administration

PASS *Pull* the safety pin, *aim* low, *squeeze* the lever, *sweep* back and forth

RACE Rescue, alarm, confine, extinguish

RRT Rapid Response Team

Safety is a basic need. Patients and residents are at great risk for accidents and falls. (See Chapter 12 for falls.) Some accidents and injuries cause death.

Common sense and simple safety measures can prevent most accidents. You must protect patients and residents, visitors, yourself, and co-workers. The safety measures in this chapter apply to everyday life. They apply to hospital, long-term care, and home settings. The care plan lists other safety measures needed by the person.

See *Focus on Long-Term Care and Home Care: Safety.*

A SAFE SETTING

In a safe setting, a person has little risk of illness or injury. The person feels safe and secure physically and mentally. The risk of infection, falls, burns, poisoning, and other injuries is low. Temperature and noise levels are comfortable. Smells are pleasant. There is enough room and light to move about safely. The person and the person's property are safe from fire and intruders. The person is not afraid. He or she has few worries and concerns.

FOCUS ON LONG-TERM CARE AND HOME CARE

Safety

LONG-TERM CARE

Ordinary and sometimes extraordinary measures are needed to prevent accidents and keep residents safe. The goal is to decrease the person's risk of accidents and injuries without limiting mobility and independence.

The Omnibus Budget Reconciliation Act of 1987 (OBRA) requires that nursing centers follow safety policies and procedures. The intent is to keep residents, visitors, and staff safe. Measures to protect residents must not interfere with their rights (Chapter 10).

The person must receive the right care and treatment. The person is protected from falls (Chapter 12), burns, poisoning, suffocation, and infection. To protect the person from harm, follow the person's care plan. Also practice the safety measures in this chapter.

See *Teamwork and Time Management: A Safe Setting*, p. 144.

ACCIDENT RISK FACTORS

Some people cannot protect themselves. They present dangers to themselves and others. They rely on others for safety. Know the factors that increase a person's risk of accidents and injuries. Follow the person's care plan.

▶ *Age.* Children and older persons are at risk for injuries. See *Focus on Children and Older Persons: Accident Risk Factor*, p. 144.

▶ *Awareness of surroundings.* People need to know their surroundings to protect themselves from injury. **Coma** is a state of being unaware of one's surroundings and being unable to react or respond to people, places, or things. A coma can occur from illness or injury. The person in a coma relies on others for protection. Confused and disoriented persons may not understand what is happening to and around them.

▶ *Agitated and aggressive behaviors.* Pain can cause these behaviors. So can confusion, decreased awareness of surroundings, and fear of what may happen.

▶ *Vision loss.* Persons with poor vision have problems seeing things. They can fall or trip over toys, rugs, equipment, furniture, and cords. Some have problems reading labels on cleaners and other containers. Poisoning can result. It also can result from taking the wrong drug or the wrong dose.

TEAMWORK AND TIME MANAGEMENT

A Safe Setting

The entire health team must provide a safe setting. You may see something unsafe. Correct the matter right away if it is something you can do. For example:

- You see a water spill. Wipe up the spill right away. Do so even if you did not cause the spill.
- You see a person sliding out of a wheelchair. Position the person correctly in the chair. Do so even if a co-worker is responsible for the person's care.
- A person is having problems holding a cup of coffee. Offer to help the person.
- Food is left unattended in a microwave oven. Turn off the device.

You cannot correct some safety issues. Follow agency policy for reporting such problems. They include:

- Electrical outlets or switches coming out of the wall
- Electrical outlets that do not work
- Water leaks from windows, doors, ceilings, pipes, faucets, tubs, showers, toilets, hot water heaters, fountains, and other water sources
- Toilets that do not work properly
- Water from faucets that does not warm up or that is very hot
- Broken windows
- Windows and doors that do not work properly
- Knobs and handles that are broken or do not work properly
- Handrails and grab bars that are loose or need repair
- Odd smells and odors
- Odd sounds
- Signs of rodents, flies, or other pests
- Broken or damaged furniture
- Lights and lamps that do not work or have burnt-out bulbs
- Flooring (carpeting, tiles) in need of repair

FOCUS ON CHILDREN AND OLDER PERSONS

Accident Risk Factors

CHILDREN

Infants are helpless. Young children have not learned the difference between safety and danger. They explore their surroundings, put objects in their mouths, and touch and feel new things. They are at risk for falls, poisoning, choking, burns, and other accidents. Practice the safety measures in Box 11-1.

OLDER PERSONS

Changes from aging increase the risk for falls and other injuries. Older persons have decreased strength and move slowly. Some are unsteady. Often balance is affected. These changes prevent quick and sudden movements to avoid dangers and prevent falls. Older persons also are less sensitive to heat and cold. They have poor vision, hearing problems, and a dulled sense of smell. Confusion, poor judgment, memory problems, and disorientation may occur (Chapter 44).

Some persons suffer from dementia. *Dementia* is the loss of cognitive and social function caused by changes in the brain (Chapter 44). Memory and the ability to think and reason are lost. Dementia is caused by diseases and injuries.

Persons with dementia are confused and disoriented. Their awareness of surroundings is reduced. They may not understand what is happening to and around them. Judgment is poor. They no longer know what is safe and what are dangers. They may access closets, cupboards, or other unsafe and unlocked areas. They may eat or drink cleaning products, drugs, or poisons. Accidents and injuries are great risks. The health team must meet all safety needs.

- *Hearing loss.* Persons with hearing loss have problems hearing explanations and instructions. They may not hear warning signals or fire alarms. Some cannot hear approaching meal carts, drug carts, stretchers, or people in wheelchairs. They do not know to move to safety.
- *Impaired smell and touch.* Illness and aging affect smell and touch. The person may not detect smoke or gas odors. When touch is reduced, burns are a risk. The person has problems sensing heat and cold. Some people have a decreased pain sense. They may be unaware of injury. For example, Mrs. Parks does not feel a blister from her shoes. She has poor circulation to her legs and feet. The blister can become a serious wound.

- *Impaired mobility.* Some diseases and injuries affect mobility. A person may know there is danger but cannot move to safety. Some persons cannot walk or propel wheelchairs. Some persons are paralyzed. **Paralysis** means loss of muscle function, loss of sensation, or loss of both muscle function and sensation. **Paraplegia** is paralysis in the legs and lower trunk. **Quadriplegia** is paralysis in the arms, legs, and trunk. **Hemiplegia** is paralysis on one side of the body.
- *Drugs.* Drugs have side effects. They include loss of balance, drowsiness, and lack of coordination. Reduced awareness, confusion, and disorientation can occur. The person may be fearful and uncooperative. Report behavior changes to the nurse. Also report the person's complaints. *Text continued on p. 148*

BOX 11-1 **Safety Measures for Infants and Children**

GENERAL SAFETY

- Do not leave infants and children unattended. Supervise them at all times.
- Avoid baby walkers on wheels.
- Use the safety strap to fasten a child in a highchair or infant carrier seat.
- Lock the highchair tray after putting the child in the chair.
- Keep highchairs away from stoves, tables, and counters.
- Do not hang items with strings, cords, or elastic cords around cribs or playpens.
- Keep child-resistant caps on drugs and other harmful substances.
- Store knives (including kitchen knives), razor blades, matches, guns, tools, and other dangerous items where children cannot reach them. Keep them in locked storage areas.
- Keep glassware, knives, dishes, appliance cords, and other objects away from counter and table edges.
- Do not prop baby bottles on a rolled towel or blanket. Hold the baby and bottle during feedings.
- Use safety gates at the top and bottom of stairs. They prevent small children from climbing up and down stairs. Make sure the child cannot get caught in the gate slats.
- Keep one hand on a child lying in a crib or on a scale, bed, table, or other surface or furniture (Fig. 11-1, p. 147).
- Keep one hand on the baby when changing a diaper.
- Read all package and label instructions. Follow the manufacturer's instructions.
- Use shopping carts safely:
  - Use the safety harness or belt to restrain a child in a shopping cart.
  - Do not let a child stand up in a shopping cart.
  - Stay close to the shopping cart.
  - Do not let a child push a shopping cart.

BEDROOM SAFETY

- Check infants often when in cribs.
- Make sure crib rails are up and locked in place when the baby is in the crib.
- Do not use a crib with loose, broken, or missing parts. This includes screws, nuts, and bolts.
- Promote bunk bed safety:
  - Make sure beds and ladders are fastened and supported properly.
  - Do not let children younger than 6 years sleep on the top bunk of bunk beds.
  - Check bunk bed guardrails. Spaces between the slats should be less than 3.5 inches. Guardrails should raise at least 5 inches above the mattress.
  - Openings on the upper and lower bunks must be small enough to prevent the child's head, torso, arm, or leg from passing through the opening.
  - Use guardrails on both sides of the upper bunk.
  - Have the child use the ladder for getting in and out of the upper bunk.
- Keep bedroom doors closed. Bedrooms of parents and older children may contain perfumes, toys, and other items that present hazards to young children. Choking, poisoning, burns, and suffocation are risks.
- See Chapter 18 for other crib safety measures.

ELECTRICAL SAFETY

- Keep electrical items away from sinks, tubs, toilets, and other water sources.
- Unplug electrical items when not in use.
- Place safety plugs in outlets (Fig. 11-2, p. 147). This includes electrical strips and surge protectors. Children cannot stick fingers or small objects into the openings.
- Keep electrical cords and electrical items out of the reach of children.

WINDOW SAFETY

- Install safety guards on windows.
- Keep cords for window coverings out of the reach of children.
- Do not place a crib, playpen, bed, or other furniture near a window. This prevents children from climbing from furniture onto a window seat or windowsill.
- Keep children away from open windows. Do not let them sit on windowsills. Window screens are not strong enough to prevent children from falling out of windows.

WATER SAFETY

- Supervise any child who is in or near water. Never leave the child alone. This includes when using tubs, toilets, sinks, buckets and containers, wading pools, swimming pools, hot tubs, spas, and whirlpools.
- Be aware of small bodies of water than can present dangers. Examples include fountains, fish ponds, ditches, rain barrels, and watering cans.
- Do not rely on bathtub seats, water wings, inner tubes, air mattresses, or other flotation devices to keep a child afloat.
- Keep bathroom doors closed to prevent drowning in toilets or bathtubs.
- Keep sinks, tubs, and basins empty when not in use.
- Keep buckets, containers, and wading pools empty and upside down when not in use.
- Keep toilet lids down. Use toilet safety locks.
- Keep diaper pails locked.
- Keep a locked safety cover on spas, hot tubs, and whirlpools when not in use.
- Remove pool, spa, hot tub, and whirlpool covers before use. The cover must be completely off. If not, the child can get trapped under the cover.
- Remove steps to above-ground pools when not in use.
- Have a phone by the pool, spa, hot tub, and whirlpool.
- Keep rescue equipment near pools.
- Promote safe swimming and diving:
  - Teach water survival when a child can crawl or walk to a pool.
  - Make sure children older than 4 years learn how to swim.
  - Do not let children swim alone.
  - Do not let children swim in areas where there are boats, fishermen, and large waves.
  - Allow children to swim at beaches only if lifeguards are present.
  - Do not let children dive into above-ground pools. They are too shallow. For safe diving, water must be 9 feet deep or greater.
  - Have children enter an in-ground pool feet first. The water is shallow.
  - Teach safe diving. Children should dive only from the diving board. They should dive with their hands in front of them.
  - Do not let children slide down a pool slide head first. Head injuries can occur.

Information from www.keepkidshealthy.com and www.usa.safekids.org.

Continued

BOX 11-1 Safety Measures for Infants and Children—cont'd

WATER SAFETY—cont'd

- Prevent hair entanglement or body part entrapment in pools, spas, hot tubs, and whirlpools. They can occur in suction and drain covers. If hair is caught, the head is kept underwater. Trapped body parts can keep the person underwater or cause serious injury.
  - Have suction and drain covers installed that meet current safety standards. Replace missing or broken covers.
  - Do not let children play near drain or suction covers.
  - Have children pin-up long hair or wear a swimming cap.
- Know where to find the power cut-off switch for pools, spas, hot tubs, or whirlpools. You must quickly turn off the electricity in an emergency.
- Keep hot tub, spa, and whirlpool temperatures no higher than 104° F. Higher temperatures can cause drowsiness, which can lead to drowning. Heat stroke and death are risks.

VEHICLE SAFETY

- Lock vehicle doors and the trunk. Keep keys where children cannot see or reach them. They can open a door or trunk with a remote control key.
- Show children how to find and use the emergency trunk release mechanism.
- Do not let children play in vehicles. They like to play hide-and-seek in cars and trunks. They can easily suffocate and die from high temperatures in the car or trunk.
- Keep any access to the trunk closed. Some vehicles have fold-down seats that give more trunk space. Children can get into the trunk from inside the car. Keep fold-down seats closed.
- Do not leave children alone in any motor vehicle, even if the windows are down. They can develop heat-related illness, suffocate, and die very quickly from high temperatures in the vehicle. It only takes a few minutes.
- Make sure all children leave the vehicle when you arrive at your destination.
- Use car safety seats correctly:
  - Use federally approved safety seats that fit the child's size and weight (Fig. 11-3). Follow the manufacturer's instructions.
  - Do not use a car safety seat that does not have the manufacturer's instructions.
  - Use a car safety seat that has a label with the manufacturer's name, model number, and the date it was made.
  - Install infant car safety seats rear-facing only (Fig. 11-4, p. 148). Infants ride this way until they are at least 20 pounds and at least 1 year old.
  - Do not use a rear-facing car or convertible seat in the front seat of a vehicle with an air bag.
  - Do not use a car safety seat that is more than 10 years old. Check the label for the date it was made.
  - Do not use a car safety seat that was involved in a crash.
  - Do not use a car safety seat that has cracks, missing parts, or torn or loose harnesses and buckles.
  - Use booster seats for children between the ages of 4 and 8 years (about 40 and 80 pounds). Secure them with lap and shoulder belts.
- Have children younger than 12 years ride in the back seat.
- Follow seat-belt laws.
- Never allow anyone to ride in the cargo bed of a pickup truck.
- Do not let children ride as passengers on tractors, mowers, mini-bikes, or all-terrain vehicles.

CLOTHING SAFETY

- Do not use pins on children's clothing.
- Remove drawstrings from jackets, coats, sweaters, swimsuits, and other clothing (Fig. 11-5, p. 148). This includes drawstrings on hoods, at the neckline, and at the waist. Drawstrings can get entangled or caught in play equipment, furniture, handrails, car or bus doors, elevators, escalators, and other moving devices.
- Do not dress children in loose clothing or clothing with drawstrings, fringe, strings, or ties if they will use playground equipment. The clothing can get caught on the equipment.
- Do not dress children in long clothing that touches or drags on the floor.
- Do not let children wear necklaces, strings, cords, or other items around the neck. These can get caught on furniture, doorknobs, and playground equipment.
- Warn children to check for hanging or dangling items from clothing and backpacks. They can catch on doors, handrails, playground equipment, furniture, and other things. Examples include key rings, scarves, belt and backpack buckles, and loose clothing.
- Make sure children wear safety shoes.
- Make sure shoelaces are tied.

TOY AND PLAY SAFETY

- Do not let children play in driveways or on streets, parking lots, or curbs.
- Do let children play behind parked cars.
- Do not let children play in piles of leaves or snow near streets.
- Keep children away from exercise bikes and equipment.
- Read all warning labels on toys.
- Check age recommendations on toys. Give children only age-appropriate toys.
- Check toys and other play equipment regularly. Look for cracks, chips, breaks, sharp edges, loose parts, and other damage. This includes playground equipment.
- Do let children play with toys that:
  - Have sharp points or edges.
  - Shoot objects into the air.
  - Make loud, sharp, or shrill noises. They could damage hearing.
  - Have long strings, straps, or cords. Strings, straps, and cords should be less than 7 inches long.
- Keep older children's toys away from infants and younger children.
- Make sure toys are too large to fit into the child's mouth. Objects should have a diameter of 1.75 inches or more.
- Do not let children use riding toys near stairs, pools, or traffic.
- Make sure children wear safety gear for bicycles, skateboards, scooters, in-line skates, and other devices with wheels. This includes helmets, elbow and knee pads, wrist guards, goggles, and reflective shoes and clothing.
- Make sure bike helmets are removed before children use playground equipment.
- Do not allow pushing, shoving, or crowding on playground equipment.

Information from www.keepkidshealthy.com and www.usa.safekids.org.

BOX 11-1 **Safety Measures for Infants and Children—cont'd**

FURNITURE SAFETY

- Prevent furniture from tipping over. Injuries and deaths can occur from children falling on, leaning on, climbing on, pulling on, sitting on, or trying to move poorly secured furniture. TV carts, bookcases, stands, chests-of-drawers, and tables present dangers.
- Prevent bookcases, shelving, and chests-of-drawers from being top heavy. If top heavy, they can tip and fall. Store heavier items on the lower shelves and in lower drawers.
- Make sure TVs, microwave ovens, and fish tanks are placed on low stands and are as far back on the stand as possible.
- Make sure that angle-braces or anchors are used to secure furniture to walls.
- Do not use tablecloths and placemats. This prevents infants and young children from pulling things off the table and onto themselves. Centerpieces, items on the table, and hot food and liquids can injure the child.
- Do not use toy chests with free-falling lids. The lid can fall on the child's head or neck. The lid should have a spring-loaded lid-support or sliding panels.

GUN SAFETY

- Store guns unloaded.
- Store guns locked up and out of the reach of children.
- Store ammunition in a separate, locked location.
- Use quality gun locks, lock boxes, or gun safes for each firearm.
- Keep gun storage keys and lock combinations hidden in a separate location.
- Teach children to never touch or play with a gun.
- Teach children to tell an adult if they find a gun.
- Teach children to call 911 if they find a gun when no adult is present.
- Do not let children visit or play in homes where gun safety is not practiced.

OTHER

- Protect the child from falls (Chapter 12).
- Protect the child from burns (p. 148).
- Protect the child from poisoning (p. 150).
- Protect the child from choking and suffocating (p. 152).
- See Chapter 47 for other infant safety measures.

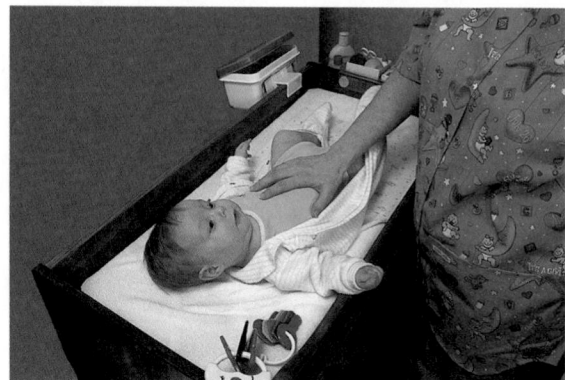

FIGURE 11-1 Keep one hand on a child lying in a crib or on a scale, bed, table, or other surface or furniture.

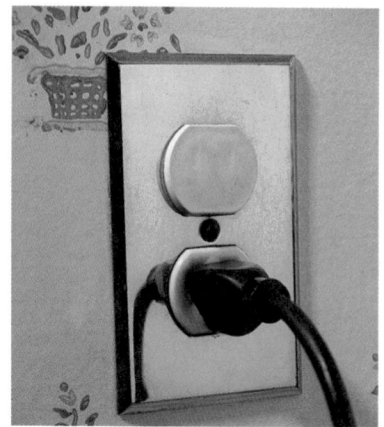

FIGURE 11-2 Safety plug in an outlet.

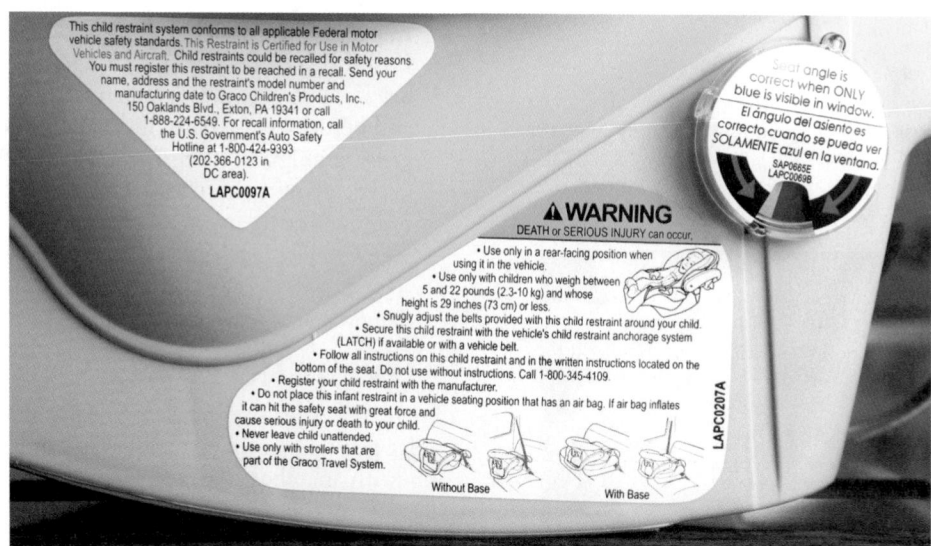

FIGURE 11-3 Federally approved car safety seats carry this label.

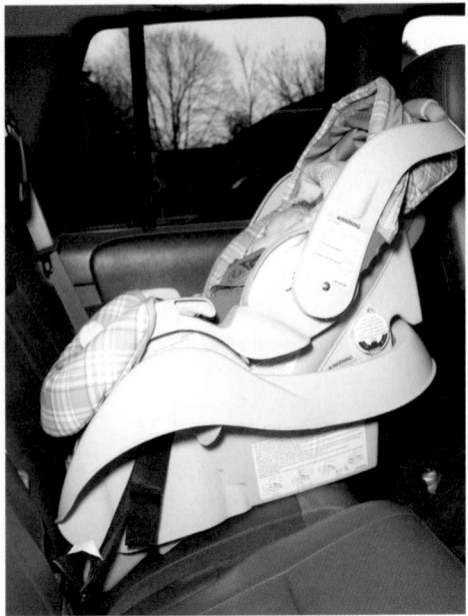

FIGURE 11-4 Infant in a car safety seat. Note that the seat is rear facing.

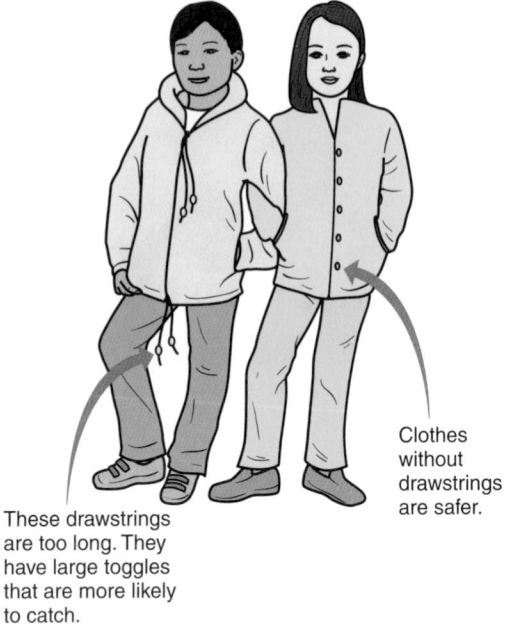

These drawstrings are too long. They have large toggles that are more likely to catch.

Clothes without drawstrings are safer.

FIGURE 11-5 Drawstrings can get caught in many things and strangle the child.

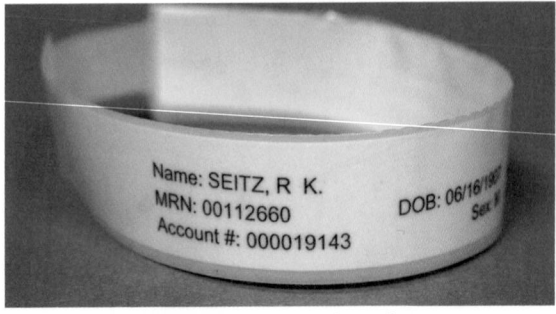

Name: SEITZ, R K.
MRN: 00112660   DOB: 06/16/19
Account #: 000019143   Sex

FIGURE 11-6 ID bracelet.

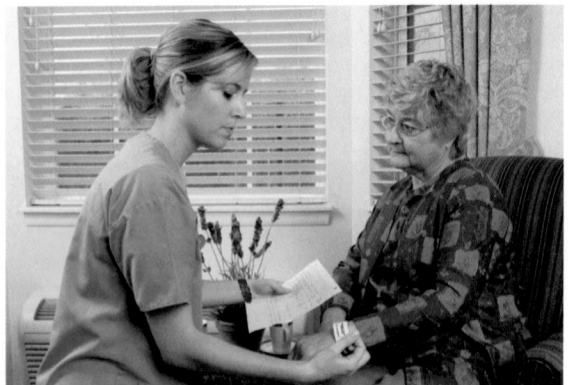

FIGURE 11-7 The ID bracelet is checked against the assignment sheet to accurately identify the person.

IDENTIFYING THE PERSON

You will care for many people. Each has different treatments, therapies, and activity limits. You must give the right care to the right person. Life and health are threatened if the wrong care is given.

The person receives an identification (ID) bracelet when admitted to the agency (Fig. 11-6). The bracelet has the person's name, room and bed number, birth date, age, doctor, and agency name. Other identifying information may include the person's ID number given by the agency. Some agencies include the person's religion.

You use the bracelet to identify the person before giving care. The assignment sheet states what care to give. To identify the person:

▶ Compare identifying information on the assignment sheet with that on the ID bracelet (Fig. 11-7). Carefully check the information. Some people have the same first and last names. For example, John Smith is a very common name.

▶ Use at least two identifiers. An identifier cannot be the person's room or bed number. Some agencies require that the person state his or her name and birth date. Others require using the person's ID number. Always follow agency policy.

▶ Call the person by name when checking the ID bracelet. This is a courtesy given as you touch the person and before giving care. Just calling the person by name is not enough to identify him or her. Confused, disoriented, drowsy, hard-of-hearing, or distracted persons may answer to any name.

See *Focus on Long-Term Care and Home Care: Identifying the Person*.

See *Promoting Safety and Comfort: Identifying the Person*.

PREVENTING BURNS

Burns are a leading cause of death among children and older persons. Smoking, spilled hot liquids, children playing with matches, barbecue grills, fireplaces, and stoves are common causes. Burns also can occur from electrical items and very hot bath or shower water. The safety measures in Box 11-2 can prevent burns.

FOCUS ON **LONG-TERM CARE** AND **HOME CARE**

Identifying the Person

LONG-TERM CARE

Alert and oriented residents may choose not to wear ID bracelets. This is noted on the person's care plan. Follow center policy and the care plan to identify the person.

Some nursing centers have photo ID systems (Fig. 11-8). The person's photo is taken on admission. Then it is placed in the person's medical record. If your center uses such a system, learn to use it safely.

PROMOTING SAFETY AND COMFORT: Identifying the Person

SAFETY

Always identify the person before you begin a task or procedure. Do not identify the person and then leave the room to collect supplies and equipment. You could go to the wrong room and give care to the wrong person. And the person for whom the care was intended would not receive it. This too could cause harm.

Sometimes ID bracelets become damaged from water, spilled food and fluids, and everyday wear and tear. Make sure you can read the information on the ID bracelet. If you cannot, tell the nurse. The nurse can have a new bracelet made for the person.

COMFORT

Make sure the person's ID bracelet is not too tight. You should be able to slide 1 or 2 fingers under the bracelet. If it is too tight, tell the nurse.

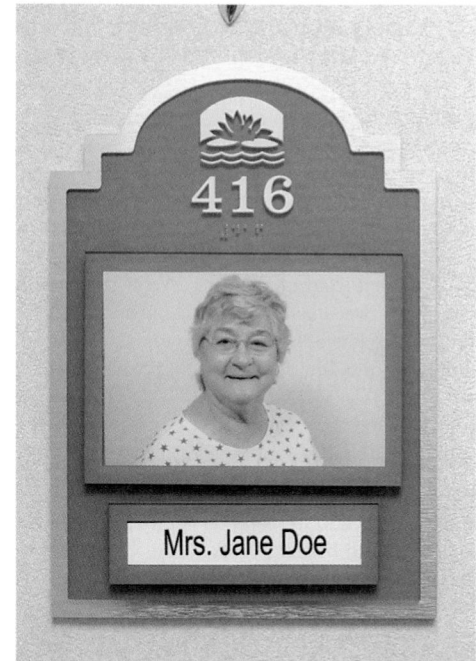

A

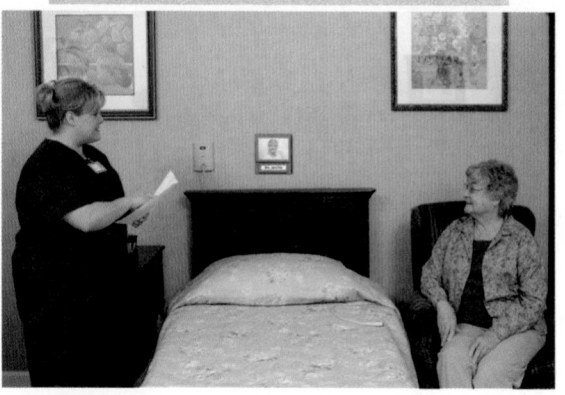

B

FIGURE 11-8 Photo ID system. **A,** The person's photo is at the room door. **B,** The person's photo is at the headboard. Her name is under the photo. The nursing assistant is using the photo to identify the person.

BOX 11-2 Safety Measures to Prevent Burns

CHILDREN
- Do not leave children home alone.
- Supervise young children at all times.
- Do not leave children alone in the kitchen, bathroom, or in a room with a fireplace.
- Store matches, lighters, lamp oils, or other flammable materials where children cannot reach them.
- Do not let children near stoves, space heaters, fireplaces, barbecue grills, radiators, registers, oil lamps, candles, and other heat sources.
- Keep space heaters and materials that can catch fire away from children.
- Teach children fire safety and fire prevention measures. Also teach the dangers of fire.
- Use the stove's back burners when infants and children are in the kitchen.

- Do not let children help you cook at the stove or in a microwave oven.
- Check metal playground equipment before children play on it. Metal surfaces exposed to sunlight can heat to high temperatures. They can burn the face, hands, arms, legs, and buttocks.
- Check car seats, seat belts, and seat belt buckles. If hot, they can burn children.
- Cover car seats with towels if you park in the sun. Also use a sun visor for the windshield.
- Do not let children play with fireworks.
- Protect children from sun exposure:
  - Use a sunscreen.
  - Cover exposed areas.
  - Limit time in the sun.

Continued

BOX 11-2 Safety Measures to Prevent Burns—cont'd

COOKING
- Point pot and pan handles so they point inward. They point away from where people stand and walk.
- Do not leave cooking utensils in pots and pans.
- Do not wear clothing with long sleeves when cooking.
- Do not put wet food into frying pans or deep-fryers. The water causes the oil to splatter.
- Use dry oven mitts and pot-holders. Water conducts heat.
- Stay near the stove, microwave, and barbecue grill when cooking. Do not leave them unattended.
- Keep hot food and liquids away from counter and table edges.
- Turn the oven and stove burners off when not in use.
- Do not pour hot liquids near a child or older person.

EATING AND DRINKING
- Assist with eating and drinking as needed. Spilled hot food or fluids can cause burns.
- Be careful when carrying hot foods and fluids near children and older persons.

WATER
- Have hot water heaters set at 120° F or less.
- Have anti-scald devices installed on faucets and shower-heads.
- Turn on cold water first, then hot water. Turn off hot water first, then cold water.
- Measure bath or shower water temperature (Chapter 19). Check it before a person gets into the tub or shower.
- Check for "hot spots" in bath water. Move your hand back and forth.

- Do not leave children unattended in bathtubs.
- Position the child facing away from faucets when bathing a child in a tub or at a sink.
- Do not let children touch faucet handles.
- Place knob covers over faucets to prevent children from turning on the water.

APPLIANCES
- See "Preventing Equipment Accidents" (p. 158).
- Do not allow the use of space heaters.
- Do not let the person sleep with a heating pad.
- Do not let the person use an electric blanket.
- Do not leave irons unattended. Keep them off when not in use.
- Keep curling irons, electric rollers, and hair dryers out of the reach of children. Turn them off when not in use.

SMOKING
- Be sure people smoke only in smoking areas.
- Do not leave smoking materials at the bedside. They are only left at the bedside if the person is trusted to smoke alone in smoking areas. Follow the care plan.
- Supervise the smoking of persons who cannot protect themselves.
- Do not allow smoking in bed.
- Do not allow smoking where oxygen is used or stored (Chapter 34).
- Be alert to ashes that may fall onto a child or older person.

OTHER
- Follow safety guidelines when applying heat and cold (Chapter 33).

PREVENTING POISONING

Poisoning also is a health hazard and a major cause of death. Children and older persons are at risk. Drugs and household products are common poisons. Poisoning in adults may be from carelessness, confusion, or poor vision when reading labels. As a result, a person may take too much of a drug. Sometimes poisoning is a suicide attempt.

Common poisons include:
- Drugs (including aspirin) and vitamins
- Household products—detergents, soaps, sprays, furniture polish, window cleaners, bleach, paint, paint thinner, toilet bowl and other cleaners, gasoline, kerosene, glue, and so on
- Personal care products—soaps, shampoos, hair conditioners, bath oils, powders, lotions, nail polish remover, sprays, makeup, perfumes, after-shave lotions, deodorants, mouthwash, and so on
- Fertilizers, insecticides, bug sprays, and so on
- Lead
- House plants
- Alcohol
- Carbon monoxide (p. 152)

To prevent poisoning, follow the safety measures in Box 11-3.

Lead Poisoning

Lead is a metal. When in the body, it interferes with normal body functions. It can injure the brain, nervous system, red blood cells, kidneys, liver, teeth, and bones. It can lower intelligence and cause learning problems and behavior problems.

Lead is found in batteries, pipes, pottery glazes, printing inks, industrial paints, and dirt. The use of lead in house-hold paint was banned in the 1970s. However, many older homes still have lead paint on walls and other surfaces.

Lead enters the body through:
- *Inhalation.* Dust in the air may contain lead. Windows may have lead-based paint. When widows are open and closed, dust is created. Dust from soil may contain lead.
- *Ingestion.* Young children can eat, chew, and suck on non-food items that may contain lead. Lead-painted surfaces—window sills and railings—are examples. They may eat paint chips. Water is a source of lead if plumbing materials contain lead.

Children between the ages of 6 months and 6 years are at risk for lead poisoning. Lead can affect almost every body system. Signs and symptoms are gradual in onset. They are not always obvious. See Box 11-4, p. 152.

BOX 11-3 Safety Measures to Prevent Poisoning

- Keep harmful products in high, locked areas (Fig. 11-9). Children and confused persons cannot see or reach them.
- Buy products with child-resistant packaging.
- Keep child-resistant caps on all harmful products.
- Use and store harmful products according to the manufacturer's instructions (p. 160).
- Do not leave harmful products unattended when in use.
- Make sure all harmful products are labeled (p. 161).
- Do not mix cleaning products.
- Read all labels carefully. Have good lighting.
- Keep harmful products in their original containers. Do not store them in food containers.
- Do not store harmful products near food.
- Discard harmful products that are outdated (p. 161).
- Use safety latches on kitchen, bathroom, utility, garage, basement, and workshop cabinets and drawers.
- Keep drugs out of purses, backpacks, briefcases, luggage, and other items where children may find them. Family and friends may keep drugs in such places. Keep children away from such items.

- Do not take drugs or vitamins in front of children.
- Never call drugs or vitamins "candy."
- Discard poisonous household plants. Or place them where persons at risk cannot reach them.
- Teach children not to eat plants and unknown foods. Teach them not to eat leaves, stems, seeds, berries, nuts, or bark.
- Place poison warning stickers ("Mr. Yuk") on harmful substances (Fig. 11-10).
- Keep all baby products and diaper-changing supplies out of the child's reach.
- Keep emergency numbers by the telephone: poison control center (1-800-222-1222), police, ambulance, hospital, and doctor.
- Supervise children when visiting family and friends. Look for harmful products on kitchen counters, kitchen tables, bathroom, and other surfaces.
- Prevent lead poisoning (p. 150).
- Prevent carbon monoxide poisoning (p. 152).

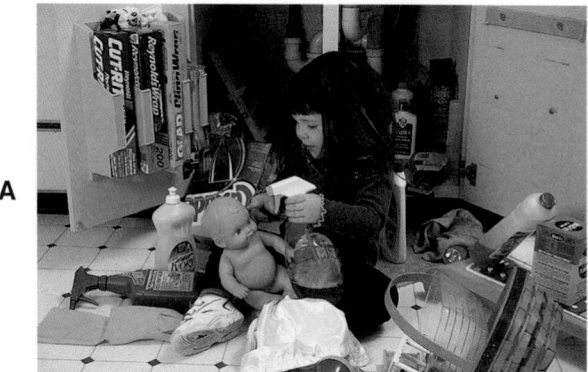 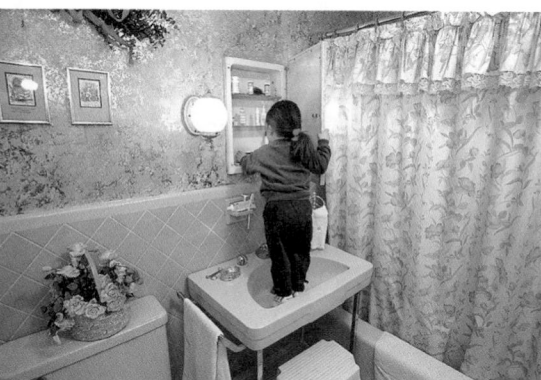

FIGURE 11-9 Harmful products must be kept in locked areas out of the reach of children. **A,** Household cleaners are within a child's reach when in low cabinets. **B,** The bathroom medicine chest holds many harmful products.

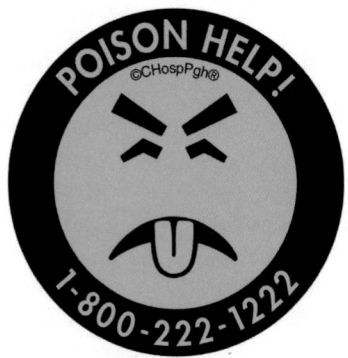

FIGURE 11-10 The "Mr. Yuk" warning sticker is placed on harmful products. (Courtesy Children's Hospital, Pittsburgh Poison Center, Pittsburgh, Pa.)

BOX 11-4 Lead Poisoning

SIGNS AND SYMPTOMS OF LEAD POISONING IN CHILDREN
- Abdominal pain
- Activity: decreased
- Appetite: poor
- Behavior problems
- Constipation
- Coordination: poor
- Diarrhea
- Fatigue
- Growth: decreased
- Headaches
- Hearing loss
- Hyperactivity
- Irritability
- Language problems
- Learning problems
- Memory problems
- Muscle weakness
- Pallor
- Reflexes: slow
- Seizures
- Sleep: increased
- Sluggishness
- Speech problems
- Vomiting
- Weight loss

SAFETY MEASURES TO PREVENT LEAD POISONING
- Prevent or discourage children from eating, chewing, or sucking on non-food items. They include:
  - Toys and furniture painted before 1976
  - Painted toys and decorations made outside the United States
  - Paint chips
  - Dirt
  - Keys
  - Pewter and lead-based figurines
  - Fishing sinkers
- Do not let children play in dirt. Have them play in grassy or sandy areas.
- Assist the child with hand washing before eating, after playing outside, and before going to bed.
- Wash toys often.
- Rinse pacifiers, baby bottles, and other items that fall to the floor.

- Prevent exposure to lead-based plumbing:
  - Let cold water run for 1 to 2 minutes before drinking water or using it for coffee or cooking. This helps flush the lead out of the plumbing.
  - Do not use hot tap water to make baby formula.
  - Do not use hot tap water for cooking or drinking.
- Prevent exposure to lead-based paint:
  - Keep children away from paint chips.
  - Keep children away from dust contaminated with lead paint.
  - Use a wet mop and wet cloths to clean up dust and paint chips.
  - Use a wet mop and wet cloths to clean furniture, window-sills, and dusty surfaces.
  - Use duct tape to cover peeling or chipping paint. This is only a temporary measure. Peeling and chipping paint must be removed.
  - Do not bump into walls or furniture that may contain lead-based paint. This prevents dust and paint chips.
  - Do not open and close windows that have lead-based paint. This prevents dust and paint chips.
  - Do not sweep or vacuum lead-based paint dust or paint chips.
- Prevent exposure to food contaminated with lead:
  - Do not use glazed pottery to cook food.
  - Do not eat foods that are stored or served in glazed pottery.
  - Do not eat foods that are canned outside the United States.
  - Wash fruits and vegetables before eating or serving them. They may have been grown in soil that contains lead.
- Prevent children from having contact with work or hobby materials that may contain lead. Children's paint sets and art supplies and welding, pottery, home building and repair, and automotive repair materials are examples.
  - Store lead-based products where children cannot see or reach them.
  - Take shoes off before entering the home.
  - Shower and change clothes before having contact with children.
  - Wash and store clothes contaminated with lead separately from others.
- Do not let children handle or play with old newspapers, magazines, or comic books. The ink may contain lead.

Modified from www.keepkidshealthy.com.

Carbon Monoxide Poisoning

Carbon monoxide is a colorless, odorless, and tasteless gas. It is produced by the burning of fuel—gas, oil, kerosene, wood, charcoal. Motor vehicles, furnaces, gas water heaters, gas stoves, and gas dryers use fuel. These devices must be in good working order and must be used correctly. Otherwise, dangerous levels of carbon monoxide may result. Instead of breathing in oxygen, the person breathes in air filled with carbon monoxide. Death can occur. See Box 11-5.

PREVENTING SUFFOCATION

Suffocation is when breathing stops from the lack of oxygen. Death occurs if the person does not start breathing. Common causes include choking, drowning, inhaling gas or smoke, strangulation, and electrical shock (p. 158).

Measures to prevent suffocation are listed in Box 11-6. Clear the airway if the person is choking.

BOX 11-5 **Carbon Monoxide Poisoning**

SIGNS AND SYMPTOMS
- Breathing problems
- Cherry-pink skin
- Confusion
- Dizziness
- Fainting
- Headache
- Nausea
- Sleepiness
- Slurred speech
- Vomiting
- Weakness

SAFETY MEASURES TO PREVENT CARBON MONOXIDE POISONING
- Have carbon monoxide detectors installed in each sleeping area.
- Have vehicle exhaust systems checked regularly.
- Have fuel-burning appliances checked regularly. This includes furnaces, gas water heaters, gas stoves and ovens, gas dryers, gas or kerosene space heaters, fireplaces, and wood stoves.

- Follow the manufacturer's instructions when using fuel-burning devices.
- Use the correct fuel when using fuel-burning devices.
- Do not idle a vehicle, lawn mower, snow blower, weed trimmer, or other device in an open or closed garage. Fumes can leak into the house.
- Have fuel-burning devices and chimneys checked when people in the same building show signs and symptoms.
- If you or others have signs and symptoms:
  - Open doors and windows.
  - Turn off appliances.
  - Leave the home.
  - Go to an emergency room.
- Open doors and windows if you notice gas odors. Turn off appliances, and leave the home.
- Have gas odors checked by trained professionals.
- Do not use a gas oven to heat a home.
- Do not use barbecue grills indoors or in a garage.

BOX 11-6 **Safety Measures to Prevent Suffocation**

ALL AGE-GROUPS
- Cut food into small, bite-sized pieces for persons who cannot do so themselves.
- Make sure dentures fit properly and are in place.
- Make sure the person can chew and swallow the food served.
- Report loose teeth or dentures.
- Check the care plan for swallowing problems before serving snacks or fluids. The person may ask for something that he or she cannot swallow.
- Tell the nurse at once if the person has swallowing problems.
- Do not give oral food or fluids to persons with feeding tubes (Chapter 24).
- Follow aspiration precautions (Chapter 23).
- Do not leave a person unattended in a bathtub or shower.
- Move all persons from the area if you smell smoke.
- Position the person in bed properly (Chapter 15).
- Use bed rails correctly (Chapter 12).
- Use restraints correctly (Chapter 13).
- Prevent entrapment in the bed system (Chapter 17).
- See "Preventing Equipment Accidents" (p. 158).

CHILDREN
- Keep plastic bags, covers, and dry-cleaning bags away from children.
- Tie large plastic bags and garment bags in knots. Then discard them.
- Place safety plugs in outlets. This includes electrical strips and surge protectors.
- Keep electrical cords and electrical items out of the reach of children.

- Position infants on their backs for sleep.
- Do not use pillows to position infants.
- Do not use pillows to prevent infants from falling off of beds and furniture.
- Remove pillows, comforters, quilts, sheepskin, stuffed toys, and other soft items from the crib when the baby is sleeping.
- Do not feed an infant while he or she is lying down.
- Do not give infants and young children hot dogs, peanuts, popcorn, grapes, raisins, hard candy, or gum.
- Use Mylar balloons instead of latex ones.
- Store latex balloons where children cannot see or reach them.
- Do not let children inflate or deflate latex balloons.
- Deflate and discard latex balloons after use.
- Pick up and discard broken balloon pieces at once. Do not let children near them.
- Check floors for small objects—buttons, coins, beads, marbles, pins, tacks, nails, screws, and so on. Keep them out of a child's reach. Pick up and store or discard such objects. Children can choke on them.
- Check toys for removable parts.
- Do not string or hang any object on or near a crib. This includes a mobile, toy, or diaper bag. The child could get caught in it and strangle.
- Never tie pacifiers or teethers around a child's neck.
- Remove bibs and necklaces whenever the child is put in a crib or playpen.
- Keep appliance doors closed—ovens, refrigerators, clothes dryers, washing machines, refrigerators, freezers, dishwashers, coolers, and so on.

♦ Choking

Foreign bodies can obstruct the airway. This is called *choking* or *foreign-body airway obstruction (FBAO)*. Air cannot pass through the air passages to the lungs. The body does not get enough oxygen. It can lead to cardiac arrest. *Cardiac arrest* is when the heart and breathing stop suddenly and without warning (Chapter 49).

Choking often occurs during eating. A large, poorly chewed piece of meat is the most common cause. Laughing and talking while eating also are common causes. So is excessive alcohol intake.

Choking can occur in the unconscious person. Common causes are aspiration of vomitus and the tongue falling back into the airway. These occur during cardiac arrest.

Foreign bodies can cause mild or severe airway obstruction. With *mild airway obstruction*, some air moves in and out of the lungs. The person is conscious. Usually the person can speak. Often forceful coughing can remove the object. The person's breathing may sound like wheezing between coughs. Encourage the person to keep coughing to expel the object.

With *severe airway obstruction*:

▶ The conscious person clutches at the throat (Fig. 11-11). Clutching at the throat is often called the "universal sign of choking."
▶ The person has difficulty breathing.
▶ The person may not be able to breathe, speak, or cough. If the person can cough, the cough is of poor quality.
▶ When the person tries to inhale, there is no noise or a high-pitched noise.
▶ Infants cannot cry.

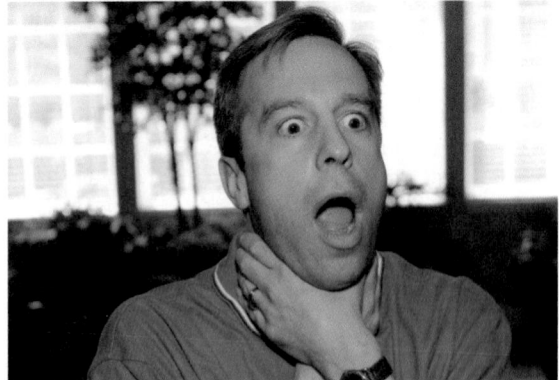

FIGURE 11-11 A choking person clutches at the throat.

▶ The person may appear pale and cyanotic (bluish color).
▶ Air does not move in and out of the lungs.

The conscious person is very frightened. If the obstruction is not removed, the person will die. Severe airway obstruction is an emergency.

Abdominal thrusts are used to relieve severe airway obstruction. The thrusts are performed with the person standing, sitting, or lying down.

Abdominal thrusts are not used for very obese persons or pregnant women. Chest thrusts are used (Box 11-7).

Call for help when an adult or child (over 1 year of age) has:

▶ Severe airway obstruction
▶ Mild airway obstruction that persists despite the person's attempts to remove the object by coughing

In an agency, activate the agency's Rapid Repsonse Team (RRT). In a public area, have someone activate the Emergency Medical Services (EMS) system by calling 911. See Chapter 49 for basic emergency care. Report and record what happened, what you did, and the person's response.

See *Focus on Children and Older Persons: Choking.*
See *Focus on Ethics and Laws: Choking.*

BOX 11-7 Obstructed Airway: Chest Thrusts for Obese or Pregnant Persons

THE PERSON IS SITTING OR STANDING
1 Stand behind the person.
2 Place your arms under the person's underarms. Wrap your arms around the person's chest.
3 Make a fist. Place the thumb side of the fist on the middle of the sternum (breastbone).
4 Grasp the fist with your other hand.
5 Give backward chest thrusts until the object is expelled or the person becomes unresponsive.
6 Activate the EMS system or the agency's RRT if the person is not responding. Start cardiopulmonary resuscitation (CPR) (Chapter 49).

THE PERSON IS LYING DOWN
1 Position the person supine.
2 Kneel next to the person.
3 Position your hands as for external chest compressions (Chapter 49).
4 Give chest thrusts until the object is expelled or the person becomes unresponsive.
5 Activate the EMS system or the agency's RRT if the person is not responding. Start CPR (Chapter 49).

FOCUS ON **CHILDREN** AND **OLDER PERSONS**

Choking

CHILDREN

Children can choke on small objects. Pieces of hot dogs, marbles, hard candy, peanuts, apples, and grapes are examples. Peanut butter and popcorn also can cause choking. So can coins and small toys and toy parts. FBAO in children is marked by the *sudden* onset of symptoms.

Respiratory infections can cause airway obstruction in infants and children. Airway structures become swollen. The airway narrows or becomes completely obstructed. Air cannot enter the airway. The child needs emergency care at once.

The procedure that follows will not relieve airway obstruction caused by an infection. Do not try it if the child has a fever, rash, respiratory congestion, hoarseness, or other signs and symptoms of infection. You will waste precious time. Give rescue breaths. Start CPR if the child is not responding, and activate the EMS system or the agency's RRT. See Chapter 49.

Abdominal thrusts are not given to infants. They can damage the liver and other organs. Back slaps (back blows) and chest thrusts are used for infants.

OLDER PERSONS

Older persons are at risk for choking. Weakness, dentures that fit poorly, dysphagia (difficulty swallowing), and chronic illness are common causes.

FOCUS ON **ETHICS** AND **LAWS**

Choking

A 32-year-old man was a patient at a developmental center. He was retarded and had a history of epilepsy. He was a patient at the center since the age of 25.

According to the facts reported in the court case, the following occurred:
- On August 28, 1978, he had a dinner of braised beef and noodles. The pieces of beef were about ½ inch wide and ¾ inch long.
- While eating dinner, he stood up, coughed out his milk, reached for his throat, and collapsed.
- Efforts were made to revive him.
- He was transported to the hospital where he died a short while later.
- His death was caused by "meat mass inhalation . . . associated with mental retardation with chronic seizure disorder. . . ."

The lawsuit claimed negligence because:
- His swallowing was affected by the dosage of a drug.
- He was not given a soft diet.
- He was not properly supervised at mealtime.

In the Court's opinion, negligent care resulted in the patient's death.

(B. Szydelko v The Department of Mental Health of the State of Illinois, 1984.)

RELIEVING CHOKING—THE RESPONSIVE ADULT OR CHILD (OVER 1 YEAR OF AGE)

1 Ask the person if he or she is choking. Help the person if he or she nods "yes" and cannot talk.

2 Call for help. Activate the EMS system (Chapter 49) or the agency's RRT.

3 *If the person is standing or sitting,* give abdominal thrusts (Fig. 11-12, p. 156):
  a Stand or kneel behind the person.
  b Wrap your arms around the person's waist.
  c Make a fist with one hand.
  d Place the thumb side of the fist against the abdomen. The fist is in the middle slightly above the navel and well below the end of the sternum (breastbone).
  e Grasp the fist with your other hand.
  f Press your fist and hand into the person's abdomen with a quick, upward thrust.
  g Repeat thrusts until the object is expelled or the person loses consciousness (is not responding).

4 *If the person is lying down,* give abdominal thrusts (Fig. 11-13, p. 156):
  a Straddle the person's thighs.
  b Place the heel of one hand against the abdomen. It is in the middle slightly above the navel and well below the end of the sternum (breastbone).
  c Place your second hand on top of your first hand.
  d Press both hands into the abdomen with a quick, upward thrust.
  e Repeat thrusts until the object is expelled or the person loses consciousness (is not responding).

5 Lower the unresponsive person to the floor or ground. Position the person supine.

6 Remove a foreign object if you see it:
  a Open the airway with the head tilt-chin lift method (Fig. 11-14, p. 156).
  b Look in the mouth for a foreign object.
  c Grasp and remove the object if it is within reach.

7 Start CPR (Chapter 49). Look for an object every time you open the airway for rescue breaths. Open the person's mouth. The mouth should be wide open. Remove the object if you see it. Use your fingers. Continue CPR if you do not see an object.

8 Do the following to relieve choking in an unresponsive person:
  a Provide 2 rescue breaths (Chapter 49).
  b Check for a pulse.
    1 If the person has no pulse and is not breathing— give chest compressions and attach an automated external defibrillator (AED) (Chapter 49).
    2 If the person has a pulse but is not breathing— continue rescue breaths. Check for a pulse every 2 minutes.
    3 If the person has a pulse and is breathing—place the person in the recovery position (Chapter 49). Continue to check the person until help arrives.

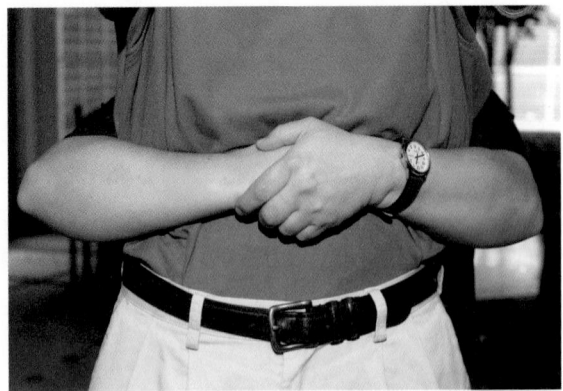

FIGURE 11-12 Abdominal thrusts with the person standing.

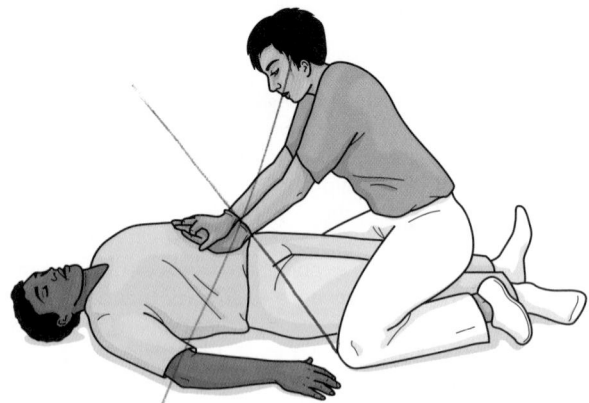

FIGURE 11-13 Abdominal thrust with the person lying down. The rescuer straddles the thighs.

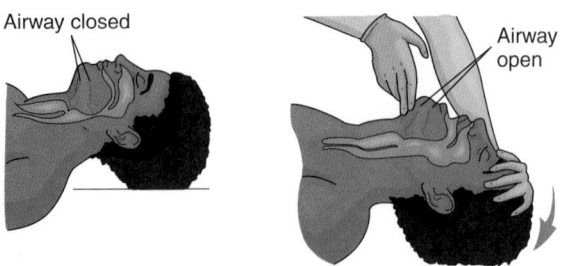

FIGURE 11-14 The head tilt-chin lift method opens the airway. One hand is on the person's forehead. Pressure is applied to lift the head back. The chin is lifted with the fingers of the other hand.

RELIEVING CHOKING IN THE INFANT

1 Kneel next to the infant. Or sit with the infant in your lap.
2 Expose the infant's chest. Perform this step if you can easily expose the chest.
3 Hold the infant face down over your forearm. (Support your arm on your thigh or lap.) The infant's head is lower than the trunk. Support the head and jaw with your hand.
4 Give up to 5 forceful back slaps (back blows) (Fig. 11-15). Use the heel of your hand. Give the back slaps between the shoulder blades. (Stop the back slaps if the object is expelled.)
5 Turn the infant as a unit:
  a Continue to support the infant's face, jaw, head, neck, and chest with one hand.
  b Support the back and the back of the infant's head with your other hand. Your palm supports the back of the head.
  c Turn the infant as a unit. The infant is in a back-lying position on your forearm. Your forearm rests on your thigh. The infant's head is lower than the trunk.

6 Give up to 5 chests thrusts (Fig. 11-16). The chest thrusts are quick and downward.
  a Locate hand position as for chest compressions (Chapter 49). The location is just below the nipple line.
  b Give chest thrusts at a rate of about 1 every second.
  c Stop chest thrusts if the object is expelled.
7 Give 5 back slaps followed by 5 chest thrusts until:
  a The object is expelled.
  b The infant becomes unresponsive.
8 Do the following if the infant becomes unresponsive:
  a Place the infant on a firm, flat surface.
  b Open the airway.
  c Look in the throat for an object.
  d Remove the object if you see it.
  e Start CPR (Chapter 49). Look for an object in the throat each time you open the airway. Remove the object if you see it.
  f Activate the EMS system or the agency's RRT after about 5 cycles of CPR (about 2 minutes).
  g Continue CPR until help arrives.

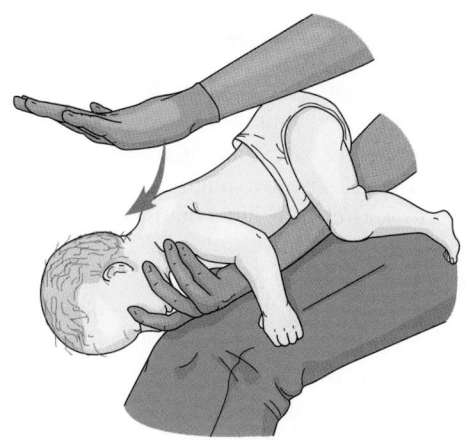

FIGURE 11-15 Back slaps (back blows). The infant is held face down and supported with one hand. The rescuer's forearm is supported on his or her thigh. Back slaps are given between the shoulder blades with the heel of one hand.

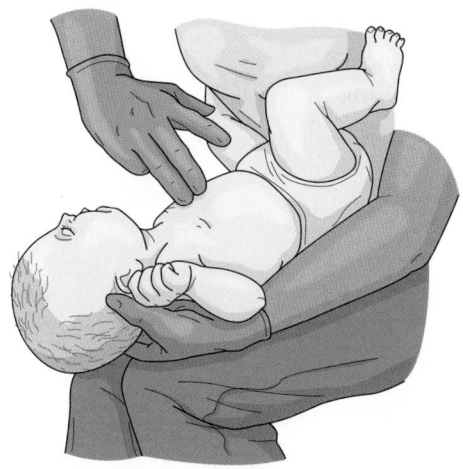

FIGURE 11-16 Chest thrusts. The infant is in the back-lying position. Hand position for chest thrusts is the same as for chest compressions (Chapter 49).

The Unresponsive Adult

You may find an adult who is unresponsive. You did not see the person lose consciousness, and you do not know the cause. Do not assume the cause is choking. Check to see if the person is responding. If not, activate the EMS system or the agency's RRT. Start CPR.

Self-Administered Abdominal Thrusts

You may choke when by yourself. You can perform abdominal thrusts to relieve the obstructed airway. To do so:
1. Make a fist with one hand.
2. Place the thumb side of the fist above your navel and below the lower end of the sternum.
3. Grasp your fist with your other hand.
4. Press inward and upward quickly.
5. Press the upper abdomen against a hard surface if the thrust did not relieve the obstruction. Use the back of a chair, a table, or railing.
6. Use as many thrusts as needed.

PREVENTING EQUIPMENT ACCIDENTS

All equipment is unsafe if broken, not used correctly, or not working properly. This includes hospital beds. Inspect all equipment before use. Check glass and plastic items for cracks, chips, and sharp or rough edges. They can cause cuts, stabs, or scratches. Follow the Bloodborne Pathogen Standard (Chapter 14).

Electrical items must work properly and be in good repair. Frayed cords (Fig. 11-17) and over-loaded electrical outlets (Fig. 11-18) can cause fires, burns, and electrical shocks. **Electrical shock** is when electrical current passes through the body. It can burn the skin, muscles, nerves, and other tissues. It can affect the heart and cause death.

Three-pronged plugs (Fig. 11-19) are used on all electrical items. Two prongs carry electrical current. The third prong is the ground. A **ground** carries leaking electricity to the earth and away from an electrical item. If a ground is not used, leaking electricity can be conducted to the person. It can cause electrical shocks and possible death. If you receive a shock, report it at once. Do not use the item.

Warning signs of a faulty electrical item include:
▶ Shocks
▶ Loss of power or a power outage
▶ Dimming or flickering lights
▶ Sparks
▶ Sizzling or buzzing sounds
▶ Burning odor
▶ Loose plugs

Do not use or give damaged items to patients or residents. Take the item to the nurse. The nurse will have you do one of the following:
▶ Discard the item following agency policy.
▶ Tag the item and send it for repair following agency policy.

Practice the safety measures in Box 11-8 when using equipment. An incident report (p. 170) is completed if a patient, resident, visitor, or staff member has an equipment-related accident. The Safe Medical Devices Act requires that agencies report equipment-related illnesses, injuries, and deaths.

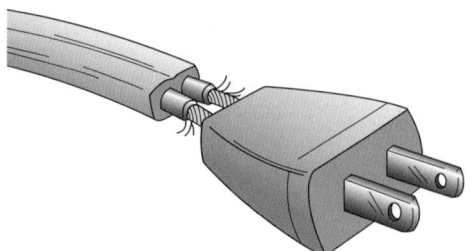

FIGURE 11-17 A frayed electrical cord.

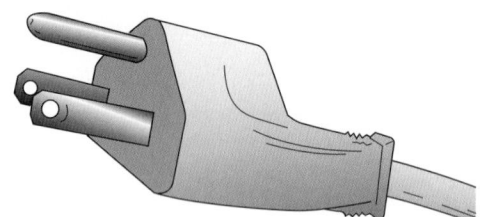

FIGURE 11-19 A three-pronged plug.

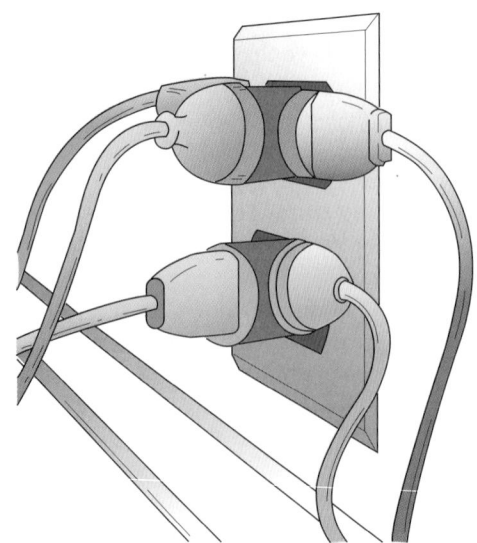

FIGURE 11-18 An over-loaded electrical outlet.

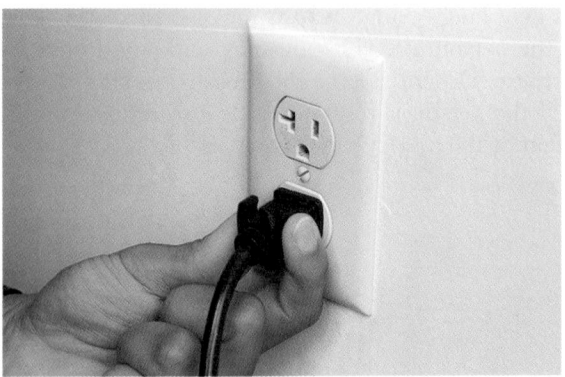

FIGURE 11-20 Hold onto the plug to remove it from an outlet.

BOX 11-8 Safety Measures to Prevent Equipment Accidents

GENERAL SAFETY
- Follow agency policies and procedures.
- Follow the manufacturer's instructions. Use equipment correctly.
- Read all caution and warning labels.
- Do not use an unfamiliar item. Ask for needed training. Also ask a nurse to supervise you the first time you use an item.
- Use an item only for its intended purpose.
- Make sure the item works before you begin.
- Make sure you have all needed equipment. For example, you need to plug in an item. There must be an outlet.
- Show a broken or damaged item to the nurse. Follow the nurse's instructions and agency policies for discarding items or sending them for repair.
- Do not try to repair broken or damaged items.
- Do not use broken or damaged items.

ELECTRICAL SAFETY
- Inspect electrical cords and appliances for damage. Make sure they are in good repair.
- Use three-pronged plugs on all electrical devices.
- Do not cover power cords with rugs, carpets, linens, or other materials. Do not run power cords under rugs.
- Connect a bed power cord directly to a wall outlet. Do not connect a bed power cord to an extension cord or outlet strip.
- Do not use electrical items owned by the person until they are safety checked. The maintenance staff does this.
- Keep electrical items away from water.
- Keep work areas clean and dry. Wipe up spills right away.
- Do not touch electrical items if you are wet, if your hands are wet, or if you are standing in water.
- Do not put a finger or any item into an outlet.
- Turn off equipment before unplugging it. Sparks occur when electrical items are unplugged while turned on.
- Hold onto the plug (not the cord) when removing it from an outlet (Fig. 11-20).
- Do not give showers or tub baths during electrical storms. Lightning can travel through pipes.
- Do not use electrical items or phones during storms.
- Do not use water to put out an electrical fire. If possible turn off or unplug the item.
- Do not touch a person who is experiencing an electrical shock. If possible, turn off or unplug the item. Call for help at once.
- Keep electrical cords away from heating vents and other heat sources.
- Turn off the device when done using the item.
- Unplug all electrical devices when not in use.

WHEELCHAIR AND STRETCHER SAFETY

Some people cannot walk or they have severe problems walking. A wheelchair may be useful (Fig. 11-21). If able, the person propels the chair using the handrims. Some use their feet to move the chair. Other wheelchairs are propelled by motors. The person moves the chair with hand, chin, mouth, or other controls. If the person cannot propel the wheelchair, another person pushes it using the handgrips/push handles.

Stretchers are used to transport persons who cannot use wheelchairs. They cannot sit up or must lie down. A stretcher is used to move the person from one area of the agency to another.

Follow the safety measures in Box 11-9 (p. 160) when using wheelchairs and stretchers. The person can fall from the wheelchair or stretcher. Or the person can fall during transfers to and from the wheelchair or stretcher.

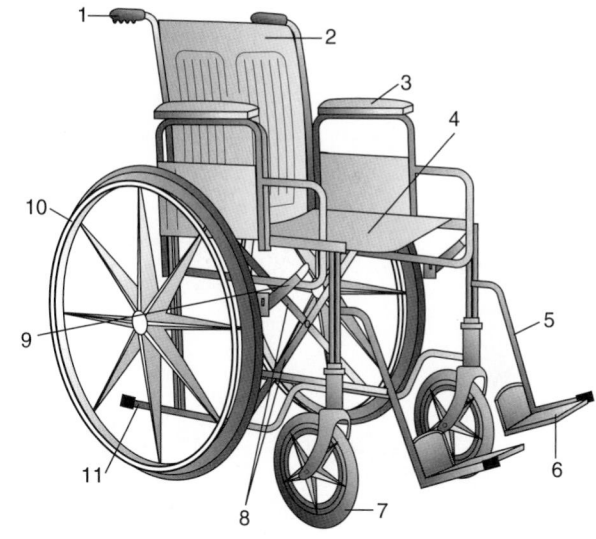

1. Handgrip/push handle
2. Back upholstery
3. Armrest
4. Seat upholstery
5. Front rigging
6. Footplate
7. Caster
8. Crossbrace
9. Wheel lock/brake
10. Wheel and handrim
11. Tipping lever

FIGURE 11-21 Parts of a wheelchair.

BOX 11-9 Wheelchair and Stretcher Safety

WHEELCHAIR SAFETY

- Check the wheel locks (brakes). Make sure you can lock and unlock them.
- Check for flat or loose tires. A wheel lock will not work on a flat or loose tire.
- Make sure the wheel spokes are intact. Damaged, broken, or loose spokes can interfere with moving the wheelchair or locking the wheels.
- Make sure the casters point forward. This keeps the wheelchair balanced and stable.
- Position the person's feet on the footplates.
- Make sure the person's feet are on the footplates before moving the chair. The person's feet must not touch or drag on the floor when the chair is moving.
- Push the chair forward when transporting the person. Do not pull the chair backward unless going through a doorway.
- Lock both wheels before you transfer a person to or from the wheelchair.
- Follow the care plan for keeping the wheels locked when not moving the wheelchair. Locking the wheels prevents the chair from moving if the person wants to move to or from the chair. (Locking the wheelchair may be considered to be a restraint. See Chapter 13.)
- Do not let the person stand on the footplates.
- Do not let the footplates fall back onto the person's legs.
- Make sure the person has needed wheelchair accessories—safety belt, pouch, tray, lapboard, cushion.

- Remove the armrests (if removable) when the person transfers to the bed, toilet, commode, tub, or car (Chapter 16).
- Swing front rigging out of the way for transfers to and from the wheelchair. Some front riggings detach for transfers.
- Clean the wheelchair according to agency policy.
- Ask a nurse or physical therapist to show you how to propel wheelchairs up steps and ramps and over curbs.
- Follow the safety measures to prevent equipment accidents, p. 158.

STRETCHER SAFETY

- Ask two co-workers to help you transfer the person to or from the stretcher (Chapter 16).
- Lock the stretcher wheels before the transfer.
- Fasten the safety straps when the person is properly positioned on the stretcher.
- Ask a co-worker to help with the transport.
- Raise the side rails. Keep them up during the transport.
- Make sure the person's arms, hands, legs, and feet do not dangle through the side rail bars.
- Stand at the head of the stretcher. Your co-worker stands at the foot of the stretcher.
- Move the stretcher feet first (Fig. 11-22).
- Do not leave the person alone.
- Follow the safety measures to prevent equipment accidents (p. 158).

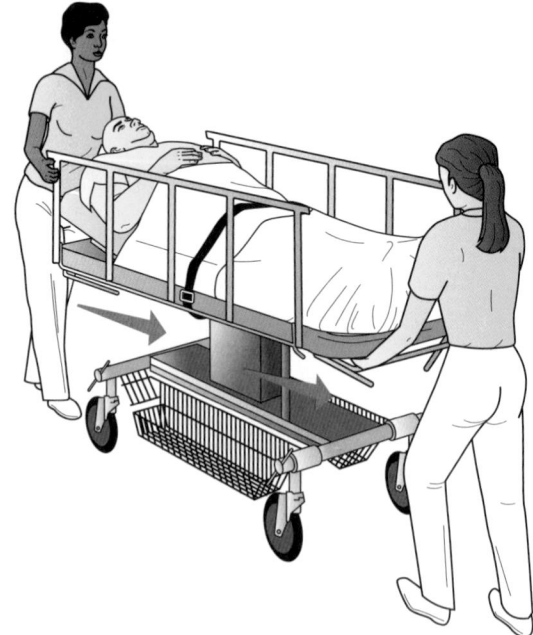

FIGURE 11-22 A person is transported by stretcher. The stretcher is moved feet first.

HANDLING HAZARDOUS SUBSTANCES

A **hazardous substance** is any chemical in the workplace that can cause harm. The Occupational Safety and Health Administration (OSHA) requires that health care employees:

▶ Understand the risks of hazardous substances
▶ Know how to safely handle them

Physical hazards can cause fires or explosions. *Health hazards* are chemicals that can cause acute or chronic health problems. Acute problems occur rapidly and last a short time. They usually occur from a short-term exposure. Chronic problems usually result from long-term exposure. They occur over a long period of time.

Health hazards can:

▶ Cause cancer
▶ Affect blood cell formation and function
▶ Damage the kidneys, nervous system, lungs, skin, eyes, or mucous membranes
▶ Cause birth defects, miscarriages, and fertility problems from reproductive system damage

Exposure to hazardous substances can occur under normal working conditions. It also can happen during certain emergencies. Such emergencies include equipment failures, container ruptures, or the uncontrolled release of a hazard into the workplace. Hazardous substances include:

- ▶ Drugs used in cancer therapy (chemotherapy, anti-cancer drugs)
- ▶ Anesthesia gases
- ▶ Gases used to sterilize equipment
- ▶ Oxygen
- ▶ Disinfectants and cleaning agents
- ▶ Radiation used for x-rays and cancer treatments
- ▶ Mercury (found in thermometers and blood pressure devices [Chapter 25])

To protect employees, OSHA requires a hazard communication program. The program includes container labeling, material safety data sheets (MSDSs), and employee training. The agency also provides eyewash and total body wash stations in areas where hazardous substances are used.

See *Focus on Ethics and Laws: Handling Hazardous Substances.*

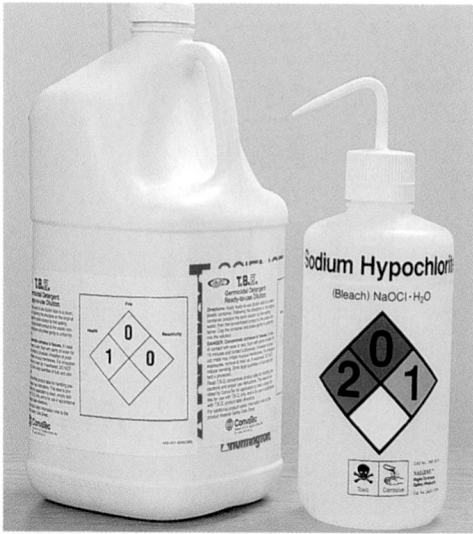

FIGURE 11-23 Warning labels on hazardous substances.

FOCUS ON ETHICS AND LAWS

Handling Hazardous Substances

The Occupational Health and Safety Administration (OSHA) is an agency of the federal government. OSHA and other federal and state agencies have the power to issue standards, rules, and regulations. These are called agency-made laws. Employers and employees must comply with them.

OSHA conducts inspections to make sure an agency is following OSHA policies. If not following them, OSHA can fine the agency. Fines can be between $5000 and $70,000 for each violation.

Labeling

Hazardous substance containers include bags, barrels, bottles, boxes, cans, cylinders, drums, and storage tanks. All need warning labels (Fig. 11-23). The manufacturer supplies all labels. Warning labels identify:

- ▶ Physical and health hazards (Health hazards include the organs affected and potential health problems.)
- ▶ Precaution measures (For example, "Do not use near open flame." Or "Avoid skin contact.")
- ▶ What personal protective equipment to wear—gown, mask, gloves, goggles, and so on
- ▶ How to use the substance safely
- ▶ Storage and disposal information

Words, pictures, and symbols communicate the warnings. A container must have a label. It must not be removed or damaged in any way. If a warning label is removed or damaged, do not use the substance. Take the container to the nurse, and explain the problem. Do not leave the container unattended.

Material Safety Data Sheets

Every hazardous substance has an MSDS. It provides detailed information about the substance:

- ▶ The chemical name and any common names
- ▶ The ingredients in the substance
- ▶ Physical and chemical characteristics (appearance, color, odor, boiling point, and others)
- ▶ Potential physical effects (fire, explosion)
- ▶ Conditions that could cause a chemical reaction
- ▶ How the chemical enters the body (inhalation, ingestion, skin contact, or absorption)
- ▶ Health hazards including signs and symptoms
- ▶ Protective measures (how to use, handle, and store the substance)
- ▶ Emergency and first aid procedures
- ▶ Explosion information and fire-fighting measures (including what type of fire extinguisher to use [p. 164])
- ▶ How to clean up a spill or leak
- ▶ Personal protective equipment needed during clean-up
- ▶ How to dispose of the hazardous substance
- ▶ Manufacturer information (name, address, and a telephone number for more information)

Employees must have ready access to MSDSs. They are in a binder at a certain place on each nursing unit (Fig. 11-24, p. 162). Or they may be on the computer. Check the MSDS before using a hazardous substance, cleaning up a leak or spill, or disposing of the substance. Tell the nurse about a leak or spill right away. Do not leave a leak or spill unattended.

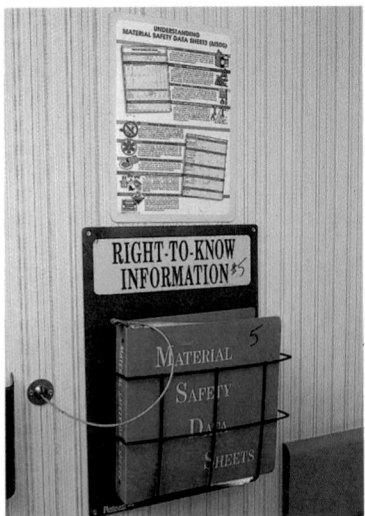

FIGURE 11-24 Material safety data sheets (MSDSs) are in binder for staff use.

BOX 11-10 Safety Measures for Hazardous Substances

- Read all warning labels.
- Follow the safety measures on the warning label and MSDS.
- Make sure each container has a warning label that is not damaged.
- Use a leak-proof container to carry or transport a hazardous substance.
- Wear personal protective equipment to clean spills and leaks. The warning label or MSDS tells you what to wear (mask, gown, gloves, eye protection, safety boots).
- Clean up spills at once. Work from clean areas to dirty areas using circular motions.
- Dispose of hazardous waste in sealed bags or containers.
- Stand behind a lead shield during x-ray or radiation therapy procedures.
- Do not enter a room while a person is having x-rays or radiation therapy.
- Wash your hands after handling hazardous substances.
- Work in well-ventilated areas to avoid inhaling gases.
- Store hazardous substances according to the MSDS.

Employee Training

Your employer provides hazardous substance training. You are told about hazards, exposure risks, and protection measures. You learn to read and use warning labels and MSDSs.

Each hazardous substance requires certain protection measures. Box 11-10 lists general rules to safely handle hazardous substances.

FOCUS ON LONG-TERM CARE AND HOME CARE

Fire Safety

HOME CARE
Fire and the Use of Oxygen
Home care patients may need oxygen therapy. Remind the patient, family, and visitors about safety measures. See Chapter 34.

Preventing Fires
Smoke detectors save lives, prevent injuries, and minimize property damage. Always locate them in a patient's home. They should be outside every sleeping area, in every bedroom, and on every floor. Make sure they are working. Tell the nurse, patient, and family if a smoke detector does not work.

Space heaters present fire hazards. Electric and fuel-burning heaters are common. Practice these safety measures:
- Follow the manufacturer's instructions. Use the recommended fuel.
- Keep heaters at least 3 feet away from window coverings, furniture, and anything that will burn.
- Do not place heaters on stairs, in doorways, or where people walk.
- Protect yourself and others from burns. Heaters are hot. Do not touch them. Keep them away from children, and persons who cannot protect themselves.
- Prevent electrocution. Keep electric heaters away from water. (Water conducts electricity.) Make sure the cord is in good repair.
- Do not leave heaters unattended.
- Store fuel in the original container. Keep the fuel container outside.
- Refill the fuel container outside.
- Do not add fuel while the heater is running or hot. Do not overfill the heater.

What to Do During a Fire
Know two exit routes from each room and two exits from the building. Keep exit routes clear. Keep furniture and heavy items away from doors and windows.

If a fire occurs, get the patient, family, and yourself out as fast as possible. Do not use elevators. In an apartment building, alert others to the fire. Use the fire alarm system and yell "FIRE" in the hallways. Call 911 or the fire department when out of the building. Do not go back into the building.

Using a Fire Extinguisher
Locate fire extinguishers in the patient's home. Read the manufacturer's instructions. Make sure the device works. Tell the nurse, patient, and family if a fire extinguisher does not work.

FIRE SAFETY

Fire is a constant danger. Faulty electrical equipment and wiring, over-loaded electrical circuits, and smoking are major causes of fires. The entire health team must prevent fires. They must act quickly and responsibly during a fire.

See *Focus on Long-Term Care and Home Care: Fire Safety.*

Fire and the Use of Oxygen

Three things are needed for a fire:

▶ A spark or flame
▶ A material that will burn
▶ Oxygen

Air has some oxygen. However, some people need extra oxygen. Doctors order oxygen therapy for them (Chapter 34). Safety measures are needed where oxygen is used and stored:

▶ "No Smoking" signs are placed on the door and near the bed.
▶ The person and visitors are reminded not to smoke in the room.
▶ Smoking materials (cigarettes, cigars, and pipes), matches, and lighters are removed from the room.
▶ Electrical items are turned off *before* being unplugged.
▶ Wool blankets and synthetic fabrics that cause static electricity are removed from the person's room.
▶ The person wears a cotton gown or pajamas.
▶ Electrical items are in good working order. This includes electric shavers, TVs, radios, and other electronic devices.
▶ Lit candles, incense, and other open flames are not allowed.
▶ Materials that ignite easily are removed from the room. They include oil, grease, nail polish remover, and so on.

Agencies have no-smoking policies and smoke-free areas. No smoking is allowed inside the buildings. Signs are posted on all entry doors. Some people ignore such rules. Remind them about the no-smoking rules.

See *Focus on Communication: Fire and the Use of Oxygen.*

FOCUS ON COMMUNICATION

Fire and the Use of Oxygen

You may have to remind a patient, resident, or visitor not to smoke inside the agency. You can simply say:

• "Mrs. Murphy, this is a smoke-free area. Here is an ashtray to put out your cigarette. If you want to smoke, I'll be happy to show you the smoking area outside."
• "Mr. Garcia, please don't smoke inside the center. We have a smoking area outside the back entrance on hallway 2. I'll be happy to show you the way."

Report to the nurse what happened, what you said, and what you did. The nurse may need to speak with the person about not smoking.

BOX 11-11 Fire Prevention Measures

• Follow the safety measures for oxygen use.
• Smoke only where allowed to do so. Do not smoke in patients' homes.
• Be sure all ashes, cigars, cigarettes, and other smoking materials are out before emptying ashtrays.
• Empty ashtrays into a metal container partially filled with sand or water. Do not empty ashtrays into plastic containers or wastebaskets lined with paper or plastic bags.
• Provide ashtrays for persons who are allowed to smoke.
• Supervise persons who smoke. This is very important for persons who are confused, disoriented, or sedated.
• Follow safety practices when using electrical items.
• Supervise the play of children.
• Keep matches, lighters, and flammable liquids and materials away from children and confused or disoriented persons.
• Do not leave cooking unattended on stoves, in ovens, in microwave ovens, or on barbecue grills.
• Store flammable liquids in their original containers. Keep the containers where children and confused or disoriented persons cannot reach them.
• Do not smoke or light matches or lighters around flammable liquids or materials.
• Do not leave candles unattended.
• Keep candles and incense away from flammable liquids and materials.
• Store fuel and flammable liquids outside.
• Keep materials that will burn away from space heaters, fireplaces, radiators, registers, candles and incense, and other heat sources.
• Follow the safety measures to prevent equipment accidents (p. 158).

Preventing Fires

Fire prevention measures were described in relation to burns, equipment accidents, and oxygen use. Other fire safety measures are listed in Box 11-11.

What To Do During a Fire

Know your agency's policies and procedures for fire emergencies. Know where to find fire alarms, fire extinguishers, and emergency exits. Fire drills are held to practice emergency fire procedures. Remember the word RACE (Fig. 11-25, p. 164):

▶ R—for *rescue*. Rescue persons in immediate danger. Move them to a safe place.
▶ A—for *alarm*. Sound the nearest fire alarm. Notify the switchboard operator.
▶ C—for *confine*. Close doors and windows to confine the fire. Turn off oxygen or electrical items used in the general area of the fire.
▶ E—for *extinguish*. Use a fire extinguisher on a small fire that has not spread to a larger area.

Clear equipment from all normal and emergency exits. *Do not use elevators if there is a fire.*

See *Promoting Safety and Comfort: What to Do During a Fire*, p. 164.

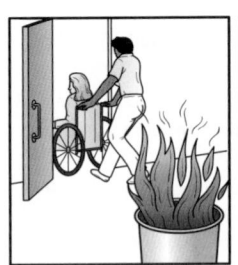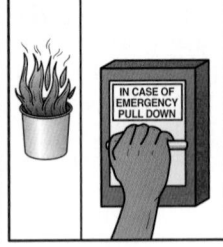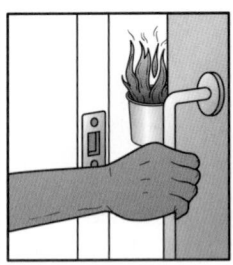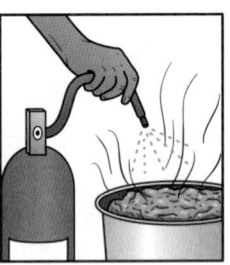

Rescue   Alarm   Confine   Extinguish

FIGURE 11-25 During a fire, RACE: **R**escue, **A**larm, **C**onfine, and **E**xtinguish.

PROMOTING SAFETY AND COMFORT: What to Do During a Fire

SAFETY

Touch doors before opening them. Do not open a hot door. Use another way out of the room or building.

If your clothing is on fire, do not run. Drop to the floor or ground. Cover your face. Roll to smother flames. If another person's clothing is on fire, get the person to the floor or ground. Roll the person, or cover the person with a blanket, bedspread, or coat. This smothers the flames.

If smoke is present, cover your nose and mouth with a damp cloth. Do the same for patients, residents, visitors, and other staff. Have everyone crawl to the nearest exit.

Do the following if you cannot get out of the building because of flames or smoke:

- Call 911 or the fire department. Tell the operator where you are. Give exact information: agency name, address, phone number, and where you are in the building or home.
- Cover your nose and mouth with a damp cloth. Do the same for patients, residents, visitors, and other staff.
- Move away from the fire. Go to a room with a window. Close the room door. Stuff wet towels, blankets, sheets, or bedspreads at the bottom of the door.
- Open the window.
- Hang something from the window (towel, sheet, blanket, clothing). This helps firefighters find you.

Using a Fire Extinguisher

Agencies require that all employees demonstrate use of a fire extinguisher. Different extinguishers are used for different kinds of fires:

- Oil and grease fires
- Electrical fires
- Paper and wood fires

A general procedure for using a fire extinguisher follows. Remember the word PASS used by the National Fire Protection Association:

- *P*—for *pull the safety pin.* Doing so unlocks the handle on many types of fire extinguishers.
- *A*—for *aim low.* Direct the hose or nozzle at the base of the fire. Do not try to spray the tops of the flames.
- *S*—for *squeeze the lever.* Squeeze or push down on the lever, handle, or button to start the stream of water. Release the lever, handle, or button to stop the stream of water.
- *S*—for *sweep back and forth.* Sweep the stream of water back and forth (side to side) at the base of the fire.

Evacuating

Agencies have evacuation policies and procedures. If evacuation is necessary, patients and residents closest to the fire are taken out first. Those who can walk are given blankets to wrap around themselves. A staff member takes them to a safe place. Figures 11-27 and 11-28, p. 166 show how to rescue persons who cannot walk. Once firefighters arrive, they direct rescue efforts.

USING A FIRE EXTINGUISHER

PROCEDURE

1 Pull the fire alarm.
2 Get the nearest fire extinguisher.
3 Carry it upright.
4 Take it to the fire.
5 Remove the safety pin (Fig. 11-26, *A*).

6 Direct the hose or nozzle at the base of the fire (Fig. 11-26, *B*).
7 Push the handle or lever down (Fig. 11-26, *C*).
8 Sweep the hose slowly back and forth at the base of the fire.

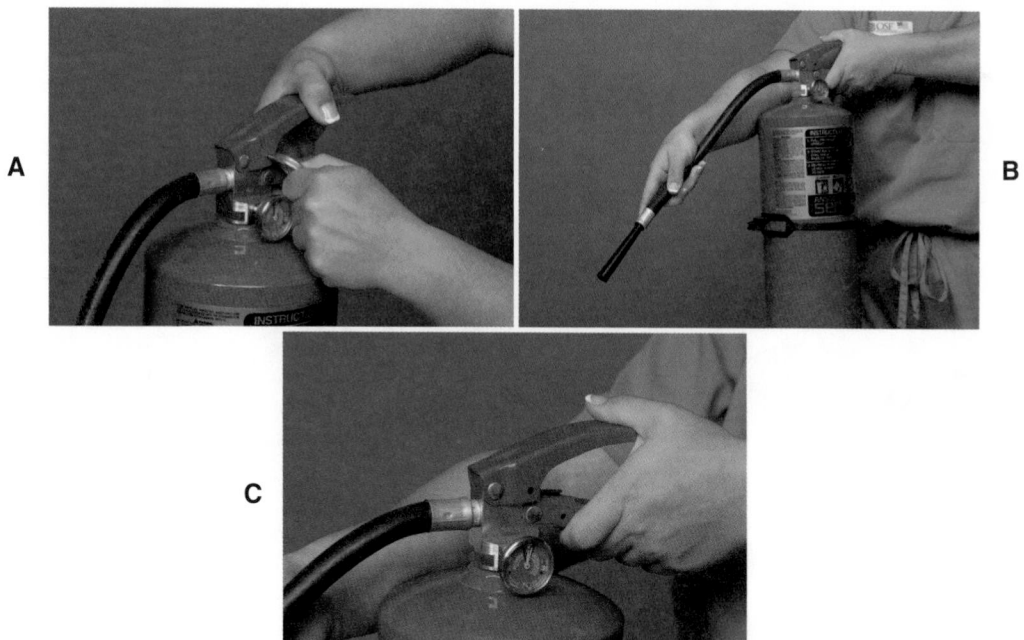

FIGURE 11-26 Using a fire extinguisher. **A,** Remove *(pull)* the safety pin. **B,** Direct *(aim)* the hose at the base of the fire. **C,** Push *(squeeze)* the top handle down (and *sweep* back and forth).

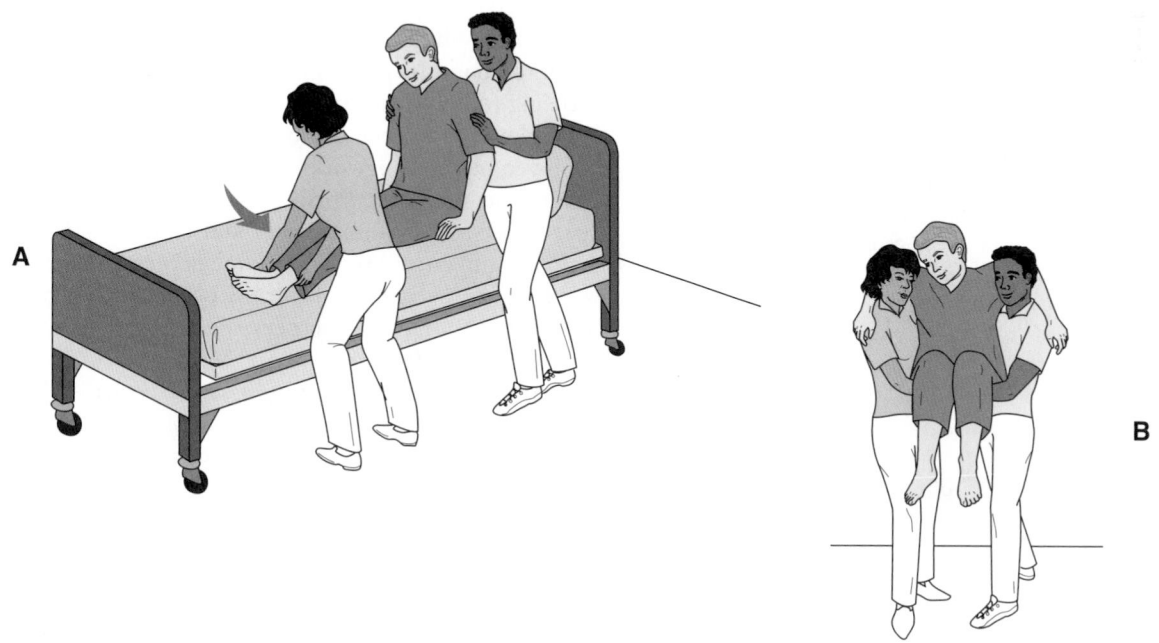

FIGURE 11-27 Swing-carry technique. **A,** Assist the person to a sitting position. A co-worker grasps the person's ankles as you both turn the person so that he sits on the side of the bed. **B,** Pull the person's arm over your shoulder. With one arm, reach across the person's back to your co-worker's shoulder. Reach under the person's knees and grasp your co-worker's arm. Your co-worker does the same.

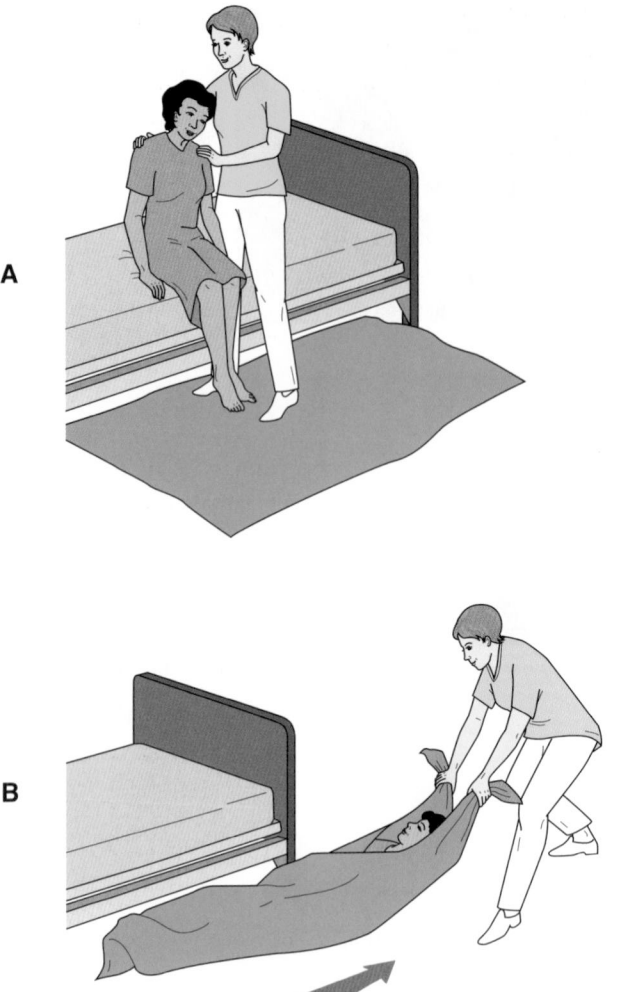

FIGURE 11-28 One-rescuer carry. **A,** Spread a blanket on the floor. Make sure the blanket will extend beyond the person's head. Assist the person to sit on the side of the bed. Grasp the person under the arms, and cross your hands over her chest. Lower the person to the floor by sliding her down one of your legs. **B,** Wrap the blanket around the person. Grasp the blanket over the head area. Pull the person to a safe area.

DISASTERS

A **disaster** is a sudden catastrophic event. People are injured and killed. Property is destroyed. Natural disasters include tornadoes, hurricanes, blizzards, earthquakes, volcanic eruptions, floods, and some fires. Human-made disasters include auto, bus, train, and airplane accidents. They also include fires, bombings, nuclear power plant accidents, riots, gas or chemical leaks, explosions, and wars.

The agency has procedures for disasters that could occur in your area. Follow them to keep patients, residents, visitors, staff, and yourself safe.

Communities, fire and police departments, and health care agencies have disaster plans. They include procedures to deal with the people needing treatment. The plan generally provides for:

▶ Discharging persons who can go home
▶ Assigning staff and equipment to emergency areas
▶ Assigning staff to transport persons from treatment areas
▶ Calling off-duty staff to work

A disaster may damage the agency. The disaster plan includes evacuation procedures.

Bomb Threats

Agencies have procedures for bomb threats. You must follow them if a caller makes a bomb threat or if you find an item that looks or sounds strange. Often bomb threats are sent by phone, mail, e-mail, messenger, or other means. Or the person can leave a bomb in the agency. If you see a stranger in the agency, tell the nurse at once. You cannot be too safe.

WORKPLACE VIOLENCE

Workplace violence is violent acts (including assault or threat of assault) directed toward persons at work or while on duty. It includes:

▶ Murders
▶ Beatings, stabbings, and shootings
▶ Rapes and sexual assaults
▶ Use of weapons—firearms, bombs, or knives
▶ Kidnapping
▶ Robbery
▶ Threats—obscene phone calls; threatening oral, written, or body language; and harassment of any nature (being followed, sworn at, or shouted at)

Workplace violence can occur in any place where an employee performs a work-related duty. It can be a permanent or temporary place. This includes buildings, parking lots, field sites, homes, and travel to and from work assignments. Workplace violence can occur anywhere in the agency. However, it occurs most often in mental health units, emergency departments, waiting rooms, and geriatric units.

According to OSHA, more assaults occur in health care settings than in other industries. Nurses and nursing assistants are at risk. They have the most contact with patients, residents, and visitors. Risk factors include:

▶ People with weapons
▶ Police holds—persons arrested or convicted of crimes
▶ Acutely disturbed and violent persons seeking health care
▶ Alcohol and drug abuse
▶ Mentally ill persons who do not take needed drugs, do not have follow-up care, and are not in hospitals unless they are an immediate threat to themselves or others
▶ Pharmacies have drugs and are a target for robberies
▶ Gang members and substance abusers are patients, residents, or visitors
▶ Upset, agitated, and disturbed family and visitors

▶ Long waits for emergency or other services
▶ Being alone with the person during care or transport to other areas
▶ Low staff levels during meals, emergencies, and at night
▶ Poor lighting in hallways, rooms, parking lots, and other areas
▶ Lack of training in recognizing and managing potentially violent situations

OSHA has guidelines for violence prevention programs. The goal is to prevent or reduce employee exposure to situations that can cause death or injury. Worksite hazards are identified. Prevention measures are developed and followed. Also, employees receive safety and health training. You need to:

▶ Understand and follow your agency's workplace violence prevention program.
▶ Understand and follow safety and security measures.
▶ Voice safety and security concerns.
▶ Report strange or suspicious persons right away.
▶ Report violent incidents promptly and accurately.
▶ Serve on health and safety committees.
▶ Attend training programs that help you recognize and manage agitation, assaultive behavior, and criminal intent.

Box 11-12 lists some measures to prevent or control workplace violence. Box 11-13, p. 168 lists personal safety practices. Follow them all the time. Complete an incident report (p. 170) as needed for workplace violence.

BOX 11-12 Measures to Prevent or Control Workplace Violence

AGITATED OR AGGRESSIVE PERSONS
- Stand away from the person. Judge the length of the person's arms and legs. Stand far enough away so that the person cannot hit or kick you.
- Stand close to the door. Do not become trapped in the room.
- Be aware of items in the room that can be used as weapons. Move away from such objects. Examples include vases, phones, radios, letter openers, paper weights, and belts.
- Know where to find panic buttons, signal lights, alarms, closed-circuit monitors, and other security devices.
- Keep your hands free.
- Stay calm. Talk to the person in a calm manner. Do not raise your voice or argue, scold, or interrupt the person.
- Be aware of your body language. Do not point a finger or glare at the person. Do not put your hands on your hips.
- Do not touch the person.
- Tell the person that you will get the nurse to speak to him or her.
- Leave the room as soon as you can. Make sure the person is safe.
- Tell the nurse or security officer about the matter. Report items in the room that can be used as weapons.

SAFETY DEVICES
- Alarm systems, closed-circuit video monitoring, panic buttons, hand-held alarms, wireless phones, two-way radios, and phone systems are installed (Fig. 11-29, p. 168). These systems have a direct line to security staff or the police.
- Metal detectors are at entrances to identify guns, knives, or other weapons.
- Curved mirrors are at hallway intersections and hard-to-see areas.
- Bullet-resistant, shatter-proof glass is at nurses' stations.
- Staff do not turn off door alarms.
- Staff do not share security codes with anyone.

WEAPONS
- Jewelry and scarves that can serve as weapons are not worn. For example, a person can grab earrings and bracelets. Or a person can strangle someone with a necklace or scarf.
- Long hair is worn up and off the collar (Chapter 4). A person can pull long hair and cause head injuries.
- Keys, scissors, pens, or other items that can serve as weapons are not visible.
- Pictures, vases, and other items that can serve as weapons are few in number.
- Tools or items left by maintenance staff or visitors are removed if they can serve as weapons.

FAMILY AND VISITORS
- Visitors sign in and receive a pass to access patient and resident areas.
- Visiting hours and policies are enforced.
- A list of "restricted visitors" is made for patients and residents with a history of violence or who are victims of violence.
- Waiting rooms and lounges are comfortable and reduce stress.
- Family and visitors are informed in a timely manner.

BUILDING SAFETY AND SECURITY
- Unused doors are locked.
- Bright lights are inside and outside buildings.
- Broken lights, windows, and door locks are replaced or repaired.
- Staff restrooms lock and prevent access to visitors.
- Access to the pharmacy and drug storage areas is controlled.
- Furniture is placed to prevent entrapment. This includes furniture in patient and resident rooms and in therapy areas, dining rooms, and lounges.
- Keys are not left unattended.

STAFF SAFETY MEASURES
- Staff members are not alone when caring for persons with agitated or aggressive behaviors.
- Staff wear ID badges that prove employment.
- A "buddy system" is used when using elevators, stairways, restrooms, and low traffic areas.
- Uniforms fit well. Tight uniforms limit running. An attacker can grab loose uniforms.
- Shoes have good soles. Shoes that cause slipping limit running.
- Vehicles are locked and in good repair.
- Security escort services are used for walking to vehicles, bus stops, or train stations.

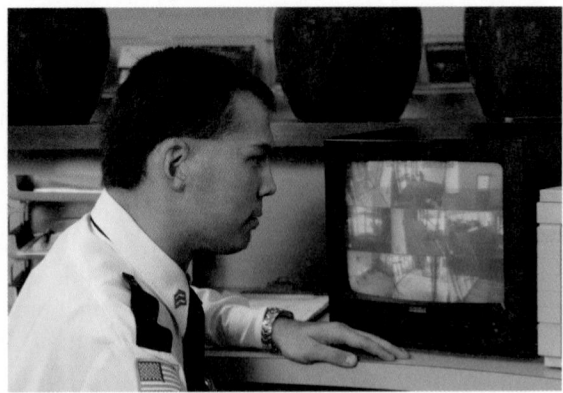

FIGURE 11-29 People entering and leaving the agency are monitored on closed-circuit TV.

BOX 11-13 Personal Safety Practices

GENERAL MEASURES

- Know the area where you are going. Ask questions about the area.
- Make a "dry run" to the area. Know the route in advance. The shortest route is not always the safest.
- Let someone know where you are at all times. Let someone know when you leave and when you arrive at your destination. If you do not call in when expected, the person knows something is wrong.
- Make it known that you do not carry drugs, needles, or syringes.
- Do not carry large amounts of money or valuables. Leave them at home or in the locked car trunk. If someone wants what you have, give it. The only thing of value is *you*.
- Carry wallets, purses, and backpacks safely. Men should carry wallets in an inside coat pocket or in a side pants pocket. Never carry a wallet in the rear pocket. Keep a firm grip on a purse. Keep it close to your body.
- Keep your wireless phone in your hand.
- Carry a whistle or shriek alarm.
- Avoid ATM machines at night.
- Be careful when getting on elevators and when entering stairways.
- Do not approach a stranger or someone acting in a suspicious manner. Report the matter right away.

HOME SETTINGS

- Keep doors and windows to the home locked at all times.
- Do not open doors to strangers. Ask for identification.
- Do not let a stranger into the home to use a phone or bathroom. Offer to call the police if the person needs help.
- Do not give personal information to callers or people at the door.

CAR SAFETY

- Have plenty of gas in your car.
- Keep your car in good working order.
- Keep these in your car—local map, flashlight with working batteries, flares, a fire extinguisher, and a first aid kit.
- Raise the hood and use the flares if the car breaks down. Stay in the car. Call the police if you have a wireless phone. If someone stops by to help, ask that person to call the police.

- Lock your car. Sometimes you may want to leave it unlocked. If you need to get in the car fast, you do not want to fumble with keys. Use your judgment. Do not leave anything in the car if you leave it unlocked.
- Have your car key ready so you can get into the car quickly. Do not fumble for keys on the way to or at the car.
- Check under the car as you approach it. A person hiding under the car can grab your ankle or leg. Leave at once if someone is under the car. The person under the car may be working with a buddy who is waiting to attack you while you are being held or injured at the ankle or leg.
- Check the back seat before getting into the car. Make sure no one is in the car. Leave at once if someone is in the car.
- Lock car doors when you get in the car. Keep windows rolled up.
- Do not open the car door or window to talk to a person approaching your car.
- Do not get out of the car to remove something from the windshield.
- Keep purses, backpacks, and other valuables under the seat or near your side. Do not leave them on the seat. They are easy targets for smash-and-grab robbers.
- Do not hitchhike or pick up hitchhikers.

PARKING YOUR CAR

- Check for places to park. Choose a well-lit area. If using a parking garage, park near entrances, exits, and on the lower level. Try to get close to the attendant if possible. The closest space to your destination is not always the safest for parking.
- Park your car so that you can leave quickly and easily. Park at street corners so no one can park in front of you. In parking lots, back in. You can see more from the front windshield than from the back window.

WALKING

- Do not wear headphones when walking. They keep you from hearing cars and people around you.
- Use well-lit and busy streets if you have to walk. Avoid vacant lots, alleys, wooded areas, and construction sites. The shortest way is not always the safest.
- Walk near the curb. Stay away from doorways, shrubs, and bushes.
- Note the location of phone booths. And carry a wireless phone. Know your location, and keep phone calls simple.
- Go to a police or fire station or a store if you think someone is following you.

Continued

BOX 11-13 Personal Safety Practices—cont'd

PUBLIC TRANSPORTATION
- Carry money for phone calls and for bus, train, or taxi fares. Have money in your pocket to avoid fumbling with a purse or wallet.
- Stand with others and near the ticket booth. Sit near the driver or conductor.
- Keep your wireless phone in your hand.

IF YOU ARE THREATENED OR ATTACKED
- Scream as loud and as long as you can. Keep screaming. Men and women should scream.
- Yell "FIRE," not "help." Most people will respond to "FIRE."

- Use your car keys as a weapon. Carry them in your strong hand. Have one key extended (Fig. 11-30). Hold the key firmly. If you are attacked, go for the person's face. Slash the person's face with the key. Do not use poking motions. Do not try for a certain target because you might miss. Do not be shy—your attacker will not be.
- Remember, you have two arms, two hands, two feet, and two knees. You can attack from more than one direction at once. Do not be shy—your attacker will not be. Push, pull, yank, and so on. You can attack a man's or woman's genitals.
- Use your thumbs as weapons. Go for the eyes and push hard.
- Carry a travel size can of aerosol hair spray. Go for the face.

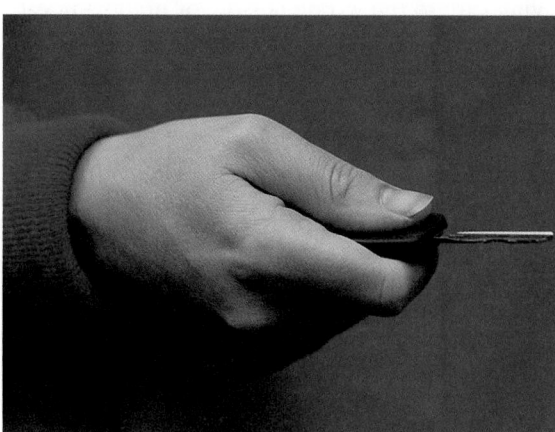

FIGURE 11-30 A car key is used as a weapon.

The nurse assesses the behavior and the behavioral history of new and transferred patients and residents. Restraints may be ordered if persons are a threat to themselves or others (Chapter 13). Persons with mental health problems are supervised as they move throughout the agency. Aggressive and agitated persons are treated in open areas. Privacy and confidentiality are maintained. Security officers deal with agitated, aggressive, or disruptive persons.

See *Focus on Long-Term Care and Home Care: Workplace Violence*.

FOCUS ON LONG-TERM CARE AND HOME CARE

Workplace Violence

HOME CARE
More measures are needed for home safety. Always keep doors locked. Do not let strangers into the home or building. Do not give information over the phone (Chapter 5). Do not let any stranger know that you are with a child or with an older, ill, or disabled person.

Child abuse, elder abuse, domestic violence, and workplace violence can occur in home settings. If you feel uncomfortable or threatened in any way, tell the nurse. Give as much information as you can. Failing to report the matter does not help you or the patient. You may feel an immediate threat to your health or well-being. Follow agency policy for what to do if you are threatened or feel threatened.

The following can threaten your safety. Report these and other threats to the nurse:
- Sexual abuse or harassment by the patient or by any person in the home (husband, wife, sister, brother, boyfriend, girlfriend, son, daughter, family, and friends). See Chapter 3.
- Hitting, kicking, slapping, spitting, biting, scratching, pinching, pushing, or other attacks by the patient or anyone in the home.
- Attacks or threatened attacks with any weapon (knife, gun, bat, rope, tool [hammer, screwdriver, and so on], razor, scissors, spray, pot, pan, cane, chair, and so on).
- Denial of meal breaks, water, bathroom use, toilet paper, or hand washing facilities.
- Denial of adequate sleeping conditions for a live-in situation.
- Inadequate heating or ventilation.
- Name calling, obscene language, or racial or cultural slurs.
- Exposure to unsafe conditions (blocked fire escapes, broken stairways, pest infestations, and so on).

RISK MANAGEMENT

Risk management involves identifying and controlling risks and safety hazards affecting the agency. The intent is to:

▶ Protect everyone in the agency—patients, residents, visitors, and staff
▶ Protect agency property from harm or danger
▶ Protect the person's valuables
▶ Prevent accidents and injuries

Risk management deals with these and other safety issues:

▶ Accident and fire prevention
▶ Negligence and malpractice
▶ Patient and resident abuse
▶ Workplace violence
▶ Federal and state requirements

Risk managers work with all agency departments. They look for patterns and trends in incident reports, patient and resident complaints, staff complaints, and accident and injury investigations. Risk managers look for and correct unsafe situations. They also make procedure changes and training recommendations as needed.

Personal Belongings

The person's belongings must be kept safe. Often they are sent home with the family. A personal belongings list is completed. Each item is listed and described. The staff member and person sign the completed list.

A valuables envelope is used for jewelry and money. Each jewelry item is listed and described on the envelope. Describe what you see. For example, describe a ring as having a white stone with six prongs in a yellow setting. Do not assume the stone is a diamond in a gold setting. For valuables:

▶ Count money with the person.
▶ Put money and each jewelry item in the envelope with the person watching. Seal the envelope. Sign the envelope like a personal belongings list.
▶ Give the envelope to the nurse. The nurse takes it to the safe, or sends it home with the family.

Dentures, eyeglasses, hearing aids, watches, some jewelry, radios, computers, and other electronic devices are kept at the bedside. Items kept at the bedside are listed in the person's record. Some people keep money for newspapers and personal items. The amount kept is noted in the person's record.

See *Focus on Long-Term Care and Home Care: Personal Belongings.*

FOCUS ON LONG-TERM CARE AND HOME CARE

Personal Belongings

LONG-TERM CARE
Clothing and shoes are labeled with the person's name. So are other items brought from home.

Reporting Incidents

An **incident** is any event that has harmed or could harm a patient, resident, visitor, or staff member. It includes accidents and errors in giving care.

Report accidents and errors at once. This includes:

▶ Accidents involving patients, residents, visitors, or staff.
▶ Errors in care. This includes giving the wrong care, giving care to the wrong person, or not giving care.
▶ Broken or lost items owned by the person. Dentures, hearing aids, and eyeglasses are examples.
▶ Lost money or clothing.
▶ Hazardous substance incidents.
▶ Workplace violence incidents.

An *incident report* is completed as soon as possible after the incident. The following information is required:

▶ Names of those involved
▶ Date and time of the accident or error
▶ Location of the accident or error
▶ A complete description of what happened
▶ Names of witnesses
▶ Any other requested information

Incident reports are reviewed by risk management and a committee of health care workers. They look for patterns and trends of accidents or errors. For example, are falls occurring on the same shift and on the same unit? Are lost or missing items being reported on the same shift or same unit? Are patients and residents being injured on the same shift or same unit? There may be new policies and procedures to prevent future incidents.

Circle the BEST answer.

1 In a safe setting, the person
   a Is not aware of surroundings
   b Has a low risk of illness or injury
   c Has no accident risk factors
   d Can see, hear, smell, and touch

2 Who provides a safe setting for patients and residents?
   a The health team
   b The nursing team
   c The administrator
   d The risk manager

3 Which is *not* a risk factor for accidents?
   a Needing eyeglasses
   b Hearing problems
   c Memory problems
   d Oriented to person, time, and place

4 A person in a coma
   a Has suffered an electrical shock
   b Has dementia
   c Is unaware of surroundings
   d Has stopped breathing

5 You are caring for infants. Which is *not* safe?
   a Checking them in cribs often
   b Laying them on their backs to sleep
   c Propping a baby bottle on a rolled towel
   d Keeping plastic bags away from them

6 The following present dangers to children *except*
   a Bicycle helmets
   b Clothes with drawstrings
   c Dangling items from backpacks
   d Necklaces

7 Which is a safety hazard for children?
   a Toilet with the lid down
   b Empty bucket
   c A crib away from the window
   d An open diaper pail

8 A person with quadriplegia is paralyzed
   a From the waist down
   b From the neck down
   c On the right side of the body
   d On the left side of the body

9 To identify a person, you
   a Call the person by name
   b Ask the person his or her name
   c Compare information on the ID bracelet against your assignment sheet
   d Ask both roommates their names

10 Burns are caused by the following *except*
   a Smoking
   b Spilled hot liquids
   c Very hot bath water
   d Oxygen

11 Safety measures to prevent poisoning include the following *except*
   a Keeping harmful products in low storage areas
   b Keeping child-resistant caps on harmful products
   c Making sure all harmful products have labels
   d Storing harmful products away from food

12 Which of the following signals a poison?
   a The "Mr. Yuk" sticker
   b The MSDS
   c RACE
   d PASS

13 Who has the greatest risk of lead poisoning?
   a Newborns
   b Infants between the ages of 1 and 6 months
   c Children between the ages of 6 months and 6 years
   d Older persons

14 A home has lead-based plumbing. You should
   a Use hot tap water for cooking and drinking
   b Use hot tap water to make baby formula
   c Let cold water run for 1 to 2 minutes before using it for cooking or drinking
   d Be alert for signs and symptoms of carbon monoxide poisoning

15 Which will *not* prevent suffocation?
   a Reporting loose teeth or dentures
   b Using electrical items that are in good repair
   c Cutting food into small, bite-size pieces
   d Over-loading an electrical outlet

16 The most common cause of choking in adults is
   a A loose denture
   b Meat
   c Marbles
   d Candy

17 If severe airway obstruction occurs, the person usually
   a Clutches at the throat
   b Can speak, cough, and breathe
   c Is calm
   d Has a seizure

18 These statements are about abdominal thrusts. Which is *false?*
   a They can be performed with the person standing, sitting, or lying down.
   b A person is unresponsive. It is assumed that the cause is choking.
   c They can be self-administered
   d CPR is started if the responsive victim loses consciousness.

19 You need to shave a new resident. Before using the person's electric shaver
   a You need to inspect it
   b The maintenance staff must do a safety check
   c You need to check for a frayed cord
   d You need an electrical outlet

20 You are using equipment. Which measure is *not* safe?
   a Following the manufacturer's instructions
   b Keeping electrical items away from water and spills
   c Pulling on the cord to remove a plug from an outlet
   d Turning off electrical items after using them

21 A person uses a wheelchair. Which measure is *not* safe?
   a The wheels are locked for transfers.
   b The chair is pulled backward to transport the person.
   c The feet are positioned on the footplates.
   d The casters point forward. *Continued*

22 Stretcher safety involves the following *except*
   a Locking the wheels for transfers
   b Fastening the safety straps
   c Raising the side rails
   d Moving the stretcher head first

23 You spilled a hazardous substance. You should do the following *except*
   a Read the material safety data sheet
   b Cover the spill and go tell the nurse
   c Wear personal protective equipment to clean up the spill
   d Complete an incident report

24 The fire alarm sounds. The following is done *except*
   a Turning off oxygen
   b Using elevators
   c Closing doors and windows
   d Moving patients and residents to a safe place

25 Your clothing is on fire. You should do the following *except*
   a Run to get help
   b Drop to the floor or ground
   c Cover your face
   d Roll to smother the flames

26 A severe weather alert was issued for your area. What should you do?
   a Take cover
   b Follow the agency's disaster plan
   c Make sure your family is safe
   d Pull the fire alarm

27 A person is agitated and aggressive. You should do the following *except*
   a Stand away from the person
   b Stand close to the door
   c Use touch to show you care
   d Talk to the person without raising your voice

28 You work the night shift. Which is *unsafe*?
   a Parking in a well-lit area
   b Locking your car
   c Finding your keys after getting into the car
   d Checking under the car and in your back seat

29 A resident brought a radio from home. Which helps prevents property loss?
   a Completing a personal belongings list
   b Labeling the radio with the person's name
   c Putting the radio in a safe
   d Using a wheelchair pouch for the radio

30 You gave a person the wrong treatment. Which is *true*?
   a Report the error at the end of the shift.
   b Take action only if the person was injured.
   c You are guilty of negligence.
   d You must complete an incident report.

Answers to these questions are on p. 779.

Preventing Falls

OBJECTIVES

- Define the key terms and key abbreviations listed in this chapter
- Identify the causes and risk factors for falls
- Describe the safety measures that prevent falls
- Explain how to use bed rails safely
- Explain the purpose of hand rails and grab bars
- Explain how to use wheel locks safely
- Describe how to use transfer/gait belts
- Explain how to the help the person who is falling
- Perform the procedures described in this chapter

PROCEDURES

- Applying A Transfer/Gait Belt
- Helping the Falling Person

KEY TERMS

bed rail A device that serves as a guard or barrier along the side of the bed; side rail

gait belt Transfer belt

transfer belt A device used to support a person who is unsteady or disabled; gait belt

The risk of falling increases with age. Persons older than 65 years are at risk. A history of falls increases the risk of falling again. Falls are the most common accidents in nursing centers.

CAUSES AND RISK FACTORS FOR FALLS

Most falls occur in patient and resident rooms and in bathrooms. Poor lighting, cluttered floors, throw rugs, and out-of-place furniture are causes. So are wet and slippery floors, bathtubs, and showers. Needing to use the bathroom, usually to urinate, is a major cause of falls. For example, Mrs. Hines has an urgent need to urinate. She falls trying to get to the bathroom.

Most falls occur between 1800 (6:00 PM) and 2100 (9:00 PM). Falls also are more likely during shift changes. During shift changes, staff are busy going off and coming on duty. Confusion can occur about who gives care and answers signal lights. Shift changes vary among agencies. They often occur between these hours:

▶ 0600 (6:00 AM) and 0800 (8:00 AM)
▶ 1400 (2:00 PM) and 1600 (4:00 PM)
▶ 2200 (10:00 PM) and 2400 (midnight)

The accident risk factors described in Chapter 11 can lead to falls. The problems listed in Box 12-1 also increase a person's risk of falling.

See *Teamwork and Time Management: Causes and Risk Factors for Falls.*

TEAMWORK AND TIME MANAGEMENT
Causes and Risk Factors for Falls

The entire health team must protect the person from harm. If you see something unsafe, tell the nurse at once. Do not assume the nurse knows or that someone is tending to the matter.

Answer all signal lights promptly. This includes the signal lights of patients and residents assigned to co-workers.

Know your role during shift changes. Nursing staff going off-duty and those of the on-coming shift must work together to prevent falls.

FALL PREVENTION PROGRAMS

Agencies have fall prevention programs. The measures listed in Box 12-2 are part of the program and the person's care plan. The care plan also lists measures for the person's specific risk factors.

Common sense and simple safety measures can prevent many falls. The health team works with the person and family to reduce the risk of falls. The goal is to prevent falls without decreasing the person's quality of life.

See *Focus on Communication: Fall Prevention Programs,* p. 176.

See *Promoting Safety and Comfort: Fall Prevention Programs,* p. 176.

BOX 12-1 Factors Increasing the Risk of Falls

- Alcohol: over-use
- Balance problems
- Blood pressure: low
- Care equipment: IV poles, drainage tubes and bags, and others
- Confusion
- Depression
- Disorientation
- Dizziness; dizziness on standing
- Drug side effects
  - Low blood pressure when standing or sitting
  - Drowsiness
  - Fainting
  - Dizziness
  - Coordination: poor
  - Unsteadiness
  - Urination: frequent
  - Diarrhea
  - Confusion and disorientation
- Elimination needs
- Falls: history of
- Foot problems
- Incontinence: urinary and fecal
- Joint pain and stiffness
- Judgment: poor
- Light-headedness
- Memory problems
- Mobility: decreased
- Muscle weakness
- Reaction time: slow
- Shoes that fit poorly
- Strange setting
- Vision problems
- Weakness
- Wheelchairs, walkers, canes, and crutches: improper use

BOX 12-2 Safety Measures to Prevent Falls

BASIC NEEDS
- Fluid needs are met.
- Eyeglasses and hearing aids are worn as needed. Reading glasses are not worn when up and about.
- Help is given with elimination needs. It is given at regular times and whenever requested. Assist the person to the bathroom. Or provide the bedpan, urinal, or commode.
- The bedpan, urinal, or commode is kept within easy reach if the person can use the device without help.
- A warm drink, soft lights, or a back massage is used to calm the person who is agitated.
- Barriers are used to prevent wandering (Fig. 12-1, p. 176).
- The person is properly positioned when in bed, a chair, or a wheelchair. Use pillows, wedge pads, or seats as the nurse and care plan direct (Chapter 15).
- Correct procedures are used for transfers (Chapter 16).

BATHROOMS AND SHOWER/TUB ROOMS
- Tubs and showers have non-slip surfaces or non-slip bath mats.
- Grab bars are in showers. They also are by tubs and toilets.
- Bathrooms have grab bars.
- Shower chairs are used (Chapter 19).
- Safety measures for tub baths and showers are followed (Chapter 19).

FLOORS
- Floors have wall-to-wall carpeting or carpeting that is tacked down.
- Scatter, area, and throw rugs are not used.
- Floor coverings are one color. Bold designs can cause dizziness in older persons.
- Floors have non-glare, non-slip surfaces.
- Non-skid wax is used on hardwood, tiled, or linoleum floors.
- Loose floor boards and tiles are reported. So are frayed rugs and carpets.
- Floors and stairs are free of clutter. They are free of items that could cause tripping—toys, cords, and other items.
- Floors are free of spills. Wipe up spills at once. Put a "Wet Floor" sign by the wet area.
- Floors are free of excess furniture and equipment.
- Electrical and extension cords are out of the way.
- Equipment and supplies are kept on one side of the hallway.

FURNITURE
- Furniture is placed for easy movement.
- Furniture is not re-arranged.
- Chairs have armrests. Armrests give support when standing or sitting.
- A phone, lamp, and personal belongings are at the bedside. They are within the person's reach.

BEDS AND OTHER EQUIPMENT
- The bed is in the lowest horizontal position, except when giving bedside care. The distance from the bed to the floor is reduced if the person falls or gets out of bed.
- Bed rails are used according to the care plan (p. 177).
- A mattress, special mat, or floor cushion is placed on the floor beside the bed (Fig. 12-2, p. 176). This reduces the chance of injury if the person falls or gets out of bed.
- Wheelchairs, walkers, canes, and crutches fit properly. Another person's equipment is not used.
- Crutches, canes, and walkers have non-skid tips.

- Correct equipment is used for transfers (Chapter 16). Follow the care plan.
- Wheelchair and stretcher safety is followed (Chapter 11).
- Wheel locks on beds (p. 178), wheelchairs, and stretchers are in working order.
- Bed wheels are locked for transfers.
- Linens are checked for sharp objects and for the person's property (dentures, eyeglasses, hearing aids, and so on.)

LIGHTING
- Rooms, hallways, and stairways have good lighting. So do bathrooms and shower/tub rooms.
- Light switches (including those in bathrooms) are within reach and easy to find.
- Night-lights are in bedrooms, hallways, and bathrooms.

SHOES AND CLOTHING
- Non-skid footwear is worn. Socks, bedroom slippers, and long shoelaces are avoided.
- Clothing fits properly. Clothing is not loose. It does not drag on the floor. Belts are tied or secured in place.

SIGNAL LIGHTS AND ALARMS
- The person is taught how to use the signal light (Chapter 17).
- The signal light is always within the person's reach. This includes when in bathrooms and tub/shower rooms.
- The person is asked to call for assistance when help is needed:
  - When getting out of bed or a chair
  - With walking
  - With getting to or from the bathroom or commode
  - With getting on or off the bedpan
- Signal lights are answered promptly. The person may need help right away. He or she may not wait for help.
- Bed and chair alarms are used. They sense when the person tries to get up (Fig. 12-3, p. 176).
- Bed and chair alarms are responded to at once.

OTHER
- The person is checked often. This may be every 15 minutes or as required by the care plan. Careful and frequent observation is important.
- Frequent checks are made on persons with poor judgment or memory. This may be every 15 minutes or as required by the care plan.
- Persons at risk of falling are in rooms close to the nurses' station.
- Hand rails are on both sides of stairs and hallways.
- The person uses hand rails when walking or using stairs.
- The person uses grab bars in bathrooms and shower/tub rooms.
- Family and friends are asked to visit during busy times. They are asked to visit during the evening and night shifts.
- Companions are provided. Sitters, companions, or volunteers are with the person.
- The person is kept involved in meaningful activities. Follow the care plan.
- Tasks and procedures are explained before and while performing them.
- Non-slip strips are on the floor next to the bed and in the bathroom. They are intact.

Continued

BOX 12-2 Safety Measures to Prevent Falls—cont'd

OTHER—cont'd
- Caution is used when turning corners, entering corridor intersections, and going through doors. You could injure a person coming from the other direction.
- Pull (do not push) wheelchairs, stretchers, carts, and other wheeled equipment through doorways. This allows you to lead the way and to see where you are going.

- A safety check is made of the room after visitors leave. (See the inside of the front book cover.) They may have lowered a bed rail, removed a signal light, or moved a walker out of reach. Or they may have brought an item that could harm the person.

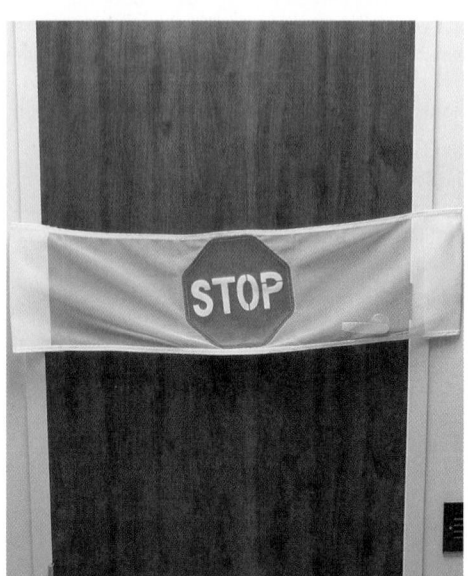

FIGURE 12-1 Barriers are used to prevent wandering.

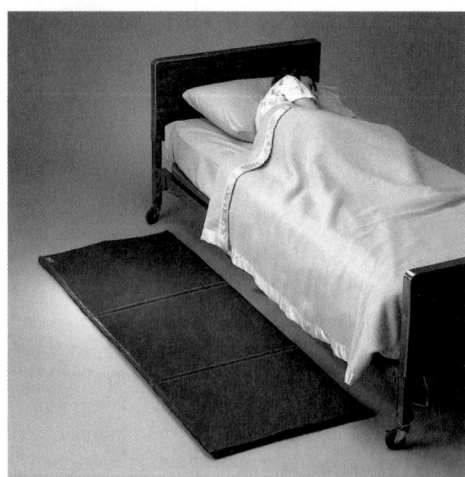

FIGURE 12-2 Floor cushion. (Image courtesy J.T. Posey Co., Arcadia, Calif.)

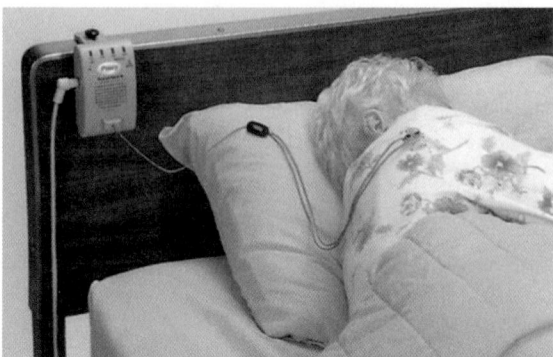

FIGURE 12-3 Bed alarm.

FOCUS ON COMMUNICATION

Fall Prevention Programs

Often falls occur when the person tries to get needed items. The person has to reach too far and falls out of bed or from a chair. Or the person tries to get up without help. Prevent falls by asking the person these questions:
- "What things would you like near you?"
- "Can I move this closer to you?"
- "Can you reach the signal light?"
- "Can you reach your cane?" (Walker and wheelchair are other examples.)
- "Do you need to use the bathroom now?"
- "Is there anything else you need before I leave the room?"

PROMOTING SAFETY AND COMFORT: Fall Prevention Programs

SAFETY

Some people are visually impaired or blind. Besides the measures in Box 12-2, other safety measures are needed to protect them from falling. See Chapter 37.

Bed Rails

A **bed rail** *(side rail)* is a device that serves as a guard or barrier along the side of the bed. Bed rails are raised and lowered (Fig. 12-4). They lock in place with levers, latches, or buttons. Bed rails are half, three quarters, or the full length of the bed. When half-length rails are used, each side may have two rails. One is for the upper part of the bed, the other for the lower part.

The nurse and care plan tell you when to raise bed rails. They are needed by persons who are unconscious or sedated with drugs. Some confused or disoriented people need them. If a person needs bed rails, keep them up at all times except when giving bedside nursing care.

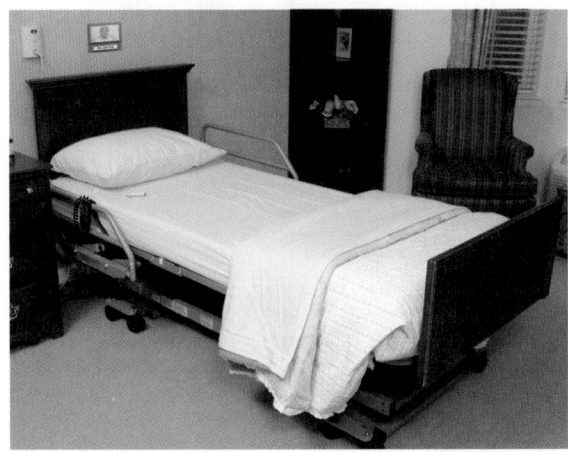

FIGURE 12-4 Bed rails. The far bed rail is raised. The near bed rail is lowered.

Bed rails present hazards. The person can fall when trying to climb over them or the person cannot get out of bed or use the bathroom. Entrapment is a risk. That is, the person can get caught, trapped, entangled, or strangled (Chapter 17).

Bedrails are considered restraints (Chapter 13) if:

▶ The person cannot get out of bed.
▶ The person cannot lower them without help.

Bed rails cannot be used unless needed to treat a person's medical symptoms. Some people feel safer with bed rails up. Others use them to change positions in bed. The person or legal representative must give consent for raised bed rails. The need for bed rails is carefully noted in the person's medical record and the care plan.

Accrediting agency standards and federal and state laws affect bed rail use. They are allowed when the person's condition requires them. Bed rails must be in the person's best interests.

The procedures in this book include using bed rails. This helps you learn to use them correctly. The nurse, the care plan, and your assignment sheet tell you which people use bed rails. If a person does not use them, omit the "raise bed rails" or "lower bed rails" steps.

If a person uses bed rails, check the person often. Report to the nurse that you checked the person. If you are allowed to chart, record when you checked the person and your observations (Fig. 12-5).

See *Focus on Children and Older Persons: Bed Rails*, p. 178.

See *Promoting Safety and Comfort: Bed Rails*, p. 178.

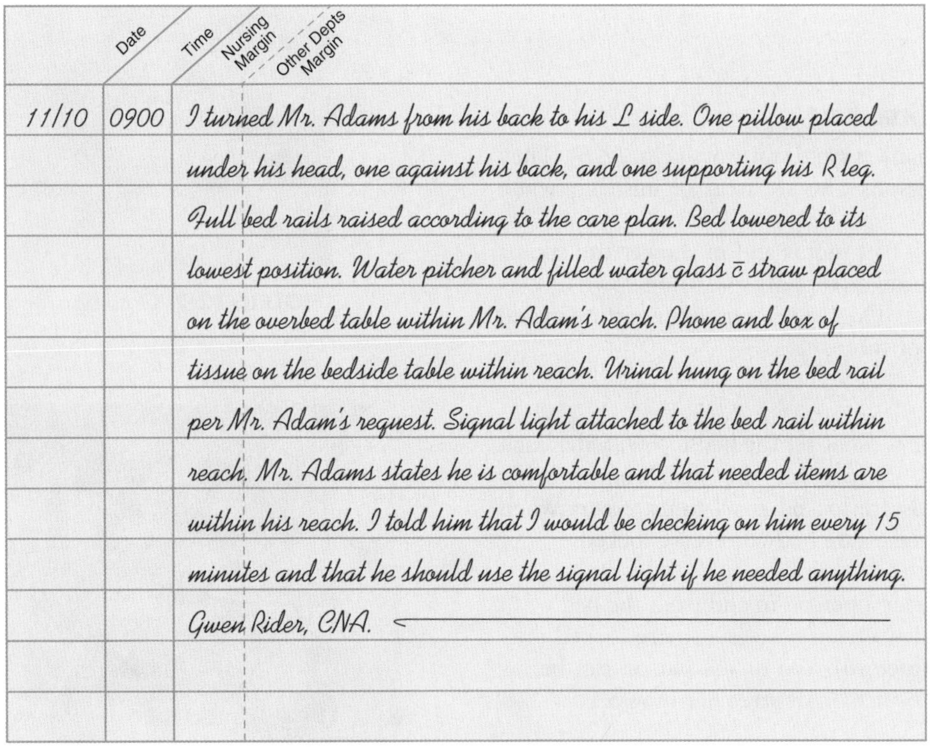

Date	Time	Nursing Margin	Other Depts Margin
11/10	0900	*I turned Mr. Adams from his back to his L side. One pillow placed under his head, one against his back, and one supporting his R leg. Full bed rails raised according to the care plan. Bed lowered to its lowest position. Water pitcher and filled water glass c̄ straw placed on the overbed table within Mr. Adam's reach. Phone and box of tissue on the bedside table within reach. Urinal hung on the bed rail per Mr. Adam's request. Signal light attached to the bed rail within reach. Mr. Adams states he is comfortable and that needed items are within his reach. I told him that I would be checking on him every 15 minutes and that he should use the signal light if he needed anything. Gwen Rider, CNA.*	

FIGURE 12-5 Charting sample.

FOCUS ON **CHILDREN** AND **OLDER PERSONS**

Bed Rails

CHILDREN

The space between the crib rail slats must be no more than 2 inches. If the space is larger, the baby's head can get caught between the slats. The baby can suffocate.

Never leave crib rails down when the baby is in the crib.

PROMOTING SAFETY AND COMFORT: Bed Rails

SAFETY

You raise the bed to give care. Follow these safety measures to prevent the person from falling:
- *For a person who uses bed rails.* Always raise the far bed rail if you are working alone. Raise both bed rails if you need to leave the bedside for any reason.
- *For the person who does not use bed rails.* Ask a co-worker to help you. The co-worker stands on the far side of the bed. This protects the person from falling.
- Never leave the person alone when the bed is raised.
- Always lower the bed to its lowest position when you are done giving care.

COMFORT

The person has to reach over raised bed rails for items on the bedside stand and overbed table. Such items include the water pitcher and cup, tissues, phone, and TV and light controls. Adjust the overbed table so it is within the person's reach. Ask if the person wants other items nearby. Place them on the overbed table too. Always make sure needed items, including the signal light, are within the person's reach.

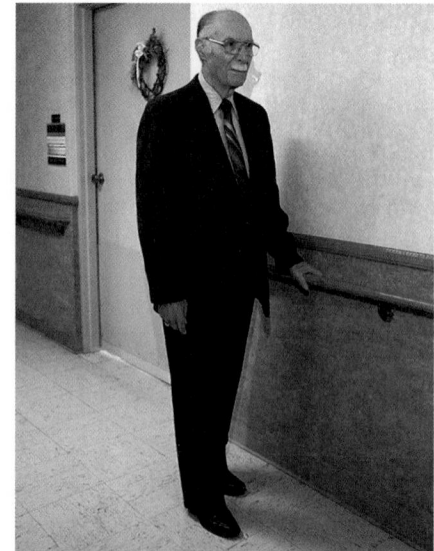

FIGURE 12-6 Hand rails provide support when walking.

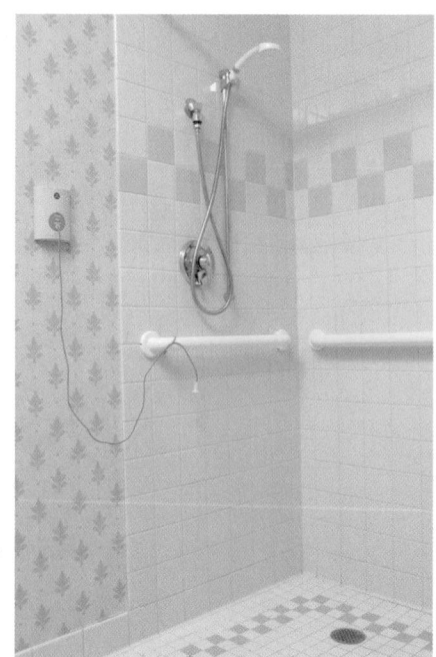

FIGURE 12-7 Grab bars in a shower.

Hand Rails and Grab Bars

Hand rails are in hallways and stairways (Fig. 12-6). They give support to persons who are weak or unsteady when walking.

Grab bars are in bathrooms and in shower/tub rooms (Fig. 12-7). They provide support for sitting down or getting up from a toilet. They also are used for getting in and out of the shower or tub.

Wheel Locks

Bed legs have wheels. They let the bed move easily. Each wheel has a lock to prevent the bed from moving (Fig. 12-8). Wheels are locked at all times except when moving the bed. Make sure bed wheels are locked:
▸ When giving bedside care
▸ When you transfer a person to and from the bed

Wheelchair and stretcher wheels also are locked during transfers (Chapter 16). You or the person can be injured if the bed, wheelchair, or stretcher moves.

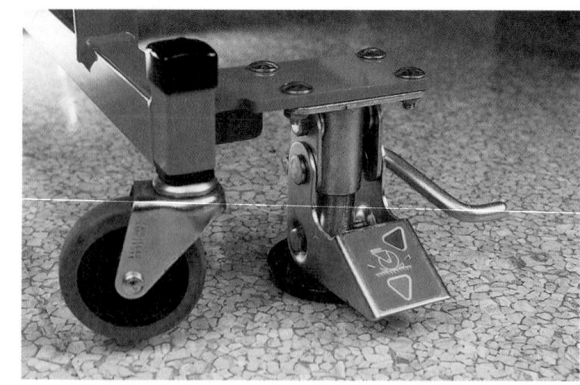

FIGURE 12-8 Lock on a bed wheel.

◆ TRANSFER/GAIT BELTS

A **transfer belt (gait belt)** is a device used to support a person who is unsteady or disabled (Fig. 12-9). It helps prevent falls and injuries. When used to transfer a person (Chapter 16), it is called a *transfer belt*. When used to help a person walk, it is called a *gait belt*.

The belt goes around the person's waist. Grasp under the belt to support the person during the transfer or when assisting the person to walk.

See *Promoting Safety and Comfort: Transfer/Gait Belts.*
See *Focus on Ethics and Laws: Transfer/Gait Belts.*

A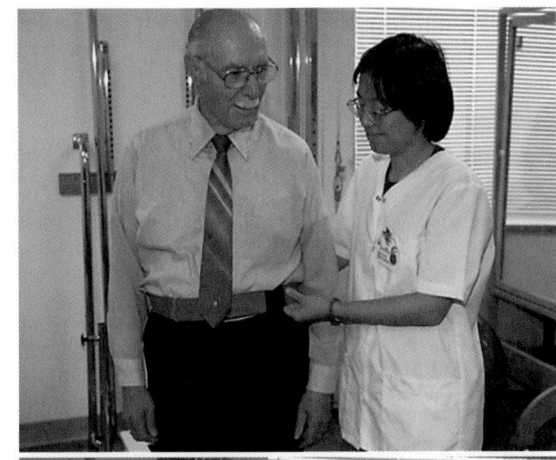

B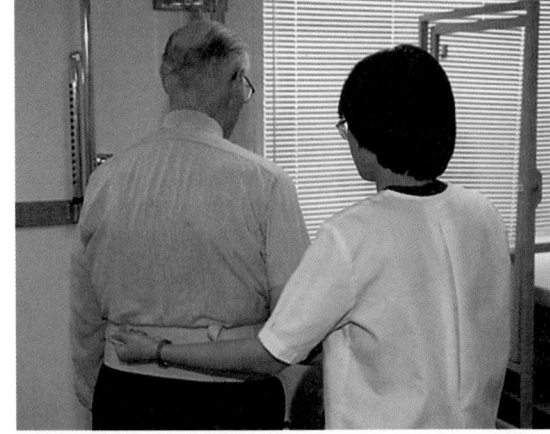

FIGURE 12-9 Transfer/gait belt. Note the different types of belts. **A,** The belt buckle is positioned off center. The nursing assistant grasps the belt from underneath. **B,** The belt buckle is not over the spine.

PROMOTING SAFETY AND COMFORT: Transfer/Gait Belts

SAFETY

Transfer/gait belts are routinely used in nursing centers. If the person needs help, a belt is required. To use one safely, always follow the manufacturer's instructions.

Some transfer/gait belts have a quick-release buckle. Position the quick-release buckle at the person's back where he or she cannot reach it. This prevents the person from releasing the buckle during the procedure. Injury could result if the buckle is released.

Do not leave excess strap dangling. Tuck the excess strap under the belt.

Remove the belt after the procedure. Do not leave the person alone while he or she is wearing a transfer/gait belt.

Using a transfer/gait belt is unsafe for some persons. The belt could cause pressure or rub against care equipment. Check with the nurse and the care plan before using a transfer/gait belt if the person has:
- An ostomy—colostomy, ileostomy, gastrostomy, urostomy (Chapters 22, 24, and 42)
- A gastric tube (Chapter 24)
- Chronic obstructive pulmonary disease (Chapter 40)
- An abdominal wound, incision, or drainage tube
- A chest wound, incision, or drainage tube
- Monitoring equipment
- A hernia
- Other conditions or care equipment involving the chest or abdomen

COMFORT

A transfer belt is always applied over clothing. It is never applied over bare skin. Also, it is applied under the breasts. Breasts must not be caught under the belt. The belt buckle is never positioned over the person's spine.

FOCUS ON **ETHICS** AND **LAWS**

Transfer/Gait Belts

A hospital patient fell and injured her right shoulder six days after knee surgery. The patient claimed that the nursing staff did not follow orders to assist with ambulation to and from the bathroom. According to the patient:
- She asked for help to raise herself from a commode to a standing position.
- She was not given assistance.
- She fell when the commode (with wheels) shifted while she tried to stand.

According to the hospital's lawyers, the staff did not use a gait belt during the transfer. Failure to use the gait belt violated hospital policy.

The case settled for $25,000.

(N. Martinez and M. Martinez v St. Catherine's Hospital, Sentry Insurance, and Wisconsin Patient Compensation Fund, 1998, Wisconsin.)

With permission from Medical Malpractice Verdicts, Settlements & Experts; Lewis Laska, Editor, 901 Church St., Nashville, TN 37203-3411, 1-800-298-6288.

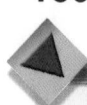

APPLYING A TRANSFER/GAIT BELT

✔**Quality of Life** *Remember to:*

- Knock before entering the person's room.
- Address the person by name.
- Introduce yourself by name and title.
- Explain the procedure to the person before beginning and during the procedure.

- Protect the person's rights during the procedure.
- Handle the person gently during the procedure.

PROCEDURE

1 See *Promoting Safety and Comfort: Transfer/Gait Belts,* p. 179.
2 Practice hand hygiene.
3 Identify the person. Check the ID bracelet against the assignment sheet. Also call the person by name.
4 Provide for privacy.
5 Assist the person to a sitting position.
6 Apply the belt around the person's waist over clothing. Do not apply it over bare skin.

7 Tighten the belt so it is snug. It should not cause discomfort or impair breathing. You should be able to slide your open, flat hand under the belt.
8 Make sure that a woman's breasts are not caught under the belt.
9 Place the buckle in the front or off-center in the back for the person's comfort (see Fig. 12-9). The buckle is not over the spine.

◆ THE FALLING PERSON

A person may start to fall when standing or walking. The person may be weak, light-headed, or dizzy. Fainting may occur. Falling may be caused by slipping or sliding on spills, waxed floors, throw rugs, or improper shoes. See p. 174 for the causes and risk factors for falls.

Do not try to prevent the fall. You could injure yourself and the person while twisting and straining to prevent the fall. Balance is lost as the person falls. If you try to prevent the fall, you could lose your balance. Thus both you and the person could fall or cause the other person to fall. Head, wrist, arm, hip, and knee injuries could occur.

If a person starts to fall, ease him or her to the floor. This lets you control the direction of the fall. You can also protect the person's head. Do not let the person move or get up before the nurse checks for injuries. Calmly explain that the nurse will check for injuries such as broken bones.

If you find a person on the floor, do not move the person. Stay with the person, and call for the nurse.

An incident report is completed after all falls. The nurse may ask you to help with the report.

See *Focus on Children and Older Persons: The Falling Person.*

FOCUS ON **CHILDREN** AND **OLDER PERSONS**

The Falling Person

OLDER PERSONS

Some older persons are confused. A confused person may not understand why you do not want him or her to move or get up after a fall. Forcing a person not to move may injure the person and you. You may need to let the person move for his or her safety and your own. Never use force to hold a person down. Stay calm, and protect the person from injury. Talk to the person in a quiet, soothing voice. Call for help.

HELPING THE FALLING PERSON

PROCEDURE

1 Stand behind the person with your feet apart. Keep your back straight.
2 Bring the person close to your body as fast as possible. Use the transfer/gait belt. Or wrap your arms around the person's waist. If necessary, you can also hold the person under the arms (Fig. 12-10, *A*).
3 Move your leg so the person's buttocks rest on it (Fig. 12-10, *B*). Move the leg near the person.
4 Lower the person to the floor. The person slides down your leg to the floor (Fig. 12-10, *C*). Bend at your hips and knees as you lower the person.
5 Call a nurse to check the person. Stay with the person.
6 Help the nurse return the person to bed. Ask other staff to help if needed.

POST-PROCEDURE

7 Provide for comfort. (See the inside of the front book cover.)
8 Place the signal light within reach.
9 Raise or lower bed rails. Follow the care plan.
10 Complete a safety check of the room. (See the inside of the front book cover.)
11 Report and record the following:
   • How the fall occurred
   • How far the person walked
   • How activity was tolerated before the fall
   • Complaints before the fall
   • How much help the person needed while walking
12 Complete an incident report.

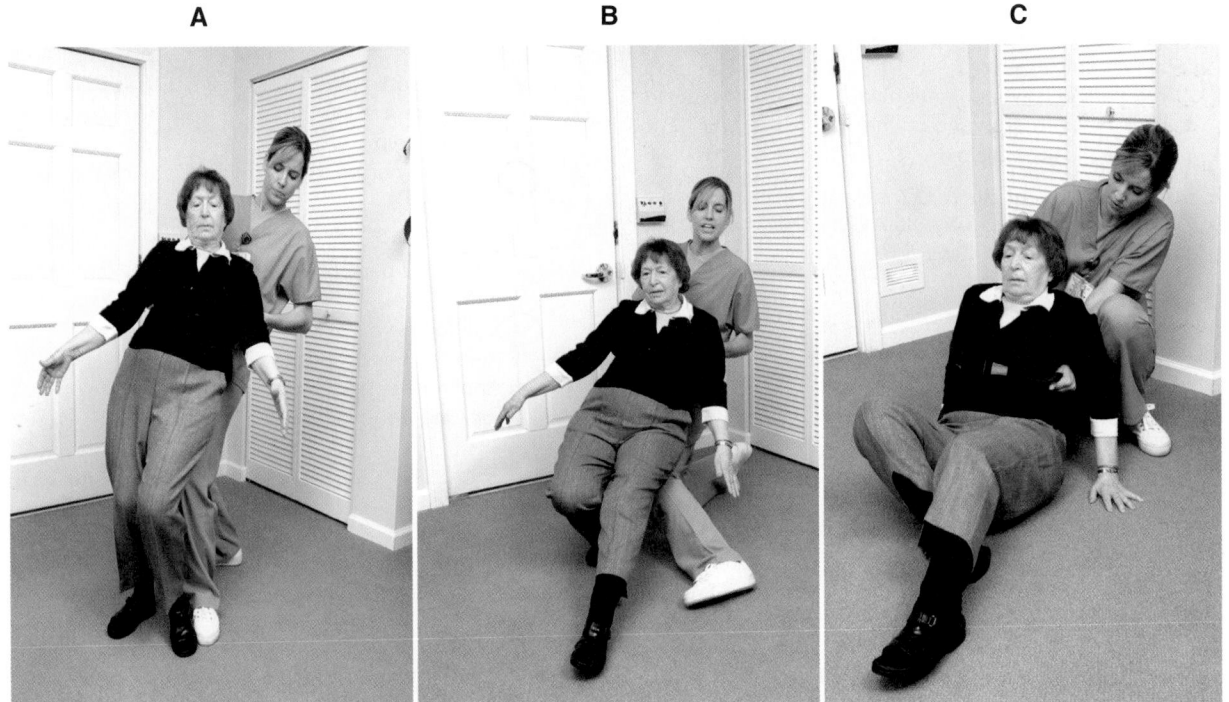

A **B** **C**

FIGURE 12-10 The falling person. **A,** The falling person is supported. **B,** The person's buttocks rest on the nursing assistant's leg. **C,** The person is eased to the floor on the nursing assistant's leg.

REVIEW QUESTIONS

Circle the BEST answer.

1 Most falls occur in
   a Patient and resident rooms and bathrooms
   b Dining rooms
   c Lounges
   d Hallways

2 Most falls occur
   a In the morning
   b At lunch time
   c In the afternoon
   d During the evening

3 A person's care plan includes fall prevention measures. Which should you question?
   a Assist with elimination needs.
   b Keep phone, lamp, and TV controls within reach.
   c Check the person every 2 hours.
   d Complete a safety check of the room after visitors leave.

4 You observe the following in the person's room. Which is *not* safe?
   a The lamp cord is by the chair.
   b The chair has armrests.
   c The night-light works.
   d The bed is in the lowest horizontal position.

5 You note the following after a person got dressed. Which is safe?
   a The person is wearing non-skid shoes.
   b Pant cuffs are dragging on the floor.
   c The belt is not fastened.
   d The shirt is too big.

6 A co-worker is helping Mr. Polk today. His chair alarm goes off. What should you do?
   a Find your co-worker.
   b Tell the nurse.
   c Assist Mr. Polk.
   d Wait for someone to respond to the alarm.

7 To help prevent falls, you need to report
   a Equipment and supplies being on one side of the hallway
   b A mattress on the floor beside the bed
   c A co-worker pulling a wheelchair through a doorway
   d Clutter on stairways

8 Bed rails are used
   a When you think they are needed
   b When the bed is raised
   c According to the care plan
   d To support persons who are weak or unsteady

9 You are going to transfer a person from the bed to a chair. Bed wheels must be locked.
   a True
   b False

10 A transfer/gait belt is applied
   a To the skin
   b Over clothing
   c Over the breasts
   d Under the robe

11 To safely use a transfer/gait belt, you must
   a Follow the manufacturer's instructions
   b Raise the bed rails
   c Lock the bed wheels
   d Set the bed alarm

12 You apply a transfer/gait belt. What should you do with the excess strap?
   a Cut it off.
   b Wrap it around the person's waist.
   c Tuck it under the belt.
   d Let it dangle.

13 A person starts to fall. Your first action is to
   a Try to prevent the fall
   b Call for help
   c Bring the person close to your body as fast as possible
   d Lower the person to the floor

14 You found a person lying on the floor. What should you do?
   a Call for the nurse.
   b Help the person back to bed.
   c Apply a transfer belt.
   d Lock the bed wheels.

Answers to these questions are on p. 780.

Promoting a Restraint-Free Environment

OBJECTIVES

- Define the key terms and key abbreviations listed in this chapter
- Describe the purpose of restraints
- Identify restraint alternatives

- Identify the complications from restraint use
- Explain the legal aspects of restraint use
- Explain how to use restraints safely
- Perform the procedure described in this chapter

PROCEDURE

- Applying Restraints

KEY TERMS

freedom of movement Any change in place or position for the body, or any part of the body, that the person is physically able to control

medical symptom An indication or characteristic of a physical or psychological condition

remove easily The manual method device, material, or equipment used to restrain the person that can be removed intentionally by the person in the same manner it was applied by the staff

restraint Any manual method or physical or mechanical device, material, or equipment attached to or near the person's body that he or she cannot remove easily and which restricts freedom of movement or normal access to one's body; a drug that is used as a restriction to manage a person's behavior or restrict the person's freedom of movement and is not a standard treatment or dosage for the person's condition

seclusion The involuntary confinement of a person alone in a room or area from which the person is physically prevented from leaving

KEY ABBREVIATIONS

CMS Centers for Medicare & Medicaid Services
FDA Food and Drug Administration

JC Joint Commission
OBRA Omnibus Budget Reconciliation Act of 1987

Chapters 11 and 12 have many safety measures. However, some persons need extra protection. They may present dangers to themselves or others.

In December 2006, the Centers for Medicare and Medicaid Services (CMS) issued new rules for the use of restraints and seclusion. The rules apply to agencies receiving Medicare and Medicaid funds—hospitals, nursing centers, rehabilitation centers, and centers for the treatment of alchol, drug dependence, or mental health problems.

Like the Omnibus Budget Reconciliation Act of 1987 (OBRA), CMS rules protect the person's rights and safety. All patients and residents have the right to be free from restraint or seclusion. Restraints or seclusion may only be used for the immediate physical safety of the person, a staff member, or others. Restraints or seclusion may only be used when less restrictive measures fail to protect the person, a staff member, or others. They must be discontinued at the earliest possible time.

To understand the CMS rules, you need to know these terms:

▶ **Restraint**—is any manual method or physical or mechanical device, material, or equipment attached to or near the person's body that he or she cannot remove easily and which restricts freedom of movement or normal access to one's body. Or it is a drug that is used as a restriction to manage a person's behavior or restrict the person's freedom of movement. The drug or its dosage is not a standard treatment for the person's condition.

▶ **Seclusion**—is the involuntary confinement of a person alone in a room, or area, from which the person is physically prevented from leaving. Seclusion can only be used to manage violent or self-destructive behavior.

▶ **Freedom of movement**—is any change in place or position for the body, or any part of the body, that the person is physically able to control.

▶ **Remove easily**—means the manual method device, material, or equipment used to restrain the person that can be removed intentionally by the person in the same manner it was applied by the staff.

HISTORY OF RESTRAINT USE

Until the late 1980s, restraints were thought to *prevent* falls. Research shows that restraints *cause* falls. Falls occur when persons try to get free of the restraints. Injuries are more serious from falls in restrained persons than in those not restrained.

Restraints also were used to prevent wandering or interfering with treatment. They were often used for persons who showed confusion, poor judgment, or behavior problems. Older persons were restrained more often than younger persons were. Restraints were viewed as necessary protective devices. Their purpose was to protect a person. However, they can cause serous harm (Box 13-1). They can even cause death.

> **BOX 13-1 Risks of Restraint Use**
>
> - Agitation
> - Anger
> - Cuts and bruises
> - Constipation
> - Dehydration
> - Depression
> - Embarrassment and humiliation
> - Fractures
> - Incontinence (Chapters 21 and 22)
> - Infections (pneumonia and urinary tract)
> - Mistrust
> - Nerve injuries
> - Pressure ulcers (Chapter 32)
> - Strangulation

Besides the CMS, the U.S. Food and Drug Administration (FDA), state agencies, and the Joint Commission (JC—an accrediting agency) have guidelines for the use of restraints and seclusion. They do not forbid the use of restraints and seclusion. However, *they require trying all other appropriate alternatives first.*

Every agency has policies and procedures about the use of restraints and seclusion. They include identifying persons at risk for harm, harmful behaviors, restraint or seclusion alternatives, and proper restraint and seclusion use. Staff training is required.

The focus of this chapter is on restraint alternatives and safe restraint use.

RESTRAINT ALTERNATIVES

Often there are causes and reasons for harmful behaviors. Knowing and treating the cause can prevent restraint use. The nurse tries to find out what the behavior means. This is very important for persons who have speech or cognitive problems. The focus is on these questions:

▶ Is the person in pain?
▶ Is the person ill or injured?
▶ Is the person short of breath? Are cells getting enough oxygen? (See Chapter 43.)
▶ Is the person afraid in a new setting?
▶ Does the person need to use the bathroom?
▶ Is a dressing tight or causing other discomfort (Chapter 32)?
▶ Is clothing tight or causing other discomfort?
▶ Is the person's position uncomfortable?
▶ Is the person too hot or too cold?
▶ Is the person hungry or thirsty?
▶ What are the person's life-long habits at this time of day?
▶ Are body fluids, secretions, or excretions causing skin irritation?
▶ Does the person have problems communicating?
▶ Is the person seeing, hearing, or feeling things that are not real (Chapter 37)?
▶ Is the person confused or disoriented (Chapter 44)?
▶ Are drugs causing the behaviors?

Restraint alternatives for the person are identified (Box 13-2). They become part of the care plan. Care plan changes are made as needed. Restraint alternatives may not protect the person. The doctor may need to order restraints.

BOX 13-2 Alternatives to Restraint Use

- Diversion is provided. This includes TV, videos, music, games, relaxation tapes, and so on.
- Life-long habits and routines are in the care plan. For example, showers before breakfast; reads in the bathroom; walks outside before lunch; watches TV after lunch, and so on.
- Family and friends make videos of themselves for the person to watch.
- Videos are made of visits with family and friends for the person to watch.
- Time is spent in supervised areas (dining room, lounge, near the nurses' station).
- Pillows, wedge cushions, and posture and positioning aids are used.
- The signal light is within reach.
- Signal lights are answered promptly.
- Food, fluid, hygiene, and elimination needs are met.
- The bedpan, urinal, or commode is within the person's reach.
- Back massages are given.
- Family, friends, and volunteers visit.
- The person has companions or sitters.
- Time is spent with the person.
- Extra time is spent with a person who is restless.
- Reminiscing is done with the person.
- A calm, quiet setting is provided.
- The person wanders in safe areas.
- The entire staff is aware of persons who tend to wander. This includes those in housekeeping, maintenance, the business office, dietary, and so on.
- Exercise programs are provided.
- Outdoor time is planned during nice weather.
- The person does jobs or tasks he or she consents to.
- Warning devices are used on beds, chairs, and doors.
- Knob guards are used on doors.
- Padded hip protectors are worn under clothing (Fig. 13-1).
- Floor cushions are placed next to beds (Chapter 12).
- Roll guards are attached to the bed frame (Fig. 13-2).
- Falls are prevented (Chapter 12).
- The person's furniture meets his or her needs (lower bed, reclining chair, rocking chair).
- Walls and furniture corners are padded.
- Observations and visits are made at least every 15 minutes.
- The person is moved to a room close to the nurses' station.
- Procedures and care measures are explained.
- Frequent explanations are given about required equipment or devices.
- Confused persons are oriented to person, time, and place. Calendars and clocks are provided.
- Light is adjusted to meet the person's basic needs and preferences.
- Staff assignments are consistent.
- Sleep is not interrupted.
- Noise levels are reduced.

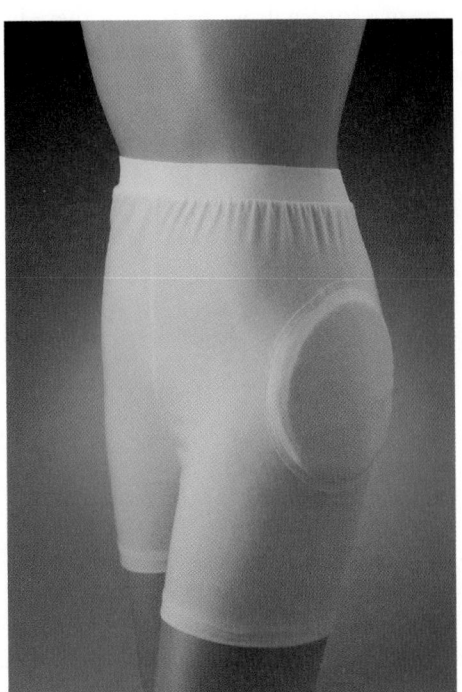

FIGURE 13-1 Hip protector. (Image courtesy J.T. Posey Co., Arcadia, Calif.)

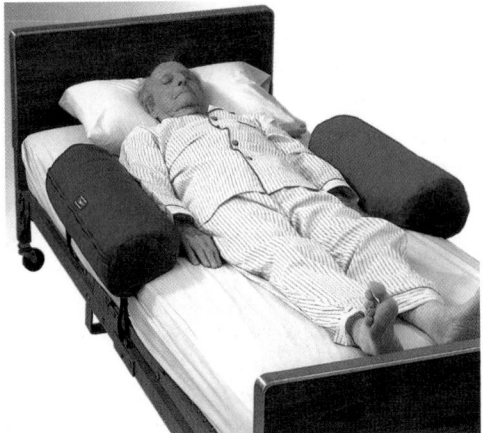

FIGURE 13-2 Roll guard. (Image courtesy J.T. Posey Co., Arcadia, Calif.)

SAFE RESTRAINT USE

Restraints can cause serious injury and even death. OBRA, CMS, FDA, and JC guidelines are followed. So are state laws. They are part of your agency's policies and procedures for restraint use.

Restraints are not used to discipline a person. They are not used for staff convenience. *Discipline* is any action that punishes or penalizes a person. *Convenience* is any action that:

▶ Controls the person's behavior
▶ Requires less effort by the center
▶ Is not in the person's best interests

Restraints are used only when necessary to treat a person's medical symptoms. The CMS defines a **medical symptom** as an indication or characteristic of a physical or psychological condition. Symptoms may relate to physical, emotional, or behavioral problems. Sometimes restraints are needed to protect the person, a staff member, or others. That is, a person may behave in ways that are harmful to self or others.

Imagine what it is like to be restrained:

▶ Your nose itches. But your hands and arms are restrained. You cannot scratch your nose.
▶ You need to use the bathroom. Your hands and arms are restrained. You cannot get up. You cannot reach your signal light. You soil yourself with urine and a bowel movement.
▶ Your phone is ringing. You cannot answer it because your hands and arms are restrained.
▶ You are not wearing your eyeglasses. You cannot identify people coming into and going out of your room. And you cannot speak because of a stroke. You have a vest restraint. You cannot move or turn in bed.
▶ You are thirsty. The water cup is within your reach but your hands and arms are restrained.
▶ You hear the fire alarm. You have on a restraint. You cannot get up to move to a safe place. You must wait until someone rescues you.

What would you try to do? Would you calmly lie or sit there? Would you try to get free from the restraint? Would you cry out for help? What would the nursing staff think? Would they think that you are uncomfortable? Or would they think that you are agitated and uncooperative? Would they think your behavior is improving or getting worse? Would you feel anger, embarrassment, or humiliation?

Try to put yourself in the person's situation. Then you can better understand how the person feels. Treat the person like you would want to be treated—with kindness, caring, respect, and dignity.

Physical and Drug Restraints

According to the CMS, *physical restraints* include these points:

▶ May be any manual method, physical or mechanical device, material, or equipment
▶ Is attached to or next to the person's body
▶ Cannot be easily removed by the person
▶ Restricts freedom of movement or access to one's body

Physical restraints are applied to the chest, waist, elbows, wrists, hands, or ankles. They confine the person to a bed or chair. Or they prevent movement of a body part. Some furniture or barriers are restraints if they prevent freedom of movement:

▶ Geriatric chairs (Geri-chairs) or chairs with attached trays (Fig. 13-3). Such chairs are often used for persons needing support to sit up.
▶ Any chair placed so close to the wall that the person cannot move.
▶ Bed rails (Chapter 12). For example, four half-length bed rails are raised. They are restraints if the person cannot lower them without help.
▶ Sheets tucked in so tightly that they restrict freedom of movement.
▶ Wheelchair locks if the person cannot release them.

Drugs or drug dosages are restraints if they:

▶ Control behavior or restrict movement
▶ Are not standard treatment for the person's condition

Drugs cannot be used for discipline or staff convenience. They cannot be used if not required for the person's treatment. They cannot be used if they affect physical or mental function.

Sometimes drugs can help persons who are confused or disoriented. They may be anxious, agitated, or aggressive. The doctor may order drugs to control these behaviors. The drugs should not make the person sleepy and unable to function at his or her highest level.

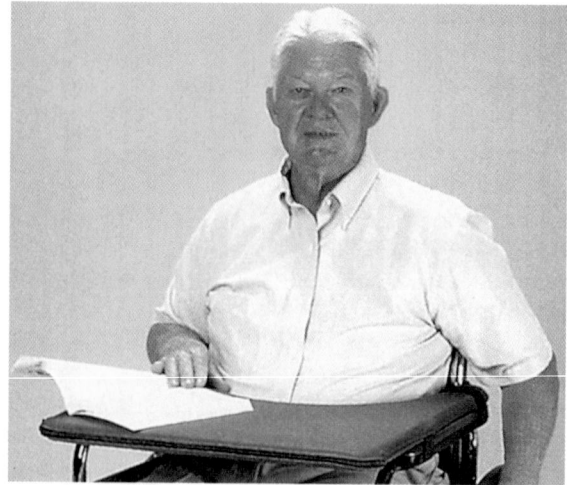

FIGURE 13-3 This lap-top tray is a restraint alternative. It is considered a restraint when used to prevent freedom of movement. (Image courtesy J.T. Posey Co., Arcadia, Calif.)

Complications of Restraint Use

Box 13-1 lists the many complications from restraints. Injuries occur as the person tries to get free of the restraint. Injuries also occur from using the wrong restraint, applying it wrong, or keeping it on too long. Cuts, bruises, and fractures are common. *The most serious risk is death from strangulation.*

There are also mental effects. Restraints affect dignity and self-esteem. Depression, anger, and agitation are common. So are embarrassment, humiliation, and mistrust.

Restraints are medical devices. The Safe Medical Device Act applies if a restraint causes illness, injury, or death. Also, CMS requires the reporting of any death that occurs:

▶ While a person is in a restraint.
▶ Within 24 hours after a restraint was removed.
▶ Within 1 week after a restraint was removed. This is done if the restraint may have contributed directly or indirectly to the person's death.

Legal Aspects

Laws applying to restraint use must be followed. Remember the following:

▶ *Restraints must protect the person.* They are not used for staff convenience or to discipline a person. Restraining someone is not easier than properly supervising and observing the person. A restrained person requires more staff time for care, supervision, and observation. A restraint is used only when it is the best safety measure for the person. Restraints are not used to punish or penalize uncooperative persons.
▶ *A doctor's order is required.* OBRA, CMS, state laws, FDA warnings, the JC and other accrediting agencies protect persons from unnecessary restraint. If restraints are needed for medical reasons, a doctor's order is required. The doctor gives the reason for the restraint, what body part to restrain, what to use for the restraint, and how long to use the restraint. This information is on the care plan and your assignment sheet.
▶ *The least restrictive method is used.* It allows the greatest amount of movement or body access possible. Some restraints attach to the person's body and to a fixed (non-movable) object. They restrict freedom of movement or body access. Vest, jacket, ankle, wrist, hand, and some belt restraints are active physical restraints. Other restraints are near but not directly attached to the person's body (bed rails or wedge cushions). They do not totally restrict freedom of movement. They allow access to certain body parts and are the least restrictive.
▶ *Restraints are used only after other measures fail to protect the person (see Box 13-2).* Some people can harm themselves or others. The care plan must include measures to protect the person and prevent harm to others. Many fall prevention measures are restraint alternatives (Chapter 12).

▶ *Unnecessary restraint is false imprisonment (Chapter 3).* You must clearly understand the reason for the restraint and its risk. If not, politely ask about its use. If you apply an unneeded restraint, you could face false imprisonment charges. See *Focus on Communication: Legal Aspects.*
▶ *Informed consent is required.* The person must understand the reason for the restraint. The person is told how the restraint will help the planned medical treatment. The person is told about the risks of restraint use. If the person cannot give consent, his or her legal representative is given the information. Either the person or the legal representative must give consent before a restraint can be used. The doctor or nurse provides the necessary information and obtains the consent.

Safety Guidelines

The restrained person must be kept safe. Follow the safety measures in Box 13-3, p. 188. Also remember these key points:

▶ *Observe for increased confusion and agitation.* Restraints can increase confusion and agitation. Whether confused or alert, people are aware of restricted movements. They may try to get out of the restraint or struggle or pull at it. Some restrained persons beg others to free or to help release them. These behaviors often are viewed as signs of confusion. Some people become more confused because they do not understand what is happening to them. Restrained persons need repeated explanations and reassurance. Spending time with them has a calming effect. See *Focus on Communication: Safety Guidelines*, p. 188.
▶ *Protect the person's quality of life.* Restraints are used for as short a time as possible. The care plan must show how to reduce restraint use. The person's needs are met with as little restraint as possible. You must meet the person's physical, emotional, and social needs. Visit with the person and explain the reason for the restraints.
▶ *Follow the manufacturer's instructions.* They explain how to apply and secure the restraint for the person's safety. The restraint must be snug and firm, but not tight. Tight restraints affect circulation and breathing. The person must be comfortable and able to move the restrained part to a limited and safe extent. You could be negligent if you do not apply or secure a restraint properly.

▶ *Apply restraints with enough help to protect the person and staff from injury.* Persons in immediate danger of harming themselves or others are restrained quickly. Combative and agitated people can hurt themselves and the staff when restraints are applied. Enough staff members are needed to complete the task safely and quickly.

▶ *Observe the person at least every 15 minutes or more often as required by the care plan.* Restraints are dangerous. Injuries and deaths can result from improper restraint use and poor observation. Prevent complications. Interferences with breathing and circulation are examples.

▶ *Remove or release the restraint, reposition the person, and meet basic needs at least every 2 hours.* The restraint is removed or released for at least 10 minutes. Provide for food, fluid, comfort, safety, hygiene, and elimination needs and give skin care. Perform range-of-motion exercises or help the person walk (Chapter 26). Follow the care plan.

▶ See *Teamwork and Time Management: Safety Guidelines.*

FOCUS ON COMMUNICATION

Safety Guidelines

Restraints can increase confusion. Remind the person why the restraint is needed and to call for help when it is needed. Repeat the following as often as needed:

- "Dr. Richards ordered this restraint for you so you don't hurt yourself. If you need to get up, please call for help. I'll check on you every 15 minutes. Other staff will check on you too."
- "How does the restraint feel? Is it too tight? Is it too loose?"
- "Please put your signal light on. I want to make sure that you can reach and use it with the restraint on."
- "Please call for help right away if the restraint is too tight."
- "Please call for help right away if you feel pain in your fingers or hands. Also call for me if you feel numbness or tingling."
- "Please call for help right away if you are having problems breathing."

TEAMWORK AND TIME MANAGEMENT

Safety Guidelines

You may not be assigned to a restrained person. However, you must still help the nursing team keep the person safe. Make sure you know who is restrained on your unit. Every time you walk past the person or the person's room, check to see if the person is safe and comfortable. Answer the person's signal light promptly.

BOX 13-3 Safety Measures for Using Restraints

BEFORE APPLYING RESTRAINTS
- Use the restraint noted in the care plan.
- Use the correct size. The nurse and care plan tell you what to use. Small restraints are tight. They cause discomfort and agitation. They also restrict breathing and circulation. Strangulation is a risk from big or loose restraints.
- Apply a restraint only after being instructed about its proper use.
- Demonstrate proper application of the restraint before applying it.
- Use only restraints that have manufacturer instructions and warning labels.
- Read the manufacturer's warning labels. Note the front and back of the restraint.
- Follow the manufacturer's instructions. Some restraints are safe for bed, chair, and wheelchair use. Others are used only with certain equipment.
- Do not use sheets, towels, tape, rope, straps, bandages, or other items to restrain a person.
- Use intact restraints. Look for tears, cuts, or frayed fabric or straps. Look for missing or loose hooks, loops, or straps or other damage.
- Do not use a restraint near a fire, a flame, or smoking materials.

APPLYING RESTRAINTS
- Do not use restraints to position a person on a toilet.
- Do not use restraints to position a person on furniture that does not allow for correct application. Follow the manufacturer's instructions.

- Follow agency policies and procedures.
- Position the person in good alignment before applying the restraint (Chapter 15).
- Pad bony areas and the skin. This prevents pressure and injury from the restraint.
- Secure the restraint. It should be snug but allow some movement of the restrained part. Follow the manufacturer's instructions to check for snugness. For example:
  - If applied to the chest or waist—Make sure that the person can breathe easily. A flat hand should slide between the restraint and the person's body (Fig. 13-4).
  - For wrist and mitt restraints—You should be able to slide 1 or 2 fingers under the restraint.
- Criss-cross vest restraints in front (Fig. 13-5). Do not criss-cross restraints in the back unless part of the manufacturer's instructions (Fig. 13-6, p. 190). Criss-crossing vests in the back can cause death from strangulation.
- Tie restraints according to agency policy. The policy should follow the manufacturer's instructions and allow for quick release in an emergency. Quick-release buckles or airline-type buckles are used (Fig. 13-7, p. 190). So are quick-release ties (Fig. 13-8, p. 190).
- Secure straps out of the person's reach.
- Leave 1 to 2 inches of slack in the straps. This allows some movement of the part.
- Secure the restraint to the movable part of the bed frame at waist level (see Fig. 13-8). For chairs, secure straps to the wheelchair or the chair frame (Fig. 13-9, p. 190).

BOX 13-3 Safety Measures for Using Restraints—cont'd

APPLYING RESTRAINTS—cont'd

- Make sure that straps will not slide in any direction. If straps slide, they change the restraint's position. The person can get suspended off the mattress or chair (Figs. 13-10, p. 190 and 13-11, p. 191). Strangulation can result.
- Never secure restraints to the bed rails. The person can reach bed rails to release knots or buckles. Also, injury to the person is likely when raising or lowering bed rails.
- Use bed rail covers or gap protectors according to the nurse's instructions (Fig. 13-12, p. 191). They prevent entrapment between the rails or the bed rail bars (see Fig. 13-10). Entrapment can occur between:
  - The bars of a bed rail
  - The space between half-length (split) bed rails
  - The bed rail and mattress
  - The headboard or footboard and mattress
- Position the person in semi-Fowler's position when using a vest, jacket, or belt restraint.
- Position the person in a chair so the hips are well to the back of the chair.
- Apply a belt restraint at a 45-degree angle over the thighs (Fig. 13-13, p. 191).

AFTER APPLYING RESTRAINTS

- Keep full bed rails up when using a vest, jacket, or belt restraint. Also use bed rail covers or gap protectors. Otherwise the person could fall off the bed and strangle on the restraint. If half-length bed rails are used, the person can get caught between them.
- Do not use back cushions when a person is restrained in a chair. If the cushion moves out of place, slack occurs in the straps. Strangulation could result if the person slides forward or down from the extra slack (see Fig. 13-11).
- Do not cover the person with a sheet, blanket, bedspread, or other covering. The restraint must be within plain view at all times.
- Check the person at least every 15 minutes for safety, comfort, and signs of injury.

- Check the person's circulation at least every 15 minutes if mitt, wrist, ankle, or elbow restraints are applied. You should feel a pulse at a pulse site below the restraint. Fingers or toes should be warm and pink. Tell the nurse at once if:
  - You cannot feel a pulse.
  - Fingers or toes are cold, pale, or blue in color.
  - The person complains of pain, numbness, or tingling in the restrained part.
  - The skin is red or damaged.
- Check the person at least every 15 minutes if a belt, jacket, or vest restraint is used. The person should be able to breathe easily. Also check the position of the restraint, especially in the front and back.
- Monitor persons in the supine position constantly. They are at great risk for aspiration if vomiting occurs (Chapter 23). Call for the nurse at once.
- Keep scissors in your pocket. In an emergency, cutting the tie may be faster than untying a knot. Never leave scissors at the bedside where the person can reach them.
- Remove or release the restraint and reposition the person every 2 hours. The restraint is removed or released for at least 10 minutes. Meet the person's basic needs. You need to:
  - Measure vital signs.
  - Meet elimination needs.
  - Offer food and fluids.
  - Meet hygiene needs.
  - Give skin care.
  - Perform range-of-motion exercises or help the person walk. Follow the care plan.
  - Provide for physical and emotional comfort. (See the inside of the front book cover.)
- Keep the signal light within the person's reach. (Chart that this was done.)
- Complete a safety check before leaving the room. (See the inside of the front book cover.)
- Report to the nurse every time you checked the person and removed or released the restraint. Report your observations and the care given. Follow agency policy for recording.

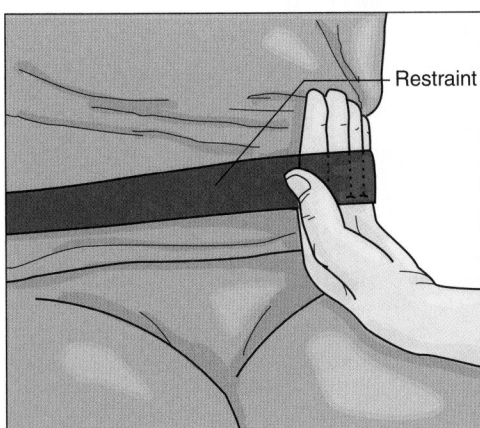

FIGURE 13-4 A flat hand slides between the restraint and the person.

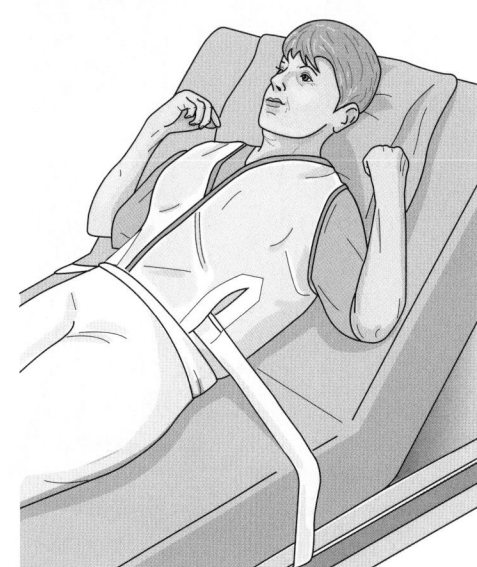

FIGURE 13-5 Vest restraint criss-crosses in front. (*NOTE:* The bed rails are raised after the restraint is applied.)

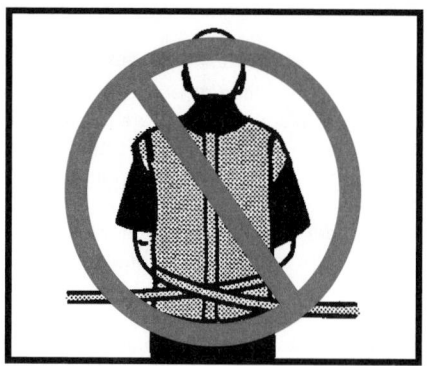

FIGURE 13-6 Never criss-cross vest or jacket straps in back. (Image courtesy J.T. Posey Co., Arcadia, Calif.)

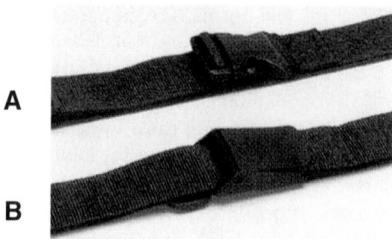

FIGURE 13-7 A, Quick-release buckle. **B,** Airline-type buckle. (Image courtesy J.T. Posey Co., Arcadia, Calif.)

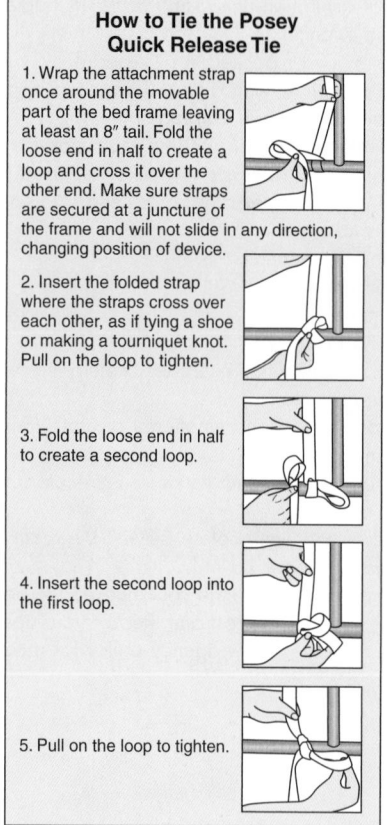

FIGURE 13-8 The Posey quick-release tie. (Image courtesy J.T. Posey Co., Arcadia, Calif.)

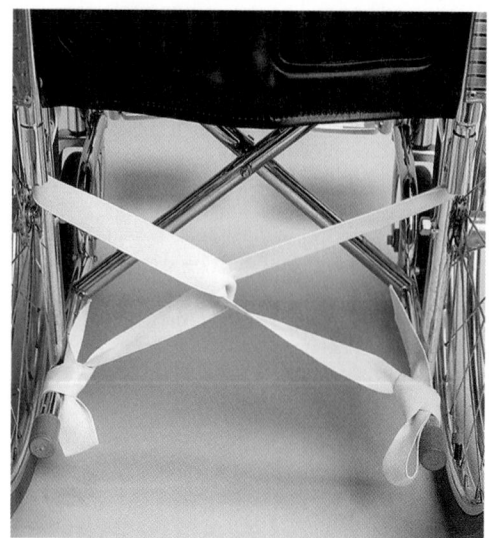

FIGURE 13-9 The restraint straps are secured to the wheelchair frame with quick-release ties. (Image courtesy J.T. Posey Co., Arcadia, Calif.)

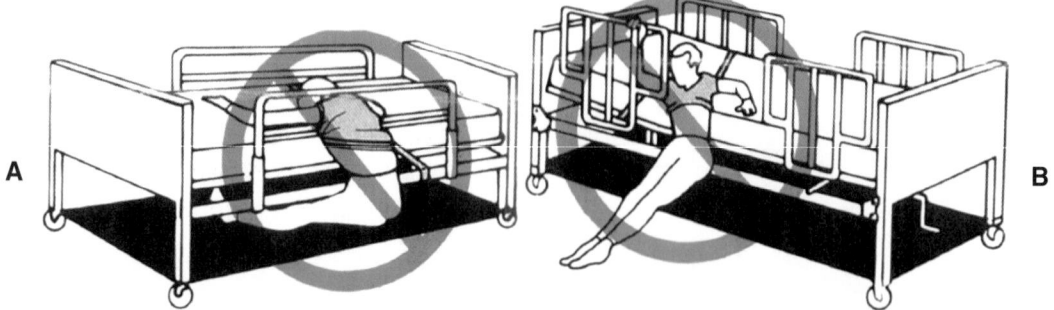

FIGURE 13-10 A, A person can get suspended and caught between bed rail bars. **B,** The person can get suspended and caught between half-length bed rails. (Images courtesy J.T. Posey Co., Arcadia, Calif.)

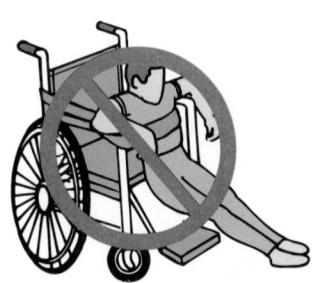

Straps to prevent sliding should always be over the thighs–NOT around the waist or chest. Straps should be at a 45° angle and secured to the chair under the seat, not behind the back. They should be snug but comfortable and not restrict breathing. If a belt or vest is too loose or applied around the waist, the person may slide partially off the seat–resulting in possible suffocation and death.

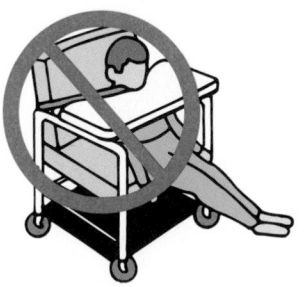

Tray tables (with or without a belt or vest) pose potential danger if the person should slide partly under the table and become caught. This could result in suffocation and death. Make sure the person's hips are positioned at the back of the chair–this may necessitate the use of an anti-slide material (Posey Grip), a pommel cushion, or a restrictive device if the person shows any tendency to slide forward.

FIGURE 13-11 Strangulation could result if the person slides forward or down because of extra slack in the restraint. (Images courtesy J.T. Posey Co., Arcadia, Calif.)

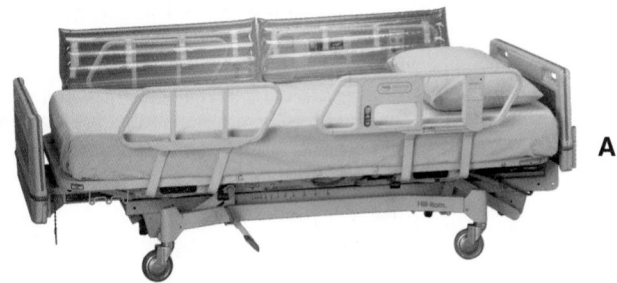

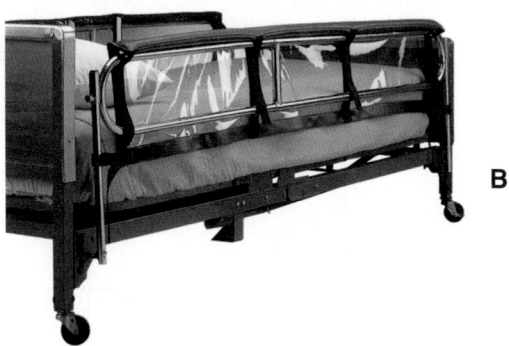

FIGURE 13-12 A, Bed rail protector. **B,** Guard rail pads. (Images courtesy J.T. Posey Co., Arcadia, Calif.)

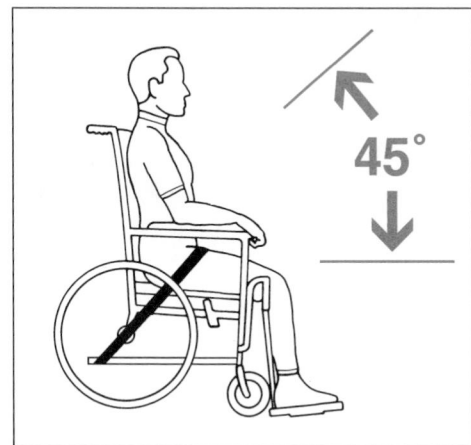

FIGURE 13-13 The safety belt is at a 45-degree angle over the thighs. (Image courtesy J.T. Posey Co., Arcadia, Calif.)

Reporting and Recording

Information about restraints is recorded in the person's medical record (Fig. 13-14, p. 192). You might apply restraints or care for a restrained person. Report and record the following:

▶ The type of restraint applied
▶ The body part or parts restrained
▶ The reason for the application
▶ Safety measures taken (for example, bed rails padded and up, signal light within reach)
▶ The time you applied the restraint
▶ The time you removed or released the restraint and for how long
▶ The person's vital signs
▶ The care given when the restraint was removed or released
▶ Skin color and condition
▶ Condition of the limbs
▶ The pulse felt in the restrained part
▶ Changes in the person's behavior
▶ Complaints of discomfort; a tight restraint; difficulty breathing; and pain, numbness, or tingling in the restrained part (Report these complaints to the nurse at once.)

RESTRAINT RELEASE RECORD
(Reference tag: F221)

PLEASE NOTE: Restrained individuals must be checked at least every 15 minutes. In addition, restraints must be released for the purpose of exercise, toileting, etc. for at least 10 minutes at least every two hours.

REASON FOR RESTRAINT	RESTRAINT ORDERED (Circle)			REMOVAL REASON CODES		
Is nonweight bearing and attempts to rise when in W/C.	Waist	Pelvic	Siderails	A- Supervised meals		F- 2-3 hrs. with periodic evaluation
	Wrist	(Belt)	2 Full	B- Supervised group activities		G- Total elimination of restraint
	Geri Chair	Vest	1 Full	C- Care provided by CNA		H- *off when in bed*
	Ankle	Bar	2 Half	D- One-to-one with volunteer		I-
	Other_____		1 Half	E- One-to-one with social worker		J-

DATE	15 MINUTE CHECK WHEN RESTRAINED			RELEASE EVERY TWO HOURS FOR PERSONAL CARE			TOTAL HOURS RELEASED PER SHIFT AND REASONS (USE REASON CODES ABOVE)			COMMENTS/ RESIDENT'S RESPONSE (Negative or Positive)
7/18	Shift Initials			Shift Initials						
Month/Year	11-7	7-3	3-11	11-7	7-3	3-11	11-7	7-3	3-11	
1	Lg	BG	MM	Lg	BG	MM	8(H)	4(A,B, C,H)	5(A,C, D,H)	No agitation – no falls no attempts to rise *Joan Grieg, RN*
2	Lg	BG	MM	Lg	BG	MM	8(H)	5(A,B, C,F,H)	6(A,C, F,H)	Doing well – no falls – *Joan Grieg, RN*
3	DL	RD	DL	ML	RD	ML	8(H)	6(A,B, C,F,H)	8(A,C, F,H)	No falls – Resident wants belt removed *Ray Lopez, RN*
4										
5										
6										

FIGURE 13-14 Charting sample. (Modified from Briggs Corp., Des Moines, Iowa.)

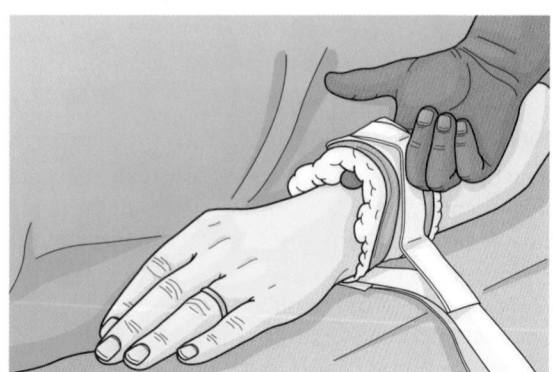

FIGURE 13-15 Wrist restraint. The soft part is toward the skin. Note that 1 finger fits between the restraint and the wrist.

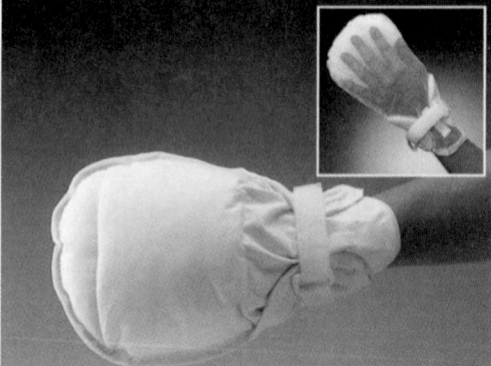

FIGURE 13-16 Mitt restraint. (Images courtesy J.T. Posey Co., Arcadia, Calif.)

◆ Applying Restraints

Restraints are made of cloth or leather. Cloth restraints (soft restraints) are mitts, belts, straps, jackets, and vests. They are applied to the wrists, ankles, hands, waist, and chest. Leather restraints are applied to the wrists and ankles. Leather restraints are used for extreme agitation and combativeness.

Wrist Restraints

Wrist restraints (limb holders) limit arm movement (Fig. 13-15). They may be used when a person continually tries to pull out tubes used for treatment (IV, feeding tube, catheter, wound drainage tubes, monitoring lines). Or the person tries to scratch at, pull at, or peel the skin, a wound, or a dressing. This can damage the skin or the wound.

Mitt Restraints

Hands are placed in mitt restraints. They prevent finger use. They do not prevent hand, wrist, or arm movements. They are used for the same reasons as wrist restraints. Most mitts are padded (Fig. 13-16).

Belt Restraints

The belt restraint (Fig. 13-17) is used when injuries from falls are risks or for positioning during a medical treatment. The person cannot get out of bed or out of a chair. However, the person can turn from side to side or sit up in bed.

The belt is applied around the waist and secured to the bed or chair. It is applied over a garment. The person can release the quick-release type. It is less restrictive than those that only staff members can release.

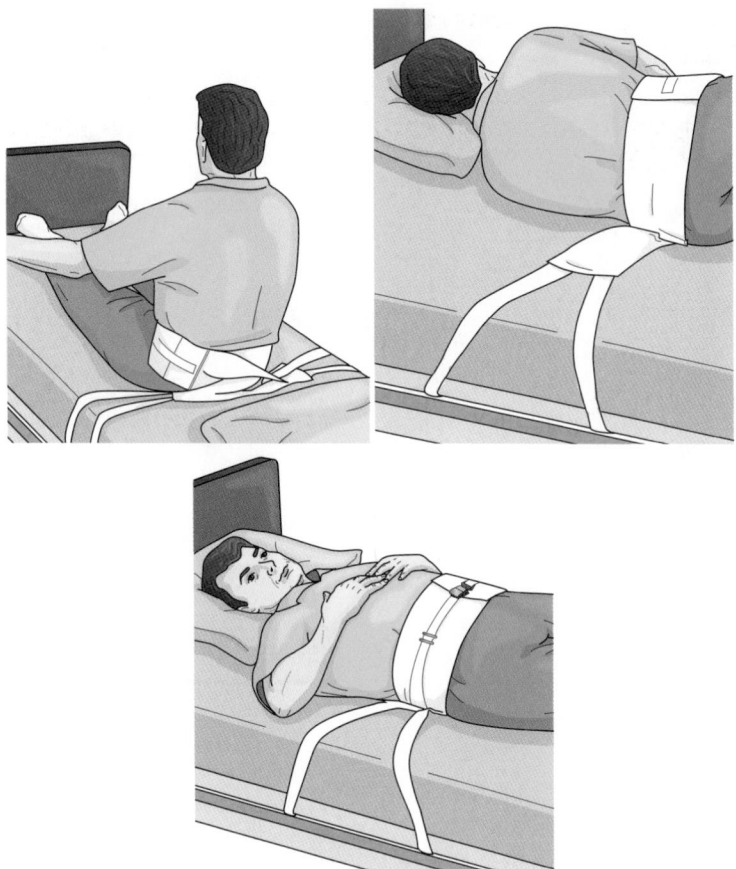

FIGURE 13-17 Belt restraint. (*NOTE:* The bed rails are raised after the restraint is applied.)

Vest Restraints and Jacket Restraints

Vest and jacket restraints are applied to the chest. They may be used to prevent injuries from falls. And they may be used for persons who need positioning for a medical treatment. The person cannot turn in bed or get out of a chair.

A jacket restraint is applied with the opening in the back. For a vest restraint, the vest crosses in front (see Fig. 13-5). *The straps of vest and jacket restraints always cross in the front.* They must *never* cross in the back. Vest and jacket restraints are never worn backward. Strangulation or other injury could occur if the person slides down in the bed or chair. The restraint is always applied over a garment. (*NOTE: A vest or jacket restraint may have a positioning slot in the back. Criss-cross the straps following the manufacturer's instructions.*)

Vest and jacket restraints have life-threatening risks. Death can occur from strangulation. If the person gets caught in the restraint, it can become so tight that the person's chest cannot expand to inhale air. The person quickly suffocates and dies. Restraints must be applied correctly. For vest and jacket restraints, this is critical. You are advised to only assist the nurse in applying them. The nurse should assume full responsibility for applying a vest or jacket restraint.

See *Focus on Children and Older Persons: Applying Restraints.*

See *Delegation Guidelines: Applying Restraints,* p. 194.

See *Promoting Safety and Comfort: Applying Restraints,* p. 194.

FOCUS ON **CHILDREN** AND **OLDER PERSONS**

Applying Restraints

OLDER PERSONS

Restraints may increase confusion and agitation in persons with dementia. They do not understand what you are doing. They may resist your efforts to apply a restraint. They may actively try to get free from the restraint. Serious injury and death are risks.

Never use force to apply a restraint. If a person is confused or agitated, ask a co-worker to help apply the restraint. Report problems to the nurse at once.

CHILDREN

Elbow restraints (elbow splints) limit arm movements. They prevent infants and children from bending their elbows (Fig. 13-18, p. 194). They are used to prevent scratching and touching incisions or pulling out tubes. Both arms are restrained to achieve the desired effect.

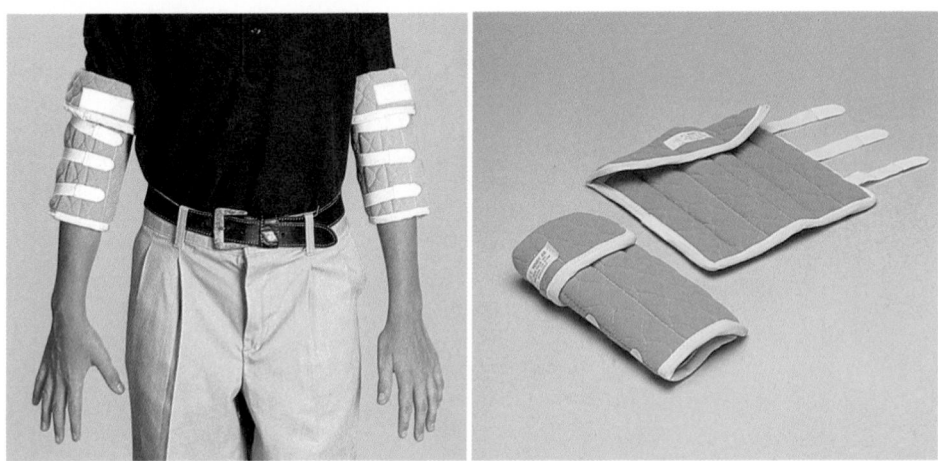

FIGURE 13-18 Elbow restraints (splints). (Images courtesy J.T. Posey Co., Arcadia, Calif.)

DELEGATION GUIDELINES: Applying Restraints

Before applying a restraint, you need this information from the nurse and the care plan:
- Why the doctor ordered the restraint
- What type and size to use
- Where to apply the restraint
- How to safely apply the restraint (Have the nurse show you how to apply it. Then demonstrate correct application back to the nurse.)
- How to correctly position the person
- What bony areas to pad and how to pad them
- If bed rail covers or gap protectors are needed
- If bed rails are up or down
- What special equipment is needed
- If the person needs to be checked more often than every 15 minutes
- When to apply and release the restraint
- What observations to report and record (p. 191)
- When to report observations
- What specific patient and resident concerns to report at once

PROMOTING SAFETY AND COMFORT: Applying Restraints

SAFETY
Restraints can cause serious harm, even death. Always follow the manufacturer's instructions. Manufacturers have many types of restraints. The instructions for one type may not apply to another. Also, the manufacturer may have specific instructions when applying restraints on persons who are agitated.

Never use force to apply a restraint. Ask a co-worker to help apply a restraint on a person who is confused and agitated. Report problems to the nurse at once.

Check the person at least every 15 minutes or more often as instructed by the nurse and the care plan. Make sure the signal light is within reach. Ask the person to use the signal light at the first sign of problems or discomfort.

Never use a restraint as a seat belt in a car or other vehicle.

COMFORT
The person's comfort is always important. It is more so when restraints are used. Remember, restraints limit the person's ability to move. This affects position changes and the ability to reach needed items. Always make sure the person is in good alignment before applying a restraint (Chapter 15). Also make sure the person can reach needed items—signal light, water, tissues, phone, bed controls, and so on.

APPLYING RESTRAINTS

✔ Quality of Life *Remember to:*

- Knock before entering the person's room.
- Address the person by name.
- Introduce yourself by name and title.
- Explain the procedure to the person before beginning and during the procedure.

- Protect the person's rights during the procedure.
- Handle the person gently during the procedure.

PRE-PROCEDURE

1 Follow *Delegation Guidelines: Applying Restraints*. See *Promoting Safety and Comfort: Applying Restraints*.
2 Collect the following as instructed by the nurse:
   - Correct type and size of restraints
   - Padding for skin and bony areas
   - Bed rail pads or gap protectors (if needed)

3 Practice hand hygiene.
4 Identify the person. Check the ID bracelet against the assignment sheet. Also call the person by name.
5 Provide for privacy.

PROCEDURE

6 Make sure the person is comfortable and in good alignment.
7 Put the bed rail pads or gap protectors (if needed) on the bed if the person is in bed. Follow the manufacturer's instructions.
8 Pad bony areas. Follow the nurse's instructions and the care plan.
9 Read the manufacturer's instructions. Note the front and back of the restraint.
10 For wrist restraints:
   a Apply the restraint following the manufacturer's instructions. Place the soft part toward the skin.
   b Secure the restraint so it is snug but not tight. Make sure you can slide 1 or 2 fingers under the restraint (see Fig. 13-15). Follow the manufacturer's instructions. Adjust the straps if the restraint is too loose or too tight. Check for snugness again.
   c Tie the straps to the movable part of the bed frame out of the person's reach. Use an agency-approved tie. Leave 1 to 2 inches of slack in the straps.
   d Repeat steps 10 a, b, and c for the other wrist.
11 For mitt restraints:
   a Make sure the person's hands are clean and dry.
   b Apply the mitt restraint. Follow the manufacturer's instructions.
   c Tie the straps to the movable part of the bed frame. Use an agency-approved tie. Leave 1 to 2 inches of slack in the straps.
   d Make sure the restraint is snug. Slide 1 or 2 fingers between the restraint and the wrist. Follow the manufacturer's instructions. Adjust the straps if the restraint is too loose or too tight. Check for snugness again.
   e Repeat steps 11 b, c, and d for the other hand.
12 For a belt restraint:
   a Assist the person to a sitting position.
   b Apply the restraint with your free hand. Follow the manufacturer's instructions.

   c Remove wrinkles or creases from the front and back of the restraint.
   d Bring the ties through the slots in the belt.
   e Help the person lie down if he or she is in bed.
   f Make sure the person is comfortable and in good alignment.
   g Secure the straps to the movable part of the bed frame out of the person's reach or to the chair or wheelchair. Use an agency-approved tie. Leave 1 or 2 inches of slack in the straps.
   h Make sure the belt is snug. Slide an open hand between the restraint and the person. Adjust the restraint if it is too loose or too tight. Check for snugness again.
13 For a vest restraint:
   a Assist the person to a sitting position.
   b Apply the restraint with your free hand. Follow the manufacturer's instructions. The "V" part of the vest crosses in front.
   c Make sure the vest is free of wrinkles in the front and back.
   d Help the person lie down if he or she is in bed.
   e Bring the straps through the slots.
   f Make sure the person is comfortable and in good alignment.
   g Secure the straps to the chair or to the movable part of the bed frame. If secured to the bed frame, the straps are secured at waist level out of the person's reach. Use an agency-approved tie. Leave 1 to 2 inches of slack in the straps.
   h Make sure the vest is snug. Slide an open hand between the restraint and the person. Adjust the restraint if it is too loose or too tight. Check for snugness again.

Continued

APPLYING RESTRAINTS—cont'd

PROCEDURE—cont'd

14 For a jacket restraint:
 a Assist the person to a sitting position.
 b Apply the restraint with your free hand. Follow the manufacturer's instructions. Remember, the jacket opening goes in the back.
 c Close the back with the zipper, ties, or hook and loop closures.
 d Make sure the side seams are under the arms. Remove any wrinkles in the front and back.
 e Help the person lie down if he or she is in bed.
 f Make sure the person is comfortable and in good alignment.
 g Secure the straps to the chair or to the movable part of the bed frame. If secured to the bed frame, the straps are secured at waist level out of the person's reach. Use an agency-approved knot. Leave 1 to 2 inches of slack in the straps.

 h Make sure the jacket is snug. Slide an open hand between the restraint and the person. Adjust the restraint if it is too loose or too tight. Check for snugness again.
15 For elbow restraints:
 a Wrap the restraint around the child's elbow. Follow the manufacturer's instructions.
 b Secure the restraint.
 c Make sure you can slide two fingers between the restraint and the child's arm. Follow the manufacturer's instructions.
 d Repeat steps 15 a, b, and c for the other arm.

POST-PROCEDURE

16 Position the person as the nurse directs.
17 Provide for comfort. (See the inside of the front book cover.)
18 Place the signal light within the person's reach.
19 Raise or lower bed rails. Follow the care plan and the manufacturer's instructions for the restraint.
20 Unscreen the person.
21 Complete a safety check of the room. (See the inside of the front book cover.)
22 Decontaminate your hands.
23 Check the person and the restraint at least every 15 minutes. Report and record your observations:
 a For wrist, mitt, and elbow restraints: check the pulse, color, and temperature of the restrained parts.
 b For vest, jacket, and belt restraints: check the person's breathing. *Call for the nurse at once if the person is not breathing or is having problems breathing.* Make sure the restraint is properly positioned in the front and back.

24 Do the following at least every 2 hours (and for at least 10 minutes):
 a Remove or release the restraint.
 b Measure vital signs.
 c Reposition the person.
 d Meet food, fluid, hygiene, and elimination needs.
 e Give skin care.
 f Perform range-of-motion exercises or help the person walk. Follow the care plan.
 g Provide for physical and emotional comfort. (See the inside of the front book cover.)
 h Reapply the restraints.
25 Complete a safety check of the room. (See the inside of the front book cover.)
26 Report and record your observations and the care given.

Circle T if the statement is true and F if the statement is false.

1 T **(F)** Restraint alternatives fail to protect a person. You can apply a restraint.

2 T **(F)** Restraints can be used for staff convenience.

3 T **(F)** A device is a restraint only if it is attached to the person's body.

4 **(T)** F Bed rails are restraints if the person cannot lower them.

5 **(T)** F Restraints are used only for specific medical symptoms.

6 **(T)** F Restraints can be used to protect the person from harming others.

7 **(T)** F Unnecessary restraint is false imprisonment.

8 **(T)** F Informed consent is needed for restraint use.

9 T **(F)** You can apply restraints when you think they are needed.

10 T **(F)** Restraints are secured within the person's reach.

11 T **(F)** You can use a vest restraint to position a person on the toilet.

12 **(T)** F Restraints are removed or released at least every 2 hours to reposition the person and give skin care.

13 T **(F)** Restraints are tied to bed rails.

14 **(T)** F A vest restraint crosses in front.

15 **(T)** F Bed rails are left down when vest restraints are used.

Circle the BEST answer.

16 These statements are about restraints. Which is *false?*
  a A restraint can be an object, device, garment, or material.
  b A restraint limits or restricts a person's freedom of movement.
  c Some drugs are restraints.
  (d) A restraint is used when the nurse thinks it is needed.

17 Which is *not* a restraint alternative?
  (a) Positioning the person's chair close to the wall
  b Answering signal lights promptly
  c Taking the person outside in nice weather
  d Padding walls and corners of furniture

18 Physical restraints
  a Control mental function
  b Control a behavior
  (c) Confine a person to a bed or chair
  d Decrease care needs

19 The following can occur because of restraints. Which is the *most* serious?
  a Fractures
  (b) Strangulation
  c Pressure ulcers
  d Urinary tract infections

20 A belt restraint is applied to a person in bed. Where should you tie the straps?
  a To the bed rails
  b To the headboard
  (c) To the movable part of the bed frame
  d To the footboard

21 A person has a restraint. You should check the person and the position of the restraint at least every
  (a) 15 minutes
  b 30 minutes
  c Hour
  d 2 hours

22 A person has mitt restraints. Which of these is especially important to report to the nurse?
  a The heart rate
  b The respiratory rate
  c Why the restraints were applied
  (d) If you felt a pulse in the restrained extremities

23 The doctor ordered mitt restraints for a person. You need the following information from the nurse *except*
  a What size to use
  b What other equipment is needed
  (c) What drugs the person is taking
  d When to apply and release the restraints

24 A person has a vest restraint. It is not too tight or too lose if you can slide
  a A fist between the vest and the person
  b One finger between the vest and the person
  (c) An open hand between the vest and the person
  d Two fingers between the vest and the person

25 The correct way to apply any restraint is to follow the
  a Nurse's directions
  b Doctor's orders
  c Care plan
  (d) Manufacturer's instructions

Answers to these questions are on p. 780.

CHAPTER 14 Preventing Infection

OBJECTIVES

- Define the key terms and key abbreviations listed in this chapter
- Identify what microbes need to live and grow
- List the signs and symptoms of infection
- Explain the chain of infection
- Describe healthcare-associated infections and the persons at risk
- Describe the practices of medical asepsis
- Describe disinfection and sterilization methods
- Explain how to care for equipment and supplies
- Explain Isolation Precautions
- Describe Standard Precautions and Transmission-Based Precautions
- Explain the Bloodborne Pathogen Standard
- Explain the principles and practices of surgical asepsis
- Perform the procedures described in this chapter

PROCEDURES

- Hand Washing
- Removing Gloves
- Donning and Removing a Gown
- Donning and Removing a Mask
- Double Bagging
- Sterile Gloving

 Procedures with this icon ⊚ are on the CDCompanion in this book; those with this icon are on the Evolve Student Resources Website.

198

KEY TERMS

antibiotic A drug that kills microbes that cause infections

asepsis Being free of disease-producing microbes

biohazardous waste Items contaminated with blood, body fluids, secretions, or excretions; *bio* means life, and *hazardous* means dangerous or harmful

carrier A human or animal that is a reservoir for microbes but does not have the signs and symptoms of infection

clean technique Medical asepsis

communicable disease A disease caused by pathogens that spread easily; a contagious disease

contagious disease Communicable disease

contamination The process of becoming unclean

disinfection The process of destroying pathogens

germicide A disinfectant applied to the skin, tissues, or non-living objects

healthcare-associated infection (HAI) An infection that develops in a person cared for in any setting where health care is given; the infection is related to receiving health care

immunity Protection against a certain disease

infection A disease state resulting from the invasion and growth of microbes in the body

infection control Practices and procedures that prevent the spread of infection

medical asepsis Practices used to remove or destroy pathogens and to prevent their spread from one person or place to another person or place; clean technique

microbe A microorganism

microorganism A small (*micro*) living plant or animal (*organism*) seen only with a microscope; a microbe

non-pathogen A microbe that does not usually cause an infection

normal flora Microbes that live and grow in a certain area

pathogen A microbe that is harmful and can cause an infection

reservoir The environment in which a microbe lives and grows; host

spore A bacterium protected by a hard shell

sterile The absence of *all* microbes

sterile field A work area free of *all* pathogens and non-pathogens (including spores)

sterile technique Surgical asepsis

sterilization The process of destroying *all* microbes

surgical asepsis The practices that keep items free of *all* microbes; sterile technique

vaccination Giving a vaccine to produce immunity against an infectious disease

vaccine A preparation containing dead or weakened microbes

KEY ABBREVIATIONS

AIDS Acquired immunodeficiency syndrome
AIIR Airborne infection isolation room
CDC Centers for Disease Control and Prevention
cm Centimeter
EPA Environmental Protection Agency
HAI Healthcare-associated infection
HBV Hepatitis B virus
HIV Human immunodeficiency virus
MDRO Multidrug-resistant organism

MSDS Material safety data sheet
MRSA Methicillin-resistant *Staphylococcus aureus*
OPIM Other potentially infectious materials
OSHA Occupational Safety and Health Administration
PPE Personal protective equipment
SARS Severe acute respiratory syndrome
TB Tuberculosis
VRE Vancomycin-resistant *Enterococcus*

Infection is a major safety and health hazard. Minor infections cause short illnesses. Some infections are serious and can cause death. Infants, older persons, and disabled persons are at risk. The health team follows certain practices and procedures to prevent the spread of infection. Called **infection control,** such practices and procedures protect patients, residents, visitors, and staff from infection.

MICROORGANISMS

A **microorganism (microbe)** is a small (*micro*) living plant or animal (*organism*). It is seen only with a microscope. Microbes are everywhere—in the mouth, nose, respiratory tract, stomach, and intestines. They are on the skin and in the air, soil, water, and food. They are on animals, clothing, and furniture.

Some microbes are harmful and can cause infections. They are called **pathogens. Non-pathogens** are microbes that do not usually cause an infection.

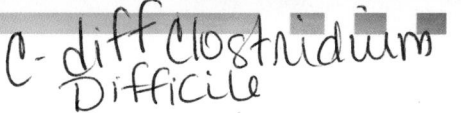

C-diff Clostridium Difficile

Types of Microbes

There are five types of microbes:

- *Bacteria*—plant life that multiples rapidly. Often called *germs*, they are one cell. They can cause an infection in any body system.
- *Fungi*—plants that live on other plants or animals. Mushrooms, yeasts, and molds are common fungi. Fungi can infect the mouth, vagina, skin, feet, and other body areas.
- *Protozoa*—one-celled animals. They can infect the blood, brain, intestines, and other body areas.
- *Rickettsiae*—found in fleas, lice, ticks, and other insects. They are spread to humans by insect bites. Rocky Mountain spotted fever is an example. The person has fever, chills, headache, rash, and other signs and symptoms.
- *Viruses*—grow in living cells. They cause many diseases. The common cold, herpes, acquired immunodeficiency syndrome (AIDS), and hepatitis are examples.

Requirements of Microbes

Microbes need a reservoir to live and grow. The **reservoir** *(host)* is the environment in which the microbe lives and grows. People, plants, animals, the soil, food, and water are common reservoirs. Microbes need *water* and *nourishment* from the reservoir. Most need *oxygen* to live. A *warm* and *dark* environment is needed. Most grow best at body temperature. They are destroyed by heat and light.

Normal Flora

Normal flora are microbes that live and grow in a certain area. Certain microbes are in the respiratory tract, in the intestines, and on the skin. They are non-pathogens when in or on a natural reservoir. When a non-pathogen is transmitted from its natural site to another site or host, it becomes a pathogen. *Escherichia coli (E. coli)* is found in the colon. If it enters the urinary system, it can cause an infection.

Multidrug-Resistant Organisms

Multidrug-resistant organisms (MDROs) are microbes that can resist the effects of antibiotics. **Antibiotics** are drugs that kill microbes that cause infections. Some microbes can change their structures. This makes them harder to kill. They can survive in the presence of antibiotics. Therefore the infections they cause are hard to treat.

MDROs are caused by doctors prescribing antibiotics when they are not needed (over-prescribing). Not taking antibiotics for the length of time prescribed also is a cause.

Two common types of MDROs are resistant to many antibiotics:

- *Methicillin-resistant Staphylococcus aureus (MRSA)*—is commonly called "staph." MRSA is normally found in the nose and on the skin. It can cause serious wound and bloodstream infections and pneumonia.
- *Vancomycin-resistant Enterococcus (VRE)*—is normally found in the intestines and is present in feces. It can be transmitted to others by contaminated hands, toilet seats, care equipment, and other items that the hands touch. When not in its natural site (the intestines), it can cause an infection. It can cause urinary tract, wound, pelvic, and other infections.

INFECTION

An **infection** is a disease state resulting from the invasion and growth of microbes in the body. A *local infection* is in a body part. A *systemic infection* involves the whole body. (Systemic means entire.) The person has some or all of the signs and symptoms listed in Box 14-1.

See *Focus on Children and Older Persons: Infection.*

BOX 14-1 Signs and Symptoms of Infection

- Fever (elevated body temperature)
- Chills
- Increased pulse and respiratory rates
- Pain or tenderness
- Fatigue and loss of energy
- Loss of appetite *(anorexia)*
- Nausea
- Vomiting
- Diarrhea
- Rash
- Sores on mucous membranes
- Redness and swelling of a body part
- Discharge or drainage from the infected area
- Heat or warmth in a body part
- Limited use of a body part
- Headache
- Muscle aches
- Joint pain
- Confusion

FOCUS ON CHILDREN AND OLDER PERSONS

Infection

OLDER PERSONS

The immune system protects the body from disease and infection (Chapter 8). Like other body systems, changes occur in the immune system with aging. When an older person has an infection, he or she may not show the signs and symptoms listed in Box 14-1. The person may have only a slight fever or no fever at all. Redness and swelling may be very slight. The person may not complain of pain. Confusion and delirium may occur (Chapter 44).

An infection can become life-threatening before the older person has obvious signs and symptoms. You must be alert to the most minor changes in the person's behavior or condition. Report any concerns to the nurse at once.

Older persons are at risk for infection. Healing takes longer than in younger persons. Therefore an infection can prolong the rehabilitation process. The person's independence and quality of life are affected.

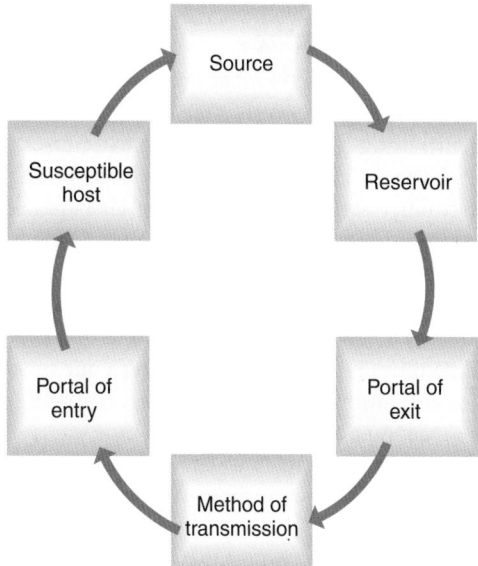

FIGURE 14-1 The chain of infection. (Redrawn from Potter PA, Perry AG: *Fundamentals of nursing: concepts, process, and practice,* ed 6, St Louis, 2004, Mosby.)

The Chain of Infection

The chain of infection (Fig. 14-1) is a process involving a:

▶ Source
▶ Reservoir
▶ Portal of exit
▶ Method of transmission
▶ Portal of entry
▶ Susceptible host

The *source* is a pathogen. It must have a *reservoir* where it can grow and multiply. Humans and animals are reservoirs. If they do not have signs and symptoms of infection, they are **carriers.** Carriers can pass the pathogen to others. To leave the reservoir, the pathogen needs a *portal of exit.* Exits are the respiratory, gastrointestinal, urinary, and reproductive tracts; breaks in the skin; and the blood.

After leaving the reservoir, the pathogen must be *transmitted* to another host (Fig. 14-2). The pathogen enters the body through a *portal of entry.* Portals of entry and exit are the same. A *susceptible host* is needed for the microbe to grow and multiply. Susceptible hosts are persons at risk for infection. They include persons who:

▶ Are very young or who are older
▶ Are ill
▶ Were exposed to the pathogen
▶ Do not follow infection control practices

The human body can protect itself from infection. The ability to resist infection relates to age, nutrition, stress, fatigue, and health. Drugs, disease, and injury also are factors.

Healthcare-Associated Infection

Community-Associated Infection

A **healthcare-associated infection (HAI)** is an infection that develops in a person cared for in any setting where health care is given. The infection is related to receiving

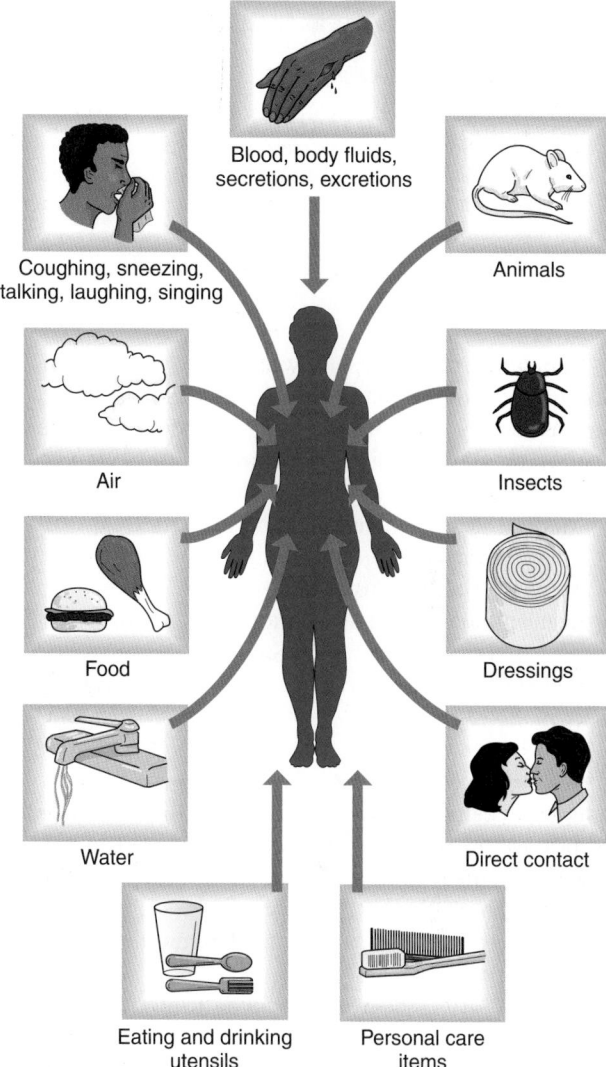

FIGURE 14-2 Methods of transmitting microbes.

health care. Hospitals, nursing centers, clinics, and home care settings are examples. HAIs also are called *nosocomial infections.* (*Nosocomial* comes from the Greek word for hospital.) HAIs are caused by normal flora. Or they are caused by microbes transmitted to the person from other sources.

For example, *E. coli* is normally in the colon. Feces (bowel movements) contain *E. coli.* Poor wiping after bowel movements can cause *E. coli* to enter the urinary system. The hands can transmit *E. coli* to other body areas. If hand washing is poor, *E. coli* spreads to any body part or anything the hands touch. It also can be transmitted to other people.

Microbes can enter the body through equipment used in treatments, therapies, and tests. Such items must be free of microbes. Staff can transfer microbes from one person to another and from themselves to others. Common sites for HAIs are:

▶ The urinary system
▶ The respiratory system
▶ Wounds
▶ The bloodstream

Patients and residents are weak from disease or injury. Some have wounds or open skin areas. Infants and older persons have a hard time fighting infections. The health team must prevent the spread of infection. HAIs are prevented by:

▶ Medical asepsis, including hand hygiene
▶ Surgical asepsis
▶ Standard Precautions
▶ Transmission-Based Precautions
▶ The Bloodborne Pathogen Standard

See *Focus on Long-Term Care and Home Care: Healthcare-Associated Infection.*

MEDICAL ASEPSIS

Asepsis is being free of disease-producing microbes. Microbes are everywhere. Measures are needed to achieve asepsis. **Medical asepsis (clean technique)** is the practices used to:

▶ Remove or destroy pathogens. The number of pathogens is reduced.
▶ Prevent pathogens from spreading from one person or place to another person or place.

Microbes cannot be present during surgery or when instruments are inserted into the body. Open wounds (cuts, burns, incisions) require the absence of microbes. They are portals of entry for microbes. **Surgical asepsis (sterile technique)** is the practices that keep items free of *all* microbes. **Sterile** means the absence of *all* microbes—pathogens and non-pathogens. **Sterilization** is the process of destroying *all* microbes (pathogens and non-pathogens).

Contamination is the process of becoming unclean. In medical asepsis, an item or area is clean when it is free of pathogens. The item or area is contaminated if pathogens are present. A sterile item or area is contaminated when pathogens or non-pathogens are present.

Common Aseptic Practices

Aseptic practices break the chain of infection. To prevent the spread of microbes, wash your hands:

▶ After urinating or having a bowel movement
▶ After changing tampons or sanitary pads
▶ After contact with your own or another person's blood, body fluids, secretions, or excretions (This includes saliva, vomitus, urine, feces, vaginal discharge, mucus, semen, wound drainage, pus, and respiratory secretions.)
▶ After coughing, sneezing, or blowing your nose
▶ Before and after handling, preparing, or eating food
▶ After smoking a cigarette, cigar, or pipe
  Also do the following:
▶ Provide all persons with their own linens and personal care items.
▶ Cover your nose and mouth when coughing, sneezing, or blowing your nose.
▶ Bathe, wash hair, and brush your teeth regularly.
▶ Wash fruits and raw vegetables before eating or serving them.
▶ Wash cooking and eating utensils with soap and water after use.

See *Focus on Children and Older Persons: Common Aseptic Practices.*

See *Focus on Long-Term Care and Home Care: Common Aseptic Practices.*

FOCUS ON LONG-TERM CARE AND HOME CARE

Common Aseptic Practices

HOME CARE

You must prevent the spread of microbes in the home. Also, protect the person from microbes brought into the home. The measures described above and others are needed. Also protect the person from foodborne illnesses (Chapter 23).

Microbes easily grow and spread in bathrooms. The entire family must help keep the bathroom clean. Aseptic measures are needed whenever the bathroom is used.

- Flush the toilet after each use.
- Rinse the sink after washing, shaving, or oral hygiene.
- Wipe out the tub or shower after each use.
- Remove and dispose of hair from the sink, tub, or shower.
- Hang towels out to dry. Or place them in a hamper.
- Wipe up water spills.

Your job may include cleaning bathrooms every day. Wear utility gloves for this task. Use a disinfectant or water and detergent to clean all surfaces:

- Toilet surfaces—bowl, seat, and all outside areas
- The floor
- The sides, walls, and curtain or door of the shower or tub
- Towel racks
- Toilet tissue, toothbrush, and soap holders
- The mirror (use a glass cleaner)
- The sink
- Windowsills

For bathroom cleaning you also need to:

- Mop uncarpeted floors. Vacuum carpeted floors.
- Empty wastebaskets.
- Put out clean towels and washcloths.
- Open bathroom windows for a short time and use air fresheners. These actions help reduce odors and give a fresh smell to the bathroom.
- Wash bath mats, the wastebasket, and the laundry hamper every week.
- Replace toilet and facial tissue as needed.

The care plan and assignment sheet tell you when to clean other areas of the home. For general housekeeping:

- Wipe up spills right away.
- Dust furniture and blinds.
- Vacuum or mop floors. Damp-mop uncarpeted floors at least weekly.
- Use a dust mop to sweep. Use a dustpan to collect dust, crumbs, and other things swept up. Sweep daily or more often if needed.
- Wash clothes and linens.

◆ Hand Hygiene

Hand hygiene is the easiest and most important way to prevent the spread of infection. Your hands are used for almost everything. They are easily contaminated. They can spread microbes to other persons or items. Practice hand hygiene before and after giving care. See Box 14-2, p. 204 for the rules of hand hygiene.

See *Promoting Safety and Comfort: Hand Hygiene.*
See *Focus on Ethics and Laws: Hand Hygiene.*

Continued

PROMOTING SAFETY AND COMFORT: Hand Hygiene

SAFETY

You use your hands in almost every task. They can pick up microbes from one person, place, or thing. Your hands transfer them to other people, places, and things. That is why hand hygiene is so very important. You must practice hand hygiene before and after giving care.

COMFORT

You will practice hand hygiene very often during your shift. Hand lotions and hand creams help prevent chapping and dry skin. Apply hand lotion or cream as often as needed.

FOCUS ON ETHICS AND LAWS

Hand Hygiene

A patient, Mr. Helman, had hip surgery (August 1) following a car accident in which he suffered many injuries. His roommate, Mr. Hagerup, had a back injury that caused paralysis from the waist down. The men shared a room for about 2 weeks.

Eight days (August 9) after Mr. Helman's hip surgery, Mr. Hagerup complained of a boil under his right arm. (A *boil* is a local skin infection. It starts in a skin gland or hair shaft. The infection is caused by *staphylococcus*.) The boil was treated with hot compresses. On August 10, there was purulent drainage from the boil. (*Purulent drainage* is thick green, yellow, or brown in color.) On the same day, a drainage specimen was sent to the laboratory. On August 13, the laboratory report showed the boil drainage contained a type of staphylococcus. Mr. Hagerup was moved at once to an isolation room.

Between August 10 and August 13, the nursing team cared for Mr. Helman and Mr. Hagerup. They "moved from one patient to the other, changed sheets, gave sponge baths, changed dressings, administered back rubs...[and] carried out the necessary hospital routine for the care of the two men. They did not observe sterile techniques . . . where infection is suspected; they did not wash their hands or leave the room between administering to the patients."

On August 13, Mr. Helman's surgical wound opened and drained a large amount of purulent drainage. Laboratory tests showed that the drainage contained the same microbe found in Mr. Hagerup's wound. Mr. Helman's wound infection destroyed bone, tissue, and ligaments. He had another surgery on October 28. His hip was fused in "a nearly immovable position." (To *fuse* means to unite two or more bones together.) He was discharged from the hospital on March 14. He needed home care and doctor's care.

In a lawsuit against the hospital, the jury returned a verdict in favor of Mr. Helman. The hospital appealed the verdict. The court hearing the appeal upheld the verdict in favor of Mr. Helman.

(George E. Helman et al v Sacred Heart Hospital, Wash, 1963.)

BOX 14-2 Rules of Hand Hygiene

- Wash your hands (with soap and water) when they are visibly dirty or soiled with blood, body fluids, secretions, or excretions.
- Wash your hands (with soap and water) before eating and after using a restroom.
- Wash your hands (with soap and water) if exposure to the anthrax spore is suspected or proven.
- Use an alcohol-based hand rub to decontaminate your hands if they are not visibly soiled. (If an alcohol-based hand rub is not available, wash your hands with soap and water.) Follow this rule in the following clinical situations:
  - Before having direct contact with a person.
  - After contact with the person's intact skin. For example, after taking a pulse or blood pressure or after moving a person.
  - After contact with body fluids or excretions, mucous membranes, non-intact skin, and wound dressings if hands are not visibly soiled.
  - When moving from a contaminated body site to a clean body site during care activities.
  - After contact with objects (including equipment) in the person's care setting.
  - After removing gloves.
- Follow these rules for washing your hands with soap and water. See procedure: *Hand Washing.*
  - Wash your hands under warm running water. Do not use hot water.
  - Stand away from the sink. Do not let your hands, body, or uniform touch the sink. The sink is contaminated (Fig. 14-3).
  - Do not touch the inside of the sink at any time.
  - Keep your hands and forearms lower than your elbows. Your hands are dirtier than your elbows and forearms. If you hold your hands and forearms up, dirty water runs from your hands to your elbows. Those areas become contaminated.
- Rub your palms together to work up a good lather (Fig. 14-4). The rubbing action helps remove microbes and dirt.
- Pay attention to areas often missed during hand washing—thumbs, knuckles, sides of the hands, little fingers, and under the nails.
- Clean fingernails by rubbing the fingertips against your palms (Fig. 14-5).
- Use a nail file or orange stick to clean under fingernails (Fig. 14-6). Microbes easily grow under the fingernails.
- Wash your hands for at least 15 seconds. Wash your hands longer if they are dirty or soiled with blood, body fluids, secretions, or excretions. Use your judgment.
- Use a clean, dry paper towel to dry your hands.
- Dry your hands starting at the fingertips. Work up to your forearms. You will dry the cleanest area first.
- Use a clean, dry paper towel for each faucet to turn water off (Fig. 14-7). Faucets are contaminated. The paper towels prevent clean hands from becoming contaminated again.
- Follow these rules when decontaminating your hands with an alcohol-based hand rub:
  - Apply the product to the palm of one hand. Follow the manufacturer's instructions for the amount to use.
  - Rub your hands together.
  - Make sure you cover all surfaces of your hands and fingers.
  - Continue rubbing your hands together until your hands are dry.
- Apply hand lotion or cream after hand hygiene. This prevents the skin from chapping and drying. Skin breaks can occur in chapped and dry skin. Skin breaks are portals of entry for microbes.

Modified from Centers for Disease Control and Prevention: Guideline for hand hygiene in health-care settings, *Morbidity Mortality Weekly Report* 51(RR-16), Oct 25, 2002.

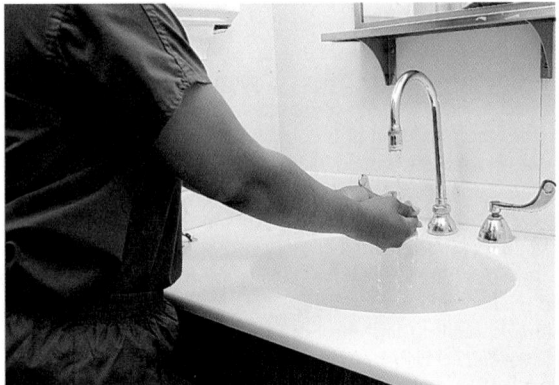

FIGURE 14-3 The uniform does not touch the sink. Soap and water are within reach. Hands are lower than the elbows. Hands do not touch the inside of the sink.

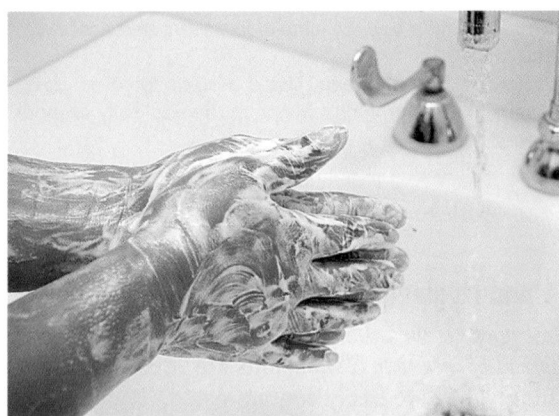

FIGURE 14-4 The palms are rubbed together to work up a good lather.

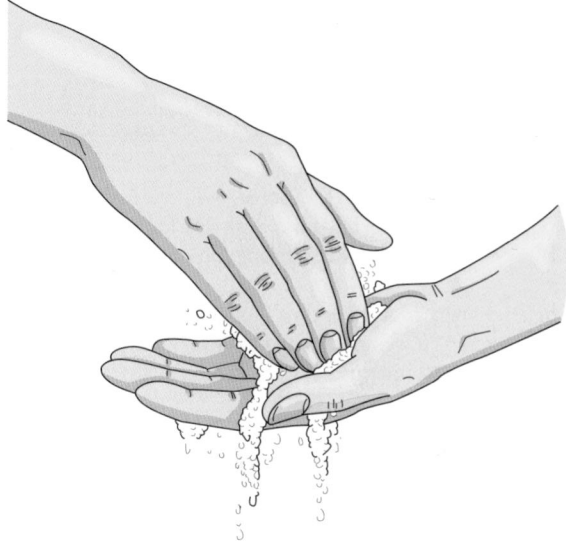

FIGURE 14-5 The fingertips are rubbed against the palms to clean under the fingernails.

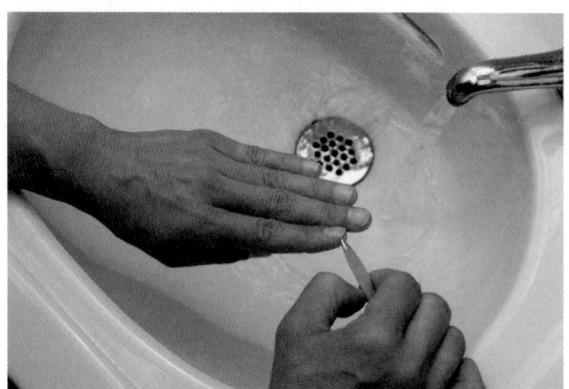

FIGURE 14-6 A nail file is used to clean under the fingernails.

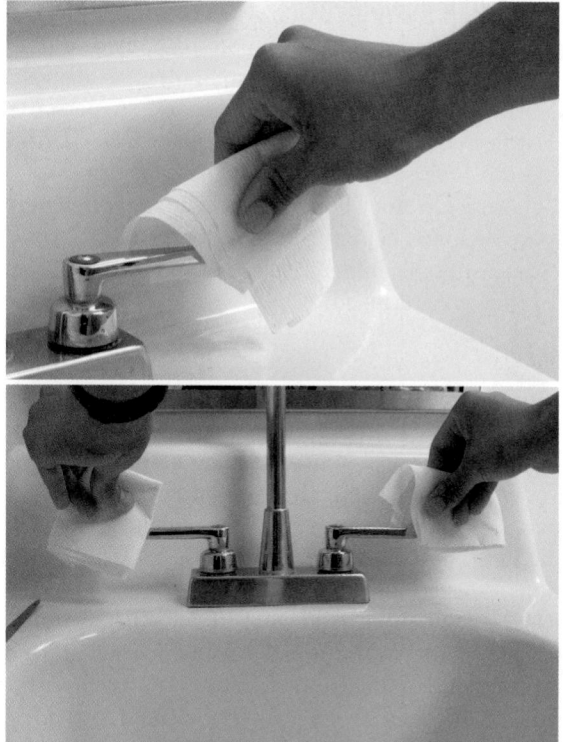

FIGURE 14-7 A paper towel is used to turn off each faucet.

HAND WASHING

PROCEDURE

1 See *Promoting Safety and Comfort: Hand Hygiene*, p. 203.
2 Make sure you have soap, paper towels, an orange stick or nail file, and a wastebasket. Collect missing items.
3 Push your watch up your arm 4 to 5 inches. If your uniform sleeves are long, push them up too.
4 Stand away from the sink so your clothes do not touch the sink. Stand so the soap and faucet are easy to reach (see Fig. 14-3). Do not touch the inside of the sink at any time.
5 Turn on and adjust the water until it feels warm.
6 Wet your wrists and hands. Keep your hands lower than your elbows. Be sure to wet the area 3 to 4 inches above your wrists.
7 Apply about 1 teaspoon of soap to your hands.
8 Rub your palms together and interlace your fingers to work up a good lather (see Fig. 14-4). This step should last at least ~~15~~ seconds. (*NOTE:* Some state competency tests require that you wash your hands for ~~20~~ seconds. Others require that you wash your hands for 1 to 2 minutes.)

9 Wash each hand and wrist thoroughly. Clean well between the fingers.
10 Clean under the fingernails. Rub your fingertips against your palms (see Fig. 14-5).
11 Clean under the fingernails with a nail file or orange stick (see Fig. 14-6). This step is done for the first hand washing of the day and when your hands are highly soiled.
12 Rinse your wrists and hands well. Water flows from the arms to the hands.
13 Repeat steps 7 through 12, if needed.
14 Dry your wrists and hands with a clean, dry paper towel. Pat dry starting at your fingertips.
15 Discard the paper towel into the wastebasket.
16 Turn off faucets with clean, dry paper towels. This prevents you from contaminating your hands (see Fig. 14-7). Use a clean paper towel for each faucet.
17 Discard the paper towels into the wastebasket.

[handwritten annotations: "ILL." and "seconds" and "15-20"]

Supplies and Equipment

Supply departments disinfect, sterilize, and distribute equipment. Most health care equipment is disposable. Single-use items are discarded after use. A person uses multi-use items many times. They include bedpans, urinals, wash basins, and water pitchers and drinking cups and glasses. Do not "borrow" them for another person. Disposable items help prevent the spread of infection.

Non-disposable items are cleaned and then disinfected. Then they are sterilized.

Cleaning

Cleaning reduces the number of microbes present. It also removes organic matter such as blood, body fluids, secretions, and excretions. When cleaning equipment:

▶ Wear personal protective equipment (PPE)—gloves, mask, gown, and goggles or a face shield—when cleaning items contaminated with blood, body fluids, secretions, or excretions.
▶ Rinse the item in cold water first. Rinsing removes organic matter. Heat causes organic matter to become thick, sticky, and hard to remove.
▶ Wash the item with soap and hot water.
▶ Scrub thoroughly. Use a brush if necessary.
▶ Rinse the item in warm water.
▶ Dry the item.
▶ Disinfect or sterilize the item.
▶ Disinfect equipment and the sink used in the cleaning procedure.
▶ Discard PPE.
▶ Practice hand hygiene.

Hospitals and nursing centers have "clean" and "dirty" utility rooms. Equipment is cleaned in the "dirty" utility room. Then it is disinfected or sterilized in the "clean" utility room.

Disinfection

Disinfection is the process of destroying pathogens. Spores are not destroyed. **Spores** are bacteria protected by a hard shell. Spores are killed by very high temperatures.

Germicides are disinfectants applied to skin, tissues, and non-living objects. Alcohol is a common germicide.

Chemical disinfectants are used to clean surfaces. Counters, tubs, and showers are examples. They also are used to clean reusable items. Such items include:

▶ Blood pressure cuffs
▶ Commodes and metal bedpans
▶ Wheelchairs and stretchers
▶ Furniture

See *Promoting Safety and Comfort: Disinfection.*
See *Focus on Long-Term Care and Home Care: Disinfection.*

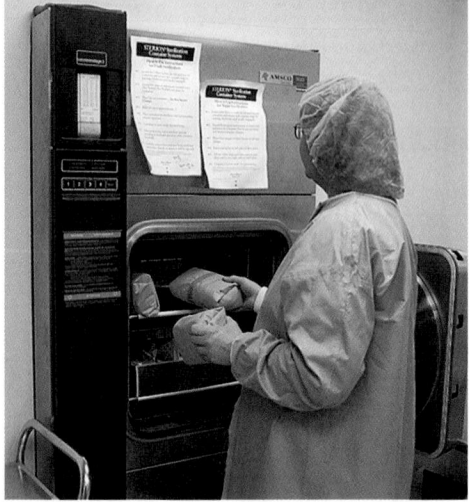

FIGURE 14-8 An autoclave.

Sterilization

Sterilizing destroys all non-pathogens and pathogens, including spores. Very high temperatures are used. Microbes are destroyed by heat.

Boiling water, radiation, liquid or gas chemicals, dry heat, and *steam under pressure* are sterilization methods. An *autoclave* (Fig. 14-8) is a pressure steam sterilizer.

Glass, surgical items, and metal objects are autoclaved. High temperatures destroy plastic and rubber items. They are not autoclaved. Steam under pressure sterilizes objects in 30 to 45 minutes.

See *Focus on Long-Term Care and Home Care: Sterilization.*

Other Aseptic Measures

Hand hygiene, cleaning, disinfection, and sterilization are important aseptic measures. So are the measures listed in Box 14-3. They are useful in home, work, and everyday life.

FOCUS ON **LONG-TERM CARE** AND **HOME CARE**

Sterilization

HOME CARE

You can use boiling water to sterilize items in the home.
- Use a pot with a lid. The pot must be large enough to hold the items.
- Wash all items to be sterilized. Use soap and hot water.
- Fill the pot with cold water. Completely cover all items with water.
- Put the lid on the pot.
- Bring the water to a full boil. Steam will escape under the lid.
- Boil the items for 5 to 15 minutes. Follow agency policy.
- Turn off the heat.
- Let the pot cool.
- Remove the items onto a clean towel. Use tongs to remove the items.
- Let the items air-dry.
- Put the items away as the family prefers or as the nurse instructs.

Many people use dishwashers to sterilize baby bottles (Fig. 14-9). However, many dishwashers do not get hot enough to actually sterilize items.

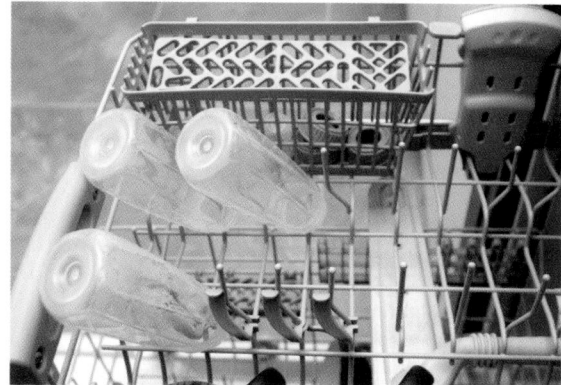

FIGURE 14-9 A dishwasher is used to sterilize these baby bottles.

BOX 14-3 **Aseptic Measures**

CONTROLLING RESERVOIRS (HOSTS—YOU OR THE PERSON)
- Provide for the person's hygiene needs (Chapter 19).
- Wash contaminated areas with soap and water. Feces, urine, and blood can contain microbes. So can body fluids, secretions, and excretions.
- Use leak-proof plastic bags for soiled tissues, linens, and other materials.
- Keep tables, counters, wheelchair trays, and other surfaces clean and dry.
- Label bottles with the person's name and the date the bottle was opened.
- Keep bottles and fluid containers tightly capped or covered.
- Keep drainage containers below the drainage site (Chapters 21 and 32).
- Empty drainage containers and dispose of drainage following agency policy. Usually drainage containers are emptied every shift. Follow the nurse's directions.

CONTROLLING PORTALS OF EXIT
- Cover your nose and mouth when coughing or sneezing.
- Provide the person with tissues to use when coughing or sneezing.
- Wear personal protective equipment as needed.

CONTROLLING TRANSMISSION
- Make sure all persons have their own personal care equipment. This includes wash basins, bedpans, urinals, commodes, and eating and drinking utensils.
- Do not take equipment from one person's room to use for another person. Even if the item is unused, do not take it from one room to another.
- Hold equipment and linens away from your uniform (Fig. 14-10, p. 208).
- Practice hand hygiene:
  - Before and after contact with every person
  - Whenever your hands are soiled
  - After contact with blood, body fluids, secretions, or excretions
  - After removing gloves
  - Before assisting with any sterile procedure
- Assist the person with hand washing:
  - Before and after eating
  - After elimination
  - After changing tampons, sanitary napkins, or other personal hygiene products
  - After contact with blood, body fluids, secretions, or excretions

Continued

BOX 14-3 Aseptic Measures—cont'd

CONTROLLING TRANSMISSION—cont'd

- Prevent dust movement. Do not shake linens or equipment. Use a damp cloth for dusting.
- Clean from the cleanest area to the dirtiest. This prevents soiling a clean area.
- Clean away from your body. Do not dust, brush, or wipe toward yourself. Otherwise you transmit microbes to your skin, hair, and clothing.
- Flush urine and feces down the toilet. Avoid splatters and splashes.
- Pour contaminated liquids directly into sinks or toilets. Avoid splashing onto other areas.
- Do not sit on the person's bed. You will pick up microbes. You will transfer them to the next surface that you sit on.
- Do not use items that are on the floor. The floor is contaminated.
- Clean tubs, showers, and shower chairs after each use. Follow the agency's disinfection procedures.
- Clean bedpans, urinals, and commodes after each use. Follow the agency's disinfection procedures.
- Report pests—ants, spiders, mice, and so on.

CONTROLLING PORTALS OF ENTRY

- Provide for good skin care (Chapter 19). This promotes intact skin.
- Provide for good oral hygiene (Chapter 19). This promotes intact mucous membranes.
- Do not let the person lie on tubes or other items. This protects the skin from injury.
- Make sure linens are dry and wrinkle-free (Chapter 18). This protects the skin from injury.
- Turn and reposition the person as directed by the nurse and care plan (Chapters 15 and 16). This protects the skin from injury.
- Assist with or clean the genital area after elimination (Chapter 19). Wipe and clean from the urethra (the cleanest area) to the rectum (the dirtiest area). This helps prevent urinary tract infections.
- Make sure drainage tubes are properly connected. This prevents microbes from entering the drainage system.

PROTECTING THE SUSCEPTIBLE HOST

- Follow the care plan to meet hygiene needs. This protects the skin and mucous membranes.
- Follow the care plan to meet nutrition and fluid needs (Chapter 23). This helps prevent infection.
- Assist with deep-breathing and coughing exercises as directed (Chapter 34). This helps prevent respiratory infections.

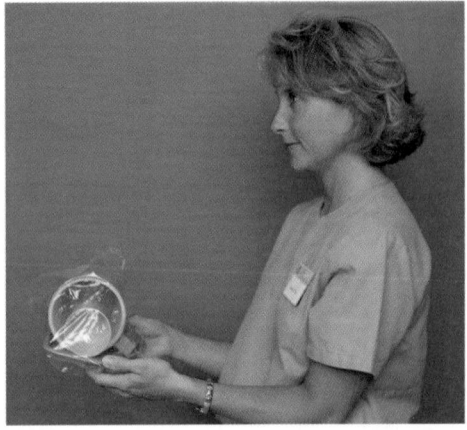

FIGURE 14-10 Hold equipment away from your uniform.

ISOLATION PRECAUTIONS

Blood, body fluids, secretions, and excretions can transmit pathogens. Sometimes barriers are needed to prevent their escape. The pathogens are kept within a certain area. Usually the area is the person's room. This requires isolation procedures.

The *Guideline for Isolation Precautions: Preventing Transmission of Infectious Agents in Healthcare Settings 2007* is followed. The guideline was issued by the Centers for Disease Control and Prevention (CDC). Isolation precautions prevent the spread of **communicable diseases** (**contagious diseases**). They are diseases caused by pathogens that spread easily. See Table 14-1 for common childhood communicable diseases.

Isolation precautions are based on *clean* and *dirty*. *Clean* areas or objects are free of pathogens. They are not contaminated. *Dirty* areas or objects are contaminated with pathogens. If a *clean* area or object has contact with something *dirty*, the clean area is now dirty. *Clean* and *dirty* also depend on how the pathogen is spread.

The CDC's isolation precautions guideline has two tiers of precautions:

▶ Standard Precautions
▶ Transmission-Based Precautions

  See *Focus on Ethics and Laws: Isolation Precautions.*
  See *Delegation Guidelines: Isolation Precautions.*
  See *Promoting Safety and Comfort: Isolation Precautions.*
  See *Teamwork and Time Management: Isolation Precautions.*
  See *Focus on Long-Term Care and Home Care: Isolation Precautions.*

FOCUS ON **ETHICS** AND **LAWS**

Isolation Precautions

The Centers for Disease Control and Prevention (CDC) is a federal agency. It serves to protect the health and safety of people in the United States. The CDC develops disease prevention and control guidelines and standards to improve health. The CDC's Hand Hygiene Guideline (p. 204) and the *Guidelines for Isolation Precautions: Preventing Transmission of Infectious Agents in Healthcare Settings 2007* are examples. Survey teams check to make sure that the agency complies with CDC guidelines and standards.

TABLE 14-1 Common Communicable Childhood Diseases

DISEASE	METHOD OF TRANSMISSION	SIGNS AND SYMPTOMS
Chickenpox *(varicella)*	Direct contact and airborne contact with respiratory secretions; direct contact with skin lesions	Fever, rash, and skin lesions
Diphtheria	Direct or indirect contact with respiratory secretions and skin lesions from the person or a carrier	Sore throat, fever, nasal discharge, enlarged lymph glands in the neck, cough, hoarseness, patches (lesions) on the tonsils, pharynx, larynx, nasal membranes, and skin
Measles *(rubeola)*	Direct or indirect contact with nasal secretions	Fever, cough, rash, inflammation of the mucous membranes of the nose, nasal discharge, bronchitis
Mumps	Direct contact with saliva droplets	Fever, headache, swollen salivary glands, earache
Whooping cough *(pertussis)*	Airborne or direct contact with droplets from the respiratory tract	Fever, sneezing, severe cough at night, coughs are short and rapid followed by a "whoop" or crowing sound with breathing in
Poliomyelitis	Airborne or direct contact with respiratory secretions; direct contact with feces	Fever, sore throat, headache, nausea and vomiting, loss of appetite, abdominal pain, neck and spinal stiffness, paralysis
German measles *(rubella)*	Airborne or direct contact with secretions from the nose and pharynx	Fever, headache, loss of appetite, nasal inflammation, sore throat, cough, rash
Scarlet fever	Airborne or direct contact with nasal and pharyngeal secretions	Fever, chills, headache, vomiting, abdominal pain, red and swollen tonsils and pharynx, rash

DELEGATION GUIDELINES: Isolation Precautions

You may assist in the care of persons who require isolation precautions. If so, review the type used with the nurse. You also need this information from the nurse and the care plan:
- What personal protective equipment (PPE) to use
- What special safety measures are needed

PROMOTING SAFETY AND COMFORT: Isolation Precautions

SAFETY
Preventing the spread of infection is important. Isolation precautions protect everyone—patients, residents, visitors, staff, and you. If you are careless, everyone's safety is at risk.

COMFORT
Persons requiring isolation precautions usually must stay in their rooms. The person may feel lonely, especially if visitors are few. You can help the person by:
- Remembering that the pathogen is undesirable, not the person
- Treating the person with respect, kindness, and dignity
- Providing newspapers, magazines, books, and other reading matter
- Providing hobby materials if possible
- Placing a clock in the room
- Urging the person to call family and friends
- Providing a current TV guide
- Organizing your work so you can stay to visit with the person
- Saying "hello" from the doorway often

Items brought into the person's room become contaminated. Disinfect or discard the items according to agency policy.

TEAMWORK AND TIME MANAGEMENT

Isolation Precautions

Donning (putting on) and removing PPE take time and effort. Once you don PPE, you must remove it before leaving the room. Therefore you need to organize your time and work so that you do not need to leave the room. Meet the needs of other patients or residents first. Ask a co-worker to answer their signal lights for you. Ask politely and thank your co-worker for helping you. Then gather the care items that you need to bring to the room. Before leaving the room, make sure the person's needs are met. Complete a safety check of the room. Also tell the person when you will return to the room.

Offer to help a co-worker if he or she will care for a person needing isolation. Bring items to the room as needed. Also answer signal lights for your co-worker. Be sure to tell the co-worker what you did for the person and what you observed.

FOCUS ON LONG-TERM CARE AND HOME CARE

Isolation Precautions

HOME CARE
Always practice Standard Precautions in home settings (p. 211). Some home care patients require Transmission-Based Precautions. The nurse tells you what measures are needed.

The nurse may have you limit the patient-care equipment brought into the home. When possible, equipment is left in the home until the person no longer needs home care services. Some equipment cannot remain in the home. Stethoscopes and blood pressure cuffs are examples. You must clean and disinfect such items before taking them out of the home. Or you can place them in a plastic bag for transport to the agency. There they will be cleaned and disinfected. The nurse tells you what to do.

BOX 14-4 Standard Precautions

KNOW

HAND HYGIENE
- Follow the rules for hand hygiene. See Box 14-2.
- Avoid unnecessary touching of surfaces close to the person. This prevents contamination of clean hands from environmental surfaces. It also prevents the transmission of pathogens from contaminated hands to other surfaces.
- Do not wear fake nails or nail extenders if you will have contact with persons at risk for infection or other adverse outcomes.

PERSONAL PROTECTIVE EQUIPMENT (PPE)
- Wear PPE when contact with blood or body fluids is likely.
- Do not contaminate your clothing or skin when removing PPE.
- Remove and discard PPE before leaving the person's room or care setting.

GLOVES
- Wear gloves when contact with the following is likely:
  - Blood
  - Potentially infectious materials (body fluids, secretions, and excretions are examples)
  - Mucous membranes
  - Non-intact skin
  - Skin that may be contaminated (for example, a person is incontinent of stool or urine)
- Wear gloves that fit and are appropriate for the task:
  - Wear disposable gloves to provide direct care to the person.
  - Wear disposable gloves or utility gloves for cleaning equipment or care settings.
- Remove gloves after contact with the person or the person's care setting. The care setting includes equipment used in the person's care.
- Remove gloves after contact with care equipment.
- Do not wear the same pair of gloves to care for more than one person. Remove gloves after contact with a person and before going to another person.
- Do not wash gloves for reuse with different persons.
- Change gloves during care if your hands will move from a contaminated body site to a clean body site.

GOWNS
- Wear a gown that is appropriate to the task.
- Wear a gown to protect your skin and clothing when contact with blood, body fluids, secretions, or excretions is likely.
- Wear a gown for direct contact with a person if he or she has uncontained secretions or excretions.
- Remove the gown and perform hand hygiene before leaving the person's room or care setting.
- Do not re-use gowns, even for repeat contacts with the same person.

MOUTH, NOSE, AND EYE PROTECTION
- Wear PPE—masks, goggles, face shields—for procedures and tasks that are likely to cause splashes and sprays of blood, body fluids, secretions, or excretions (Fig. 14-11).
- Wear PPE—mask, goggles, face shield—appropriate for the procedure or task.
- Wear gloves, a gown, and one of the following for procedures that are likely to cause sprays of respiratory secretions:
  - A face shield that fully covers the front and sides of the face
  - A mask with attached shield
  - A mask and goggles

RESPIRATORY HYGIENE/COUGH ETIQUETTE
- Instruct persons with respiratory symptoms to:
  - Cover the nose and mouth when coughing or sneezing.
  - Use tissues to contain respiratory secretions.
  - Dispose of tissues in the nearest waste container after use.
  - Perform hand hygiene after contact with respiratory secretions.
  - Provide visitors with masks according to agency policy.

CARE EQUIPMENT
- Wear appropriate PPE when handling care equipment that is visibly soiled with blood, body fluids, secretions, or excretions.
- Wear appropriate PPE when handling care equipment that may have been in contact with blood, body fluids, secretions, or excretions.
- Remove organic material before disinfection and sterilization procedures. Use cleaning agents according to agency policy.

CARE OF THE ENVIRONMENT
- Follow agency policies and procedures for cleaning and maintaining surfaces. Environmental surfaces and care equipment are examples. Surfaces near the person may need more frequent cleaning and maintenance—door knobs, bed rails, toilet surfaces and areas, and so on.
- Clean and disinfect multi-use electronic equipment according to ageny policy. This includes:
  - Items used by patients and residents
  - Items used to give care
  - Mobile devices that are moved in and out of patient or resident rooms.
- Follow these rules for toys used by pediatric patients or child play toys in waiting areas:
  - Select play toys that can be easily cleaned and disinfected.
  - Do not allow use of stuffed furry toys if they will be shared.
  - Clean and disinfect large stationary toys (for example, climbing equipment) at least weekly and whenever visibly soiled.
  - Rinse toys with water after disinfection if they are likely to be mouthed by children. Or wash them in a dishwasher.
  - Clean and disinfect a toy immediately when it requires cleaning. Or store the toy in a labeled container away from toys that are clean and ready for use.

TEXTILES AND LAUNDRY
- Handle used textiles and fabrics (linens) with minimum agitation. This is done to avoid contamination of air, surfaces, and other persons.

WORKER SAFETY
- Protect yourself and others from exposure to bloodborne pathogens. This includes how to handle needles and other sharps. Follow federal and state standards and guidelines. See the Bloodborne Pathogen Standard (p. 221).
- Use a mouthpiece, resuscitation bag, or other ventilation device during resuscitation to prevent contact with the person's mouth and oral secretions. See Chapter 49.

PATIENT OR RESIDENT PLACEMENT
- A private room is preferred if the person is at risk for transmitting the infection to others.
- Follow the nurse's instructions if a private room is not available.

Modified from Siegel JD, Rhinehart E, Jackson M, Chiarello L, and the Healthcare Infection Control Practices Advisory Committee, *2007 Guideline for Isolation Precautions: Preventing Transmission of Infectious Agents in Healthcare Settings,* Centers for Disease Control and Prevention, June 2007.

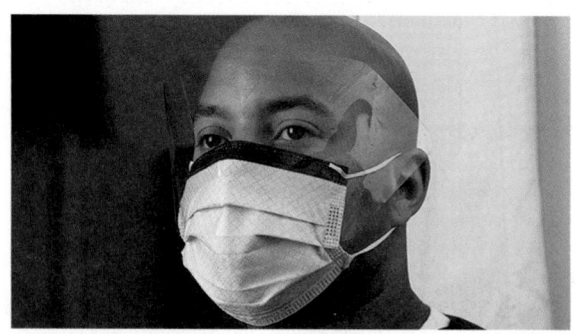

FIGURE 14-11 This mask has an eye shield. The eyes and the mucous membranes of the mouth and nose are protected.

Standard Precautions

Standard Precautions are part of the CDC's isolation precautions (Box 14-4). They reduce the risk of spreading pathogens. They also reduce the risk of spreading known and unknown infections. *Standard Precautions are used for all persons whenever care is given.* They prevent the spread of infection from:

▶ Blood
▶ All body fluids, secretions, and excretions (except sweat) even if blood is not visible

▶ Non-intact skin (skin with open breaks)
▶ Mucous membranes

Transmission-Based Precautions

Some infections require Transmission-Based Precautions (Box 14-5). You must understand how certain infections are spread (see Fig. 14-2). This helps you understand the types of Transmission-Based Precautions.

In December 2005, the CDC issued new guidelines for preventing the spread of tuberculosis (TB). TB is a bacterial infection affecting the lungs (Chapter 40). Airborne Precautions are needed.

Some agencies have airborne infection isolation rooms (AIIRs). An AIIR is a private (single-person) room with a private bathroom. AIIR practices include:

▶ All persons entering the room wear a TB respirator.
▶ The room door is kept closed except when someone enters or leaves the room.
▶ Treatments and procedures are done in the room.
▶ The person wears a mask during transport.

See *Focus on Long-Term Care and Home Care: Transmission-Based Precautions*, p. 212.

BOX 14-5 Transmission-Based Precautions

CONTACT PRECAUTIONS
- Used for persons with known or suspected infections or conditions that increase the risk of contact transmission.
- Patient or resident placement:
  - A single room is preferred.
  - Do the following if a room is shared with another person who is not infected with the same agent:
    - Keep the privacy curtain between the beds closed.
    - Change PPE and perform hand hygiene between contact with persons in the same room. Do so regardless of whether one or both persons are on Contact Precautions.
- Gloves:
  - Don gloves upon entering the person's room or care settting.
  - Wear gloves whenever touching the person's intact skin.
  - Wear gloves whenever touching surfaces or items near the person.
- Gowns:
  - Wear a gown whenever clothing may have direct contact with the person.
  - Wear a gown whenever contact is likely with surfaces or equipment near the person.
  - Don the gown upon entering the person's room or care setting.
  - Remove the gown and perform hand hygiene before leaving the person's room or care setting.
  - After removing the gown, make sure your clothing and skin do not touch potentially contaminated surfaces.
- Patient or resident transport:
  - Limit transport and movement of the person outside of the room to medically-necessary purposes.
  - Cover the area of the person's body that is infected.
  - Remove and discard contaminated PPE and perform hand hygiene before transporting the person.
  - Don clean PPE to handle the person at the transport destination.
- Care equipment:
  - Follow Standard Precautions.

- Use disposable equipment when possible. If possible, leave non-disposable equipment in the person's room.
- Clean and disinfect non-disposable and multiple-use equipment before use on another person.
- For home care settings:
  - Limit the amount of non-disposable care items brought into the home. Leave them in the home as long as they are needed.
  - Clean and disinfect items that cannot be left in the home. Stethoscopes and blood pressure cuffs are examples. Clean and disinfect care items before taking them from the home. Or place them in a plastic bag for transport for later cleaning and disinfection.

DROPLET PRECAUTIONS
- Used for persons known or suspected to be infected with pathogens transmitted by respiratory droplets. Such droplets are generated by a person who is coughing, sneezing, or talking.
- Patient or resident placement:
  - A single room is preferred.
  - Do the following if a room is shared with another person who is not infected with the same agent:
    - Keep the privacy curtain between the beds closed.
    - Change PPE and perform hand hygiene between contact with persons in the same room. Do so regardless of whether one or both persons are on Droplet Precautions.
- Personal protective equipment:
  - Don a mask upon entering the person's room or care setting.
- Patient or resident transport:
  - Limit transport and movement of the person outside of the room to medically-necessary purposes.
  - Have the person wear a mask.
  - Instruct the person to follow Respiratory Hygiene/Cough Etiquette (see "Standard Precautions").
  - No mask is required for health team members transporting the person.

Modified from Siegel JD, Rhinehart E, Jackson M, Chiarello L, and the Healthcare Infection Control Practices Advisory Committee, *2007 Guideline for Isolation Precautions: Preventing Transmission of Infectious Agents in Healthcare Settings*, Centers for Disease Control and Prevention, June 2007.

Continued

BOX 14-5 Transmission-Based Precautions—cont'd

AIRBORNE PRECAUTIONS
- Used for persons known or suspected to be infected with pathogens transmitted by person-to-person by the airborne route. Tuberculosis, measles, chickenpox, smallpox, and severe acute respiratory syndrome (SARS) are examples.
- The patient or resident is placed in an AIIR. If one is not available, the person is transferred to an agency with an AIIR.
- Health team members susceptible to the infection are restricted from entering the room. This is if immune staff members are available.
- Personal protective equipment:
  - An approved respirator is worn on entering the room or home of a person with tuberculosis.
  - Repsiratory protection is recommended for all health team members when caring for persons with smallpox.

- Patient or resident transport:
  - Limit transport and movement of the person outside of the room to medically-necessary purposes.
  - Have the person wear a surgical mask.
  - Instruct the person to follow Respiratory Hygiene/Cough Etiquette (see "Standard Precautions").
  - Cover skin lesions infected with the microbe.
  - No mask or respirator is required for health team members transporting the person if:
    —The person is wearing a mask or respirator
    —Skin lesions are covered

Modified from Siegel JD, Rhinehart E, Jackson M, Chiarello L, and the Healthcare Infection Control Practices Advisory Committee, *2007 Guideline for Isolation Precautions: Preventing Transmission of Infectious Agents in Healthcare Settings,* Centers for Disease Control and Prevention, June 2007.

FOCUS ON LONG-TERM CARE AND HOME CARE

Transmission-Based Precautions

LONG-TERM CARE
According to the CDC, persons with suspected or confirmed TB should not be treated in a long-term care setting. Such settings include skilled nursing facilities and hospices. Persons with suspected or confirmed TB can be treated in such settings if:
- Administrative and environmental controls are in place
- The agency has a respiratory-protection program

Cough-inducing procedures are not performed unless appropriate infection controls are in place. Or such procedures are done outside.

Standard Precautions and Airborne Precautions are followed. The person wears a mask during transport to other areas, in waiting areas, and when others are present.

HOME CARE
The nurse teaches the person with TB and household members about taking drugs, respiratory hygiene and cough etiquette, and the need for proper medical care. The person may have to stay at home until tests are negative for TB or the person is no longer infectious.

Wear a TB respirator to enter the home of a person with suspected or confirmed TB. Also wear a TB respirator if you need to transport the person in a vehicle. The person wears a mask during transport to other areas, in waiting areas, and when others are present.

As with long-term care, cough-inducing procedures are not performed unless appropriate infection controls are in place. Or such procedures are done outside.

Protective Measures

Agency policies may differ from those in this text. The rules in Box 14-6 (p. 215) are a guide for giving safe care when using isolation precautions.

Isolation precautions involve wearing PPE—gloves, a gown, a mask, and goggles or a face shield.

Removing linens, trash, and equipment from the room may require double bagging. Follow agency procedures when collecting specimens and transporting persons.

See *Promoting Safety and Comfort: Protective Measures.*

PROMOTING SAFETY AND COMFORT: Protective Measures

SAFETY
The PPE needed for Standard Precautions depends on what tasks, procedures, and care measures you will do while in the room. The PPE needed also depends on the type of Transmission-Based Precautions ordered for the person. Sometimes only gloves are needed. The nurse tells you when other PPE are needed.

According to the CDC's isolation guideline, gloves are always worn when gowns are worn. Sometimes other PPE are needed when gowns are worn. The isolation guideline shows PPE donned and removed in the following order (Fig. 14-12):
- Donning PPE
  - Gown
  - Mask or respirator
  - Eyewear (goggles or face shield)
  - Gloves
- Removing PPE (removed at the doorway before leaving the person's room) (Fig. 14-12, *B*, p. 214)
  - Gloves
  - Goggles or face shield
  - Gown
  - Mask or respirator

**Donning Personal
Protective Equipment (PPE)
DONNING PPE**

GOWN
- Fully cover torso from neck to knees, arms to end of wrist, and wrap around the back
- Fasten in back at neck and waist

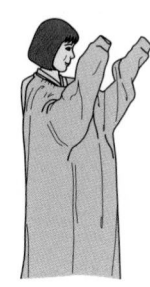

MASK OR RESPIRATOR
- Secure ties or elastic band at middle of head and neck
- Fit flexible band to nose bridge
- Fit snug to face and below chin
- Fit-check respirator

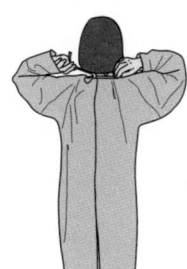

A

GOGGLES/FACE SHIELD
- Put over face and eyes and adjust to fit

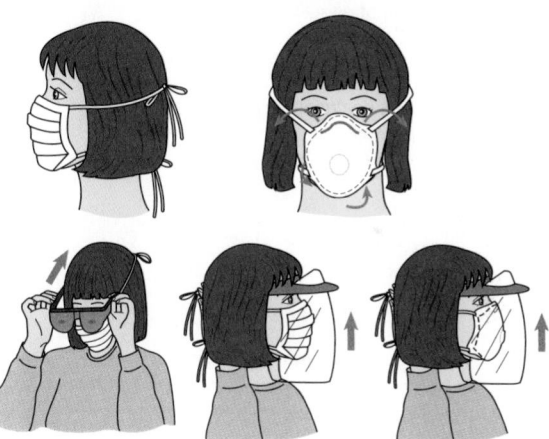

GLOVES
- Use non-sterile for isolation
- Select according to hand size
- Extend to cover wrist of isolation gown

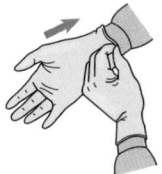

SAFE WORK PRACTICES
- Keep hands away from face
- Work from clean to dirty
- Limit surfaces touched
- Change when torn or heavily contaminated
- Perform hand hygiene

FIGURE 14-12 A, Donning personal protective equipment. (Redrawn from Centers for Disease Control and Prevention: *Guideline for isolation precautions: preventing transmission of infectious agents in healthcare settings 2007,* Atlanta, Ga).

Continued

REMOVING PPE

Remove PPE at doorway before leaving patient room or in anteroom

GLOVES
- Outside of gloves are contaminated!
- Grasp outside of glove with opposite gloved hand; peel off.
- Hold removed glove in gloved hand.
- Slide fingers of ungloved hand under remaining glove at wrist.

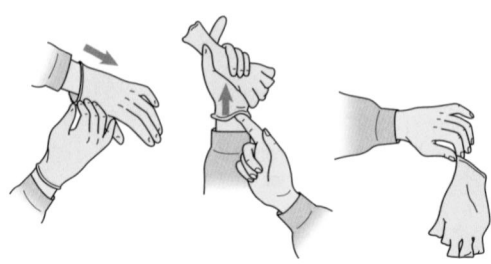

GOGGLES/FACE SHIELD
- Outside of goggles or face shield is contaminated!
- To remove, handle by "clean" head band or ear pieces.
- Place in designated receptacle for reprocessing or in waste container.

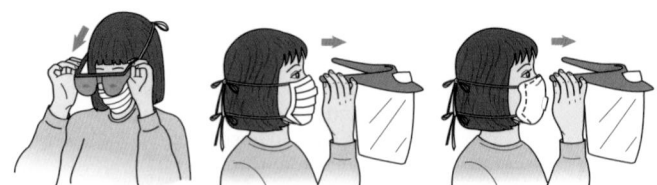

B

GOWN
- Gown and front and sleeves are contaminated!
- Unfasten neck, the waist ties.
- Remove gown using a peeling motion; pull gown from each shoulder toward the same hand.
- Gown will turn inside out.
- Hold removed gown away from body, roll into a bundle and discard into waste or linen receptacle.

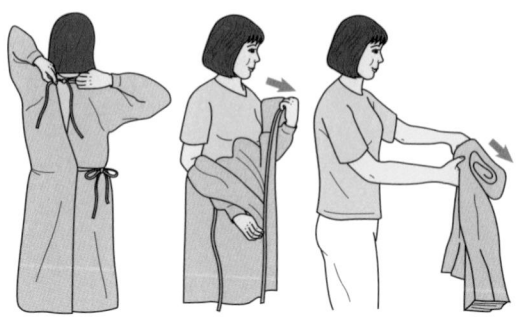

MASK OR RESPIRATOR
- Front of mask/respirator is contaminated – DO NOT TOUCH!
- Grasp ONLY bottom then top ties/elastics and remove.
- Discard in waste container.

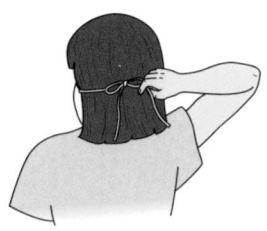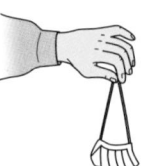

HAND HYGIENE

Perform immediately after removing all PPE!

FIGURE 14-12, cont'd B, Removing personal protective equipment. (Redrawn from Centers for Disease Control and Prevention: *Guideline for isolation precautions: preventing transmission of infectious agents in healthcare settings 2007*, Atlanta, Ga).

BOX 14-6 Rules for Isolation Precautions

- Collect all needed items before entering the room.
- Prevent contamination of equipment and supplies. Floors are contaminated. So is any object on the floor or that falls to the floor.
- Use mops wetted with a disinfectant solution to clean floors. Floor dust is contaminated.
- Prevent drafts. Some microbes are carried in the air by drafts.
- Use paper towels to handle contaminated items.
- Remove items from the room in leak-proof plastic bags.
- Double bag items if the outer part of the bag is or can be contaminated (p. 219).
- Follow agency policy for removing and transporting disposable and reusable items.
- Return reusable dishes, drinking vessels, eating utensils, and trays to the food service (dietary) department. Discard disposable dishes, drinking vessels, eating utensils, and trays in the waste container in the person's room.

- Do not touch your hair, nose, mouth, eyes, or other body parts.
- Do not touch any clean area or object if your hands are contaminated.
- Wash your hands if they are visibly dirty or contaminated with blood, body fluids, secretions, or excretions.
- Place clean items on paper towels.
- Do not shake linens.
- Use paper towels to turn faucets on and off.
- Use a paper towel to open the door to the person's room. Discard it as you leave.
- Tell the nurse if you have any cuts, open skin areas, a sore throat, vomiting, or diarrhea.

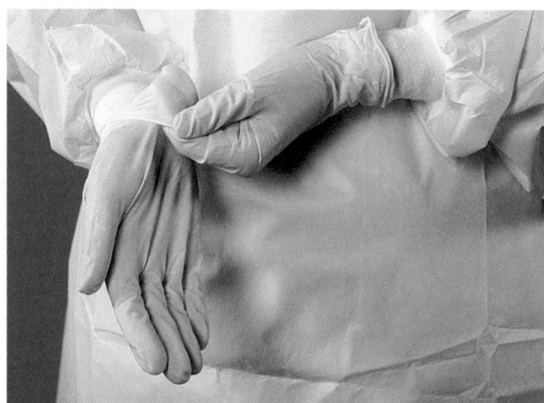

FIGURE 14-13 The gloves cover the cuffs of the gown.

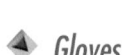 Gloves

The skin is a natural barrier. It prevents microbes from entering the body. Small skin breaks on the hands and fingers are common. Some are very small and hard to see. Disposable gloves act as a barrier. They protect you from pathogens in the person's blood, body fluids, secretions, and excretions. They also protect the person from microbes on your hands.

Wear gloves whenever contact with blood, body fluids, secretions, excretions, mucous membranes, and non-intact skin is likely. Contact may be direct. Or contact may be with items or surfaces contaminated with blood, body fluids, secretions, or excretions.

Wearing gloves is the most common protective measure used with Standard Precautions and Transmission-Based Precautions. Remember the following when using gloves:

- ▶ The outside of gloves is contaminated.
- ▶ Gloves are easier to put on when your hands are dry.
- ▶ Do not tear gloves when putting them on. Carelessness, long fingernails, and rings can tear gloves. Blood, body fluids, secretions, and excretions can enter the glove through the tear. This contaminates your hand.
- ▶ You need a new pair for every person.

- ▶ Remove and discard torn, cut, or punctured gloves at once. Practice hand hygiene. Then put on a new pair.
- ▶ Wear gloves once. Discard them after use.
- ▶ Put on clean gloves just before touching mucous membranes or non-intact skin.
- ▶ Put on new gloves whenever gloves become contaminated with blood, body fluids, secretions, or excretions. A task may require more than one pair of gloves.
- ▶ Change gloves whenever moving from a contaminated body site to a clean body site.
- ▶ Change gloves if interacting with the person involves touching portable computer keyboards or other mobile equipment that is transported from room to room.
- ▶ Put on gloves last when worn with other PPE.
- ▶ Make sure gloves cover your wrists. If you wear a gown, gloves cover the cuffs (Fig. 14-13).
- ▶ Remove gloves so the inside part is on the outside. The inside is *clean*.
- ▶ Decontaminate your hands after removing gloves. See *Promoting Safety and Comfort: Gloves.*

PROMOTING SAFETY AND COMFORT: Gloves

SAFETY
No special method is needed to put on gloves. To remove gloves, see procedure: *Removing Gloves*, p. 216.

Some gloves are made of latex (a rubber product). Latex allergies are common. They can cause skin rashes. Asthma and shock are more serious problems. Report skin rashes and breathing problems to the nurse at once.

You may have a latex allergy. Some patients and residents are allergic to latex. This information is on the care plan and your assignment sheet. Latex-free gloves are worn for latex allergies.

COMFORT
Many nurses and nursing assistants wear gloves for every patient or resident contact. Remember, gloves are needed whenever contact with blood, body fluids, secretions, excretions, mucous membranes, and non-intact skin is likely. You do not need to wear gloves when such contact is not likely. Back massages and brushing and combing hair are examples. Wearing gloves only when needed helps reduce exposure to latex.

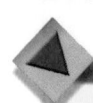

REMOVING GLOVES

PROCEDURE

1 See *Promoting Safety and Comfort: Gloves*, p. 215.
2 Make sure that glove touches only glove.
3 Grasp a glove just below the cuff (Fig. 14-14, *A*). Grasp it on the outside.
4 Pull the glove down over your hand so it is inside out (Fig. 14-14, *B*).
5 Hold the removed gloved with your other gloved hand.

6 Reach inside the other glove. Use the first two fingers of the ungloved hand (Fig. 14-14, *C*).
7 Pull the glove down (inside out) over your hand and the other glove (Fig. 14-14, *D*).
8 Discard the gloves. Follow agency policy.
9 Decontaminate your hands.

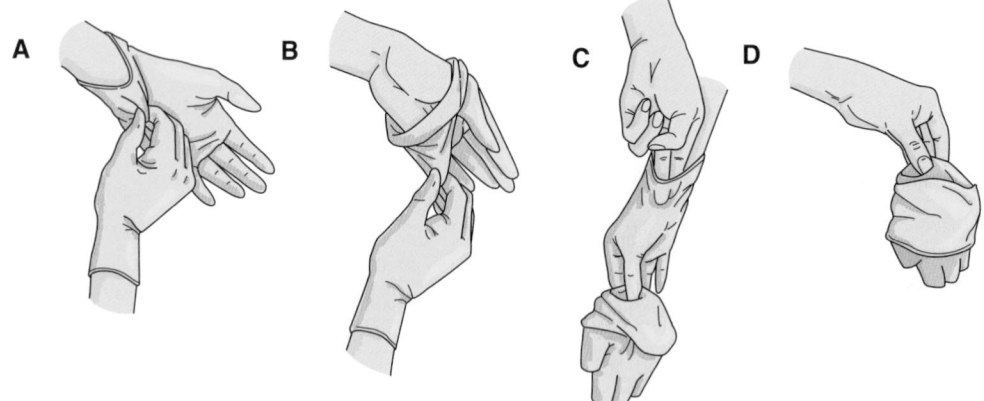

FIGURE 14-14 Removing gloves, **A,** Grasp the glove below the cuff. **B,** Pull the glove down over the hand. The glove is inside out. **C,** Insert the fingers of the ungloved hand inside the other glove. **D,** Pull the glove down and over the other hand and glove. The glove is inside out.

 ## Gowns

Gowns prevent the spread of microbes. They protect your clothes and body from contact with blood, body fluids, secretions, and excretions. They also protect against splashes and sprays.

Gowns must completely cover you from your neck to your knees. The long sleeves have tight cuffs. The gown opens at the back. It is tied at the neck and waist. The gown front and sleeves are considered to be *contaminated*.

Gowns are used once. A wet gown is contaminated. It is removed and a dry one put on. Disposable gowns are made of paper. They are discarded after use.

DONNING AND REMOVING A GOWN

PROCEDURE

1 Remove your watch and all jewelry.
2 Roll up uniform sleeves.
3 Practice hand hygiene.
4 Hold a clean gown out in front of you. Let it unfold. Do not shake the gown.
5 Put your hands and arms through the sleeves (Fig. 14-15, *A*).
6 Make sure the gown covers you from your neck to your knees. It must cover your arms to the end of your wrists.
7 Tie the strings at the back of the neck (Fig. 14-15, *B*).
8 Overlap the back of the gown. Make sure it covers your uniform. The gown should be snug, not loose (Fig. 14-15, *C*).
9 Tie the waist strings. Tie them at the back or the side. Do not tie them in front.
10 Put on the gloves. Put on other PPE. Provide care.
   a Mask or respirator (if needed)
   b Goggles or face shield (if needed)
   c Gloves

11 Remove and discard the gloves. Decontaminate your hands.
12 Remove and discard the goggles or face shield if worn.
13 Remove the gown:
   a Untie the neck and waist strings. Do not touch the front of the gown.
   b Pull the gown down from each shoulder toward the same hand.
   c Turn the gown inside out as it is removed. Hold it at the inside shoulder seams, and bring your hands together (Fig. 14-15, *D*).
14 Hold and roll up the gown away from you. Keep it inside out.
15 Discard the gown. Follow agency policy.
16 Remove and discard the mask if worn.
17 Decontaminate your hands.

put on: mask, gown, gloves
put off: gloves, gown, mask

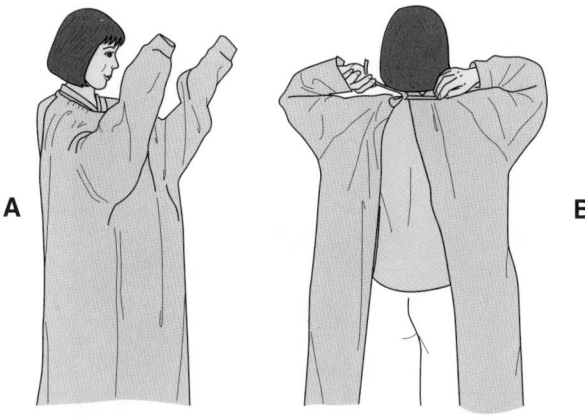

Masks and Respiratory Protection

You wear masks for these reasons:

► For protection from contact with infectious materials from the patient or resident. Respiratory secretions and sprays of blood or body fluids are examples.
► During sterile procedures to protect the person from infectious agents carried in your nose and mouth.

Masks are disposable. A wet or moist mask is contaminated. Breathing can cause masks to become wet or moist. Apply a new mask when contamination occurs.

A mask fits snugly over your nose and mouth. Practice hand hygiene before putting on a mask. When removing a mask, touch only the ties or the elastic bands. The front of the mask is contaminated.

Tuberculosis respirators (Fig. 14-16) are worn when caring for persons with TB (Chapter 40).

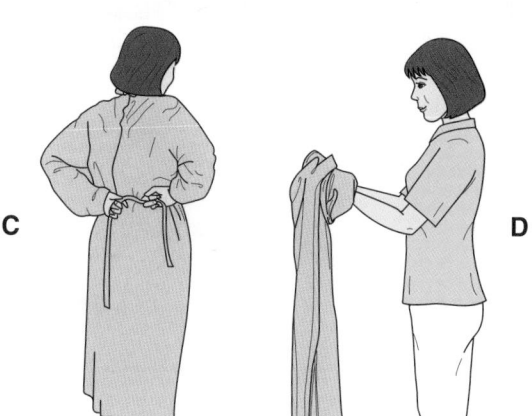

FIGURE 14-15 Donning and removing a gown. **A,** The arms and hands are put through the sleeves. **B,** The strings are tied at the back of the neck. **C,** The gown is overlapped in the back to cover the entire uniform. The ties are secured in the back. **D,** The gown is turned inside out as it is removed.

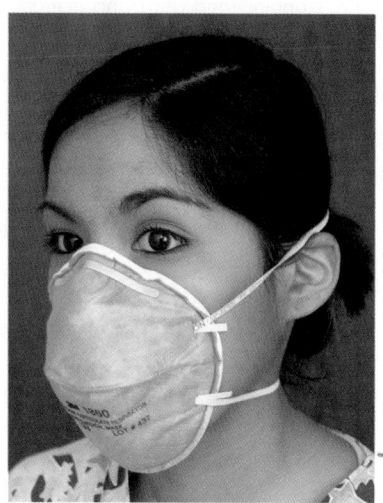

FIGURE 14-16 Tuberculosis respirator.

DONNING AND REMOVING A MASK

PROCEDURE

1 Practice hand hygiene.
2 Put on a gown if required.
3 Pick up a mask by its upper ties. Do not touch the part that will cover your face.
4 Place the mask over your nose and mouth (Fig. 14-17, *A*).
5 Place the upper strings above your ears. Tie them at the back in the middle of your head (Fig. 14-17, *B*).
6 Tie the lower strings at the back of your neck (Fig. 14-17, *C*). The lower part of the mask is under your chin.
7 Pinch the metal band around your nose. The top of the mask must be snug over your nose. If you wear eyeglasses, the mask must be snug under the bottom of the eyeglasses.
8 Make sure the mask is snug over your face and under your chin.
9 Put on goggles or a face shield if needed and if not part of the mask.
10 Put on gloves.
11 Provide care. Avoid coughing, sneezing, and unnecessary talking.
12 Change the mask if it becomes wet or contaminated.
13 Remove the mask.
  a Remove the gloves. Practice hand hygiene.
  b Remove the goggles or face shield and gown if worn.
  c Untie the lower strings of the mask.
  d Untie the top strings.
  e Hold the top strings. Remove the mask.
14 Discard the mask. Follow agency policy.
15 Decontaminate your hands.

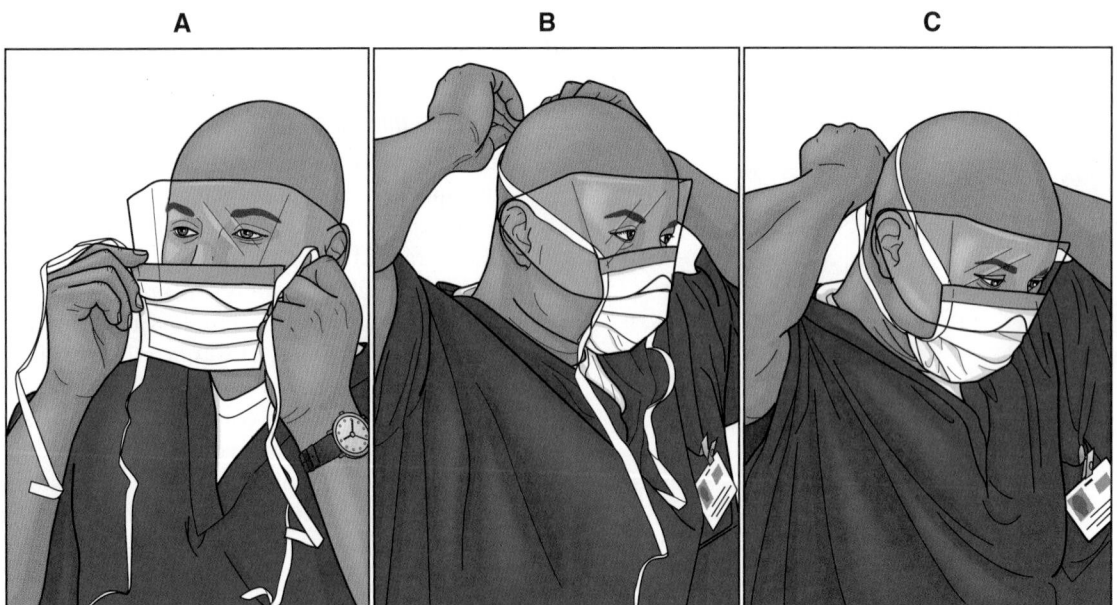

FIGURE 14-17 Donning and removing a mask. **A,** The mask covers the nose and mouth. **B,** Upper strings are tied at the back of the head. **C,** Lower strings are tied at the back of the neck.

Goggles and Face Shields

Goggles and face shields protect your eyes, mouth, and nose from splashing or spraying of blood, body fluids, secretions, and excretions (see Fig. 14-11). Splashes and sprays can occur when giving care, cleaning items, or disposing of fluids.

The front of goggles or a face shield is contaminated. The ties, earpieces, or headband used to secure the device are considered "clean." Use them to remove the device after practicing hand hygiene. They are safe to touch with bare hands.

Discard disposable goggles or face shields after use. Reusable eyewear is cleaned before reuse following agency procedures.

See *Promoting Safety and Comfort: Goggles and Face Shields.*

PROMOTING SAFETY AND COMFORT: Goggles and Face Shields

Safety

Eyeglasses and contact lenses do not provide adequate eye protection. If you wear eyeglasses, use a face shield that fits over your glasses with minimal gaps.

Goggles do not provide splash or spray protection to other parts of your face.

◆ Bagging Items

Contaminated items are bagged to remove them from the person's room. Leak-proof plastic bags are used. They have the *BIOHAZARD* symbol (Fig. 14-18). Items contaminated with blood, body fluids, secretions, or excretions are called **biohazardous waste.** (*Bio* means life. *Hazardous* means dangerous or harmful.)

Bag and transport linens following agency policy. All linen bags need a *BIOHAZARD* symbol. Melt-away bags are common. They dissolve in hot water. Once soiled linen is bagged, no one needs to handle it. Do not overfill the bag. Tie the bag securely. Then place it in a laundry hamper lined with a biohazard plastic bag.

Trash is placed in a container labeled with the *BIOHAZARD* symbol. Follow agency policy for bagging and transporting trash, equipment, and supplies.

Usually one bag is needed. Double bagging involves two bags. Double bagging is not needed unless the outside of the bag is soiled.

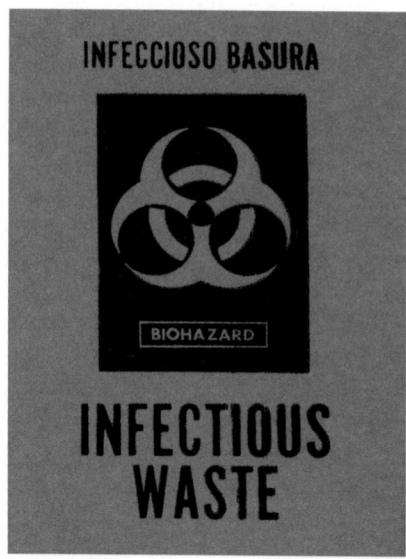

FIGURE 14-18 *BIOHAZARD* symbol.

DOUBLE BAGGING

PROCEDURE

1 Ask a co-worker to help you.
2 Place soiled linen, reusable items, disposable supplies, and trash in the right containers. Containers are lined with leak-proof biohazard bags.
3 Seal the bags securely.
4 Ask your co-worker to make a wide cuff on the clean bag. It is held wide open. The cuff protects the hands from contamination (Fig. 14-19, *A*).

5 Place the contaminated bag into the clean bag (Fig. 14-19, *B*). Do not touch the outside of the clean bag.
6 Ask your co-worker to seal the bag. Have the bag labeled according to agency policy.
7 Repeat steps 4, 5, and 6 for other contaminated bags.
8 Ask your co-worker to take or send the bags to the appropriate department for disposal, disinfection, or sterilization.

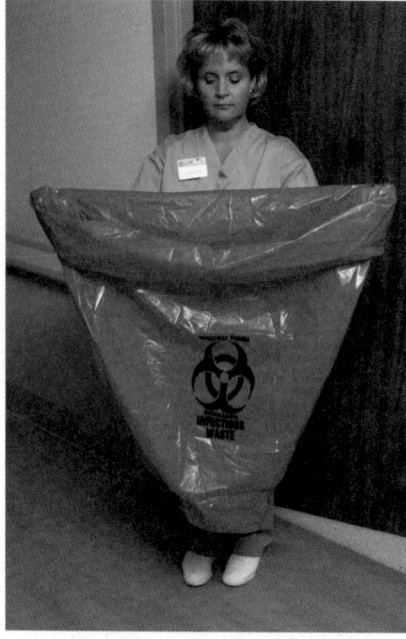
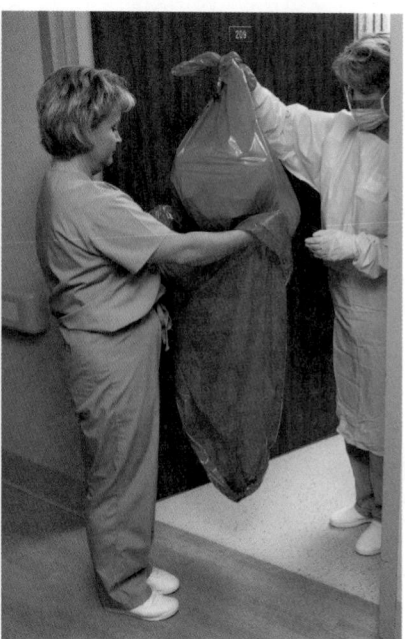

FIGURE 14-19 Double bagging. **A,** A cuff is made on a clean bag. **B,** One nursing assistant is in the room by the doorway. The other is outside the doorway. The "dirty" bag is placed inside the "clean" bag.

Collecting Specimens

Blood, body fluids, secretions, and excretions often require laboratory testing (Chapter 30). Specimens are transported to the laboratory in biohazard specimen bags. To collect a specimen:

▶ Label the specimen container and biohazard specimen bag. Apply warning labels according to agency policy.
▶ Don personal protective equipment as required. Gloves are worn.
▶ Put the specimen container and lid in the person's bathroom. Put them on a paper towel.
▶ Collect the specimen. Do not contaminate the outside of the container. Also avoid contamination when transferring the specimen from the collecting vessel to the specimen container.
▶ Put the lid on securely.
▶ Remove the gloves. Decontaminate your hands.
▶ Use a paper towel to pick up and take the container outside the room.
▶ Put the container in the biohazard bag.
▶ Discard the paper towels.
▶ Follow agency policy for storing the specimen.
▶ Decontaminate your hands.

Transporting Persons

Persons on Transmission-Based Precautions usually do not leave their rooms. Sometimes they go to other areas for treatments or tests.

Transporting procedures vary among agencies. Some require transport by bed. This prevents contaminating wheelchairs and stretchers. Others use wheelchairs and stretchers.

A safe transport means that other persons are protected from the infection. Follow agency procedures and these guidelines:

▶ Have the person wear a clean gown or pajamas and an isolation gown.
▶ Have the person wear a mask as required by the Transmission-Based Precautions used.
▶ Cover any draining wounds.
▶ Give the person tissues and a leak-proof bag. Used tissues are placed in the bag.
▶ Wear PPE as required.
▶ Place an extra layer of sheets and absorbent pads on the stretcher or wheelchair. This protects against draining body fluids.
▶ Do not let anyone else on the elevator. This reduces exposure to infection.
▶ Alert staff in the receiving area about the Transmission-Based Precautions. They wear PPE as needed.
▶ Disinfect the stretcher or wheelchair after use.

Meeting Basic Needs

The person has love, belonging, and self-esteem needs. Often they are unmet when Transmission-Based Precautions are used. Visitors and staff often avoid the person. They may need to put on gowns, masks, goggles or face shields, and gloves. These tasks take extra effort before entering the room. Some are not sure what they can touch. They may fear getting the disease.

The person may feel lonely, unwanted, and rejected. Self-esteem suffers. The person knows the disease can be spread to others. He or she may feel dirty and undesirable. Without intending to, visitors and staff can make the person feel ashamed and guilty for having a contagious disease.

The nurse helps the person, visitors, and staff understand the need for Transmission-Based Precautions and how they affect the person. You can help meet love, belonging, and self-esteem needs. (See *Promoting Safety and Comfort: Isolation Precautions*, p. 209.)

See *Focus on Children and Older Persons: Meeting Basic Needs.*

See *Focus on Communication: Meeting Basic Needs.*

FOCUS ON **CHILDREN** AND **OLDER PERSONS**

Meeting Basic Needs

CHILDREN

Infants and children do not understand isolation. Goggles, face shields, masks, and gowns may scare them. Parents and staff look different. Gloves and gowns prevent skin-to-skin contact with parents. Because of likely contamination, toys and comfort items (blankets, stuffed animals) may be kept from the child. This adds to the child's distress.

The nurse prepares the child and family for isolation. Simple explanations are given to the child. If appropriate for his or her age, the child is given a mask and goggles or face shield to touch and play with.

Children need to see the faces of people entering the room. Let the child see your face before putting on a mask and goggles or a face shield. Say "hello" to the child, and state your name.

OLDER PERSONS

Persons with poor vision need to know who you are. Let them see your face before you put on a mask or goggles or a face shield. State your name and explain what you are going to do. Then put on PPE.

Persons with dementia do not understand the need for isolation precautions. Masks, gowns, goggles, and face shields may increase confusion and cause fear and agitation. These measures can help:

• Let the person see your face before putting on PPE.
• Tell the person who you are and what you are going to do.
• Use a calm, soothing voice.
• Do not hurry the person.
• Use touch to reassure the person.
• Follow the care plan and the nurse's instructions for other measures to help the person.
• Report signs of increased confusion or behavior changes.

Meeting Basic Needs

Without intending to, people can make the person feel ashamed and guilty for having a contagious disease. Be careful what you say. For example, do *not* say:
- "What were you doing?"
- "How did you get that?"
- "I'm afraid to touch you."
- "Don't breathe on me."
  Always treat the person with respect, kindness, and dignity.

BLOODBORNE PATHOGEN STANDARD

The human immunodeficiency virus (HIV) and the hepatitis B virus (HBV) are major health concerns (Chapters 38 and 41). The health team is at risk for exposure to these viruses. The Bloodborne Pathogen Standard is intended to protect them from exposure. It is a regulation of the Occupational Safety and Health Administration (OSHA). See Box 14-7 for terms used in the standard.

HIV and HBV are found in the blood. They are bloodborne pathogens. They exit the body through blood. They are spread to others by blood. Other potentially infectious materials (OPIM) also spread the viruses (see Box 14-7).

BOX 14-7 **Bloodborne Pathogen Standard Terms**

blood Human blood, human blood components, and products made from human blood

bloodborne pathogens Pathogens present in human blood and that can cause disease in humans; they include but are not limited to the hepatitis B virus (HBV) and human immunodeficiency virus (HIV)

contaminated The presence or reasonably anticipated presence of blood or other potentially infectious materials on an item or surface

contaminated laundry Laundry soiled with blood or other potentially infectious materials or that may contain sharps

contaminated sharps Any contaminated object that can penetrate the skin—needles, scalpels, broken glass, broken capillary tubes, exposed ends of dental wires, and so on

decontamination The use of physical or chemical means to remove, inactivate, or destroy bloodborne pathogens on a surface or item to the point where infectious particles can no longer be transmitted and the surface or item is safe for handling, use, or disposal

engineering controls Controls that isolate or remove the bloodborne pathogen hazard from the workplace (sharps disposal containers, self-sheathing needles)

exposure incident Eye, mouth, other mucous membrane, non-intact skin, or parenteral contact with blood or other potentially infectious materials that results from an employee's duties

hand washing facilities The adequate supply of running water, soap, single-use towels, or hot-air drying machines

HBV Hepatitis B virus

HIV Human immunodeficiency virus

occupational exposure Reasonably anticipated skin, eye, mucous membrane, or parenteral contact with blood or other potentially infectious materials that may result from an employee's duties

other potentially infectious materials (OPIM):
- Human body fluids—semen, vaginal secretions, cerebrospinal fluid, synovial fluid, pleural fluid, pericardial fluid,

peritoneal fluid, amniotic fluid, saliva in dental procedures, any body fluid that is visibly contaminated with blood, and all body fluids when it is difficult or impossible to differentiate between them

- Any tissue or organ (other than intact skin) from a human (living or dead)

- HIV-containing cell or tissue cultures, organ cultures, and HIV- or HBV-containing culture medium or other solutions; blood, organs, or other tissues from experimental animals infected with HIV or HBV

parenteral Piercing mucous membranes or the skin barrier through needle-sticks, human bites, cuts, abrasions, and so on

personal protective equipment (PPE) The clothing or equipment worn by an employee for protection against a hazard

regulated waste:
- Liquid or semi-liquid blood or OPIM
- Contaminated items that would release blood or OPIM in a liquid or semi-liquid state if compressed
- Items caked with dried blood or OPIM that can release these materials during handling
- Contaminated sharps
- Pathological and microbiological wastes containing blood or OPIM

source individual Any person (living or dead) whose blood or OPIM may be a source of occupational exposure to employees; examples include but are not limited to:
- Hospital and clinic patients
- Clients in agencies for the developmentally disabled
- Trauma victims
- Clients of drug and alcohol treatment agencies
- Hospice and nursing center residents
- Human remains
- Persons who donate or sell blood or blood components

sterilize The use of a physical or chemical procedure to destroy all microbes, including spores

work practice controls Controls that reduce the likelihood of exposure by changing the way the task is performed

Exposure Control Plan

The agency must have an exposure control plan. It identifies staff at risk for exposure to blood or OPIM. All caregivers and the laundry, central supply, and housekeeping staffs are at risk. The plan includes actions to take for an exposure incident.

Staff at risk receive free training. Training occurs upon employment and yearly. Training is also required for new or changed tasks involving exposure to bloodborne pathogens. Training must include:

▶ An explanation of the standard and where to get a copy
▶ The causes, signs, and symptoms of bloodborne diseases
▶ How bloodborne pathogens are spread
▶ An explanation of the exposure control plan and where to get a copy
▶ How to know which tasks might cause exposure
▶ The use and limits of safe work practices, engineering controls, and personal protective equipment
▶ Information about the hepatitis B vaccination
▶ Who to contact and what to do in an emergency
▶ Information on reporting an exposure incident, post-exposure evaluation, and follow-up
▶ Information on warning labels and color-coding

Preventive Measures

Preventive measures reduce the risk of exposure. Such measures follow.

Hepatitis B Vaccination

Hepatitis B is a liver disease. It is caused by the hepatitis B virus (HBV). HBV is spread by blood and sexual contact.

The hepatitis B vaccine produces immunity against hepatitis B. **Immunity** means that a person has protection against a certain disease. He or she will not get the disease.

A **vaccination** involves giving a vaccine to produce immunity against an infectious disease. A **vaccine** is a preparation containing dead or weakened microbes. The hepatitis B vaccination involves 3 injections (shots). The second injection is given 1 month after the first. The third injection is given 6 months after the second one. The vaccination can be given before or after exposure to HBV.

You can receive the hepatitis B vaccination within 10 working days of being hired. The agency pays for it. You can refuse the vaccination. If so, you must sign a statement refusing the vaccine. You can have the vaccination at a later date.

Engineering and Work Practice Controls

Engineering controls reduce employee exposure in the workplace. Special containers for contaminated sharps (needles, broken glass) and specimens remove and isolate the hazard from staff. Containers are puncture-resistant, leak-proof, and color-coded in red. They have the *BIOHAZARD* symbol.

Work practice controls also reduce exposure risks. All tasks involving blood or OPIM are done in ways to limit splatters, splashes, and sprays. Producing droplets also is avoided. OSHA requires these work practice controls:

▶ Do not eat, drink, smoke, apply cosmetics or lip balm, or handle contact lenses in areas of occupational exposure.
▶ Do not store food or drinks where blood or OPIM are kept.
▶ Practice hand hygiene after removing gloves.
▶ Wash hands as soon as possible after skin contact with blood or OPIM.
▶ Never recap, bend, or remove needles by hand. When recapping, bending, or removing contaminated needles is required, use mechanical means (forceps) or a one-handed method.
▶ Never shear or break contaminated needles.
▶ Discard contaminated needles and sharp instruments (such as razors) in containers that are closable, puncture-resistant, and leak-proof. Containers are color-coded in red and have the *BIOHAZARD* symbol. Containers must be upright and not allowed to overfill.

Personal Protective Equipment (PPE)

This includes gloves, goggles, face shields, masks, laboratory coats, gowns, shoe covers, and surgical caps. Blood or OPIM must not pass through them. They protect your clothes, undergarments, skin, eyes, mouth, and hair.

PPE is free to employees. Correct sizes are available. The agency makes sure that PPE is cleaned, laundered, repaired, replaced, or discarded. OSHA requires these measures for the safe handling and use of PPE.

▶ Remove PPE before leaving the work area.
▶ Remove PPE when a garment becomes contaminated.
▶ Place used PPE in marked areas or containers when being stored, washed, decontaminated, or discarded.
▶ Wear gloves when you expect contact with blood or OPIM.
▶ Wear gloves when handling or touching contaminated items or surfaces.
▶ Replace worn, punctured, or contaminated gloves.
▶ Never wash or decontaminate disposable gloves for reuse.
▶ Discard utility gloves that show signs of cracking, peeling, tearing, or puncturing. Utility gloves are decontaminated for reuse if the process will not ruin them.

Equipment

Contaminated equipment is cleaned and decontaminated. Decontaminate work surfaces with a proper disinfectant:

▶ Upon completing tasks
▶ At once when there is obvious contamination
▶ After any spill of blood or OPIM
▶ At the end of the work shift when surfaces became contaminated since the last cleaning

Use a brush and dustpan or tongs to clean up broken glass. Never pick up broken glass with your hands, not even with gloves. Discard broken glass into a puncture-resistant container.

Waste

Special measures are used to discard regulated waste:

▶ Liquid or semi-liquid blood or OPIM
▶ Items contaminated with blood or OPIM
▶ Items caked with blood or OPIM
▶ Contaminated sharps

Closable, puncture-resistant, and leak-proof containers are used. Containers are color-coded in red. They have the *BIOHAZARD* symbol.

See *Focus on Long-Term Care and Home Care: Waste.*

Housekeeping

The agency must be kept clean and sanitary. A cleaning schedule is required. It includes decontamination methods and the tasks and procedures to be done.

Laundry

OSHA requires these measures for contaminated laundry:

▶ Handle it as little as possible.
▶ Wear gloves or other needed PPE.
▶ Bag contaminated laundry where it is used.
▶ Mark laundry bags or containers with the *BIOHAZARD* symbol for laundry sent off-site.
▶ Place wet, contaminated laundry in leak-proof containers before transport. The containers are color-coded in red or have the *BIOHAZARD* symbol.

Exposure Incidents

An *exposure incident* is any eye, mouth, other mucous membrane, non-intact skin, or parenteral contact with blood or OPIM. *Parenteral* means piercing the mucous membranes or the skin barrier. Piercing occurs through needle-sticks, human bites, cuts, and abrasions.

Report exposure incidents at once. Medical evaluation, follow-up, and required tests are free. Your blood is tested for HIV and HBV. If you refuse testing, the blood sample is kept for at least 90 days. Testing is done later if you change your mind.

Confidentiality is important. You are told of the evaluation results. You also are told of any medical conditions that may need treatment. You receive a written opinion of the medical evaluation within 15 days after its completion.

The *source individual* is the person whose blood or body fluids are the source of an exposure incident. His or her blood is tested for HIV or HBV. State laws vary about releasing the results. The agency informs you about laws affecting the source's identity and test results.

SURGICAL ASEPSIS

Surgical asepsis (sterile technique) is the practice that keeps equipment and supplies free of *all* microbes. **Sterile** means the absence of *all* microbes, including spores. Surgical asepsis is required any time the skin or sterile tissues are entered.

Surgery and labor and delivery areas require surgical asepsis. So do many tests and nursing procedures. If a break occurs in sterile technique, microbes can enter the body. Infection is a risk.

FOCUS ON **LONG-TERM CARE** AND **HOME CARE**

Waste

HOME CARE

Dressings, gloves, and other care items are used in home care. So are syringes, needles, and other sharps (such as razors). You will not use syringes, needles, and other sharps. However, you assist the family in disposing of them. Proper disposal is needed to:

• Protect neighbors, children, pets, janitors, housekeepers, trash handlers, and sewage treatment workers from injury and infection
• Prevent needle sharing and the re-use of sharps
• Protect the environment
  According to the Environmental Protection Agency (EPA):
• Do not throw loose needles, syringes, or sharps into the garbage.
• Do not flush needles, syringes, or sharps down the toilet.
• Do not put needles, syringes, or sharps in recycling containers.

You must properly store used needles, syringes, and sharps. Put them into a commercial or household sharps container at once after use. A household container can be a hard plastic bottle with a screw-on lid. A plastic bleach or detergent bottle with a screw-on lid is an example. Securing the lid in place with heavy tape gives added protection. The container must be puncture-resistant. Do not use soda cans, milk cartons, glass bottles, coffee cans, or other containers that are not puncture resistant.

Many cities and towns have disposal options. The nurse and care plan tell you what is used at the person's address. The EPA describes these disposal options:

• *Drop-off collection sites.* The filled sharps container is taken to a collection site. Hospitals, doctors' offices, clinics, pharmacies, health departments, and police and fire stations are examples.
• *Household hazardous waste collection sites.* The sharps container is taken to a hazardous waste collection site. The container is placed in a sharps collection bin.
• *Residential special waste pickup services.* Used sharps are placed in a special container. It is like a recycling container. The container is placed outside the home for collection by special waste handlers. Some programs have regular pickup schedules. Other programs require the customer to call for a pickup.
• *Mail-back programs.* Used sharps are placed in a special container. The container is mailed to a collection site. U.S. Postal Service procedures are followed.
• *Syringe exchange programs.* Used needles and syringes are exchanged for new ones. The agency operating the program disposes of those used.
• *Home destruction devices.* Such devices clip, melt, or burn the needle. The syringe and destroyed needle are placed in the garbage.

Dressings, gloves, soiled bed protectors, and other care items also need proper disposal.

• Place them in plastic bags.
• Close the bags securely.
• Label each plastic bag with a "Not for Recycling" label.
• Place the bags in a garbage can with a lid.
• Make sure animals cannot get into the garbage can. Trash scents can attract animals.

Assisting With Sterile Procedures

You can assist nurses with sterile procedures. Some states let nursing assistants perform certain sterile procedures. A sterile dressing change is an example.

See *Focus on Long-Term Care and Home Care: Assisting With Sterile Procedures.*

See *Delegation Guidelines: Assisting With Sterile Procedures.*

See *Promoting Safety and Comfort: Assisting With Sterile Procedures.*

FOCUS ON LONG-TERM CARE AND HOME CARE

Assisting With Sterile Procedures

HOME CARE
You may need to clean a work surface before you practice surgical asepsis. Use soap and water. Follow Standard Precautions and the Bloodborne Pathogen Standard. Clean from the cleanest area to the dirtiest. Also clean away from your body and uniform. Dry the surface after cleaning.

DELEGATION GUIDELINES: Assisting With Sterile Procedures

A nurse may ask you to assist with a sterile procedure. If so, you need this information from the nurse:
- The name of the procedure and the reason for it
- What gloves to wear—sterile or disposable
- What you are expected to do
- When to report observations
- What you can and cannot touch
- What specific patient or resident concerns to report at once

PROMOTING SAFETY AND COMFORT: Assisting With Sterile Procedures

SAFETY
Do not perform a sterile procedure unless:
- Your state allows you to perform the procedure
- The procedure is in your job description
- You received the necessary education and training
- You review the procedure with the nurse
- A nurse is available for questions and guidance

Principles of Surgical Asepsis

All items in contact with the person are kept sterile. If an item is contaminated, infection is a risk. A sterile field is needed. A **sterile field** is a work area free of *all* pathogens and non-pathogens (including spores). Box 14-8 lists the principles and practices of surgical asepsis. Follow them to maintain a sterile field.

BOX 14-8 **Principles and Practices for Surgical Asepsis**

- A sterile item can touch only another sterile item:
  - If a sterile item touches a clean item, the sterile item is contaminated.
  - If a clean item touches a sterile item, the sterile item is contaminated.
  - A sterile package that is open, torn, punctured, wet, or moist is contaminated.
  - A sterile package is contaminated when the expiration date has passed.
  - Place only sterile items on a sterile field.
  - Use sterile gloves or sterile forceps to handle other sterile items (Fig. 14-20).
  - Consider any item as contaminated if unsure of its sterility.
  - Do not use contaminated items. They are discarded or re-sterilized.
- A sterile field or sterile items are always kept within your vision and above your waist:
  - If you cannot see an item, the item is contaminated.
  - If the item is below your waist, the item is contaminated.
  - Keep sterile-gloved hands above your waist and within your sight.
  - Do not leave a sterile field unattended.
  - Do not turn your back on a sterile field.
- Airborne microbes can contaminate sterile items or a sterile field:
  - Prevent drafts. Close the door, and avoid extra movements. Ask other staff in the room to avoid extra movements.
  - Avoid coughing, sneezing, talking, or laughing over a sterile field. Turn your head away from the sterile field if you must talk.
  - Wear a mask if you need to talk during the procedure.
  - Do not perform or assist with sterile procedures if you have a respiratory infection.
  - Do not reach over a sterile field.
- Fluid flows downward, in the direction of gravity:
  - Hold wet items down (see Fig. 14-20). If held up, fluid flows down into a contaminated area. The contaminated fluid flows back into the sterile field when the item is held down.
- The sterile field is kept dry, unless the area below it is sterile:
  - The sterile field is contaminated if it gets wet and the area below it is not sterile.
  - Avoid spilling and splashing when pouring sterile fluids into sterile containers.
- The edges of a sterile field are contaminated:
  - A 1-inch (2.5 centimeter [cm]) margin around the sterile field is considered contaminated (Fig. 14-21).
  - Place all sterile items inside the 1-inch (2.5 cm) margin of the sterile field.
  - Items outside the 1-inch (2.5 cm) margin are contaminated.
- Honesty is essential to sterile technique:
  - You know when you contaminate an item or sterile field. Be honest with yourself even if other staff members are not present.
  - Remove the contaminated item, and correct the matter. If necessary, start over with sterile supplies.
  - Report the contamination to the nurse.

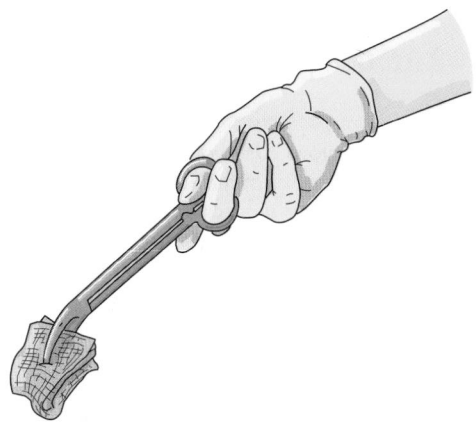

FIGURE 14-20 Sterile forceps are used to handle sterile items.

FIGURE 14-21 A 1-inch (2.5 cm) margin around the sterile field is considered contaminated. The shading and slash marks show that the 1-inch margin is contaminated.

◆ Sterile Gloving

You might need sterile gloves when assisting with a sterile procedure. The sterile field is set up first. Then sterile gloves are put on. After sterile gloves are on, you can handle sterile items within the sterile field. Do not touch anything outside the sterile field.

Sterile gloves are disposable. They come in many sizes so they fit snugly. The insides are powdered for ease in donning the gloves. The right and left gloves are marked on the package.

See *Promoting Safety and Comfort: Sterile Gloving.*

PROMOTING SAFETY AND COMFORT: Sterile Gloving

SAFETY

Always keep sterile gloved hands above your waist and within your vision. Touch only items within the sterile field. If you contaminate the gloves, remove them. Tell the nurse what happened. Decontaminate your hands, and put on a new pair. Replace gloves that are torn, cut, or punctured.

STERILE GLOVING

PROCEDURE

1 Follow *Delegation Guidelines: Assisting With Sterile Procedures.* See *Promoting Safety and Comfort:*
   • *Assisting With Sterile Procedures*
   • *Sterile Gloving*
2 Practice hand hygiene.
3 Inspect the package of sterile gloves for sterility.
   a Check the expiration date.
   b See if the package is dry.
   c Check for tears, holes, punctures, and watermarks.
4 Arrange a work surface.
   a Make sure you have enough room.
   b Arrange the work surface at waist level and within your vision.
   c Clean and dry the work surface.
   d Do not reach over or turn your back on the work surface.

5 Open the package. Grasp the flaps. Gently peel them back.
6 Remove the inner package. Place it on your work surface.
7 Read the manufacturer's instructions on the inner package. It may be labeled with *left, right, up,* and *down.*
8 Arrange the inner package for left, right, up, and down. The left glove is on your left. The right glove is on your right. The cuffs are near you with the fingers pointing away from you.
9 Grasp the folded edges of the inner package. Use the thumb and index finger of each hand.
10 Fold back the inner package to expose the gloves (Fig. 14-22, *A,* p. 226). Do not touch or otherwise contaminate the inside of the package or the gloves. The inside of the inner package is a sterile field.

Continued

STERILE GLOVING—cont'd

PROCEDURE—cont'd

11 Note that each glove has a cuff about 2 to 3 inches wide. The cuffs and insides of the gloves are *not considered sterile.*

12 Put on the right glove if you are right-handed. Put on the left glove if you are left-handed.
   a Pick up the glove with your other hand. Use your thumb and index and middle fingers (Fig. 14-22, *B*).
   b Touch only the cuff and inside of the glove.
   c Turn the hand to be gloved palm side up.
   d Lift the cuff up. Slide your fingers and hand into the glove (Fig. 14-22, *C*).
   e Pull the glove up over your hand. If some fingers get stuck, leave them that way until the other glove is on. *Do not use your ungloved hand to straighten the glove. Do not let the outside of the glove touch any non-sterile surface.*
   f Leave the cuff turned down.

13 Put on the other glove. Use your gloved hand.
   a Reach under the cuff of the second glove. Use the four fingers of your gloved hand (Fig. 14-22, *D*). Keep your gloved thumb close to your gloved palm.
   b Pull on the second glove (Fig. 14-22, *E*). Your gloved hand cannot touch the cuff or any surface. Hold the thumb of your first gloved hand away from the gloved palm.

14 Adjust each glove with the other hand. The gloves should be smooth and comfortable (Fig. 14-22, *F*).

15 Slide your fingers under the cuffs to pull them up (Fig. 14-22, *G*).

16 Touch only sterile items.

17 Remove the gloves. See Figure 14-14.

18 Decontaminate your hands.

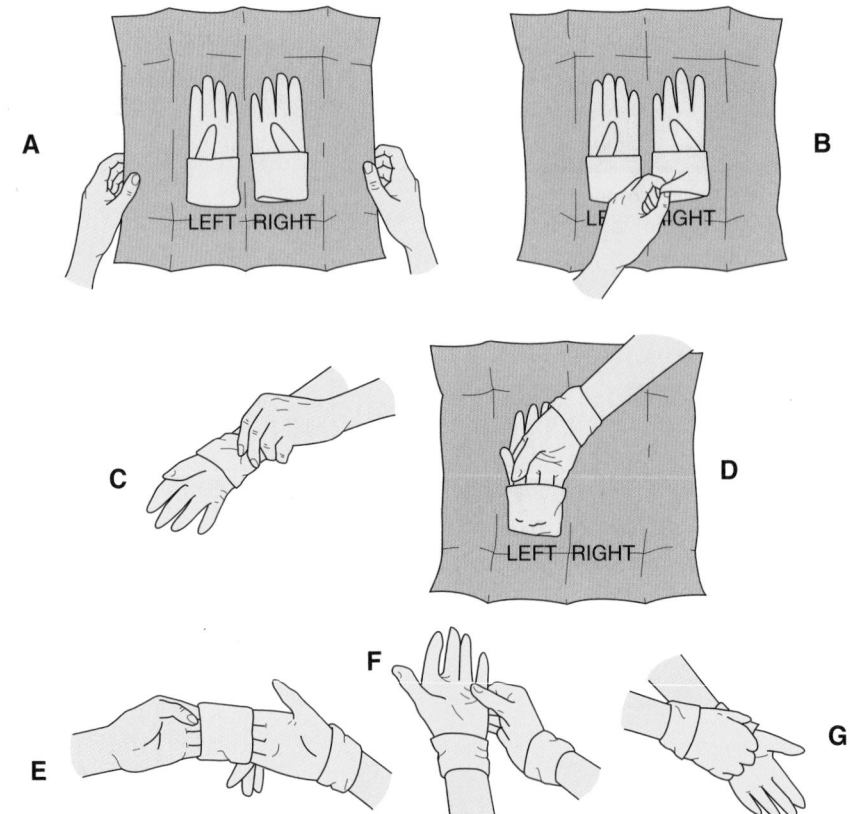

FIGURE 14-22 Sterile gloving. **A,** Open the inner wrapper to expose the gloves. **B,** Pick up the glove at the cuff with your thumb and index and middle fingers. **C,** Slide your fingers and hand into the glove. **D,** Reach under the cuff of the other glove with your fingers. **E,** Pull on the second glove. **F,** Adjust each glove for comfort. **G,** Slide your fingers under the cuffs to pull them up.

REVIEW QUESTIONS

Circle T if the statement is true and F if it is false.

1 T **(F)** Microbes are pathogens in their natural sites.

2 **(T)** F A pathogen can cause an infection.

3 **(T)** F An infection results when microbes invade and grow in the body.

4 T **(F)** An item is sterile if non-pathogens are present.

5 T **(F)** You hold your hands and forearms up during hand washing.

6 T **(F)** Unused items in the person's room are used for another person.

7 T **(F)** A person received the hepatitis B vaccine. The person will develop the disease.

8 **(T)** F The 1-inch edge around a sterile field is considered contaminated.

9 **(T)** F The inside and cuffs of sterile gloves are considered contaminated.

Circle the BEST answer.

10 Most pathogens need the following to grow *except*
   a Water
   b Light
   c Oxygen
   d Nourishment

11 Signs and symptoms of infection include the following *except*
   a Fever, nausea, vomiting, rash, and/or sores
   b Pain or tenderness, redness, and/or swelling
   c Fatigue, loss of appetite, and/or a discharge
   d A wound and/or bleeding

12 Which is *not* a portal of exit?
   a Respiratory tract
   b Blood
   c Reproductive system
   d Intact skin

13 Which does *not* prevent healthcare-associated infections?
   a Hand hygiene before and after giving care
   b Sterilizing all care items
   c Surgical asepsis
   d Standard Precautions

14 Your hands are soiled with blood. What should you do?
   a Wash your hands.
   b Decontaminate your hands.
   c Rinse your hands.
   d Tell the nurse.

15 During care, you move from a contaminated body site to a clean body site. What should you do?
   a Wash your hands.
   b Decontaminate your hands.
   c Rinse your hands.
   d Put on sterile gloves.

16 You are going to decontaminate your hands with an alcohol-based hand rub. Which action is *not* correct?
   a Wash your hands before applying the hand rub.
   b Rub your hands together.
   c Cover all surfaces of your hands and fingers.
   d Rub your hands together until your hands are dry.

17 When cleaning equipment, do the following *except*
   a Rinse the item in cold water before cleaning
   b Wash the item with soap and hot water
   c Use a brush if necessary
   d Work from dirty to clean areas

18 Isolation precautions
   a Prevent infection
   b Destroy pathogens
   c Keep pathogens within a certain area
   d Destroy all microbes

19 Standard Precautions
   a Are used for all persons
   b Prevent the spread of pathogens through the air
   c Require gowns, masks, gloves, and goggles
   d Require a doctor's order

20 You wear utility gloves for contact with
   a Blood
   b Body fluids
   c Secretions and excretions
   d Cleaning solutions

21 A mask
   a Can be reused
   b Is clean on the inside
   c Is contaminated when moist
   d Should fit loosely for breathing

22 These statements are about personal protective equipment (PPE). Which is *false*?
   a Wash disposable gloves for reuse.
   b Remove PPE before leaving the work area.
   c Discard cracked or torn utility gloves.
   d Wear gloves when touching contaminated items or surfaces.

23 Contaminated surfaces are cleaned at the following times *except*
   a After completing a task
   b When there is obvious contamination
   c After blood is spilled
   d After removing gloves

24 Goggles or a face shield is worn
   a When using Standard Precautions
   b When splashing body fluids is likely
   c If you have an eye infection
   d When assisting with sterile procedures

25 The Bloodborne Pathogen Standard involves the following *except*
   a Wearing gloves
   b Discarding sharp items into a biohazard container
   c Storing food and blood in different places
   d Eating and drinking in care settings

26 You were exposed to a bloodborne pathogen. Which is *true*?

a You do not have to report the exposure.

b You pay for required tests.

c You can refuse HIV and HBV testing.

d The source individual can refuse testing.

27 These statements are about surgical asepsis. Which is *false*?

a A sterile item can touch only another sterile item.

b Wet items are held up.

c If you cannot see an item, it is considered contaminated.

d Sterile items are kept above your waist.

28 You have on sterile gloves. You can touch

a Anything on the sterile field

b Anything on your work surface

c Anything below your waist

d Any part of your uniform

Answers to these questions are on p. 780.

Body Mechanics

OBJECTIVES

- Define the key terms and key abbreviations listed in this chapter
- Explain the purpose and rules of body mechanics
- Explain how ergonomics can prevent work-related injuries
- Identify the causes, signs, and symptoms of back injuries
- Position persons in the basic bed positions and in a chair

KEY TERMS

base of support The area on which an object rests

body alignment The way the head, trunk, arms, and legs are aligned with one another; posture

body mechanics Using the body in an efficient and careful way

dorsal recumbent position The back-lying or supine position

ergonomics The science of designing a job to fit the worker

Fowler's position A semi-sitting position; the head of the bed is raised between 45 and 60 degrees

lateral position The person lies on one side or the other; side-lying position

posture Body alignment

prone position Lying on the abdomen with the head turned to one side

semi-prone side position Sims' position

side-lying position The lateral position

Sims' position A left side-lying position in which the upper leg is sharply flexed so it is not on the lower leg and the lower arm is behind the person; semi-prone side position

supine position The back-lying or dorsal recumbent position

KEY ABBREVIATIONS

OSHA Occupational Safety and Health Administration
WMSD Work-related musculoskeletal disorder

Body mechanics means using the body in an efficient and careful way. It involves good posture, balance, and using your strongest and largest muscles for work. Fatigue, muscle strain, and injury can result from improper use and positioning of the body during activity or rest. Focus on the person's and your own body mechanics. Good body mechanics reduces the risk of injury.

See Box 15-1 for a review of the musculoskeletal system. Or review Chapter 8.

BOX 15-1 Musculoskeletal System: Body Structure and Function

The musculoskeletal system:
- Provides the framework for the body
- Lets the body move
- Protects the body
- Gives the body shape

Bones
Bones are hard, rigid structures. They are made up of living cells.
- *Long bones* bear the body's weight. Leg bones are long bones.
- *Short bones* allow skill and ease in movement. Bones in the wrists, fingers, ankles, and toes are short bones.
- *Flat bones* protect the organs. They include the ribs, skull, pelvic bones, and shoulder blades.
- *Irregular bones* are the vertebrae in the spinal column. They allow various degrees of movement and flexibility.

Joints
A *joint* is the point at which two or more bones meet. Joints allow movement. There are three types of joints (Fig. 15-1):
- *Ball-and-socket joint* allows movement in all directions. The joints of the hips and shoulders are ball-and-socket joints.
- *Hinge joint* allows movement in one direction. The elbow is a hinge joint.
- *Pivot joint* allows turning from side to side. A pivot joint connects the skull to the spine.

Muscles
The human body has more than 500 *muscles* (Fig. 15-2).
- *Voluntary muscles* can be consciously controlled. Muscles attached to bones *(skeletal muscles)* are voluntary. Arm muscles do not work unless you move your arm; likewise for leg muscles.
- *Involuntary muscles* work automatically. You cannot control them. They control the action of the stomach, intestines, blood vessels, and other body organs.
- *Cardiac muscle* is in the heart. It is an involuntary muscle.
Muscles have three functions:
- Movement of body parts
- Maintenance of posture
- Production of body heat
Some muscles constantly contract to maintain the body's posture. When muscles contract, they burn food for energy. Heat is produced. The more muscle activity, the greater the amount of heat produced. Shivering is how the body produces heat when exposed to cold. Shivering is from rapid, general muscle contractions.

PRINCIPLES OF BODY MECHANICS

Body alignment (posture) is the way the head, trunk, arms, and legs are aligned with one another. Good alignment lets the body move and function with strength and efficiency. Standing, sitting, and lying down require good alignment.

Base of support is the area on which an object rests. A good base of support is needed for balance (Fig. 15-3). When standing, your feet are your base of support. Stand with your feet apart for a wider base of support and more balance.

Your strongest and largest muscles are in the shoulders, upper arms, hips, and thighs. Use these muscles to handle and move persons and heavy objects. Otherwise, you place strain and exertion on smaller and weaker muscles. This causes fatigue and injury. *Back injuries are a major risk.* For good body mechanics:

▶ Bend your knees and squat to lift a heavy object (Fig. 15-4, p. 232). Do not bend from your waist. Bending from the waist places strain on small back muscles.

▶ Hold items close to your body and base of support (see Fig. 15-4). This involves upper arm and shoulder muscles. Holding objects away from your body places strain on small muscles in your lower arms.

All activities require good body mechanics. You must safely and efficiently handle and move persons and heavy objects. Follow the rules in Box 15-2, p. 232.

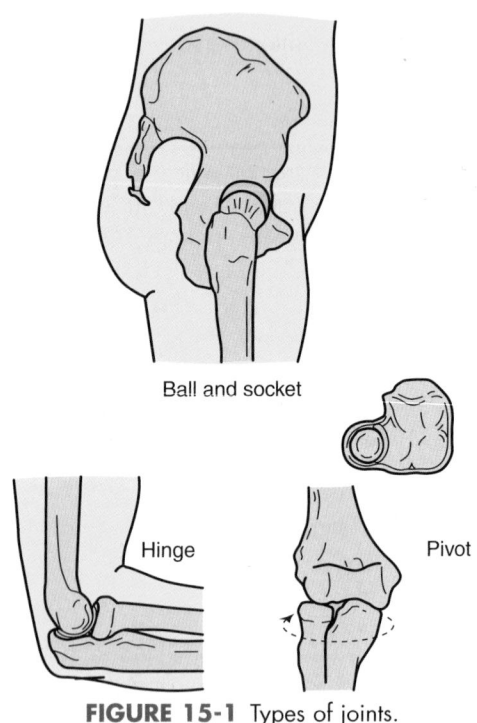

Ball and socket

Hinge

Pivot

FIGURE 15-1 Types of joints.

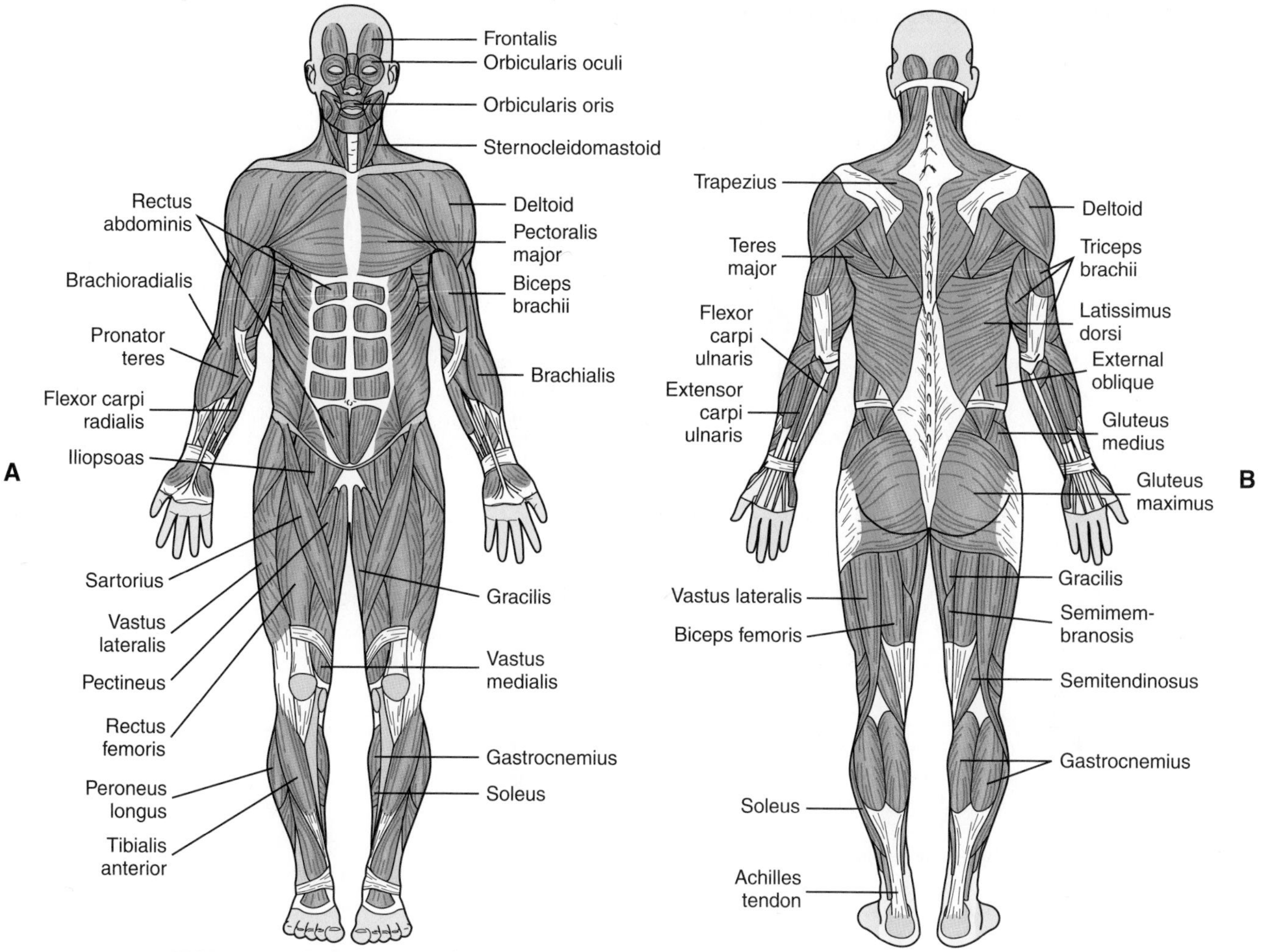

A

- Frontalis
- Orbicularis oculi
- Orbicularis oris
- Sternocleidomastoid
- Rectus abdominis
- Deltoid
- Pectoralis major
- Brachioradialis
- Biceps brachii
- Pronator teres
- Brachialis
- Flexor carpi radialis
- Iliopsoas
- Sartorius
- Gracilis
- Vastus lateralis
- Pectineus
- Vastus medialis
- Rectus femoris
- Peroneus longus
- Gastrocnemius
- Soleus
- Tibialis anterior

B

- Trapezius
- Deltoid
- Teres major
- Triceps brachii
- Flexor carpi ulnaris
- Latissimus dorsi
- Extensor carpi ulnaris
- External oblique
- Gluteus medius
- Gluteus maximus
- Vastus lateralis
- Gracilis
- Biceps femoris
- Semimembranosis
- Semitendinosus
- Gastrocnemius
- Soleus
- Achilles tendon

FIGURE 15-2 A, Anterior (front) view of the muscles. **B,** Posterior (back) view of the muscles.

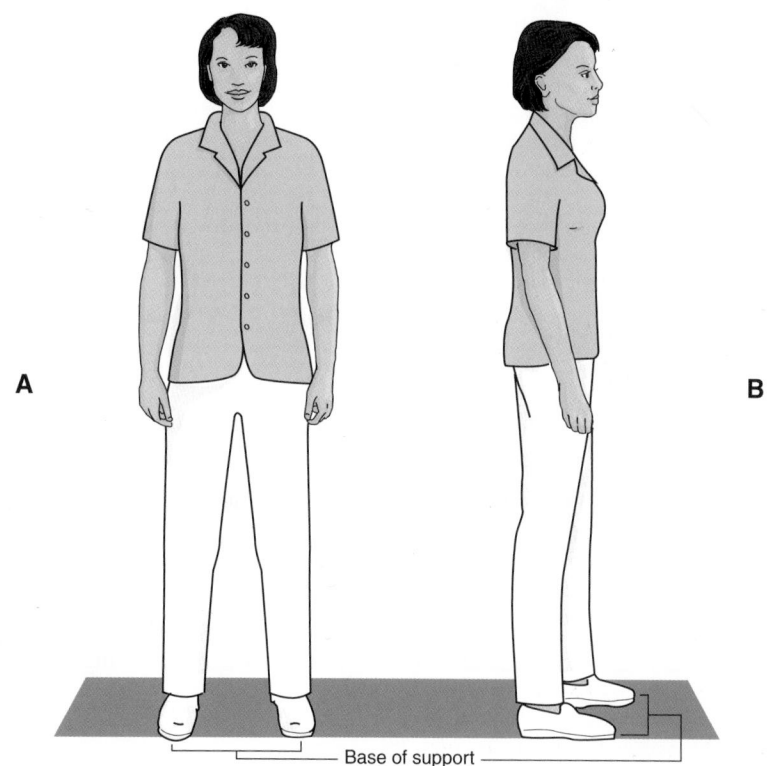

Base of support

A

B

FIGURE 15-3 A, Anterior (front) view of an adult in good body alignment. The feet are apart for a wide base of support. **B,** Lateral (side) view of an adult with good posture and alignment.

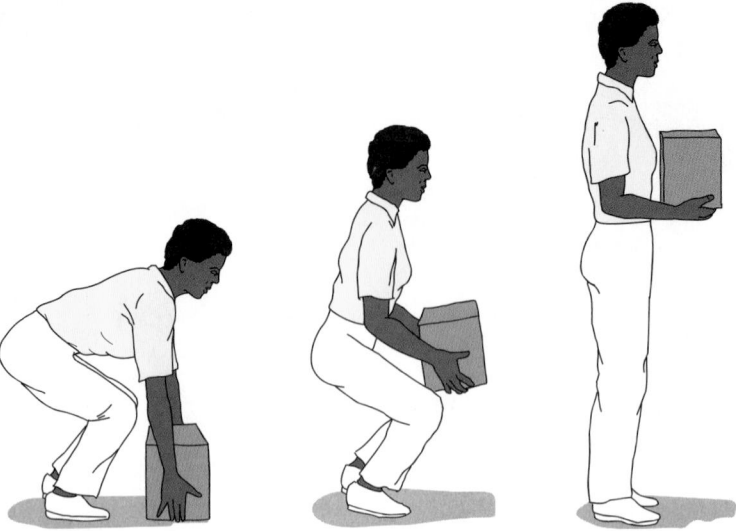

FIGURE 15-4 Picking up a box using good body mechanics.

BOX 15-2 Rules for Body Mechanics

- Keep your body in good alignment with a wide base of support.
- Use an upright working posture. Bend your legs. Do not bend your back.
- Use the stronger and larger muscles in your shoulders, upper arms, thighs, and hips.
- Keep objects close to your body when you lift, move, or carry them (see Fig. 15-4).
- Avoid unnecessary bending and reaching. Raise the bed so it is close to your waist. Adjust the overbed table so it is at your waist level.
- Face your work area. This prevents unnecessary twisting.
- Push, slide, or pull heavy objects whenever you can rather than lifting them. Pushing is easier than pulling.
- Widen your base of support when pushing or pulling. Move your front leg forward when pushing. Move your rear leg back when pulling (Fig. 15-5).
- Use both hands and arms to lift, move, or carry objects.
- Turn your whole body when changing the direction of your movement. Move and turn your feet in the direction of the turn instead of twisting your body.
- Work with smooth and even movements. Avoid sudden or jerky motions.
- Do not lean over a person to give care.
- *Get help from a co-worker to move heavy objects. Do not lift or move them by yourself.*
- Bend your hips and knees to lift heavy objects from the floor (see Fig. 15-4). Straighten your back as the object reaches thigh level. Your leg and thigh muscles work to raise the item off the floor and to waist level.
- Do not lift objects higher than chest level. Do not lift above your shoulders. Use a step stool or ladder to reach an object higher than chest level.

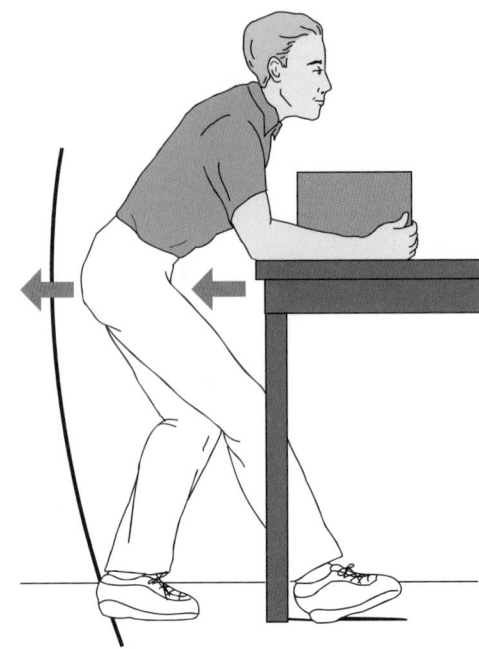

FIGURE 15-5 Move your rear leg back when pulling an item.

ERGONOMICS

Ergonomics is the science of designing a job to fit the worker. (*Ergo* means work. *Nomos* means law.) It involves changing the task, work station, equipment, and tools to help reduce stress on the worker's body. The goal is to eliminate a serious and disabling work-related musculoskeletal disorder (WMSD). WMSDs are caused or made worse by the work setting.

WMSDs are injuries and disorders of the muscles, tendons, ligaments, joints, and cartilage. They also can involve the nervous system. The arms and back are often affected. So are the hands, fingers, neck, wrists, legs, and shoulders. WMSDs are painful and disabling. They can develop slowly over weeks, months, and years. Or they can occur from one event. Pain, numbness, tingling, stiff joints, difficulty moving, and muscle loss can occur. Sometimes there is paralysis.

WMSDs are workplace health hazards. Early signs and symptoms include pain, limited joint movement, or soft tissue swelling. Time off work is often needed. According to the U.S. Department of Labor, nursing assistants are at great risk.

Always report a work-related injury as soon as possible. Early attention can help prevent the problem from becoming worse. Also, injuries are often less serious and less costly to treat if they receive early attention. In later stages, the problem can become more serious and harder and more costly to treat.

The following nursing tasks are known to be high risk for WMSDs:

- Transfers—to and from beds, chairs, wheelchairs, Geri-chairs, toilets, stretchers, and bathtubs
- Trying to stop a person from falling
- Picking up a person from the floor to the bed
- Lifting alone
- Lifting persons who are confused or uncooperative
- Lifting persons who cannot support their own weight
- Lifting heavy persons
- Weighing a person
- Moving a person up in bed
- Repositioning a person in a bed or in a chair
- Changing an incontinence product
- Making beds
- Dressing and undressing a person
- Feeding a person in bed
- Giving a bed bath
- Applying anti-embolism stockings

The Occupational Safety and Health Administration (OSHA) has identified risk factors for WMSDs in nursing team members. WMSDs result from these risk factors. The risk of a WMSD increases if risk factors combine. For example, a task involves both force and repeating actions.

- Force—the amount of physical effort needed to perform a task. Lifting or transferring heavy patients and residents, preventing falls, and unexpected or sudden motions are examples.
- Repeating action—performing the same motion or series of motions continually or frequently. Repositioning patients and residents and transfers to and from beds, chairs, and commodes without adequate rest breaks are examples. So is the frequent cranking of manual beds.

- Awkward postures—assuming positions that place stress on the body. Examples include reaching above shoulder height, kneeling, squatting, leaning over a bed, bending, or twisting the torso while lifting.
- Heavy lifting—manually lifting patients and residents who cannot move themselves.

OSHA requires that employers provide employees with a safe work setting. The setting must be free of recognized hazards that are causing or likely to cause death or serious physical harm to employees. The employer must make reasonable attempts to prevent or reduce the hazard. The OSHA inspection team enforces this law.

See *Focus on Ethics and Laws: Ergonomics.*

Back Injuries

Back injuries are major threats. Back injuries can occur from repeated activities or from one event. Signs and symptoms include:

- Pain when trying to assume a normal posture
- Decreased mobility
- Pain when standing or rising from a seated position
These and other factors can lead to back disorders:
- Reaching while lifting
- Poor posture when sitting or standing
- Staying in one position too long
- Poor body mechanics when lifting, pushing, pulling, or carrying objects
- Poor physical condition—not having the strength or endurance to perform tasks without strain
- Repeated lifting of awkward items, equipment, or persons
- Shifting weight when a person loses balance or strength while moving
- Twisting while lifting
- Bending while lifting
- Maintaining a bent posture such as leaning over a bed

▶ Reaching over raised bed rails
▶ Working in a confined, crowded, or cluttered area (rooms, bathrooms, hallways)
▶ Fatigue
▶ Poor footing such as on slippery floors
▶ Lifting with forceful movement

Follow the rules in Box 15-2. They help prevent back injuries. Also, be extra careful when performing tasks that are associated with back injuries.

See *Promoting Safety and Comfort: Back Injuries.*

POSITIONING THE PERSON

The person must be properly positioned at all times. Regular position changes and good alignment promote comfort and well-being. Breathing is easier. Circulation is promoted. Pressure ulcers and contractures are prevented.

You move and turn when in bed or a chair for your comfort. Many patients and residents do too. Some need reminding to adjust their positions. Other need help. Still others depend entirely on the nursing team for position changes.

Whether in bed or chair, the person is repositioned at least every 2 hours. Some people are repositioned more often. You must follow the nurse's instructions and the care plan. Follow these guidelines to safely position a person:

▶ Use good body mechanics.
▶ Ask a co-worker to help you if needed.
▶ Explain the procedure to the person.
▶ Be gentle when moving the person.
▶ Provide for privacy.
▶ Use pillows as directed by the nurse for support and alignment.
▶ Provide for comfort after positioning. (See the inside of the front book cover.)
▶ Place the signal light within reach after positioning.
▶ Complete a safety check before leaving the room. (See the inside of the front book cover.)

See *Focus on Children and Older Persons: Positioning the Person.*

See *Delegation Guidelines: Positioning the Person.*

See *Promoting Safety and Comfort: Positioning the Person.*

PROMOTING SAFETY AND COMFORT: Back Injuries

SAFETY
According to OSHA, these activities are associated with back injuries in nursing centers:
• Moving a person who totally depends on others for care
• Moving a person who is combative
• Transferring a person who is on the floor to the bed or a chair
• Repositioning a person in bed or in a chair
• Transferring a person from bed to chair or from chair to bed
• Transferring a person from one chair to another (includes transfers to and from the wheelchair and toilet)
• Bending to bathe, dress, or feed a person
• Bending to make a bed or change linens
• Weighing a person
• Changing an incontinence product
• Trying to stop a person from falling
Use good body mechanics to protect yourself from injury. Do not work alone. Avoid lifting whenever possible.

FOCUS ON CHILDREN AND OLDER PERSONS

Positioning the Person

OLDER PERSONS
Most older persons do not tolerate the prone position. They have limited range of motion in their necks. The Sims' position usually is not comfortable for them. Check with the nurse before placing any older person in the prone position or Sims' position.

DELEGATION GUIDELINES: Positioning the Person

You are often delegated tasks that involve positioning and repositioning. You need this information from the nurse and the care plan:
• Position or positioning limits ordered by the doctor
• How often to turn and reposition the person
• How many staff members need to help you
• What assist devices to use (Chapter 16)
• What skin care measures to perform (Chapter 19)
• What range-of-motion exercises to perform (Chapter 26)
• Where to place pillows
• What positioning devices are needed and how to use them (Chapter 26)
• What observations to report and record
• When to report observations
• What specific patient or resident concerns to report at once

Fowler's Position

Fowler's position is a semi-sitting position. The head of the bed is raised between 45 and 60 degrees (Fig. 15-6). The knees may be slightly elevated. For good alignment:
- The spine is straight.
- The head is supported with a small pillow.
- The arms are supported with pillows.

The nurse may ask you to place small pillows under the lower back, thighs, and ankles. Persons with heart and respiratory disorders usually breathe easier in Fowler's position.

Supine Position

The **supine position (dorsal recumbent position)** is the back-lying position (Fig. 15-7). For good alignment:
- The bed is flat.
- The head and shoulders are supported on a pillow.
- Arms and hands are at the sides. You can support the arms with regular pillows. Or you can support the hands on small pillows with the palms down.

The nurse may ask you to place a folded or rolled towel under the lower back and a small pillow under the thighs. A pillow under the lower legs lifts the heels off of the bed. This prevents them from rubbing on the sheets.

Prone Position

A person in the **prone position** lies on the abdomen with the head turned to one side. For good alignment:
- The bed is flat.
- Small pillows are placed under the head, abdomen, and lower legs (Fig. 15-8).
- Arms are flexed at the elbows with the hands near the head.

You also can position a person with the feet hanging over the end of the mattress (Fig. 15-9, p. 236). A pillow is not needed under the feet.

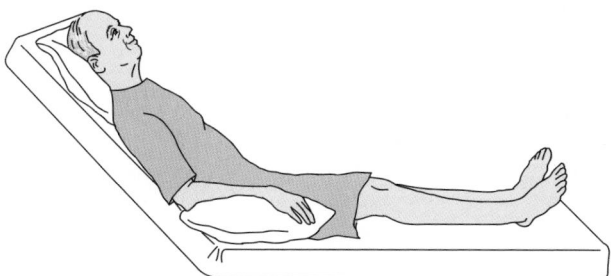
FIGURE 15-6 Fowler's position.

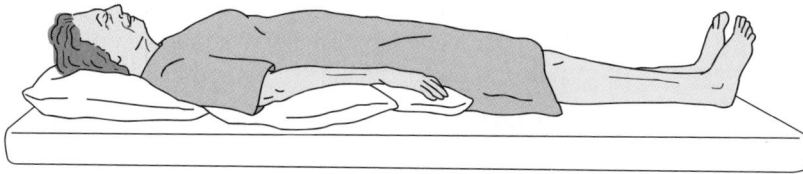
FIGURE 15-7 Supine position.

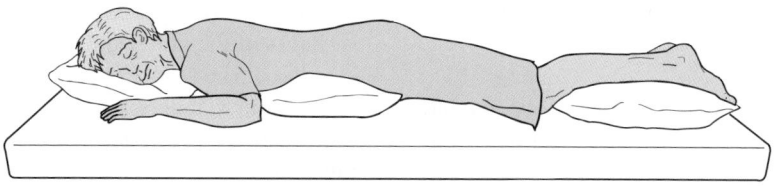
FIGURE 15-8 Prone position.

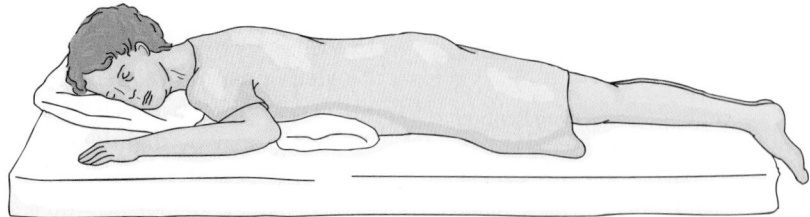

FIGURE 15-9 Prone position with the feet hanging over the edge of the mattress.

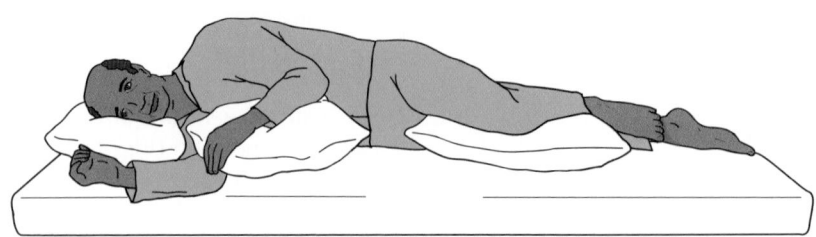

FIGURE 15-10 Lateral position.

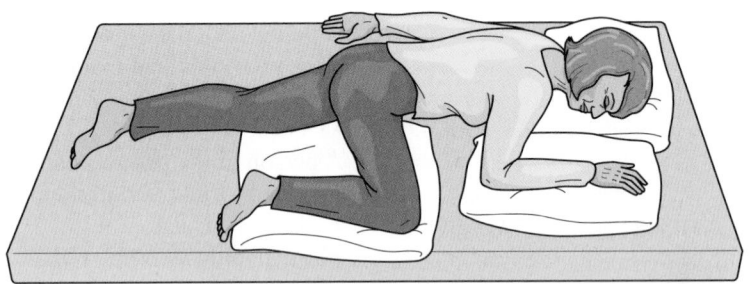

FIGURE 15-11 Sims' position.

Lateral Position

A person in the **lateral position (side-lying position)** lies on one side or the other (Fig. 15-10):

- The bed is flat.
- A pillow is under the head and neck.
- The upper leg is in front of the lower leg. (The nurse may ask you to position the upper leg behind the lower leg, not on top of it.)
- The ankle, upper leg, and thigh are supported with pillows.
- A small pillow is positioned against the person's back. The person rolls back against the pillow so that his or her back is at a 45-degree angle with the mattress.
- A small pillow is under the upper hand and arm.

Sims' Position

The **Sims' position (semi-prone side position)** is a left side-lying position. The upper leg is sharply flexed so it is not on the lower leg. The lower arm is behind the person (Fig. 15-11).

For good alignment:

- The bed is flat.
- A pillow is under the person's head and shoulder.
- The upper leg is supported with a pillow.
- A pillow is under the upper arm and hand.

Chair Position

Persons who sit in chairs must hold their upper bodies and heads erect. If not, poor alignment results. For good alignment:

- The person's back and buttocks are against the back of the chair.
- Feet are flat on the floor or wheelchair footplates. Never leave feet unsupported.
- Backs of the knees and calves are slightly away from the edge of the seat (Fig. 15-12).

The nurse may ask you to put a small pillow between the person's lower back and the chair. This supports the lower back. *Remember, a pillow is not used behind the back if restraints are used (Chapter 13).*

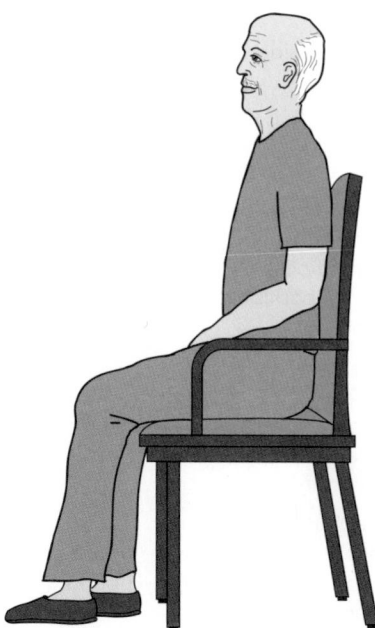

FIGURE 15-12 The person is positioned in a chair. The person's feet are flat on the floor; the calves do not touch the chair. The back is straight and against the back of the chair.

Paralyzed arms are supported on pillows. Some persons have positioners (Fig. 15-13). Ask the nurse about their proper use. Wrists are positioned at a slight upward angle.

Some people require postural supports if they cannot keep their upper bodies erect (Fig. 15-14). Postural supports help keep them in good alignment. The health team selects the best product for the person's needs. The person's safety, dignity, and function are considered.

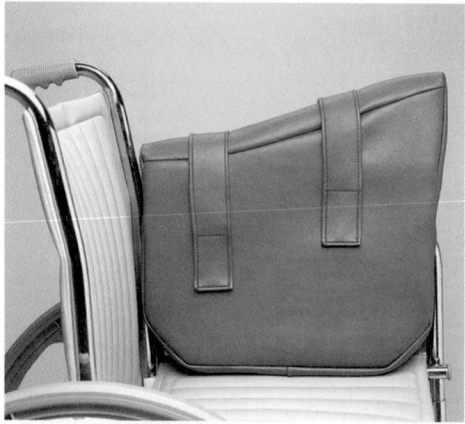

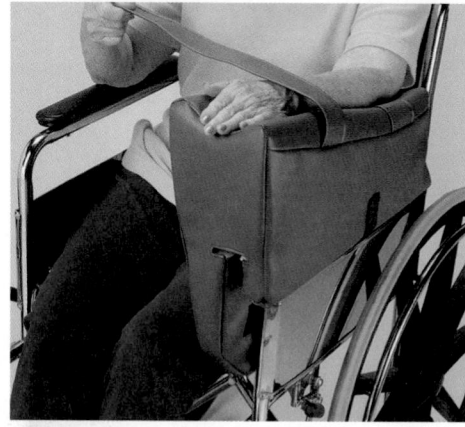

FIGURE 15-13 Elevated armrest. (Images courtesy J.T. Posey Co., Arcadia, Calif.)

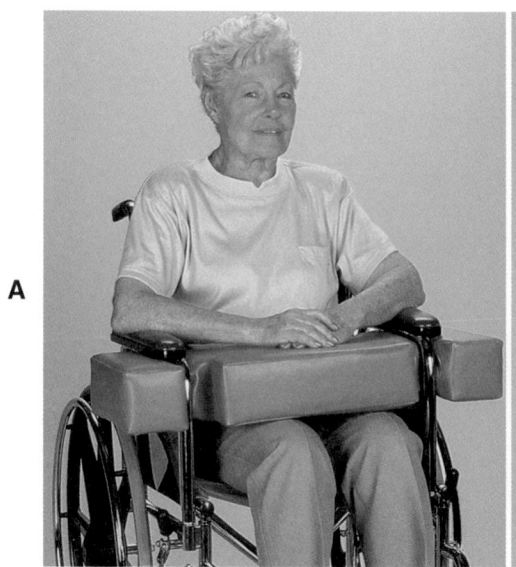

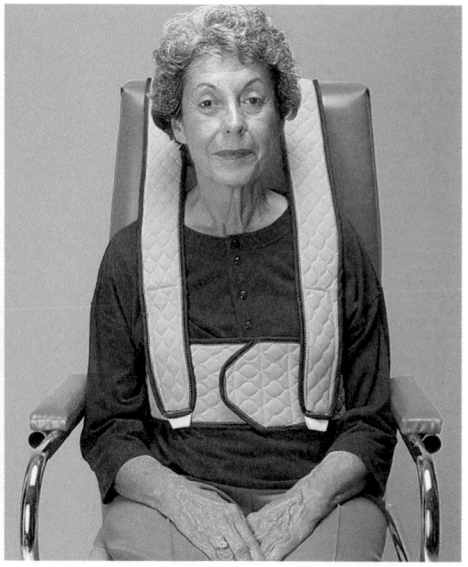

FIGURE 15-14 Postural supports. **A,** Pelvic holder. **B,** Torso support. (Images courtesy J.T. Posey Co., Arcadia, Calif.)

Circle the BEST answer.

1 Good body mechanics involves the following *except*
 a Good posture
 b Balance
 c Using the strongest and largest muscles
 d Having the job fit the worker

2 Good alignment means
 a The area on which an object rests
 b Having the head, trunk, arms, and legs aligned with one another
 c Using muscles, tendons, ligaments, and joints correctly
 d The back-lying or supine position

3 These statements are about body mechanics. Which statement is *not* correct?
 a Hold objects away from your body when lifting, moving, or carrying them.
 b Face the direction you are working to prevent twisting.
 c Push, pull, or slide heavy objects.
 d Use both hands and arms to lift, move, or carry heavy objects.

4 Which action is easier?
 a Pushing
 b Pulling
 c Sliding
 d Lifting

5 The purpose of ergonomics is to
 a Reduce stress on the worker's body
 b Safely position a person
 c Promote quality of life
 d Use good body mechanics

6 Risk factors for work-related musculoskeletal disorders include the following *except*
 a Repeating actions
 b Awkward postures
 c Bending your hips and knees
 d Force

7 Patients and residents are repositioned at least every
 a 30 minutes
 b 1 hour
 c 2 hours
 d 3 hours

8 The back-lying position is called
 a Fowler's position
 b The supine position
 c The prone position
 d Sims' position

9 Breathing is usually easier in
 a Fowler's position
 b The supine position
 c The lateral position
 d Sims' position

10 For Fowler's position
 a The bed is flat
 b The head of the bed is raised between 45 and 60 degrees
 c The person's head is turned toward one side
 d The person's feet hang over the edge of the mattress

11 A pillow is placed against the person's back in
 a Fowler's position
 b The prone position
 c The lateral position
 d Sims' position

12 A person is positioned in a chair. The feet
 a Must be flat on the floor
 b Are positioned on footplates
 c Dangle
 d Are positioned on pillows

Answers to these questions are on p. 780.

Safely Handling, Moving, and Transferring the Person

OBJECTIVES

- Define the key terms and key abbreviations listed in this chapter
- Identify comfort and safety measures for handling, moving, and transferring the person
- Explain how to prevent work-related injuries when handling, moving, and transferring persons
- Describe four levels of dependence
- Identify the information needed from the nurse and care plan before handling, moving, and transferring persons
- Perform the procedures described in this chapter

PROCEDURES

- Raising the Person's Head and Shoulders
- Moving the Person Up in Bed
- Moving the Person Up in Bed With an Assist Device
- Moving the Person to the Side of the Bed
- Turning and Repositioning the Person
- Logrolling the Person
- Sitting On the Side of the Bed (Dangling)

- Transferring the Person to a Chair or Wheelchair
- Transferring the Person From a Chair or Wheelchair to Bed
- Transferring the Person Using a Mechanical Lift
- Transferring the Person To and From the Toilet
- Moving the Person to a Stretcher

Procedures with this icon ⊙ are on the CDCompanion in this book; those with this icon [View Video] are on the Evolve Student Resources Website.

KEY TERMS

friction The rubbing of one surface against another
logrolling Turning the person as a unit, in alignment, with one motion

shearing When skin sticks to a surface while muscles slide in the direction the body is moving
transfer Moving the person from one place to another

KEY ABBREVIATIONS

OSHA Occupational Safety and Health Administration

You will turn and reposition persons often. You move them in bed. You transfer them to and from beds, chairs, wheelchairs, stretchers, and toilets. To **transfer** a person means moving the person from one place to another. During these and other tasks, you must use your body correctly. This protects you and the person from injury.

See *Promoting Safety and Comfort: Safely Handling, Moving, and Transferring the Person.*

See *Focus on Communication: Safely Handling, Moving, and Transferring the Person.*

See *Teamwork and Time Management: Safely Handling, Moving, and Transferring the Person.*

FOCUS ON COMMUNICATION

Safely Handling, Moving, and Transferring the Person

Handling, moving, and transfers can be very painful following an injury or surgery. Many older persons have painful joints. You must make sure the person is comfortable and that you are not causing pain. You can say:
- "Am I hurting you?"
- "Please tell me when you feel pain or discomfort."
- "Do you need a pillow adjusted?"
- "Are you comfortable?"
- "How can I help make you more comfortable?"

PROMOTING SAFETY AND COMFORT: Safely Handling, Moving, and Transferring the Person

SAFETY

Many older persons have osteoporosis or arthritis (Chapter 39). They have fragile bones and joints. To prevent injuries:
- Follow the rules of body mechanics (Chapter 15).
- Always have help when moving a person.
- Move the person carefully to prevent injury or pain.
- Keep the person in good alignment.
- Position the person in good alignment after handling, moving, or transferring him or her. Make sure his or her face, nose, or mouth is not obstructed by a pillow or other device.

COMFORT

To promote mental comfort when handling, moving, or transferring the person:
- Always explain what you are going to do and how the person can help.
- Always screen and cover the person to protect the right to privacy.
  To promote physical comfort:
- Keep the person in good alignment.
- Make sure the person's head does not hit the headboard when he or she is moved up in bed. If the person can be without a pillow, place it upright against the headboard.
- Use pillows to position the person as directed by the nurse and the care plan. If a pillow is allowed under the person's head, make sure it is under the head and shoulders.
- Use other positioning devices as directed by the nurse and the care plan.

TEAMWORK AND TIME MANAGEMENT

Safely Handling, Moving, and Transferring the Person

Patients and residents need to be moved, turned, transferred, and repositioned. These tasks and procedures are best done by at least 2 staff members.

Friendships are common among co-workers. And some working relationships are better than others. Do not just ask your friends or those with whom you work well to help you. Include all co-workers. Do not just help your friends or those with whom you work well. Assist anyone who asks for your help. This includes new staff members and those from other units.

PREVENTING WORK-RELATED INJURIES

You must prevent work-related injuries when handling, moving, and transferring patients and residents. Follow the rules in Box 16-1. The Occupational Safety and Health Administration (OSHA) recommends that:
- Manual lifting be minimized in all cases.
- Manual lifting be eliminated when possible.

To safely handle, move, and transfer the person, the nurse and health team determine:

▶ *The person's dependence level.* Dependence levels relate to the ability to move without help. Some persons do not need help moving. Others totally depend on the staff. You need to know the person's dependence level before you handle, move, or transfer a person. See Box 16-2, p. 242.

▶ *The amount of assistance needed.* This depends on the person's height, weight, cognitive function, and dependence level. Some persons only need help from one staff member. Others need help from at least 2 or 3 staff members.

▶ *What procedure to use.* This chapter includes handling, moving, and transfer procedures. The nurse and care plan tell you what procedure to use.

▶ *The equipment needed.* Assist equipment and devices are useful to safely handle, move, and transfer persons. They are presented throughout this chapter. The nurse and care plan tell you what to use. Always follow the manufacturer's instructions. Ask for any needed training to use the equipment and devices safely.

See *Focus on Children and Older Persons: Preventing Work-Related Injuries,* p. 243.

See *Teamwork and Time Management: Preventing Work-Related Injuries,* p. 243.

See *Delegation Guidelines: Preventing Work-Related Injuries,* p. 244.

See *Promoting Safety and Comfort: Preventing Work-Related Injuries,* p. 244.

See *Focus on Ethics and Laws: Preventing Work-Related Injuries,* p. 244.

Text continued on p. 244

BOX 16-1 Preventing Work-Related Injuries

GENERAL GUIDELINES
- Wear shoes that provide good traction. Avoid shoes with worn-down soles. Good traction can help prevent slips or falls.
- Use assist equipment and devices whenever possible instead of lifting and moving the person manually. Follow the person's care plan.
- Get help from other staff. The nurse and care plan tell you how many staff members are needed to complete the task.
- Plan and prepare for the task. For example, know what equipment you will need, where to place chairs or wheelchairs, and what side of the bed to work on.
- Schedule harder tasks early in your shift.
- Balance lighter and harder tasks. Plan your work so that you can complete a lighter task after a harder one.
- Tell the person what he or she can do to help. Give clear, simple instructions. Give the person time to respond.
- Do not hold or grab the person under the underarms.
- Do not let the person hold or grasp you around your neck.

MANUAL LIFTING
- Use good body mechanics.
  - Stand with good posture. Keep your back straight.
  - Bend your legs, not your back.
  - Use your legs to do the work.
  - Face the person.
  - Do not twist or turn. Pick up your feet, and pivot your whole body in the direction of the move.
- Try to keep what you are moving close to you—the person, equipment, or supplies.
- Move the person toward you, not away from you.
- Use slides and lateral transfers instead of manual lifting.
- Use a wide, balanced base of support. Stand with one foot slightly ahead of the other.
- Lower the person slowly by bending your legs. Do not bend your back. Return to an erect position as soon as possible.
- Use smooth, even movements. Avoid jerking movements.
- Lift on the "count of 3" when lifting with others. Everyone should lift at the same time.

LATERAL TRANSFERS
- Position surfaces as close as possible to each other (bed and chair; bed and stretcher).
- Adjust surfaces so that they are at about waist height. The receiving surface should be slightly lower to take advantage of gravity. For example, when transferring the person from bed to a chair, the chair surface is lower than the bed.
- Make sure bed rails are down. Make sure side rails on stretchers are down.
- Use drawsheets, turning pads, large incontinence pads, or other friction-reducing devices. Such devices include slide boards, slide sheets, and low-friction mattress covers.
- Get a good hand-hold. Roll up drawsheets, turning pads, and incontinence pads. Or use assist devices with handles.
- Kneel on the bed or stretcher. This helps prevent extended reaches and bending the back.
- Have staff on both sides of the bed or other surface. Move the person on the "count of 3." Use a smooth, push-pull motion. Do not reach across the person.

GAIT/TRANSFER BELTS
- Keep the person as close to you as possible.
- Avoid bending, reaching, or twisting when:
  - Attaching or removing a belt
  - Lowering the person to a chair, the bed, toilet, or the floor
  - Assisting the person with ambulation
- Use a gentle rocking motion to assist the person to stand. The rocking motion gives strength and force as you pull the person to a standing position.
- See Chapter 11.

STAND-PIVOT TRANSFERS
- Use assist devices as directed. Follow the care plan.
- Use a gait/transfer belt with handles.
- Keep your feet at least shoulder width apart.
- Lower the bed so the person can place his or her feet on the floor.
- Plan the transfer so that the person moves his or her strong side first.

(Modified from *A back injury prevention guide for health care providers,* Cal/OSHA, revised November 1997, Sacramento, Calif. as referenced in *Ergonomics: guidelines for nursing homes,* Occupational Health and Safety Administration, September 12, 2005.)

Continued

BOX 16-1 Preventing Work-Related Injuries—cont'd

STAND-PIVOT TRANSFERS—cont'd
- Get the person close to the edge of the bed or the chair. Ask the person to lean forward as he or she stands.
- Block the person's weak leg with your legs or knees. If the position is awkward, do the following:
  - Use a transfer belt with handles.
  - Straddle your legs around the person's weak leg.
- Bend your legs. Do not bend your back.
- Pivot with your feet to turn.
- Use a gentle rocking motion to assist the person to stand. The rocking motion gives strength and force as you pull the person to a standing position.

LIFTING OR MOVING THE PERSON IN BED
- Adjust the height of the bed, stretcher, or other surface so that it is at waist level.
- Lower the bed rail or the stretcher side rail.
- Work on the side where the person will be closest to you.
- Place equipment or other items close to you and at waist level.
- Use drawsheets, turning pads, large incontinence pads, or slide sheets.

TRANSPORTING PATIENTS, RESIDENTS, AND EQUIPMENT
- Push, do not pull.
- Keep the load close to your body.
- Use an upright posture.
- Push with your whole body, not just your arms.
- Move down the center of the hallway. This helps avoid collisions.
- Watch out for door handles and high thresholds on floors. These can cause abrupt stops.

TRANSFERRING THE PERSON FROM THE FLOOR
- Use a mechanical lift if possible (p. 264). If not, place a sling, blanket, drawsheet, cot, or other assist device under the person as directed by the nurse.
- Position at least two staff members on each side of the person. More staff is needed if the person is large.
- Bend at your knees, not your back. Do not twist.
- Roll the person onto his or her side to position the assist device. Do not reach across the person.
- Lower the hoist (if using a mechanical lift) to attach the sling. The hoist should be low enough to that you can easily attach the sling.
- Do the following for a manual lift:
  - Kneel on one knee.
  - Grasp the blanket, drawsheet, cot, or other device.
  - Lift smoothly with your legs as you stand on the "count of 3." Do not bend your back.

(Modified from *A back injury prevention guide for health care providers*, Cal/OSHA, revised November 1997, Sacramento, Calif. as referenced in *Ergonomics: guidelines for nursing homes*, Occupational Health and Safety Administration, September 12, 2005.)

BOX 16-2 Levels of Dependence

Code 4: Total Dependence. The person cannot help with the transfer. The task or procedure is done by the staff.
- The person should be lifted and transferred using a full-sling mechanical lift (Fig. 16-1). The mechanical lift is used for transfers between beds, chairs, and toilets. It is also used for transfers to and from bathtubs and weighing scales.

Code 3: Extensive Assistance. The person can bear some weight, can sit up with help, and may be able to pivot to transfer.
- The person should be lifted and transferred using a mechanical lift. The mechanical lift is used for transfers between beds, chairs, and toilets. It is also used for transfers to and from bathtubs and weighing scales. The type of lift to use is noted on the person's care plan—full-sling mechanical lift or stand-assist lift (Fig. 16-2).

Code 2: Limited Assistance. The person is highly involved in the moving or transfer procedure. He or she needs some help moving the legs. The person can stand (bear weight). The person has upper body strength and can sit up. He or she is able to pivot transfer.
- Stand-assist devices may be needed. These can be attached to the bed or chair (Fig. 16-3). Other stand-assist devices include walkers (Chapter 26) and gait/transfer belts with handles (Chapter 11)
- Sliding boards are useful for transfers to and from beds and chairs (Fig. 16-4).

Code 1: Supervision. The staff needs to look after, encourage, or cue the person. To cue means to remind the person what to do.
- The assist devices for Code 2 may be needed.

Code 0: Independent. The person can walk without help. Sometimes the person may need limited assistance.
- Mechanical assistance is not normally required for transfers, lifting, or repositioning.

(Modified from Nelson AL: *Patient care ergonomics resource guide: safe patient handling and movement*, Patient Safety Center of Inquiry (Tampa, Fla), Veterans Health Administration and Department of Defense, April 2005.)

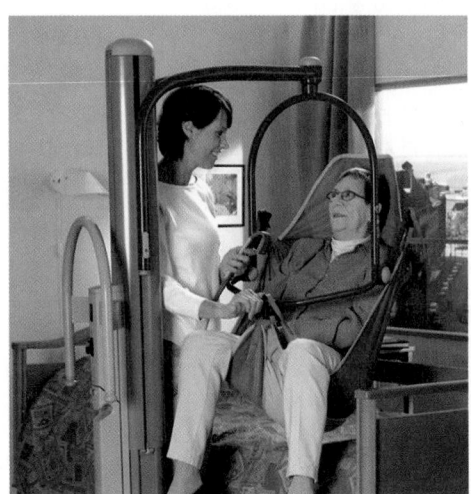

FIGURE 16-1 Full-sling mechanical lift. (Courtesy ARJO, Inc., Roselle, Ill. (800)323-1245.)

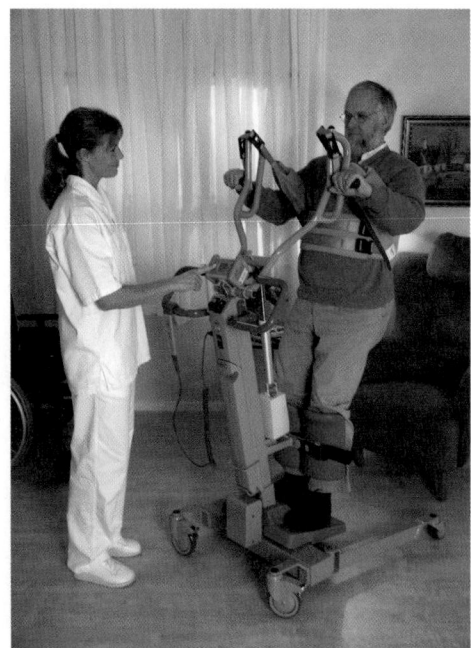

FIGURE 16-2 Stand-assist lift. (Courtesy ARJO, Inc., Roselle, Ill. (800)323-1245.)

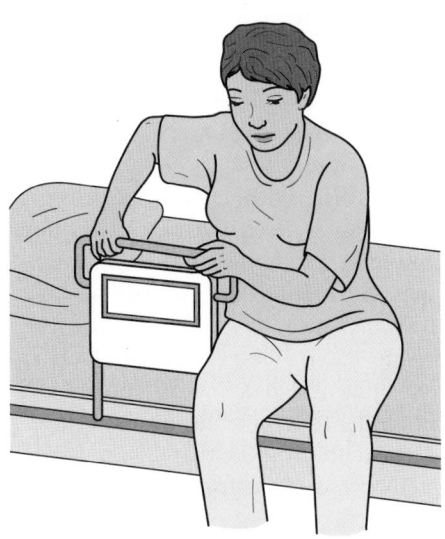

FIGURE 16-3 Stand-assist bed attachment.

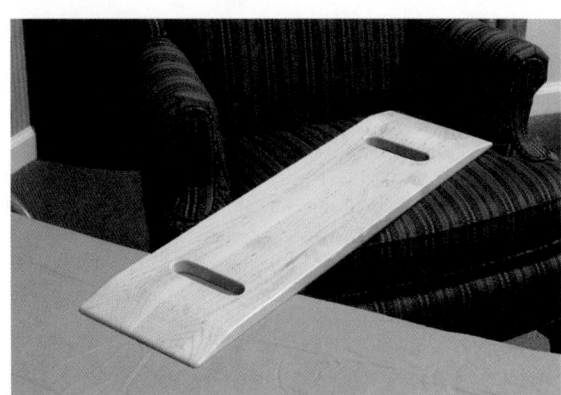

FIGURE 16-4 Slide board for transferring to and from surfaces.

FOCUS ON **CHILDREN** AND **OLDER PERSONS**

Preventing Work-Related Injuries

OLDER PERSONS

Some older persons have dementia. They may not understand what you are doing. They may resist your handling, moving, and transfer efforts. The person may shout at you, grab you, or try to hit you. Always get a co-worker to help you. Do not force the person. The rules and guidelines in Box 16-1 apply. The person's care plan also has measures for providing safe care. For example:

- Proceed slowly
- Use a calm, pleasant voice
- Divert the person's attention

Tell the nurse at once if you have problems handling, moving, or transferring the person.

TEAMWORK AND TIME MANAGEMENT

Preventing Work-Related Injuries

Some agencies have "lift teams." These teams perform most of the lifting, moving, and transfer procedures. They use assist equipment and do not manually lift or move patients and residents unless necessary.

The nurse advises the lift team of scheduled procedures. The team is called by beeper, pager, or other device for unscheduled transfers.

Do not assume that the lift team will lift, move, or transfer your assigned patients and residents. Follow agency policy for checking or adding to the lift team's schedule. Do not neglect or omit a procedure because the agency has a lift team. If the person is on the team's schedule, always check to make sure that the procedure was done. Sometimes the team can get delayed because of unscheduled or unexpected events. Always thank the team for the work that they do. Their work protects patients, residents, and you from injury.

DELEGATION GUIDELINES: Preventing Work-Related Injuries

Many delegated tasks involve handling, moving, and transferring persons. Before doing so, you need this information from the nurse and the care plan:
- The person's height and weight
- The person's dependence level (see Box 16-2)
- The person's physical abilities (For example, can the person sit up, stand up, or walk without help? Does the person have strength in his or her arms?)
- If the person has a weak side (If yes, what side?)
- If the person has a medical condition that increases the risk of injury (Dizziness, confusion, hearing or vision problems, recent surgery, and fragile skin are examples.)
- If there are any doctor's orders for handling, moving, or transferring the person
- The person's ability to follow directions
- If behavior problems are likely (Combative, agitated, uncooperative, and unpredictable behaviors are examples.)
- The amount of assistance needed
- How many staff members are needed to complete the task safely
- What procedure to use
- What equipment to use

PROMOTING SAFETY AND COMFORT: Preventing Work-Related Injuries

SAFETY

Decide how to move the person before starting the procedure. If you need help from other staff members, ask them to help before you begin. Also plan how to protect drainage tubes or containers connected to the person.

Beds are raised to move persons in bed (Chapter 17). This reduces bending and reaching. You must:
- Use the bed correctly.
- Protect the person from falling when the bed is raised.
- Follow the rules of body mechanics (Chapter 15).

FOCUS ON ETHICS AND LAWS

Preventing Work-Related Injuries

The Occupational Safety and Health Act requires that employers provide employees with a safe work setting. The setting must be free of recognized hazards that are causing or likely to cause death or serious physical harm to employees. The employer must reasonably try to prevent or reduce the hazard. OSHA inspection teams enforce this law.

DELEGATION GUIDELINES: Moving Persons in Bed

Many delegated tasks involve moving the person in bed. Before moving a person, you need this information from the nurse and the care plan:
- What procedure to use
- How many workers are needed to safely move the person
- Position limits and restrictions
- How far you can lower the head of the bed
- Any limits in the person's ability to move or be repositioned
- What pillows can be removed before moving the person
- What equipment is needed—trapeze, lift sheet, slide sheet, mechanical lift
- How to position the person
- If the person uses bed rails
- What observations to report and record:
  - Who helped you with the procedure
  - How much help the person needed
  - How the person tolerated the procedure
  - How you positioned the person
  - Complaints of pain or discomfort
- When to report observations
- What specific patient or resident concerns to report at once

MOVING PERSONS IN BED

Some persons can move and turn in bed. Others need help from at least one person. Those who are weak, unconscious, paralyzed, or in casts need help. Sometimes 2 or 3 people or a mechanical lift is needed. OSHA recommends the following:

▶ If the person has a dependence level of *Code 4: Total Dependence*—use a mechanical lift or friction-reducing device. At least 2 staff members are needed.
▶ If the person has a dependence level of *Code 3: Extensive Assistance*—use a mechanical lift or friction-reducing device. At least 2 staff members are needed.
▶ If the person weighs less than 200 pounds—2 to 3 staff members and a friction-reducing device are needed.
▶ If the person weighs more than 200 pounds—at least 3 staff members and a friction-reducing device are needed.

See *Delegation Guidelines: Moving Persons in Bed.*

Protecting the Skin

Protect the person's skin during handling, moving, and transfer procedures. Friction and shearing injure the skin. Both cause infection and pressure ulcers (Chapter 32).

▶ **Friction** is the rubbing of one surface against another. When moved in bed, the person's skin rubs against the sheet.
▶ **Shearing** is when the skin sticks to a surface while muscles slide in the direction the body is moving (Fig. 16-5). It occurs when the person slides down in bed or is moved in bed.

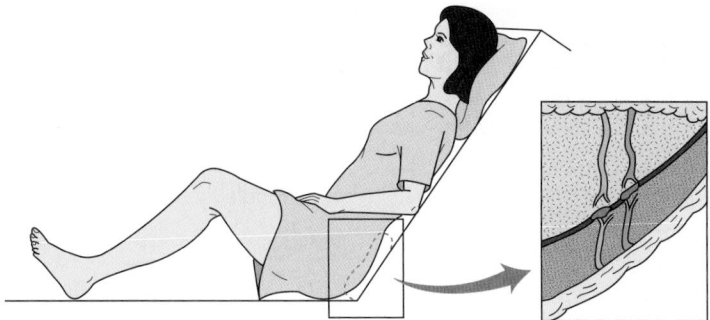

FIGURE 16-5 When the head of the bed is raised to a sitting position, skin on the buttocks stays in place. However, internal structures move forward as the person slides down in bed. This causes the skin to be pinched between the mattress and the hip bones.

Protecting the Skin

OLDER PERSONS

Older persons are at great risk for shearing. Their skin is fragile and easily torn. Many have arthritis and osteoporosis (Chapter 39). They have fragile bones and joints. Protect them from pain and injury.

Ask a co-worker to help you move older persons. Use a friction-reducing device. Move older persons carefully and gently. Persons with dementia may try to resist your efforts. Do not force the person. Proceed slowly. Use a calm voice. Divert the person's attention if necessary.

Reduce friction and shearing when moving the person in bed. Do so by:
▶ Rolling the person.
▶ Using friction-reducing devices. Such devices include a lift sheet (turning sheet). A cotton drawsheet (Chapter 18) serves as a lift sheet (turning sheet). Turning pads, large incontinence products, slide boards, and slide sheets are other friction-reducing devices.

See *Focus on Children and Older Persons: Protecting the Skin.*

Raising the Person's Head and Shoulders

You may have to raise the person's head and shoulders to give care. Simply turning or removing a pillow requires this procedure. You can raise the person's head and shoulders easily and safely by locking arms with the person. *Do not pull on the person's arm or shoulder.* It is best to have help with older persons and with those who are heavy or hard to move. This protects the person and you from injury.

See *Focus on Ethics and Laws: Raising the Person's Head and Shoulders.*

FOCUS ON ETHICS AND LAWS

Raising the Person's Head and Shoulders

A patient sued the hospital for a shoulder injury. Admitted to the hospital for a respiratory problem, the patient had a history of shoulder injuries and surgeries. A nurse positioned the patient in a sitting position. The patient testified that she had immediate pain and heard a "popping sound in her arm."

In her lawsuit, the patient claimed that:
• A large sign warned the staff not to touch her arms. The sign was posted by her husband.
• The nurse was negligent for not reading the sign and the patient's chart.
The hospital claimed that:
• There was no sign.
• The nurse did not pull on the patient's arm.
• The patient caused her own injury.
The jury found in favor of the hospital. The hospital did not have to pay damages (Chapter 3) to the patient.

(*Theresa J. Rosen v Verdugo Hills Hospital,* Calif, 1999.) With permission from Medical Malpractice Verdicts, Settlements & Experts; Lewis Laska, Editor, 901 Church St., Nashville, TN 37203-3411, 1-800-298-6288.

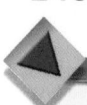

RAISING THE PERSON'S HEAD AND SHOULDERS

✔ Quality of Life *Remember to:*

- Knock before entering the person's room.
- Address the person by name.
- Introduce yourself by name and title.
- Explain the procedure to the person before beginning and during the procedure.

- Protect the person's rights during the procedure.
- Handle the person gently during the procedure.

PRE-PROCEDURE

1 Follow *Delegation Guidelines:*
   - *Preventing Work-Related Injuries,* p. 244
   - *Moving Persons in Bed,* p. 244
   See *Promoting Safety and Comfort:*
   - *Safely Handling, Moving, and Transferring the Person,* p. 240
   - *Preventing Work-Related Injuries,* p. 244
2 Ask a co-worker to assist if you need help.

3 Practice hand hygiene.
4 Identify the person. Check the ID bracelet against the assignment sheet. Also call the person by name.
5 Provide for privacy.
6 Lock the bed wheels.
7 Raise the bed for proper body mechanics. Bed rails are up if used.

PROCEDURE

8 Ask your co-worker to stand on the other side of the bed. Lower the bed rails if up.
9 Ask the person to put the near arm under your near arm and behind your shoulder. His or her hand rests on top of your shoulder. If you are standing on the right side, the person's right hand rests on your shoulder (Fig. 16-6, *A*). The person does the same with your co-worker. The person's left hand rests on your co-worker's left shoulder (Fig. 16-7, *A*).
10 Put your arm nearest to the person under his or her arm. Your hand is on the person's shoulder. Your co-worker does the same.

11 Put your free arm under the person's neck and shoulders (Fig. 16-6, *B*). Your co-worker does the same (Fig. 16-7, *B*).
12 Help the person raise to a sitting or semi-sitting position on the "count of 3" (Figs. 16-6, *C* and 16-7, *C*).
13 Use the arm and hand that supported the person's neck and shoulders to give care (Fig. 16-6, *D*). Your co-worker supports the person (Fig. 16-7, *D*).
14 Help the person lie down. Provide support with your locked arm. Support the person's neck and shoulders with your other arm. Your co-worker does the same.

POST-PROCEDURE

15 Provide for comfort. (See the inside of the front book cover.)
16 Place the signal light within reach.
17 Lower the bed to its lowest position.
18 Raise or lower bed rails. Follow the care plan.

19 Unscreen the person.
20 Complete a safety check of the room. (See the inside of the front book cover.)
21 Decontaminate your hands.
22 Report and record your observations.

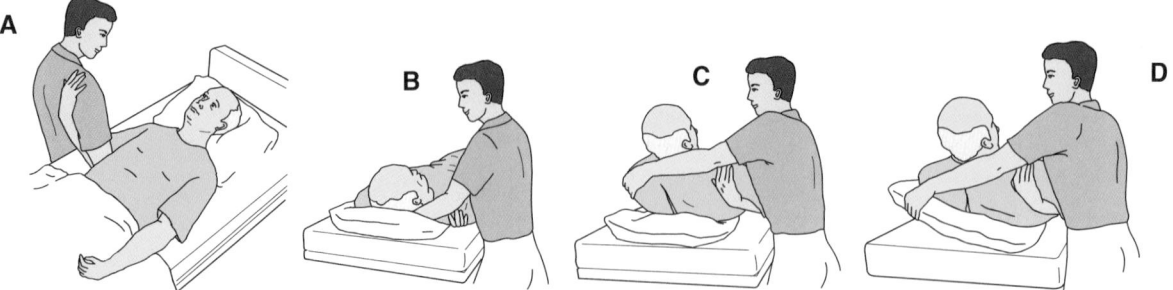

FIGURE 16-6 Raising the person's head and shoulders by locking arms with the person. **A,** The person's near arm is under the nursing assistant's near term and behind the shoulder. **B,** The nursing assistant's far arm is under the person's neck and shoulders, with the near arm under the person's nearest arm. **C,** The person is raised to a semi-sitting position by locking arms. **D,** The nursing assistant lifts the pillow while the person is in a semi-sitting position.

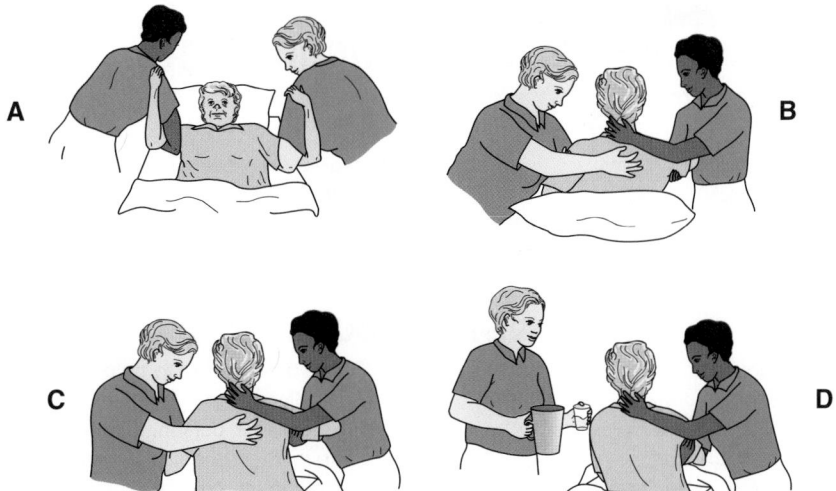

FIGURE 16-7 Raising the person's head and shoulders with a co-worker. **A,** Two nursing assistants lock arms with the person. **B,** The nursing assistants have their arms under the person's head and neck. **C,** The nursing assistants raise the person to a semi-sitting position. **D,** One nursing assistant supports the person in the semi-sitting position while the other gives care.

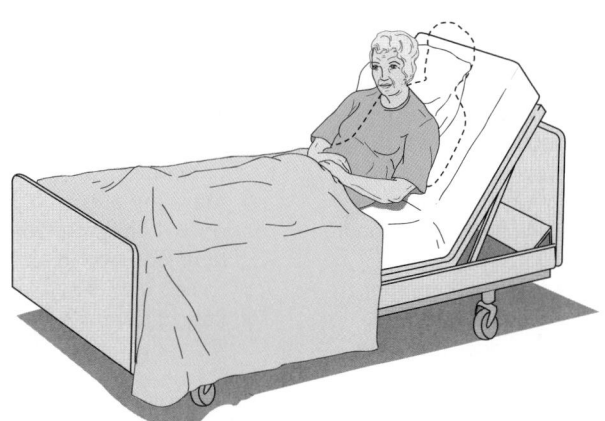

FIGURE 16-8 A person in poor alignment after sliding down in bed.

◆ Moving the Person Up in Bed

When the head of the bed is raised, it is easy to slide down toward the middle and foot of the bed (Fig. 16-8). The person is moved up in bed for good alignment and comfort.

You can usually move small children up in bed alone. You can sometimes move lightweight adults up in bed alone if they can assist and use a trapeze. However, it is best to have help and to use an assist device—lift sheet, large incontinence product, slide sheet (p. 249). Two or more staff members are needed to move heavy, weak, and very old persons up in bed. Always protect the person and yourself from injury.

See *Promoting Safety and Comfort: Moving the Person Up in Bed.*

PROMOTING SAFETY AND COMFORT: Moving the Person Up in Bed

SAFETY

This procedure is best done with at least two staff members. Assist devices are used as directed by the nurse and the care plan.

Perform this procedure alone *only if:*
- The person is small in size.
- The person can follow directions.
- The person can assist with much of the moving.
- The person uses a trapeze.
- The person can push against the mattress with his or her feet.
- The nurse says it is safe to do so.
- You are comfortable doing so.

Follow the nurse's directions and the care plan. Ask any questions before you begin the procedure.

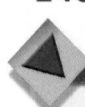

MOVING THE PERSON UP IN BED

✔ Quality of Life *Remember to:*

- Knock before entering the person's room.
- Address the person by name.
- Introduce yourself by name and title.
- Explain the procedure to the person before beginning and during the procedure.

- Protect the person's rights during the procedure.
- Handle the person gently during the procedure.

PRE-PROCEDURE

1 Follow *Delegation Guidelines:*
  - *Preventing Work-Related Injuries,* p. 244
  - *Moving Persons in Bed,* p. 244
  See *Promoting Safety and Comfort:*
  - *Safely Handling, Moving, and Transferring the Person,* p. 240
  - *Preventing Work-Related Injures,* p. 244
  - *Moving the Person Up in Bed,* p. 247

2 Ask a co-worker to help you.
3 Practice hand hygiene.
4 Identify the person. Check the ID bracelet against the assignment sheet. Also call the person by name.
5 Provide for privacy.
6 Lock the bed wheels.
7 Raise the bed for proper body mechanics. Bed rails are up if used.

PROCEDURE

8 Lower the head of the bed to a level appropriate for the person. It is as flat as possible.
9 Stand on one side of the bed. Your co-worker stands on the other side.
10 Lower the bed rails if up.
11 Remove pillows as directed by the nurse. Place a pillow upright against the headboard if the person can be without it.
12 Stand with a wide base of support. Point your foot near the head of the bed toward the head of the bed. Face the head of the bed.
13 Bend your hips and knees. Keep your back straight.
14 Place one arm under the person's shoulder and one arm under the thighs. Your co-worker does the same. Grasp each other's forearms (Fig. 16-9).

15 Ask the person to grasp the trapeze.
16 Have the person flex both knees.
17 Explain the following:
  a You will count "1, 2, 3."
  b The move will be on "3."
  c On "3," the person pushes against the bed with the feet if able. And the person pulls up with the trapeze.
18 Move the person to the head of the bed on the count of "3." Shift your weight from your rear leg to your front leg (see Fig. 16-9). Your co-worker does the same.
19 Repeat steps 12 through 18 if necessary.

POST-PROCEDURE

20 Put the pillow under the person's head and shoulders. Straighten linens.
21 Position the person in good alignment.
22 Provide for comfort. (See the inside of the front book cover.)
23 Place the signal light within reach.
24 Raise the head of the bed to a level appropriate for the person.

25 Lower the bed to its lowest position.
26 Raise or lower bed rails. Follow the care plan.
27 Unscreen the person.
28 Complete a safety check of the room. (See the inside of the front book cover.)
29 Decontaminate your hands.
30 Report and record your observations.

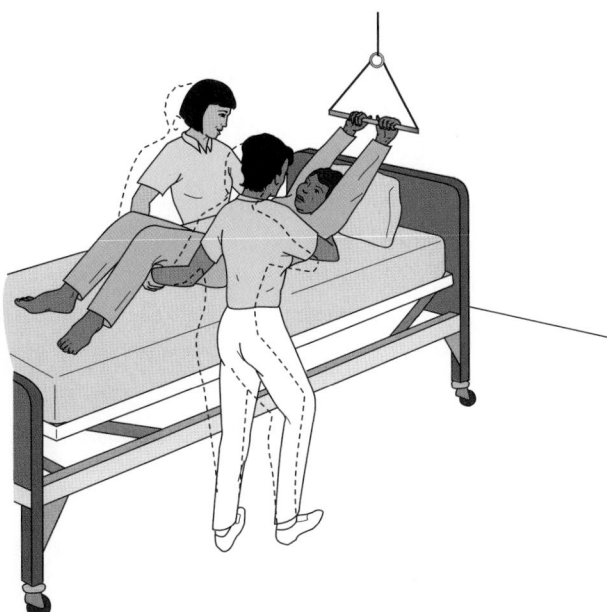

FIGURE 16-9 A person is moved up in bed by two nursing assistants. Each has one arm under the person's shoulders and the other under the thighs. They have locked arms under the person. The person grasps the trapeze and flexes the knees. The nursing assistants shift their weight from the rear leg to the front leg as the person is moved up in bed.

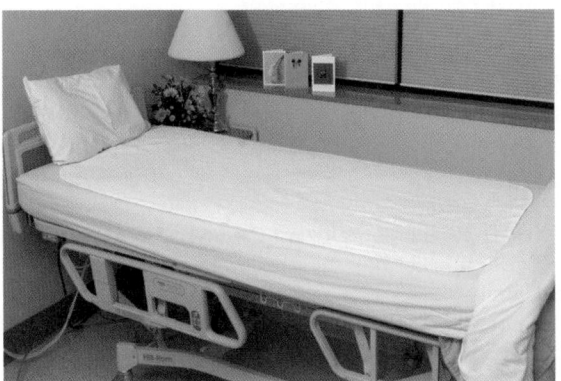

FIGURE 16-10 Turning pad.

Moving the Person Up in Bed With an Assist Device

Assist devices are used to move some persons up in bed. Such assist devices include a drawsheet (lift sheet), flat sheet folded in half, turning pad (Fig. 16-10), slide sheet (Fig. 16-11), and large incontinence product. With these devices, the person is moved more evenly. And the devices reduce shearing and friction.

The device is placed under the person from the head to above the knees or lower. At least two staff members are needed. This procedure is used for most patients and residents. It is used:

▶ Following OSHA recommendations (p. 244)
▶ For persons recovering from spinal cord surgery or spinal cord injuries
▶ For older persons

See *Promoting Safety and Comfort: Moving the Person Up in Bed With an Assist Device.*

PROMOTING SAFETY AND COMFORT: Moving the Person Up in Bed With an Assist Device

SAFETY

Not all incontinence products can be used as assist devices. Disposable, single-use underpads are not strong enough to hold the person's weight during the move. Reusable underpads are stronger. For safety, the underpad must:

• Be strong enough to support the person's weight
• Extend from under the person's head to above the knees or lower
• Be wide enough for you and other staff to get a firm grip for the move

Check with the nurse to make sure the person's underpad is safe to use as an assist device.

If using a slide sheet, you will need to place it under the person. See procedure: *Making an Occupied Bed* in Chapter 18 for this step. After moving the person up in bed, remove the slide sheet. The person is in danger of sliding down in bed or off the bed if the slide sheet is not removed.

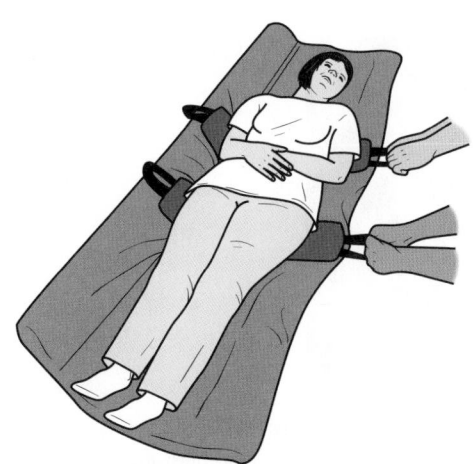

FIGURE 16-11 Slide sheet.

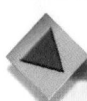

MOVING THE PERSON UP IN BED WITH AN ASSIST DEVICE

✔ **Quality of Life** *Remember to:*

- Knock before entering the person's room.
- Address the person by name.
- Introduce yourself by name and title.
- Explain the procedure to the person before beginning and during the procedure.

- Protect the person's rights during the procedure.
- Handle the person gently during the procedure.

PRE-PROCEDURE

1 Follow *Delegation Guidelines:*
   - *Preventing Work-Related Injuries,* p. 244
   - *Moving Persons in Bed,* p. 244
   See *Promoting Safety and Comfort:*
   - *Safely Handling, Moving, and Transferring the Person,* p. 240
   - *Preventing Work-Related Injuries,* p. 244
   - *Moving the Person Up in Bed,* p. 247
   - *Moving the Person Up in Bed With an Assist Device,* p. 249

2 Ask a co-worker to help you.
3 Practice hand hygiene.
4 Identify the person. Check the ID bracelet against the assignment sheet. Also call the person by name.
5 Provide for privacy.
6 Lock the bed wheels.
7 Raise the bed for proper body mechanics. Bed rails are up if used.

PROCEDURE

8 Lower the head of the bed to a level appropriate for the person. It is as flat as possible.
9 Stand on one side of the bed. Your co-worker stands on the other side.
10 Lower the bed rails if up.
11 Remove pillows as directed by the nurse. Place a pillow upright against the headboard if the person can be without it.
12 Stand with a broad base of support. Point your foot near the head of the bed toward the head of the bed. Face that direction.

13 Roll the sides of the assist device up close to the person. (*NOTE:* Omit this step if the device has handles.)
14 Grasp the rolled-up assist device firmly near the person's shoulders and hips (Fig. 16-12). Or grasp it by the handles. Support the head.
15 Bend your hips and knees.
16 Move the person up in bed on the count of "3." Shift your weight from your rear leg to your front leg.
17 Repeat steps 12 through 16 if necessary.
18 Unroll the assist device. (*NOTE:* Omit this step if the device has handles.)

POST-PROCEDURE

19 Put the pillow under the person's head and shoulders.
20 Position the person in good alignment.
21 Provide for comfort. (See the inside of the front book cover.)
22 Place the signal light within reach.
23 Raise the head of the bed to a level appropriate for the person.

24 Lower the bed to its lowest position.
25 Raise or lower bed rails. Follow the care plan.
26 Unscreen the person.
27 Complete a safety check of the room. (See the inside of the front book cover.)
28 Decontaminate your hands.
29 Report and record your observations.

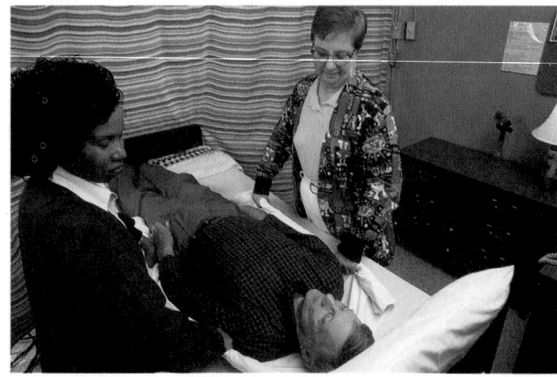

FIGURE 16-12 A drawsheet is used to move the person up in bed. It extends from the person's head to above the knees. Rolled close to the person, the drawsheet is held near the shoulders and hips.

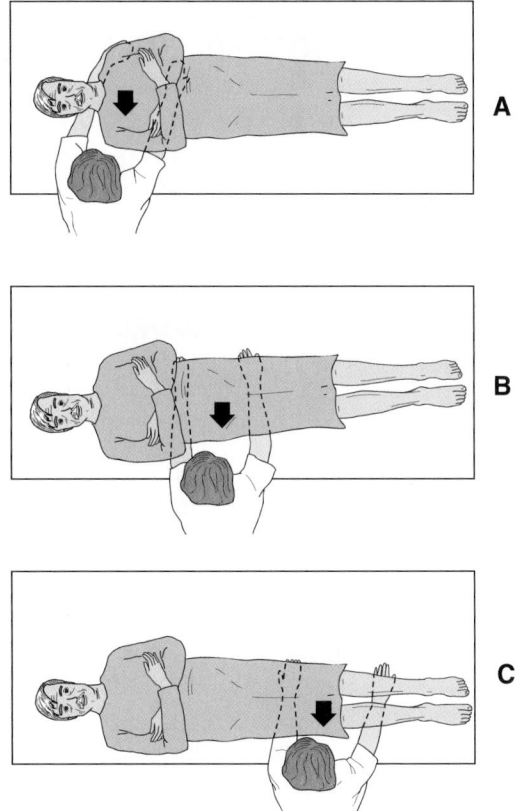

FIGURE 16-13 Moving the person to the side of the bed in segments. **A,** The upper part of the body is moved. **B,** The lower part of the body is moved. **C,** The legs and feet are moved.

Moving the Person to the Side of the Bed

Repositioning and care procedures require moving the person to the side of the bed. The person is moved to the side of the bed before turning. Otherwise, after turning, the person lies on the side of the bed—not in the middle.

Sometimes you have to reach over the person. Giving a bed bath is an example. You reach less if the person is close to you.

One method involves moving the person in segments (Fig. 16-13). Sometimes one person can do this. Use a mechanical lift (p. 264) or the assist device method:

▶ Following OSHA recommendations (p. 244)
▶ For older persons
▶ For persons with arthritis
▶ For persons recovering from spinal cord injuries or spinal cord surgery

Assist devices for this procedure include a drawsheet (lift sheet), flat sheet folded in half, turning pad, slide sheet, slide board, and large incontinence product. Using an assist device helps prevent pain and skin damage. It also helps prevent injury to the bones, joints, and spinal cord.

See *Promoting Safety and Comfort: Moving the Person to the Side of the Bed.*

PROMOTING SAFETY AND COMFORT: Moving the Person to the Side of the Bed

SAFETY

Use the method and equipment that are best for the person. Get this information from the nurse and the care plan when delegated tasks that involve moving the person to the side of the bed. Such tasks include repositioning, bedmaking, bathing, and range-of-motion exercises.

The wrong method could seriously injure a person. This is very important for persons who are very old, have arthritis, or have spinal cord involvement.

When using an assist device, you need at least 1 co-worker to help you. Depending on the person's size, 3 staff members may be needed. You will need to ask 2 co-workers to help you.

If using a slide board or slide sheet, you will need to place it under the person. After moving the person up in bed, remove the device.

To move the person in segments, move the person toward you, not away from you. This helps protect you from injury.

COMFORT

After moving the person to the side of the bed, move the pillow too. Make sure the pillow is positioned correctly. It should be under the person's head and shoulders.

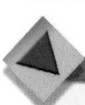

MOVING THE PERSON TO THE SIDE OF THE BED

✔ **Quality of Life** *Remember to:*

- Knock before entering the person's room.
- Address the person by name.
- Introduce yourself by name and title.
- Explain the procedure to the person before beginning and during the procedure.

- Protect the person's rights during the procedure.
- Handle the person gently during the procedure.

PRE-PROCEDURE

1 *Follow Delegation Guidelines:*
   - *Preventing Work-Related Injuries, p. 244*
   - *Moving Persons in Bed, p. 244*
   See *Promoting Safety and Comfort:*
   - *Safely Handling, Moving, and Transferring the Person, p. 240*
   - *Preventing Work-Related Injuries, p. 244*
   - *Moving the Person to the Side of the Bed, p. 251*

2 Ask a co-worker to help you if using an assist device.
3 Practice hand hygiene.
4 Identify the person. Check the ID bracelet against the assignment sheet. Also call the person by name.
5 Provide for privacy.
6 Lock the bed wheels.
7 Raise the bed for proper body mechanics. Bed rails are up if used.

PROCEDURE

8 Lower the head of the bed to a level appropriate for the person. It is as flat as possible.
9 Stand on the side of the bed to which you will move the person.
10 Lower the bed rail near you if bed rails are used. (Both bed rails are lowered for step 15.)
11 Remove pillows as directed by the nurse.
12 Stand with your feet about 12 inches apart. One foot is in front of the other. Flex your knees.
13 Cross the person's arms over the person's chest.
14 *Method 1: Moving the person in segments:*
   a Place your arm under the person's neck and shoulders. Grasp the far shoulder.
   b Place your other arm under the mid-back.
   c Move the upper part of the person's body toward you. Rock backward and shift your weight to your rear leg (see Fig. 16-13, *A*).
   d Place one arm under the person's waist and one under the thighs.

e Rock backward to move the lower part of the person toward you (see Fig. 16-13, *B*).
f Repeat the procedure for the legs and feet (see Fig. 16-13, *C*). Your arms should be under the person's thighs and calves.
15 *Method 2: Moving the person with a drawsheet:*
   a Roll up the drawsheet close to the person (see Fig. 16-12).
   b Grasp the rolled-up drawsheet near the person's shoulders and hips. Your co-worker does the same. Support the person's head.
   c Rock backward on the count of "3," moving the person toward you. Your co-worker rocks backward slightly and then forward toward you while keeping the arms straight.
   d Unroll the drawsheet. Remove any wrinkles.

POST-PROCEDURE

16 Position the person in good alignment.
17 Provide for comfort. (See the inside of the front book cover.)
18 Place the signal light within reach.
19 Lower the bed to its lowest position.
20 Raise or lower bed rails. Follow the care plan.

21 Unscreen the person.
22 Complete a safety check of the room. (See the inside of the front book cover.)
23 Decontaminate your hands.
24 Report and record your observations.

Turning Persons

OLDER PERSONS

Many older persons suffer from arthritis in their spines, hips, and knees. When turning these persons, logrolling is preferred (p. 255). Logrolling may be less painful for these persons.

DELEGATION GUIDELINES: Turning Persons

Before turning and repositioning a person, you need this information from the nurse and the care plan:

- The person's dependency level (see Box 16-2)
- How much help the person needs
- How many staff members are needed to safely complete the procedure
- The person's comfort level and what body parts are painful
- Which procedure to use
- What assist devices to use
- What supportive devices are needed for positioning (Chapter 26)
- Where to place pillows
- What observations to report and record:
  - Who helped you with the procedure
  - How much help the person needed
  - How the person tolerated the procedure
  - How you positioned the person
  - Complaints of pain or discomfort
- When to report observations
- What specific patient or resident concerns to report at once

◆ TURNING PERSONS

Turning persons onto their sides helps prevent complications from bedrest (Chapter 26). Certain procedures and care measures also require the side-lying position. The person is turned toward you or away from you. The direction depends on the person's condition and the situation.

After the person is turned, position him or her in good alignment. Use pillows to support the person in the side-lying position.

Some persons can turn and reposition themselves in bed. Others need help. Some totally depend on the nursing staff for care.

See *Focus on Children and Older Persons: Turning Persons.*
See *Delegation Guidelines: Turning Persons.*
See *Promoting Safety and Comfort: Turning Persons.*

PROMOTING SAFETY AND COMFORT: Turning Persons

SAFETY

Use good body mechanics when turning a person in bed (Chapter 15). Follow the rules in Box 16-1.

The person must be in good alignment. Otherwise, musculoskeletal injuries, skin breakdown, or pressure ulcers could occur.

If using an assist device, ask a co-worker to help you.

Do not turn a person away from you with the far bed rail down. Raise the bed rail on the side near you. Then go to the other side of the bed. Lower that bed rail if up. Turn the person toward you.

COMFORT

After turning, position the person in good alignment. Use pillows as directed to support the person in the side-lying position (Chapter 15). Make sure the person's face, nose, or mouth is not obstructed by a pillow or other device.

NNAAP™ Skill

TURNING AND REPOSITIONING THE PERSON

✔ **Quality of Life** *Remember to:*

- Knock before entering the person's room.
- Address the person by name.
- Introduce yourself by name and title.
- Explain the procedure to the person before beginning and during the procedure.

- Protect the person's rights during the procedure.
- Handle the person gently during the procedure.

PRE-PROCEDURE

1 Follow *Delegation Guidelines:*
- *Preventing Work-Related Injuries, p. 244*
- *Moving Persons in Bed, p. 244*
- *Turning Persons*
See *Promoting Safety and Comfort:*
- *Safely Handling, Moving, and Transferring the Person, p. 240*
- *Preventing Work-Related Injuries, p. 244*
- *Moving the Person to the Side of the Bed, p. 251*
- *Turning Persons*

2 Practice hand hygiene.
3 Identify the person. Check the ID bracelet against the assignment sheet. Also call the person by name.
4 Provide for privacy.
5 Lock the bed wheels.
6 Raise the bed for proper body mechanics. Bed rails are up if used.

Continued

TURNING AND REPOSITIONING THE PERSON—cont'd

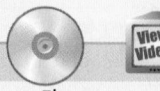

PROCEDURE

7 Lower the head of the bed to a level appropriate for the person. It is as flat as possible.

8 Stand on the side of the bed opposite to where you will turn the person. The far bed rail is up if used.

9 Lower the bed rail near you if used.

10 Move the person to the side near you. (See procedure: *Moving the Person to the Side of the Bed,* p. 252.)

11 Cross the person's arms over the person's chest. Cross the leg near you over the far leg.

12 *Turning the person away from you:*
  a Stand with a wide base of support. Flex the knees.
  b Place one hand on the person's shoulder. Place the other on the hip near you.
  c Push the person gently toward the other side of the bed (Fig. 16-14, *A*). Shift your weight from your rear leg to your front leg.

13 *Turning the person toward you:*
  a Raise the bed rail if used.
  b Go to the other side of the bed. Lower the bed rail if used.

  c Stand with a wide base of support. Flex your knees.
  d Place one hand on the person's far shoulder. Place the other on the far hip.
  e Roll the person toward you gently (Fig. 16-14, *B*).

14 Position the person. Follow the nurse's directions and the care plan. The following is common:
  a Place a pillow under the head and neck.
  b Adjust the shoulder. The person should not lie on an arm.
  c Place a small pillow under the upper hand and arm.
  d Position a pillow against the back.
  e Flex the upper knee. Position the upper leg in front of the lower leg.
  f Support the upper leg and thigh on pillows. Make sure the ankle is supported.

POST-PROCEDURE

15 Provide for comfort. (See the inside of the front book cover.)

16 Place the signal light within reach.

17 Lower the bed to its lowest position.

18 Raise or lower bed rails. Follow the care plan.

19 Unscreen the person.

20 Complete a safety check of the room. (See the inside of the front book cover.)

21 Decontaminate your hands.

22 Report and record your observations.

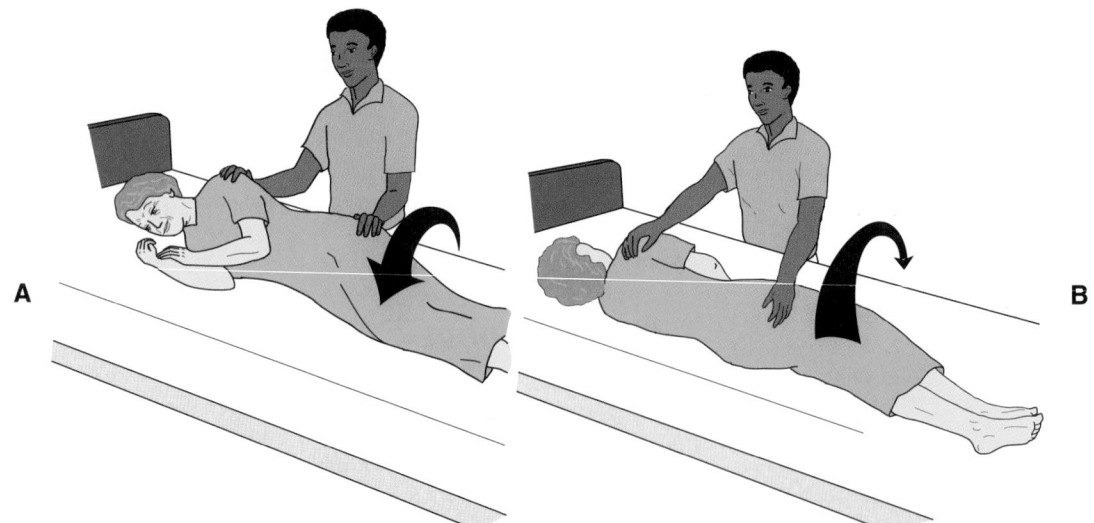

FIGURE 16-14 Turning the person. **A,** Turning the person away from you. **B,** Turning the person toward you.

◀ Logrolling

Logrolling is turning the person as a unit, in alignment, with one motion. The spine is kept straight. The procedure is used to turn:

▶ Older persons with arthritic spines or knees
▶ Persons recovering from hip fractures
▶ Persons with spinal cord injuries (the spine is kept straight at all times after spinal cord injury)
▶ Persons recovering from spinal surgery (the spine is kept straight all times after spinal surgery)
  See *Promoting Safety and Comfort: Logrolling.*

PROMOTING SAFETY AND COMFORT: Logrolling

SAFETY
Two or three staff members are needed to logroll a person. Three are needed if the person is tall or heavy. Sometimes an assist device is needed—drawsheet, turning pad, large incontinence product, slide sheet.

COMFORT
After spinal cord injury or surgery, the spine must be kept straight. This includes the person's neck. Therefore, *usually a pillow is not allowed under the head and neck.* Follow the nurse's directions and the care plan for positioning the person and using pillows.

LOGROLLING THE PERSON

✔ Quality of Life *Remember to:*

- Knock before entering the person's room.
- Address the person by name.
- Introduce yourself by name and title.
- Explain the procedure to the person before beginning and during the procedure.

- Protect the person's rights during the procedure.
- Handle the person gently during the procedure.

PRE-PROCEDURE

1 Follow *Delegation Guidelines:*
  • *Preventing Work-Related Injuries,* p. 244
  • *Moving Persons in Bed,* p. 244
  • *Turning Persons,* p. 253
  See *Promoting Safety and Comfort:*
  • *Safely Handling, Moving, and Transferring the Person,* p. 240
  • *Preventing Work-Related Injuries,* p. 244
  • *Turning Persons,* p. 253
  • *Logrolling*

2 Ask a co-worker to help you.
3 Practice hand hygiene.
4 Identify the person. Check the ID bracelet against the assignment sheet. Also call the person by name.
5 Provide for privacy.
6 Lock the bed wheels.
7 Raise the bed for proper body mechanics. Bed rails are up if used.

PROCEDURE

8 Make sure the bed is flat.
9 Stand on the side opposite to which you will turn the person. Your co-worker stands on the other side.
10 Lower the bed rails if used.
11 Move the person as a unit to the side of the bed near you. Use the assist device.
12 Place the person's arms across the chest. Place a pillow between the knees.
13 Raise the bed rail if used.
14 Go to the other side.
15 Stand near the shoulders and chest. Your co-worker stands near the hips and thighs.
16 Stand with a broad base of support. One foot is in front of the other.

17 Ask the person to hold his or her body rigid.
18 Roll the person toward you (Fig. 16-15, A, p. 256). Or use the assist device (Fig. 16-15, B, p. 256). Turn the person as a unit.
19 Position the person in good alignment. Use pillows as directed by the nurse and the care plan. The following is common (unless the spinal cord is involved):
  • One pillow against the back for support
  • One pillow under the head and neck if allowed
  • One pillow or a folded bath blanket between the legs
  • A small pillow under the upper arm and hand

POST-PROCEDURE

20 Provide for comfort. (See the inside of the front book cover.)
21 Place the signal light within reach.
22 Lower the bed to its lowest position.
23 Raise or lower bed rails. Follow the care plan.

24 Unscreen the person.
25 Complete a safety check of the room. (See the inside of the front book cover.)
26 Decontaminate your hands.
27 Report and record your observations.

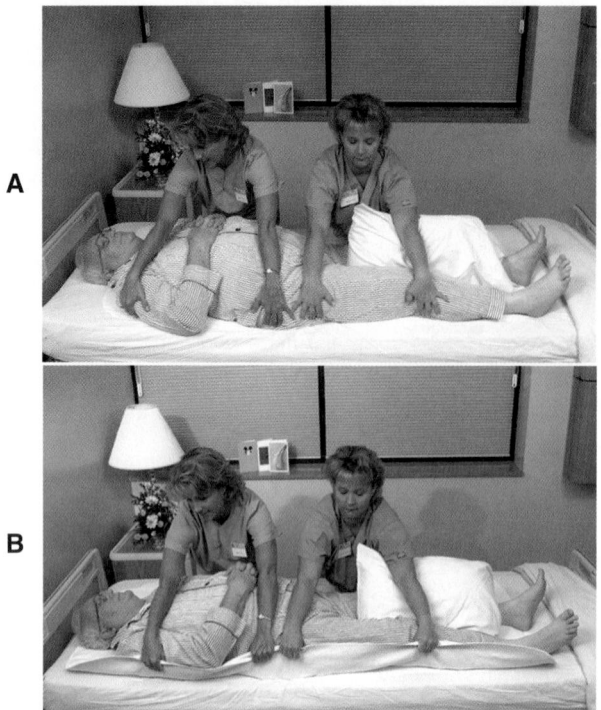

FIGURE 16-15 Logrolling. **A,** A pillow is between the person's legs. The arms are crossed on the chest. The person is on the far side of the bed. **B,** The assist device is used to logroll the person.

◆ SITTING ON THE SIDE OF THE BED (DANGLING)

Residents sit on the side of the bed *(dangle)* for many reasons. Many older persons become dizzy or faint when getting out of bed too fast. They may need to sit on the side of the bed for 1 to 5 minutes before walking or transferring. Some persons increase activity in stages—bedrest, to sitting on the side of the bed, and then to sitting in a chair. Walking is the next step.

While dangling the legs, the person coughs and deep breathes. He or she moves the legs back and forth in circles. This stimulates circulation.

Two staff members may be needed. Persons with balance and coordination problems need support. If dizziness or fainting occurs, lay the person down.

See *Focus on Children and Older Persons: Dangling.*
See *Delegation Guidelines: Dangling.*
See *Promoting Safety and Comfort: Dangling.*

FOCUS ON **CHILDREN** AND **OLDER PERSONS**

Dangling

Many older persons have circulatory changes. They may become dizzy or faint when getting up too fast. They may need to sit on the side of the bed for a few minutes before a transfer or walking.

DELEGATION GUIDELINES: Dangling

The nurse may ask you to help a person sit on the side of the bed. The procedure is part of other tasks—assisting the person to stand, transferring from bed to chair, partial bath, and others. When delegated the dangling procedure or tasks that involve dangling, you need this information from the nurse and the care plan:
- Areas of weakness (For example, if the person's arms are weak, he or she cannot hold onto the side of the mattress for support. If the left side is weak, turn the person onto the stronger right side. The person can use the right arm to help move from the lying to sitting position.)
- The person's dependence level (see Box 16-2)
- The amount of help the person needs
- If you need a co-worker to help you
- How long the person needs to sit on the side of the bed
- What exercises the person needs to perform while dangling:
  - Leg and foot exercises (Chapter 31)
  - Range-of-motion exercises (Chapter 26)
  - Deep-breathing and coughing exercises (Chapter 34)
- If the person will walk or transfer to a chair after dangling
- What observations to report and record (Fig. 16-16):
  - Pulse and respiratory rates (Chapter 25)
  - Pale or bluish skin color (cyanosis)
  - Complaints of dizziness, light-headedness, or difficulty breathing
  - How well the activity was tolerated
  - The length of time the person dangled
  - The amount of help needed
  - Other observations and complaints
- When to report observations
- What specific patient or resident concerns to report at once

PROMOTING SAFETY AND COMFORT: Dangling

SAFETY
This procedure is not used for persons with these dependence levels:
- Code 4: Total Dependence
- Code 3: Extensive Assistance

Problems with sitting and balance often occur after illness, injury, surgery, and bedrest. Some persons who are disabled also have problems sitting and with balance. Provide support when the person is sitting on the side of the bed. This protects the person from falling and other injuries.

COMFORT
Provide for the person's warmth during the dangling procedure. Help the person put on a robe. Or cover the person's shoulders and back with a bath blanket.

The person may want to perform simple hygiene measures while sitting on the side of the bed. Oral hygiene and washing the face and hands are examples (Chapter 19). These measures refresh the person and stimulate circulation. Follow the nurse's directions and the care plan.

	Date	Time	Nursing Margin	Other Depts Margin	
	9/9	0900			Assisted to sit on the side of the bed with assistance of one.
					Active leg exercises performed. Tolerated procedure without
					complaints of pain or discomfort. No c/o dizziness. BP-130/78 L
					arm sitting, P-74 regular rate and rhythm, R-20 unlabored. Color
					good. Assisted to lie down after 5 minutes. Positioned on L side.
					Bed in low position, signal light within reach. Adam Aims, CNA ———

FIGURE 16-16 Charting sample.

SITTING ON THE SIDE OF THE BED (DANGLING)

✔ Quality of Life *Remember to:*

- Knock before entering the person's room.
- Address the person by name.
- Introduce yourself by name and title.
- Explain the procedure to the person before beginning and during the procedure.

- Protect the person's rights during the procedure.
- Handle the person gently during the procedure.

PRE-PROCEDURE

1 Follow *Delegation Guidelines:*
   - *Preventing Work-Related Injuries,* p. 244
   - *Dangling*
   See *Promoting Safety and Comfort:*
   - *Safely Handling, Moving, and Transferring the Person,* p. 240
   - *Preventing Work-Related Injuries,* p. 244
   - *Dangling*
2 Practice hand hygiene.

3 Identify the person. Check the ID bracelet against the assignment sheet. Also call the person by name.
4 Provide for privacy.
5 Decide what side of the bed to use.
6 Move furniture to provide moving space.
7 Lock the bed wheels.
8 Raise the bed for proper body mechanics. Bed rails are up if used.

PROCEDURE

9 Lower the bed rail if up.
10 Position the person in a side-lying position facing you. The person lies on the strong side.
11 Raise the head of the bed to a sitting position.
12 Stand by the person's hips. Face the foot of the bed.
13 Stand with your feet apart. The foot near the head of the bed is in front of the other foot.
14 Slide one arm under the person's neck and shoulders. Grasp the far shoulder. Place your other hand over the thighs near the knees (Fig. 16-17, A, p. 258).
15 Pivot toward the foot of the bed while moving the person's legs and feet over the side of the bed. As the legs go over the edge of the mattress, the trunk is upright (Fig. 16-17, B, p. 258).
16 Ask the person to hold onto the edge of the mattress. This supports the person in the sitting position.

17 Do not leave the person alone. Provide support if necessary.
18 Check the person's condition:
   - Ask how the person feels. Ask if the person feels dizzy or light-headed.
   - Check the pulse and respirations.
   - Check for difficulty breathing.
   - Note if the skin is pale or bluish in color *(cyanosis).*
19 Help the person lie down if necessary.
20 Reverse the procedure to return the person to bed.
21 Lower the head of the bed after the person returns to bed. Help him or her move to the center of the bed.
22 Position the person in good alignment.

POST-PROCEDURE

23 Provide for comfort. (See the inside of the front book cover.)
24 Place the signal light within reach.
25 Lower the bed to its lowest position.
26 Raise or lower bed rails. Follow the care plan.
27 Return furniture to its proper place.

28 Unscreen the person.
29 Complete a safety check of the room. (See the inside of the front book cover.)
30 Decontaminate your hands.
31 Report and record your observations.

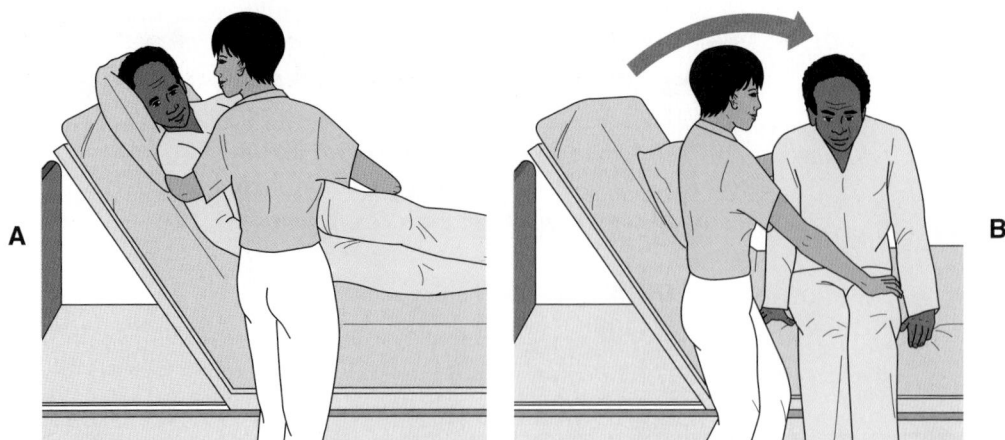

FIGURE 16-17 Helping the person sit on the side of the bed. **A,** The person's shoulders and thighs are supported. **B,** The person sits upright as the legs and feet are pulled over the edge of the bed.

TRANSFERRING PERSONS

Patients and residents are moved to and from beds, chairs, wheelchairs, shower chairs, commodes, toilets, and stretchers. The amount of help needed and the method used vary with the person's dependency level (see Box 16-2). Some persons transfer by themselves or need little help. Some persons need help from at least 1, 2, or 3 people.

The rules of body mechanics apply to transfers (Chapter 15). So do guidelines in Box 16-1. Arrange the room so there is enough space for a safe transfer. Correct placement of the chair, wheelchair, or other device also is needed for a safe transfer.

See *Delegation Guidelines: Transferring Persons.*

See *Promoting Safety and Comfort: Transferring Persons.*

See *Teamwork and Time Management: Transferring Persons.*

Transfer Belts

Transfer belts were discussed in Chapter 11. Also called gait belts, they are used to support patients and residents during transfers. They also are used to reposition persons in chairs and wheelchairs (p. 270).

Wider belts have padded handles. They are easier to grip and allow better control should the person fall.

DELEGATION GUIDELINES: Transferring Persons

When delegated transferring procedures, you need this information from the nurse and the care plan:
* What procedure to use.
* The person's dependency level (Box 16-2).
* The amount of help the person needs.
* What equipment to use—transfer belt, wheelchair, mechanical assist device, positioning devices, wheelchair cushion, or other.
* The person's height and weight.
* How many staff members are needed to complete the transfer safely.
* Areas of weakness. For example, if the person's arms are weak, the person cannot hold onto the mattress for support. If the person has a weak left side, he or she gets out of bed on the stronger right side. The person uses the right arm to help move from the lying to the sitting position.
* What observations to report and record:
    * Pulse rate before and after the transfer (Chapter 25)
    * Complaints of light-headedness, pain, discomfort, difficulty breathing, weakness, or fatigue
    * The amount of help needed to transfer the person
    * How the person helped with the transfer
* When to report observations.
* What specific patient or resident concerns to report at once.

PROMOTING SAFETY AND COMFORT: Transferring Persons

SAFETY

The person wears non-skid footwear for transfers. Such footwear protects the person from falls. Slipping and sliding are prevented. Remember to securely tie shoelaces. Otherwise, the person can trip and fall.

Lock bed, wheelchair, stretcher, or other assist device wheels. This prevents the bed and the device from moving during the transfer. Otherwise, the person can fall. You also are at risk for injury.

COMFORT

After the transfer, position the person in good alignment. Make sure needed items are within reach.

TEAMWORK AND TIME MANAGEMENT

Transferring Persons

Mechanical assist devices are used to transfer some residents. After using such a device, return it to the storage area. It needs to be available for use by other staff. Do not leave a device in a person's room or other care setting. Your co-workers should not have to assume that an assist device is in use or take time looking for one.

Many mechanical assist devices are battery-operated. The battery must be charged for the device to work properly. Follow agency policy for charging or replacing batteries.

You may need help from 1 or 2 co-workers to safely transfer a person. Politely ask co-workers to help you. Tell them what time you need the help and for how long. This helps them plan their own work. Always thank your co-workers for helping you. Willingly help them when asked.

◆ Bed to Chair or Wheelchair Transfers

Safety is important for chair, wheelchair, commode, and shower chair transfers. Help the person out of bed on his or her strong side. If the left side is weak and the right side strong, get the person out of bed on the right side. In transferring, the strong side moves first. It pulls the weaker side along. Transfers from the weak side are awkward and unsafe.

The following stand and pivot transfers are used if:
▶ The person's legs are strong enough to bear some or all of his or her weight.
▶ The person is cooperative and can follow directions.
▶ The person can assist with the transfer.

See *Focus on Children and Older Persons: Bed to Chair or Wheelchair Transfers.*

See *Promoting Safety and Comfort: Bed to Chair or Wheelchair Transfers.*

FOCUS ON **CHILDREN** AND **OLDER PERSONS**

Bed to Chair or Wheelchair Transfers: Older Persons

Some residents cannot assist in transfers to or from chairs or wheelchairs. For those residents, a mechanical lift is used (p. 264).

PROMOTING SAFETY AND COMFORT: Bed to Chair or Wheelchair Transfers

SAFETY

The chair, wheelchair, or other device must support the person's weight. The number of staff members needed for a transfer depends on the person's abilities, condition, and size. For some persons, you will need to use mechanical assist devices (p. 264). Full-sling lifts or stand-assist lifts are examples.

The person must not put his or her arms around your neck. Otherwise, the person can pull you forward or cause you to lose your balance. Neck, back, and other injuries from falls are possible. Bed and wheelchair wheels are locked for a safe transfer.

If not using a mechanical assist device, using a gait/transfer belt is the preferred method for chair or wheelchair transfers. It is safer for the person and you. Putting your arms around the person and grasping the shoulder blades is the other method. It can cause the person discomfort. And it can be stressful for you. Use this method *only* if instructed to do so by the nurse and the care plan.

Wheelchair wheels are locked for a safe transfer. After the transfer, unlock the wheels to position the wheelchair as the person prefers. After positioning the chair, lock the wheels or keep them unlocked according to the care plan. Locked wheels may be considered to be restraints if the person cannot unlock them to move the wheelchair (Chapter 13). However, falls and other injuries are risks if the person tries to stand when the wheelchair wheels are unlocked.

COMFORT

Most wheelchairs and bedside chairs have vinyl seats and backs. Vinyl holds body heat. The person becomes warm and perspires more. You can cover the back and seat with a folded bath blanket. This increases the person's comfort in the chair. Some people have wheelchair cushions or positioning devices. Ask the nurse how to use and place the devices. Also follow the manufacturer's instructions.

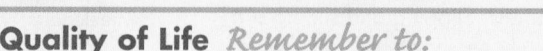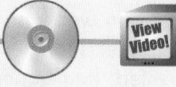

TRANSFERRING THE PERSON TO A CHAIR OR WHEELCHAIR

✔ Quality of Life *Remember to:*

- Knock before entering the person's room.
- Address the person by name.
- Introduce yourself by name and title.
- Explain the procedure to the person before beginning and during the procedure.

- Protect the person's rights during the procedure.
- Handle the person gently during the procedure.

PRE-PROCEDURE

1 Follow *Delegation Guidelines:*
- *Preventing Work-Related Injuries,* p. 244
- *Transferring Persons,* p. 258

See *Promoting Safety and Comfort:*
- *Transfer/Gait Belts* (Chapter 11)
- *Safely Handling, Moving, and Transferring the Person,* p. 240
- *Preventing Work-Related Injuries,* p. 244
- *Transferring Persons,* p. 259
- *Bed to Chair or Wheelchair Transfers,* p. 259

2 Collect:
- Wheelchair or arm chair
- Bath blanket

- Lap blanket
- Robe and non-skid footwear
- Paper or sheet
- Transfer belt (if needed)
- Seat cushion (if needed)

3 Practice hand hygiene.

4 Identify the person. Check the ID bracelet against the assignment sheet. Also call the person by name.

5 Provide for privacy.

6 Decide which side of the bed to use. Move furniture for a safe transfer.

PROCEDURE

7 Place the chair near the bed on the person's strong side. The arm of the chair should almost touch the bed.

8 Place a folded bath blanket or cushion on the seat (if needed).

9 Lock the wheelchair wheels. Raise the footplates. Remove or swing the front rigging out of the way.

10 Lower the bed to its lowest position. Lock the bed wheels.

11 Fan-fold top linens to the foot of the bed.

12 Place the paper or sheet under the person's feet. Put footwear on the person.

13 Help the person sit on the side of the bed (p. 256). His or her feet touch the floor.

14 Help the person put on a robe.

15 Apply the transfer belt if needed (Chapter 11).

16 *Method 1: Using a transfer belt:*
- **a** Stand in front of the person.
- **b** Have the person hold onto the mattress.
- **c** Make sure the person's feet are flat on the floor.
- **d** Have the person lean forward.
- **e** Grasp the transfer belt at each side. Grasp the handles or grasp the belt from underneath.
- **f** Prevent the person from sliding or falling by doing one of the following:
  - (1) Brace your knees against the person's knees. Block his or her feet with your feet (Fig. 16-18).
  - (2) Use the knee and foot of one leg to block the person's weak leg or foot. Place your other foot slightly behind you for balance.
  - (3) Straddle your legs around the person's weak leg.

- **g** Explain the following:
  - (1) You will count "1, 2, 3."
  - (2) The move will be on "3."
  - (3) On "3," the person pushes down on the mattress and stands.
- **h** Ask the person to push down on the mattress and to stand on the count of "3."
- **i** Pull the person to a standing position as you straighten your knees (Fig. 16-19).

17 *Method 2: No transfer belt:* (NOTE: Use this method only if directed by the nurse and the care plan.)
- **a** Follow steps 16 a-c.
- **b** Place your hands under the person's arms. Your hands are around the person's shoulder blades (Fig. 16-20, p. 262).
- **c** Have the person lean forward.
- **d** Prevent the person from sliding or falling by doing one of the following:
  - (1) Brace your knees against the person's knees. Block his or her feet with your feet.
  - (2) Use the knee and foot of one leg to block the person's weak leg or foot. Place your other foot slightly behind you for balance.
  - (3) Straddle your legs around the person's weak leg.
- **e** Explain the "count of 3." See step 16-g.
- **f** Ask the person to push down on the mattress and to stand on the count of "3." Pull the person up into a standing position as you straighten your knees.

TRANSFERRING THE PERSON
TO A CHAIR OR WHEELCHAIR—cont'd

PROCEDURE—cont'd

18 Support the person in the standing position. Hold the transfer belt, or keep your hands around the person's shoulder blades. Continue to prevent the person from sliding or falling.

19 Turn the person so he or she can grasp the far arm of the chair. The legs will touch the edge of the chair (Fig. 16-21, p. 262).

20 Continue to turn the person until the other armrest is grasped.

21 Lower him or her into the chair as you bend your hips and knees. The person assists by leaning forward and bending the elbows and knees (Fig. 16-22, p. 262).

22 Make sure the buttocks are to the back of the seat. Position the person in good alignment.

23 Attach the wheelchair front rigging. Position the person's feet on the wheelchair footplates.

24 Cover the person's lap and legs with a lap blanket. Keep the blanket off the floor and the wheels.

25 Remove the transfer belt if used.

26 Position the chair as the person prefers. Lock the wheelchair wheels according to the care plan.

POST-PROCEDURE

27 Provide for comfort. (See the inside of the front book cover.)

28 Place the signal light and other needed items within reach.

29 Unscreen the person.

30 Complete a safety check of the room. (See the inside of the front book cover.)

31 Decontaminate your hands.

32 Report and record your observations.

33 See procedure: *Transferring the Person From a Chair or Wheelchair to Bed* (p. 263) to return the person to bed.

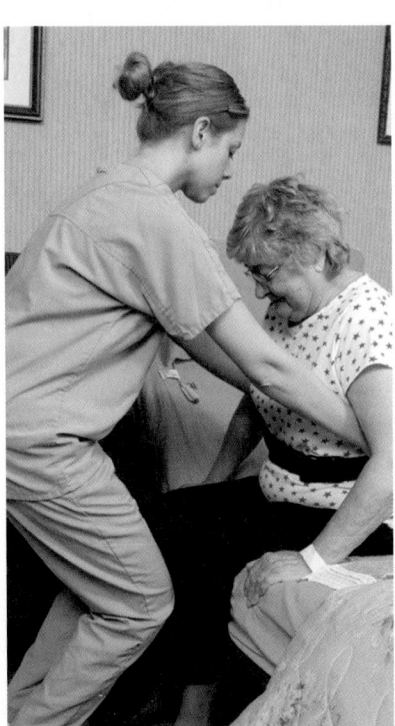

FIGURE 16-18 Transferring the person to a chair using a transfer belt. The person's feet and knees are blocked by the nursing assistant's feet and knees. This prevents the person from sliding or falling.

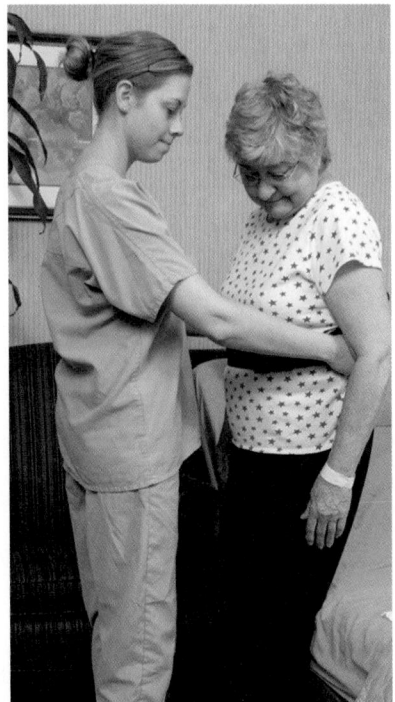

FIGURE 16-19 The person is pulled up to a standing position and supported by holding the transfer belt and blocking the person's knees and feet.

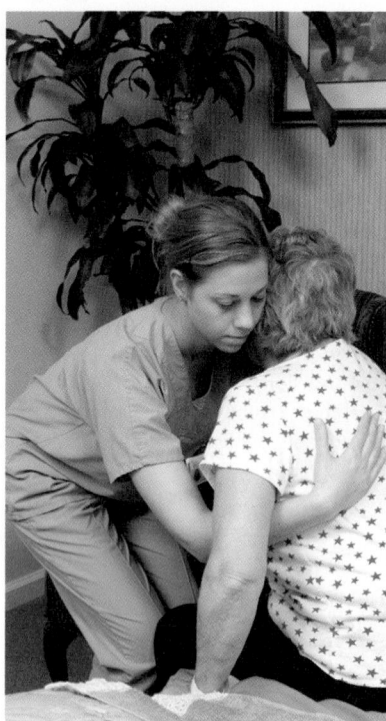

FIGURE 16-20 The person is being prepared to stand. The hands are placed under the person's arms and around the shoulder blades.

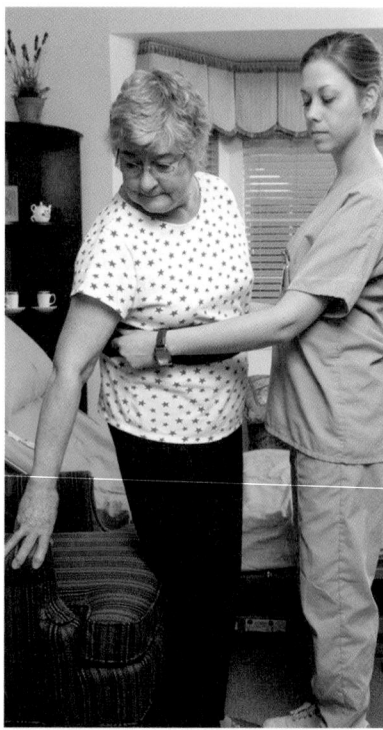

FIGURE 16-21 The person is supported as he or she grasps the far arm of the chair. The legs are against the chair.

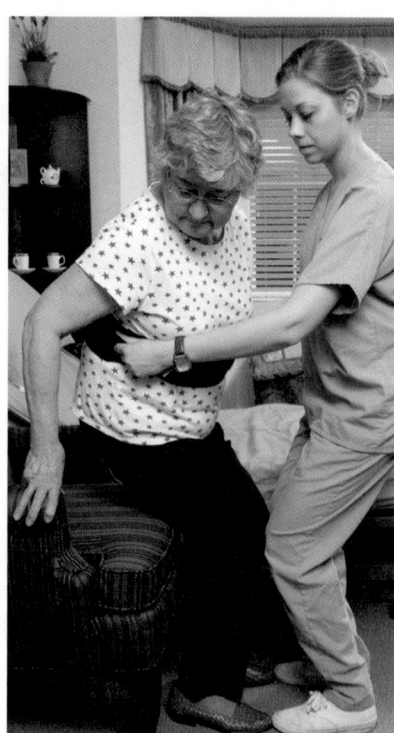

FIGURE 16-22 The person holds the armrests, leans forward, and bends the elbows and knees while being lowered into the chair.

◆ Chair or Wheelchair to Bed Transfers

Chair or wheelchair to bed transfers have the same rules as bed to chair transfers. If the person is weak on one side, transfer the person so that the strong side moves first. Therefore the person is transferred to bed on the opposite side from which the person transferred out of bed. Or the chair or wheelchair is positioned so the strong side is near the bed so it moves first.

For example, Mrs. Lee's right side is weak. Her left side is strong. To transfer her from bed to chair, the chair was on the left side of the bed. This allowed her left side (strong side) to move first. Now you will transfer Mrs. Lee back to bed. If the chair is on the left side of the bed, her right side—the weak side—is near the bed. It is unsafe to move the weak side first. You need to move the chair to the other side of the bed or turn the chair around. Mrs. Lee's stronger left side will be near the bed. The stronger side moves first for a safe transfer.

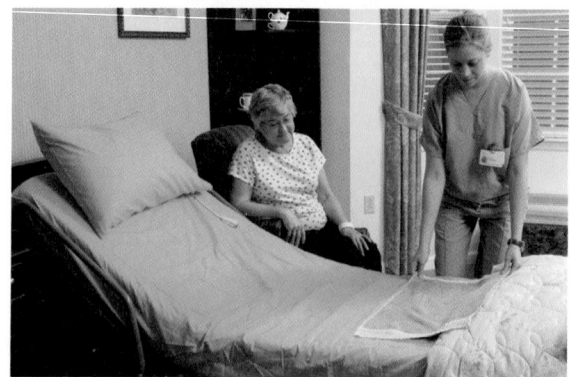

FIGURE 16-23 The chair is on the person's strong side.

TRANSFERRING THE PERSON FROM A CHAIR OR WHEELCHAIR TO BED

✔ Quality of Life *Remember to:*

- Knock before entering the person's room.
- Address the person by name.
- Introduce yourself by name and title.
- Explain the procedure to the person before beginning and during the procedure.

- Protect the person's rights during the procedure.
- Handle the person gently during the procedure.

PRE-PROCEDURE

1 Follow *Delegation Guidelines:*
  - *Preventing Work-Related Injuries,* p. 244
  - *Transferring Persons,* p. 258
  See *Promoting Safety and Comfort:*
  - *Transfer/Gait Belts* (Chapter 11)
  - *Safely Handling, Moving, and Transferring the Person,* p. 240
  - *Preventing Work-Related Injuries,* p. 244

  - *Transferring Persons,* p. 259
  - *Bed to Chair or Wheelchair Transfers,* p. 259
2 Collect a transfer belt if needed.
3 Practice hand hygiene.
4 Identify the person. Check the ID bracelet against the assignment sheet. Also call the person by name.
5 Provide for privacy.

PROCEDURE

6 Move furniture for moving space.
7 Raise the head of the bed to a sitting position. The bed is in the lowest position.
8 Move the signal light so it is on the strong side when the person is in bed.
9 Position the chair or wheelchair so the person's strong side is next to the bed (Fig. 16-23). Have a co-worker help you if necessary.
10 Lock the wheelchair and bed wheels.
11 Remove and fold the lap blanket.
12 Remove the person's feet from the footplates. Raise the footplates. Remove or swing the front rigging out of the way.
13 Apply the transfer belt (if needed).
14 Make sure the person's feet are flat on the floor.
15 Stand in front of the person.
16 Ask the person to hold onto the armrests. Or place your arms under the person's arms. Your hands are around the shoulder blades.
17 Have the person lean forward.
18 Grasp the transfer belt on each side if using it. Grasp underneath the belt.

19 Prevent the person from sliding or falling by doing one of the following:
  a Brace your knees against the person's knees. Block his or her feet with your feet.
  b Use the knee and foot of one leg to block the person's weak leg or foot. Place your other foot slightly behind you for balance.
  c Straddle your legs around the person's weak leg.
20 Explain the "count of 3." (See procedure: *Transferring the Person to a Chair or Wheelchair,* p. 260.)
21 Ask the person to push down on the armrests on the count of "3." Pull the person into a standing position as you straighten your knees.
22 Support the person in the standing position. Hold the transfer belt, or keep your hands around the person's shoulder blades. Continue to prevent the person from sliding or falling.
23 Turn the person so he or she can reach the edge of the mattress. The legs will touch the mattress.
24 Continue to turn the person until he or she can reach the mattress with both hands.
25 Lower him or her onto the bed as you bend your hips and knees. The person assists by leaning forward and bending the elbows and knees.
26 Remove the transfer belt.
27 Remove the robe and footwear.
28 Help the person lie down.

POST-PROCEDURE

29 Provide for comfort. (See the inside of the front book cover.)
30 Place the signal light and other needed items within reach.
31 Raise or lower bed rails. Follow the care plan.
32 Arrange furniture to meet the person's needs.

33 Unscreen the person.
34 Complete a safety check of the room. (See the inside of the front book cover.)
35 Decontaminate your hands.
36 Report and record your observations.

Mechanical Lifts

Persons who cannot help themselves are transferred with mechanical lifts. So are persons too heavy for the staff to transfer. The devices are used for transfers to and from beds, chairs, stretchers, tubs, shower chairs, toilets, commodes, whirlpools, or vehicles.

There are manual, battery-operated, and electric lifts. Some lifts are mounted on the ceiling.

Slings

The type of sling used depends on the person's size, condition, and other needs. Slings are padded, unpadded, or made of mesh.

▶ Standard full sling—used for normal transfers.
▶ Extended length sling—used for persons with extra large thighs.
▶ Bathing sling—used to transfer the person directly from the bed or chair into a bathtub. The sling is left in placed and attached to the lift during the bath.
▶ Toileting sling—the sling bottom is open. For infection control, each person should have his or her own toileting sling.
▶ Amputee sling—used for the person who has had both legs amputated (double amputee).

Follow agency policy and the manufacturer's instructions for washing slings. Also follow agency policy for handling and washing contaminated slings. A sling is considered contaminated when the sling:

▶ Has any visible sign of blood, body fluids, secretions, or excretions
▶ Is used on a person's bare skin
▶ Is used to bathe a person

◀ Using a Mechanical Lift

Before using a lift:
▶ You must be trained in its use.
▶ It must work.
▶ The sling, straps, hooks, and chains must be in good repair.
▶ The person's weight must not exceed the lift's capacity.
▶ At least two staff members are needed.

There are different types of mechanical lifts. Always follow the manufacturer's instructions. The following procedure is used as a guide.

See *Delegation Guidelines: Using Mechanical Lifts.*

See *Promoting Safety and Comfort: Using Mechanical Lifts.*

DELEGATION GUIDELINES: Using Mechanical Lifts

When you are delegated tasks that involve using a mechanical lift, you need this information from the nurse and the care plan:

• The person's dependency level (see Box 16-2)
• What lift to use
• What sling to use—full, extended length, bathing, toileting, amputee
• If you should use a padded, unpadded, or mesh sling
• How many staff members are needed to perform the task safely

---

PROMOTING SAFETY AND COMFORT: Using Mechanical Lifts

SAFETY
Mechanical lifts vary among manufacturers. Also, manufacturers have different models. Knowing how to use one lift does not mean that you know how to use others. Always follow the manufacturer's instructions.

If you have questions, ask the nurse. If you have not used a certain lift before, ask for needed training. Ask the nurse to help you use it the first time and until you are comfortable using the lift.

Mechanical lifts must be in good working order. Tell the nurse when a lift needs repair or is not working properly.

Some mechanical lifts are powered by batteries. The batteries must be well-charged. Follow the manufacturer's instructions.

COMFORT
The person will be lifted up and off the bed or chair. Falling from the lift is a common fear. To promote the person's mental comfort, always explain the procedure before you begin. Also show the person how the lift works.

TRANSFERRING THE PERSON USING A MECHANICAL LIFT

✔ Quality of Life *Remember to:*

- Knock before entering the person's room.
- Address the person by name.
- Introduce yourself by name and title.
- Explain the procedure to the person before beginning and during the procedure.

- Protect the person's rights during the procedure.
- Handle the person gently during the procedure.

PRE-PROCEDURE

1 Follow *Delegation Guidelines:*
- *Preventing Work-Related Injuries,* p. 244
- *Transferring Persons,* p. 258
- *Using Mechanical Lifts*

See *Promoting Safety and Comfort:*
- *Safely Handling, Moving, and Transferring the Person,* p. 240
- *Preventing Work-Related Injuries,* p. 244
- *Transferring Persons,* p. 258
- *Using Mechanical Lifts*

2 Ask a co-worker to help you.

3 Collect:
- Mechanical lift
- Armchair or wheelchair
- Footwear
- Bath blanket or cushion
- Lap blanket

4 Practice hand hygiene.

5 Identify the person. Check the ID bracelet against the assignment sheet. Also call the person by name.

6 Provide for privacy.

PROCEDURE

7 Raise the bed for proper body mechanics. Bed rails are up if used.

8 Lower the head of the bed to a level appropriate for the person. It is as flat as possible.

9 Stand on one side of the bed. Your co-worker stands on the other side.

10 Lower the bed rails if up.

11 Center the sling under the person (Fig. 16-24, *A*, p. 266). To position the sling, turn the person from side to side as if making an occupied bed (Chapter 18). Position the sling according to the manufacturer's instructions.

12 Position the person in semi-Fowler's position.

13 Place the chair at the head of the bed. It is even with the headboard and about 1 foot away from the bed. Place a folded bath blanket or cushion in the chair.

14 Lock the bed wheels. Lower the bed to its lowest position.

15 Raise the lift so you can position it over the person.

16 Position the lift over the person (Fig. 16-24, *B*, p. 266).

17 Lock the lift wheels in position.

18 Attach the sling to the swivel bar (Fig. 16-24, *C*, p. 266).

19 Raise the head of the bed to a sitting position.

20 Cross the person's arms over the chest. He or she can hold onto the straps or chains but not the swivel bar.

21 Raise the lift high enough until the person and sling are free of the bed (Fig. 16-24, *D*, p. 266).

22 Have your co-worker support the person's legs as you move the lift and the person away from the bed (Fig. 16-24, *E*, p. 266).

23 Position the lift so the person's back is toward the chair.

24 Position the chair so you can lower the person into it.

25 Lower the person into the chair. Guide the person into the chair (Fig. 16-24, *F*, p. 266).

26 Lower the swivel bar to unhook the sling. Remove the sling from under the person unless otherwise indicated.

27 Put footwear on the person. Position the person's feet on the wheelchair footplates.

28 Cover the person's lap and legs with a lap blanket. Keep it off the floor and wheels.

29 Position the chair as the person prefers. Lock the wheelchair wheels according to the care plan.

POST-PROCEDURE

30 Provide for comfort. (See the inside of the front book cover.)

31 Place the signal light and other needed items within the person's reach.

32 Unscreen the person.

33 Complete a safety check of the room. (See the inside of the front book cover.)

34 Decontaminate your hands.

35 Report and record your observations.

36 Reverse the procedure to return the person to bed.

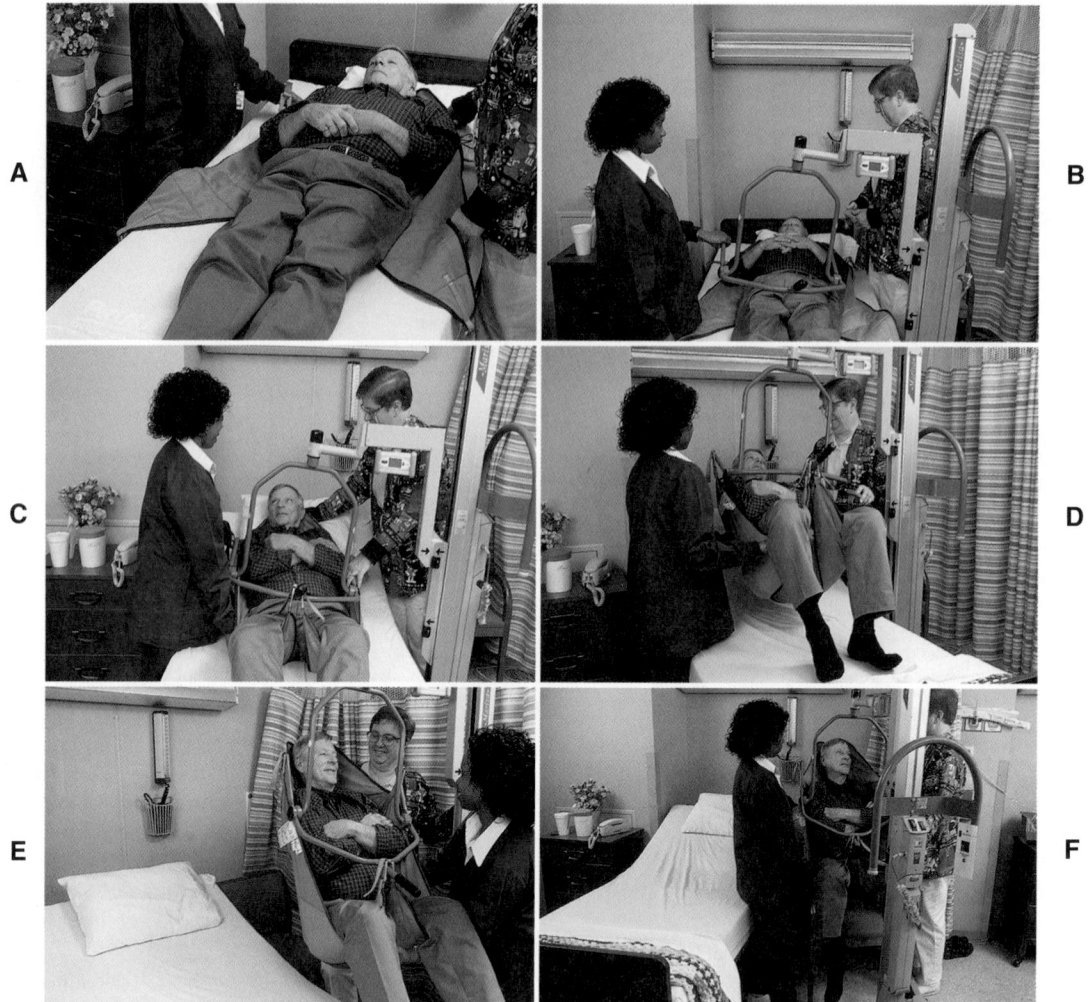

FIGURE 16-24 Using a mechanical lift. **A,** The sling is positioned under the person. **B,** The lift is over the person. **C,** The sling is attached to a swivel bar. **D,** The lift is raised until the sling and person are off of the bed. **E,** The person's legs are supported as the person and lift are moved away from the bed. **F,** The person is guided into a chair.

◆ Transferring the Person To and From the Toilet

Using the bathroom for elimination promotes dignity, self-esteem, and independence. It also is more private than using a bedpan, urinal, or bedside commode. However, getting to the toilet is hard for persons who use wheelchairs. Bathrooms are often small. There is little room for you or a wheelchair. Therefore transfers involving wheelchairs and toilets are often hard. Falls and work-related injuries are risks.

Sometimes mechanical lifts are used to transfer the person to and from a toilet. A slide board (see Fig. 16-4) may be used if:

▶ The wheelchair armrests are removable.
▶ The person has upper body strength.
▶ The person has good sitting balance.
▶ There is enough room to position the wheelchair next to the toilet.

The following procedure can be used if the person can stand and pivot from the wheelchair to the toilet.

See *Promoting Safety and Comfort: Transferring the Person to and from a Toilet.*

PROMOTING SAFETY AND COMFORT: Transferring the Person To and From a Toilet

SAFETY

Make sure the person has a raised toilet seat. The toilet seat and wheelchair are at the same level.

Check the grab bars by the toilet. If they are loose, tell the nurse. Do not transfer the person to the toilet if the grab bars are not secure.

TRANSFERRING THE PERSON TO AND FROM THE TOILET

✔ Quality of Life *Remember to:*

- Knock before entering the person's room.
- Address the person by name.
- Introduce yourself by name and title.
- Explain the procedure to the person before beginning and during the procedure.

- Protect the person's rights during the procedure.
- Handle the person gently during the procedure.

PRE-PROCEDURE

1 Follow *Delegation Guidelines:*
   - *Preventing Work-Related Injuries*, p. 244
   - *Transferring Persons*, p. 258
   See *Promoting Safety and Comfort:*
   - *Transfer/Gait Belts* (Chapter 11)
   - *Safely Handling, Moving, and Transferring the Person*, p. 240

   - *Preventing Work-Related Injuries*, p. 244
   - *Transferring Persons*, p. 258
   - *Bed to Chair or Wheelchair Transfers*, p. 259
   - *Transferring the Person To and From a Toilet.*
2 Practice hand hygiene.

PROCEDURE

3 Have the person wear non-skid footwear.
4 Position the wheelchair next to the toilet if there is enough room. If not, position the chair at a right angle (90-degree angle) to the toilet (Fig. 16-25, p. 268). It is best if the person's strong side is near the toilet.
5 Lock the wheelchair wheels.
6 Raise the footplates. Remove or swing the front rigging out of the way.
7 Apply the transfer belt.
8 Help the person unfasten clothing.
9 Use the transfer belt to help the person stand and to turn to the toilet. (See procedure: *Transferring the Person to a Chair or Wheelchair*, p. 260.) The person uses the grab bars to turn to the toilet.
10 Support the person with the transfer belt while he or she lowers clothing. Or have the person hold onto the grab bars for support. Lower the person's pants and undergarments.
11 Use the transfer belt to lower the person onto the toilet seat. Make sure he or she is properly positioned on the toilet.
12 Remove the transfer belt.
13 Tell the person you will stay nearby. Remind the person to use the signal light or call for you when help is needed. Stay with the person if required by the care plan.

14 Close the bathroom door to provide for privacy.
15 Stay near the bathroom. Complete other tasks in the person's room. Check on the person every 5 minutes.
16 Knock on the bathroom door when the person calls for you.
17 Help with wiping, perineal care (Chapter 19), flushing, and hand washing as needed. Wear gloves and practice hand hygiene after removing the gloves.
18 Apply the transfer belt.
19 Use the transfer belt to help the person stand.
20 Help the person raise and secure clothing.
21 Use the transfer belt to transfer the person to the wheelchair. (See procedure: *Transferring the Person to a Chair or Wheelchair*, p. 260.)
22 Make sure the person's buttocks are to the back of the seat. Position the person in good alignment.
23 Position the person's feet on the footplates.
24 Cover the person's lap and legs with a lap blanket. Keep the blanket off the floor and wheels.
25 Position the chair as the person prefers. Lock the wheelchair wheels according to the care plan.

POST-PROCEDURE

26 Provide for comfort. (See the inside of the front book cover.)
27 Place the signal light and other need items within the person's reach.
28 Unscreen the person.

29 Complete a safety check of the room. (See the inside of the front book cover.)
30 Practice hand hygiene.
31 Report and record your observations.

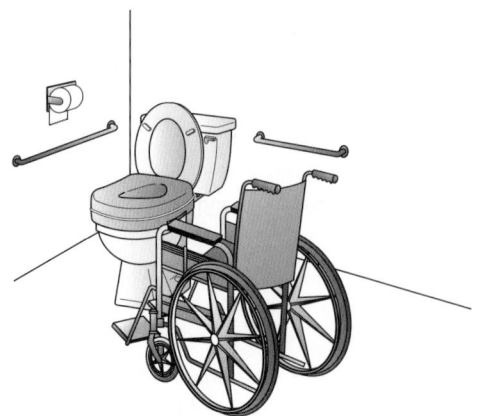

FIGURE 16-25 The wheelchair is placed at a right angle (90-degree angle) to the toilet.

◀ Moving the Person to a Stretcher

Stretchers (gurneys) are used to transport persons to other areas. They are used for persons who:

▶ Cannot sit up

▶ Must stay in a lying position

▶ Are seriously ill

The stretcher is covered with a folded flat sheet or bath blanket. A pillow and extra blankets are on hand. With the nurse's permission, raise the head of the stretcher to a Fowler's or semi-Fowler's position (Chapter 17). This increases the person's comfort.

A drawsheet, turning pad, large incontinence underpad, slide sheet, or slide board is used. At least 2 or 3 staff members are needed for a safe transfer. OSHA recommends the following:

▶ If the person weighs less than 100 pounds—use a lateral sliding aid and 2 staff members

▶ If the person weighs 100 to 200 pounds—use a lateral sliding aid or a friction-reducing device and 2 staff members

▶ If the person weighs more than 200 pounds, use one of the following:

   ▶ A lateral sliding aid and 3 staff members

   ▶ A friction-reducing device or lateral transfer device and 2 staff members

   ▶ A mechanical lateral transfer device with a built-in slide board

Safety straps are used when the person is on the stretcher. The stretcher side rails are kept up during the transport. The stretcher is moved feet first. This is so the staff member at the head of the stretcher can watch the person's breathing and color during the transport. Never leave a person on a stretcher alone.

See *Promoting Safety and Comfort: Moving the Person to a Stretcher.*

PROMOTING SAFETY AND COMFORT: Moving the Person to a Stretcher

SAFETY

Protect yourself and the person from injury:

• Position the stretcher and bed surfaces as close as possible to each other.

• Avoid extended reaches and bending your back. You may need to kneel on the bed or stretcher.

• Follow the rules for stretcher safety (Chapter 11).

• Make sure the bed and stretcher wheels are locked.

• Practice good body mechanics (Chapter 15) and follow the guidelines in Box 16-1.

• Keep the person in good alignment.

• Make sure you have enough help.

• Hold the person securely. You must not drop the person onto the floor.

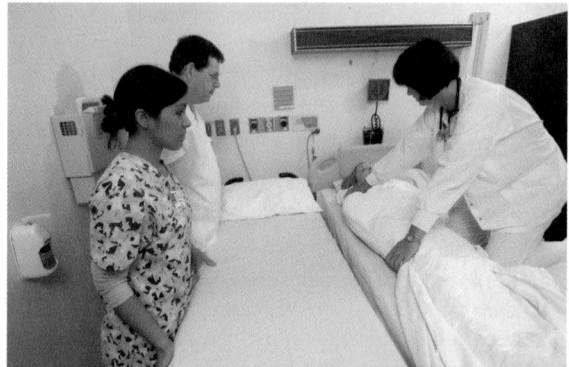

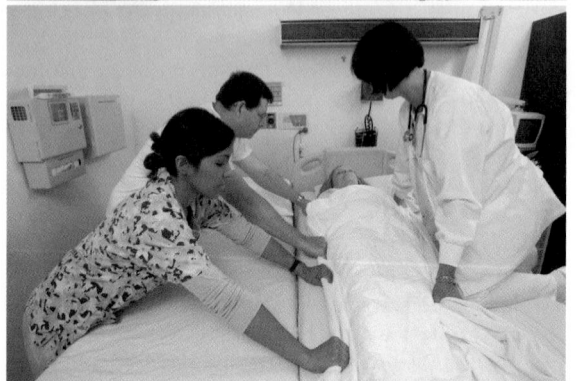

FIGURE 16-26 Transferring the person to a stretcher. **A,** The stretcher is against the bed and is held in place. **B,** A drawsheet is used to transfer the person from the bed to a stretcher.

MOVING THE PERSON TO A STRETCHER

✔ Quality of Life *Remember to:*

- Knock before entering the person's room.
- Address the person by name.
- Introduce yourself by name and title.
- Explain the procedure to the person before beginning and during the procedure.

- Protect the person's rights during the procedure.
- Handle the person gently during the procedure.

PRE-PROCEDURE

1 Follow *Delegation Guidelines:*
   - *Preventing Work-Related Injuries,* p. 244
   - *Transferring Persons,* p. 259
   See *Promoting Safety and Comfort:*
   - *Safely Handling, Moving, and Transferring the Person,* p. 240
   - *Preventing Work-Related Injuries,* p. 244
   - *Transferring Persons,* p. 258
   - *Moving the Person to a Stretcher*
2 Ask 1 or 2 staff members to help you.
3 Collect:
   - Stretcher covered with a sheet or bath blanket
   - Bath blanket

   - Pillow(s) if needed
   - Slide sheet, slide board, drawsheet, or other assist device
4 Practice hand hygiene.
5 Identify the person. Check the ID bracelet against the assignment sheet. Also call the person by name.
6 Provide for privacy.
7 Raise the bed and stretcher for proper body mechanics.

PROCEDURE

8 Position yourself and co-workers:
   a One or two workers stand on the side of the bed where the stretcher will be.
   b One worker stands on the other side of the bed.
9 Lower the head of the bed. It is as flat as possible.
10 Lower the bed rails if used.
11 Cover the person with a bath blanket. Fan-fold top linens to the foot of the bed.
12 Position the assist device. Or loosen the drawsheet on each side.
13 Use the assist device to move the person to the side of the bed. This is the side where the stretcher will be.
14 Protect the person from falling. Hold the far arm and leg.

15 Have your co-workers position the stretcher next to the bed. They stand behind the stretcher (Fig. 16-26, A).
16 Lock the bed and stretcher wheels.
17 Grasp the assist device (Fig. 16-26, B).
18 Transfer the person to the stretcher on the count of "3." Center the person on the stretcher.
19 Place a pillow or pillows under the person's head and shoulders if allowed. Raise the head of the stretcher if allowed.
20 Cover the person. Provide for comfort.
21 Fasten the safety straps. Raise the side rails.
22 Unlock the stretcher wheels. Transport the person.

POST-PROCEDURE

23 Decontaminate your hands.
24 Report and record:
   - The time of the transport
   - Where the person was transported to

   - Who went with him or her
   - How the transfer was tolerated
25 Reverse the procedure to return the person to bed.

REPOSITIONING IN A CHAIR OR WHEELCHAIR

The person can slide down into the chair. For good alignment and safety, the person's back and buttocks must be against the back of the chair.

Some persons can help with repositioning. Others need help. If the person cannot help, a mechanical lift is needed to reposition the person. Follow the nurse's directions and the care plan for the best way to reposition a person in a chair or wheelchair. *Do not pull the person from behind the chair or wheelchair.*

If the person's chair reclines, do the following:

▶ Ask a co-worker to help you.
▶ Lock the wheels.
▶ Recline the chair.
▶ Position a friction-reducing device (drawsheet or slide sheet) under the person.
▶ Use the device to move the person up. See procedure: *Moving the Person Up in Bed With an Assist Device,* p. 250.

This method can be used if the person is alert and co-operative. The person must be able to follow directions. And the person must have the strength to help.

▶ Lock the wheelchair wheels.
▶ Remove or swing the front rigging out of the way.
▶ Position the person's feet flat on the floor.
▶ Apply a transfer belt.
▶ Position the person's arms on the armrests.
▶ Stand in front of the person. Block his or her knees and feet with your knees and feet.
▶ Grasp the transfer belt on each side while the person leans forward.
▶ Ask the person to push with his or her feet and arms on the count of "3."
▶ Move the person back into the chair on the count of "3" as the person pushes with his or her feet and arms (Fig. 16-27).

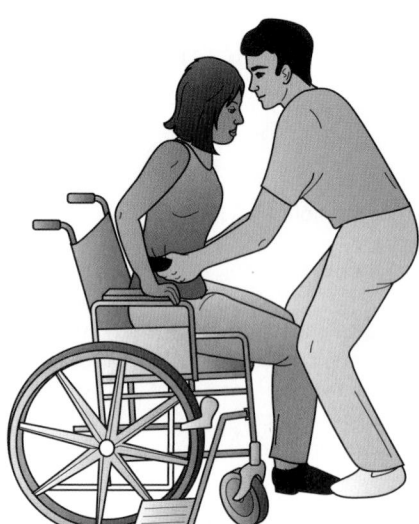

FIGURE 16-27 Repositioning the person in a wheelchair. A transfer belt is used to move the person to the back of the chair.

REVIEW QUESTIONS

Circle the BEST answer.

1 A person's skin rubs against the sheet. This is called
   a Shearing
   b Friction
   c Ergonomics
   d Posture

2 Which occurs when a person slides down in bed?
   a Shearing
   b Friction
   c Ergonomics
   d Posture

3 Which protects the skin when moving the person in bed?
   a Rolling the person
   b Sliding the person up in bed
   c Moving the mattress
   d Using ergonomics

4 Whenever you handle, move, or transfer a person, you must
   a Allow personal choice
   b Protect the person's privacy
   c Use pillows for support
   d Get help from a co-worker

5 You are delegated tasks that involve moving persons in bed. Which is *true*?
   a The nurse tells you how to position the person.
   b You decide which procedure to use.
   c Bed rails are used at all times.
   d Three workers are needed to complete the task safely.

6 You are using a drawsheet as an assist device. It is placed so that it
   a Covers the person's body
   b Is under the person from the head to above the knees
   c Extends from the mid-back to mid-thigh level
   d Covers the entire mattress

7 Before turning a person onto his or her side, you
   a Move the person to the side of the bed
   b Move the person to the middle of the bed
   c Lock arms with the person
   d Position pillows for comfort

8 The logrolling procedure
   a Is used after spinal cord injuries or surgeries
   b Requires a transfer belt
   c Requires a mechanical lift
   d Involves a stretcher and a drawsheet

9 When getting ready to dangle a person, you need to know
   a Which side is stronger
   b If bed rails are used
   c If a mechanical lift is needed
   d If a transfer belt is needed

10 For chair and wheelchair transfers, the person must
    a Wear non-skid footwear
    b Have the bed rails up
    c Use a mechanical lift
    d Have a drawsheet or other assist device

11 Before transferring a person to or from a bed, you must
    a Have the person wear non-skid footwear
    b Lock the bed wheels
    c Apply a transfer belt
    d Position pillows for support

12 When transferring the person to a bed, a chair, or the toilet
    a The person's strong side moves first
    b The weak side moves first
    c Pillows are used for support
    d The transfer belt is removed

13 You are going to use a mechanical lift. You must do the following *except*
    a Follow the manufacturer's instructions
    b Make sure the lift works
    c Compare the person's weight to the lift's weight limit
    d Use a transfer belt

14 To safely transfer a person with a mechanical lift, at least
    a 1 worker is needed
    b 2 workers are needed
    c 3 workers are needed
    d 4 workers are needed

15 These statements are about transfers to and from a toilet. Which is *false*?
    a The person wears non-skid footwear.
    b Wheelchair wheels must be locked.
    c The person uses the towel bars for support.
    d A transfer belt is used.

16 These statements are about transfers to and from a stretcher? Which is *false*?
    a The bed and stretcher wheels must be locked.
    b The stretcher's side rails are raised when the person is on the stretcher.
    c Once on the stretcher, the person can be left alone.
    d At least 2 workers are needed for a safe transfer.

Answers to these questions are on p. 780.

The Person's Unit

OBJECTIVES

- Define the key terms and key abbreviations listed in this chapter
- Identify the room temperatures required by OBRA
- Describe how to protect the person from drafts
- List ways to prevent or reduce odors and noise
- Explain how lighting affects comfort
- Describe the basic bed positions
- Identify the persons at risk for entrapment in the hospital bed system
- Identify hospital bed system entrapment zones
- Explain how to use the furniture and equipment in the person's unit
- Describe how a bathroom is equipped for the person's use
- Describe how to provide safety, privacy, and comfort in the person's unit
- Explain how to maintain the person's unit
- Describe the OBRA requirements for resident rooms

KEY TERMS

Fowler's position A semi-sitting position; the head of the bed is raised between 45 and 60 degrees

full visual privacy Having the means to be completely free from public view while in bed

high-Fowler's position A semi-sitting position; the head of the bed is raised 60 to 90 degrees

reverse Trendelenburg's position The head of the bed is raised and the foot of the bed is lowered

semi-Fowler's position The head of the bed is raised 30 degrees; or the head of the bed is raised 30 degrees and the knee portion is raised 15 degrees

Trendelenburg's position The head of the bed is lowered and the foot of the bed is raised

KEY ABBREVIATIONS

CNA Certified Nursing Assistant
F Fahrenheit
FDA Food and Drug Administration

IV Intravenous
OBRA Omnibus Budget Reconciliation Act of 1987

The *person's unit* is the personal space, furniture, and equipment provided for the person by the agency (Fig. 17-1). The person's room is a private area.

Many agencies have private rooms. A private room is for one person. Semi-private rooms are for two people. Some agencies have rooms that are shared by four people. Patient and resident rooms are designed to provide comfort, safety, and privacy.

See *Focus on Long-Term Care and Home Care: The Person's Unit.*

COMFORT

Age, illness, and activity affect comfort. So do temperature, ventilation, noise, odors, and lighting. These factors are controlled to meet the person's needs.

Temperature and Ventilation

Heating and air conditioning systems maintain a comfortable temperature. Most healthy people are comfortable when the temperature is 68° F to 74° F. This range may be too hot or too cold for others. Infants, older persons, and those who are ill may need higher temperatures for comfort. Therefore hospitals and nursing centers usually have higher room temperatures.

Persons who are less active usually do not like cool areas. Nor do those who need help moving about. They must be dressed warmly. They also need warm room temperatures. You may find the rooms rather warm.

Stale room air and lingering odors affect comfort and rest. Ventilation systems provide fresh air and move room air. Drafts occur as air moves. Infants, older persons, and persons who are ill are sensitive to drafts. To protect them from drafts:

► Make sure they wear the correct clothing.
► Make sure they wear enough clothing.
► Offer lap robes to those in chairs and wheelchairs. Lap robes cover the legs.
► Provide enough blankets for warmth.
► Cover them with bath blankets when giving care.
► Move them from drafty areas.

See *Focus on Long-Term Care and Home Care: Temperature and Ventilation.*

See *Focus on Children and Older Persons: Temperature and Ventilation.*

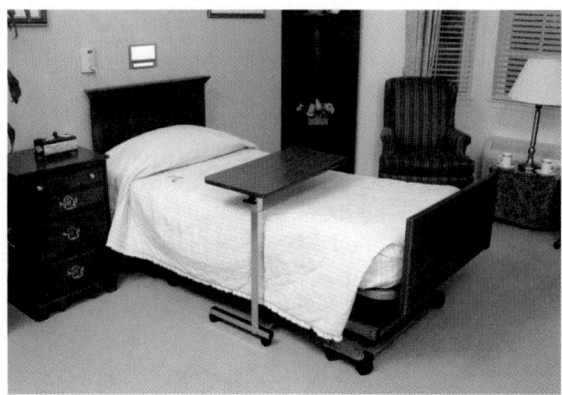

FIGURE 17-1 Furniture and equipment in a resident's unit.

FOCUS ON **LONG-TERM CARE** AND **HOME CARE**

The Person's Unit

LONG-TERM CARE

The resident's unit is treated like the person's home. The Omnibus Budget Reconciliation Act of 1987 (OBRA) requires that resident units be as personal and home-like as possible. Residents are allowed to bring and use some furniture and personal items from home. This promotes dignity and self-esteem.

As space allows, the person chooses where to place personal items. However, a resident cannot take or use another person's space. Doing so violates the other person's rights.

FOCUS ON **LONG-TERM CARE** AND **HOME CARE**

Temperature and Ventilation

OLDER PERSONS

OBRA requires that nursing centers maintain a temperature range of 71° F to 81° F.

FOCUS ON **CHILDREN** AND **OLDER PERSONS**

Temperature and Ventilation

OLDER PERSONS

Poor circulation and loss of the skin's fatty tissue layer occur with aging. Therefore older persons are sensitive to cold (Chapter 10). They must wear enough clothing. Many wear sweaters in warm weather. Respect the person's wishes and choices.

Odors

Many odors occur in health care agencies. Food aromas and flower scents are pleasant. Bowel movements and urine have embarrassing odors. So do draining wounds and vomitus. Body, breath, and smoking odors may offend others.

Some people are very sensitive to odors. They may become nauseated. Good nursing care, ventilation, and housekeeping practices help prevent odors. To reduce odors:

▶ Empty, clean, and disinfect bedpans, urinals, commodes, and kidney basins promptly.
▶ Check to make sure toilets are flushed.
▶ Check incontinent persons often (Chapters 21 and 22).
▶ Clean persons who are wet or soiled from urine, feces, vomitus, or wound drainage.
▶ Change wet or soiled linens and clothing promptly.
▶ Keep laundry containers closed.
▶ Follow agency policy for wet or soiled linens and clothing.
▶ Dispose of incontinence and ostomy products promptly (Chapters 21 and 22).
▶ Provide good hygiene to prevent body and breath odors (Chapter 19).
▶ Use room deodorizers as needed and allowed by agency policy. Sometimes odors remain after removing the cause. Do not use sprays around persons with breathing problems. Ask the nurse if you are unsure.

Smoke odors present special problems. Patients, residents, and staff smoke only in the areas allowed. If you smoke, follow the agency's policy. Practice hand washing after handling smoking materials and before giving care. Give careful attention to your uniforms, hair, and breath because of smoke odors.

Noise

Ill and many older persons are sensitive to noises and sounds. Common health care sounds may disturb them. Examples include:

▶ The clanging of equipment
▶ The clatter of dishes and meal trays
▶ Loud voices, TVs, and radios
▶ Ringing phones
▶ Intercom systems and signal lights
▶ Equipment needing repair
▶ Wheels on stretchers, wheelchairs, carts, and other items needing oil

Loud talking and laughter in hallways and at the nurses' station are common. Patients and residents may think that the staff are talking and laughing about them.

People want to know the cause and meaning of new sounds. This relates to safety and security needs. Patients and residents may find sounds dangerous, frightening, or irritating. They may become upset, anxious, and uncomfortable. What is noise to one person may not be noise to another. For example, a teenager enjoys loud music. It may bother adults.

Health care agencies are designed to reduce noise. Window coverings, carpets, and acoustical tiles absorb noise. Plastic items make less noise than metal equipment (bedpans, urinals, wash basins). To decrease noise:

▶ Control your voice.
▶ Handle equipment carefully.
▶ Keep equipment in good working order.
▶ Answer phones, signal lights, and intercoms promptly. See *Focus on Children and Older Persons: Noise.*

Lighting

Good lighting is needed for safety and comfort. Glares, shadows, and dull lighting can cause falls, headaches, and eyestrain. A bright room is cheerful. Dim light is better for relaxing and rest.

Adjust lighting to meet the person's changing needs. Window coverings are adjusted as needed. The overbed light can provide soft, medium, or bright lighting. Some agencies have ceiling lights. They provide soft to very bright light.

Persons with poor vision need bright light. This is very important at mealtime and when moving about in the room and agency. Bright lighting also helps the staff perform procedures.

Always keep light controls within the person's reach. This protects the right to personal choice.

See *Focus on Children and Older Persons: Lighting.*

ROOM FURNITURE AND EQUIPMENT

Rooms are furnished and equipped to meet basic needs. The room has furniture and equipment for comfort, sleep, elimination, nutrition, hygiene, and activity. There is equipment to communicate with staff, family, and friends. The right to privacy is considered.

FOCUS ON CHILDREN AND OLDER PERSONS

Noise

OLDER PERSONS

Persons with dementia do not understand what is happening around them. They do not react to common, everyday sounds as other people do. For example, a ringing phone may frighten a person with dementia. The person may not know or understand the sound. He or she may have an extreme reaction to the sound (Chapter 44). The reaction may be more severe at night. This is likely when the sound awakens the person suddenly. A dark, strange room can make the problem worse.

FOCUS ON CHILDREN AND OLDER PERSONS

Lighting

OLDER PERSONS

In dementia care units, lighting is adjusted to help control agitated and aggressive behaviors. Soft, non-glare lights are relaxing. They can decrease agitation. Brighter lighting may improve orientation. This is because the person can see surroundings more clearly.

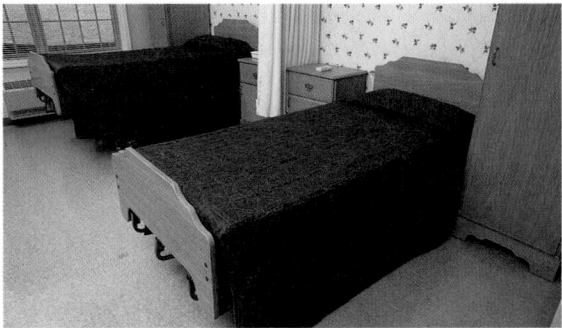

FIGURE 17-2 One bed is in the highest horizontal position. The other bed is in the lowest horizontal position.

The Bed

Beds have electrical or manual controls. Beds are raised horizontally to give care. This reduces bending and reaching. The lowest horizontal position lets the person get out of bed with ease (Fig. 17-2). The head of the bed is flat or raised varying degrees.

Electric beds are common. Controls are on a side panel, bed rail, or the footboard (Fig. 17-3, *A*). Some controls are hand-held devices (Fig. 17-3, *B*). Patients and residents are taught to use the controls safely. They are warned not to raise the bed to the high position or to adjust the bed to harmful positions. They are told of any position limits or restrictions.

Most electric beds "lock" into any position by the staff. The person cannot adjust the bed to unsafe positions. Persons restricted to certain positions may need their beds locked. So may persons with confusion or dementia.

Manual beds have cranks at the foot of the bed (Fig. 17-4):

▶ Left crank—raises or lowers the head of the bed
▶ Right crank—adjusts the knee portion
▶ Center crank—raises or lowers the entire bed horizontally

The cranks are pulled up for use. They are kept down at all other times. Cranks in the "up" position are safety hazards. Anyone walking past may bump into them.

See *Promoting Safety and Comfort: The Bed.*
See *Focus on Long-Term Care and Home Care: The Bed.*

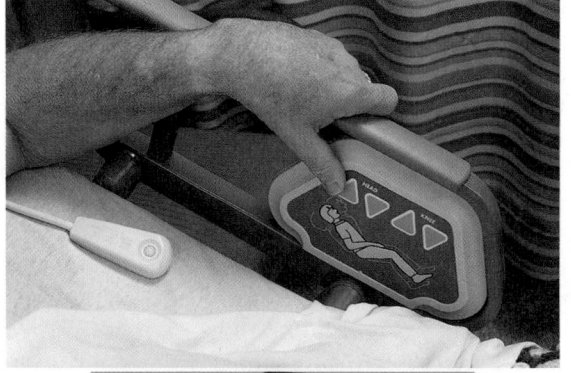
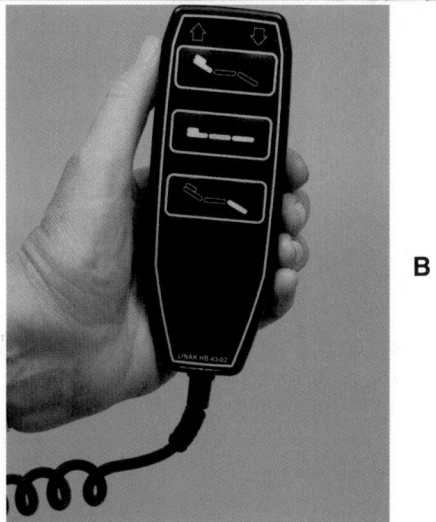

FIGURE 17-3 Controls for an electric bed. **A,** Controls in the bed rail. **B,** Hand-held bed control.

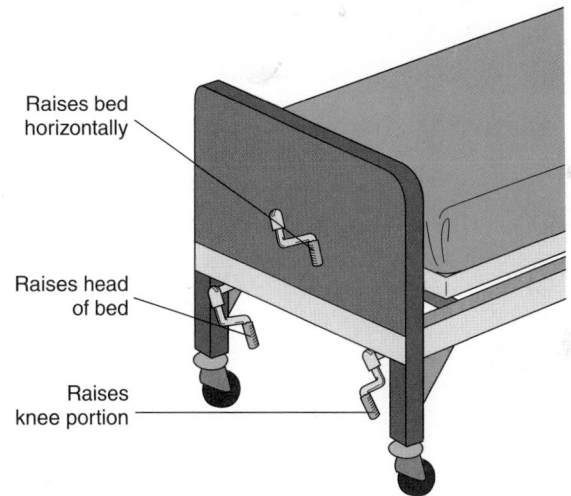

Raises bed horizontally
Raises head of bed
Raises knee portion

FIGURE 17-4 Manually operated hospital bed.

PROMOTING SAFETY AND COMFORT: The Bed

SAFETY
Beds have bed rails and wheels (Chapter 11). Bed wheels are locked at all times except when moving the bed. They must be locked when you:
• Give bedside care.
• Transfer the person to and from the bed. The person can be injured if the bed moves. So can you.
Use bed rails as the nurse and care plan direct. Otherwise the person could suffer injury or harm.

COMFORT
Some persons spend a lot of time in bed. Make sure the bed is adjusted to meet the person's needs. Tell the nurse if the person complains about the bed or mattress.

FOCUS ON LONG-TERM CARE AND HOME CARE

The Bed

HOME CARE
Some home care patients have hospital beds. Others use their regular beds. You cannot raise regular beds to give care. Therefore you will bend more when giving care. To avoid injuring yourself, use good body mechanics.

Bed Positions

The six basic bed positions are:

▶ *Flat*—This is the usual sleeping position. The position is used after spinal cord injury or surgery and for cervical traction.

▶ *Fowler's position*—**Fowler's position** is a semi-sitting position. The head of the bed is raised between 45 and 60 degrees (Fig. 17-5). See Chapter 15.

▶ *High-Fowler's position*—**High-Fowler's position** is a semi-sitting position. The head of the bed is raised 60 to 90 degrees (Fig. 17-6).

▶ *Semi-Fowler's position*—In **semi-Fowler's position**, the head of the bed is raised 30 degrees (Fig. 17-7). Some agencies define semi-Fowler's position as when the head of the bed is raised 30 degrees and the knee portion is raised 15 degrees. This position is comfortable and prevents sliding down in bed. However, raising the knee portion can interfere with circulation in the legs. To give safe care, know the definition used by your agency Also check with the nurse before using this position.

▶ *Trendelenburg's position*—In the **Trendelenburg's position**, the head of the bed is lowered and the foot of the bed is raised (Fig. 17-8). A doctor orders the position. Blocks are placed under the legs at the foot of the bed. Or the bed frame is tilted.

▶ *Reverse Trendelenburg's position*—In the **reverse Trendelenburg's position**, the head of the bed is raised and the foot of the bed is lowered (Fig. 17-9). Blocks are placed under the legs at the head of the bed. Or the bed frame is tilted. This position requires a doctor's order.

See *Focus on Long-Term Care and Home Care: Bed Positions.*

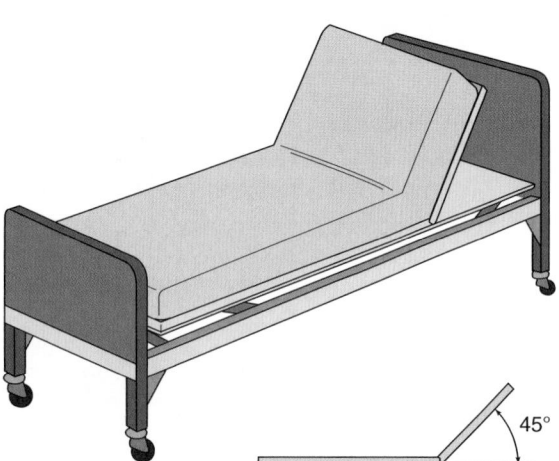

FIGURE 17-5 Fowler's position.

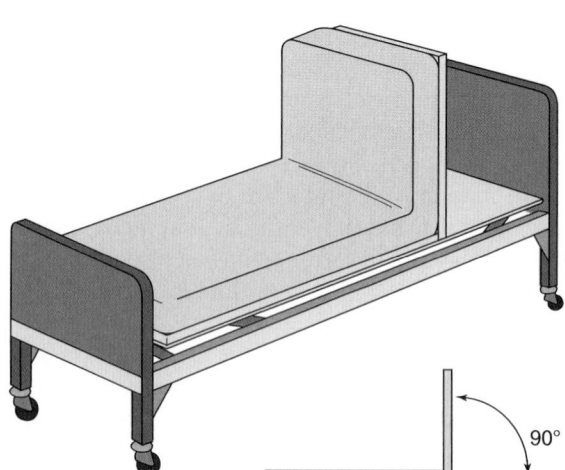

FIGURE 17-6 High-Fowler's position.

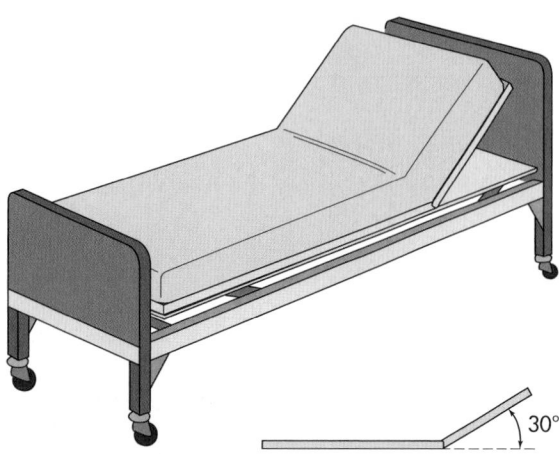

FIGURE 17-7 Semi-Fowler's position.

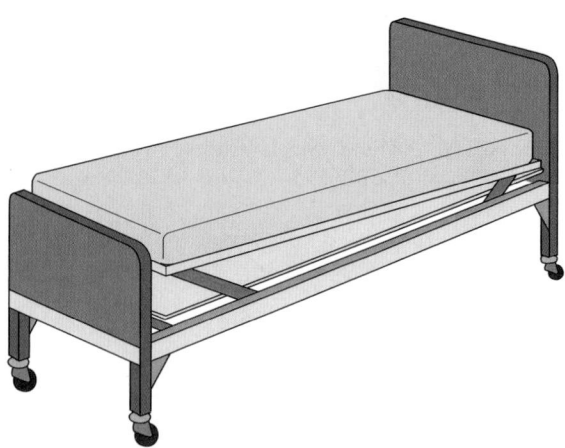

FIGURE 17-8 Trendelenburg's position.

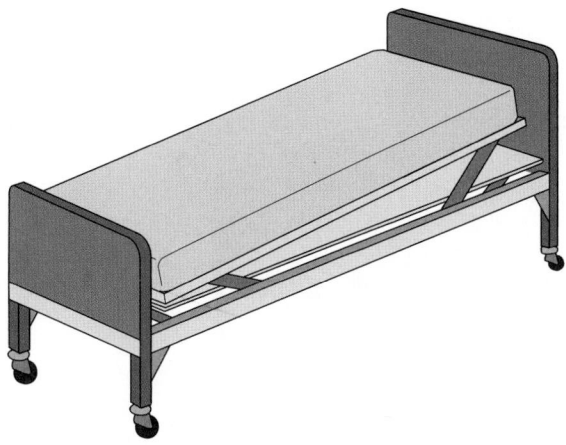

FIGURE 17-9 Reverse Trendelenburg's position.

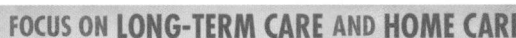

Bed Safety

Bed safety involves the *hospital bed system.* The Food and Drug Administration (FDA) defines the hospital bed system as the bed frame and its parts. The parts include the mattress, bed rails, headboard and footboard, and bed attachments. *Entrapment* within parts of the hospital bed system is a risk. That is, the person can get caught, trapped, or entangled in spaces created by bed rails, the mattress, the bed frame, the headboard, or footboard. Serious injuries and deaths have occurred from head, neck, and chest entrapment. Arm and leg entrapment also can occur. Persons at greatest risk include persons who:

- Are older
- Are frail
- Are confused or disoriented
- Are restless
- Have uncontrolled body movements
- Have poor muscle control
- Are small in size
- Are restrained (Chapter 13)

Hospital bed systems have seven entrapment zones (Fig. 17-11, p. 278):

- *Zone 1:* Within the bed rail (Fig. 17-12, *A*, p. 279)
- *Zone 2:* Between the top of the compressed mattress and the bottom of the bed rail and between the rail supports (Fig. 17-12, *B*, p. 279)
- *Zone 3:* Between the bed rail and the mattress (Fig. 17-12, *C*, p. 279)

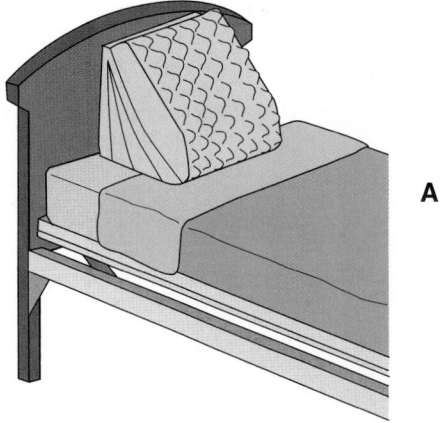

A

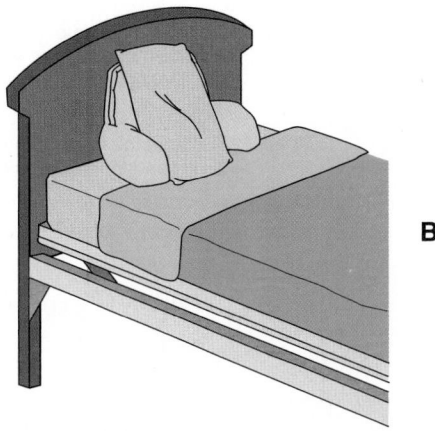

B

FIGURE 17-10 Backrests for regular beds. **A,** Wedge pillow. **B,** Study pillow (dorm pillow) with armrests. A pillow is added for additional support.

- *Zone 4:* Between the top of the compressed mattress and the bottom of the bed rail and at the end of the bed rail (Fig. 17-12, *D*, p. 279)
- *Zone 5:* Between the split bed rails (Fig. 17-12, *E*, p. 279)
- *Zone 6:* Between the end of the bed rail and the side edge of the headboard or footboard (Fig. 17-12, *F*, p. 279)
- *Zone 7:* Between the headboard or footboard and the end of the mattress (Fig. 17-12, *G*, p. 279)

You may feel that a person is at risk for entrapment. Report your concerns to the nurse at once. Also, always check the person for entrapment. If a person is caught, trapped, or entangled in the bed or any of its parts, try to release the person. Also call for the nurse at once.

See *Focus on Children and Older Persons: Bed Safety,* p. 278.

The Overbed Table

The overbed table (see Fig. 17-1) is placed over the bed by sliding the base under the bed. It is raised or lowered for the person in bed or in a chair. Turn the handle or lever to adjust the table. It is used for meals, writing, reading, and other activities.

Many overbed tables have a storage area under the top. The storage area often is used for beauty, hair care,

Zone 1: Within the rail

Zone 2: Between the top of the compressed mattress and the bottom of the rail, between the supports

Zone 3: Between the rail and the mattress

Zone 4: Between the top of the compressed mattress and the bottom of the rail, at the end of the rail

Zone 5: Between the split bed rails

Zone 6: Between the end of the rail and the side edge of the headboard or footboard

Zone 7: Between the head or foot board and the mattress end

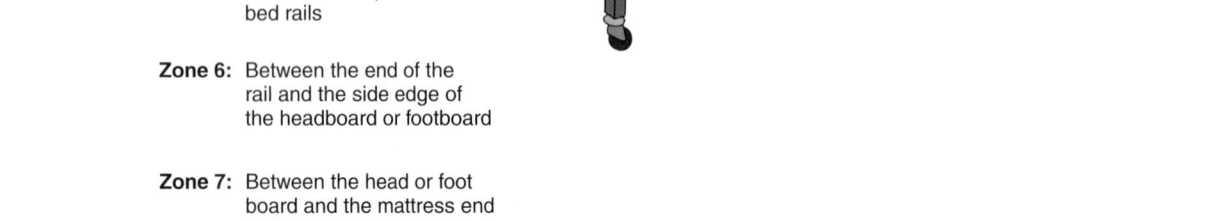

FIGURE 17-11 Hospital bed system entrapment zones. (Redrawn from *Guidance for industry and FDA staff: hospital bed system dimensional and assessment guidance to reduce entrapment,* March 10, 2006, Food and Drug Administration.)

---

shaving, or other personal items. Many also have a flip-up mirror for grooming.

The nursing team uses the overbed table as a work area. Only clean and sterile items are placed on the table. Never place bedpans, urinals, or soiled linen on the overbed table. Clean the table after using it for a work surface.

The Bedside Stand

The bedside stand is next to the bed. It is used to store personal items and personal care equipment. It has a top drawer and a lower cabinet with shelves or drawers (Fig. 17-13, p. 280). The top drawer is used for money, eyeglasses, books, and other items.

The top shelf or middle drawer is used for the wash basin. The wash basin can hold personal items—soap and soap dish, powder, lotion, deodorant, towels, washcloth, bath blanket, and a clean gown or pajamas. An emesis basin or kidney basin (shaped like a kidney) can hold oral hygiene items. The kidney basin is stored in the top drawer, in the middle drawer, or on the top shelf. The bedpan and its cover, the urinal, and toilet paper are stored on the lower shelf or in the bottom drawer.

The top of the stand is often used for tissues and other personal items. The person may put a radio, clock, photos, phone, flowers, cards, gifts, and other things there. Some stands have a side or back rod for towels and washcloths.

Place only clean and sterile items on top of the bedside stand. Never place bedpans, urinals, or soiled linen on the top of the stand. If you use the bedside stand for a work surface, clean it when you are done.

Chairs

The person's unit always has at least one chair for personal and visitor use (see Fig. 17-1). The chair is usually upholstered with armrests. It must be comfortable and sturdy. It must not move or tip during transfers. The person should be able to get in and out of the chair with ease. It should not be too low or too soft. Nursing center residents may bring chairs from home.

Privacy Curtains

Rooms have privacy curtains. The curtain is pulled around the bed to provide privacy for the person (Chapter 3). Rooms with more than one bed have a privacy curtain between the units. *Always* pull the curtain completely around the bed before giving care.

Privacy curtains prevent others from seeing the person. They do not block sound or conversations. Others in the room can hear sounds or talking behind the curtain.

See *Focus on Long-Term Care and Home Care: Privacy Curtains,* p. 280.

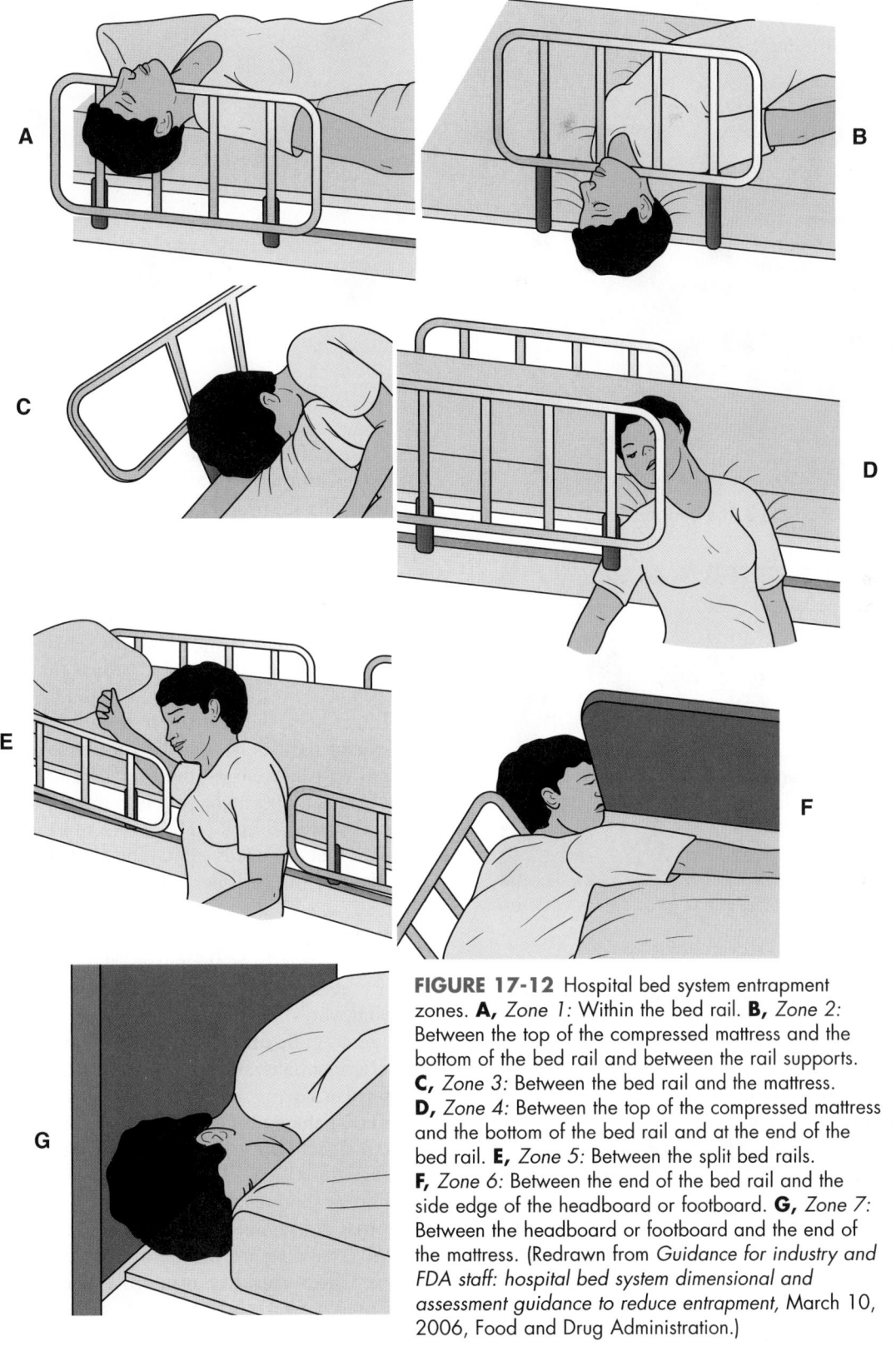

FIGURE 17-12 Hospital bed system entrapment zones. **A,** Zone 1: Within the bed rail. **B,** Zone 2: Between the top of the compressed mattress and the bottom of the bed rail and between the rail supports. **C,** Zone 3: Between the bed rail and the mattress. **D,** Zone 4: Between the top of the compressed mattress and the bottom of the bed rail and at the end of the bed rail. **E,** Zone 5: Between the split bed rails. **F,** Zone 6: Between the end of the bed rail and the side edge of the headboard or footboard. **G,** Zone 7: Between the headboard or footboard and the end of the mattress. (Redrawn from *Guidance for industry and FDA staff: hospital bed system dimensional and assessment guidance to reduce entrapment,* March 10, 2006, Food and Drug Administration.)

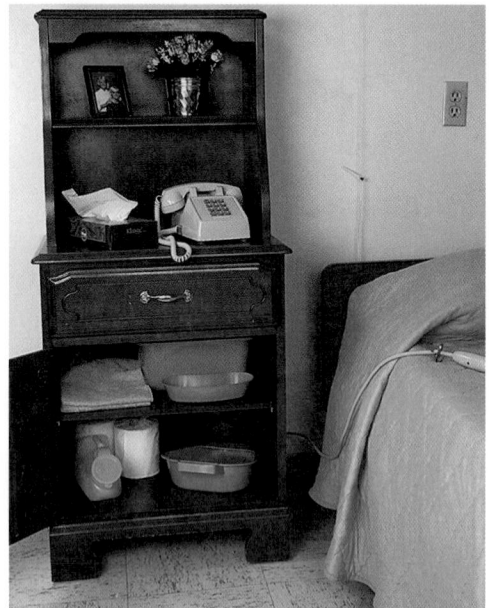

FIGURE 17-13 The bedside stand.

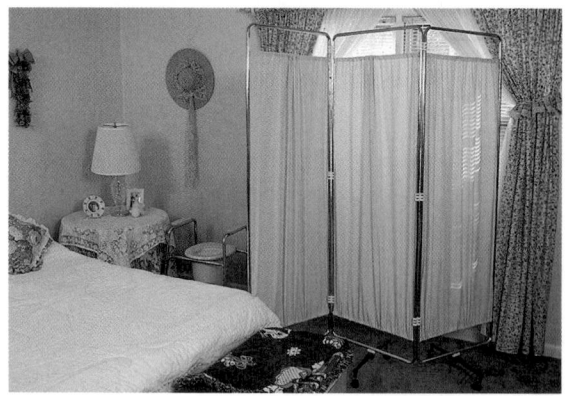

FIGURE 17-14 A portable screen provides privacy in the home.

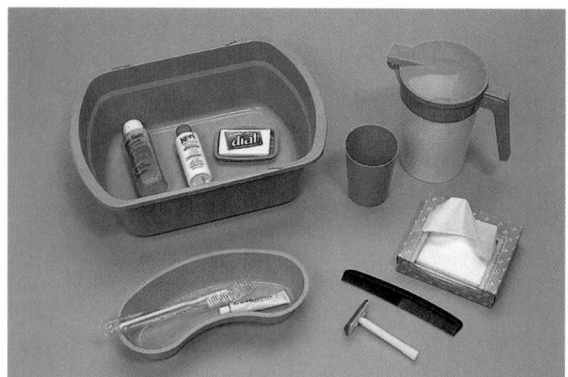

FIGURE 17-15 Personal care items.

FOCUS ON LONG-TERM CARE AND HOME CARE

Privacy Curtains

LONG-TERM CARE

According to OBRA, each person has the right to full visual privacy. **Full visual privacy** is having the means to be completely free from public view while in bed. The privacy curtain helps provide full visual privacy.

HOME CARE

Portable screens help provide privacy in the home setting (Fig. 17-14). Decorator screens provide color and are pleasant to look at.

Personal Care Items

Personal care items are used for hygiene and elimination. A bedpan and urinal are provided. The agency also provides a wash basin, kidney basin, water pitcher and cup, and soap and a soap dish (Fig. 17-15). Some provide powder, lotion, toothbrush, toothpaste, mouthwash, tissues, and a comb.

Some persons bring their own oral hygiene equipment, hair care supplies, and deodorant. Some also prefer their own soap, lotion, and powder. Respect the person's choices in personal care products.

The Call System

The call system lets the person signal for help. The signal light is at the end of a long cord (Fig. 17-16). It attaches to the bed or chair. Always keep the signal light within the person's reach—in the room, bathroom, and shower or tub room.

To get help, the person presses a button at the end of the signal light. The signal light at the bedside is connected to a light above the room door. The signal light also connects to a light panel or intercom system at the nurses' station (Fig. 17-17). These tell the nursing team that the person needs help. The staff member shuts off the light at the bedside when responding to the call for help.

An intercom system lets a nursing team member talk with the person from the nurses' station. The person tells what is needed. Then the light is turned off at the station. Persons who are hard of hearing may have problems using an intercom. Be careful when using an intercom. Remember confidentiality. Persons nearby can hear what you and the person say.

Some persons have limited hand mobility. They may need a signal light that is turned on by tapping it with a hand or fist (Fig. 17-18).

The person is taught how to use the call system when admitted to the agency. Some people cannot use signal lights. Examples are persons who are confused or in a coma. Check the care plan for special communication measures. Check these persons often. Make sure their needs are met.

The phrase "signal light" is used in this book when referring to the call system. You must:

▶ Keep the signal light within the person's reach. Even if the person cannot use the signal light, keep it within reach for use by visitors and staff. They may need to signal for help.

▶ Place the signal light on the person's strong side.

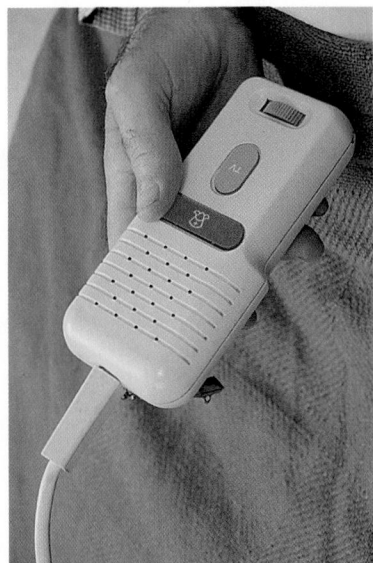

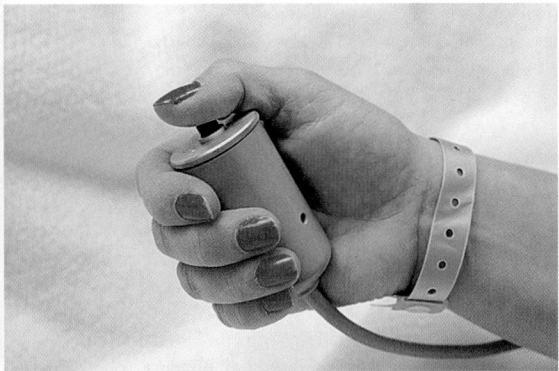

FIGURE 17-16 The signal light button is pressed when help is needed. *NOTE:* There are different types of signal lights.

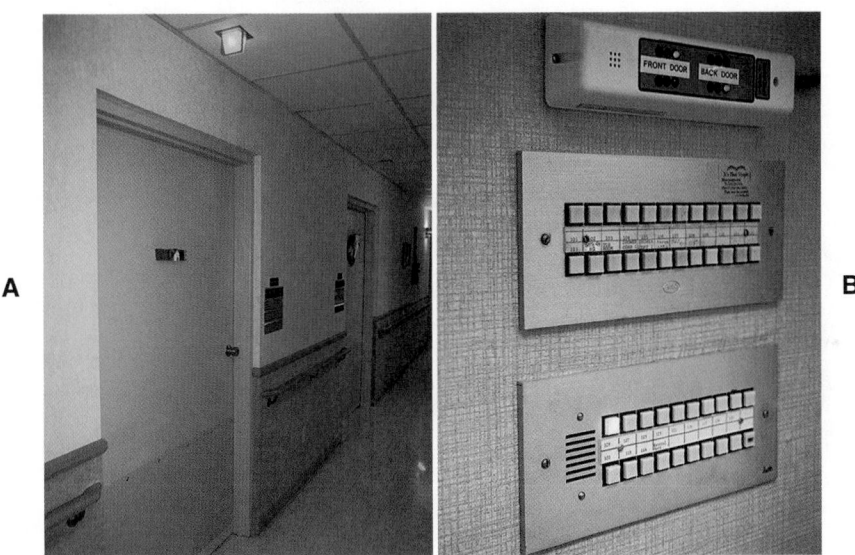

FIGURE 17-17 A, Light above the room door. **B,** Light panel and intercom at the nurses' station.

▶ Remind the person to signal when help is needed.
▶ Answer signal lights promptly. The person signals when help is needed. For example, the person may have an urgent need to use the bathroom. You can prevent embarrassing problems by promptly helping the person to the bathroom. You also help prevent infection, skin breakdown, pressure ulcers, and falls.
▶ Answer bathroom and shower or tub room signal lights at once.

See *Focus on Long-Term Care and Home Care: The Call System*, p. 282.

See *Teamwork and Time Management: The Call System*, p. 282.

See *Focus on Communication: The Call System*, p. 282.

See *Focus on Ethics and Laws: The Call System*, p. 282.

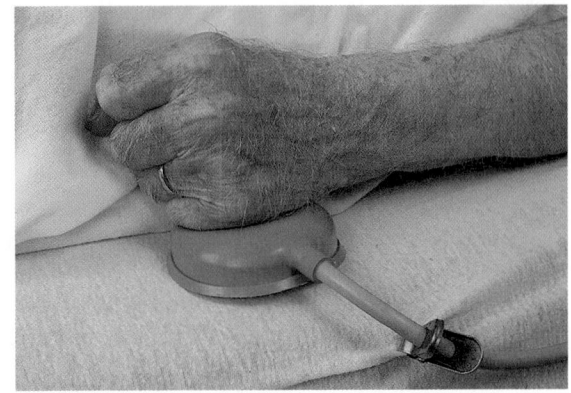

FIGURE 17-18 Signal light for a person with limited hand mobility.

FOCUS ON LONG-TERM CARE AND HOME CARE

The Call System

HOME CARE

Some home care patients stay in bed or in a certain part of the home. They need a way to call for help. Tap bells, dinner bells, baby monitors, and other devices are useful (Fig. 17-19.) Or you can give the person a small can with a few coins inside. Children's toys with bells, horns, and whistles may be useful.

TEAMWORK AND TIME MANAGEMENT

The Call System

Patients and residents use their signal lights when they need help. A person may turn on a signal light when you are assisting another person. The same may happen to another nursing team member. If nursing team members answer signal lights for each other, lights are answered promptly. Patients and residents receive quality care. Everyone is responsible for answering signal lights even if not assigned to the person.

FOCUS ON COMMUNICATION

The Call System

You will answer signal lights for co-workers. Therefore it is possible that you do not know their patients and residents and that they do not know you. To promote quality of life and promote safe care, you can say:

- "My name is Kate Hines. I'm a nursing assistant. How can I help you?"
- "Mrs. Janz, I'll need to check your care plan before I bring you more salt. I'll be right back, but is there anything else I can do before I leave?"
- "Mr. Duncan, I'll be happy to take your meal tray. I'll tell your nursing assistant what you ate."
- "Mrs. Palmer, do you use the bathroom or the bedpan?"

The Bathroom

Many agencies have a bathroom in each room. Some have a bathroom between two rooms. A toilet, sink, call system, and mirror are standard equipment (Fig. 17-20). Some bathrooms have showers.

Grab bars are by the toilet for the person's safety. The person uses them for support when lowering to or raising from the toilet. Some bathrooms have raised toilet seats. The higher toilets make wheelchair transfers easier. They also are helpful for persons with joint problems.

Towel racks, toilet paper, soap, paper towel dispenser, and a wastebasket are in the bathroom. They are placed within easy reach of the person.

FOCUS ON ETHICS AND LAWS

The Call System

A certified nursing assistant (CNA) worked at a nursing home in Arizona. In February 2002, she was counseled to improve her attendance and to stop having negative outbursts. In August 2002, it was noted that she gave poor care:

- Residents were not turned and/or briefs were not changed every 2 hours according to facility policy.
- She continued to have negative outbursts.

In November 2003, the CNA was terminated from employment for resident abuse. It was reported to the Arizona State Board of Nursing that she abused a resident for failure to provide care and by not meeting his needs.

- The resident was described as alert, paralyzed, on a ventilator for chronic respiratory failure, and totally dependent for all needs.
- The CNA was in his room many times during the night. She did not provide the care he requested.
- The CNA placed the signal light out of his reach. He used his head to use the signal light for assistance.

The CNA was hired by another agency in December 2003. She worked there until March 2004. On March 17 she was counseled for:

- Telling a resident that if she did not speak English she should go back to her country
- Being rough, rude, and verbally abusive to residents
- Refusing to work on a nursing unit "because all patients stink"
- Being critical and judgmental with new staff
- Leaving residents soaking wet at the end of her shift
- Telling a resident to "pee in your britches" rather than helping him to the bathroom

Her employment was terminated on March 19, 2004.

In January 2004, the Arizona State Board of Nursing sent the CNA a questionnaire for her to complete. It was returned to the Board as undeliverable. The CNA failed to notify the Board of an address change within the past 30 days as required by law.

The Board revoked the CNA's certificate for unprofessional conduct. She violated the following aspects of the state's Nurse Practice Act:

- Conduct or practice that is or might be harmful or dangerous to the health of a patient or the public
- Failing to follow an employer's policies and procedures designed to safeguard the client
- Failing to respect client rights and dignity
- Neglecting or abusing a client physically, verbally, or financially
- Practicing in any other manner that gives the Board reasonable cause to believe that the health of a client or the public may be harmed
- Failing to notify the board in writing within 30 days of any address change

She could apply for re-instatement of her certificate after a 5-year period.

(Arizona State Board of Nursing, May 18, 2006. NOTE: Names withheld by request of the Arizona State Board of Nursing.)

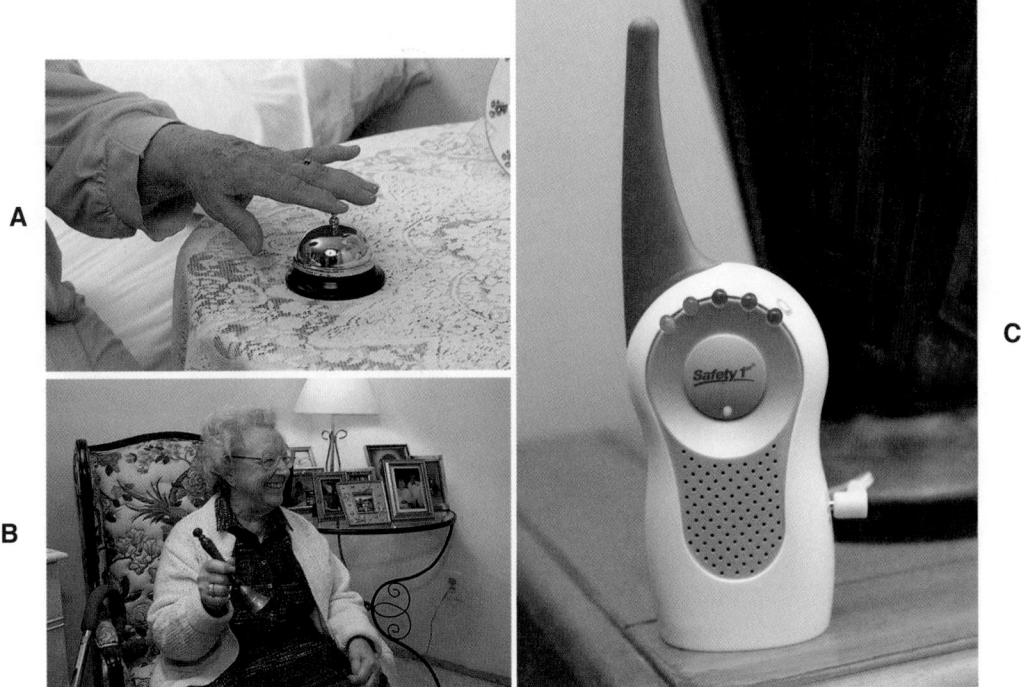

FIGURE 17-19 A, Tap bell. **B,** Dinner bell. **C,** Baby monitor.

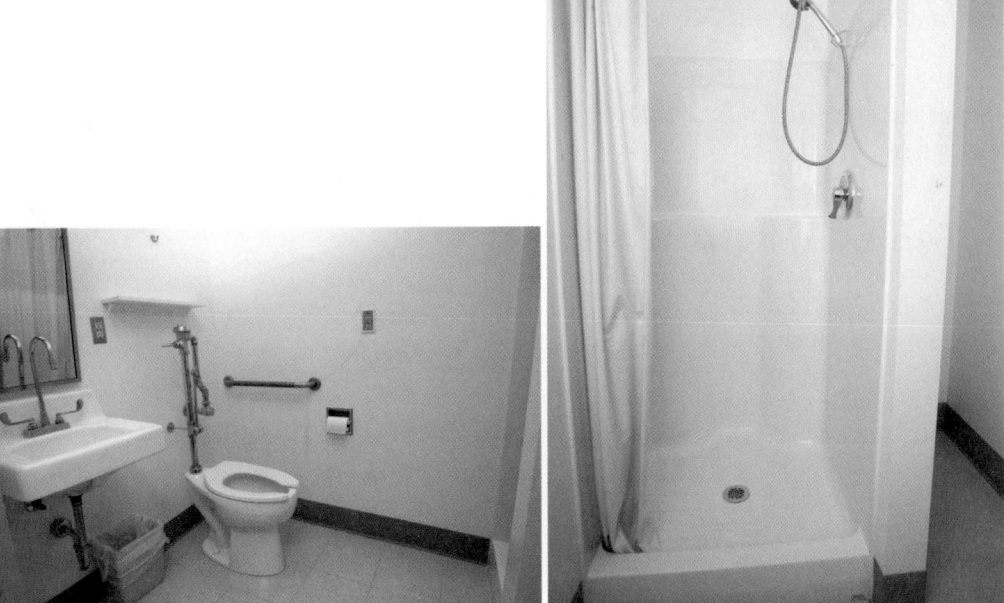

FIGURE 17-20 Bathroom in a nursing center.

Usually the signal light is next to the toilet. Pressing a button or pulling a cord turns on the signal light. When the bathroom signal light is used, the light flashes above the room door and at the nurses' station. The sound at the nurses' station is different from signal lights in rooms. These differences alert the nursing team that the person is in the bathroom. Someone must respond at once when a person needs help in a bathroom.

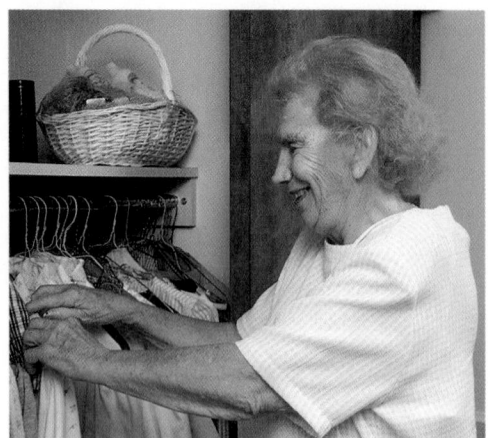

FIGURE 17-21 The resident can reach items in her closet.

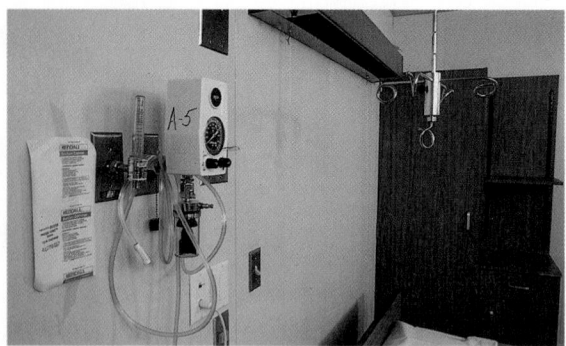

FIGURE 17-22 This room has an IV pole and oxygen and suction outlets.

Closet and Drawer Space

Closet and drawer space are provided for clothing. OBRA requires that nursing centers provide each person with closet space. The closet space must have shelves and a clothes rack (Fig. 17-21). The person must have free access to the closet and its contents.

Items in closets and drawers are the person's private property. You must have the person's permission to open or search closets or drawers.

Sometimes people hoard items—drugs, napkins, straws, food, sugar, salt, pepper, and so on. Hoarding can cause safety or health risks. Agency staff can inspect a person's closet or drawers if hoarding is suspected. The person is informed of the inspection. He or she is present when it takes place.

See *Promoting Safety and Comfort: Closet and Drawer Space.*

Other Equipment

Many agencies furnish rooms with other equipment. A TV, radio, and clock provide comfort and relaxation. Many rooms have phones, a computer, and Internet access.

Blood pressure equipment is often mounted on walls. There also are wall outlets for oxygen and suction (Fig. 17-22). Oxygen tanks and portable suction equipment are common in nursing centers and home care settings. For an intravenous (IV) infusion, an IV pole (IV standard) is used to hang IV bags or feeding bags.

See *Focus on Long-Term Care and Home Care: Other Equipment.*

PROMOTING SAFETY AND COMFORT: Closet and Drawer Space

SAFETY

The nurse may ask you to inspect a person's closet, drawers, or personal items. If so, the person must be present. Also have a co-worker with you. Your co-worker is a witness to what you are doing. This protects you if the person claims that something was stolen or damaged.

FOCUS ON LONG-TERM CARE AND HOME CARE

Other Equipment

LONG-TERM CARE

Nursing center residents have left their homes. Each had furniture, appliances, a private bathroom, and many personal belongings and treasures. Now the person lives in a strange place. He or she probably shares a room with another person. Leaving one's home is a hard part of growing old with poor health. It is important to make the person's unit as home-like as possible.

Residents may bring some furniture and personal items from home. A chair, footstool, lamp, and small table are often allowed. They can bring photos, religious items, and books. Some have plants to care for.

The resident is allowed personal choice in arranging items. The choices must be safe and not cause falls or other accidents. Also, the person's choices must not interfere with the rights of others. You may have to help the person choose the best place for personal items.

The center is now the person's home. You must help the person feel safe, secure, and comfortable. A home-like setting is important for quality of life. OBRA serves to promote quality of life. Box 17-1 lists OBRA requirements for resident rooms.

GENERAL RULES

The person's unit is kept clean, neat, safe, and comfortable. This is the responsibility of everyone involved in the person's care. The rules in Box 17-2 are followed to maintain the person's unit.

BOX 17-1 OBRA Requirements for Resident Rooms

- Designed for 1 to 4 persons
- Direct access to an exit corridor
- Full visual privacy—privacy curtain that extends around the bed, movable screens, doors
- At least one window to the outside
- Closet space with racks and shelves for each person
- Toilet facilities in the room or nearby (includes bathing facilities)
- Call system in the room and in toilet/bathing areas
- Bed of proper height and size
- Clean, comfortable mattress
- Bed linens are appropriate to the weather and climate
- Furniture for clothing, personal items, and a chair for visitors
- Clean and orderly room
- Odor-free room
- Room temperature between 71° and 81° F
- Acceptable noise level
- Adequate ventilation and room humidity
- Appropriate lighting
- No glares from floors, windows, and lighting
- Clean, orderly drawers, shelves, and personal items
- Pest-free room
- Hand rails in needed areas
- Bed rails only if needed
- Clean, dry floor
- Pathways are free of clutter and furniture
- Bed in low position
- Bed wheels are locked
- Personal supplies and items labeled and stored appropriately
- Drawers are free of unwrapped food
- Items within reach for use in bed or bathroom
- Space for wheelchair or walker use
- Raised toilet seat (if needed)
- Stool and skid-proof tub or shower

BOX 17-2 Maintaining the Person's Unit

- Keep the signal light within the person's reach at all times.
- Meet the needs of persons who cannot use the call system.
- Make sure the person can reach the overbed table and the bedside stand.
- Arrange personal items as the person prefers. Make sure they are easily reached.
- Make sure the person can reach the phone, TV, bed, and light controls.
- Provide the person with enough tissues and toilet paper.
- Adjust lighting, temperature, and ventilation for the person's comfort.
- Handle equipment carefully to prevent noise.
- Explain the causes of strange noises.
- Empty wastebaskets in the person's room and bathroom. They are emptied at least once a day. In some agencies they are emptied every shift.
- Respect the person's belongings. An item may not have importance or value to you. Yet it has great meaning for the person. Even a scrap of paper can have great meaning to the person.
- Do not throw away any items belonging to the person.
- Do not move furniture or the person's belongings. Persons with poor vision rely on memory or feel for the location of items.
- Straighten bed linens and towels as often as needed.
- Complete a safety check before leaving the room. (See the inside of the front book cover.)

REVIEW QUESTIONS

Circle the BEST answer.

1 Which temperature range is required by OBRA?
a 61° to 68° F
b 68° to 74° F
c 71° to 81° F
d 76° to 81° F

2 Which does *not* protect a person from drafts?
a Wearing enough clothing
b Being covered with enough blankets
c Being moved from a drafty area
d Sitting by a fan

3 Which does *not* prevent or reduce odors?
a Placing flowers in the room
b Emptying bedpans promptly
c Using room deodorizers
d Practicing good hygiene

4 To prevent odors, you need to do the following *except*
a Check incontinent persons often
b Dispose of ostomy products at the end of your shift
c Keep laundry containers closed
d Clean persons who are wet or soiled

5 Which does *not* control noise?
a Using plastic items
b Handling dishes with care
c Speaking softly
d Talking with others in the hallway

6 Beds are raised horizontally to
a Prevent bending and reaching when giving care
b Let the person get in and out of bed with ease
c Raise the head of the bed
d Lock the bed in position

Continued

7 The head of the bed is raised 30 degrees. This is called
   a Fowler's position
   b Semi-Fowler's position
   c Trendelenburg's position
   d Reverse Trendelenburg's position

8 These statements are about hospital bed system entrapment. Which is *false*?
   a Serious injuries and death can occur.
   b Older, frail, and confused persons are at risk.
   c The head, neck, and chest are areas of entrapment.
   d Bed rails present the only risk for entrapment.

9 The overbed table is *not* used
   a For eating
   b As a working surface
   c For the urinal
   d To store shaving items

10 The bedpan is stored in the
   a Closet
   b Bedside stand
   c Overbed table
   d Bathroom

11 Signal lights are answered
   a When you have time
   b At the end of your shift
   c Promptly
   d When you are near the person's room

12 To maintain the person's unit, you can do the following *except*
   a Save items that do not look important
   b Provide enough tissues and toilet paper
   c Place personal items as you choose
   d Straighten bed linens as needed

Circle T if the statement is true and F if the statement is false.

13 T F The person's unit is considered private.

14 T F Persons with dementia may have extreme reactions to strange sounds.

15 T F The privacy curtain prevents others from hearing conversations.

16 T F Soft, dim lighting is relaxing.

17 T F The signal light must always be within the person's reach.

18 T F The overbed table and bedside stand should be within the person's reach.

19 T F You should explain the cause of strange noises.

20 T F The person must be able to reach items in the closet.

21 T F You can adjust the person's room temperature for your comfort.

22 T F You can look through a person's closet and drawers.

Answers to these questions are on p. 780.

Bedmaking

OBJECTIVES

- Define the key terms listed in this chapter
- Describe open, closed, occupied, and surgical beds
- Explain when to change linens
- Explain how to use drawsheets
- Handle linens following the rules of medical asepsis
- Perform the procedures described in this chapter

PROCEDURES

- Making a Closed Bed
- Making an Open Bed
- Making an Occupied Bed
- Making a Surgical Bed

KEY TERMS

cotton drawsheet A drawsheet made of cotton; it helps keep the mattress and bottom linens clean

drawsheet A small sheet placed over the middle of the bottom sheet

plastic drawsheet A waterproof drawsheet made of plastic placed between the bottom sheet and the cotton drawsheet to protect the mattress and bottom linens from dampness and soiling; waterproof drawsheet

Procedures with this icon are on the CDCompanion in this book; those with this icon ![View Video!] are on the Evolve Student Resources Website.

Beds are made every day. Clean, dry, and wrinkle-free linens promote comfort. They also prevent skin breakdown and pressure ulcers (Chapter 32).

Beds are usually made in the morning after baths. Or they are made while the person is in the shower, up in the chair, or out of the room. Beds are made and rooms straightened before visitors arrive.

Do the following to keep beds neat and clean:

▶ Straighten linens whenever loose or wrinkled.
▶ Straighten loose or wrinkled linens at bedtime.
▶ Check for and remove food and crumbs after meals.
▶ Check linens for dentures, eyeglasses, hearing aids, sharp objects, and other items.
▶ Change linens whenever they become wet, soiled, or damp.
▶ Follow Standard Precautions and the Bloodborne Pathogen Standard. Contact with blood, body fluids, secretions, or excretions is likely.

TYPES OF BEDS

Beds are made in these ways:

▶ A *closed bed* is not in use. Top linens are not folded back (Fig. 18-1). The bed is ready for a new patient or resident. In nursing centers, closed beds are made for residents who are up during the day.
▶ An *open bed* is in use. Top linens are fan-folded back so the person can get into bed. A closed bed becomes an open bed by fan-folding back the top linens (Fig. 18-2).
▶ An *occupied bed* is made with the person in it (Fig. 18-3).
▶ A *surgical bed* is made to transfer a person from a stretcher (Fig. 18-4). This bed also is made for persons who arrive by ambulance.

LINENS

When handling linens and making beds, practice medical asepsis. Your uniform is considered dirty. Always hold linens away from your body and uniform (Fig. 18-5). Never shake linens. Shaking them spreads microbes. Place clean linens on a clean surface. Never put clean or dirty linens on the floor.

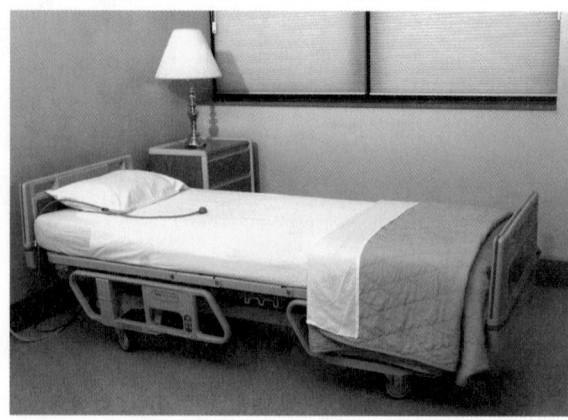

FIGURE 18-2 Open bed. Top linens are fan-folded to the foot of the bed.

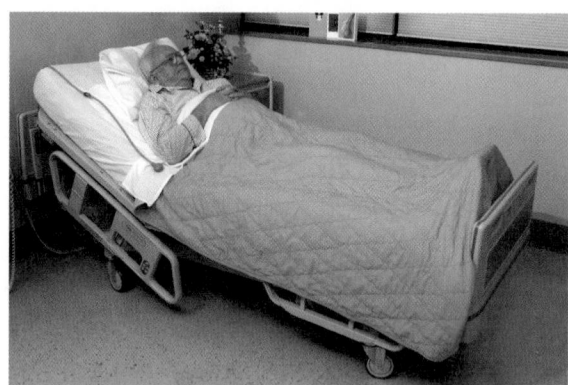

FIGURE 18-3 Occupied bed.

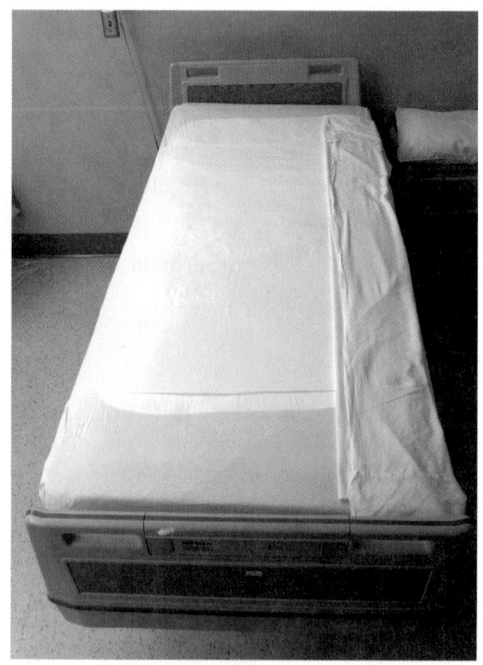

FIGURE 18-4 Surgical bed.

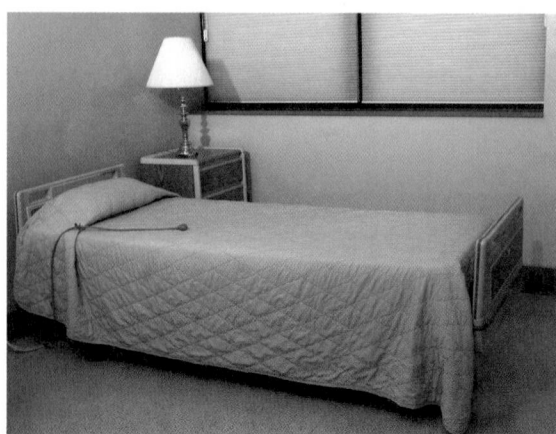

FIGURE 18-1 Closed bed.

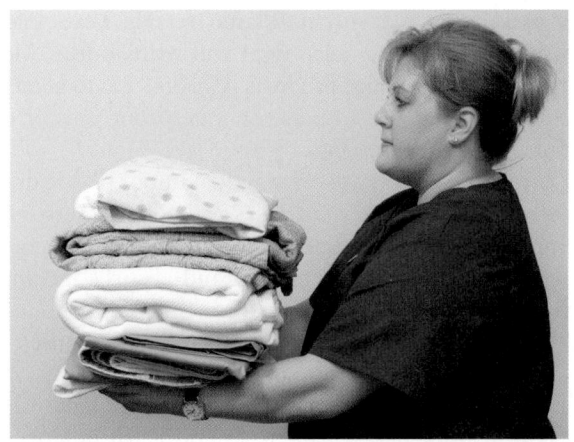

FIGURE 18-5 Hold linens away from your body and uniform.

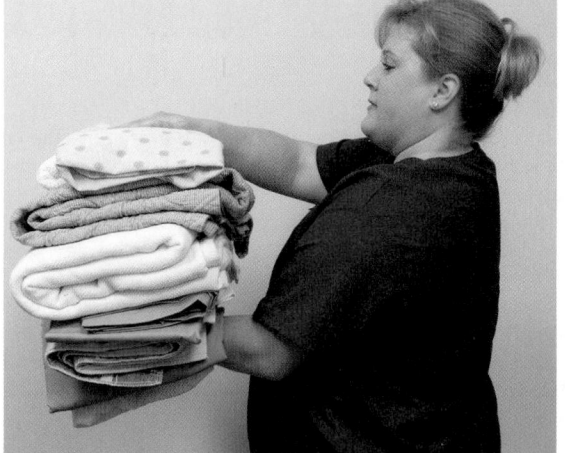

A

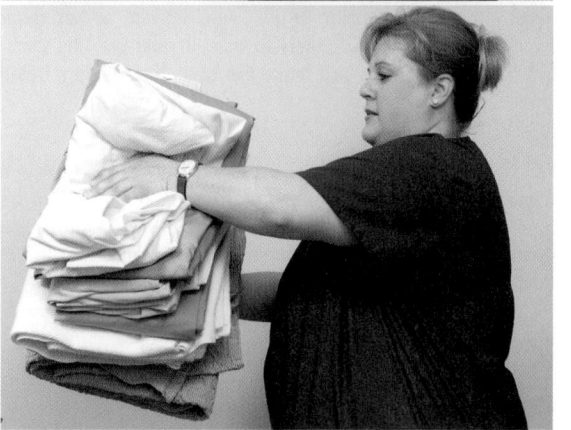

B

FIGURE 18-6 Collecting linens. **A,** The arm is placed over the top of the stack of linens. **B,** The stack of linens is turned onto the arm. Note that the linens are held away from the body.

Collect enough linens. If the person has two pillows, get two pillowcases. The person may need extra blankets for warmth. Do not bring unneeded linens to a person's room. Once in the person's room, extra linen is considered contaminated. It is not used for another person.

Collect linens in the order you will use them:
▶ Mattress pad (if needed)
▶ Bottom sheet (flat or fitted)
▶ Plastic drawsheet (waterproof drawsheet) or waterproof pad (if needed)
▶ Cotton drawsheet (if needed)
▶ Top sheet
▶ Blanket
▶ Bedspread
▶ Pillowcase(s)
▶ Bath towel(s)
▶ Hand towel
▶ Washcloth
▶ Gown or pajamas
▶ Bath blanket

Use one arm to hold the linens. Use your other hand to pick them up. The item you will use first is at the bottom of your stack. (You picked up the mattress pad first. It is at the bottom. The bath blanket is on top.) You need the mattress pad first. To get it on top, place your arm over the bath blanket. Then turn the stack over onto the arm on the bath blanket (Fig. 18-6). The arm that held the linens is now free. Place the clean linen on a clean surface.

Remove dirty linen one piece at a time. Roll each piece away from you. The side that touched the person is inside the roll and away from you (Fig. 18-7).

In hospitals, top and bottom sheets, the cotton drawsheet, and pillowcases are changed daily. The mattress pad, plastic drawsheet, blanket, and bedspread are reused for the same person. They are not reused if soiled, wet, or wrinkled. Wet, damp, or soiled linens are changed right away. Wear gloves and follow Standard Precautions and the Bloodborne Pathogen Standard.

See *Focus on Long-Term Care and Home Care: Linens,* p. 290.

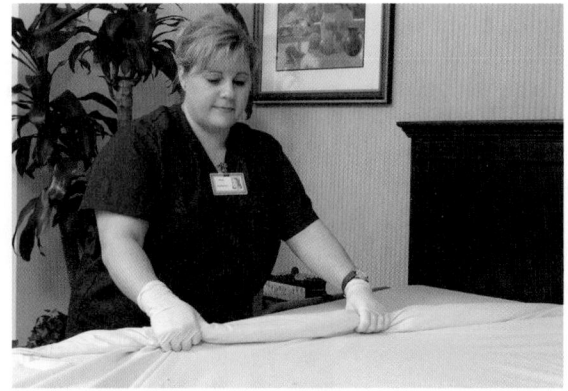

FIGURE 18-7 Roll dirty linen away from you.

FOCUS ON **LONG-TERM CARE** AND **HOME CARE**

Linens

LONG-TERM CARE

In nursing centers, linens are not changed every day. The center is the person's home. People do not change linens every day at home. A complete linen change is usually done weekly on the person's bath day. Pillowcases, top and bottom sheets, and drawsheets (if used) may be changed twice a week. Linens are always changed if wet, damp, soiled, or very wrinkled.

Some residents bring bedspreads, pillows, blankets, quilts, or afghans from home. Use them to make the bed. These items are the person's property. Make sure the items are labeled with the person's name. This prevents loss or confusion with another person's property.

Some centers have colored or printed linens. If so, let the person choose what color to use. Also let him or her decide how many pillows or blankets to use. If possible, the person chooses the time when you make the bed. The resident has the right to personal choice.

HOME CARE

Linen changes in the home are usually done weekly. Follow the person's routine. Change linens more often if the person asks you to do so. Always change linens that are wet, damp, soiled, or very wrinkled. Contact the nurse if the person refuses to have linens changed.

Drawsheets

A **drawsheet** is a small sheet place over the middle of the bottom sheet.

▶ A **cotton drawsheet** is made of cotton. It helps keep the mattress and bottom linens clean.
▶ A **plastic drawsheet** (waterproof drawsheet) is waterproof. Made of plastic, it is placed between the bottom sheet and cotton drawsheet. It protects the mattress and bottom linens from dampness and soiling.

The cotton drawsheet protects the person from contact with plastic and absorbs moisture. However, discomfort and skin breakdown may occur. Plastic retains heat. Plastic drawsheets are hard to keep tight and wrinkle-free. Many centers use incontinence products (Chapter 21) to keep the person and linens dry. Others use waterproof pads or disposable bed protectors (Fig. 18-8).

Cotton drawsheets are often used without plastic drawsheets. Plastic-covered mattresses cause some persons to perspire heavily. This increases discomfort. A cotton drawsheet reduces heat retention and absorbs moisture. Cotton drawsheets are often used as assist devices to move and transfer persons in bed (Chapter 16). When used for this purpose, do not tuck them in at the sides.

The bedmaking procedures that follow include plastic and cotton drawsheets. This is so you learn how to use them. Ask the nurse about their use in your agency.

See *Focus on Long-Term Care and Home Care: Drawsheets.*

FOCUS ON **LONG-TERM CARE** AND **HOME CARE**

Drawsheets

HOME CARE

A flat sheet folded in half can serve as a cotton drawsheet. A twin-size sheet is easier to use for this purpose. The nurse tells you what to use.

Medical supply stores sell plastic drawsheets and waterproof pads. The nurse discusses the need for these items with the person and family.

Some people use plastic mattress protectors. They protect mattresses. They do not protect bottom linens (cotton drawsheet, bottom sheet, and mattress pad). Some people place plastic under the drawsheet. The nurse tells you what is safe for the person.

Do not use plastic trash bags or dry-cleaning bags. They are not strong enough to protect the linens and mattress. They slide easily and can move out of place. Suffocation is a risk if the bag covers the person's nose and mouth.

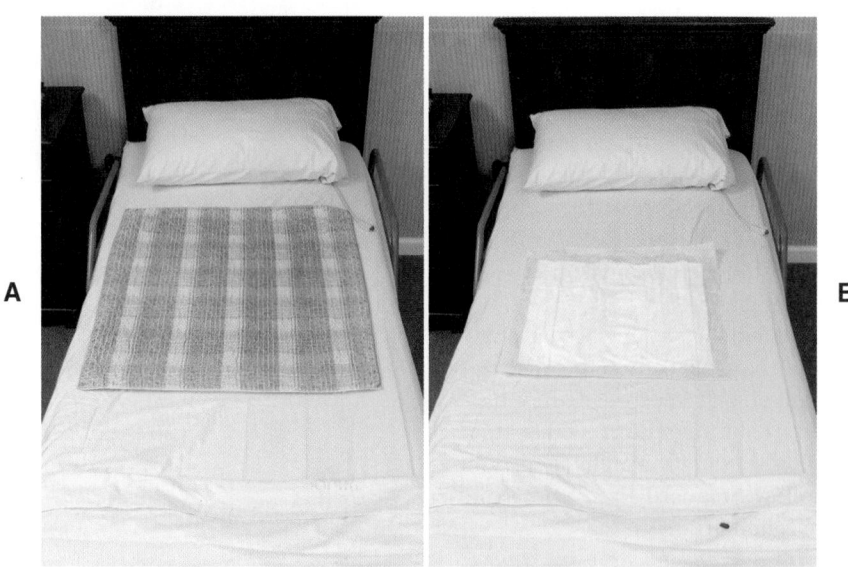

FIGURE 18-8 A, Waterproof pad. **B,** Disposable bed protector.

MAKING BEDS

When making beds, safety and medical asepsis are important. Follow the rules in Box 18-1.

See *Focus on Long-Term Care and Home Care: Making Beds.*

See *Focus on Children and Older Persons: Making Beds.*

See *Delegation Guidelines: Making Beds*, p. 292.

See *Promoting Safety and Comfort: Making Beds*, p. 292.

See *Teamwork and Time Management: Making Beds*, p. 292.

See *Focus on Ethics and Laws: Making Beds*, p. 292.

BOX 18-1 Rules for Bedmaking

- Use good body mechanics at all times (Chapter 15).
- Follow the rules in Chapter 16 to safely handle, move, and transfer the person.
- Follow the rules of medical asepsis.
- Follow Standard Precautions and the Bloodborne Pathogen Standard.
- Practice hand hygiene before handling clean linen.
- Practice hand hygiene after handling dirty linen.
- Bring enough linen to the person's room. Do not bring extra linens.
- Bring only the linens that you will need. Extra linens cannot be used for another person.
- Place clean linen on a clean surface. You can use the bedside chair, overbed table, or bedside stand. Place a barrier (towel, paper towels) between the clean surface and the linens if required by agency policy.
- Do not use extra linen in the person's room for another patient or resident. Extra linen is considered contaminated. Put it with the dirty laundry.
- Do not use torn or frayed linen.
- Never shake linens. Shaking linens spreads microbes.
- Hold linens away from your body and uniform. Dirty and clean linen must not touch your uniform.
- Never put dirty linens on the floor or on clean linens. Follow agency policy for dirty linen.
- Keep bottom linens tucked in and wrinkle-free.
- Cover a plastic drawsheet with a cotton drawsheet. A plastic drawsheet must not touch the person's body.
- Straighten and tighten loose sheets, blankets, and bedspreads as needed.
- Make as much of one side of the bed as possible before going to the other side. This saves time and energy.
- Change wet, damp, and soiled linens right away.

Making Beds

CHILDREN

Cribs and crib linens present safety hazards. Mattresses, linens, and bumper pads pose many dangers. They can cause strangulation and suffocation. Report any hazard to the nurse. Follow these safety measures and those in Chapters 11 and 17.

- The crib mattress must be firm. A soft mattress can cover the baby's nose and mouth. This prevents breathing.
- The mattress must fit tight into the crib. If not, the baby can get caught between the mattress and the crib. There must be no gaps between the mattress and the crib.
- Do not use plastic trash bags, dry-cleaning bags, or plastic packaging materials to protect the mattress. The plastic can cling to the baby's face, nose, and mouth. This prevents breathing and causes suffocation.
- The space between the crib rail slats must be no more than 2 inches. If the space is larger, the baby's head can get caught between the slats. The baby can suffocate.
- The mattress must be at least 26 inches lower than the top of the crib rails. This prevents the baby from falling out of the crib. The mattress is lowered to the lowest position when the baby starts to stand in the crib.
- The headboard and footboard must not have cut-outs.
- Bumper pads:
  - Must cover the entire inside of the crib.
  - Must fit snugly against the slats. If not, the baby's head can get caught between the bumper pads and the slats.
  - Tie or snap in place. At least 6 ties or straps are needed.
  - Are placed so the ties or straps are away from the baby.
  - Must not have long ties or straps. Extra length in the ties or straps is cut off. The baby can get entangled in long ties or straps.
  - Are removed from the crib when the baby starts to stand.
- The mattress is covered with a crib sheet. The crib sheet fits snugly.
- Only crib sheets are used in cribs. Sheets for twin, regular, queen, king, and other beds are not used.
- Sheets are not used if they are frayed, worn, or have loose threads or stitching.
- Pillows, blankets, comforters, quilts, sheepskin, and pillow-like stuffed toys and other soft products are not placed in the crib.

Making Beds

HOME CARE

Many home care patients do not have hospital beds. You will use twin-, regular-, queen-, and king-sized beds. Water beds, sofa sleepers, cots, and recliners are common. Make the bed as the person wishes. Follow the rules in Box 18-1. If the person's wishes are not safe, contact the nurse.

Your assignment may include doing laundry. Wash linen when soiling is fresh to help prevent staining. Urine, feces, vomit, and blood can stain linens. Follow these guidelines:

- Wear gloves. Linens may contain blood, body fluids, secretions, or excretions.
- Rinse the item in cold water to remove the substance.

- Treat the stain. The person may use a stain-removing agent. Read and follow the manufacturer's instructions. Or the nurse may direct you to soak the item for 30 minutes in an ammonia solution:
  - 1 quart warm water
  - ½ teaspoon liquid dishwashing detergent
  - 1 tablespoon ammonia
- Rinse the item with cool water after soaking.
- Machine-wash the item with a detergent.

Ammonia is a poison. Do not inhale the fumes or let the ammonia have contact with your skin or eyes. Follow the manufacturer's instructions. Do not mix ammonia with bleach or other chemicals. Deadly fumes will result.

DELEGATION GUIDELINES: Making Beds

Before making a bed, you need this information from the nurse and the care plan:

- What type of bed to make—closed, open, occupied, or surgical.
- If you need to use a cotton drawsheet.
- If you need to use a plastic drawsheet, waterproof pad, or incontinence product.
- Position restrictions or limits in the person's movement or activity.
- If the person uses bed rails.
- The person's treatment, therapy, and activity schedule. For example, Mr. Smith needs a treatment in bed. Change linens after the treatment. Mrs. Jones goes to physical therapy. Make the bed while she is away from the room.
- How to position the person and the positioning devices needed.
- If the bed needs to be locked into a certain position (Chapter 17).

PROMOTING SAFETY AND COMFORT: Making Beds

SAFETY

You need to raise the bed for good body mechanics. The bed also must be flat. If the bed is locked, unlock it. Then adjust the bed. Return the bed to the desired position when you are done. Then lock the bed.

Wear gloves when removing linen from the person's bed. Also follow other aspects of Standard Precautions and the Bloodborne Pathogen Standard. Linens may contain blood, body fluids, secretions, or excretions.

After making a bed, lower the bed to its lowest position. For an occupied bed, raise or lower bed rails according to the care plan.

COMFORT

For an occupied bed, cover the person with a bath blanket before removing the top sheet. Do not leave the person uncovered when making the bed. The bath blanket provides for warmth and privacy.

If the person uses a pillow, adjust it as needed during the procedure. After the procedure, position the person as directed by the nurse and the care plan. Always make sure linens are straight and wrinkle-free.

TEAMWORK AND TIME MANAGEMENT

Making Beds

To save time and energy, make beds with a co-worker. Make one side of the bed while your co-worker makes the other.

Making beds with a co-worker is faster, easier, and safer for patients and residents, you, and your co-worker. Remember to thank your co-worker for helping you. Also help your co-worker make beds when asked to do so.

⬥ The Closed Bed

The closed bed is made after a person is discharged. It is made for a new patient or resident. The bed is made after the bed frame and mattress are cleaned and disinfected. Clean linens are needed for the entire bed.

See *Focus on Long-Term Care and Home Care: The Closed Bed.*

Text continued on p. 297

FOCUS ON ETHICS AND LAWS

Making Beds

On August 2, 1990, a patient had back surgery. She was on complete bedrest until August 4 when the doctor changed the order. The new order was "increase activity up as tolerated with assist." According to the facts reported in the court case, the following occurred between the patient and a nurse:

- On August 5 the patient was awakened when the nurse bumped into her bed. The nurse told the patient that she had to get up and have her bed made. The patient explained that she had an uncomfortable night, could not sleep, and wanted to rest. Despite pleas to stay in bed, the nurse told the patient that she [the nurse] had to make the bed.
- The nurse then pulled the patient by her arm. The patient pleaded with the nurse to leave her alone because she wanted to sleep. The patient also told the nurse that it hurt to have her arm pulled that way.
- The nurse let go of the patient's arm. The patient laid down in bed.
- The nurse then pulled the patient's feet off of the bed. In extreme pain, the patient "started to yell, to plead with the nurse not to do what she was doing and told her that it hurt."
- The nurse insisted that the patient had to get up. The nurse insisted that she had to make the bed. The nurse forced the patient into a standing position. The patient, in pain, told the nurse that she was going to "throw up or faint."
- The nurse shoved the patient "into a straight back chair using her hands to press down hard on the [patient's] shoulders."
- In extreme pain, the patient pleaded with the nurse and said that she was going to faint.
- The nurse then forced the patient's head between her knees down to her lap. The patient felt extreme pain in the middle of her back.
- The nurse then raised the patient's back. In extreme pain, the patient could not get up when she tried to do so. The patient continued to plead with the nurse to put her back to bed.
- The nurse again told the patient that she had to make the bed. The nurse "ripped the sheet off the bed and used it to tie [the patient] in the chair with a knot towards the back."
- The patient "tried to reach forward to push the nurse's call button . . . [The nurse] kicked and pushed the table out at the same time, away and out of the [patient's] grasp." The patient said that she wanted to call a nurse.
- The nurse left the room for 10 minutes. "She came back and made the bed with a laboratory technician." After making the bed, they put the patient back in bed. The patient was crying.

The Appellate Court of Illinois reviewing the case said the "negligence here was . . . grossly apparent . . . ." The case was sent back to the trial court for a full trial.

(R. Prairie v University of Chicago Hospitals, 1998.)

FOCUS ON LONG-TERM CARE AND HOME CARE

The Closed Bed

LONG-TERM CARE

In nursing centers, closed beds are made for residents who are up for most or all of the day. Top linens are folded back at bedtime. Clean linens are used as needed.

HOME CARE

A closed bed means that linens are not folded back. Closed beds are made for patients who are up for most or all of the day. Clean linens are used as needed.

MAKING A CLOSED BED

- Knock before entering the person's room.
- Address the person by name.
- Introduce yourself by name and title.
- Explain the procedure to the person before beginning and during the procedure.

- Protect the person's rights during the procedure.
- Handle the person gently during the procedure.

PRE-PROCEDURE

1 Follow *Delegation Guidelines: Making Beds.* See *Promoting Safety and Comfort: Making Beds.*
2 Practice hand hygiene.
3 Collect clean linen:
- Mattress pad (if needed)
- Bottom sheet (flat sheet or fitted sheet)
- Plastic drawsheet or waterproof pad (if needed)
- Cotton drawsheet (if needed)
- Top sheet
- Blanket
- Bedspread

- A pillowcase for each pillow
- Bath towel(s)
- Hand towel
- Washcloth
- Gown
- Bath blanket
- Gloves
- Laundry bag

4 Place linen on a clean surface.
5 Raise the bed for good body mechanics.

PROCEDURE

6 Put on the gloves.
7 Remove linen. Roll each piece away from you. Place each piece in a laundry bag. (*NOTE:* Discard incontinence products or disposable bed protectors in the trash. Do not put them in the laundry bag.)
8 Clean the bed frame and mattress if this is part of your job.
9 Remove and discard gloves. Decontaminate your hands.
10 Move the mattress to the head of the bed.
11 Put the mattress pad on the mattress. It is even with the top of the mattress.
12 Place the bottom sheet on the mattress pad (Fig. 18-9, p. 294):
   a Unfold it lengthwise.
   b Place the center crease in the middle of the bed.
   c Position the lower edge even with the bottom of the mattress.
   d Place the large hem at the top and the small hem at the bottom.
   e Face hem-stitching downward, away from the person.
13 Open the sheet. Fan-fold it to the other side of the bed (Fig. 18-10, p. 294).
14 Tuck the top of the sheet under the mattress. The sheet is tight and smooth.
15 Make a mitered corner if using a flat sheet (Fig. 18-11, p. 295).
16 Place the plastic drawsheet on the bed. It is in the middle of the mattress. Or put the waterproof pad on the bed.
17 Open the plastic drawsheet. Fan-fold it to the other side of the bed.
18 Place a cotton drawsheet over the plastic drawsheet. It covers the entire plastic drawsheet (Fig. 18-12, p. 295).
19 Open the cotton drawsheet. Fan-fold it to the other side of the bed.

20 Tuck both drawsheets under the mattress. Or tuck each in separately.
21 Go to the other side of the bed.
22 Miter the top corner of the flat bottom sheet.
23 Pull the bottom sheet tight so there are no wrinkles. Tuck in the sheet.
24 Pull the drawsheets tight so there are no wrinkles. Tuck both in together or separately (Fig. 18-13, p. 295).
25 Go to the other side of the bed.
26 Put the top sheet on the bed:
   a Unfold it lengthwise.
   b Place the center crease in the middle.
   c Place the large hem even with the top of the mattress.
   d Open the sheet. Fan-fold it to the other side.
   e Face hem-stitching outward, away from the person.
   f Do not tuck the bottom in yet.
   g Never tuck top linens in on the sides.
27 Place the blanket on the bed:
   a Unfold it so the center crease is in the middle.
   b Put the upper hem about 6 to 8 inches from the top of the mattress.
   c Open the blanket. Fan-fold it to the other side.
   d If steps 33 and 34 are not done, turn the top sheet down over the blanket. Hem-stitching is down, away from the person.
28 Place the bedspread on the bed:
   a Unfold it so the center crease is in the middle.
   b Place the upper hem even with the top of the mattress.
   c Open and fan-fold the spread to the other side.
   d Make sure the spread facing the door is even. It covers all top linens.
29 Tuck in top linens together at the foot of the bed. They should be smooth and tight. Make a mitered corner.
30 Go to the other side.
31 Straighten all top linen. Work from the head of the bed to the foot.

Continued

MAKING A CLOSED BED—cont'd

PROCEDURE—cont'd

32 Tuck in top linens together at the foot of the bed. Make a mitered corner.

33 Turn the top hem of the spread under the blanket to make a cuff (Fig. 18-14).

34 Turn the top sheet down over the spread. Hem-stitching is down. (Steps 33 and 34 are not done in some agencies. The spread covers the pillow. If so, tuck the spread under the pillow.)

35 Put the pillowcase on the pillow as in Figure 18-15, p. 296 or Figure 18-16, p. 296. Fold extra material under the pillow at the seam end of the pillowcase.

36 Place the pillow on the bed. The open end of the pillowcase is away from the door. The seam is toward the head of the bed.

POST-PROCEDURE

37 Provide for comfort. (See the inside of the front book cover.) *NOTE:* Omit this step if the bed is prepared for a new patient or resident.

38 Attach the signal light to the bed. Or place it within the person's reach.

39 Lower the bed to its lowest position. Lock the bed wheels.

40 Put the towels, washcloth, gown or pajamas, and bath blanket in the bedside stand.

41 Complete a safety check of the room. (See the inside of the front book cover.)

42 Follow agency policy for dirty linen.

43 Decontaminate your hands.

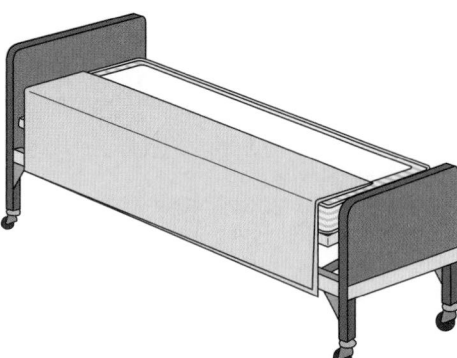

FIGURE 18-9 The bottom sheet is on the bed with the center crease in the middle. The lower edge of the sheet is even with the bottom of the mattress.

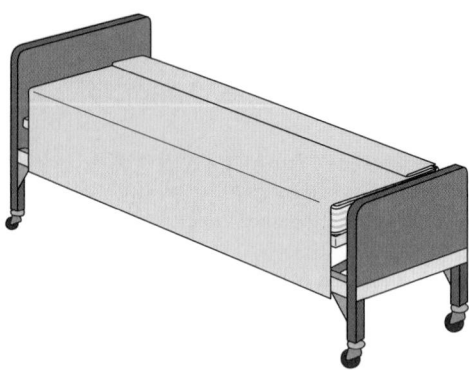

FIGURE 18-10 The bottom sheet is fan-folded to the other side of the bed.

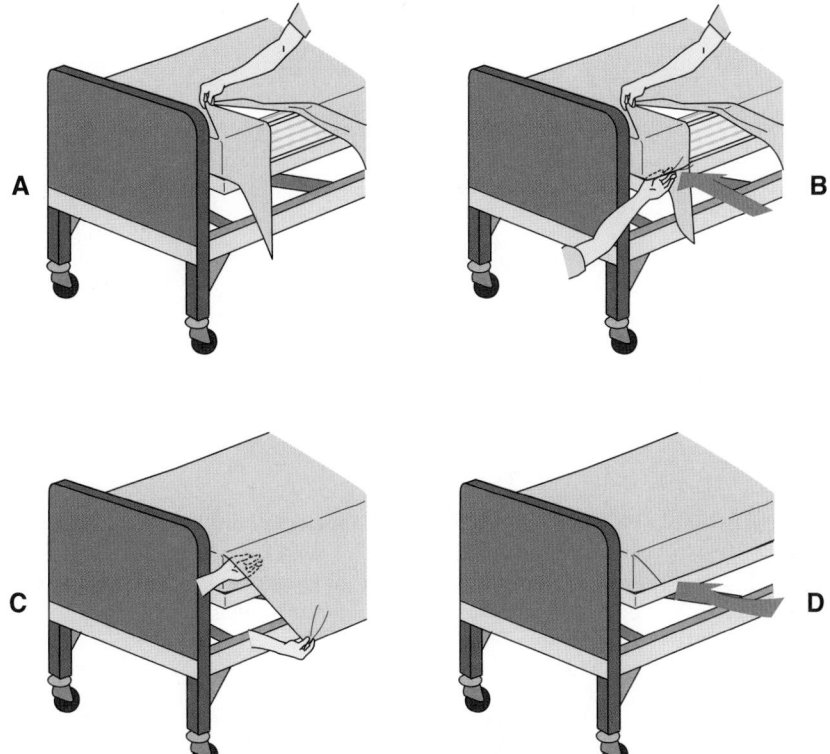

FIGURE 18-11 Making a mitered corner. **A,** The bottom sheet is tucked under the mattress at the head of the bed. The side of the sheet is raised onto the mattress. **B,** The remaining portion of the sheet is tucked under the mattress. **C,** The raised portion of the sheet is brought off the mattress. **D,** The entire side of the sheet is tucked under the mattress.

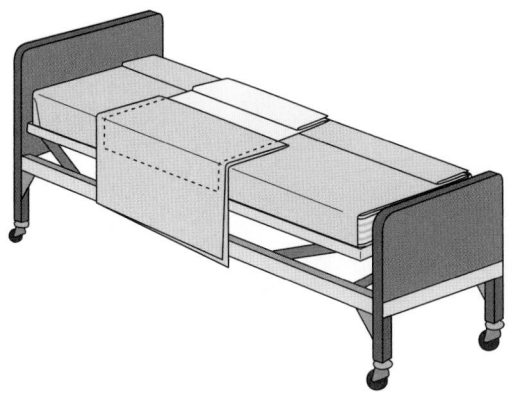

FIGURE 18-12 A cotton drawsheet is over the plastic drawsheet. The cotton drawsheet completely covers the plastic drawsheet.

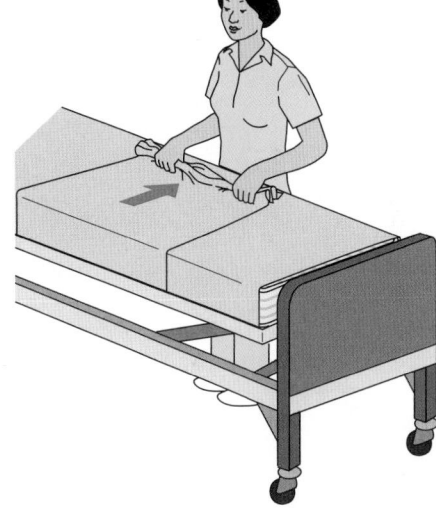

FIGURE 18-13 The drawsheet is pulled tight to remove wrinkles.

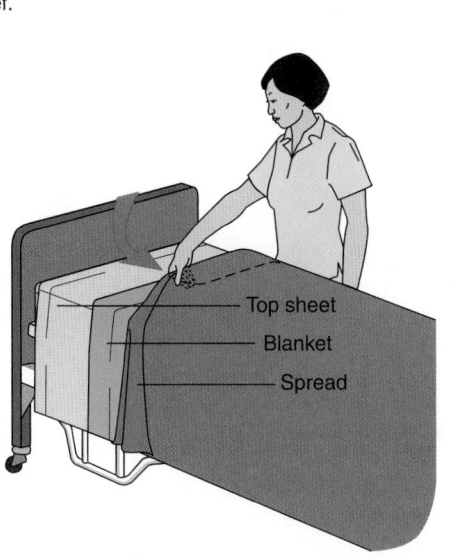

- Top sheet
- Blanket
- Spread

FIGURE 18-14 The top hem of the bedspread is turned under the top hem of the blanket to make a cuff.

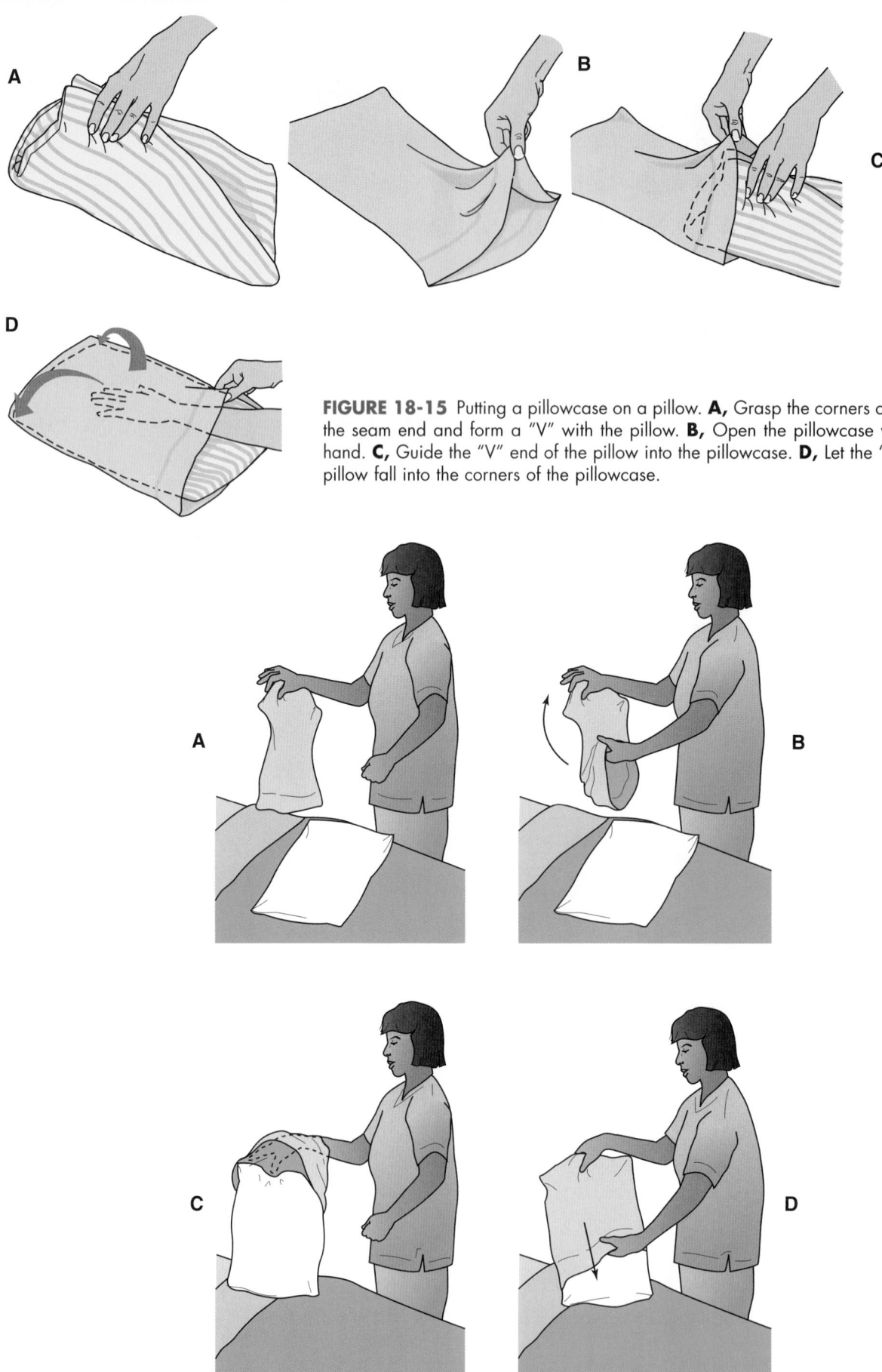

FIGURE 18-15 Putting a pillowcase on a pillow. **A,** Grasp the corners of the pillow at the seam end and form a "V" with the pillow. **B,** Open the pillowcase with your free hand. **C,** Guide the "V" end of the pillow into the pillowcase. **D,** Let the "V" end of the pillow fall into the corners of the pillowcase.

FIGURE 18-16 Putting a pillowcase on a pillow. **A,** Grasp the closed end of the pillowcase. **B,** Using your other hand, gather up the pillowcase. The pillowcase should cover your hand holding the closed end. **C,** Grasp the pillow with the hand covered by the pillowcase. **D,** Pull the pillowcase down over the pillow with your other hand.

◆ The Open Bed

A closed bed becomes an open bed by fan-folding back the top linen. The open bed lets the person get into bed with ease. Make this bed for:

▸ Newly admitted persons arriving by wheelchair
▸ Persons who are getting ready for bed
▸ Persons who are out of bed for a short time

MAKING AN OPEN BED

✔ Quality of Life *Remember to:*

- Knock before entering the person's room.
- Address the person by name.
- Introduce yourself by name and title.
- Explain the procedure to the person before beginning and during the procedure.

- Protect the person's rights during the procedure.
- Handle the person gently during the procedure.

PROCEDURE

1 Follow *Delegation Guidelines: Making Beds,* p. 292. See *Promoting Safety and Comfort: Making Beds,* p. 292.
2 Practice hand hygiene.
3 Collect linen for a closed bed.
4 Make a closed bed. See procedure: *Making a Closed Bed,* p. 293.

5 Fan-fold top linens to the foot of the bed (see Fig. 18-2).
6 Attach the signal light to the bed.
7 Lower the bed to its lowest position.
8 Put towels, washcloth, gown or pajamas, and the bath blanket in the bedside stand.

POST-PROCEDURE

9 Provide for comfort. (See the inside of the front book cover.)
10 Place the signal light within the person's reach.
11 Complete a safety check of the room. (See the inside of the front book cover.)

12 Follow agency policy for dirty linen.
13 Decontaminate your hands.

◆ The Occupied Bed

You make an occupied bed when the person stays in bed. Keep the person in good alignment. Follow restrictions or limits in the person's movement or position.

Explain each procedure step to the person before it is done. This is important even if the person cannot respond to you or is in a coma.

See *Focus on Communication: The Occupied Bed.*
See *Promoting Safety and Comfort: The Occupied Bed.*

Text continued on p. 300

FOCUS ON COMMUNICATION

The Occupied Bed

After making an occupied bed, make sure the person is comfortable. You can ask:

- "Are you comfortable?"
- "What can I do to make you more comfortable?"
- "Are you warm enough?"
- "Can I adjust your pillow?"

After making the bed, thank the person for cooperating.

PROMOTING SAFETY AND COMFORT: The Occupied Bed

SAFETY

The person lies on one side of the bed and then the other. Protect the person from falling out of bed. If the person uses bed rails, the far bed rail is up. If the person does not use bed rails, have another person help you. You work on one side of the bed. Your co-worker works on the other.

COMFORT

To make an occupied bed, the person lays on his or her side. You tuck dirty bottom linens under the person. Then you put clean linens on the bed. These, too, are tucked under the person. The tucked linens create a "bump" in the middle of the bed. To make the other side, the person rolls over the "bump" to the other side of the bed. For the person's comfort, try to make the "bump" as low as possible. Do this by fan-folding dirty and clean bottom linens neatly and flatly.

MAKING AN OCCUPIED BED

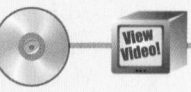

✔ **Quality of Life** *Remember to:*

- Knock before entering the person's room.
- Address the person by name.
- Introduce yourself by name and title.

- Explain the procedure to the person before beginning and during the procedure.
- Protect the person's rights during the procedure.
- Handle the person gently during the procedure.

PROCEDURE

1 Follow *Delegation Guidelines: Making Beds,* p. 292. See *Promoting Safety and Comfort:*
  - *Making Beds,* p. 292
  - *The Occupied Bed,* p. 297
2 Practice hand hygiene.
3 Collect the following:
  - Gloves
  - Laundry bag
  - Clean linen (see procedure: *Making a Closed Bed,* p. 293)

4 Place linen on a clean surface.
5 Identify the person. Check the ID bracelet against the assignment sheet. Also call the person by name.
6 Provide for privacy.
7 Remove the signal light.
8 Raise the bed for good body mechanics. Bed rails are up.
9 Lower the head of the bed. It is as flat as possible.

PROCEDURE

10 Decontaminate your hands. Put on gloves.
11 Loosen top linens at the foot of the bed.
12 Remove the bedspread (Fig. 18-17). Then remove the blanket. Place each over the chair.
13 Cover the person with a bath blanket. Use the blanket in the bedside stand.
  a Unfold a bath blanket over the top sheet.
  b Ask the person to hold onto the bath blanket. If he or she cannot, tuck the top part under the person's shoulders.
  c Grasp the top sheet under the bath blanket at the shoulders. Bring the sheet down to the foot of the bed. Remove the sheet from under the blanket (Fig. 18-18, p. 300).
14 Lower the bed rail near you.
15 Position the person on the side of the bed away from you. Adjust the pillow for comfort.
16 Loosen bottom linens from the head to the foot of the bed.
17 Fan-fold bottom linens one at a time toward the person. Start with the cotton drawsheet (Fig. 18-19, p. 300). If reusing the mattress pad, do not fan-fold it.
18 Place a clean mattress pad on the bed. Unfold it lengthwise. The center crease is in the middle. Fan-fold the top part toward the person. If reusing the mattress pad, straighten and smooth any wrinkles.
19 Place the bottom sheet on the mattress pad. Hem-stitching is away from the person. Unfold the sheet so the crease is in the middle. The small hem is even with the bottom of the mattress. Fan-fold the top part toward the person.
20 Make a mitered corner at the head of the bed. Tuck the sheet under the mattress from the head to the foot.
21 Pull the plastic drawsheet toward you over the bottom sheet. Tuck excess material under the mattress. Do the following for a clean plastic drawsheet (Fig. 18-20, p. 300):
  a Place the plastic drawsheet on the bed. It is in the middle of the mattress.

  b Fan-fold the top part toward the person.
  c Tuck in excess fabric.
22 Place the cotton drawsheet over the plastic draw-sheet. It covers the entire plastic drawsheet. Fan-fold the top part toward the person. Tuck in excess fabric.
23 Raise the bed rail. Go to the other side, and lower the bed rail.
24 Explain to the person that he or she will roll over a "bump." Assure the person that he or she will not fall.
25 Help the person turn to the other side. Adjust the pillow for comfort.
26 Loosen bottom linens. Remove one piece at a time. Place each piece in the laundry bag. (NOTE: Discard disposable bed protectors and incontinence products in the trash. Do not put them in the laundry bag.)
27 Remove and discard the gloves. Decontaminate your hands.
28 Straighten and smooth the mattress pad.
29 Pull the clean bottom sheet toward you. Make a mitered corner at the top. Tuck the sheet under the mattress from the head to the foot of the bed.
30 Pull the drawsheets tightly toward you. Tuck both under together or separately.
31 Position the person supine in the center of the bed. Adjust the pillow for comfort.
32 Put the top sheet on the bed. Unfold it lengthwise. The crease is in the middle. The large hem is even with the top of the mattress. Hem-stitching is on the outside.
33 Ask the person to hold onto the top sheet so you can remove the bath blanket. Or tuck the top sheet under the person's shoulders. Remove the bath blanket.
34 Place the blanket on the bed. Unfold it so the crease is in the middle and it covers the person. The upper hem is 6 to 8 inches from the top of the mattress.
35 Place the bedspread on the bed. Unfold it so the center crease is in the middle and it covers the person. The top hem is even with the mattress top.

MAKING AN OCCUPIED BED—cont'd

PROCEDURE—cont'd

36 Turn the top hem of the spread under the blanket to make a cuff.

37 Bring the top sheet down over the spread to form a cuff.

38 Go to the foot of the bed.

39 Make a toe pleat. Make a 2-inch pleat across the foot of the bed. The pleat is about 6 to 8 inches from the foot of the bed.

40 Lift the mattress corner with one arm. Tuck all top linens under the mattress. Make a mitered corner.

41 Raise the bed rail. Go to the other side, and lower the bed rail.

42 Straighten and smooth top linens.

43 Tuck all top linens under the mattress. Make a mitered corner.

44 Change the pillowcase(s).

POST-PROCEDURE

45 Provide for comfort. (See the inside of the front book cover.)

46 Place the signal light within reach.

47 Lower the bed to its lowest position. Lock the bed wheels.

48 Raise or lower bed rails. Follow the care plan.

49 Put the towels, washcloth, gown or pajamas, and bath blanket in the bedside stand.

50 Unscreen the person.

51 Complete a safety check of the room. (See the inside of the front book cover.)

52 Follow agency policy for dirty linen.

53 Decontaminate your hands.

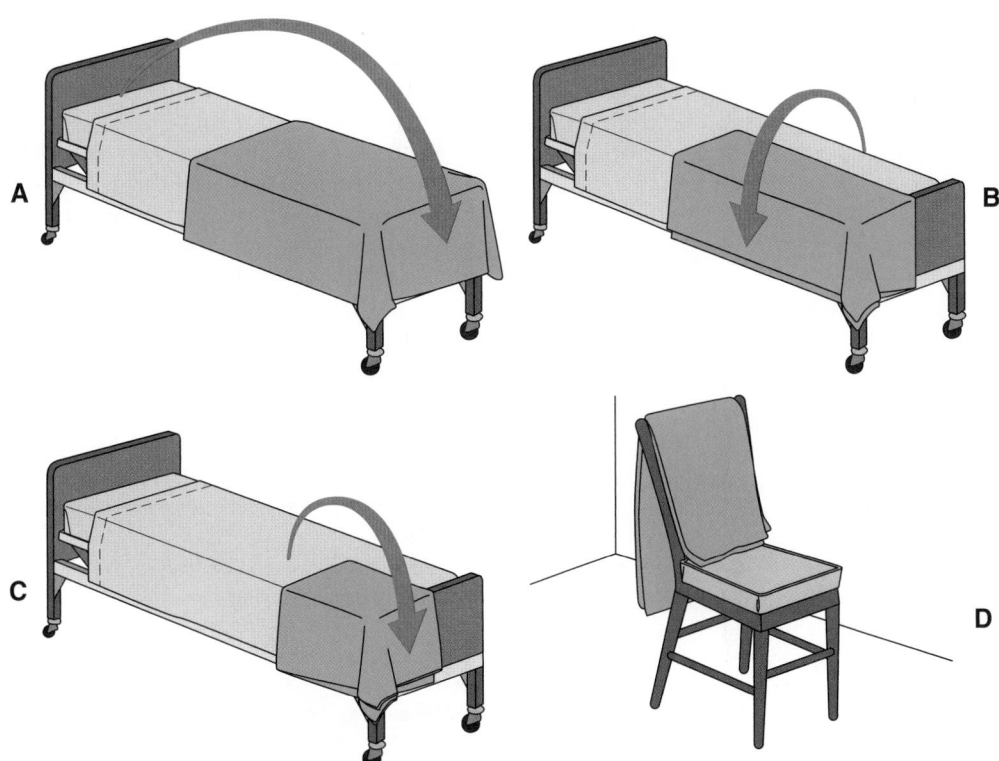

FIGURE 18-17 Folding linen for reuse. **A,** Fold the top edge of the bedspread down to the bottom edge. **B,** Fold the bedspread from the far side of the bed to the near side. **C,** Fold the top edge of the bedspread down to the bottom edge again. **D,** Place the folded bedspread over the back of the chair.

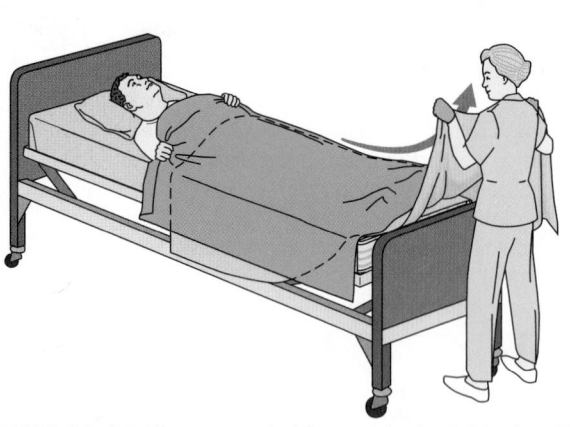

FIGURE 18-18 The person holds onto the bath blanket. The top sheet is removed from under the bath blanket.

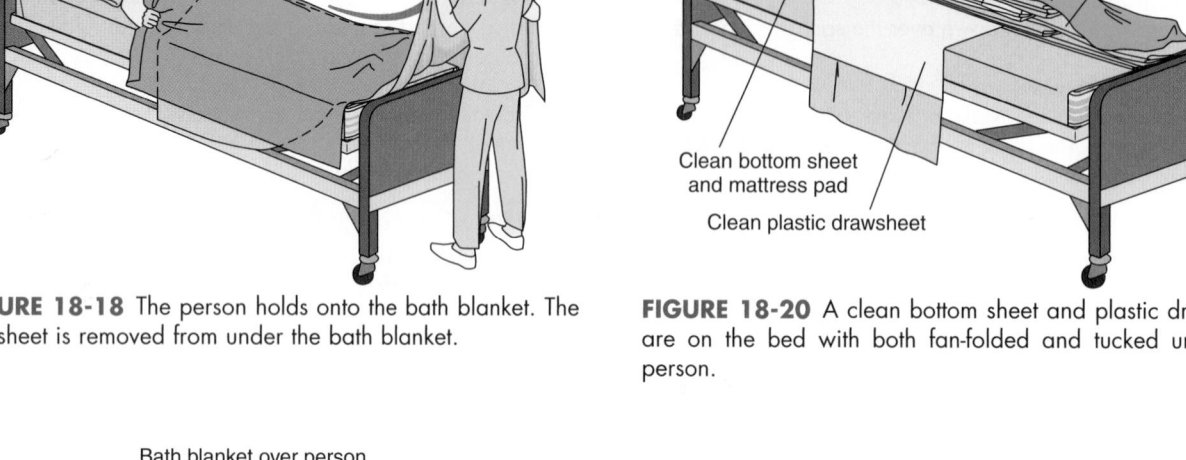

FIGURE 18-20 A clean bottom sheet and plastic drawsheet are on the bed with both fan-folded and tucked under the person.

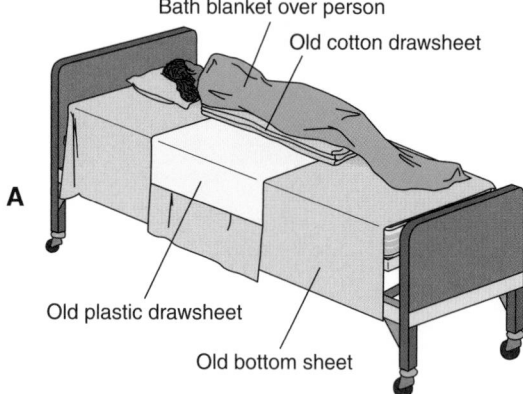

A

Bath blanket over person

Old cotton drawsheet

Old plastic drawsheet

Old bottom sheet

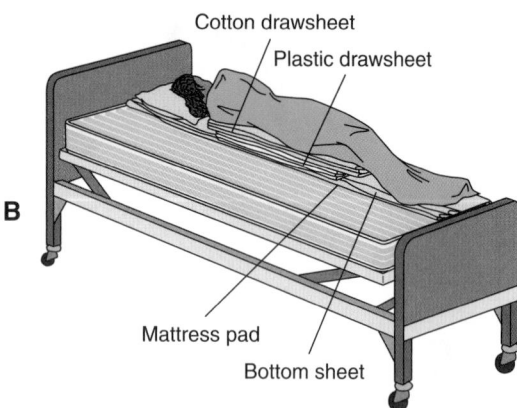

B

Cotton drawsheet

Plastic drawsheet

Mattress pad

Bottom sheet

FIGURE 18-19 Occupied bed. **A,** The cotton drawsheet is fan-folded and tucked under the person. **B,** All bottom linens are tucked under the person.

◆ The Surgical Bed

The surgical bed also is called a *recovery bed* or *post-operative bed.* It is a form of the open bed. Top linens are folded to transfer the person from a stretcher to the bed. These beds are made for persons:

▶ Returning to their rooms from surgery. A complete linen change is needed.

▶ Who arrive at the agency by ambulance. A complete linen change is needed if the person is a new patient or resident or is returning to the center from the hospital.

▶ Who are taken by stretcher to treatment or therapy areas. A complete linen change is not needed.

▶ Using portable tubs. Because the person will have a bath, a complete linen change is needed.
  See *Promoting Safety and Comfort: The Surgical Bed.*

PROMOTING SAFETY AND COMFORT: The Surgical Bed

SAFETY

To safely transfer a person from a stretcher to a surgical bed, see procedure: *Moving the Person to a Stretcher* (Chapter 16). Also follow the rules for stretcher safety (Chapter 11). After the transfer, lower the bed to its lowest position. Make sure the bed wheels are locked. Raise or lower bed rails according to the care plan.

MAKING A SURGICAL BED

PROCEDURE

1 Follow *Delegation Guidelines: Making Beds,* p. 292. See *Promoting Safety and Comfort:*
   • *Making Beds,* p. 292
   • *The Surgical Bed*
2 Practice hand hygiene.
3 Collect the following:
   • Clean linen (see procedure: *Making a Closed Bed,* p. 293)
   • Gloves
   • Laundry bag
   • Equipment requested by the nurse
4 Place linen on a clean surface.
5 Remove the signal light.
6 Raise the bed for good body mechanics.
7 Remove all linen from the bed. Wear gloves. Decontaminate your hands after removing gloves.
8 Make a closed bed (see procedure: *Making a Closed Bed,* p. 293). Do not tuck top linens under the mattress.
9 Fold all top linens at the foot of the bed back onto the bed. The fold is even with the edge of the mattress (Fig. 18-21, *A*).

10 Fan-fold linen lengthwise to the side of the bed farthest from the door (Fig. 18-21, *B*).
11 Put the pillowcase(s) on the pillow(s).
12 Place the pillow(s) on a clean surface.
13 Leave the bed in its highest position.
14 Leave both bed rails down.
15 Put the towels, washcloth, gown or pajamas, and bath blanket in the bedside stand.
16 Move furniture away from the bed. Allow room for the stretcher and the staff.
17 Do not attach the signal light to the bed.
18 Complete a safety check of the room. (See the inside of the front book cover.)
19 Follow agency policy for soiled linen.
20 Decontaminate your hands.

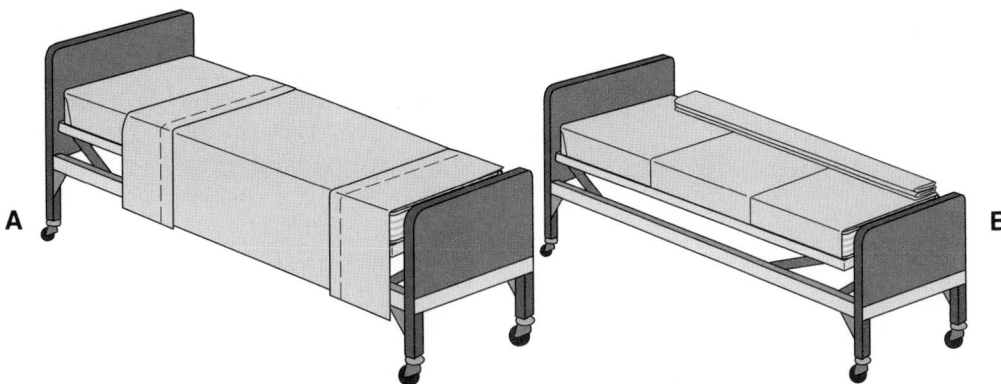

FIGURE 18-21 Surgical bed. **A,** The bottom of the top linens is folded back onto the bed. The fold is even with the bottom edge of the mattress. **B,** Top linens are fan-folded lengthwise to the opposite side of the bed.

REVIEW QUESTIONS

Circle T if the statement is true and F if the statement is false.

1 T **(F)** In nursing centers, complete linen changes are required for closed beds and surgical beds.

2 **(T)** F The hem-stitching of the bottom sheet is placed away from the person.

3 T **(F)** To remove crumbs from the bed, you shake linens in the air.

4 **(T)** F The upper hem of the bedspread is even with the top of the mattress.

5 **(T)** F Top linens are fan-folded to the foot of the bed for an open bed.

6 T **(F)** A cotton drawsheet is used only with a plastic drawsheet.

7 T **(F)** Nursing centers usually allow residents to bring bed coverings from home.

Circle the BEST answer.

8 Which requires a linen change?
   a The person will have visitors
   (b) Wet linen
   c Wrinkled linen
   d Crumbs in the bed

9 You will transfer a person from a stretcher to the bed. Which bed should you make?
   a A closed bed
   b An open bed
   c An occupied bed
   (d) A surgical bed

10 When handling linens
    a Put dirty linens on the floor
    (b) Hold linens away from your body and uniform
    c Shake linens to unfold them
    d Take extra linen to another person's room

11 A resident is out of the bed most of the day. Which bed should you make?
    (a) A closed bed
    b An open bed
    c An occupied bed
    d A surgical bed

12 A complete linen change is done when
    a The bottom linens are wet or soiled
    (b) The bed is made for a new person
    c The person will transfer from a stretcher to a bed
    d Linens are loose or wrinkled

13 You are using a plastic drawsheet. Which is *true*?
    (a) A cotton drawsheet must completely cover the plastic drawsheet.
    b Waterproof pads are needed.
    c The person's consent is needed.
    d The plastic is in contact with the person's skin.

14 When making an occupied bed, you do the following *except*
    a Cover the person with a bath blanket
    b Screen the person
    c Raise the far bed rail
    (d) Fan-fold top linens to the foot of the bed

15 A surgical bed is kept
    a In Fowler's position
    b In the lowest position
    (c) In the highest position
    d In the supine position

Answers to these questions are on p. 780.

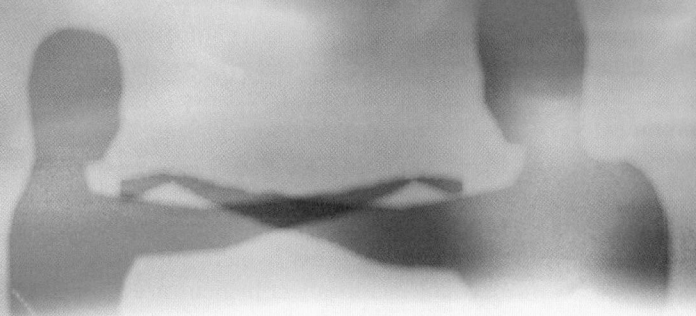

Personal Hygiene

OBJECTIVES

- Define the key terms listed in this chapter
- Explain why personal hygiene is important
- Describe the care given before and after breakfast, after lunch, and in the evening
- Describe the rules for bathing
- Identify safety measures for tub baths and showers
- Explain the purposes of a back massage
- Explain the purposes of perineal care
- Identify the observations to report and record while assisting with hygiene
- Perform the procedures described in this chapter

PROCEDURES

- Assisting the Person to Brush and Floss the Teeth
- Brushing and Flossing the Person's Teeth
- Providing Mouth Care for the Unconscious Person
- Providing Denture Care
- Giving a Complete Bed Bath

- Assisting With the Partial Bath
- Assisting With a Tub Bath or Shower
- Giving a Back Massage
- Giving Female Perineal Care
- Giving Male Perineal Care

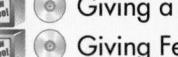 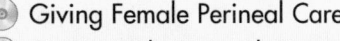

 Procedures with this icon are on the CDCompanion in this book; those with this icon are on the Evolve Student Resources Website.

KEY TERMS

AM care Early morning care

aspiration Breathing fluid, food, vomitus, or an object into the lungs

denture An artificial tooth or a set of artificial teeth

early morning care Care given before breakfast; AM care

evening care Care given in the evening at bedtime; PM care

morning care Care given after breakfast; hygiene measures are more thorough at this time

oral hygiene Mouth care

pericare Perineal care

perineal care Cleaning the genital and anal areas; pericare

plaque A thin film that sticks to the teeth; it contains saliva, microbes, and other substances

PM care Evening care

tartar Hardened plaque

Hygiene promotes comfort, safety, and health. The skin is the body's first line of defense against disease. Intact skin prevents microbes from entering the body and causing an infection. Likewise, mucous membranes of the mouth, genital area, and anus must be clean and intact. Besides cleansing, good hygiene prevents body and breath odors. It is relaxing and increases circulation. (Review the structures and functions of the skin and teeth in Box 19-1.)

Culture and personal choice affect hygiene. See *Caring About Culture: Personal Hygiene.* Some people take showers. Others take tub baths. Some bathe at bedtime. Others bathe in the morning. Bathing frequency also varies. Some bathe one or two times a day—before work and after work or exercise. Some people do not have water for bathing. Others cannot afford soap, deodorant, shampoo, toothpaste, or other hygiene products.

Many factors affect hygiene needs—perspiration, elimination, vomiting, drainage from wounds or body openings, bedrest, and activity. Illness and aging changes can affect self-care abilities. Some people need help with hygiene. The nurse uses the nursing process to meet the person's hygiene needs. Follow the nurse's directions and the care plan.

See *Focus on Children and Older Persons: Personal Hygiene.*
See *Focus on Communication: Personal Hygiene.*

BOX 19-1 Teeth, Gums, and Skin: Body Structure and Function

THE TEETH AND GUMS

The teeth cut, chop, and grind food into small bits for digestion and swallowing. A tooth has three main parts: the crown, neck, and root (Fig. 19-1). The crown is the outer part. It is covered by enamel. The neck is surrounded by gums (gingivae). The root fits into the bone of the lower or upper jaw.

THE SKIN

The skin is the largest system. It is the body's natural covering. There are two layers: the epidermis and the dermis (Fig. 19-2). The *epidermis* is the outer layer. It contains living and dead cells. Dead cells constantly flake off and are replaced by living cells. Living cells also die and flake off. The epidermis has no blood vessels and few nerve endings. The *dermis* is the inner layer. It is made up of connective tissue. Blood vessels, nerves, sweat and oil glands, and hair roots are found in the dermis.

Sweat glands help regulate body temperature. Sweat is secreted through the skin's pores. The body is cooled as sweat evaporates. Oil glands secrete an oily substance into the space near the hair shaft. Oil travels to the skin surface. The oil helps keep the hair and skin soft and shiny.

The skin has these functions:

- Provides the body's protective covering. Intact skin prevents bacteria and other substances from entering the body.
- Prevents large amounts of water from leaving the body.
- Protects the organs from injury.
- Nerve endings in the skin sense both pleasant and unpleasant stimulation. Cold, pain, touch, and pressure are sensed.
- Helps regulate body temperature. Blood vessels dilate (widen) when temperature outside the body is high. More blood is brought to the body surface for cooling during evaporation. When blood vessels constrict (narrow), the body retains heat because less blood reaches the skin.

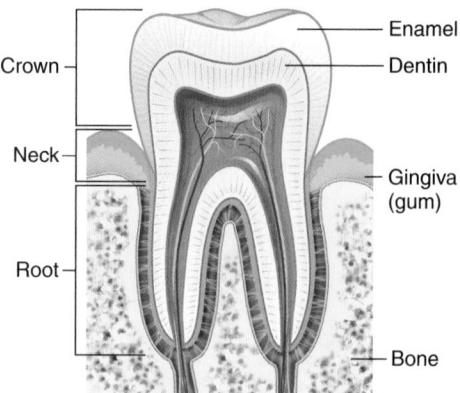

FIGURE 19-1 Parts of the tooth. (From Thibodeau GA, Patton KT: *The human body in health & disease*, ed 4, St Louis, 2005, Mosby.)

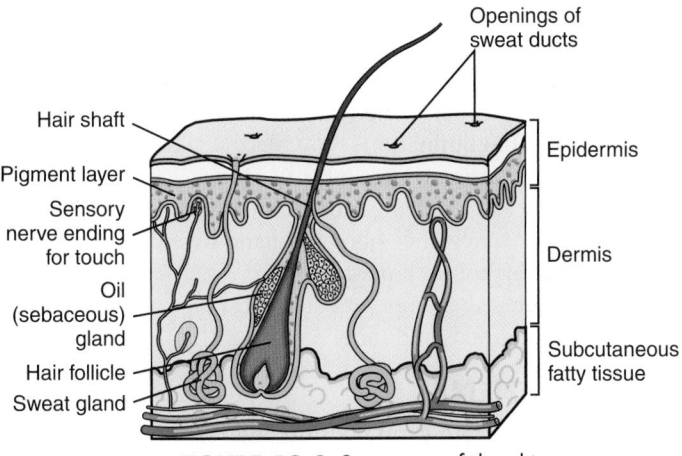

FIGURE 19-2 Structures of the skin.

Openings of sweat ducts

Hair shaft

Pigment layer

Sensory nerve ending for touch

Oil (sebaceous) gland

Hair follicle

Sweat gland

Epidermis

Dermis

Subcutaneous fatty tissue

FOCUS ON CHILDREN AND OLDER PERSONS

Personal Hygiene

OLDER PERSONS

Some older persons resist your efforts to assist with hygiene. Illness, disability, dementia, and personal choice are common reasons. Follow the care plan to meet the person's needs.

Older and disabled persons may have a hard time bending and reaching. Some have weak hand grips. They cannot hold onto soap or a washcloth. To maintain independence, the person may use an adaptive device for hygiene (Fig. 19-3). Remember, the person should do as much for himself or herself as safely possible.

CARING ABOUT CULTURE

Personal Hygiene

Personal hygiene is very important to *East Indian Hindus.* Their religion requires at least one bath a day. Some believe it is harmful to bathe after a meal. Another Hindu belief is that a cold bath prevents blood disease. Some believe that eye injuries can occur if a bath is too hot. Hot water can be added to cold water. However, cold water is not added to hot water. After bathing, the body is carefully dried with a towel.

From Giger JN, Davidhizar RE: *Transcultural nursing: assessment and intervention,* ed 4, St Louis, 2004, Mosby.

FOCUS ON COMMUNICATION

Personal Hygiene

During hygiene procedures, you must make sure that the person is warm enough. You can ask:
* "Is the water warm enough?" "Is it too hot?" "Is it too cold?"
* "Are you warm enough?"
* "Do you need another bath blanket?"
* "Is the water starting to cool?"
* "Is the room warm enough?"

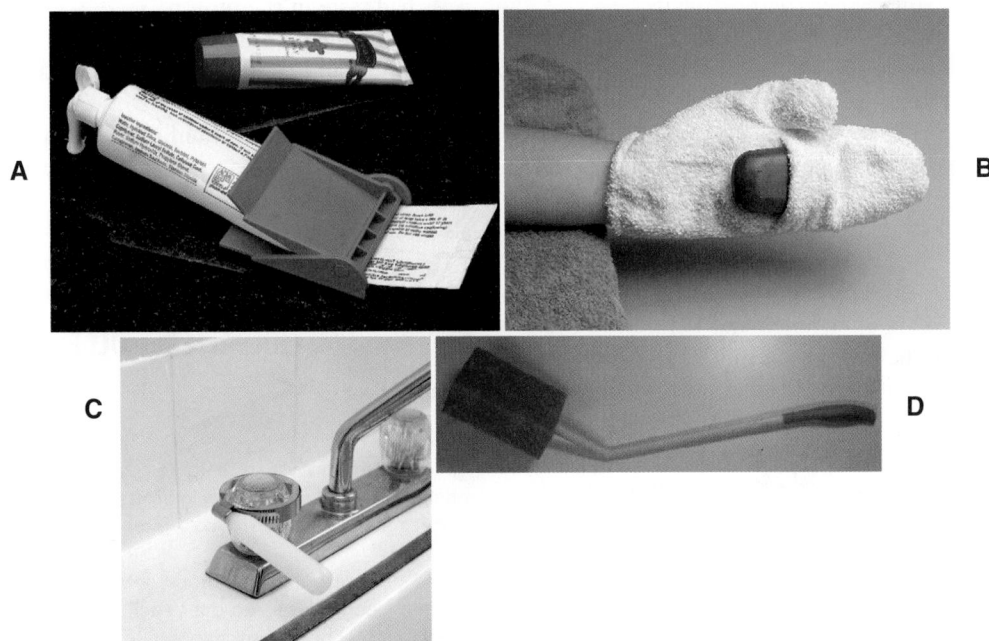

FIGURE 19-3 Adaptive devices for hygiene. **A,** Tube squeezer for toothpaste. **B,** The wash mitt holds a bar of soap. **C,** A tap turner makes round knobs easy to turn. **D,** A long-handled sponge is used for hard to reach body parts. (Courtesy ElderStore, Alpharetta, Ga.)

DAILY CARE

Most people have hygiene routines and habits. For example, teeth are brushed and face and hands washed after sleep. These and other hygiene measures are often done before and after meals and at bedtime.

Infants and young children need help with hygiene. So do some weak or disabled adults. Routine care is given during the day and evening. You assist with hygiene whenever it is needed. You must protect the person's right to privacy and to personal choice.

Before Breakfast

Routine care given before breakfast is called **early morning care** or **AM care**. Night shift or day shift staff members give AM care. They get patients and residents ready for breakfast or morning tests. AM care includes:

▶ Assisting with elimination
▶ Cleaning incontinent persons
▶ Changing wet or soiled linens and garments
▶ Assisting with hygiene—face and hand washing and oral hygiene
▶ Assisting with dressing and hair care
▶ Positioning persons for breakfast—dining room, bedside chair, or in bed
▶ Making beds and straightening units

After Breakfast

Morning care is given after breakfast. Hygiene measures are more thorough at this time. They usually involve:

▶ Assisting with elimination
▶ Cleaning incontinent persons
▶ Changing wet or soiled linens and garments
▶ Assisting with hygiene—face and hand washing, oral hygiene, bathing, back massage, and perineal care
▶ Assisting with grooming—hair care, shaving, dressing, and undressing
▶ Assisting with activity—range-of-motion exercises and ambulation
▶ Making beds and straightening units

Afternoon Care

Routine hygiene is done after lunch and before the evening meal. It is done before the person takes a nap, has visitors, or attends activity programs. Afternoon care involves:

▶ Assisting with elimination before and after naps
▶ Cleaning incontinent persons before and after naps
▶ Changing wet or soiled linen before and after naps
▶ Changing wet or soiled garments before and after naps
▶ Assisting with hygiene and grooming—face and hand washing, oral hygiene, and hair care
▶ Assisting with activity—range-of-motion exercises and ambulation
▶ Straightening beds and units

Evening Care

Care given in the evening at bedtime is called **evening care** or **PM care**. Evening care is relaxing and promotes comfort. Measures performed before sleep include:

▶ Assisting with elimination
▶ Cleaning incontinent persons
▶ Changing wet or soiled linens and garments
▶ Assisting with hygiene—face and hand washing, oral hygiene, and back massages
▶ Helping persons change into sleepwear
▶ Straightening beds and units

ORAL HYGIENE

Oral hygiene (mouth care) does the following:

▶ Keeps the mouth and teeth clean
▶ Prevents mouth odors and infections
▶ Increases comfort
▶ Makes food taste better
▶ Reduces the risk for *cavities (dental caries)* and *periodontal disease*

Periodontal disease (*gum disease, pyorrhea*) is an inflammation of tissues around the teeth. Plaque and tartar build up from poor oral hygiene. **Plaque** is a thin film that sticks to teeth. It contains saliva, microbes, and other substances. Plaque causes tooth decay *(cavities)*. When plaque hardens, it is called **tartar**. Tartar builds up at the gum line near the neck of the tooth. Tartar buildup causes periodontal disease. The gums are red and swollen and bleed easily. As the disease progresses, bone is destroyed and teeth loosen. Tooth loss is common.

Illness, disease, and some drugs often cause:

▶ A bad taste in the mouth
▶ A whitish coating in the mouth and on the tongue
▶ Redness and swelling in the mouth and on the tongue
▶ Dry mouth (Dry mouth also is common from oxygen, smoking, decreased fluid intake, and anxiety.)

The nurse assesses the person's need for mouth care. The speech/language pathologist and the dietitian may also do so.

See *Focus on Children and Older Persons: Oral Hygiene.*

FOCUS ON CHILDREN AND OLDER PERSONS

Oral Hygiene

CHILDREN

Infants need mouth care to remove food and bacteria. This helps prevent *baby bottle tooth decay (early childhood tooth caries [cavities]).* It can occur in all teeth. It is most common in the upper teeth.

To prevent baby bottle tooth decay, wipe the baby's gums with a clean gauze pad after each feeding. After the first baby tooth erupts, begin brushing with a child's soft toothbrush.

Children learn to brush their teeth around 3 years of age. They may not be thorough. They need help brushing. Older children can do a thorough job. Remind them when to brush.

FOCUS ON **CHILDREN** AND **OLDER PERSONS**

Flossing

CHILDREN

By age 2½ years, all baby teeth have erupted. Flossing begins at this time. You need to floss for pre-schoolers. Older children can floss themselves. They may need reminding and some supervision.

OLDER PERSONS

Flossing was not a common oral hygiene measure many years ago. Therefore some older persons do not floss their teeth. Follow the care plan.

Flossing

Flossing removes plaque and tartar from the teeth. These substances cause periodontal disease. Flossing also removes food from between the teeth. Usually done after brushing, it can be done at other times. Some people floss after meals. If done once a day, bedtime is the best time to floss. You need to floss for persons who cannot do so themselves.

See *Focus on Children and Older Persons: Flossing.*

Equipment

A toothbrush, toothpaste, dental floss, and mouthwash are needed. The toothbrush should have soft bristles. Persons with dentures need a denture cleaner, denture cup, and denture brush or toothbrush. Use only denture cleaning products. Otherwise, you could damage dentures.

Sponge swabs are used for persons with sore, tender mouths. They also are used for unconscious persons. Use sponge swabs with care. Check the foam pad to make sure it is tight on the stick. The person could choke on the foam pad if it comes off the stick.

You also need a kidney basin, water glass or cup, straw, tissues, towels, and gloves. Many persons bring oral hygiene equipment from home.

See *Delegation Guidelines: Oral Hygiene.*
See *Promoting Safety and Comfort: Oral Hygiene.*

DELEGATION GUIDELINES: Oral Hygiene

To assist with oral hygiene you need this information from the nurse and the care plan:
- The type of oral hygiene to give:
  - *Assisting the Person to Brush and Floss the Teeth*
  - *Brushing and Flossing the Person's Teeth*
  - *Providing Mouth Care for the Unconscious Person*
  - *Providing Denture Care*
- If flossing is needed
- What cleaning agent and equipment to use
- If lubricant is applied to the lips; if so what lubricant to use
- How often to give oral hygiene
- How much help the person needs
- What observations to report and record:
  - Dry, cracked, swollen, or blistered lips
  - Mouth or breath odor
  - Redness, swelling, irritation, sores, or white patches in the mouth or on the tongue
  - Bleeding, swelling, or redness of the gums
  - Loose teeth
  - Rough, sharp, or chipped areas on dentures
- When to report observations
- What specific patient or resident concerns to report at once

PROMOTING SAFETY AND COMFORT: Oral Hygiene

SAFETY

Follow Standard Precautions and the Bloodborne Pathogen Standard when giving oral hygiene. You have contact with the person's mucous membranes. Gums may bleed during mouth care. Also, the mouth has many microbes. Pathogens spread through sexual contact may be in the mouths of some persons.

COMFORT

Assist with oral hygiene after sleep, after meals, and at bedtime. Many people practice oral hygiene before meals. Some persons need mouth care every 2 hours or more often. Always follow the care plan.

◆ Brushing and Flossing Teeth

Many people perform oral hygiene themselves. Others need help gathering and setting up equipment. You may have to brush the teeth of persons who:
▶ Are very weak
▶ Cannot use or move their arms
▶ Are too confused to brush their teeth

Text continued on p. 310

ASSISTING THE PERSON TO BRUSH AND FLOSS THE TEETH

✔ Quality of Life *Remember to:*

- Knock before entering the person's room.
- Address the person by name.
- Introduce yourself by name and title.
- Explain the procedure to the person before beginning and during the procedure.

- Protect the person's rights during the procedure.
- Handle the person gently during the procedure.

Continued

ASSISTING THE PERSON TO BRUSH AND FLOSS THE TEETH—cont'd

PRE-PROCEDURE

1 Follow *Delegation Guidelines: Oral Hygiene*, p. 307. See *Promoting Safety and Comfort: Oral Hygiene*, p. 307.
2 Practice hand hygiene.
3 Collect the following:
   - Toothbrush
   - Toothpaste
   - Mouthwash (or solution noted on the care plan)
   - Dental floss (if used)
   - Water glass with cool water
   - Straw
   - Kidney basin
   - Hand towel
   - Paper towels
   - Gloves
4 Place the paper towels on the overbed table. Arrange items on top of them.
5 Identify the person. Check the ID bracelet against the assignment sheet. Also call the person by name.
6 Provide for privacy.
7 Position the person so he or she can brush with ease.

PROCEDURE

8 Lower the bed rail near you if up.
9 Place the towel over the person's chest. This protects garments and linens from spills.
10 Adjust the overbed table in front of the person.
11 Let the person perform oral hygiene. This includes brushing the teeth, rinsing the mouth, flossing, and using mouthwash or other solution.
12 Remove the towel when the person is done.
13 Move the overbed table to the side of the bed.

POST-PROCEDURE

14 Provide for comfort. (See the inside of the front book cover.)
15 Place the signal light within reach.
16 Raise or lower bed rails. Follow the care plan.
17 Clean and return items to their proper place. Wear gloves.
18 Wipe off the overbed table with the paper towels. Discard the paper towels.
19 Remove the gloves. Decontaminate your hands.
20 Unscreen the person.
21 Complete a safety check of the room. (See the inside of the front book cover.)
22 Follow agency policy for dirty linen.
23 Decontaminate your hands.
24 Report and record your observations.

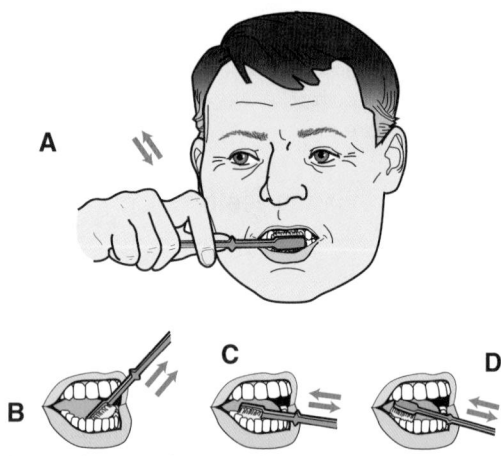

FIGURE 19-4 Brushing teeth. **A,** The brush is held at a 45-degree angle to the gums. Teeth are brushed with short strokes. **B,** The brush is at a 45-degree angle against the inside of the front teeth. Teeth are brushed from the gum to the crown of the tooth with short strokes. **C,** The brush is held horizontally against the inner surfaces of the teeth. The teeth are brushed back and forth. **D,** The brush is positioned on the biting surfaces of the teeth. The teeth are brushed back and forth.

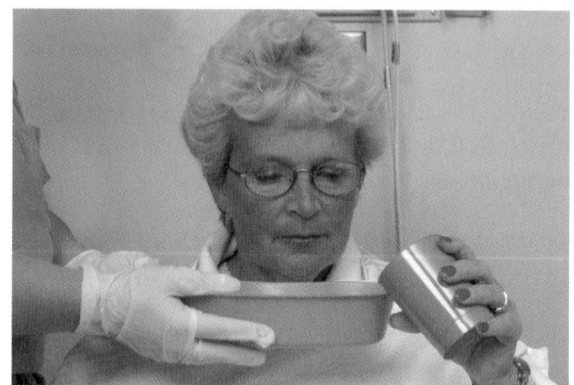

FIGURE 19-5 The kidney basin is held under the person's chin.

BRUSHING AND FLOSSING THE PERSON'S TEETH

✔ Quality of Life *Remember to:*

- Knock before entering the person's room.
- Address the person by name.
- Introduce yourself by name and title.

- Explain the procedure to the person before beginning and during the procedure.
- Protect the person's rights during the procedure.
- Handle the person gently during the procedure.

PRE-PROCEDURE

1 Follow *Delegation Guidelines: Oral Hygiene,* p. 307. See *Promoting Safety and Comfort: Oral Hygiene,* p. 307.
2 Practice hand hygiene.
3 Collect the items listed in procedure: *Assisting the Person to Brush and Floss the Teeth.*

4 Place the paper towels on the overbed table. Arrange items on top of them.
5 Identify the person. Check the ID bracelet against the assignment sheet. Also call the person by name.
6 Provide for privacy.
7 Raise the bed for good body mechanics. Bed rails are up if used.

PROCEDURE

8 Lower the bed rail near you if up.
9 Assist the person to a sitting position or to a side-lying position near you.
10 Place the towel across the person's chest.
11 Adjust the overbed table so you can reach it with ease.
12 Decontaminate your hands. Put on the gloves.
13 Hold the toothbrush over the kidney basin. Pour some water over the brush.
14 Apply toothpaste to the toothbrush.
15 Brush the teeth gently (Fig. 19-4).
16 Brush the tongue gently.
17 Let the person rinse the mouth with water. Hold the kidney basin under the person's chin (Fig. 19-5). Repeat this step as needed.
18 Floss the person's teeth (optional):
  a Break off an 18-inch piece of floss from the dispenser.
  b Hold the floss between the middle fingers of each hand (Fig. 19-6, A).

c Stretch the floss with your thumbs.
d Start at the upper back tooth on the right side. Work around to the left side.
e Move the floss gently up and down between the teeth (Fig. 19-6, B). Move the floss up and down against the side of the tooth. Work from the top of the crown to the gum line.
f Move to a new section of floss after every second tooth.
g Floss the lower teeth. Use up and down motions as for the upper teeth. Start on the right side. Work around to the left side.
19 Let the person use mouthwash or other solution. Hold the kidney basin under the chin.
20 Wipe the person's mouth. Remove the towel.
21 Remove and discard the gloves. Decontaminate your hands.

POST-PROCEDURE

22 Provide for comfort. (See the inside of the front book cover.)
23 Place the signal light within reach.
24 Lower the bed to its lowest position.
25 Raise or lower bed rails. Follow the care plan.
26 Clean and return equipment to its proper place. Wear gloves.
27 Wipe off the overbed table with the paper towels. Discard the paper towels.

28 Remove the gloves. Decontaminate your hands.
29 Unscreen the person.
30 Complete a safety check of the room. (See the inside of the front book cover.)
31 Follow agency policy for dirty linen.
32 Decontaminate your hands.
33 Report and record your observations.

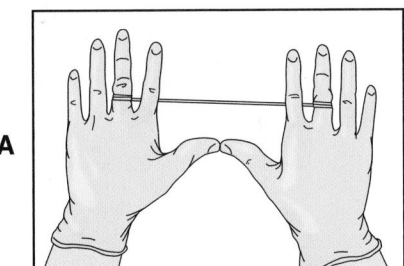
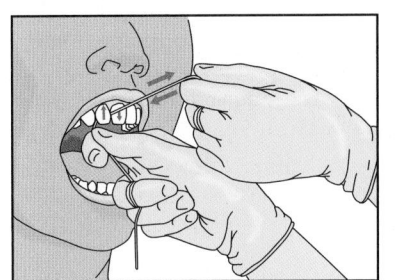

FIGURE 19-6 Flossing. **A,** Floss is wrapped around the middle fingers. **B,** Floss is moved in up-and-down motions between the teeth. Floss is moved up and down from the crown to the gum line.

◆ Mouth Care for the Unconscious Person

Unconscious persons cannot eat or drink. They may breathe with their mouths open. Many receive oxygen. These factors cause mouth dryness. They also cause crusting on the tongue and mucous membranes. Oral hygiene keeps the mouth clean and moist. It also helps prevent infection.

The care plan tells you what cleaning agent to use. Use sponge swabs to apply the cleaning agent. Apply a lubricant (check the care plan) to the lips after cleaning. It prevents cracking of the lips.

Unconscious persons usually cannot swallow. Protect them from choking and aspiration. **Aspiration** is breathing fluid, food, vomitus, or an object into the lungs. It can cause pneumonia and death. To prevent aspiration:

▶ Position the person on one side with the head turned well to the side (Fig. 19-7). In this position, excess fluid runs out of the mouth.

▶ Use only a small amount of fluid to clean the mouth. Sometimes oral suctioning (Chapter 35) is needed.

▶ Do not insert dentures. Dentures are not worn when the person is unconscious.

Keep the person's mouth open with a padded tongue blade (Fig. 19-8). Do not use your fingers. The person can bite down on them. The bite breaks the skin and creates a portal of entry for microbes. Infection is a risk.

Unconscious persons cannot speak or respond to you. However, some can hear. Always assume that unconscious persons can hear. Explain what you are doing step by step. Also tell the person when you are done, when you are leaving the room, and when you will return.

Mouth care is given at least every 2 hours. Follow the nurse's directions and the care plan.

See *Promoting Safety and Comfort: Mouth Care for the Unconscious Person.*

PROMOTING SAFETY AND COMFORT: Mouth Care for the Unconscious Person

SAFETY
Use sponge swabs with care. Make sure the sponge pad is tight on the stick. The person could choke or aspirate on the sponge if it comes off the stick.

COMFORT
Unconscious persons are repositioned at least every 2 hours. To promote comfort, combine mouth care with skin care, repositioning, and other comfort measures.

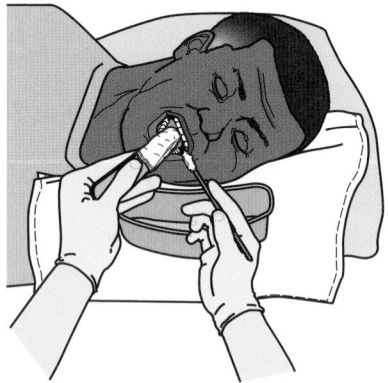

FIGURE 19-7 The unconscious person's head is turned well to the side to prevent aspiration. A padded tongue blade is used to keep the mouth open while cleaning the mouth with swabs.

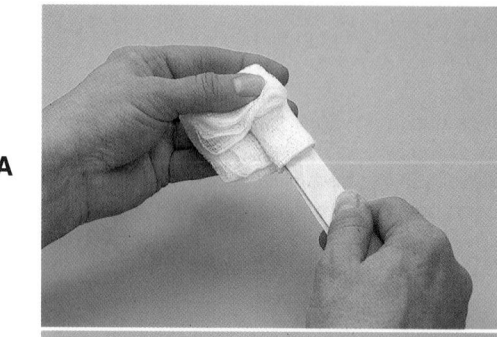

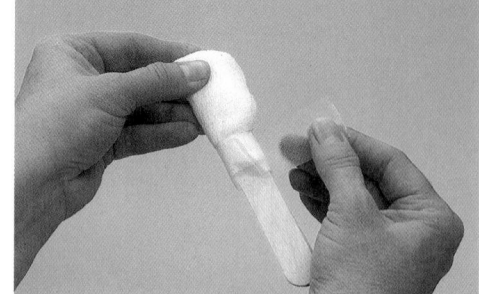

FIGURE 19-8 Making a padded tongue blade. **A,** Place two wooden tongue blades together. Wrap gauze around the top half. **B,** Tape the gauze in place.

PROVIDING MOUTH CARE
FOR THE UNCONSCIOUS PERSON

✔ **Quality of Life** *Remember to:*

- Knock before entering the person's room.
- Address the person by name.
- Introduce yourself by name and title.
- Explain the procedure to the person before beginning and during the procedure.

- Protect the person's rights during the procedure.
- Handle the person gently during the procedure.

PRE-PROCEDURE

1 Follow *Delegation Guidelines: Oral Hygiene*, p. 307. See *Promoting Safety and Comfort:*
  - *Oral Hygiene*, p. 307
  - *Mouth Care for the Unconscious Person*
2 Practice hand hygiene.
3 Collect the following:
  - Cleaning agent (check the care plan)
  - Sponge swabs
  - Padded tongue blade
  - Water glass or cup with cool water
  - Hand towel

- Kidney basin
- Lip lubricant
- Paper towels
- Gloves

4 Place the towels on the overbed table. Arrange items on top of them.
5 Identify the person. Check the ID bracelet against the assignment sheet. Also call the person by name.
6 Provide for privacy.
7 Raise the bed for good body mechanics. Bed rails are up if used.

PROCEDURE

8 Lower the bed rail near you if up.
9 Decontaminate your hands. Put on the gloves.
10 Position the person in a side-lying position near you. Turn his or her head well to the side.
11 Place the towel under the person's face.
12 Place the kidney basin under the chin.
13 Separate the upper and lower teeth. Use the padded tongue blade. Be gentle. Never use force. If you have problems, ask the nurse for help.
14 Clean the mouth using sponge swabs moistened with the cleaning agent (see Fig. 19-7).
  a Clean the chewing and inner surfaces of the teeth.
  b Clean the gums and outer surfaces of the teeth.

c Swab the roof of the mouth, inside of the cheeks, and the lips.
d Swab the tongue.
e Moisten a clean swab with water. Swab the mouth to rinse.
f Place used swabs in the kidney basin.
15 Apply lubricant to the lips.
16 Remove the kidney basin and supplies.
17 Wipe the person's mouth. Remove the towel.
18 Remove and discard the gloves. Decontaminate your hands.

POST-PROCEDURE

19 Provide for comfort. (See the inside of the front book cover.)
20 Place the signal light within reach.
21 Lower the bed to its lowest position.
22 Raise or lower bed rails. Follow the care plan.
23 Clean and return equipment to its proper place. Discard disposable items. (Wear gloves.)
24 Wipe off the overbed table with paper towels. Discard the paper towels.

25 Remove the gloves. Decontaminate your hands.
26 Unscreen the person.
27 Complete a safety check of the room. (See the inside of the front book cover.)
28 Tell the person that you are leaving the room. Tell him or her when you will return.
29 Follow agency policy for dirty linen.
30 Decontaminate your hands.
31 Report and record your observations.

◆ Denture Care

A **denture** is an artificial tooth or a set of artificial teeth. Some people call them "false teeth" (Fig. 19-9, p. 312). Dentures replace missing teeth. People lose teeth because of gum disease, tooth decay, or injury. Full and partial dentures are common:

▸ *Full denture.* The person has no upper or lower natural teeth. Dentures replace the upper or lower teeth.
▸ *Partial denture.* The person has some natural teeth. The partial denture replaces the missing teeth.

Mouth care is given and dentures cleaned as often as natural teeth. Dentures are slippery when wet. They easily break or chip if dropped onto a hard surface (floors, sinks, counters). Hold them firmly. During cleaning, firmly hold them over a basin of water lined with a towel. This prevents them from falling onto a hard surface.

To use a cleaning agent, follow the manufacturer's instructions. They tell how to use the cleaning agent and what water temperature to use. Hot water causes dentures to lose their shape (warp). If not worn after cleaning, store dentures in a container with cool water or a denture soaking solution. Otherwise, they can dry out and warp.

Dentures are usually removed at bedtime. Some people do not wear their dentures. Others wear dentures for eating and remove them after meals. Remind them not to wrap dentures in tissues or napkins. Otherwise, they are easily discarded.

Many people clean their own dentures. Some need help collecting items used to clean dentures. They may need help getting to the bathroom. You clean dentures for those who cannot do so.

See *Promoting Safety and Comfort: Denture Care.*

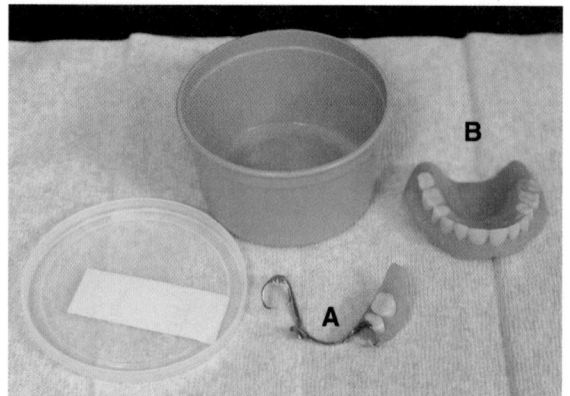

FIGURE 19-9 Dentures. **A,** Partial denture. **B,** Full denture.

PROMOTING SAFETY AND COMFORT: Denture Care

SAFETY
Dentures are the person's property. They are costly. Handle them very carefully. Label the denture cup with the person's name and room and bed number. Report lost or damaged dentures to the nurse at once. Losing or damaging dentures is negligent conduct.

COMFORT
Many people do not like being seen without their dentures. Privacy is important. Allow privacy when the person cleans dentures. If you clean dentures, return them to the person as quickly as possible.

Persons with dentures may have some natural teeth. They need to brush and floss the natural teeth. See procedure: *Assisting the Person to Brush and Floss the Teeth*, p. 307. Or see procedure: *Brushing and Flossing the Person's Teeth*, p. 309.

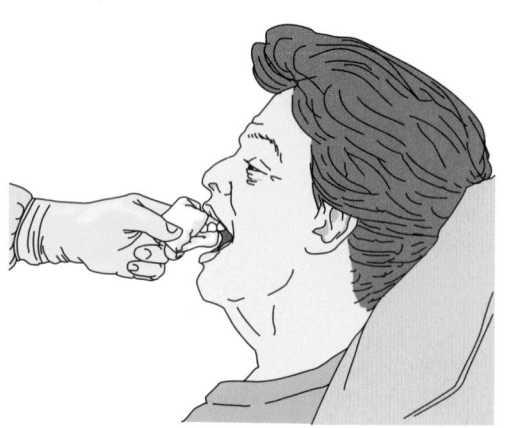

FIGURE 19-10 Remove the upper denture by grasping it with the thumb and index finger of one hand. Use a piece of gauze to grasp the slippery denture.

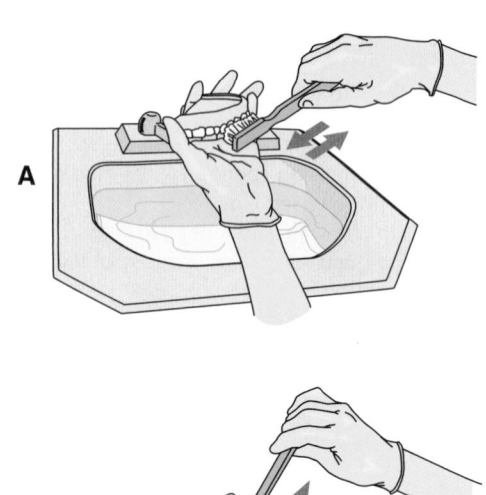
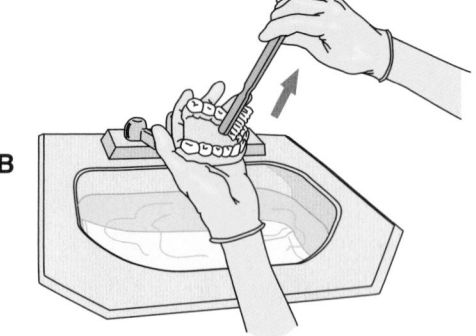

FIGURE 19-11 Cleaning dentures. **A,** Outer surfaces of the denture are brushed with back-and-forth motions. Note that the denture is held over the sink. The sink is filled halfway with water and is lined with a towel. **B,** Position the brush vertically to clean the inner surfaces of the denture. Use upward strokes.

PROVIDING DENTURE CARE

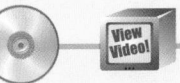

✔ **Quality of Life** *Remember to:*

- Knock before entering the person's room.
- Address the person by name.
- Introduce yourself by name and title.
- Explain the procedure to the person before beginning and during the procedure.

- Protect the person's rights during the procedure.
- Handle the person gently during the procedure.

PRE-PROCEDURE

1 Follow *Delegation Guidelines: Oral Hygiene*, p. 307. See *Promoting Safety and Comfort:*
   - *Oral Hygiene*, p. 307
   - *Denture Care*
2 Practice hand hygiene.
3 Collect the following:
   - Denture brush or toothbrush (for cleaning dentures)
   - Denture cup labeled with the person's name and room and bed number
   - Denture cleaning agent
   - Soft-bristled toothbrush or sponge swabs (for oral hygiene)
   - Toothpaste
   - Water glass with cool water
   - Straw
   - Mouthwash (or other noted solution)
   - Kidney basin
   - Two hand towels
   - Gauze squares
   - Paper towels
   - Gloves

4 Place the paper towels on the overbed table. Arrange items on top of them.
5 Identify the person. Check the ID bracelet against the assignment sheet. Also call the person by name.
6 Provide for privacy.
7 Raise the bed for good body mechanics.

PROCEDURE

8 Lower the bed rail near you if used.
9 Decontaminate your hands. Put on the gloves.
10 Place a towel over the person's chest.
11 Ask the person to remove the dentures. Carefully place them in the kidney basin.
12 Remove the dentures if the person cannot do so. Use gauze squares to get a good grip on the slippery dentures.
   a Grasp the denture with your thumb and index finger (Fig. 19-10). Move it up and down slightly to break the seal. Gently remove the denture. Place it in the kidney basin.
   b Grasp and remove the lower denture with your thumb and index finger. Turn it slightly, and lift it out of the person's mouth. Place it in the kidney basin.
13 Follow the care plan for raising bed rails.
14 Take the kidney basin, denture cup, denture brush, and denture cleaning agent to the sink.
15 Line the sink with a towel. Fill the sink halfway with water.
16 Rinse each denture under cool running water.
17 Return dentures to the kidney basin or denture cup.
18 Apply the denture cleaning agent to the brush.
19 Brush the dentures as in Figure 19-11.
20 Rinse the dentures under running water. Use warm or cool water as directed by the cleaning agent manufacturer. (Some state competency tests require cool water.)

21 Rinse the denture cup. Place dentures in the denture cup. Cover the dentures with cool water.
22 Clean the kidney basin.
23 Take the denture cup and kidney basin to the overbed table.
24 Lower the bed rail if up.
25 Position the person for oral hygiene.
26 Clean the person's gums and tongue, using toothpaste and the toothbrush (or sponge swabs).
27 Have the person use mouthwash (or noted solution). Hold the kidney basin under the chin.
28 Ask the person to insert the dentures. Insert them if the person cannot.
   a Hold the upper denture firmly with your thumb and index finger. Raise the upper lip with the other hand. Insert the denture. Gently press on the denture with your index fingers to make sure it is in place.
   b Hold the lower denture with your thumb and index finger. Pull the lower lip down slightly. Insert the denture. Gently press down on it to make sure it is in place.
29 Place the denture cup in the top drawer of the bedside stand if the dentures are not worn. The dentures must be in water or in a denture soaking solution.
30 Wipe the person's mouth. Remove the towel.
31 Remove the gloves. Decontaminate your hands.

Continued

PROVIDING DENTURE CARE—cont'd
POST-PROCEDURE

32 Assist with hand washing.
33 Provide for comfort. (See the inside of the front book cover.)
34 Place the signal light within reach.
35 Lower the bed to its lowest position.
36 Raise or lower bed rails. Follow the care plan.
37 Clean and return equipment to its proper place. Discard disposable items. Wear gloves for this step.
38 Wipe off the overbed table with the paper towels. Discard the paper towels.

39 Remove the gloves. Decontaminate your hands.
40 Unscreen the person.
41 Complete a safety check of the room. (See the inside of the front book cover.)
42 Follow agency policy for dirty linen.
43 Decontaminate your hands.
44 Report and record your observations.

BATHING

Bathing cleans the skin. It also cleans the mucous membranes of the genital and anal areas. Microbes, dead skin, perspiration, and excess oils are removed. A bath is refreshing and relaxing. Circulation is stimulated and body parts exercised. Observations are made, and you have time to talk to the person.

Complete or partial baths, tub baths, or showers are given. The method depends on the person's condition, self-care abilities, and personal choice. In hospitals, bathing is common after breakfast. In nursing centers, bathing usually occurs after breakfast or the evening meal. The person's choice of bath time is respected whenever possible.

Bathing frequency is a personal matter. Some people bathe daily. Others bathe once or twice a week. Personal choice, weather, activity, and illness affect bathing frequency. Ill persons may have fevers and perspire heavily. They need frequent bathing. Other illnesses and dry skin may limit bathing to every 2 or 3 days.

The rules for bed baths, showers, and tub baths are listed in Box 19-2. Table 19-1 describes common skin care products.

See *Focus on Children and Older Persons: Bathing.*
See *Delegation Guidelines: Bathing,* p. 316.
See *Promoting Safety and Comfort: Bathing,* p. 316.

BOX 19-2 Rules for Bathing

- Follow the care plan for bathing method and skin care products.
- Allow personal choice whenever possible.
- Follow Standard Precautions and the Bloodborne Pathogen Standard.
- Collect needed items before starting the procedure.
- Provide for privacy. Screen the person. Close doors and window coverings—drapes, shades, blinds, shutters, and so on.
- Assist the person with elimination. Bathing stimulates the need to urinate. Comfort and relaxation increase if urination needs are met.
- Cover the person for warmth and privacy.
- Reduce drafts. Close doors and windows.
- Protect the person from falling.
- Use good body mechanics at all times.
- Follow the rules to safely handle, move, and transfer the person (Chapter 16).
- Know what water temperature to use. See *Delegation Guidelines: Bathing,* p. 316.
- Keep bar soap in the soap dish between latherings. This prevents soapy water. It also reduces the chances of slipping and falls in showers and tubs.
- Wash from the cleanest areas to the dirtiest areas.
- Encourage the person to help as much as is safely possible.
- Rinse the skin thoroughly. You must remove all soap.
- Pat the skin dry to avoid irritating or breaking the skin. Do not rub the skin.
- Dry under the breasts, between skin folds, in the perineal area, and between the toes.
- Bathe skin when urine or feces is present. This prevents skin breakdown and odors.

TABLE 19-1 Skin Care Products

TYPE	PURPOSE	CARE CONSIDERATIONS
Soaps	Clean the skin Remove dirt, dead skin, skin oil, some microbes, and perspiration	Tend to dry and irritate the skin Dry skin is easily injured and causes itching and discomfort Skin must be thoroughly rinsed to remove all soap Not needed for every bath; plain water can clean the skin Plain water is often used for older persons because of dry skin People with dry skin may prefer soaps containing bath oils Not used if a person has very dry skin
Bath oils	Keep the skin soft Prevent dry skin	Some soaps contain bath oil Liquid bath oil can be added to bath water Showers and tubs become slippery from bath oils; safety measures are needed to prevent falls
Creams and lotions	Protect the skin from the drying effect of air and evaporation	Do not feel greasy but leave an oily film on the skin Lotion is applied to bony areas after bathing to prevent skin breakdown (back, elbows, knees, and heels) Lotion is used for back massages Most are scented
Powders	Absorb moisture Prevent friction when two skin surfaces rub together	Usually applied under the breasts, under the arms, and in the groin area, and sometimes between the toes Applied to dry skin in a thin, even layer Excessive amounts cause caking and crusts that can irritate the skin
Deodorants	Mask and control body odors	Applied to the underarms Not applied to irritated skin Do not take the place of bathing
Antiperspirants	Reduce the amount of perspiration	Applied to the underarms Not applied to irritated skin Do not take the place of bathing

FOCUS ON **CHILDREN** AND **OLDER PERSONS**

Bathing

CHILDREN

The nurse collects information about the child's bathing practices on admission. The care plan reflects the child's normal practices and needs during illness.

Many older children enjoy showers. The nurse tells you how much help and supervision the child needs. Remember, independence and privacy are important to older children.

OLDER PERSONS

Dry skin occurs with aging. Soap also dries the skin. Dry skin is easily damaged. Therefore older persons usually need a complete bath or shower twice a week. Partial baths are taken the other days. Some bathe daily but not with soap. Thorough rinsing is needed when using soap. Lotions and oils help keep the skin soft.

Bathing procedures can threaten persons with dementia. They do not understand what is happening or why. And they may fear harm or danger. Confusion can increase. Therefore they may resist care and become agitated and combative. They may shout at you and cry out for help. You must be calm, patient, and soothing.

The nurse assesses the person's behaviors and routines. The person may be calmer and less confused or agitated during a certain time of the day. Bathing is scheduled for the person's calm times. The nurse decides if a bed bath, tub bath, shower, or towel bath (p. 320) is best for the person.

The rules in Box 19-1 apply when bathing these persons. The care plan also includes measures to help the person through the bath. Such measures may include:

- Use terms such as "cleaned up" or "washed" rather than "shower" or "bath."
- Complete pre-procedure activities. For example, get supplies and linens ready. Make sure you have everything that you will need.
- Provide for warmth. Increase the room temperature before starting the bath or shower. Have extra towels and a robe nearby.
- Provide for safety. Use a hand-held shower nozzle. Have the person use a shower chair or shower bench. Do not leave the person alone in the tub or shower.
- Draw bath water ahead of time. Test the water temperature. Add more warm or cold water as necessary.
- Tell the person what you are doing step-by-step. Use clear, simple statements.
- Let the person help as much as possible. For example, give the person a washcloth. Ask him or her to wash the arms. If the person does not know what to do, still let the person hold the washcloth if it is safe to do so.
- Do not rush the person.
- Use a calm, pleasant voice.
- Divert the person's attention if necessary (Chapter 44).
- Calm the person.
- Handle the person gently.
- Try giving a partial bath if a shower or tub bath agitates the person.
- Try the bath later if the person continues to resist care.

Delegation Guidelines: Bathing

To assist with bathing, you need this information from the nurse and the care plan:
- What bath to give—complete bed bath, partial bath, tub bath, shower, towel bath, or bag bath.
- How much help the person needs.
- The person's activity or position limits.
- What water temperature to use. Bath water in a basin cools rapidly. Heat is lost to the overbed table, the washcloth, and your hands.Therefore water temperature for complete bed baths and partial bed baths is usually between 110° and 115° F (43.3° and 46.1° C) for adults. Infants and young children have fragile skin. So do older persons. They need lower water temperatures.
- What skin care products to use and what the person prefers.
- What observations to report and record:
  - The color of the skin, lips, nail beds, and sclera (whites of the eyes)
  - The location and description of rashes
  - Dry skin
  - Bruises or open skin areas
  - Pale or reddened areas, particularly over bony parts
  - Drainage or bleeding from wounds or body openings
  - Swelling of the feet and legs
  - Corns or calluses on the feet
  - Skin temperature
  - Complaints of pain or discomfort
- When to report observations.
- What specific patient or resident concerns to report at once.

◆ The Complete Bed Bath

The *complete bed bath* involves washing the person's entire body in bed. You give complete bed baths to persons who cannot bathe themselves. Bed baths are usually needed by persons who are:
▶ Unconscious
▶ Paralyzed
▶ In casts or traction
▶ Weak from illness or surgery

A bed bath is new to some people. Some are embarrassed to have others see their bodies. Some fear exposure. Explain how the bed bath is given. Also explain how you cover the body for privacy.

See *Focus on Children and Older Persons: The Complete Bed Bath.* *Text continued on p. 320*

PROMOTING SAFETY AND COMFORT: Bathing

SAFETY

Hot water can burn delicate and fragile skin. Measure water temperature according to agency policy. If unsure if the water is too hot, ask the nurse to check it.

Protect the person from falls and other injuries. Practice the safety measures presented in Chapters 11 and 12. Also protect the person from drafts.

Use caution when applying powder. Do not use powders near persons with respiratory disorders. Inhaling powder can irritate the airway and lungs. Before applying powder, check with the nurse and the care plan. Do not shake or sprinkle powder onto the person. To safely apply powder:
- Turn away from the person.
- Sprinkle a small amount of powder onto your hands or a cloth.
- Apply the powder in a thin layer.
- Make sure powder does not get on the floor. Powder is slippery and can cause falls.

Beds are made after baths. After making the bed, lower the bed to its lowest position. Then lock the bed wheels. For an occupied bed, raise or lower bed rails according to the care plan.

Protect the person and yourself from infection. When giving baths and making beds, contact with blood, body fluids, secretions, and excretions is likely. Follow Standard Precautions and the Bloodborne Pathogen Standard.

COMFORT

Before bathing, allow the person to use the bathroom, commode, bedpan, or urinal. Bathing stimulates the need to urinate. The person is more comfortable if his or her bladder is empty. Also, bathing is not interrupted.

Many people perform oral hygiene as part of their bathing routine. Some do so before the bathing procedure; others do so after. Allow personal choice and follow the person's care plan.

Provide for warmth. Cover the person with a bath blanket. Make sure the water is warm enough for the person. Cool water causes chilling.

Remove the person's gown or pajamas after washing the eyes, face, ears, and neck. Waiting to remove sleepwear at this time helps the person feel less exposed and more comfortable with the bath. If the person prefers, you can remove the sleepwear before washing the eyes, face, ears, and neck.

FOCUS ON CHILDREN AND OLDER PERSONS

The Complete Bed Bath

CHILDREN

See Chapter 47 for bathing infants. Follow the adult procedure for bathing toddlers and older children. Infants and young children have fragile skin. Lower water temperatures are used. Ask the nurse what water temperature to use.

OLDER PERSONS

Older persons have fragile skin. Lower water temperatures are used. Ask the nurse what water temperature to use.

GIVING A COMPLETE BED BATH

✔ Quality of Life *Remember to:*

- Knock before entering the person's room.
- Address the person by name.
- Introduce yourself by name and title.
- Explain the procedure to the person before beginning and during the procedure.

- Protect the person's rights during the procedure.
- Handle the person gently during the procedure.

PRE-PROCEDURE

1 Follow *Delegation Guidelines: Bathing.* See *Promoting Safety and Comfort: Bathing.*
2 Practice hand hygiene.
3 Identify the person. Check the ID bracelet against the assignment sheet. Also call the person by name.
4 Collect clean linen for a closed bed. See procedure: *Making a Closed Bed* in Chapter 18. Place linen on a clean surface.
5 Collect the following:
   - Wash basin
   - Soap
   - Bath thermometer
   - Orange stick or nail file
   - Washcloth
   - Two bath towels and two hand towels

- Bath blanket
- Clothing or sleepwear
- Lotion
- Powder
- Deodorant or antiperspirant
- Brush and comb
- Other grooming items as requested
- Paper towels
- Gloves

6 Cover the overbed table with paper towels. Arrange items on the overbed table. Adjust the height as needed.
7 Provide for privacy.
8 Raise the bed for good body mechanics. Bed rails are up if used.

PROCEDURE

9 Remove the signal light.
10 Decontaminate your hands. Put on gloves.
11 Cover the person with a bath blanket. Remove top linens (see procedure: *Making an Occupied Bed* in Chapter 18).
12 Lower the head of the bed. It is as flat as possible. The person has at least one pillow.
13 Fill the wash basin ⅔ (two-thirds) full with water. Water temperature is usually 110° to 115° F (43.3° to 46.1° C) for adults. Measure water temperature. Use the bath thermometer. Or test the water by dipping your elbow or inner wrist into the basin.
14 Place the basin on the overbed table.
15 Lower the bed rail near you if up.
16 Place a hand towel over the person's chest.
17 Make a mitt with the washcloth (Fig. 19-12, p. 318). Use a mitt for the entire bath.
18 Wash around the person's eyes with water. Do not use soap.
   a Clean the far eye. Gently wipe from the inner to the outer aspect of the eye with a corner of the mitt (Fig. 19-13, p. 319).
   b Clean around the eye near you. Use a clean part of the washcloth for each stroke.
19 Ask the person if you should use soap to wash the face.
20 Wash the face, ears, and neck. Rinse and pat dry with the towel on the chest.
21 Help the person move to the side of the bed near you.
22 Remove the sleepwear. Do not expose the person.
23 Place a bath towel lengthwise under the far arm.

24 Support the arm with your palm under the person's elbow. His or her forearm rests on your forearm.
25 Wash the arm, shoulder, and underarm. Use long, firm strokes (Fig. 19-14, p. 319). Rinse and pat dry.
26 Place the basin on the towel. Put the person's hand into the water (Fig. 19-15, p. 319). Wash it well. Clean under the fingernails with an orange stick or nail file.
27 Have the person exercise the hand and fingers.
28 Remove the basin. Dry the hand well. Cover the arm with the bath blanket.
29 Repeat steps 23 to 28 for the near arm.
30 Place a bath towel over the chest crosswise. Hold the towel in place. Pull the bath blanket from under the towel to the waist.
31 Lift the towel slightly, and wash the chest (Fig. 19-16, p. 319). Do not expose the person. Rinse and pat dry, especially under the breasts.
32 Move the towel lengthwise over the chest and abdomen. Do not expose the person. Pull the bath blanket down to the pubic area.
33 Lift the towel slightly, and wash the abdomen (Fig. 19-17, p. 319). Rinse and pat dry.
34 Pull the bath blanket up to the shoulders, covering both arms. Remove the towel.
35 Change soapy or cool water. Measure bath water temperature as in step 13. If bed rails are used, raise the bed rail near you before leaving the bedside. Lower it when you return.
36 Uncover the far leg. Do not expose the genital area. Place a towel lengthwise under the foot and leg.
37 Bend the knee, and support the leg with your arm. Wash it with long, firm strokes. Rinse and pat dry.

Continued

GIVING A COMPLETE BED BATH—cont'd

PROCEDURE—cont'd

38 Place the basin on the towel near the foot.

39 Lift the leg slightly. Slide the basin under the foot.

40 Place the foot in the basin (Fig. 19-18, p. 320). Use an orange stick or nail file to clean under toenails if necessary. If the person cannot bend the knees:

  a Wash the foot. Carefully separate the toes. Rinse and pat dry.

  b Clean under the toenails with an orange stick or nail file if necessary.

41 Remove the basin. Dry the leg and foot. Apply lotion to the foot if directed by the nurse and care plan. Cover the leg with the bath blanket. Remove the towel.

42 Repeat steps 36 to 41 for the near leg.

43 Change the water. Measure water temperature as in step 13. If bed rails are used, raise the bed rail near you before leaving the bedside. Lower it when you return.

44 Turn the person onto the side away from you. The person is covered with the bath blanket.

45 Uncover the back and buttocks. Do not expose the person. Place a towel lengthwise on the bed along the back.

46 Wash the back. Work from the back of the neck to the lower end of the buttocks. Use long, firm, continuous strokes (Fig. 19-19, p. 320). Rinse and dry well.

47 Give a back massage (p. 326). The person may want the back massage after the bath.

48 Turn the person onto his or her back.

49 Change the water for perineal care (p. 329). See step 13 for how to measure water temperature. (Some state competency tests also require changing gloves and hand hygiene at this time). If bed rails are used, raise the bed rail near you before leaving the bedside. Lower it when you return.

50 Let the person wash the genital area. Adjust the overbed table so he or she can reach the wash basin, soap, and towels with ease. Place the signal light within reach. Ask the person to signal when finished. Make sure the person understands what to do.

51 Remove the gloves. Decontaminate your hands.

52 Answer the signal light promptly. Knock before entering the room. Provide perineal care if the person cannot do so (p. 329). (Decontaminate your hands and wear gloves for perineal care.)

53 Give a back massage if you have not already done so.

54 Apply deodorant or antiperspirant. Apply lotion and powder as requested. See *Promoting Safety and Comfort: Bathing.*

55 Put clean garments on the person.

56 Comb and brush the hair (Chapter 20).

57 Make the bed.

POST-PROCEDURE

58 Provide for comfort. (See the inside of the front book cover.)

59 Place the signal light within reach.

60 Lower the bed to its lowest position.

61 Raise or lower bed rails. Follow the care plan.

62 Empty and clean the wash basin. Return it and other supplies to their proper place.

63 Wipe off the overbed table with paper towels. Discard the paper towels.

64 Unscreen the person.

65 Complete a safety check of the room. (See the inside of the front book cover.)

66 Follow agency policy for dirty linen.

67 Decontaminate your hands.

68 Report and record your observations.

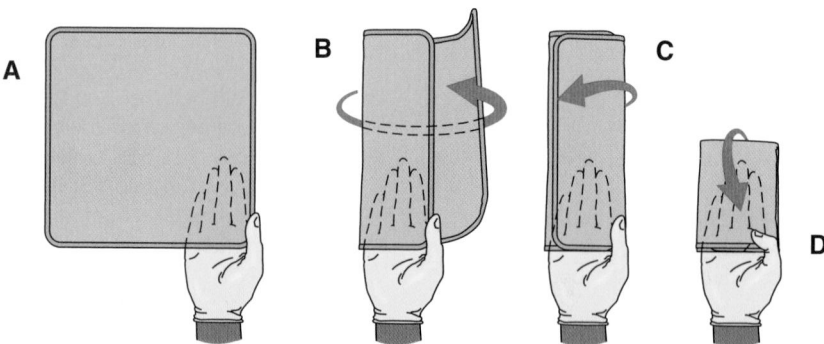

FIGURE 19-12 Making a mitted washcloth. **A,** Grasp the near side of the washcloth with your thumb. **B,** Bring the washcloth around and behind your hand. **C,** Fold the side of the washcloth over your palm as you grasp it with your thumb. **D,** Fold the top of the washcloth down and tuck it under next to your palm.

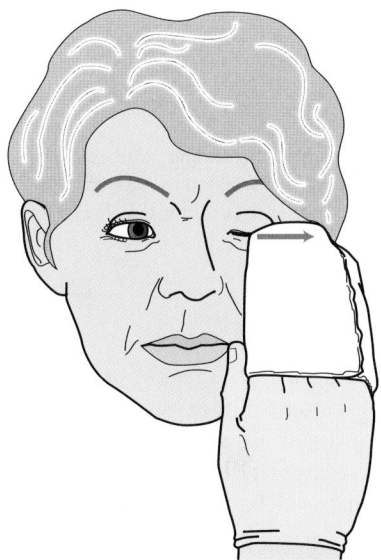

FIGURE 19-13 Wash around the person's eyes with a mitted washcloth. Wipe from the inner to the outer aspect of the eye.

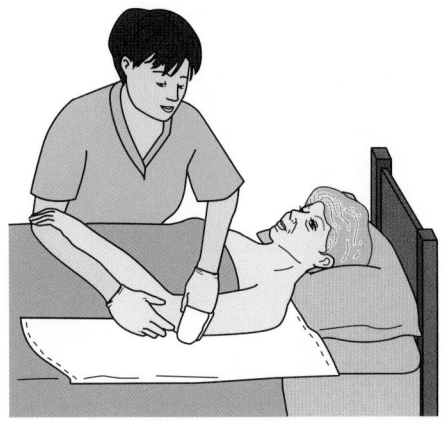

FIGURE 19-14 The person's arm is washed with firm, long strokes using a mitted washcloth.

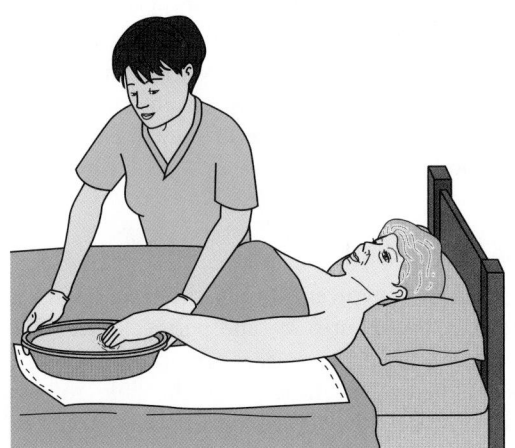

FIGURE 19-15 The person's hands are washed by placing the wash basin on the bed.

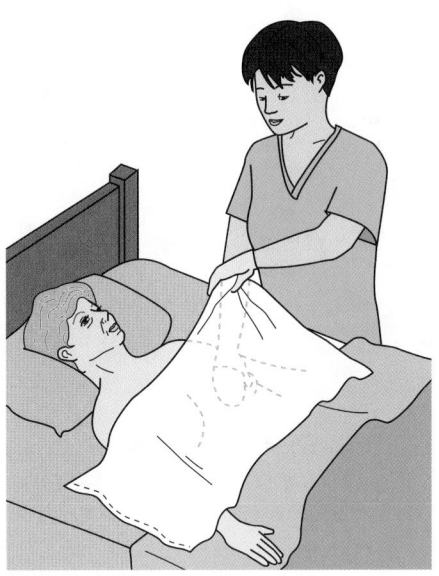

FIGURE 19-16 The person's breasts are not exposed during the bath. A bath towel is placed horizontally over the chest area. The towel is lifted slightly to reach under to wash the breasts and chest.

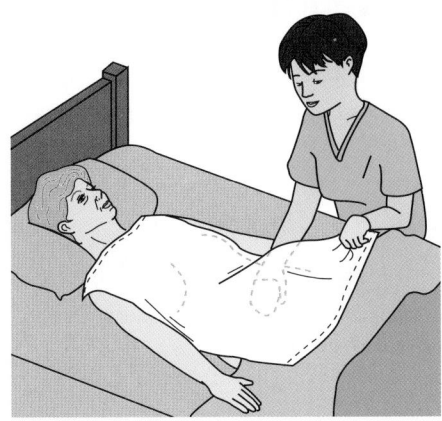

FIGURE 19-17 The bath towel is turned so that it is vertical to cover the breasts and abdomen. The towel is lifted slightly to bathe the abdomen. The bath blanket covers the pubic area.

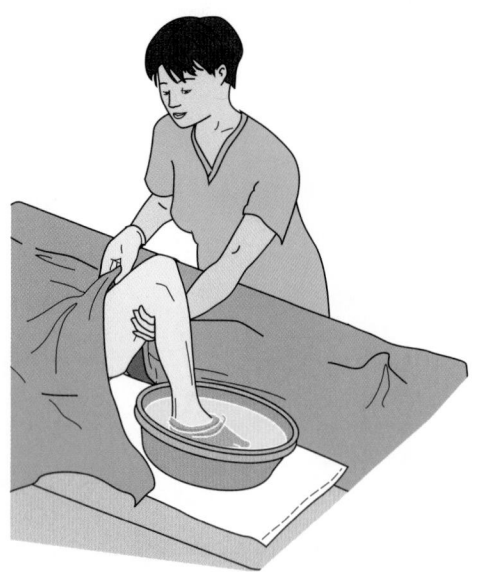

FIGURE 19-18 The foot is washed by placing it in the wash basin on the bed.

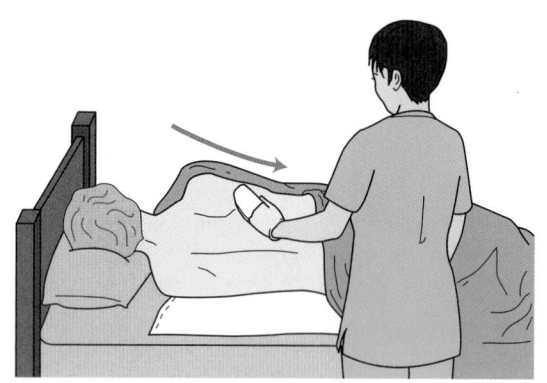

FIGURE 19-19 The back is washed with long, firm, continuous strokes. Note that the person is in a side-lying position. A towel is placed lengthwise on the bed to protect the linens from water.

> ### FOCUS ON **CHILDREN** AND **OLDER PERSONS**
> Towel Baths
>
> **OLDER PERSONS**
> The towel bath is quick, soothing, and relaxing. Persons with dementia often respond well to this type of bath. The nurse and care plan tell you when to use the towel bath.

Towel Baths

For a towel bath, an over-sized towel is used. It covers the body from the neck to the feet. The towel is completely wet with a cleansing solution—water, cleaning agent, and skin-softening agent. It also has a drying agent so the person's body dries fast. The nurse and care plan tell you when to use a towel bath. To give a towel bath, follow agency policy.

See *Focus on Children and Older Persons: Towel Baths.*

Bag Baths

Bag baths are commercially prepared or prepared at the agency. There are 8 to 10 washcloths in a plastic bag. They are moistened with a cleaning agent that does not need rinsing. The washcloths are warmed in a microwave oven. (The nurse and manufacturer's instructions tell you what microwave setting to use.) A new washcloth is used for each body part. The skin air-dries. Towels are not needed.

◆ The Partial Bath

The *partial bath* involves bathing the face, hands, axillae (underarms), back, buttocks, and perineal area. Odors or discomfort occurs if these areas are not clean. Some persons bathe themselves in bed or at the sink. You assist as needed. Most need help washing the back. You give partial baths to persons who cannot bathe themselves.

The rules for bathing apply (see Box 19-2). So do the complete bed bath considerations.

ASSISTING WITH THE PARTIAL BATH

✔ Quality of Life *Remember to:*

- Knock before entering the person's room.
- Address the person by name.
- Introduce yourself by name and title.
- Explain the procedure to the person before beginning and during the procedure.

- Protect the person's rights during the procedure.
- Handle the person gently during the procedure.

PRE-PROCEDURE

1 Follow *Delegation Guidelines: Bathing*, p. 316. See *Promoting Safety and Comfort: Bathing*, p. 316.

2 Follow steps 2 through 7 in procedure: *Giving a Complete Bed Bath*, p. 317.

ASSISTING WITH THE PARTIAL BATH—cont'd

PROCEDURE

3 Make sure the bed is in the lowest position.
4 Decontaminate your hands, Put on gloves.
5 Cover the person with a bath blanket. Remove top linens.
6 Fill the wash basin ⅔ (two-thirds) full with water. Water temperature is 110° to 115° F (43.3° to 46.1° C) or as directed by the nurse. Measure water temperature with the bath thermometer. Or test bath water by dipping your elbow or inner wrist into the basin.
7 Place the basin on the overbed table.
8 Position the person in Fowler's position. Or assist him or her to sit at the bedside.
9 Adjust the overbed table so the person can reach the basin and supplies.
10 Help the person undress. Provide for privacy and warmth with the bath blanket.
11 Ask the person to wash easy to reach body parts (Fig. 19-20). Explain that you will wash the back and areas the person cannot reach.
12 Place the signal light within reach. Ask him or her to signal when help is needed or bathing is complete.

13 Leave the room after decontaminating your hands.
14 Return when the signal light is on. Knock before entering. Decontaminate your hands.
15 Change the bath water. Measure bath water temperature as in step 6.
16 Raise the bed for good body mechanics. The far bed rail is up if used.
17 Ask what was washed. Put on gloves. Wash and dry areas the person could not reach. The face, hands, underarms, back, buttocks, and perineal area are washed for the partial bath.
18 Remove the gloves. Decontaminate your hands.
19 Give a back massage (p. 326).
20 Apply lotion, powder, and deodorant or antiperspirant as requested.
21 Help the person put on clean garments.
22 Assist with hair care and other grooming needs.
23 Assist the person to a chair. (Lower the bed if the person transfers to a chair.) Or turn the person onto the side away from you.
24 Make the bed. (Raise the bed for good body mechanics.)

POST-PROCEDURE

25 Provide for comfort. (See the inside of the front book cover.)
26 Place the signal light within reach.
27 Lower the bed to its lowest position.
28 Raise or lower bed rails. Follow the care plan.
29 Empty and clean the basin. Return the basin and supplies to their proper place.
30 Wipe off the overbed table with the paper towels. Discard the paper towels.

31 Unscreen the person.
32 Complete a safety check of the room. (See the inside of the front book cover.)
33 Follow agency policy for dirty linen.
34 Decontaminate your hands.
35 Report and record your observations.

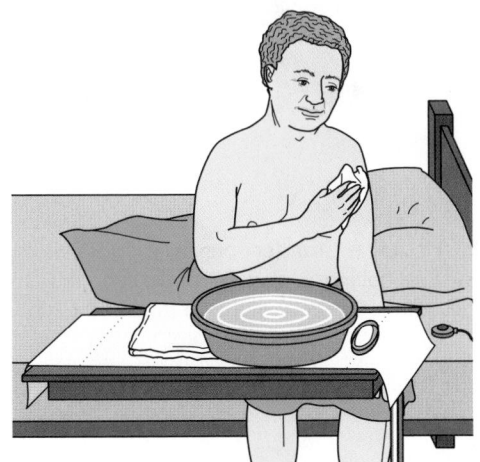

FIGURE 19-20 The person is bathing himself while sitting on the side of the bed. Necessary equipment is within his reach.

◀ Tub Baths and Showers

Some people like tub baths. Others prefer showers. Falls, burns, and chilling from water are risks. Safety is important (Box 19-3, p. 322). The measures in Box 19-2 also apply. If other measures are needed, follow the nurse's directions and the care plan.

Some bathrooms have showers. If not, reserve the shower or tub room for the person.

Tub Baths

Tub baths are relaxing. A tub bath can cause a person to feel faint, weak, or tired. These are greater risks for person who were on bedrest. A tub bath lasts no longer than 20 minutes.

BOX 19-3 Safety Measures for Tub Baths and Showers

- Know what water temperature to use. See *Delegation Guidelines: Tub Baths and Showers*, p. 324.
- Clean and disinfect the tub or shower before and after use.
- Dry the tub or shower room floor.
- Check handrails, grab bars, hydraulic lifts, and other safety aids. They must be in working order.
- Place a bath mat in the tub or on the shower floor. This is not needed if there are non-skid strips or a non-skid surface.
- Cover the person for warmth and privacy. This includes during transport to and from the shower or tub room.
- Place needed items within the person's reach.
- Place the signal light within the person's reach.
- Show the person how to use the signal light in the shower or tub room.
- Have the person use the grab bars when getting in and out of the tub. The person must not use towel bars for support.
- Turn cold water on first, then hot water. Turn hot water off first, then the cold water.
- Adjust water temperature and pressure to prevent chilling or burns. Do this before the person gets into the shower. If a shower chair is used, position it first.
- Direct water away from the person while adjusting water temperature and pressure.

- Fill the tub before the person gets into it.
- Measure the water temperature. For showers and tub baths, use the digital display. Or you can use a bath thermometer for a tub bath.
- Keep the water spray directed toward the person during the shower. This helps keep him or her warm. (*NOTE:* Do not direct the water spray toward the person's face. This can frighten the person.)
- Keep bar soap in the soap dish between latherings. This prevents soapy water. It reduces the risk of slipping and falls in showers and tubs.
- Avoid using bath oils. They make tub and shower surfaces slippery.
- Do not leave weak or unsteady persons unattended.
- Stay within hearing distance if the person can be left alone. Wait outside the shower curtain or door. You will be nearby if the person calls for you or has an accident.
- Drain the tub before the person gets out of the tub. Turn off the shower before the person gets out of the shower. Cover him or her to provide privacy and prevent chilling.

The person may need one of these devices to get in and out of the tub:

▶ Transfer bench (Fig. 19-21).
▶ A tub with a side entry door (Fig. 19-22).
▶ Wheelchair or stretcher lift. The person is transferred to the tub room by wheelchair or stretcher. Then the device and person are lifted into the tub (Fig. 19-23).
▶ Mechanical lift (Chapter 16).

Whirlpool tubs have a cleansing action. You wash the upper body. Carefully wash under the breasts and between skin folds. Also wash the perineal area. Pat dry the person with towels after the bath.

Showers

Some people can stand and use a regular shower. Have them use the grab bars for support during the shower. Like tubs, showers have non-skid surfaces. If not, a bath mat is used. Never let weak or unsteady persons stand in the shower. They may need to use one of the following:

▶ *Shower chairs.* Water drains through an opening (Fig. 19-24). The chair is used to transport the person to and from the shower. The wheels are locked during the shower to prevent the chair from moving.
▶ *Shower stalls or cabinets.* The person walks into the device or is wheeled in on a wheelchair (Fig. 19-25). Hand-held shower nozzles are used.
▶ *Shower trolleys.* These devices allow the person to have a shower lying down (Fig. 19-26). They also are called portable tubs. The sides are lowered to transfer the person from the bed to the trolley. The sides are raised after the transfer. Then the person is transported to the tub or shower room. A hand-held nozzle is used to give the shower in the usual manner.

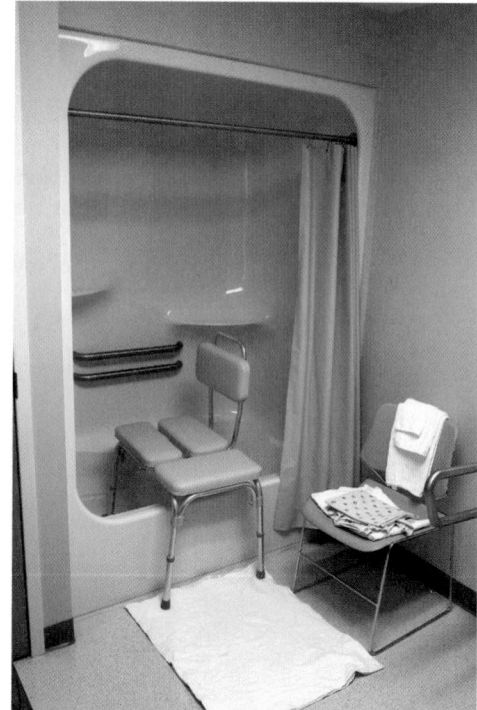

FIGURE 19-21 A transfer bench is positioned for the person's use in getting in and out of the tub. The tub is filled halfway with water. A floor mat is in front of the tub.

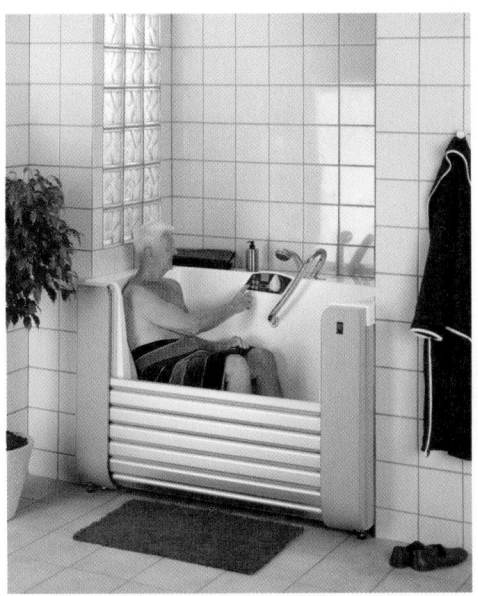

FIGURE 19-22 Tub with a side entry door. (Courtesy ARJO, Inc., Roselle, Ill. (800)323-1245.)

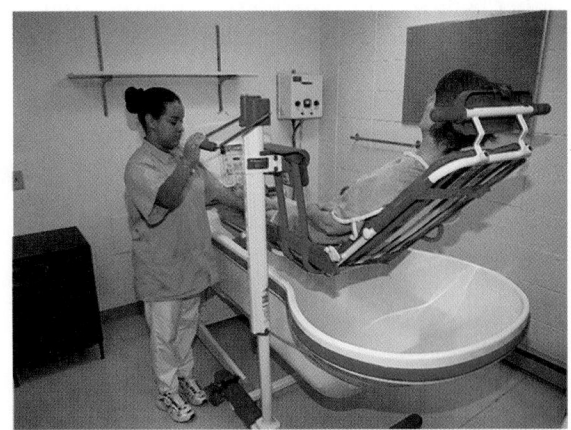

FIGURE 19-23 The stretcher and person are lowered into the tub.

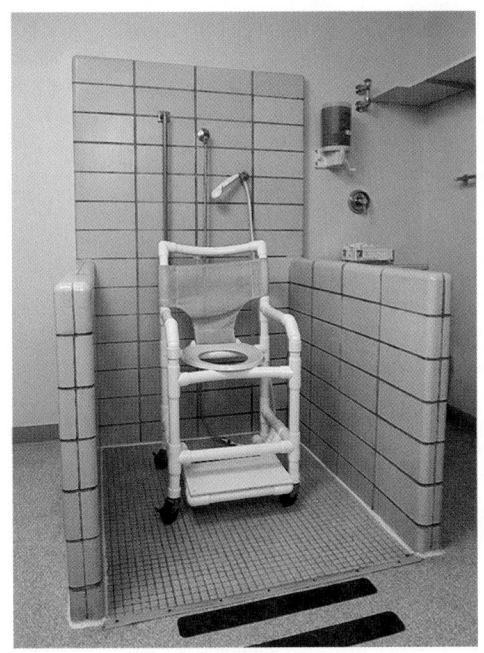

FIGURE 19-24 A shower chair in a shower stall.

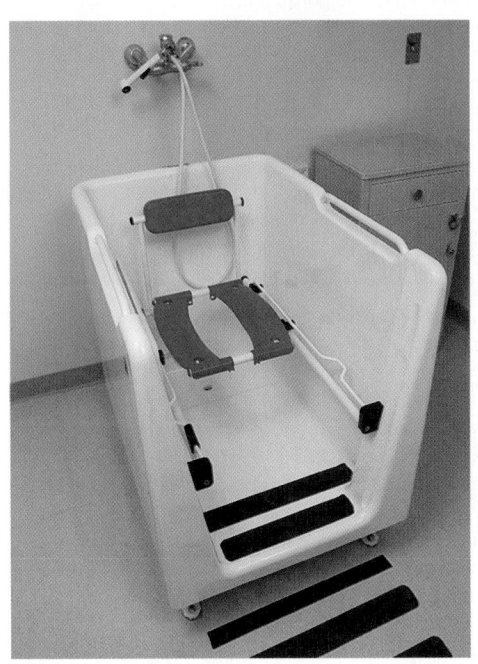

FIGURE 19-25 A shower cabinet.

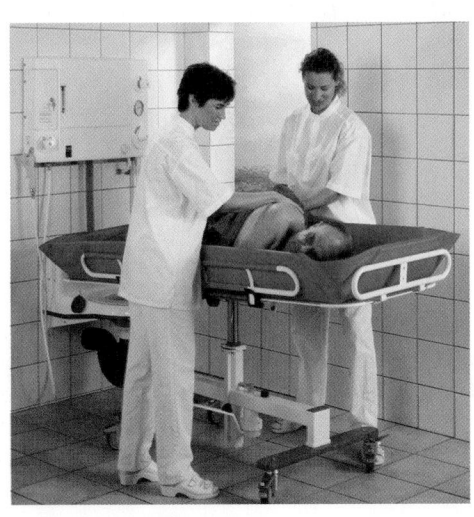

FIGURE 19-26 Shower trolley. The sides are lowered for transfers into and out of the trolley. (Courtesy ARJO, Inc., Roselle, Ill. (800)323-1245.)

Some shower rooms have two or more stations. Protect the person's privacy. The person has the right not to have his or her body seen by others. Properly screen and cover the person. Also close doors and the shower curtain.

See *Focus on Long-Term Care and Home Care: Showers.*

See *Delegation Guidelines: Tub Baths and Showers.*

See *Promoting Safety and Comfort: Tub Baths and Showers.*

See *Teamwork and Time Management: Tub Baths and Showers.*

See *Focus on Ethics and Laws: Tub Baths and Showers.*

Showers

HOME CARE

Many homes have shower stalls or bathtub-shower units. If the person has to step into the tub or shower, grab bars are needed for the person's use. Assist the person in getting into and out of the shower as needed.

The person can buy or rent a shower chair. Or a sturdy chair can be used. A sturdy lawn chair is an example. The nurse helps the person and family find a safe chair for shower use.

The bathtub unit may not have a shower. A hand-held shower nozzle can be installed.

DELEGATION GUIDELINES: Tub Baths and Showers

Before assisting with a tub bath or shower, you need this information from the nurse and the care plan:
- If the person takes a tub bath or shower
- What water temperature to use (usually 105° F; 40.5° C)
- What equipment is needed—shower chair, shower cabinet, shower trolley, and so on
- If the person uses adaptive devices (p. 305)
- How much help the person needs
- If the person can bathe unattended
- What observations to report and record:
  - Dizziness
  - Light-headedness
  - See *Delegation Guidelines: Bathing*, p. 316
  - When to report observations
- What specific patient or resident concerns to report at once

PROMOTING SAFETY AND COMFORT: Tub Baths and Showers

SAFETY

Some persons are very weak. At least two persons are needed to safely assist them with tub baths and showers. If the person is heavy, 3 staff members may be needed.

The person may use a tub with a side entry door, a shower chair, a shower trolley, or other device. Always follow the manufacturer's instructions.

Protect the person from falls, chilling, and burns. Follow the safety measures in Chapters 11 and 12. Remember to measure water temperature.

Clean and disinfect the tub or shower before and after use. This prevents the spread of microbes and infection.

COMFORT

Warmth and privacy promote comfort during tub baths and showers. You need to:
- Make sure the tub or shower room is warm.
- Provide for privacy. Close the room door, screen the person, and close window coverings.
- Make sure the water temperature is warm enough for the person.
- Have the person remove his or her clothing or robe and footwear just before getting into the tub or shower. Do not let the person remain exposed longer than necessary.
- Leave the room if the person can be alone.

TEAMWORK AND TIME MANAGEMENT

Tub Baths and Showers

Many agencies do not have tub and shower equipment for each person. You need to reserve the room and needed equipment for the person. Your co-workers do the same for their patients and residents. Consider the needs of others. For example, you reserve the shower room from 0945 to 1030 (9:45 to 10:30 AM). Do your very best to follow the schedule. Make sure the shower room is clean and ready for the next person. Or you and a co-worker schedule something for the same time. Discuss the matter with your co-worker to plan a new schedule.

All bed linens are changed on the person's bath or shower day. Ask co-workers to make the person's bed while you are assisting with the tub bath or shower. Also ask them to straighten the person's unit. The person returns to a clean bed and unit. Remember to return the favor when your co-workers are assisting with tub baths, showers, or other care measures.

■ ■ ■ ■ ━━━━━━━━━━━━━━━

FOCUS ON **ETHICS** AND **LAWS**

Tub Baths and Showers

A patient (Mr. Genza) was paralyzed on his right side because of a stroke. He could not walk or talk. He could stand with difficulty. He died at age 51 from burns suffered during a shower.

A wrongful death suit was filed for what was claimed to be negligent care. According to the facts reported in the court case, the following occurred:

- On December 7, 1965, an attendant took the patient to the shower. He was taken in a wheelchair.
- The attendant undressed the patient. The patient was placed on a chair and under running water in the shower.
- The attendant claimed that he tested the water.
- The shower room was supervised by an RN. The RN testified that an attendant was required to be present at all times while a paralyzed patient was receiving a shower.
- The attendant stated that he washed the patient's back and head. Then he went to attend to another patient 5 or 6 feet from the shower. A tub was between the attendant and Mr. Genza.
- When the attendant asked if he wanted to get out of the shower, Mr. Genza indicated that he did not.
- Two minutes later, the attendant was getting another patient out of the tub. The attendant heard Mr. Genza shout and saw that the shower handle was moved from its original setting.
- Two days later, Mr. Genza died from burns.
- On the day of the accident, the hot water gauge read 171° F. It tested at 158° to 159° F.
- An expert witness stated that 110° F is hot enough for shower room use.

In the Court's opinion, the home was grossly negligent for:

- Failing to provide the supervision needed by a helpless person
- Providing water facilities that were dangerous and a threat to the lives of anyone using them

In another case, a daughter filed a complaint for the wrongful death of her mother. According to the complaint, on August 29, 1993, a nurse's aide ran water in a whirlpool bath for the nursing home resident. The nurse's aide tested the water with her bare arm and hand. She found the water satisfactory. The resident also tested the water by putting her foot in the water, which showed that the water was okay. Using a lift chair, the resident was transferred into the tub.

After the bath, the nurse's aide asked two co-workers to help her get the resident out of the tub. After getting her out, a co-worker noted a small spot on the resident's left hip. The resident had no burns on her body before the bath. However, redness of her extremities was noted over the next 30 minutes. Blisters began and continued to form.

The resident had second and third degree burns from her mid-back down over the buttocks, the perineal area, and lower extremities. (Author note: a *first degree burn* means the epidermis is damaged. A *second degree burn* involves the epidermis and part of the dermis. A *third degree burn* involves the epidermis and the entire dermis.) The resident was transferred to the hospital. She died on September 1, 1993.

The daughter sued the county, the nursing home and hospital, the nursing home administrator, hospital board members, and the nurse's aide. The trial court dismissed the case on a legal technicality. However, the Appellate Court reversed the dismissal by the trial court and returned the case to court for trial.

(D. Burton v Choctaw County, Mississippi, Choctaw Hospital d/b/a Choctaw County Nursing Home; and others, 1997.)

(M. Lewinski v State of Illinois, 1967.)

━━━━━━━━━━━━━━━ ■ ■ ■ ■

ASSISTING WITH A TUB BATH OR SHOWER

✔ **Quality of Life** *Remember to:*

- Knock before entering the person's room.
- Address the person by name.
- Introduce yourself by name and title.
- Explain the procedure to the person before beginning and during the procedure.

- Protect the person's rights during the procedure.
- Handle the person gently during the procedure.

PRE-PROCEDURE

1 Follow *Delegation Guidelines:*
   - *Bathing,* p. 316
   - *Tub Baths and Showers*
   See *Promoting Safety and Comfort:*
   - *Bathing,* p. 316
   - *Tub Baths and Showers*
2 Reserve the bathtub or shower.
3 Practice hand hygiene.
4 Identify the person. Check the ID bracelet against the assignment sheet. Also call the person by name.
5 Collect the following:

- Washcloth and two bath towels
- Soap
- Bath thermometer (for a tub bath)
- Clothing or sleepwear
- Grooming items as requested
- Robe and non-skid footwear
- Rubber bath mat if needed
- Disposable bath mat
- Gloves
- Wheelchair, shower chair, transfer bench, and so on as needed

Continued

ASSISTING WITH A TUB BATH OR SHOWER—cont'd

PROCEDURE

6 Place items in the tub or shower room. Use the space provided or a chair.
7 Clean and disinfect the tub or shower.
8 Place a rubber bath mat in the tub or on the shower floor. Do not block the drain.
9 Place the disposable bath mat on the floor in the front of the tub or shower.
10 Put the OCCUPIED sign on the door.
11 Return to the person's room. Provide for privacy. Decontaminate your hands.
12 Help the person sit on the side of the bed.
13 Help the person put on a robe and non-skid footwear. Or the person can leave on clothing.
14 Assist or transport the person to the tub room or shower.
15 Have the person sit on a chair if he or she walked to the tub or shower room.
16 Provide for privacy.
17 *For a tub bath:*
   a Fill the tub halfway with warm water (105° F; 40.5° C).
   b Measure water temperature with the bath thermometer. Or check the digital display.
18 *For a shower:*
   a Turn on the shower.
   b Adjust water temperature and pressure. Check the digital display.
19 Help the person undress and remove footwear.

20 Help the person into the tub or shower. Position the shower chair, and lock the wheels.
21 Assist with washing as necessary. Wear gloves.
22 Ask the person to use the signal light when done or when help is needed. Remind the person that a tub bath lasts no longer than 20 minutes.
23 Place a towel across the chair.
24 Leave the room if the person can bathe alone. If not, stay in the room or nearby. Remove your gloves and decontaminate your hands if you will leave the room.
25 Check the person at least every 5 minutes.
26 Return when he or she signals for you. Knock before entering. Decontaminate your hands.
27 Turn off the shower, or drain the tub. Cover the person while the tub drains.
28 Help the person out of the shower or tub and onto the chair.
29 Help the person dry off. Pat gently. Dry under the breasts, between skin folds, in the perineal area, and between the toes.
30 Assist with lotion and other grooming items as needed.
31 Help the person dress and put on footwear.
32 Help the person return to the room. Provide for privacy.
33 Assist the person to a chair or into bed.
34 Provide a back massage if the person returns to bed.
35 Assist with hair care and other grooming needs.

POST-PROCEDURE

36 Provide for comfort. (See the inside of the front book cover.)
37 Place the signal light within reach.
38 Raise or lower bed rails. Follow the care plan.
39 Unscreen the person.
40 Complete a safety check of the room. (See the inside of the front book cover.)

41 Clean and disinfect the tub or shower. Remove soiled linen. Wear gloves for this step.
42 Discard disposable items. Put the UNOCCUPIED sign on the door. Return supplies to their proper place.
43 Follow agency policy for dirty linen.
44 Decontaminate your hands.
45 Report and record your observations.

◆ THE BACK MASSAGE

The back massage (back rub) relaxes muscles and stimulates circulation. Massages are given after the bath and with evening care. You also can give back massages at other times. Examples include after repositioning or when helping the person to relax.

Back massages last 3 to 5 minutes. Observe the skin before the massage. Look for breaks in the skin, bruises, reddened areas, and other signs of skin breakdown.

Lotion reduces friction during the back massage.

It is warmed before being applied. To warm lotion, do one of the following:

▶ Rub some lotion between your hands.
▶ Place the bottle in the bath water.
▶ Hold the bottle under warm water.

Use firm strokes. Also keep your hands in contact with the person's skin. After the massage, apply some lotion to the elbows, knees, and heels. This keeps the skin soft. Bony areas are at risk for skin breakdown.

See *Delegation Guidelines: The Back Massage.*
See *Promoting Safety and Comfort: The Back Massage.*

DELEGATION GUIDELINES: The Back Massage

Before giving a back massage, you need this information from the nurse and the care plan:

- If the person can have a back massage (see *Promoting Safety and Comfort: The Back Massage*)
- How to position the person
- If the person has position limits
- When the person should receive a back massage
- If the person needs frequent back massages for comfort and relaxation
- What observations to report and record:
  - Breaks in the skin
  - Bruising
  - Reddened areas
  - Signs of skin breakdown
- When to report observations
- What specific patient or resident concerns to report at once

PROMOTING SAFETY AND COMFORT: The Back Massage

SAFETY

Back massages are dangerous for persons with certain heart diseases, back injuries, back surgeries, skin diseases, and lung disorders. Check with the nurse and the care plan before giving back massages to persons with these conditions.

Do not massage reddened bony areas. Reddened areas signal skin breakdown and pressure ulcers. Massage can lead to more tissue damage.

Wear gloves if the person's skin is not intact. Always follow Standard Precautions and the Bloodborne Pathogen Standard.

COMFORT

The prone position is best for a massage. The side-lying position is often used. Older and disabled persons usually find the side-lying position more comfortable.

GIVING A BACK MASSAGE

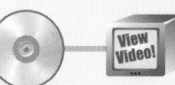

✔ **Quality of Life** *Remember to:*

- Knock before entering the person's room.
- Address the person by name.
- Introduce yourself by name and title.
- Explain the procedure to the person before beginning and during the procedure.

- Protect the person's rights during the procedure.
- Handle the person gently during the procedure.

PRE-PROCEDURE

1 Follow *Delegation Guidelines: The Back Massage.* See *Promoting Safety and Comfort: The Back Massage.*
2 Practice hand hygiene.
3 Identify the person. Check the ID bracelet against the assignment sheet. Also call the person by name.

4 Collect the following:
- Bath blanket
- Bath towel
- Lotion
5 Provide for privacy.
6 Raise the bed for good body mechanics. Bed rails are up if used.

PROCEDURE

7 Lower the bed rail near you if up.
8 Position the person in the prone or side-lying position. The back is toward you.
9 Expose the back, shoulders, upper arms, and buttocks. Cover the rest of the body with the bath blanket.
10 Lay the towel on the bed along the back. (This step is done if the person is in a side-lying position.)
11 Warm the lotion.
12 Explain that the lotion may feel cool and wet.
13 Apply lotion to the lower back area.
14 Stroke up from the buttocks to the shoulders. Then stroke down over the upper arms. Stroke up the upper arms, across the shoulders, and down the back to the buttocks (Fig. 19-27, p. 328). Use firm strokes. Keep your hands in contact with the person's skin.

15 Repeat step 14 for at least 3 minutes.
16 Knead the back (Fig. 19-28, p. 328):
  a Grasp the skin between your thumb and fingers.
  b Knead half of the back. Start at the buttocks and move up to the shoulder. Then knead down from the shoulder to the buttocks.
  c Repeat on the other half of the back.
17 Apply lotion to bony areas. Use circular motions with the tips of your index and middle fingers. (Do not massage reddened bony areas.)
18 Use fast movements to stimulate. Use slow movements to relax the person.
19 Stroke with long, firm movements to end the massage. Tell the person you are finishing.
20 Straighten and secure clothing or sleepwear.
21 Cover the person. Remove the towel and bath blanket.

Continued

GIVING A BACK MASSAGE—cont'd

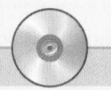

POST-PROCEDURE

22 Provide for comfort. (See the inside of the front book cover.)
23 Place the signal light within reach.
24 Lower the bed to its lowest position.
25 Raise or lower bed rails. Follow the care plan.
26 Return lotion to its proper place.

27 Unscreen the person.
28 Complete a safety check of the room. (See the inside of the front book cover.)
29 Follow agency policy for dirty linen.
30 Decontaminate your hands.
31 Report and record your observations.

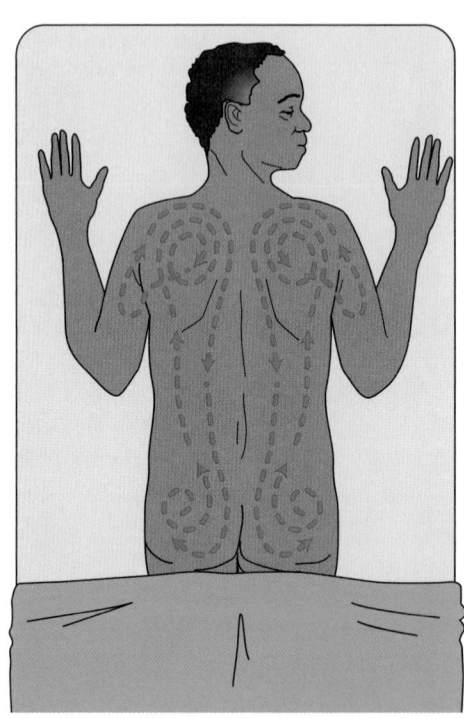

FIGURE 19-27 The person lies in the prone position for a back massage. Stroke upward from the buttocks to the shoulders, down over the upper arms, back up the upper arms, across the shoulders, and down the back to the buttocks.

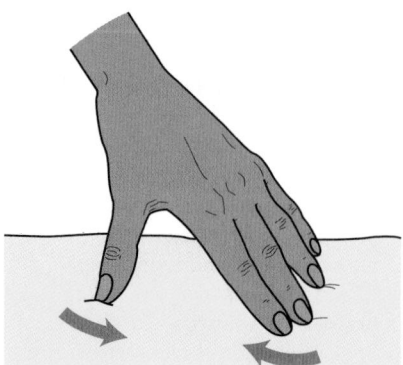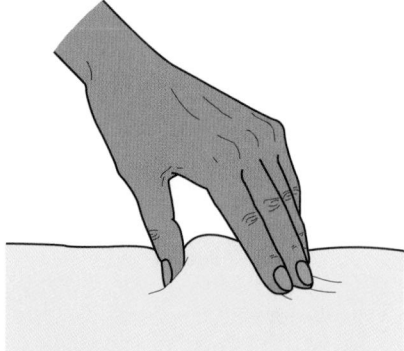

FIGURE 19-28 Kneading is done by picking up tissue between the thumb and fingers.

◆ PERINEAL CARE

Perineal care (pericare) involves cleaning the genital and anal areas. These areas provide a warm, moist, and dark place for microbes to grow. Cleaning prevents infection and odors, and it promotes comfort.

Perineal care is done daily during the bath. It also is done whenever the area is soiled with urine or feces. Perineal care is very important for persons who:

▶ Have urinary catheters (Chapter 21).
▶ Have had rectal or genital surgery.
▶ Have given birth (Chapter 47).
▶ Are menstruating (Chapter 8).
▶ Are incontinent of urine or feces.
▶ Are uncircumcised. Being *circumcised* means that the fold of skin (foreskin) covering the head of the penis was surgically removed. Being *uncircumcised* means that the person has foreskin covering the head of the penis.

The person does perineal care if able. Otherwise, it is given by the nursing staff. This procedure embarrasses many people and nursing staff, especially when it involves the other sex.

Perineal and *perineum* are not common terms. Most people understand *privates*, *private parts*, *crotch*, *genitals*, or the *area between the legs*. Use terms the person understands. The term must be in good taste professionally.

Standard Precautions, medical asepsis, and the Bloodborne Pathogen Standard are followed. Work from the cleanest area to the dirtiest. This is commonly called cleaning from "front to back." The urethral area (the front) is the cleanest. The anal area (the back) is the dirtiest. Therefore clean from the urethra to the anal area. This prevents the transmission of bacteria from the anal area to the vagina and urinary system.

The perineal area is delicate and easily injured. Use warm water, not hot. Use washcloths, towelettes, cotton balls, or swabs according to agency policy. Rinse thoroughly. Pat dry after rinsing. This reduces moisture and promotes comfort.

See *Focus on Children and Older Persons: Perineal Care.*
See *Delegation Guidelines: Perineal Care.*
See *Promoting Safety and Comfort: Perineal Care.*

Text continued on p. 332

FOCUS ON **CHILDREN** AND **OLDER PERSONS**
Perineal Care

CHILDREN

All children need perineal care. When diapers are worn, the perineal area is exposed to urine and feces. Poor wiping after urinating and bowel movements is a common problem in younger children. Older children may hesitate to clean the genital and anal areas.

DELEGATION GUIDELINES: Perineal Care

Before giving perineal care, you need this information from the nurse and the care plan:
• When to give perineal care.
• What terms the person understands—perineum, privates, private parts, crotch, genitals, area between the legs, and so on.
• How much help the person needs.
• What water temperature to use—usually 105° to 109° F (40.5° to 42.7° C). Water in a basin cools rapidly.
• What cleaning agent to use.
• Any position restrictions or limits.
• What observations to report and record:
  • Odors
  • Redness, swelling, discharge, bleeding, or irritation
  • Complaints of pain, burning, or other discomfort
  • Signs of urinary or fecal incontinence
• When to report observations.
• What specific patient or resident concerns to report at once.

PROMOTING SAFETY AND COMFORT: Perineal Care

SAFETY

Hot water can burn delicate perineal tissues. To prevent burns, measure water temperature according to agency policy. If the water seems too hot, ask the nurse to check it.

Protect yourself and the person from infection. Contact with blood, body fluids, secretions, or excretions is likely during perineal care. Follow Standard Precautions and the Bloodborne Pathogen Standard.

Persons who are incontinent need perineal care. You must protect the person and dry garments and linens from the wet or soiled items. After cleaning and drying the perineal area, remove the wet or soiled incontinence products, garments, and linen. Then apply clean, dry ones.

COMFORT

To avoid embarrassment, it is best if the person does perineal care. If you provide this care, explain how privacy is protected. Act in a professional manner at all times.

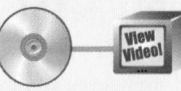

GIVING FEMALE PERINEAL CARE

✔ **Quality of Life** *Remember to:*

- Knock before entering the person's room.
- Address the person by name.
- Introduce yourself by name and title.

- Explain the procedure to the person before beginning and during the procedure.
- Protect the person's rights during the procedure.
- Handle the person gently during the procedure.

PRE-PROCEDURE

1 Follow *Delegation Guidelines: Perineal Care,* p. 329. See *Promoting Safety and Comfort: Perineal Care,* p. 329.
2 Practice hand hygiene.
3 Collect the following:
  - Soap or other cleaning agent as directed
  - At least 4 washcloths
  - Bath towel
  - Bath blanket
  - Bath thermometer
  - Wash basin

  - Waterproof pad
  - Gloves
  - Paper towels
4 Cover the overbed table with paper towels. Arrange items on top of them.
5 Identify the person. Check the ID bracelet against the assignment sheet. Also call her by name.
6 Provide for privacy.
7 Raise the bed for good body mechanics. Bed rails are up if used.

PROCEDURE

8 Lower the bed rail near you if up.
9 Decontaminate your hands. Put on gloves.
10 Cover the person with a bath blanket. Move top linens to the foot of the bed.
11 Position the person on her back.
12 Drape her as in Figure 19-29.
13 Raise the bed rail if used.
14 Fill the wash basin. Water temperature is about 105° to 109° F (40.5° to 42.7° C). Measure water temperature according to agency policy.
15 Place the basin on the overbed table.
16 Lower the bed rail if up.
17 Help the person flex her knees and spread her legs. Or help her spread her legs as much as possible with the knees straight.
18 Place a waterproof pad under her buttocks. Protect the person and dry linen from the wet or soiled incontinence product.
19 Fold the corner of the bath blanket between her legs onto her abdomen.
20 Wet the washcloths.
21 Squeeze out excess water from a washcloth. Make a mitted washcloth. Apply soap.
22 Separate the labia. Clean downward from front to back with one stroke (Fig. 19-30).
23 Repeat steps 21 and 22 until the area is clean. Use a clean part of the washcloth for each stroke. Use more than one washcloth if needed.

24 Rinse the perineum with a clean washcloth. Separate the labia. Stroke downward from front to back. Repeat as necessary. Use a clean part of the washcloth for each stroke. Use more than one washcloth if needed.
25 Pat the area dry with the towel. Dry from front to back.
26 Fold the blanket back between her legs.
27 Help the person lower her legs and turn onto her side away from you.
28 Apply soap to a mitted washcloth.
29 Clean the rectal area. Clean from the vagina to the anus with one stroke (Fig. 19-31).
30 Repeat steps 28 and 29 until the area is clean. Use a clean part of the washcloth for each stroke. Use more than one washcloth if needed.
31 Rinse the rectal area with a washcloth. Stroke from the vagina to the anus. Repeat as necessary. Use a clean part of the washcloth for each stroke. Use more than one washcloth if needed.
32 Pat the area dry with the towel. Dry from front to back.
33 Remove any wet or soiled incontinence product. Remove the waterproof pad.
34 Remove and discard the gloves. Decontaminate your hands. Put on clean gloves.
35 Provide clean and dry linens and incontinence products as needed.

POST-PROCEDURE

36 Cover the person. Remove the bath blanket.
37 Provide for comfort. (See the inside of the front book cover.)
38 Place the signal light within reach.
39 Lower the bed to its lowest position.
40 Raise or lower bed rails. Follow the care plan.
41 Empty and clean the wash basin.
42 Return the basin and supplies to their proper place.

43 Wipe off the overbed table with the paper towels. Discard the paper towels.
44 Remove the gloves. Decontaminate your hands.
45 Unscreen the person.
46 Complete a safety check of the room. (See the inside of the front book cover.)
47 Follow agency policy for dirty linen.
48 Decontaminate your hands.
49 Report and record your observations.

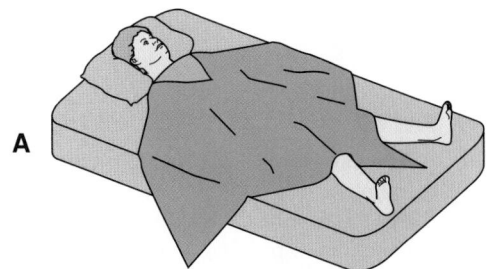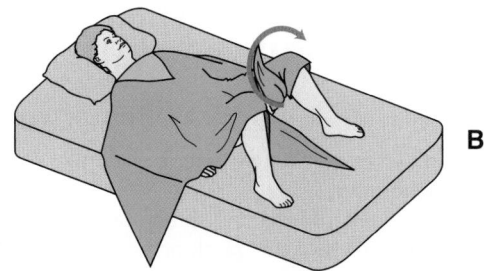

FIGURE 19-29 Draping for perineal care. **A,** Position the bath blanket like a diamond: one corner is at the neck, there is a corner at each side, and one corner is between the person's legs. **B,** Wrap the blanket around the leg by bringing the corner around under the leg and over the top. Tuck the corner under the hip.

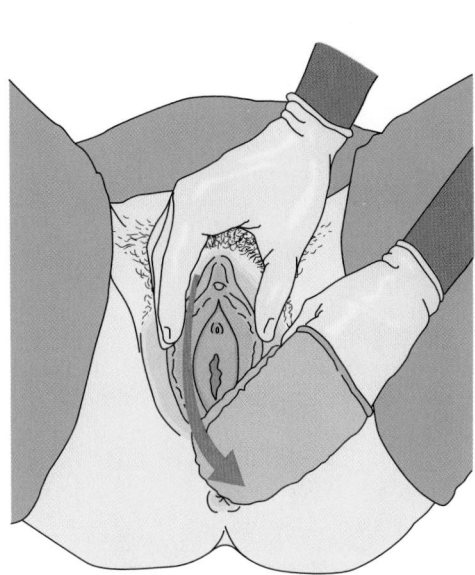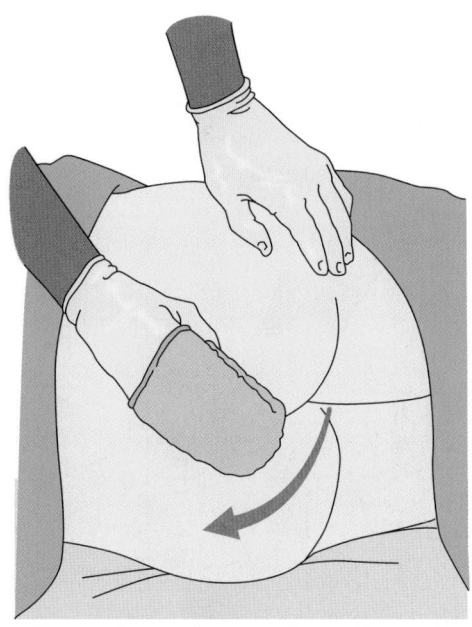

FIGURE 19-30 Separate the labia with one hand. Use a mitted washcloth to cleanse between the labia with downward strokes.

FIGURE 19-31 The rectal area is cleaned by wiping from the vagina to the anus. The side-lying position allows the anal area to be cleaned more thoroughly.

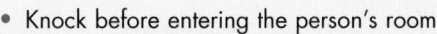 **NNAAP™ Skill**

GIVING MALE PERINEAL CARE

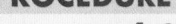

✔ **Quality of Life** *Remember to:*

- Knock before entering the person's room.
- Address the person by name.
- Introduce yourself by name and title.
- Explain the procedure to the person before beginning and during the procedure.

- Protect the person's rights during the procedure.
- Handle the person gently during the procedure.

PROCEDURE

1 Follow steps 1 through 16 in procedure: *Giving Female Perineal Care.* Drape the person as in Figure 19-29.
2 Place a waterproof pad under his buttocks. Protect the person and dry linen from the wet or soiled incontinence product.
3 Retract the foreskin if the person is uncircumcised (Fig. 19-32, p. 332).

4 Grasp the penis.
5 Clean the tip. Use a circular motion. Start at the meatus of the urethra, and work outward (Fig. 19-33, p. 332). Repeat as needed. Use a clean part of the washcloth each time.
6 Rinse the area with another washcloth.
7 Return the foreskin to its natural position.

Continued

GIVING MALE PERINEAL CARE — cont'd

PROCEDURE — cont'd

8 Clean the shaft of the penis. Use firm downward strokes. Rinse the area.

9 Help the person flex his knees and spread his legs. Or help him spread his legs as much as possible with his knees straight.

10 Clean the scrotum. Rinse well. Observe for redness and irritation of the skin folds.

11 Pat dry the penis and the scrotum. Use the towel.

12 Fold the bath blanket back between his legs.

13 Help him lower his legs and turn onto his side away from you.

14 Clean the rectal area (see procedure: *Giving Female Perineal Care*, p. 330). Rinse and dry well.

15 Remove any wet or soiled incontinence product. Remove the waterproof pad.

16 Remove and discard the gloves. Decontaminate your hands. Put on clean gloves.

17 Provide clean and dry linens and incontinence products.

POST-PROCEDURE

18 Follow steps 36 through 49 in procedure: *Giving Female Perineal Care*, p. 330.

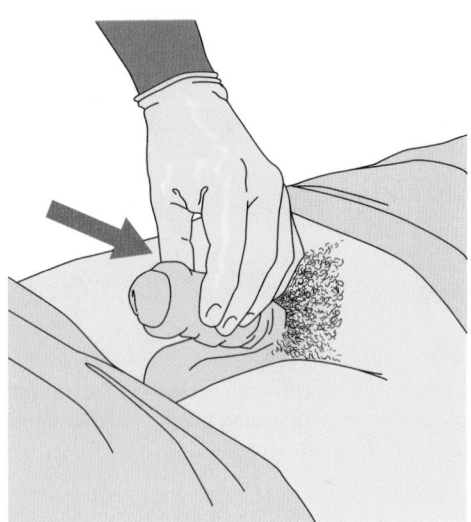

FIGURE 19-32 The foreskin of the uncircumcised male is pulled back for perineal care. It is returned to the normal position immediately after cleaning.

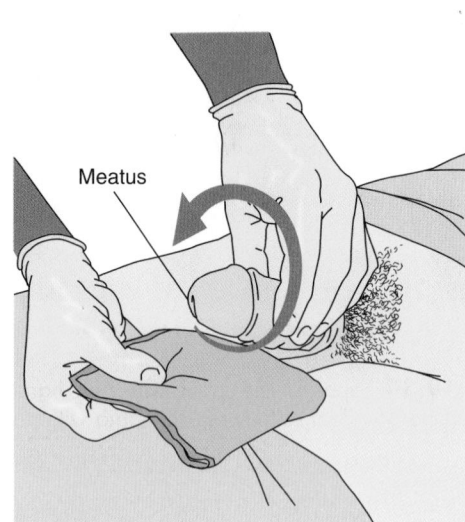

Meatus

FIGURE 19-33 The penis is cleaned with circular motions starting at the meatus.

REPORTING AND RECORDING

You make many observations while assisting with hygiene. Report the following at once:

▶ Bleeding

▶ Signs of skin breakdown

▶ Discharge from the vagina or urinary tract

▶ Unusual odors

▶ Changes from prior observations

Also report and record the care given. (See the "Activities of Daily Living" flow sheet in Chapter 5.) If care is not recorded, it is assumed that care was not given. This can cause serious legal problems.

REVIEW QUESTIONS

Circle T if the statement is true and F if it is false.

1 (T) F Hygiene is needed for comfort, safety, and health.

2 (T) F After lunch Mrs. Bell asks for a back massage. You can give the back massage.

3 T (F) A toothbrush has hard bristles. They are good for oral hygiene.

4 T (F) Unconscious persons are supine for mouth care.

5 T (F) You use your fingers to keep an unconscious person's mouth open for oral hygiene.

6 T (F) A person has a lower denture. It is cleaned over a counter.

7 T (F) Bath oils cleanse and soften the skin.

8 (T) F Powders absorb moisture and prevent friction.

9 T (F) Deodorants reduce the amount of perspiration.

10 T (F) A tub bath lasts 30 minutes.

11 T (F) You can give permission for showers but not tub baths.

12 T (F) Weak persons are left alone in the shower if they are sitting.

13 (T) F A back massage relaxes muscles and stimulates circulation.

14 (T) F Perineal care helps prevent infection.

15 (T) F Foreskin is returned to its normal position immediately after cleaning.

Circle the BEST answer.

16 Oral hygiene does the following *except*
  a Prevent mouth odors
  b Prevent infection
  c Increase comfort
  (d) Coat and dry the mouth

17 You brush a person's teeth and note the following. Which is *not* reported to the nurse?
  a Bleeding, swelling, or redness of the gums
  b Irritations, sores, or white patches in the mouth or on the tongue
  c Lips that are dry, cracked, swollen, or blistered
  (d) Food between the teeth

18 Which is *not* a purpose of bathing?
  a Increasing circulation
  (b) Promoting drying of the skin
  c Exercising body parts
  d Refreshing and relaxing the person

19 Soaps do the following *except*
  a Remove dirt and dead skin
  (b) Soften the skin
  c Remove skin oil
  d Dry the skin

20 Which action is *wrong* when bathing a person?
  a Covering the person for warmth and privacy
  b Rinsing the skin thoroughly to remove all soap
  (c) Washing from the dirtiest to the cleanest area
  d Patting the skin dry

21 Water for a complete bed bath is at least
  a 100° F
  b 105° F
  (c) 110° F
  d 120° F

22 You are going to give a back massage. Which is *false?*
  a It should last 3 to 5 minutes.
  (b) Lotion is warmed before being applied.
  c Your hands are always in contact with the skin.
  (d) The side-lying position is best.

Answers to these questions are on p. 780.

OBJECTIVES

- Define the key terms and key abbreviations listed in this chapter
- Explain why grooming is important
- Identify the factors that affect hair care
- Explain how to care for matted and tangled hair
- Describe how to shampoo hair
- Describe the measures practiced when shaving a person
- Explain why nail and foot care is important
- Describe the rules for changing clothing and gowns
- Perform the procedures described in this chapter

PROCEDURES

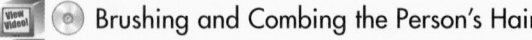 Brushing and Combing the Person's Hair

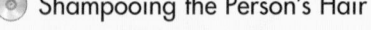 Shampooing the Person's Hair

Shaving the Person's Face With a Safety Razor

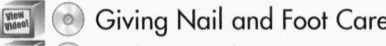 Giving Nail and Foot Care

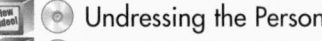 Undressing the Person

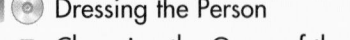 Dressing the Person

Changing the Gown of the Person With an IV

Procedures with this icon ⊚ are on the CDCompanion in this book; those with this icon 📺 are on the Evolve Student Resources Website.

KEY TERMS

alopecia Hair loss
dandruff Excessive amounts of dry, white flakes from the scalp
hirsutism Excessive body hair
lice Pediculosis
mite A very small spider-like organism

pediculosis Infestation with wingless insects; lice
pediculosis capitis Infestation of the scalp (*capitis*) with lice
pediculosis corporsis Infestation of the body (*corporsis*) with lice
pediculosis pubis Infestation of the pubic (*pubis*) hair with lice

KEY ABBREVIATIONS

ADEAR Alzheimer's Disease Education and Referral Center
C Centigrade

F Fahrenheit
IV Intravenous

Hair care, shaving, and nail and foot care are important to many people. Like hygiene, these grooming measures prevent infection and promote comfort. They also affect love, belonging, and self-esteem needs.

People differ in their grooming measures. Some want only clean hair. Others want a certain hairstyle. Some want only clean hands. Others want clean, manicured, and polished nails. Many men shave and groom their beards. Likewise, many women shave their legs and underarms. Some women have facial hair. They may shave or use other hair removal methods.

As with hygiene, the person should tend to grooming measures to the extent possible. This promotes the person's independence and quality of life. The person may use adaptive devices for hair care and dressing. See Figure 20-1 for examples.

See *Teamwork and Time Management: Grooming*.

HAIR CARE

How the hair looks and feels affects mental well-being. Some people cannot perform hair care. You assist with hair care whenever needed.

The nursing process reflects the person's culture, personal choice, skin and scalp condition, health history, and self-care ability.

See *Focus on Long-Term Care and Home Care: Hair Care*.

Skin and Scalp Conditions

Skin and scalp conditions include hair loss, excessive body hair, dandruff, lice, and scabies.

Alopecia, Hirsutism, and Dandruff

Alopecia means hair loss. Hair loss may be complete or partial. Male pattern baldness occurs with aging. It results from heredity. Hair also thins in some women with aging. Cancer treatments (radiation therapy to the head and chemotherapy) often cause alopecia in males and females. Skin disease is another cause. Stress, poor nutrition, pregnancy, some drugs, and hormone changes are other causes. Except for hair loss from aging, hair usually grows back.

Hirsutism is excessive body hair. It can occur in women and children. It results from heredity and abnormal amounts of male hormones.

TEAMWORK AND TIME MANAGEMENT

Grooming

Some equipment for grooming procedures is shared among patients and residents. Shampoo trays, electric shavers, and whirlpool foot baths are examples. Let other team members know when you need to use an item. Schedule use of the item following agency policy. After the procedure, clean and promptly return the item to its proper place. A co-worker should not have to clean or look for an item after you use it.

FOCUS ON LONG-TERM CARE AND HOME CARE

Hair Care

LONG-TERM CARE

Many nursing centers have beauty and barber shops for residents. Residents can have their hair shampooed, cut, and styled. Men also can have their mustaches and beards groomed.

Dandruff is the excessive amount of dry, white flakes from the scalp. Itching often occurs. Sometimes eyebrows and ear canals are involved. Medicated shampoos correct the problem.

Lice

Pediculosis (lice) is the infestation with wingless insects (*lice*). *Infestation* means being in or on a host. **Pediculosis capitis** is the infestation of the scalp (*capitis*) with lice. The lice attach their eggs (*nits*) to hair shafts. Nits are oval and yellow to white in color. They hatch in about one week.

After hatching, lice must feed on blood to live. Therefore they bite the scalp or skin. Adult lice are about the size of a sesame seed. They are tan to grayish-white in color. Lice bites cause severe itching in the affected body area.

▶ **Pediculosis pubis**—the infestation of the pubic (*pubis*) hair with lice. This form of lice is also called "crabs."
▶ **Pediculosis corporis**—the infestation of the body (*corporis*) with lice. Nits attach to clothing and furniture.

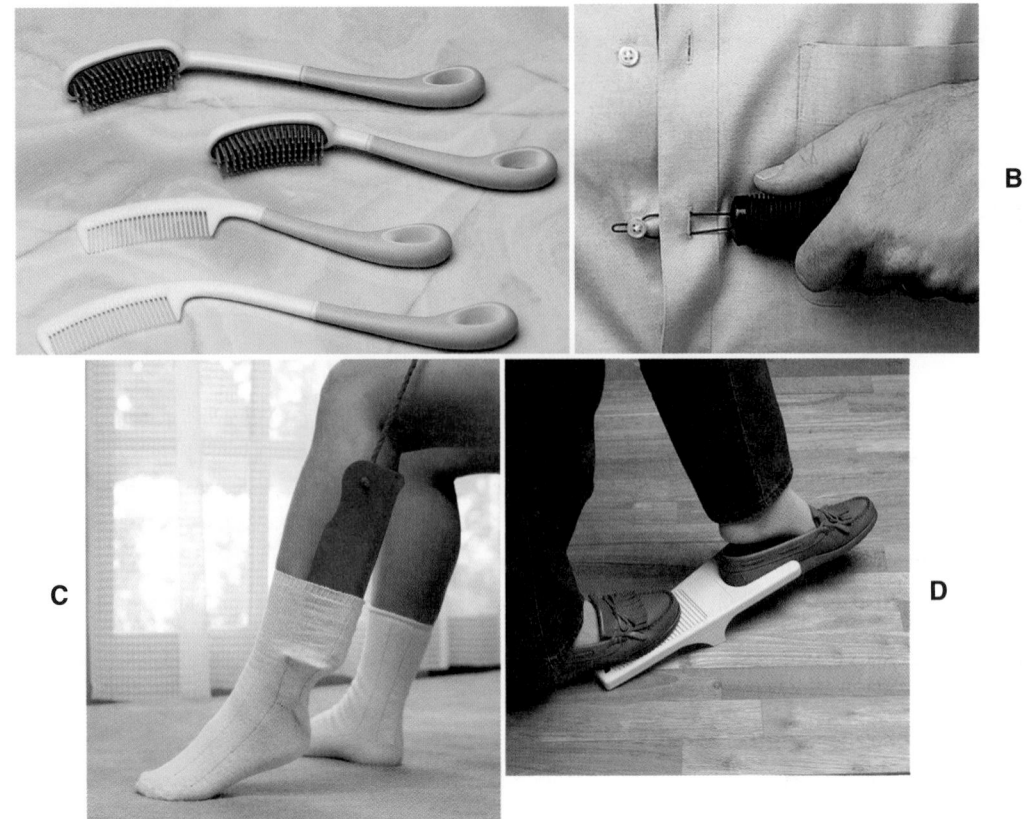

FIGURE 20-1 Grooming aids. **A,** Long-handled combs and brushes for hair care. **B,** A button hook is used to button and zip clothing. **C,** A sock assist is used to pull on socks and stockings. **D,** A shoe remover is used to take off shoes. (From North Coast Medical Inc., Morgan Hill, Calif.)

Lice easily spread to others through clothing, head coverings, furniture, beds, towels, bed linen, and sexual contact. They also are spread by sharing combs and brushes. Medicated shampoos, lotions, and creams are used to treat lice. Thorough bathing is needed. So is washing clothing and linens in hot water.

Report signs and symptoms of lice to the nurse at once:

- Complaints of a tickling feeling or something moving in the hair
- Itching
- Irritability
- Sores on the head or body caused by scratching
- Rash

Scabies

Scabies is a skin disorder caused by a female mite. A **mite** is a very small spider-like organism. The female mite burrows into the skin and lays eggs. When the eggs hatch, the females produce more eggs. The person becomes infested with mites.

The person has a rash and intense itching. Common sites are between the fingers, around the wrists, in the underarm area, on the thighs, and in the genital area. Other sites include the breasts, waist, and buttocks.

Scabies is highly contagious. It is transmitted to others by close contact. Persons living in crowded living settings are at risk. So are persons with weakened immune systems. Special creams are ordered to kill the mites. The person's room is cleaned. Clothing and linens are washed in hot water.

◆ Brushing and Combing Hair

Brushing and combing hair are part of early morning care, morning care, and afternoon care. Some people brush and comb their hair at bedtime too. Brushing and combing also are done whenever needed. Make sure you complete hair care before visitors arrive.

Encourage patients and residents to do their own hair care. Assist as needed. Perform hair care for those who cannot do so. The person chooses how to brush, comb, and style hair.

Brushing increases blood flow to the scalp. It also brings scalp oils along the hair shaft. Scalp oils help keep hair soft and shiny. Brushing and combing prevent tangled and matted hair. When brushing and combing hair, start at the scalp. Then brush or comb to the hair ends.

Long hair easily mats and tangles. Daily brushing and combing prevent the problem. So does braiding. Do not braid hair without the person's consent. *Never cut matted or tangled hair. Never cut hair for any reason.* Tell the nurse if the person has matted or tangled hair. The nurse may have you comb or brush through the matting and tangling.

Special measures are needed for curly, coarse, and dry hair. Use a wide-tooth comb for curly hair. Start at the neckline. Working upward, lift and fluff hair outward. Continue to the forehead. Wet hair or apply conditioner or petroleum jelly as directed. This makes combing easier.

The person may have certain hair care practices and hair care products. They are part of the care plan. Also, the person can guide you when giving hair care.

See *Caring about Culture: Brushing and Combing Hair.*

See *Focus on Children and Older Persons: Brushing and Combing Hair.*

See *Delegation Guidelines: Brushing and Combing Hair.*

See *Promoting Safety and Comfort: Brushing and Combing Hair.*

CARING ABOUT CULTURE

Brushing and Combing Hair

Styling hair in small braids is a common practice of some cultural groups. The braids are left intact for shampooing. To undo these braids, the nurse obtains the person's consent.

FOCUS ON CHILDREN AND OLDER PERSONS

Brushing and Combing Hair

CHILDREN

Hairstyles are important to older children and teenagers. Do not make judgments about the child's hairstyle. Style hair in a way that pleases the child and parents. Do not style hair according to your standards or customs.

DELEGATION GUIDELINES: Brushing and Combing Hair

Before brushing and combing hair, you need this information from the nurse and the care plan:
- How much help the person needs
- What to do if hair is matted or tangled
- What measures are needed for curly, coarse, or dry hair
- What hair care products to use
- The person's preferences and routine hair care measures
- What observations to report and record:
  - Scalp sores
  - Flaking
  - Itching
  - The presence of nits or lice
  - Patches of hair loss
  - Very dry or very oily hair
  - Matted or tangled hair
- When to report observations
- What specific patient or resident concerns to report at once

PROMOTING SAFETY AND COMFORT: Brushing and Combing Hair

SAFETY

Sharp bristles can injure the scalp. So can a comb with sharp or broken teeth. Tell the nurse if you have concerns about the person's brush or comb.

COMFORT

When giving hair care, place a towel across the person's back and shoulders to protect garments from falling hair. If the person is in bed, give hair care before changing linens and the pillowcase. If done after a linen change, place a towel across the pillow to collect falling hair.

BRUSHING AND COMBING THE PERSON'S HAIR

✔ **Quality of Life** *Remember to:*

- Knock before entering the person's room.
- Address the person by name.
- Introduce yourself by name and title.
- Explain the procedure to the person before beginning and during the procedure.
- Protect the person's rights during the procedure.
- Handle the person gently during the procedure.

PRE-PROCEDURE

1 Follow *Delegation Guidelines: Brushing and Combing Hair.* See *Promoting Safety and Comfort: Brushing and Combing Hair.*
2 Practice hand hygiene.
3 Identify the person. Check the ID bracelet against the assignment sheet. Also call the person by name.
4 Ask the person how to style hair.
5 Collect the following:
- Comb and brush
- Bath towel
- Other hair care items as requested
6 Arrange items on the bedside stand.
7 Provide for privacy.

Continued

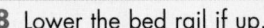
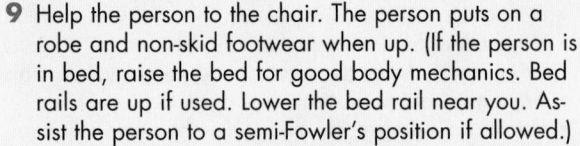

PROCEDURE

8 Lower the bed rail if up.
9 Help the person to the chair. The person puts on a robe and non-skid footwear when up. (If the person is in bed, raise the bed for good body mechanics. Bed rails are up if used. Lower the bed rail near you. Assist the person to a semi-Fowler's position if allowed.)
10 Place a towel across the person's back and shoulders or across the pillow.
11 Ask the person to remove eyeglasses. Put them in the eyeglass case. Put the case inside the bedside stand.
12 *Brush and comb hair that is not matted or tangled:*
   a Use the comb to part the hair.
      (1) Part hair down the middle into 2 sides (Fig. 20-2, *A*).
      (2) Divide one side into 2 smaller sections (Fig. 20-2, *B*).

   b Brush one of the small sections of hair. Start at the scalp, and brush toward the hair ends (Fig. 20-3). Do the same for the other small section of hair.
   c Repeat steps 12a(2) and 12b for the other side.
13 *Brush and comb matted and tangled hair:*
   a Take a small section of hair near the ends.
   b Comb or brush through to the hair ends.
   c Add small sections of hair as you work up to the scalp.
   d Comb or brush through each longer section to the hair ends.
   e Brush or comb from the scalp to the hair ends.
14 Style the hair as the person prefers.
15 Remove the towel.
16 Let the person put on the eyeglasses.

POST-PROCEDURE

17 Provide for comfort. (See the inside of the front book cover.)
18 Place the signal light within reach.
19 Lower the bed to its lowest position.
20 Raise or lower bed rails. Follow the care plan.
21 Clean and return hair care items to their proper place.

22 Unscreen the person.
23 Complete a safety check of the room. (See the inside of the front book cover.)
24 Follow agency policy for dirty linen.
25 Decontaminate your hands.

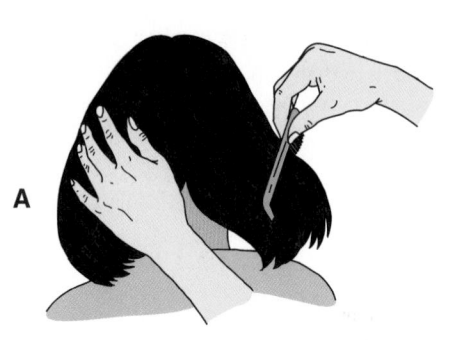
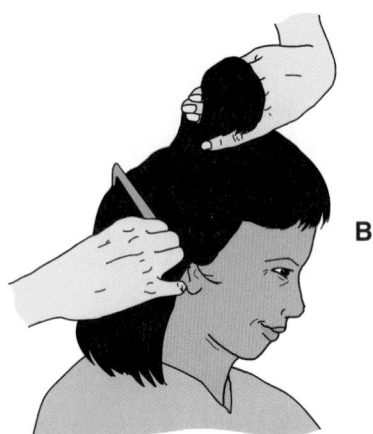

FIGURE 20-2 Part hair. **A,** Part hair down the middle. Divide it into two sides. **B,** Then part one side into two smaller sections.

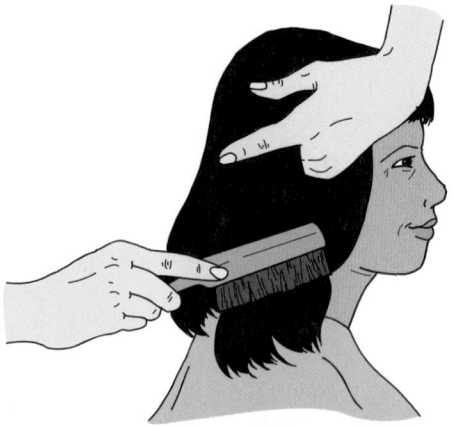

FIGURE 20-3 Brush hair by starting at the scalp. Brush down to the hair ends.

◆ SHAMPOOING

Most people shampoo at least once a week. Some shampoo two or three times a week. Others shampoo every day. Many factors affect frequency. They include the condition of the hair and scalp, hairstyle, and personal choice.

Some persons use certain shampoos and conditioners. Others used medicated products ordered by the doctor.

The person may need help shampooing. Do not shampoo a person's hair unless the nurse tells you to do so. The nurse tells you what method to use. The shampoo method depends on the person's condition, safety factors, and personal choice.

▶ *Shampoo during the shower or tub bath.* The person shampoos in the shower. A hand-held nozzle is used for those using shower chairs or taking tub baths. A spray of water is directed to the hair.

▶ *Shampoo at the sink.* The person sits facing away from the sink. A folded towel is placed over the sink edge to protect the neck. The person's head is tilted back over the edge of the sink. A water pitcher or hand-held nozzle is used to wet and rinse the hair.

▶ *Shampoo on a stretcher.* The stretcher is in front of the sink. A towel is under the neck. The head is tilted over the edge of the sink (Fig. 20-4). A water pitcher or hand-held nozzle is used to wet and rinse the hair.

▶ *Shampoo in bed.* The person's head and shoulders are moved to the edge of the bed if possible. A shampoo tray is under the head to protect the linens and mattress from water (Fig. 20-5). The tray also drains into a basin placed on a chair by the bed. Use a water pitcher to wet and rinse the hair. This method is used for persons who need complete bed baths. It also is used for persons who cannot use a chair, wheelchair, or stretcher.

Hair is dried and styled as quickly as possible after the shampoo. Women may want hair curled or rolled up before drying. Check with the nurse before doing so.

See *Focus on Children and Older Persons: Shampooing.*
See *Focus on Long-Term Care and Home Care: Shampooing.*
See *Delegation Guidelines: Shampooing,* p. 340.
See *Promoting Safety and Comfort: Shampooing,* p. 340.

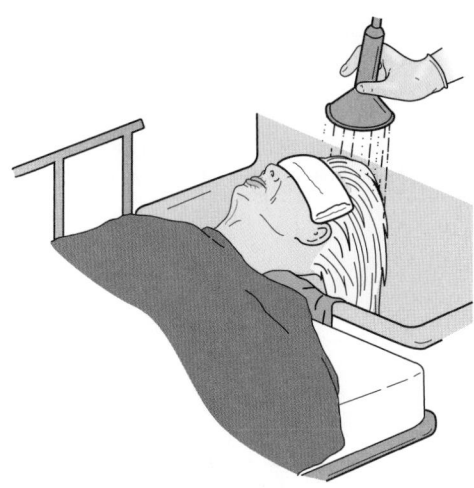

FIGURE 20-4 Shampooing while the person is on a stretcher. The stretcher is in front of the sink.

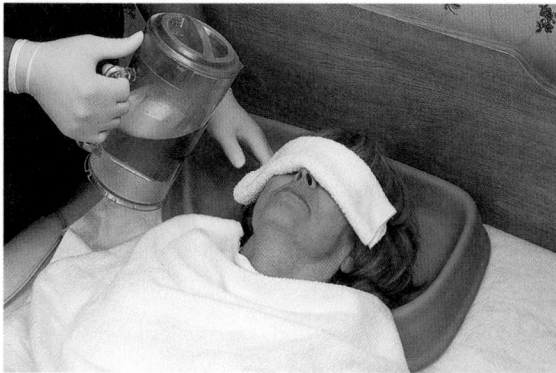

FIGURE 20-5 A shampoo tray is used to shampoo a person in bed. The tray is directed to the side of the bed so water drains into a collecting basin.

FOCUS ON **CHILDREN** AND **OLDER PERSONS**

Shampooing

CHILDREN
Oil gland secretion increases with puberty. Therefore adolescents tend to have oily hair. Frequent shampooing is often needed.

OLDER PERSONS
Oil gland secretion decreases with aging. Therefore older persons have dry hair. They may shampoo less often than younger adults do.

When shampooing during the tub bath or shower, the person tips his or her head back to keep shampoo and water out of the eyes. Support the back of the head with one hand as you shampoo with the other. Some older people cannot tip their heads back. They lean forward and hold a washcloth over the eyes. Support the forehead with one hand as you shampoo with the other. Make sure the person can breathe easily.

Many older persons have limited range of motion in their necks. They cannot tolerate shampooing at the sink or on a stretcher.

FOCUS ON **LONG-TERM CARE** AND **HOME CARE**

Shampooing

LONG-TERM CARE
Shampooing is usually done weekly on the person's bath or shower day. If a woman's hair is done by a beautician, do not shampoo her hair. She wears a shower cap during the tub bath or shower.

HOME CARE
You can make a shampoo trough from a plastic shower curtain or tablecloth. Or use a sturdy plastic drop cloth for painting. Do not use plastic trash bags. They slip and slide easily and are not sturdy.

Place the plastic under the person's head. Make a raised edge around the plastic to prevent water from spilling over the sides. Direct the ends of the plastic into a basin. Water flows into the basin.

DELEGATION GUIDELINES: Shampooing

Before shampooing a person, you need this information from the nurse and the care plan:
- When to shampoo the person's hair
- What method to use
- What shampoo and conditioner to use
- The person's position restrictions or limits
- What water temperature to use—usually 105° F (40.5° C)
- If hair is curled or rolled up before drying
- What observations to report and record
  - Scalp sores
  - Flaking
  - Itching
  - The presence of nits or lice
  - Patches of hair loss
  - Hair falling out in patches
  - Very dry or very oily hair
  - Matted or tangled hair
  - How the person tolerated the procedure
- When to report observations
- What specific patient or resident concerns to report at once

PROMOTING SAFETY AND COMFORT: Shampooing

SAFETY
Keep shampoo away from and out of the eyes. Have the person hold a washcloth over the eyes. When rinsing, cup your hand at the person's forehead. This keeps soapy water from running down the person's forehead and into the eyes.

Return medicated products to the nurse. Never leave them at the bedside unless instructed to do so.

Wear gloves if the person has scalp sores. Follow Standard Precautions and the Bloodborne Pathogen Standard.

For a shampoo on a stretcher, follow the rules for stretcher use (Chapter 11). To safely transfer the person to and from the stretcher, see procedure: *Moving the Person to a Stretcher* in Chapter 16. Remember to lock the stretcher wheels and use the safety straps and side rails. The far side rail is raised during the procedure.

Some people can shampoo themselves during a tub bath or shower. Place an extra towel, shampoo, and hair conditioner within the person's reach. Assist as needed.

COMFORT
When shampooing during the tub bath or shower, the person tips his or her head back to keep shampoo and water out of the eyes. Support the back of the person's head with one hand. Shampoo with your other hand. Some persons cannot tip their heads back. They lean forward and hold a folded washcloth over the eyes. Support the forehead with one hand as you shampoo with the other. Make sure that the person can breathe easily.

Many people have limited range of motion in their necks. They are not shampooed at the sink or on a stretcher.

SHAMPOOING THE PERSON'S HAIR

✔ Quality of Life *Remember to:*

- Knock before entering the person's room.
- Address the person by name.
- Introduce yourself by name and title.
- Explain the procedure to the person before beginning and during the procedure.

- Protect the person's rights during the procedure.
- Handle the person gently during the procedure.

PRE-PROCEDURE

1 Follow *Delegation Guidelines: Shampooing*. See *Promoting Safety and Comfort: Shampooing*.
2 Practice hand hygiene.
3 Collect the following:
  - Two bath towels
  - Washcloth
  - Shampoo
  - Hair conditioner (if requested)
  - Bath thermometer
  - Pitcher or hand-held nozzle (if needed)
  - Shampoo tray (if needed)
  - Basin (if needed)

  - Waterproof pad (if needed)
  - Gloves (if needed)
  - Comb and brush
  - Hair dryer
4 Arrange items nearby.
5 Identify the person. Check the ID bracelet against the assignment sheet. Also call the person by name.
6 Provide for privacy.
7 Raise the bed for good body mechanics for a shampoo in bed. Bed rails are up if used.
8 Decontaminate your hands.

SHAMPOOING THE PERSON'S HAIR—cont'd

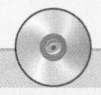

PROCEDURE

9 Lower the bed rail near you if up.
10 Cover the person's chest with a bath towel.
11 Brush and comb the hair to remove snarls and tangles.
12 Position the person for the method you will use. To shampoo the person in bed:
   a Lower the head of the bed and remove the pillow.
   b Place the waterproof pad and shampoo tray under the head and shoulders. Position the basin.
   c Support the head and neck with a folded towel if necessary.
13 Raise the bed rail if used.
14 Obtain water. Water temperature usually is 105° F (40.5° C). Test water temperature according to agency policy. Adjust water as needed.
15 Lower the bed rail near you if up.
16 Put on gloves (if needed).
17 Ask the person to hold a washcloth over the eyes. It should not cover the nose and mouth. (NOTE: A damp washcloth is easier to hold. It will not slip. However, some state competency tests require a dry washcloth.)
18 Use the pitcher or nozzle to wet the hair.

19 Apply a small amount of shampoo.
20 Work up a lather with both hands. Start at the hairline. Work toward the back of the head.
21 Massage the scalp with your fingertips. Do not scratch the scalp.
22 Rinse the hair until the water runs clear.
23 Repeat steps 19 through 22.
24 Apply conditioner. Follow directions on the container.
25 Squeeze water from the person's hair.
26 Cover the hair with a bath towel.
27 Remove the shampoo tray, basin, and waterproof pad.
28 Dry the person's face with the towel. Use the towel on the person's chest.
29 Help the person raise the head if appropriate. For the person in bed, raise the head of the bed.
30 Rub the hair and scalp with the towel. Use the second towel if the first one is wet.
31 Comb the hair to remove snarls and tangles.
32 Dry and style hair as quickly as possible.
33 Remove and discard the gloves (if used). Decontaminate your hands.

POST-PROCEDURE

34 Provide for comfort. (See the inside of the front book cover.)
35 Place the signal light within reach.
36 Lower the bed to its lowest position.
37 Raise or lower bed rails. Follow the care plan.
38 Unscreen the person.
39 Complete a safety check of the room. (See the inside of the front book cover.)

40 Clean and return equipment to its proper place. Remember to clean the brush and comb. Discard disposable items.
41 Follow agency policy for dirty linen.
42 Decontaminate your hands.
43 Report and record your observations.

◆ SHAVING

Many men shave for comfort and mental well-being. Many women shave their legs and underarms. Women with coarse facial hair may shave. Or they may use other hair removal methods. See Box 20-1 for shaving rules.

Safety razors or electric shavers are used. Patients and residents may have their own electric shavers. If the agency's shaver is used, clean it after every use. Follow the manufacturer's instructions for brushing out whiskers. Also follow agency policy for cleaning electric shavers.

Safety razors (blade razors) involve razor blades. They can cause nicks and cuts. Older persons with wrinkled skin are at risk for nicks and cuts. Therefore safety razors are not used on persons who have healing problems or for those who take anticoagulant drugs. An *anticoagulant* prevents or slows down *(anti)* blood clotting *(coagulate)*. Bleeding occurs easily and is hard to stop. A nick or cut can cause serious bleeding. Electric shavers are used.

Soften the beard before using an electric shaver or safety razor. Do so by applying a moist, warm washcloth or towel for a few minutes. Then pat dry the face and apply talcum

BOX 20-1 Rules for Shaving

- Use electric shavers for persons taking anticoagulant drugs. Never use safety razors.
- Protect bed linens. Place a towel under the part being shaved. Or place a towel across the person's chest and shoulders to protect clothing.
- Soften the skin before shaving. Apply a wet washcloth or towel to the face for a few minutes.
- Encourage the person to do as much as safely possible.
- Hold the skin taut as needed.
- Shave in the correct direction:
  - Shaving the face with a safety razor—shave in the direction of hair growth.
  - Shaving the underarms with a safety razor—shave in the direction of hair growth.
  - Shaving the legs with a safety razor—shave up from the ankles. This is against hair growth.
  - Using an electric shaver—shave against the direction of hair growth. If using a rotary-type shaver, move the shaver in small circles over the face.
- Do not cut, nick, or irritate the skin.
- Rinse the body part thoroughly.
- Apply direct pressure to nicks or cuts (Chapter 49).
- Report nicks, cuts, or irritation to the nurse at once.

powder if using an electric shaver. If using a safety razor, lather the face with soap and water or shaving cream.

See *Focus on Children and Older Persons: Shaving.*
See *Delegation Guidelines: Shaving.*
See *Promoting Safety and Comfort: Shaving.*
See *Focus on Ethics and Laws: Shaving.*

FOCUS ON CHILDREN AND OLDER PERSONS

Shaving

OLDER PERSONS
Safety razors are not used to shave persons with dementia. They may not understand what you are doing. They may resist care and move suddenly. Serious nicks and cuts can occur. Use electric shavers for these persons.

DELEGATION GUIDELINES: Shaving

Before shaving a person, you need this information from the nurse and the care plan:
• What shaver to use—electric or safety
• If the person takes anticoagulant drugs
• When to shave the person
• What facial hair to shave
• The location of tender or sensitive areas on the person's face
• What observations to report and record:
  • Nicks (report at once)
  • Cuts (report at once)
  • Bleeding (report at once)
  • Irritation
• When to report observations
• What specific patient or resident concerns to report at once

PROMOTING SAFETY AND COMFORT: Shaving

SAFETY
Safety razors are very sharp. Protect the person and yourself from nicks or cuts. Prevent contact with blood. If using an electric shaver, follow safety measures for electrical equipment (Chapter 11).

Rinse the safety razor often during the shaving procedure. Rinsing removes whiskers and lather. Then wipe the razor. Protect yourself from cuts by:
• Placing several thicknesses of tissues or paper towels on the overbed table. Do not hold them in your hand.
• Wiping the razor on the tissues or paper towels.

Follow Standard Precautions and the Bloodborne Pathogen Standard. Discard used razor blades and disposable shavers in the sharps container. Do not recap the razor.

COMFORT
Some men have tender and sensitive skin. Usually the neck area below the jaw is tender and sensitive. Some electric shavers become very warm or hot while in use. Such heat can irritate the skin. Shave tender areas first while the shaver is cool. Then move to the other areas of the face.

Some people apply lotion or after-shave to the skin after shaving. Lotion softens the skin. After-shave closes skin pores. Heat is applied before shaving to soften the skin. It also opens pores.

FOCUS ON ETHICS AND LAWS

Shaving

A nurse told a patient that she was going to cut his hair and trim his beard. The patient repeatedly stated that he did not want a haircut or his beard trimmed. The patient protested and resisted the nurse's actions. She continued her actions while two other staff members restrained the patient.

The patient reported the incident to his social worker. An internal investigation was conducted.

The nurse lost her job. The United States Court of Appeals agreed that the nurse's termination was warranted because of:
• The nature and seriousness of the offense
• The restraint of the patient after he repeatedly objected

(*L. Taylor v Department of Veterans Affairs,* 2006.)

Caring for Mustaches and Beards

Mustaches and beards need daily care. Food can collect in the whiskers. So can mouth and nose drainage. Daily washing and combing are needed. Ask the person how to groom his mustache or beard. *Never trim a mustache or beard without the person's consent.*

Shaving Legs and Underarms

Many women shave their legs and underarms. This practice varies among cultures. Some women shave only the lower legs. Others shave to mid-thigh or the entire leg.

Legs and underarms are shaved after bathing. The skin is soft at this time. Soap and water, shaving cream, or lotion is used for lather. Collect shaving items with bath items. Use the kidney basin to rinse the razor. Do not use the bath water. Follow the rules in Box 20-1.

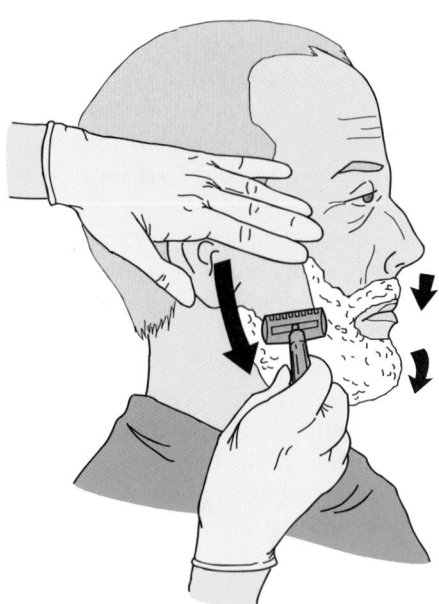

FIGURE 20-6 Shave in the direction of hair growth. Use longer strokes on the larger areas of the face. Use short strokes around the chin and lips.

SHAVING THE PERSON'S FACE WITH A SAFETY RAZOR

✔ Quality of Life *Remember to:*

- Knock before entering the person's room.
- Address the person by name.
- Introduce yourself by name and title.
- Explain the procedure to the person before beginning and during the procedure.

- Protect the person's rights during the procedure.
- Handle the person gently during the procedure.

PRE-PROCEDURE

1 Follow *Delegation Guidelines: Shaving.* See *Promoting Safety and Comfort: Shaving.*
2 Practice hand hygiene.
3 Collect the following:
   - Wash basin
   - Bath towel
   - Hand towel
   - Washcloth
   - Safety razor
   - Mirror
   - Shaving cream, soap, or lotion
   - Shaving brush
   - After-shave or lotion
   - Tissues or paper towels
   - Paper towels
   - Gloves
4 Arrange paper towels and supplies on the overbed table.
5 Identify the person. Check the ID bracelet against the assignment sheet. Also call the person by name.
6 Provide for privacy.
7 Raise the bed for good body mechanics. Bed rails are up if used.

PROCEDURE

8 Fill the wash basin with warm water.
9 Place the basin on the overbed table.
10 Lower the bed rail near you if up.
11 Decontaminate your hands. Put on gloves.
12 Assist the person to semi-Fowler's position if allowed or to the supine position.
13 Adjust lighting to clearly see the person's face.
14 Place the bath towel over the person's chest and shoulders.
15 Adjust the overbed table for easy reach.
16 Tighten the razor blade to the shaver.
17 Wash the person's face. Do not dry.
18 Wet the washcloth or towel. Wring it out.
19 Apply the washcloth or towel to the face for a few minutes.
20 Apply shaving cream with your hands. Or use a shaving brush to apply lather.
21 Hold the skin taut with one hand.
22 Shave in the direction of hair growth. Use shorter strokes around the chin and lips (Fig. 20-6).
23 Rinse the razor often. Wipe it with tissues or paper towels.
24 Apply direct pressure to any bleeding areas (Chapter 49).
25 Wash off any remaining shaving cream or soap. Pat dry with a towel.
26 Apply after-shave or lotion if requested. (If there are nicks or cuts, do not apply after-shave lotion.)
27 Remove the towel and gloves. Decontaminate your hands.

POST-PROCEDURE

28 Provide for comfort. (See the inside of the front book cover.)
29 Place the signal light within reach.
30 Lower the bed to its lowest position.
31 Raise or lower bed rails. Follow the care plan.
32 Clean and return equipment and supplies to their proper place. Discard a razor blade or a disposable razor into the sharps container. Discard other disposable items. Wear gloves.
33 Wipe off the overbed table with paper towels. Discard the paper towels.
34 Remove the gloves. Decontaminate your hands.
35 Unscreen the person.
36 Complete a safety check of the room. (See the inside of the front book cover.)
37 Follow agency policy for dirty linen.
38 Decontaminate your hands.
39 Report nicks, cuts, irritation, or bleeding to the nurse at once. Also report and record other observations.

◆ NAIL AND FOOT CARE

Nail and foot care prevents infection, injury, and odors. Hangnails, ingrown nails (nails that grow in at the side), and nails torn away from the skin cause skin breaks. These breaks are portals of entry for microbes. Long or broken nails can scratch skin or snag clothing.

The feet are easily infected and injured. Dirty feet, socks, or stockings harbor microbes and cause odors. Shoes and socks provide a warm, moist environment for the growth of microbes. Injuries occur from stubbing toes, stepping on sharp objects, or being stepped on. Shoes that fit poorly cause blisters.

Poor circulation prolongs healing. Diabetes and vascular diseases are common causes of poor circulation. Infections or foot injuries are very serious for older persons and persons with circulatory disorders. Gangrene and amputation are serious complications (Chapter 39). Trimming and clipping toenails can easily result in injuries.

Nails are easier to trim and clean right after soaking or bathing. Use nail clippers to cut fingernails. *Never use scissors.* Use extreme caution to prevent damage to nearby tissues.

Some agencies do not let nursing assistants cut or trim toenails. Follow agency policy.

See *Focus on Long-Term Care and Home Care: Nail and Foot Care.*

See *Delegation Guidelines: Nail and Foot Care.*

See *Promoting Safety and Comfort: Nail and Foot Care.*

See *Teamwork and Time Management: Nail and Foot Care.*

FOCUS ON **LONG-TERM CARE** AND **HOME CARE**

Nail and Foot Care

HOME CARE

The feet soak during a tub bath. Or the person can sit on the side of the tub and soak the feet. Make sure the person can step into and out of the tub. Otherwise, soak the feet in a basin or a whirlpool foot bath.

If comfortable for the person, he or she can soak the fingers in the sink. Or use a bowl if a small basin is not available.

DELEGATION GUIDELINES: Nail and Foot Care

Before giving nail and foot care, you need this information from the nurse and the care plan:
- What water temperature to use
- How long to soak fingernails (usually 5 to 10 minutes)
- How long to soak feet (usually 15 to 20 minutes)
- What observations to report and record:
  - Reddened, irritated, or callused areas
  - Breaks in the skin
  - Corns on top of and between the toes
  - Very thick nails
  - Loose nails
- When to report observations
- What specific patient or resident concerns to report at once

---

PROMOTING SAFETY AND COMFORT: Nail and Foot Care

SAFETY

You do not cut or trim toenails if a person:
- Has diabetes
- Has poor circulation to the legs and feet
- Takes drugs that affect blood clotting
- Has very thick nails or ingrown toenails

The RN or podiatrist (foot *[pod]* doctor) cuts toenails and provides foot care for these persons.

Check between the toes for cracks and sores. These areas are often overlooked. If left untreated, a serious infection could occur.

The feet are easily burned. Persons with decreased sensation or circulatory problems may not feel hot temperatures.

After soaking, apply lotion or petroleum jelly to the feet. This can cause slippery feet. Help the person put on non-skid footwear before you transfer the person or let the person walk.

Breaks in the skin and bleeding can occur. Follow Standard Precautions and the Bloodborne Pathogen Standard.

COMFORT

Sometimes just the fingernails are trimmed. Sometimes just foot care is given. Sometimes both are done. When both are done, the person sits at the overbed table. Make sure the person is warm and comfortable.

Promote your own comfort when giving nail and foot care. Sit in front of the overbed table when cleaning and trimming fingernails. When giving foot care, rest the person's lower leg and foot on your lap. Or you can kneel on the floor. Lay a towel across your lap or on the floor to protect your uniform. Remember to use good body mechanics. However you position yourself, you must support the person's foot and ankle when giving foot care.

TEAMWORK AND TIME MANAGEMENT

Nail and Foot Care

Use your time well when giving nail and foot care. The fingernails soak for 5 to 10 minutes. The feet soak for 15 to 20 minutes. You can make the person's bed or straighten the person's unit while the fingernails and feet soak. Or you could assist with brushing and combing hair. Check your assignment sheet for other ways to meet the person's needs.

GIVING NAIL AND FOOT CARE

✓ **Quality of Life** *Remember to:*

- Knock before entering the person's room.
- Address the person by name.
- Introduce yourself by name and title.
- Explain the procedure to the person before beginning and during the procedure.

- Protect the person's rights during the procedure.
- Handle the person gently during the procedure.

PRE-PROCEDURE

1 Follow *Delegation Guidelines: Nail and Foot Care.* See *Promoting Safety and Comfort: Nail and Foot Care.*
2 Practice hand hygiene.
3 Collect the following:
   - Wash basin or whirlpool foot bath
   - Soap
   - Bath thermometer
   - Bath towel
   - Hand towel
   - Washcloth
   - Kidney basin
   - Nail clippers
   - Orange stick

   - Emery board or nail file
   - Lotion for the hands
   - Lotion or petroleum jelly for the feet
   - Paper towels
   - Bath mat
   - Gloves

4 Arrange paper towels and other items on the overbed table.
5 Identify the person. Check the ID bracelet against the assignment sheet. Also call the person by name.
6 Provide for privacy.
7 Assist the person to the bedside chair. Place the signal light within reach.

PROCEDURE

8 Place the bath mat under the feet.
9 Fill the wash basin or whirlpool foot bath ⅔ (two-thirds) full with water. The nurse tells you what water temperature to use. (Measure water temperature with a bath thermometer. Or test it by dipping your elbow or inner wrist into the basin. Follow agency policy.)
10 Place the basin or foot bath on the bath mat.
11 Help the person put the feet into the basin or foot bath. Make sure both feet are completely covered by water.
12 Adjust the overbed table in front of the person.
13 Fill the kidney basin ⅔ (two-thirds) full with water. See step 9 for water temperature.
14 Place the kidney basin on the overbed table.
15 Place the person's fingers into the basin. Position the arms for comfort (Fig. 20-7, p. 346).
16 Let the fingers soak for 5 to 10 minutes. Let the feet soak for 15 to 20 minutes. Rewarm water as needed.
17 Decontaminate your hands. Put on gloves.
18 Remove the kidney basin.
19 Clean under the fingernails with the orange stick. Use a towel to wipe the orange stick after each nail.

20 Dry the hands and between the fingers thoroughly.
21 Clip fingernails straight across with the nail clippers (Fig. 20-8, p. 346).
22 Shape nails with an emery board or nail file. Nails are smooth with no rough edges.
23 Push cuticles back with the orange stick or a washcloth (Fig. 20-9, p. 346).
24 Apply lotion to the hands. Warm lotion before applying it.
25 Move the overbed table to the side.
26 Wash the feet and between the toes with soap and a washcloth. Rinse the feet and between the toes.
27 Remove the feet from the basin or foot bath. Dry thoroughly, especially between the toes.
28 Apply lotion or petroleum jelly to the tops and soles of the feet. Do not apply between the toes. Warm lotion or petroleum jelly before applying it. Remove excess lotion or petroleum jelly with a towel.
29 Remove and discard the gloves. Decontaminate your hands.
30 Help the person put on non-skid footwear.

POST-PROCEDURE

31 Provide for comfort. (See the inside of the front book cover.)
32 Place the signal light within reach.
33 Raise or lower bed rails. Follow the care plan.
34 Clean and return equipment and supplies to their proper place. Discard disposable items. Wear gloves for this step.

35 Remove the gloves. Decontaminate your hands.
36 Unscreen the person.
37 Complete a safety check of the room. (See the inside of the front book cover.)
38 Follow agency policy for dirty linen.
39 Decontaminate your hands.
40 Report and record your observations.

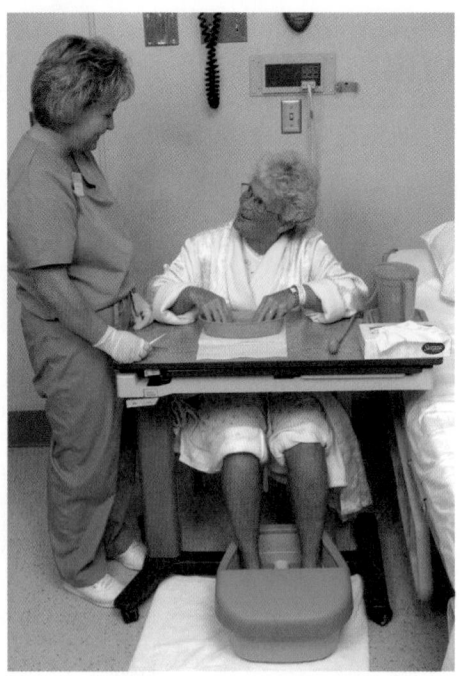

FIGURE 20-7 Nail and foot care. The feet soak in a whirlpool foot bath. The fingers soak in a kidney basin.

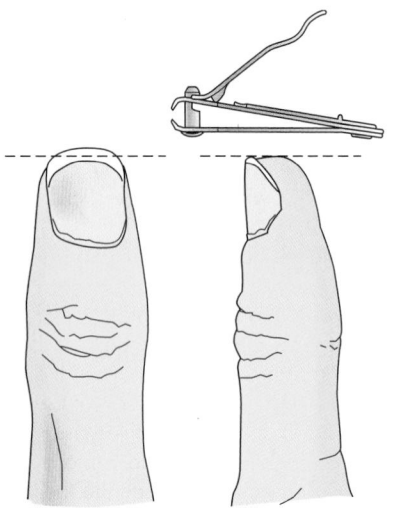

FIGURE 20-8 Clip fingernails straight across. Use a nail clipper.

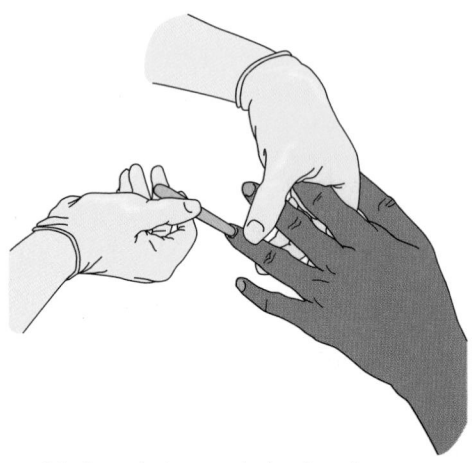

FIGURE 20-9 Push the cuticle back with an orange stick.

CHANGING CLOTHING AND HOSPITAL GOWNS

Gowns or pajamas are changed after the bath and when wet or soiled. Some people wear street clothes. They change from sleepwear into clothing after morning care. They undress and put on sleepwear at bedtime. Garments are changed whenever wet or soiled.

You may need to assist with changing clothes and hospital gowns. Follow these rules:

▶ Provide for privacy. Do not expose the person.
▶ Encourage the person to do as much as possible.
▶ Let the person choose what to wear. Make sure the right undergarments are chosen.
▶ Remove clothing from the strong or "good" side first. This is often call the *unaffected side*.
▶ Put clothing on the weak side first. This is often called the *affected side*.
▶ Support the arm or leg when removing or putting on a garment.

◆ Dressing and Undressing

Clothing changes are usually necessary on admission and discharge. Some people enter and leave the agency in a gown or pajamas. Most wear street clothes.

See *Focus on Children and Older Persons: Dressing and Undressing.*

See *Focus on Long-Term Care and Home Care: Dressing and Undressing.*

See *Focus on Communication: Dressing and Undressing.*

See *Delegation Guidelines: Dressing and Undressing.*

Text continued on p. 351

Dressing and Undressing

OLDER PERSONS

Persons with dementia may not want to change clothes. Or they may not know how. For example, a person may try to put slacks on over his or her head. The Alzheimer's Disease Education and Referral Center (ADEAR) suggests the following:

- Try to assist with dressing at the same time each day. The person will learn to expect dressing as a part of his or her daily routine.
- Let the person dress himself or herself to the extent possible. Allow extra time for this task. Do not rush the person.
- Let the person choose what to wear from 2 or 3 outfits. If the person has a favorite outfit, the family may buy several of the same outfits. This makes dressing easier if the person insists on wearing the same outfit.
- Choose clothes that are comfortable to wear and easy to get on and off. Garments with elastic waistbands and Velcro closures are examples. The person does not have to handle zippers, buttons, hooks, snaps, or other closures.
- Stack clothes in the order that they will be put on. The person sees one item at a time. For example, underpants or undershorts are put on first. The item is on top of the stack.
- Give clear, simple, step-by-step directions.

Dressing and Undressing

LONG-TERM CARE

Most residents wear street clothes during the day. Some dress and undress themselves. Others need help. Personal choice is a resident right. Let the person choose what to wear.

HOME CARE

Patients often wear street clothes during the day. Or sleepwear and robes are worn. The procedures that follow apply to sleepwear, robes, and street clothes.

Dressing and Undressing

Make sure you allow for personal choice and independence when assisting with dressing and undressing. You can ask:
- "What would you like to wear today?"
- "There's a concert today in the lounge. Do you want to wear something special?"
- "Can I help you with those buttons?"
- "Would you like me to help you with that zipper?"

Before assisting with dressing and undressing, you need this information from the nurse and the care plan:
- How much help the person needs
- Which side is the person's strong side
- If the person needs to wear certain garments
- What observations to report and record:
  - How much help was given
  - How the person tolerated the procedure
  - Any complaints by the person
  - Any changes in the person's behavior
- When to report observations
- What specific patient or resident concerns to report at once

UNDRESSING THE PERSON

✔ **Quality of Life** *Remember to:*

- Knock before entering the person's room.
- Address the person by name.
- Introduce yourself by name and title.
- Explain the procedure to the person before beginning and during the procedure.
- Protect the person's rights during the procedure.
- Handle the person gently during the procedure.

PRE-PROCEDURE

1 Follow *Delegation Guidelines: Dressing and Undressing.*
2 Practice hand hygiene.
3 Collect a bath blanket and clothing requested by the person.
4 Identify the person. Check the ID bracelet against the assignment sheet. Also call the person by name.
5 Provide for privacy.
6 Raise the bed for good body mechanics. Bed rails are up if used.
7 Lower the bed rail on the person's weak side.
8 Position him or her supine.
9 Cover the person with a bath blanket. Fan-fold linens to the foot of the bed.

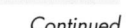

Continued

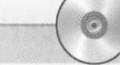

PROCEDURE

10 Remove garments that open in the back.

   a Raise the head and shoulders. Or turn him or her onto the side away from you.

   b Undo buttons, zippers, ties, or snaps.

   c Bring the sides of the garment to the sides of the person (Fig. 20-10). If he or she is in a side-lying position, tuck the far side under the person. Fold the near side onto the chest (Fig. 20-11).

   d Position the person supine.

   e Slide the garment off the shoulder on the strong side. Remove it from the arm (Fig. 20-12).

   f Repeat step 10e for the weak side.

11 Remove garments that open in the front:

   a Undo buttons, zippers, ties, or snaps.

   b Slide the garment off the shoulder and arm on the strong side.

   c Assist the person to sit up or raise the head and shoulders. Bring the garment over to the weak side (Fig. 20-13).

   d Lower the head and shoulders. Remove the garment from the weak side.

   e If you cannot raise the head and shoulders:

     (1) Turn the person toward you. Tuck the removed part under the person.

     (2) Turn him or her onto the side away from you.

     (3) Pull the side of the garment out from under the person. Make sure he or she will not lie on it when supine.

     (4) Return the person to the supine position.

     (5) Remove the garment from the weak side.

12 Remove pullover garments:

   a Undo any buttons, zippers, ties, or snaps.

   b Remove the garment from the strong side.

   c Raise the head and shoulders. Or turn the person onto the side away from you. Bring the garment up to the person's neck (Fig. 20-14).

   d Remove the garment from the weak side.

   e Bring the garment over the person's head.

   f Position him or her in the supine position.

13 Remove pants or slacks:

   a Remove footwear and socks.

   b Position the person supine.

   c Undo buttons, zippers, ties, snaps, or buckles.

   d Remove the belt.

   e Ask the person to lift the buttocks off the bed. Slide the pants down over the hips and buttocks (Fig. 20-15). Have the person lower the hips and buttocks.

   f If the person cannot raise the hips off the bed:

     (1) Turn the person toward you.

     (2) Slide the pants off the hip and buttock on the strong side (Fig. 20-16).

     (3) Turn the person away from you.

     (4) Slide the pants off the hip and buttock on the weak side (Fig. 20-17).

   g Slide the pants down the legs and over the feet.

14 Dress the person. See procedure: *Dressing the Person*, p. 350.

POST-PROCEDURE

15 Provide for comfort. (See the inside of the front book cover.)

16 Place the signal light within reach.

17 Lower the bed to its lowest position.

18 Raise or lower bed rails. Follow the care plan.

19 Unscreen the person.

20 Complete a safety check of the room. (See the inside of the front book cover.)

21 Follow agency policy for soiled clothing.

22 Decontaminate your hands.

23 Report and record your observations.

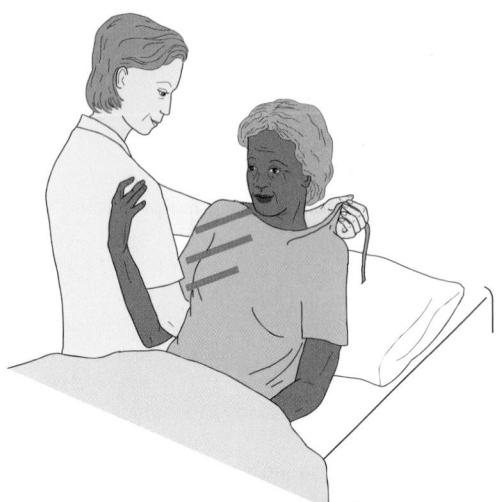

FIGURE 20-10 The sides of the garment are brought from the back to the sides of the person. (Note that the "weak" side is *indicated by slash marks*.)

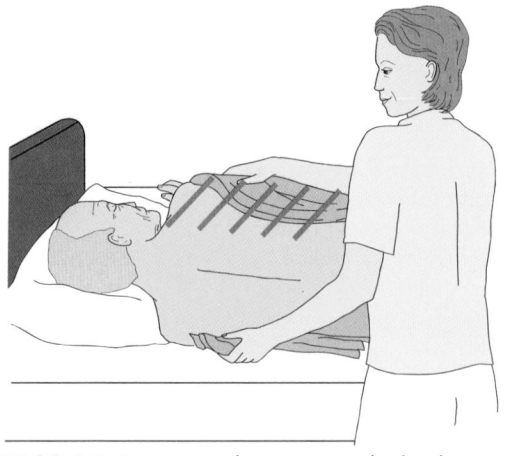

FIGURE 20-11 A garment that opens in the back is removed from the person in the side-lying position. The far side of the garment is tucked under the person. The near side is folded onto the person's chest. (Note that the "weak" side is *indicated by slash marks*.)

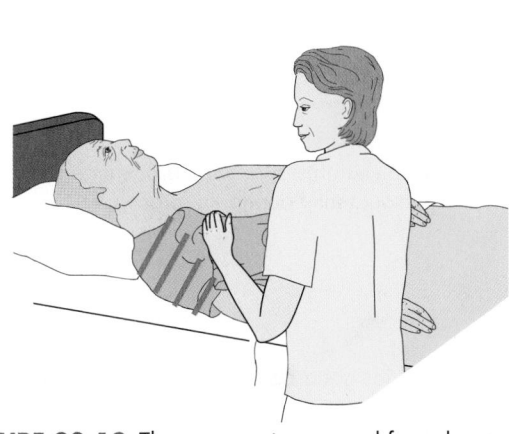

FIGURE 20-12 The garment is removed from the strong side first. (Note that the "weak" side is *indicated by slash marks*.)

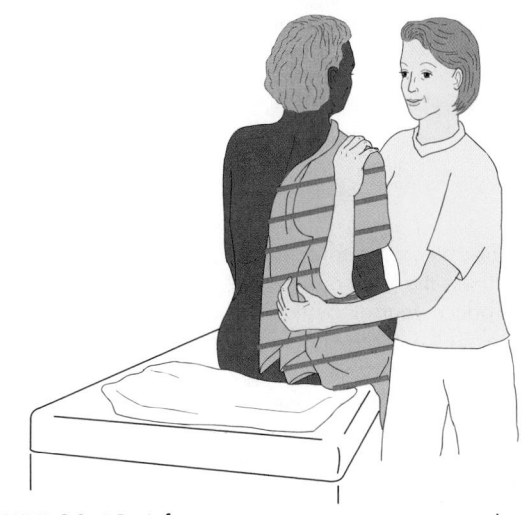

FIGURE 20-13 A front-opening garment is removed with the person's head and shoulders raised. The garment is removed from the strong side first. Then it is brought around the back to the weak side. (Note that the "weak" side is *indicated by slash marks*.)

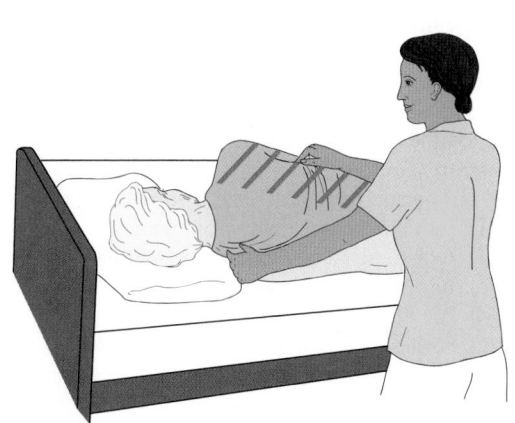

FIGURE 20-14 A pullover garment is removed from the strong side first. Then the garment is brought up to the person's neck so that it can be removed from the weak side. (Note that the "weak" side is *indicated by slash marks*.)

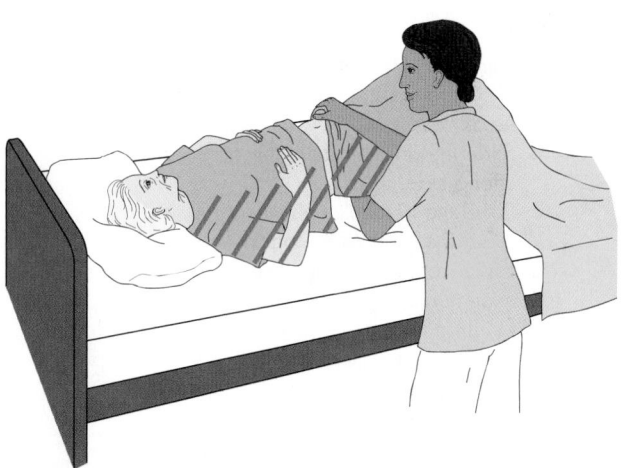

FIGURE 20-15 The person lifts the hips and buttocks for removing the pants. The pants are slid down over the hips and buttocks. (Note that the "weak" side is *indicated by slash marks*.)

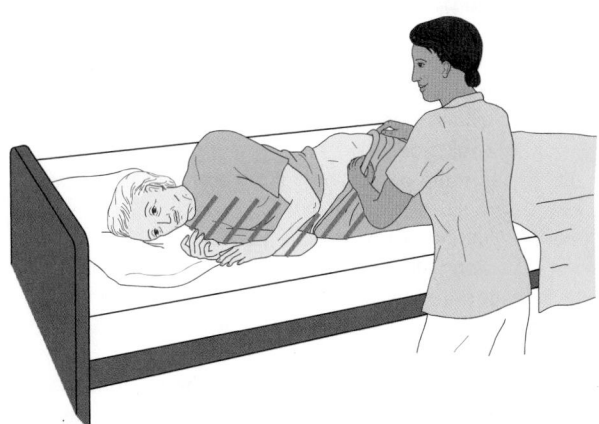

FIGURE 20-16 Pants are removed in the side-lying position. They are removed from the strong side first. They are slid over the hip and buttock. (Note that the "weak" side is *indicated by slash marks*.)

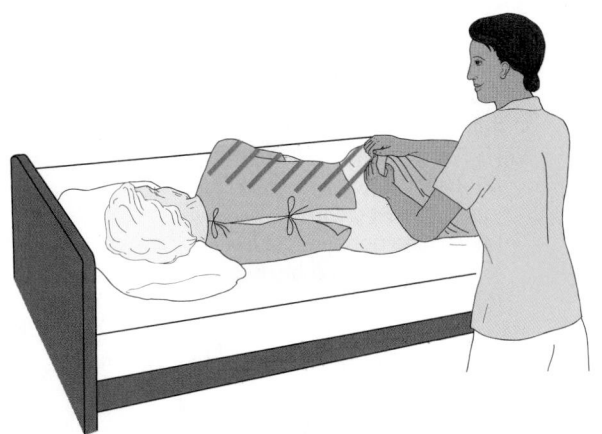

FIGURE 20-17 The person is turned onto the strong side. The pants are removed from the weak side. (Note that the "weak" side is *indicated by slash marks*.)

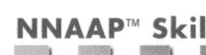

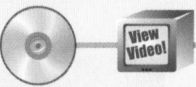

DRESSING THE PERSON

✔ Quality of Life *Remember to:*

- Knock before entering the person's room.
- Address the person by name.
- Introduce yourself by name and title.
- Explain the procedure to the person before beginning and during the procedure.

- Protect the person's rights during the procedure.
- Handle the person gently during the procedure.

PRE-PROCEDURE

1 Follow *Delegation Guidelines: Dressing and Undressing,* p. 347.
2 Practice hand hygiene.
3 Ask the person what he or she would like to wear.
4 Get a bath blanket and clothing requested by the person.
5 Identify the person. Check the ID bracelet against the assignment sheet. Also call the person by name.
6 Provide for privacy.

7 Raise the bed for good body mechanics. Bed rails are up if used.
8 Lower the bed rail (if up) on the person's strong side.
9 Position the person supine.
10 Cover the person with a bath blanket. Fan-fold linens to the foot of the bed.
11 Undress the person. (See procedure: *Undressing the Person.*)

PROCEDURE

12 Put on garments that open in the back:
  a Slide the garment onto the arm and shoulder of the weak side.
  b Slide the garment onto the arm and shoulder of the strong side.
  c Raise the person's head and shoulders.
  d Bring the sides to the back.
  e If you cannot raise the person's head and shoulders:
    (1) Turn the person toward you.
    (2) Bring one side of the garment to the person's back (Fig. 20-18, *A*).
    (3) Turn the person away from you.
    (4) Bring the other side to the person's back (Fig. 20-18, *B*).
  f Fasten buttons, zippers, snaps, or other closures.
  g Position the person supine.
13 Put on garments that open in the front:
  a Slide the garment onto the arm and shoulder on the weak side.
  b Raise the head and shoulders. Bring the side of the garment around to the back. Lower the person down. Slide the garment onto the arm and shoulder of the strong arm.
  c If the person cannot raise the head and shoulders:
    (1) Turn the person away from you.
    (2) Tuck the garment under him or her.
    (3) Turn the person toward you.
    (4) Pull the garment out from under him or her.
    (5) Turn the person back to the supine position.
    (6) Slide the garment over the arm and shoulder of the strong arm.
  d Fasten buttons, zippers, ties, snaps, or other closures.
14 Put on pullover garments:
  a Position the person supine.
  b Bring the neck of the garment over the head.

  c Slide the arm and shoulder of the garment onto the weak side.
  d Raise the person's head and shoulders.
  e Bring the garment down.
  f Slide the arm and shoulder of the garment onto the strong side.
  g If the person cannot assume a semi-sitting position:
    (1) Turn the person away from you.
    (2) Tuck the garment under the person.
    (3) Turn the person toward you.
    (4) Pull the garment out from under him or her.
    (5) Position the person supine.
    (6) Slide the arm and shoulder of the garment onto the strong side.
  h Fasten buttons, zippers, ties, snaps, or other closures.
15 Put on pants or slacks:
  a Slide the pants over the feet and up the legs.
  b Ask the person to raise the hips and buttocks off the bed.
  c Bring the pants up over the buttocks and hips.
  d Ask the person to lower the hips and buttocks.
  e If the person cannot raise the hips and buttocks:
    (1) Turn the person onto the strong side (away from you).
    (2) Pull the pants over the buttock and hip on the weak side.
    (3) Turn the person onto the weak side (toward you).
    (4) Pull the pants over the buttock and hip on the strong side.
    (5) Position the person supine.
  f Fasten buttons, zippers, ties, snaps, a belt buckle, or other closures.
16 Put socks and non-skid footwear on the person. Make sure socks are up all the way and smooth.
17 Help the person get out of bed. If the person will stay in bed, cover the person. Remove the bath blanket.

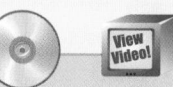

DRESSING THE PERSON—cont'd
POST-PROCEDURE

18 Provide for comfort. (See the inside of the front book cover.)

19 Place the signal light within reach.

20 Lower the bed to its lowest position.

21 Raise or lower bed rails. Follow the care plan.

22 Unscreen the person.

23 Complete a safety check of the room. (See the inside of the front book cover.)

24 Follow agency policy for soiled clothing.

25 Decontaminate your hands.

26 Report and record your observations.

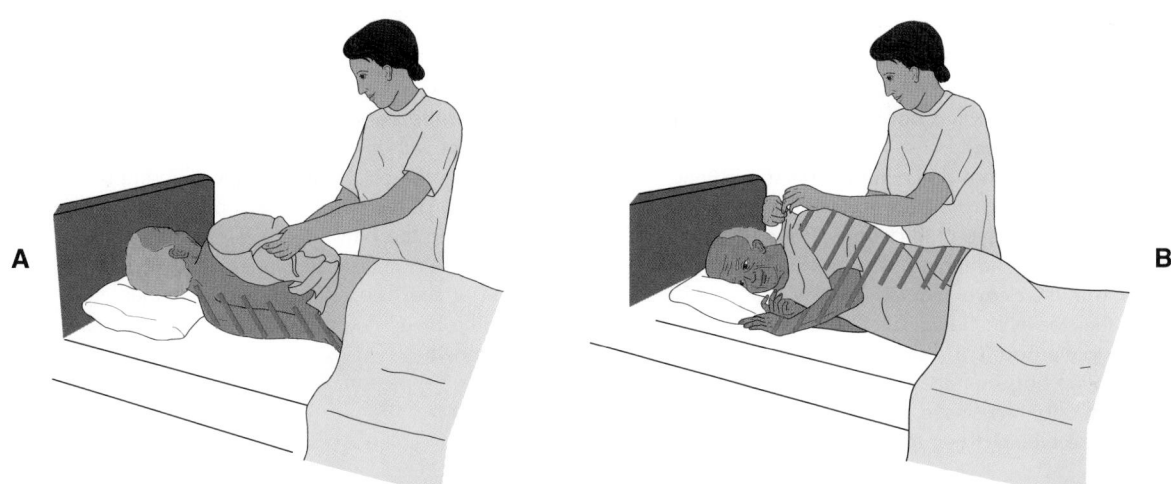

FIGURE 20-18 Dressing a person. **A,** The side-lying position can be used to put on garments that open in the back. Turn the person toward you after the garment is put on the arms. The side of the garment is brought to the person's back. **B,** Then turn the person away from you. The other side of the garment is brought to the back and fastened. (Note that the "weak" side is *indicated by slash marks.*)

◆ Changing Hospital Gowns

Many hospital patients wear gowns. So do some nursing center residents. Gowns are usually worn for IV (intravenous) therapy (Chapter 24). Some agencies have special gowns for IV therapy. They open along the sleeve and close with ties, snaps, or Velcro. Sometimes standard gowns are used.

If there is injury or paralysis, the gown is removed from the strong arm first. Support the weak arm while removing the gown. Put the clean gown on the weak arm first and then on the strong arm.

See *Delegation Guidelines: Changing Hospital Gowns.*

See *Promoting Safety and Comfort: Changing Hospital Gowns.*

DELEGATION GUIDELINES: Changing Hospital Gowns

Before changing a gown, you need this information from the nurse and the care plan:
- Which arm has the IV
- If the person has an IV pump (see *Promoting Safety and Comfort: Changing Hospital Gowns*)

PROMOTING SAFETY AND COMFORT: Changing Hospital Gowns

SAFETY

IV pumps control how fast fluid enters a vein. This is called the *flow rate*. If the person has an IV pump and a standard gown, do not use the following procedure. The arm with the IV is not put through the sleeve.

If the person has an IV, changing the gown can cause the flow rate to change (Chapter 24). Always ask the nurse to check the flow rate after you change a gown.

Do not disconnect or remove any part of the IV set-up. See Chapter 24.

COMFORT

Some hospital gowns are secured with ties at the upper back. The back and buttocks are exposed when the person stands. Other gowns overlap in the back and tie at the side. These gowns provide more privacy. Because they tie at the side, uncomfortable bows and knots at the back are avoided.

CHANGING THE GOWN OF THE PERSON WITH AN IV

✔ **Quality of Life** *Remember to:*

- Knock before entering the person's room.
- Address the person by name.
- Introduce yourself by name and title.
- Explain the procedure to the person before beginning and during the procedure.

- Protect the person's rights during the procedure.
- Handle the person gently during the procedure.

PRE-PROCEDURE

1 Follow *Delegation Guidelines: Changing Hospital Gowns*, p. 351. See *Promoting Safety and Comfort: Changing Hospital Gowns*, p. 351.
2 Practice hand hygiene.
3 Get a clean gown and a bath blanket.

4 Identify the person. Check the ID bracelet against the assignment sheet. Also call the person by name.
5 Provide for privacy.
6 Raise the bed for good body mechanics. Bed rails are up if used.

PROCEDURE

7 Lower the bed rail near you (if up).
8 Cover the person with a bath blanket. Fan-fold linens to the foot of the bed.
9 Untie the gown. Free parts that the person is lying on.
10 Remove the gown from the arm with *no IV.*
11 Gather up the sleeve of the arm *with the IV.* Slide it over the IV site and tubing. Remove the arm and hand from the sleeve (Fig. 20-19, *A*).
12 Keep the sleeve gathered. Slide your arm along the tubing to the bag (Fig. 20-19, *B*).
13 Remove the bag from the pole. Slide the bag and tubing through the sleeve (Fig. 20-19, *C*). Do not pull on the tubing. Keep the bag above the person.

14 Hang the IV bag on the pole.
15 Gather the sleeve of the clean gown that will go on the arm with the IV infusion.
16 Remove the bag from the pole. Slip the sleeve over the bag at the shoulder part of the gown (Fig. 20-19, *D*). Hang the bag.
17 Slide the gathered sleeve over the tubing, hand, arm, and IV site. Then slide it onto the shoulder.
18 Put the other side of the gown on the person. Fasten the gown.
19 Cover the person. Remove the bath blanket.

POST-PROCEDURE

20 Provide for comfort. (See the inside of the front book cover.)
21 Place the signal light within reach.
22 Lower the bed to its lowest position.
23 Raise or lower bed rails. Follow the care plan.
24 Unscreen the person.

25 Complete a safety check of the room. (See the inside of the front book cover.)
26 Follow agency policy for dirty linen.
27 Decontaminate your hands.
28 Ask the nurse to check the flow rate.
29 Report and record your observations.

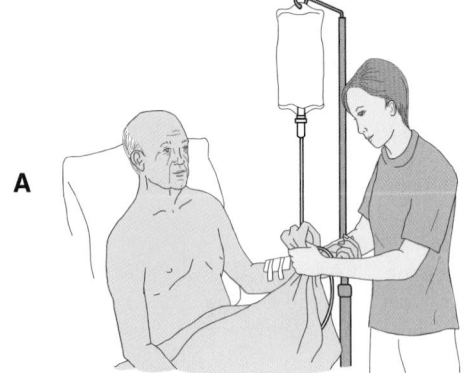
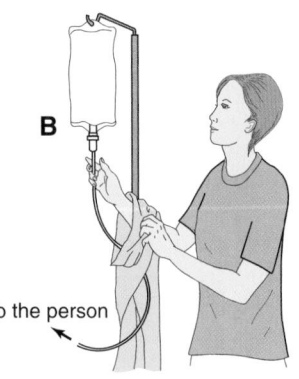
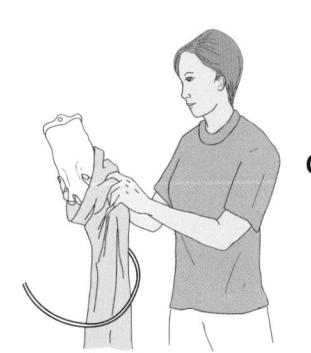
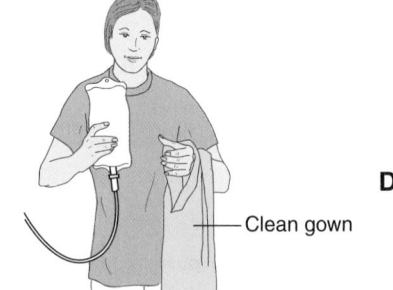

To the person

Clean gown

FIGURE 20-19 Changing a gown. **A,** The gown is removed from the arm with no IV. The sleeve on the arm with the IV is gathered up, slipped over the IV site and tubing, and removed from the arm and hand. **B,** The gathered sleeve is slipped along the IV tubing to the bag. **C,** The IV bag is removed from the pole and passed through the sleeve. **D,** The gathered sleeve of the clean gown is slipped over the IV bag at the shoulder part of the gown.

REVIEW QUESTIONS

Circle the BEST answer.

1 A person has alopecia. This is
 a Excessive body hair
 b Dry, white flakes from the scalp
 c An infestation with lice
 d Hair loss

2 Which prevents hair from matting and tangling?
 a Bedrest
 b Daily brushing and combing
 c Daily shampooing
 d Cutting hair

3 A person's hair is not matted or tangled. When brushing hair, start at
 a The forehead and brush backward
 b The hair ends
 c The scalp
 d The back of the neck and brush forward

4 Brushing keeps the hair
 a Soft and shiny
 b Clean
 c Free of lice
 d Long

5 A person requests a shampoo. You should
 a Shampoo the hair during the person's shower
 b Shampoo hair at the sink
 c Shampoo the person in bed
 d Follow the care plan

6 When shaving a person's face, do the following *except*
 a Practice Standard Precautions
 b Follow the Bloodborne Pathogen Standard
 c Shave in the direction of hair growth
 d Shave when the skin is dry

7 A person is nicked during shaving. Your first action is to
 a Wash your hands
 b Apply direct pressure
 c Tell the nurse
 d Apply a bandage

8 Fingernails are cut with
 a An emery board
 b Scissors
 c A nail file
 d Nail clippers

9 Fingernails are trimmed
 a Before soaking
 b After soaking
 c Before trimming toenails
 d After trimming toenails

Circle T if the statement is true and F if the statement is false.

10 T **F** Mr. Polk has a mustache and beard. To promote his comfort, you can shave his beard and mustache.

11 **T** F Clothing is removed from the strong side first.

12 **T** F The person chooses what to wear.

13 T **F** A person has poor circulation in the legs and feet. You can cut and trim the person's toenails.

14 T **F** You can cut matted hair.

Answers to these questions are on p. 780.

353

21 Urinary Elimination

OBJECTIVES

- Define the key terms and key abbreviations listed in this chapter
- Describe normal urine
- Describe the rules for normal urinary elimination
- Identify the observations to report to the nurse
- Describe urinary incontinence and the care required

- Describe straight, indwelling, and condom catheters
- Explain why catheters are used
- Explain how to care for persons with catheters
- Explain how to remove indwelling catheters
- Describe two methods of bladder training
- Perform the procedures described in this chapter

PROCEDURES

 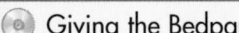 Giving the Bedpan
- Giving the Urinal
- Helping the Person to the Commode

 Giving Catheter Care

- Changing a Leg Bag to a Drainage Bag
- Emptying a Urinary Drainage Bag
- Removing an Indwelling Catheter
- Applying a Condom Catheter

KEY TERMS

catheter A tube used to drain or inject fluid through a body opening

catheterization The process of inserting a catheter

dysuria Painful or difficult *(dys)* urination *(uria)*

Foley catheter An indwelling or retention catheter

functional incontinence The person has bladder control but cannot use the toilet in time

hematuria Blood *(hemat)* in the urine *(uria)*

Continued

 Procedures with this icon are on the CDCompanion in this book; those with this icon ![View Video!] are on the Evolve Student Resources Website.

KEY TERMS—cont'd

indwelling catheter A catheter left in the bladder so urine drains constantly into a drainage bag; retention or Foley catheter

micturition Urination or voiding

mixed incontinence Having more than one type of incontinence

nocturia Frequent urination *(uria)* at night *(noct)*

oliguria Scant amount *(olig)* of urine *(uria);* less than 500 mL in 24 hours

overflow incontinence Small amounts of urine leak from a bladder that is always full

polyuria Abnormally large amounts *(poly)* of urine *(uria)*

reflex incontinence The loss of urine at predictable intervals when the bladder is full

retention catheter A Foley or indwelling catheter

straight catheter A catheter that drains the bladder and then is removed

stress incontinence When urine leaks during exercise and certain movements that cause pressure on the bladder

urge incontinence The loss of urine in response to a sudden, urgent need to void; the person cannot get to a toilet in time

urinary frequency Voiding at frequent intervals

urinary incontinence The loss of bladder control

urinary urgency The need to void at once

urination The process of emptying urine from the bladder; micturition or voiding

voiding Urination or micturition

KEY ABBREVIATIONS

ADEAR Alzheimer's Disease Education and Referral Center
I&O Intake and Output

IV Intravenous
mL Milliliter

Eliminating waste is a physical need. The respiratory, digestive, integumentary, and urinary systems remove body wastes. The digestive system rids the body of solid wastes. The lungs remove carbon dioxide. Sweat contains water and other substances. Blood contains waste products from body cells burning food for energy. The urinary system removes waste products from the blood. It also maintains the body's water balance. See Box 21-1 for a review of the urinary system.

NORMAL URINATION

The healthy adult produces about 1500 mL (milliliters), or 3 pints of urine a day. Many factors affect urine production. They include age, disease, the amount and kinds of fluid ingested, dietary salt, body temperature, perspiration, and drugs. Some substances increase urine production—coffee, tea, alcohol, and some drugs. A diet high in salt causes the body to retain water. When water is retained, less urine is produced.

Urination, micturition, and **voiding** mean the process of emptying urine from the bladder. The amount of fluid intake, habits, and available toilet facilities affect frequency. So do activity, work, and illness. People usually void at bedtime, after sleep, and before meals. Some people void every 2 to 3 hours. The need to void at night disturbs sleep.

Some persons need help getting to the bathroom. Others use bedpans, urinals, or commodes. Follow the rules in Box 21-2 (p. 356) and the person's care plan.

See *Focus on Children and Older Persons: Normal Urination.*

See *Focus on Communication: Normal Urination,* p. 356.

See *Teamwork and Time Management: Normal Urination,* p. 356.

BOX 21-1 The Urinary System: Body Structure and Function

The two kidneys (Fig. 21-1, p. 356) lie in the upper abdomen against the muscles of the back on each side of the spine. Blood passes through the two kidneys. Urine is formed in the kidneys.

Urine consists of wastes and excess fluids filtered out of the blood. Urine flows through the two ureters to the urinary bladder. Urine is stored in the bladder. The urethra connects the bladder to the outside of the body. Urine passes from the body through the urethra. Urination, micturition, and voiding mean the process of emptying the bladder.

See Chapter 8 for more information.

FOCUS ON CHILDREN AND OLDER PERSONS

Normal Urination

CHILDREN

Infants produce 200 to 300 mL of urine a day. The amount increases as the baby grows older. An infant can have 6 to 20 wet diapers a day. Tell the nurse at once if an infant does not have a wet diaper for several hours. This signals dehydration. It is very serious in infants.

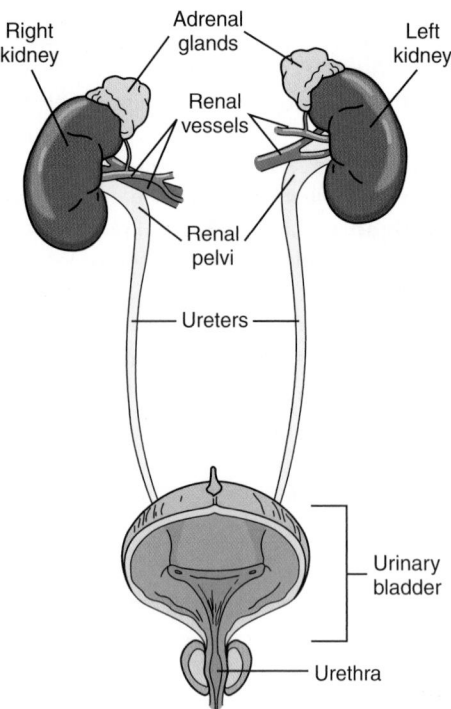

FIGURE 21-1 The urinary system.

Normal Urination

Patients and residents may not use "voiding" or "urinating" terms. The person may not understand what you are saying. Do not ask: "Do you need to void?" or "Do you need to urinate?" Instead, ask these questions:
- "Do you need to use the bathroom?"
- "Do you need to use the bedpan?"
- "Do you need to pass urine?"
- "Do you need to pee?"

TEAMWORK AND TIME MANAGEMENT

Normal Urination

A person's need to void may be urgent. Answer signal lights promptly. Also answer signal lights for co-workers. Otherwise incontinence may result. The person is wet and embarrassed. He or she is at risk for skin breakdown and infection. Your co-worker has extra work—changing linens and garments. You like help when you are busy. So do your co-workers.

Observations

Normal urine is pale yellow, straw-colored, or amber. It is clear with no particles. A faint odor is normal. Observe urine for color, clarity, odor, amount, and particles.

Some foods affect urine color. Red food dyes, beets, blackberries, and rhubarb cause red-colored urine. Carrots and sweet potatoes cause bright yellow urine. Certain drugs change urine color. Asparagus causes a urine odor.

Ask the nurse to observe urine that looks or smells abnormal. Report complaints of urgency, burning on urination, or painful or difficult urination. Also report the problems in Table 21-1. The nurse uses the information for the nursing process.

◆ Bedpans

Bedpans are used by persons who cannot be out of bed. Women use bedpans for voiding and bowel movements. Men use them for bowel movements.

The *standard bedpan* is shown in Figure 21-2. A *fracture pan* has a thin rim. It is only about ½-inch deep at one end (see Fig. 21-2). The smaller end is placed under the buttocks (Fig. 21-3). Fracture pans are used:
▶ By persons with casts
▶ By persons in traction
▶ By persons with limited back motion
▶ After spinal cord injury or surgery
▶ After a hip fracture
▶ After hip replacement surgery

See *Focus on Children and Older Persons: Bedpans.*
See *Delegation Guidelines: Bedpans*, p. 358.
See *Promoting Safety and Comfort: Bedpans.*
See *Focus on Ethics and Laws: Bedpans.*

BOX 21-2 Rules for Normal Urination

- Practice medical asepsis.
- Follow Standard Precautions and the Bloodborne Pathogen Standard.
- Provide fluids as the nurse and care plan direct.
- Follow the person's voiding routines and habits. Check with the nurse and the care plan.
- Help the person to the bathroom when the request is made. Or provide the commode, bedpan, or urinal. The need to void may be urgent.
- Help the person assume a normal position for voiding if possible. Women sit or squat. Men stand.
- Warm the bedpan or urinal.
- Cover the person for warmth and privacy.
- Provide for privacy. Pull the curtain around the bed, close room and bathroom doors, and close window coverings. Leave the room if the person can be alone.
- Tell the person that running water, flushing the toilet, or playing music can mask voiding sounds. Voiding with others close by embarrasses some people.
- Stay nearby if the person is weak or unsteady.
- Place the signal light and toilet tissue within reach.
- Allow enough time. Do not rush the person.
- Promote relaxation. Some people like to read.
- Run water in a sink if the person cannot start the stream. Or place the person's fingers in warm water.
- Provide perineal care as needed (Chapter 19).
- Assist with hand washing after voiding. Provide a wash basin, soap, washcloth, and towel.
- Assist the person to the bathroom or offer the bedpan, urinal, or commode at regular times. Some people are embarrassed or are too weak to ask for help.

TABLE 21-1 **Common Urinary Elimination Problems**

PROBLEM	DEFINITION	CAUSES
Dysuria	Painful or difficult (dys) urination (uria)	Urinary tract infection, trauma, urinary tract obstruction
Hematuria	Blood (hemat) in the urine (uria)	Kidney disease, urinary tract infection, trauma
Nocturia	Frequent urination (uria) at night (noct)	Excess fluid intake, kidney disease, prostate disease
Oliguria	Scant amount (olig) of urine (uria); less than 500 mL in 24 hours	Poor fluid intake, shock, burns, kidney disease, heart failure
Polyuria	Abnormally large amounts (poly) of urine (uria)	Drugs, excess fluid intake, diabetes, hormone imbalance
Urinary frequency	Voiding at frequent intervals	Excess fluid intake, bladder infections, pressure on the bladder, drugs
Urinary incontinence	The loss of bladder control	Trauma, disease, urinary tract infections, reproductive or urinary tract surgeries, aging, fecal impaction, constipation, not getting to the bathroom in time
Urinary urgency	The need to void at once	Urinary tract infection, fear of incontinence, full bladder, stress

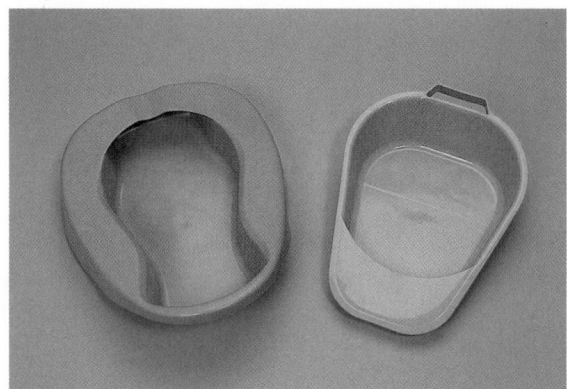

FIGURE 21-2 Standard bedpan (left) and the fracture pan (right).

FOCUS ON **CHILDREN** AND **OLDER PERSONS**

Bedpans

OLDER PERSONS

Osteoporosis and arthritis are common in older persons (Chapter 39). Osteoporosis causes fragile bones. Arthritis causes painful joints. Fracture pans provide more comfort than standard bedpans.

DELEGATION GUIDELINES: Bedpans

Before assisting with a bedpan, you need this information from the nurse and the care plan:
- What bedpan to use—standard bedpan or fracture pan
- Position or activity limits
- If you can leave the room or if you need to stay with the person
- If the nurse needs to observe the results before disposing of the contents
- What observations to report and record:
  - Urine color, clarity, and odor
  - Amount
  - Presence of particles
  - Complaints of urgency, burning, dysuria, or other problems (see Table 21-1)
  - For bowel movements, see Chapter 22
- When to report observations
- What specific patient or resident concerns to report at once

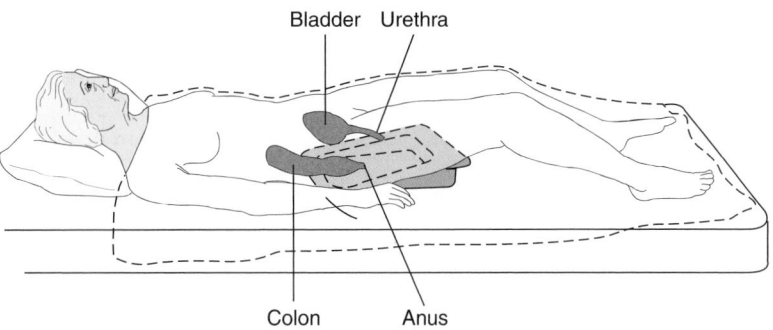

FIGURE 21-3 A person positioned on a fracture pan. The small end is under the buttocks.

PROMOTING SAFETY AND COMFORT: Bedpans

SAFETY

Urine and bowel movements may contain blood and microbes. Microbes can live and grow in dirty bedpans. Follow Standard Precautions and the Bloodborne Pathogen Standard when handling bedpans and their contents. Thoroughly clean and disinfect bedpans after use.

Remember to raise the bed as needed for good body mechanics. Lower the bed before leaving the room. Raise or lower the bed rails according to the care plan.

COMFORT

The person must not sit on a bedpan for a long time. Bedpans are uncomfortable. And they can lead to pressure ulcers from prolonged pressure (Chapter 32).

FOCUS ON ETHICS AND LAWS

Bedpans

A patient was admitted to the hospital with a diagnosis of mild pneumonia. He was to be in the hospital for 24 to 48 hours. While in the hospital, he was left on a bedpan for 4 hours. Pressure ulcers resulted. He died of pneumonia after 41 days in the hospital.

His family sued the hospital. The jury awarded the family $800,000.

(Estate of D. Roberts v William Beaumont Hospital, Mich, 2002.)

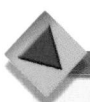

NNAAP™ Skill

GIVING THE BEDPAN

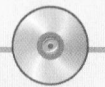

✔ Quality of Life *Remember to:*

- Knock before entering the person's room.
- Address the person by name.
- Introduce yourself by name and title.
- Explain the procedure to the person before beginning and during the procedure.

- Protect the person's rights during the procedure.
- Handle the person gently during the procedure.

PRE-PROCEDURE

1 Follow *Delegation Guidelines: Bedpans,* p. 357. See *Promoting Safety and Comfort: Bedpans.*
2 Provide for privacy.
3 Practice hand hygiene.
4 Put on gloves.

5 Collect the following:
- Bedpan
- Bedpan cover
- Toilet tissue
- Waterproof pad (if required by the agency)
6 Arrange equipment on the chair or bed.

PROCEDURE

7 Lower the bed rail near you if up.
8 Position the person supine. Raise the head of the bed slightly.
9 Fold the top linens and gown out of the way. Keep the lower body covered.
10 Ask the person to flex the knees and raise the buttocks by pushing against the mattress with his or her feet.
11 Slide your hand under the lower back. Help raise the buttocks. If using a waterproof pad, place it under the person's buttocks.
12 Slide the bedpan under the person (Fig. 21-4).

13 If the person cannot assist in getting on the bedpan:
  a If using a waterproof pad, place it under the person's buttocks.
  b Turn the person onto the side away from you.
  c Place the bedpan firmly against the buttocks (Fig. 21-5, A, p. 360).
  d Push the bedpan down and toward the person (Fig. 21-5, B, p. 360).
  e Hold the bedpan securely. Turn the person onto his or her back.
  f Make sure the bedpan is centered under the person.

GIVING THE BEDPAN—cont'd

PROCEDURE—cont'd

14 Cover the person.
15 Raise the head of the bed so the person is in a sitting position (Fowler's position) if the person is using a standard bedpan.
16 Make sure the person is correctly positioned on the bedpan (Fig. 21-6, p. 360).
17 Raise the bed rail if used.
18 Place the toilet tissue and signal light within reach.
19 Ask the person to signal when done or when help is needed.
20 Remove the gloves. Practice hand hygiene.
21 Leave the room, and close the door.
22 Return when the person signals. Or check on the person ever 5 minutes. Knock before entering.
23 Decontaminate your hands. Put on gloves.
24 Raise the bed for good body mechanics. Lower the bed rail (if used) and the head of the bed.
25 Ask the person to raise the buttocks. Remove the bedpan. Or hold the bedpan and turn him or her onto the side away from you.

26 Clean the genital area if the person cannot do so. Clean from front (urethra) to back (anus) with toilet tissue. Use fresh tissue for each wipe. Provide perineal care if needed. Remove and discard the waterproof pad if using one.
27 Cover the bedpan. Take it to the bathroom. Raise the bed rail (if used) before leaving the bedside.
28 Note the color, amount, and character of urine or feces.
29 Empty the bedpan contents into the toilet and flush.
30 Rinse the bedpan. Pour the rinse into the toilet and flush.
31 Clean the bedpan with a disinfectant.
32 Removed soiled gloves. Practice hand hygiene, and put on clean gloves.
33 Return the bedpan and clean cover to the bedside stand.
34 Help the person with hand washing. (Wear gloves for this step.)
35 Remove the gloves. Practice hand hygiene.

POST-PROCEDURE

36 Provide for comfort. (See the inside of the front book cover.)
37 Place the signal light within reach.
38 Lower the bed to its lowest position.
39 Raise or lower bed rails. Follow the care plan.
40 Unscreen the person.

41 Complete a safety check of the room. (See the inside of the front book cover.)
42 Follow agency policy for soiled linen.
43 Practice hand hygiene.
44 Report and record your observations.

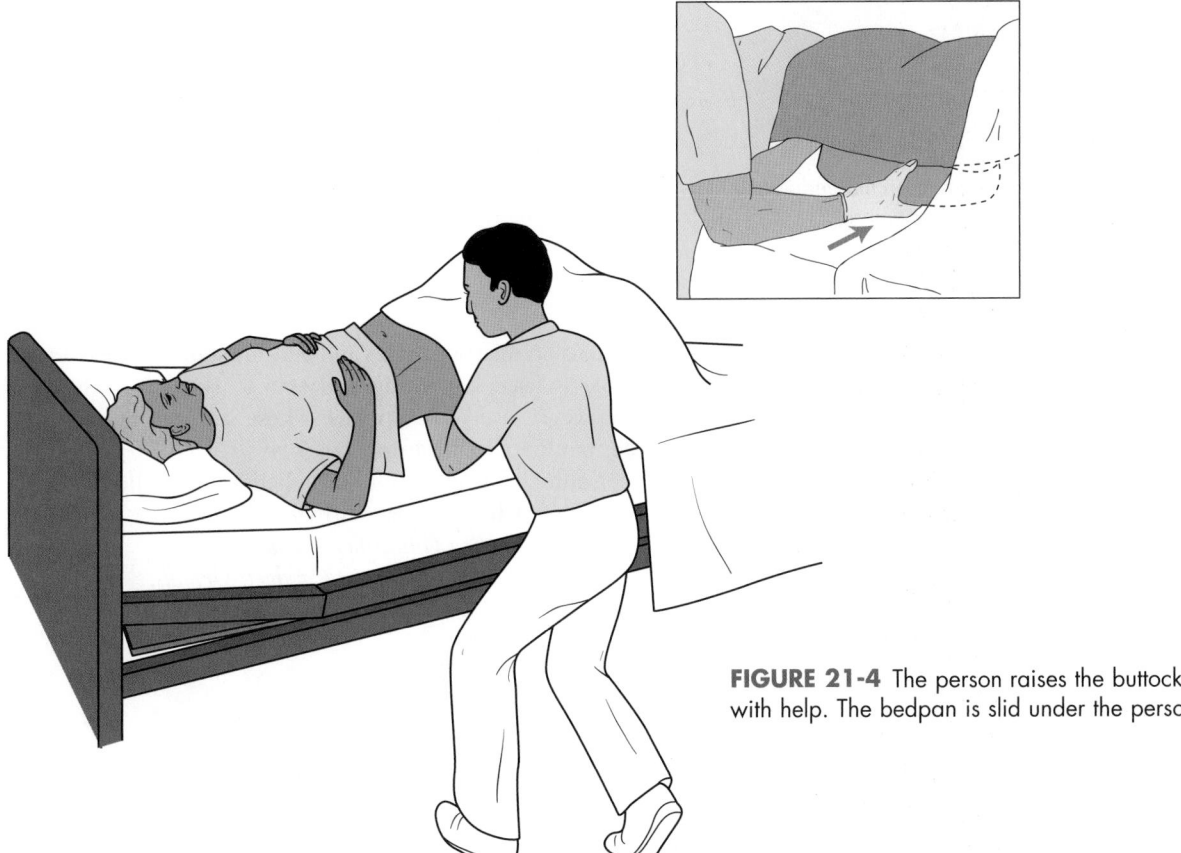

FIGURE 21-4 The person raises the buttocks off the bed with help. The bedpan is slid under the person.

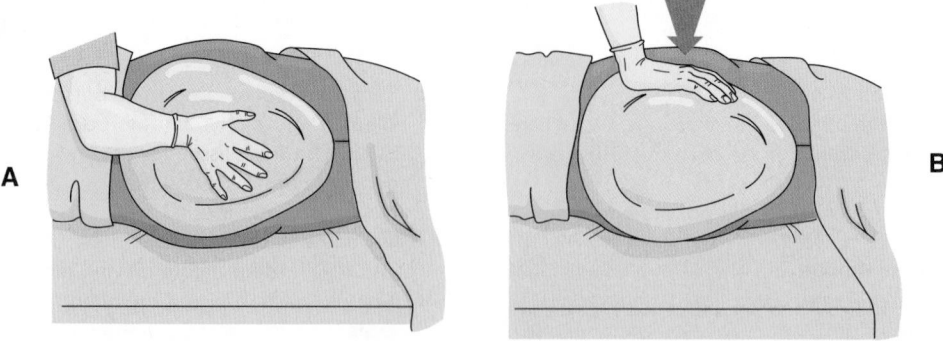

FIGURE 21-5 Giving a bedpan. **A,** Position the person on one side. Place the bedpan firmly against the buttocks. **B,** Push downward on the bedpan and toward the person.

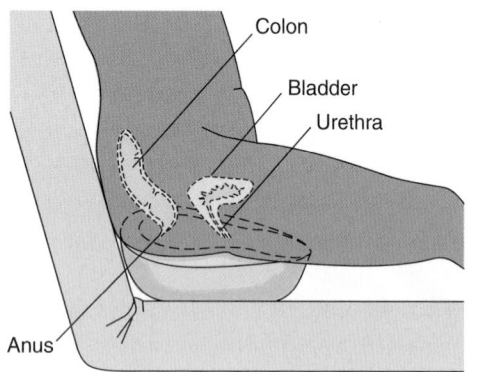

FIGURE 21-6 The person is positioned on the bedpan so the urethra and anus are directly over the opening.

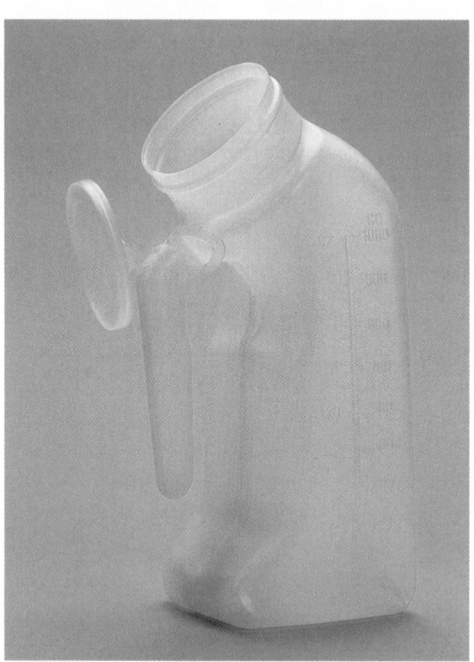

FIGURE 21-7 Male urinal.

◆ Urinals

Men use urinals to void (Fig. 21-7). Plastic urinals have caps and hook-type handles. The urinal hooks to the bed rail within the man's reach. He stands to use the urinal if possible. Or he sits on the side of the bed or lies in bed to use it. Some men need support when standing. You may have to place and hold the urinal for some men.

After voiding, the urinal cap is closed. This prevents urine spills. Remind men to hang urinals on bed rails and to signal after using them. Remind them not to place urinals on overbed tables and bedside stands. The overbed table is used for eating and as a work surface. Bedside stands are used for supplies. These surfaces must not be contaminated with urine.

Some beds may not have bed rails. Follow agency policy for where to place urinals.

See *Delegation Guidelines: Urinals.*

See *Promoting Safety and Comfort: Urinals.*

DELEGATION GUIDELINES: Urinals

Before assisting with urinals, you need this information from the nurse and the care plan:
- How the urinal is used—standing, sitting, or lying in bed
- If help is needed with placing or holding the urinal
- If the man needs support to stand (If yes, how many staff members are needed.)
- If you can leave the room or if you need to stay with the person
- If the nurse needs to observe the urine before its disposal
- What observations to report and record (see *Delegation Guidelines: Bedpans,* p. 357)
- When to report observations
- What specific patient or resident concerns to report at once

PROMOTING SAFETY AND COMFORT: Urinals

SAFETY
Follow Standard Precautions and the Bloodborne Pathogen Standard when handling urinals and their contents. Empty them promptly to prevent odors and the spread of microbes. A filled urinal spills easily, causing safety hazards. Also, it is an unpleasant sight and a source of odor. Urinals are cleaned like bedpans.

COMFORT
You may have to place the urinal for some men. This means that you have to place the penis in the urinal. This may embarrass both the person and you. Act in a professional manner at all times.

GIVING THE URINAL

✔ Quality of Life *Remember to:*

- Knock before entering the person's room.
- Address the person by name.
- Introduce yourself by name and title.
- Explain the procedure to the person before beginning and during the procedure.
- Protect the person's rights during the procedure.
- Handle the person gently during the procedure.

PRE-PROCEDURE

1 Follow *Delegation Guidelines: Urinals.* See *Promoting Safety and Comfort: Urinals.*
2 Provide for privacy.
3 Determine if the man will stand, sit, or lie in bed.
4 Practice hand hygiene.
5 Put on gloves.
6 Collect the following:
   - Urinal
   - Non-skid footwear if the person will stand to void

PROCEDURE

7 Give him the urinal if he is in bed. Remind him to tilt the bottom down to prevent spills.
8 If he is going to stand:
   a Help him sit on the side of the bed.
   b Put non-skid footwear on him.
   c Help him stand. Provide support if he is unsteady.
   d Give him the urinal.
9 Position the urinal if necessary. Position his penis in the urinal if he cannot do so.
10 Place the signal light within reach. Ask him to signal when done or when he needs help.
11 Provide for privacy.
12 Remove the gloves. Practice hand hygiene.
13 Leave the room, and close the door.
14 Return when he signals for you. Or check on him every 5 minutes. Knock before entering.
15 Decontaminate your hands. Put on gloves.
16 Close the cap on the urinal. Take it to the bathroom.
17 Note the color, amount, and character of urine.
18 Empty the urinal into the toilet and flush.
19 Rinse the urinal with cold water. Pour rinse into the toilet and flush.
20 Clean the urinal with a disinfectant.
21 Return the urinal to its proper place.
22 Remove soiled gloves. Practice hand hygiene, and put on clean gloves.
23 Assist with hand washing.
24 Remove the gloves. Practice hand hygiene.

POST-PROCEDURE

25 Provide for comfort. (See the inside of the front book cover.)
26 Place the signal light within reach.
27 Raise or lower bed rails. Follow the care plan.
28 Unscreen him.
29 Complete a safety check of the room. (See the inside of the front book cover.)
30 Follow agency policy for soiled linen.
31 Practice hand hygiene.
32 Report and record your observations.

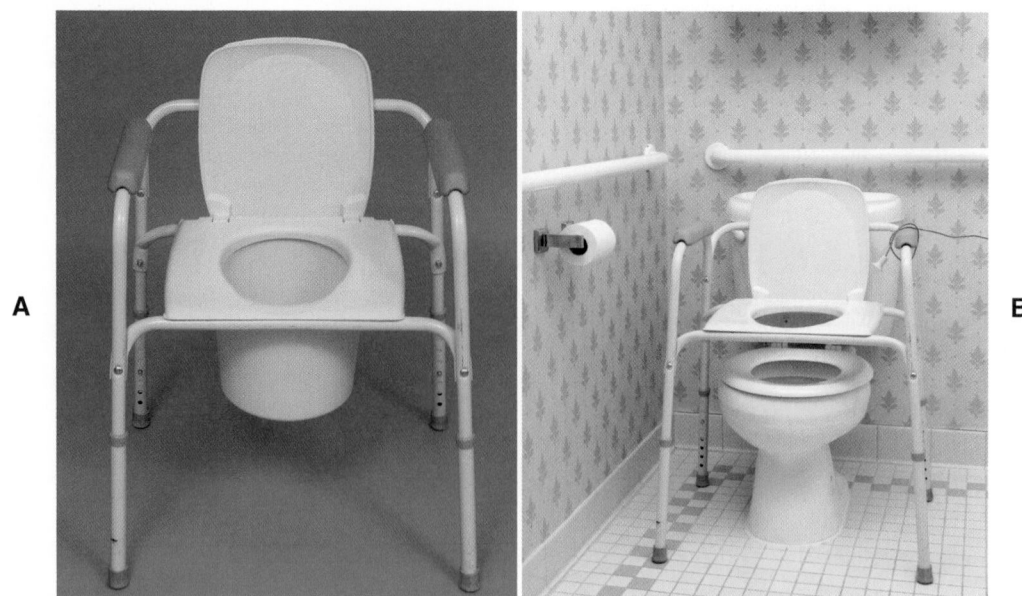

FIGURE 21-8 A, The commode has a toilet seat with a container. The container slides out from under the seat for emptying. **B,** The container is removed. The commode chair is placed over the toilet.

◆ Commodes

A commode is a chair or wheelchair with an opening for a container (Fig. 21-8). Persons unable to walk to the bathroom often use commodes. The commode allows a normal position for elimination. The commode arms and back provide support and help prevent falls.

Some commodes are wheeled into bathrooms and placed over toilets. They are useful for persons who need support when sitting. The container is removed if the commode is used with the toilet. Wheels are locked after the commode is positioned over the toilet.

See *Delegation Guidelines: Commodes.*
See *Promoting Safety and Comfort: Commodes.*
See *Focus on Ethics and Laws: Commodes.*

PROMOTING SAFETY AND COMFORT: Commodes

SAFETY
For commode use, transfer the person from bed, chair, or wheelchair to the commode. Practice safe transfer procedures (Chapter 16). Use the transfer belt, and lock the wheels.

Urine and feces may contain blood and microbes. Follow Standard Precautions and the Bloodborne Pathogen Standard. Thoroughly clean and disinfect the commode container after use. Clean and disinfect the seat and other commode parts if necessary.

COMFORT
After the person transfers to the commode, cover his or her lap and legs with a bath blanket. This provides warmth and promotes privacy.

DELEGATION GUIDELINES: Commodes

You need this information from the nurse and care plan when assisting with commodes:
- If the commode is used at the bedside or over the toilet
- How much help the person needs
- If you can leave the room or if you need to stay with the person
- If the nurse needs to observe urine or bowel movements
- What observations to report and record (see *Delegation Guidelines: Bedpans,* p. 357)
- When to report observations
- What specific patient or resident concerns to report at once

FOCUS ON **ETHICS** AND **LAWS**

Commodes

A patient was treated in the hospital for a stroke. She was paralyzed on her left side. After hospital care for 9 days, she was transferred to the rehabilitation section of the hospital. She was left on the commode the next day. The commode had arm rails. The patient was instructed:
- Not to reach for the toilet paper
- To call when ready

The patient fell off the commode when reaching for the toilet paper. The patient claimed that the fall damaged a nerve in her leg "resulting in drop foot." (Author note: the person with drop foot [commonly called *footdrop*] cannot bend the toes and foot up at the ankle. See Chapter 26.)

The patient sued the hospital. The jury returned a verdict in favor of the patient. The jury awarded the patient $325,000. The amount was reduced to $178,750 because the patient's actions contributed to the injury.

(M. Naya v Mercy Medical Center, NY, 2003.)

HELPING THE PERSON TO THE COMMODE

✔ Quality of Life *Remember to:*

- Knock before entering the person's room.
- Address the person by name.
- Introduce yourself by name and title.
- Explain the procedure to the person before beginning and during the procedure.

- Protect the person's rights during the procedure.
- Handle the person gently during the procedure.

PRE-PROCEDURE

1 Follow *Delegation Guidelines: Commodes*. See *Promoting Safety and Comfort: Commodes*.
2 Provide for privacy.
3 Practice hand hygiene.
4 Put on gloves.

5 Collect the following:
  - Commode
  - Toilet tissue
  - Bath blanket
  - Transfer belt
  - Robe and non-skid footwear

PROCEDURE

6 Bring the commode next to the bed. Remove the chair seat and container lid.
7 Help the person sit on the side of the bed. Lower the bed rail if used.
8 Help him or her put on a robe and non-skid footwear.
9 Assist the person to the commode. Use the transfer belt.
10 Cover the person with a bath blanket for warmth.
11 Place the toilet tissue and signal light within reach.
12 Ask him or her to signal when done or when help is needed. (Stay with the person if necessary. Be respectful. Provide as much privacy as possible.)
13 Remove the gloves. Practice hand hygiene.
14 Leave the room. Close the door.
15 Return when the person signals. Or check on the person every 5 minutes. Knock before entering.
16 Decontaminate your hands. Put on the gloves.
17 Help the person clean the genital area as needed. Remove the gloves, and practice hand hygiene.

18 Help the person back to bed using the transfer belt. Remove the robe, transfer belt, and footwear. Raise the bed rail if used.
19 Put on clean gloves. Remove and cover the commode container. Clean the commode.
20 Take the container to the bathroom.
21 Observe urine and feces for color, amount, and character.
22 Empty the container contents into the toilet and flush.
23 Rinse the container. Pour the rinse into the toilet and flush.
24 Clean and disinfect the container.
25 Return the container to the commode. Return other supplies to their proper place.
26 Remove soiled gloves. Practice hand hygiene, and put on clean gloves.
27 Assist with hand washing.
28 Remove the gloves. Practice hand hygiene.

POST-PROCEDURE

29 Provide for comfort. (See the inside of the front book cover.)
30 Place the signal light within reach.
31 Raise or lower bed rails. Follow the care plan.
32 Unscreen the person.

33 Complete a safety check of the room. (See the inside of the front book cover.)
34 Follow agency policy for dirty linen.
35 Practice hand hygiene.
36 Report and record your observations.

URINARY INCONTINENCE

Urinary incontinence is the loss of bladder control. It may be temporary or permanent. The basic types of incontinence are:

▶ **Stress incontinence.** Urine leaks during exercise and certain movements that cause pressure on the bladder. Urine loss is small (less than 50 mL). Often called *dribbling*, it occurs with laughing, sneezing, coughing, lifting, or other activities. Obesity and late pregnancy also are causes. The problem is common in women and may begin during menopause. Pelvic muscles weaken from pregnancies and with aging.

▶ **Urge incontinence.** Urine is lost in response to a sudden, urgent need to void. The person cannot get to a toilet in time. Urinary frequency, urinary urgency, and night-time voidings are common. Causes include urinary tract infections, Alzheimer's disease, nervous system disorders, bladder cancer, and an enlarged prostate.

▶ **Overflow incontinence.** Small amounts of urine leak from a bladder that is always full. The person feels like the bladder is not empty. The person only dribbles or has a weak urine stream. Diabetes, enlarged prostate, and some drugs are causes. So are spinal cord injuries.

▶ **Functional incontinence.** The person has bladder control but cannot use the toilet in time. Immobility, restraints, unanswered signal lights, no signal light within reach, and not knowing where to find the bathroom are causes. So is difficulty removing clothing. Confusion and disorientation are other causes.

▶ **Reflex incontinence.** Urine is lost at predictable intervals when the bladder is full. The person does not feel the need to void. Nervous system disorders and injuries are common causes.

▶ **Mixed incontinence.** A person can have more than one type of incontinence. Stress and urge incontinence often occur together.

Sometimes incontinence results from intestinal, rectal, and reproductive system surgeries. Incontinence may result from a physical illness. If incontinence is a new problem, tell the nurse at once.

Incontinence is embarrassing. Garments get wet, and odors develop. The person is uncomfortable. Skin irritation, infection, and pressure ulcers are risks. Falling is a risk when trying to get to the bathroom quickly. The person's pride, dignity, and self-esteem are affected. Social isolation, loss of independence, and depression are common. Quality of life suffers.

The person's care plan may include some of the measures listed in Box 21-3. *Good skin care and dry garments and linens are essential.* Promoting normal urinary elimination prevents incontinence in some people (see Box 21-2). Others need bladder training (p. 374). Sometimes catheters are needed.

Incontinence products help keep the person dry (Fig. 21-9). They have two layers and a waterproof back. Fluid passes through the first layer. It is absorbed by the lower layer. The nurse selects products that best meet the person's needs. Follow the manufacturer's instructions and agency procedures when using them.

Incontinence is linked to abuse, mistreatment, and neglect. Caring for persons with incontinence is stressful. They need frequent care. They may wet again right after skin care and changing wet garments and linens. Remember, incontinence is beyond the person's control. It is not something the person chooses to do. Be patient. The person's needs are great. If you find yourself becoming

---

BOX 21-3 Nursing Measures for Persons With Urinary Incontinence

- Record the person's voidings. This includes incontinent times and successful use of the toilet, commode, bedpan, or urinal.
- Answer signal lights promptly. The need to void may be urgent.
- Promote normal urinary elimination (see Box 21-2).
- Promote normal bowel elimination (Chapter 22).
- Encourage voiding at scheduled intervals.
- Follow the person's bladder training program (p. 374).
- Have the person wear easy-to-remove clothing. Incontinence can occur while trying to deal with buttons, zippers, other closures, and undergarments.
- Encourage the person to do pelvic muscle exercises as instructed by the nurse.
- Help prevent urinary tract infections:
  - Promote fluid intake as the nurse directs.
  - Have the person wear cotton underwear.
  - Keep the perineal area clean and dry.
- Decrease fluid intake at bedtime.
- Provide good skin care.
- Apply a barrier cream as directed by the nurse. The cream prevents irritation and skin damage.
- Provide dry garments and linens.
- Observe for signs of skin breakdown (Chapter 32).
- Use incontinence products as the nurse directs. Follow the manufacturer's instructions.
- Provide perineal care as needed (Chapter 19). Remember to:
  - Use a safe and comfortable water temperature.
  - Follow Standard Precautions and the Bloodborne Pathogen Standard.
  - Protect the person and dry garments and linen from the wet incontinence product.
  - Expose only the perineal area.
  - Wash, rinse, and dry the perineal area and buttocks.
  - Remove wet incontinence products, garments, and linen. Apply clean, dry ones.

---

short-tempered and impatient, talk to the nurse at once. The person has the right to be free from abuse, mistreatment, and neglect. Kindness, empathy, understanding, and patience are needed.

See *Focus on Children and Older Persons: Urinary Incontinence.*

See *Focus on Long-Term Care and Home Care: Urinary Incontinence.*

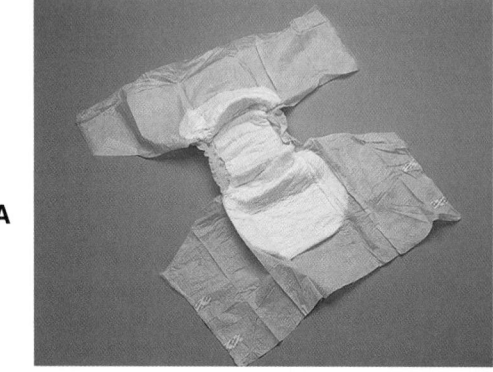
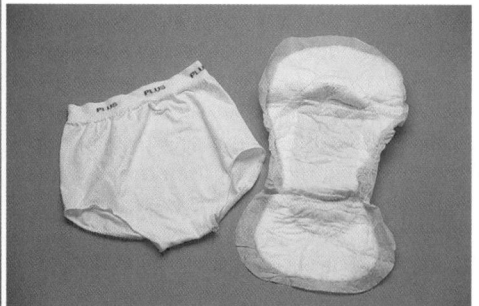

FIGURE 21-9 Disposable garment protectors. **A,** Complete incontinence brief. **B,** Pant liner and undergarment.

FOCUS ON **CHILDREN** AND **OLDER PERSONS**

Urinary Incontinence

CHILDREN

Urinary incontinence is common in children. Night-time wetting occurs more often in boys. Day-time wetting is more common in girls.

Waiting for incontinence to disappear naturally is one treatment. This usually happens after age 5. The bladder grows in size and can hold more urine. The child learns to respond to the body's signal that it is time to void. Sometimes incontinence is caused by stress and anxiety. As the child grows older, stressful and anxiety-producing events may pass.

Other treatments include diet changes, moisture alarms, drugs, and bladder training.

OLDER PERSONS

Urinary incontinence is common in older persons. They are at risk for nervous, endocrine, and reproductive system disorders. Dementia, tumors, and poor mobility are risks.

Complications from incontinence pose serious problems for older persons. These include falls, pressure ulcers, and urinary tract infections. Long hospital or long-term care stays are often necessary. The resulting health care costs are high.

Persons with dementia may develop incontinence. They may void in the wrong places. Trash cans, planters, heating vents, and closets are examples. Some persons remove incontinence products and throw them on the floor or in the toilet. Other persons resist staff efforts to keep them clean and dry.

You must must provide safe care for these persons. The care plan lists needed measures. The care plan may include these measures recommended by the Alzheimer's Disease Education and Referral Center (ADEAR):

- Follow the person's bathroom routine as closely as possible. For example, take the person to the bathroom every 3 hours during the day. Do not wait for the person to ask.
- Observe for signs that the person may need to void. Restlessness and pulling at clothes are examples. Respond quickly.
- Stay calm when the person is incontinent. Reassure the person if he or she becomes upset.
- Tell the nurse when the person is incontinent. Report the time, what the person was doing, and other observations. There may be a pattern to the person's incontinence. If so, measures can be taken to prevent the problem.
- Prevent episodes of incontinence during sleep. Limit the type and amount of fluids in the evening. Follow the care plan.
- Plan ahead if the person will leave the agency. Have the person wear clothing that is easy to remove. Pack an extra set of clothing. Know where to find restrooms.

You may need a co-worker's help to keep the person clean and dry. If you have questions, ask the nurse for help.

Remember, everyone has the right to safe care. They also have the right to be treated with dignity and privacy.

FOCUS ON **LONG-TERM CARE** AND **HOME CARE**

Urinary Incontinence

HOME CARE

Incontinence is stressful for the family. They often have problems coping with the person's incontinence. It is a common reason for long-term care.

◆ CATHETERS

A **catheter** is a tube used to drain or inject fluid through a body opening. Inserted through the urethra into the bladder, a urinary catheter drains urine.

- A **straight catheter** drains the bladder and then is removed.
- An **indwelling catheter (retention or Foley catheter)** is left in the bladder. Urine drains constantly into a drainage bag. A balloon near the tip is inflated with sterile water after the catheter is inserted. The balloon prevents the catheter from slipping out of the bladder (Fig. 21-10). Tubing connects the catheter to the drainage bag.

Catheterization is the process of inserting a catheter. It is done by a doctor or nurse. With the proper education and supervision, some states and agencies let nursing assistants insert and remove catheters.

Catheters often are used before, during, and after surgery. They keep the bladder empty. This reduces the risk of bladder injury during surgery. After surgery, a full bladder causes pressure on nearby organs. Such pressure can lead to pain or discomfort.

Some people are too weak or disabled to use the bedpan, urinal, commode, or toilet. Dying persons are examples. For them, catheters can promote comfort and prevent incontinence. Catheters can protect wounds and pressure ulcers from contact with urine. They also allow

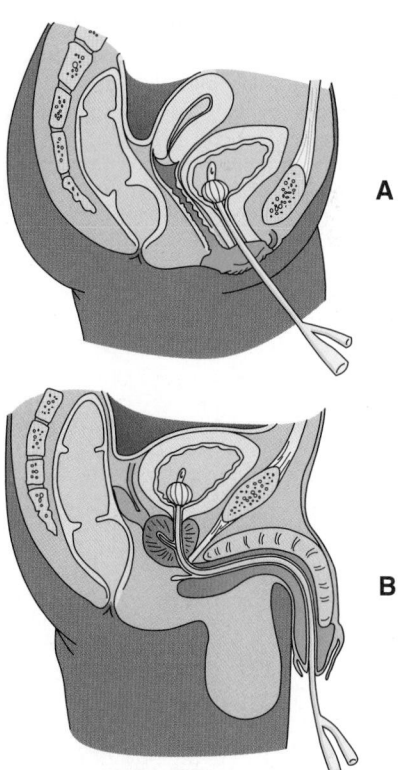

FIGURE 21-10 Indwelling catheter. **A,** Indwelling catheter in the female bladder. The inflated balloon at the tip prevents the catheter from slipping out through the urethra. **B,** Indwelling catheter with the balloon inflated in the male bladder.

hourly urinary output measurements. However, they are a last resort for incontinence. Catheters do not treat the cause of incontinence.

Catheters also have diagnostic uses:

▶ To collect sterile urine specimens.
▶ To measure the amount of urine left in the bladder after the person voids. This is called *residual urine*.

You will care for persons with indwelling catheters. The risk of infection is high. Follow the rules in Box 21-4 to promote safety and comfort.

See *Delegation Guidelines: Catheters*.
See *Promoting Safety and Comfort: Catheters*.

BOX 21-4 Caring for Persons With Indwelling Catheters

- Follow the rules of medical asepsis.
- Follow Standard Precautions and the Bloodborne Pathogen Standard.
- Allow urine to flow freely through the catheter or tubing. Tubing should not have kinks. The person should not lie on the tubing.
- Keep the catheter connected to the drainage tubing. Follow the measures on p. 369 if the catheter and drainage tube are disconnected.
- Keep the drainage tube below the bladder. This prevents urine from flowing backward into the bladder.
- Move the bag to the other side of the bed when the person is turned and repositioned on his or her other side.
- Attach the drainage bag to the bed frame, back of the chair, or lower part of an IV (intravenous) pole. *Never attach the drainage bag to the bed rail.* Otherwise it is higher than the bladder when the bed rail is raised.
- Do not let the drainage bag rest on the floor. This can contaminate the system.
- Coil the drainage tubing on the bed. Secure it to the bottom linen (Fig. 21-11). Follow agency policy. Use a clip, bed sheet clamp, tape, safety pin with rubber band, or other device as directed by the nurse. Tubing must not loop below the drainage bag.

- Secure the catheter to the inner thigh (see Fig. 21-11). Or secure it to the man's abdomen. This prevents excess catheter movement and friction at the insertion site. Secure the catheter with a tube holder, tape, or other devices as the nurse directs.
- Check for leaks. Check the site where the catheter connects to the drainage bag. Report any leaks to the nurse at once.
- Provide catheter care daily or twice a day, after bowel movements, and when vaginal discharge is present. (See procedure: *Giving Catheter Care*). Some agencies consider perineal care to be sufficient. Follow the care plan.
- Provide perineal care daily, after bowel movements, and when there is vaginal drainage. Follow the care plan.
- Empty the drainage bag at the end of the shift or as the nurse directs. Measure and record the amount of urine (see procedure: *Emptying a Urinary Drainage Bag*, p. 371). Report an increase or decrease in the amount of urine.
- Use a separate measuring container for each person. This prevents the spread of microbes from one person to another.
- Do not let the drain on the drainage bag touch any surface.
- Report complaints to the nurse at once—pain, burning, the need to void, or irritation. Also report the color, clarity, and odor of urine and the presence of particles.
- Encourage fluid intake as directed by the nurse and the care plan.

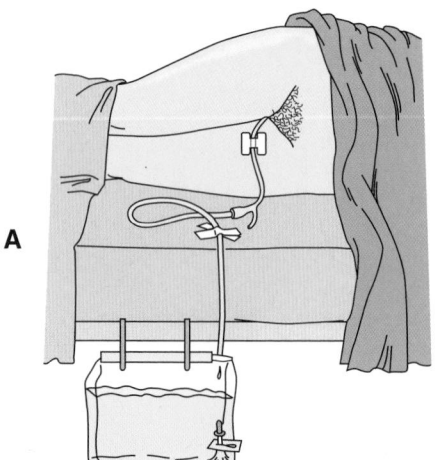 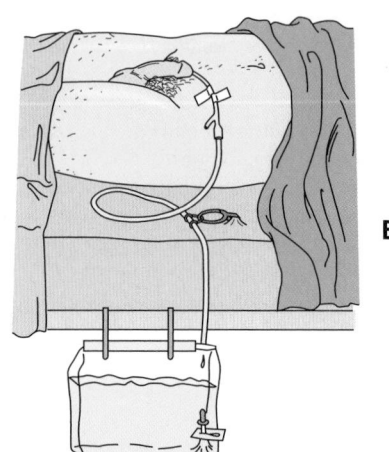

FIGURE 21-11 Securing catheters. **A,** The drainage tube is coiled on the bed and secured to the bottom linens. The catheter is secured to the inner thigh with a tube holder. Drainage tubing is secured to bottom linens with tape. **B,** The catheter is secured to the man's abdomen with tape. Drainage tubing is secured to bottom linens with a clamp.

DELEGATION GUIDELINES: Catheters

The nurse may delegate catheter care to you. If so, you need this information from the nurse and the care plan:
- When to give catheter care—daily, twice a day, after bowel movements, or when vaginal discharge is present
- Where to secure the catheter—thigh or abdomen
- How to secure the catheter—tube holder, tape, or other device
- How to secure drainage tubing—clip, bed sheet clamp, tape, safety pin with rubber band, or other device
- What observations to report and record:
  - Complaints of pain, burning, irritation, or the need to void (report at once)
  - Crusting, abnormal drainage, or secretions
  - The color, clarity, and odor of urine
  - Particles in the urine
  - Urine leaking at the insertion site
  - Drainage system leaks
- When to report observations
- What specific patient or resident concerns to report at once

PROMOTING SAFETY AND COMFORT: Catheters

SAFETY
Urine may contain microbes and blood. Follow Standard Precautions and the Bloodborne Pathogen Standard.

Be very careful when using a safety pin and rubber band to secure the drainage tubing to the bottom linens:
- The safety pin must work properly. It must not be stretched out of shape.
- The rubber band must be intact. It should not be frayed or over-stretched.
- Do not insert the pin through the catheter.
- Point the pin away from the person.

COMFORT
The catheter must not pull at the insertion site. This causes discomfort and irritation. Hold the catheter securely during catheter care. Then properly secure the catheter. Make sure the tubing is not under the person. Besides obstructing urine flow, laying on the tubing is uncomfortable. It can also cause skin breakdown. To promote comfort, see Box 21-4.

GIVING CATHETER CARE

✔ **Quality of Life** *Remember to:*

- Knock before entering the person's room.
- Address the person by name.
- Introduce yourself by name and title.
- Explain the procedure to the person before beginning and during the procedure.
- Protect the person's rights during the procedure.
- Handle the person gently during the procedure.

PRE-PROCEDURE

1 Follow *Delegation Guidelines: Catheters.* See *Promoting Safety and Comfort: Catheters.*
2 Practice hand hygiene.
3 Collect the following:
  - Items for perineal care (Chapter 19)
  - Gloves
  - Bath blanket

4 Identify the person. Check the ID bracelet against the assignment sheet. Also call the person by name.
5 Provide for privacy.
6 Raise the bed for good body mechanics. Bed rails are up if used.

PROCEDURE

7 Lower the bed rail near you if up.
8 Decontaminate your hands. Put on the gloves.
9 Cover the person with a bath blanket. Fan-fold top linens to the foot of the bed.
10 Drape the person for perineal care. (See Chapter 19.)
11 Fold back the bath blanket to expose the genital area.
12 Place the waterproof pad under the buttocks. Ask the person to flex the knees and raise the buttocks off the bed.
13 Separate the labia (female). In an uncircumcised male, retract the foreskin (Fig. 21-12, p. 368). Check for crusts, abnormal drainage, or secretions.
14 Give perineal care. (See Chapter 19.)
15 Apply soap to a clean, wet washcloth.
16 Hold the catheter near the meatus.

17 Clean the catheter from the meatus down the catheter about 4 inches (Fig. 21-13, p. 368). Clean downward, away from the meatus with 1 stroke. Do not tug or pull on the catheter. Repeat as needed with a clean area of the washcloth. Use a clean washcloth if needed.
18 Rinse the catheter with a clean washcloth. Rinse from the meatus down the catheter about 4 inches. Rinse downward, away from the meatus with 1 stroke. Do not tug or pull on the catheter. Repeat as needed with a clean area of the washcloth. Use a clean washcloth if needed.
19 Pat dry the perineal area. Dry from front to back.
20 Return the foreskin to its natural position.
21 Secure the catheter. Coil and secure tubing (see Fig. 21-11).
22 Remove the waterproof pad.
23 Cover the person. Remove the bath blanket.
24 Remove the gloves. Practice hand hygiene.

Continued

GIVING CATHETER CARE—cont'd

POST-PROCEDURE

25 Provide for comfort. (See the inside of the front book cover.)

26 Place the signal light within reach.

27 Lower the bed to its lowest position.

28 Raise or lower bed rails. Follow the care plan.

29 Clean and return equipment to its proper place. Discard disposable items. (Wear gloves for this step.)

30 Remove the gloves. Practice hand hygiene.

31 Unscreen the person.

32 Complete a safety check of the room. (See the inside of the front book cover.)

33 Follow agency policy for soiled linen.

34 Practice hand hygiene.

35 Report and record your observations (Fig. 21-14).

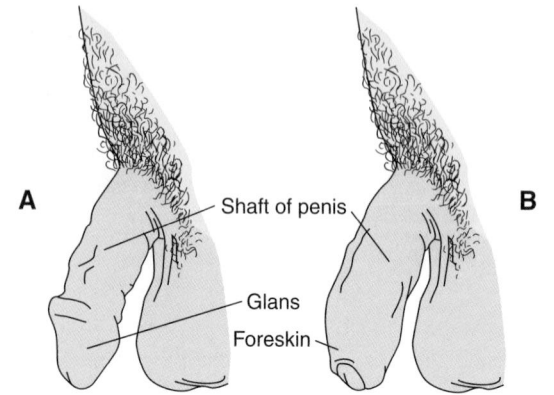

FIGURE 21-12 A, Circumcised male. **B,** Uncircumcised male.

Labels: Shaft of penis, Glans, Foreskin

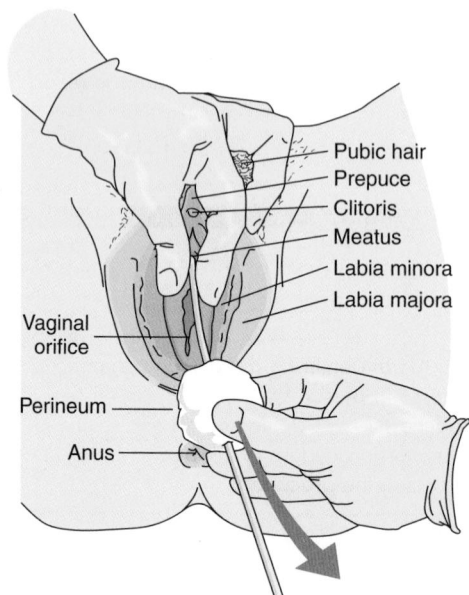

FIGURE 21-13 The catheter is cleaned starting at the meatus. About 4 inches of the catheter is cleaned.

Labels: Pubic hair, Prepuce, Clitoris, Meatus, Labia minora, Labia majora, Vaginal orifice, Perineum, Anus

Date	Time	Nursing Margin	Other Depts Margin
12/21	0900	Catheter care given. No drainage from around the catheter. Resident denies discomfort. Clear amber urine flowing freely. Catheter secured to abdomen with tape. Drainage tubing attached to bed with clip. Resident positioned on L side. Bed in low position. Signal light within reach. Adam Aims, CNA ————	

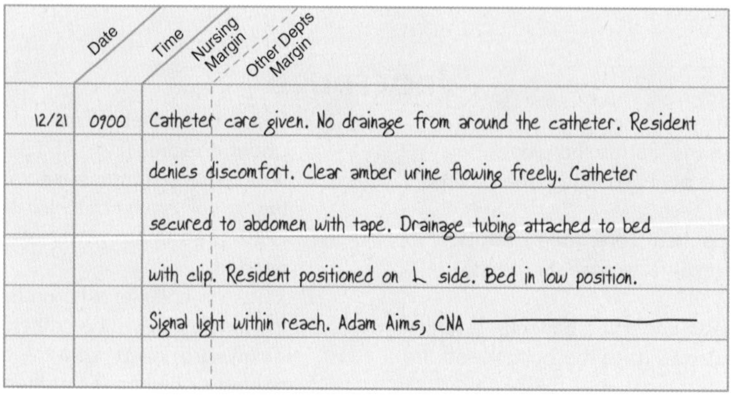

FIGURE 21-14 Charting sample.

◆ Drainage Systems

A closed drainage system is used for indwelling catheters. Nothing can enter the system from the catheter to the drainage bag. The urinary system is sterile. Infection can occur if microbes enter the drainage system. The microbes travel up the tubing or catheter into the bladder and kidneys. A urinary tract infection can threaten health and life.

The drainage system has tubing and a drainage bag. Tubing attaches at one end to the catheter. At the other end, it attaches to the drainage bag.

The bag hangs from the bed frame, chair, or wheelchair. It must not touch the floor. The bag is always kept lower than the person's bladder (see Fig. 21-11). Some people wear leg bags when up. The leg bag attaches to the thigh or calf (p. 374).

Microbes can grow in urine. If the drainage bag is higher than the bladder, urine can flow back into the bladder. An infection can occur. *Therefore do not hang the drainage bag on a bed rail.* Otherwise when the bed rail is raised, the bag is higher than bladder level. When the person walks, the bag is held lower than the bladder.

Sometimes drainage systems are disconnected accidentally. If that happens, tell the nurse at once. Do not touch the ends of the catheter or tubing. Do the following:

▶ Practice hand hygiene. Put on gloves.
▶ Wipe the end of the tube with an antiseptic wipe.
▶ Wipe the end of the catheter with another antiseptic wipe.
▶ Do not put the ends down. Do not touch the ends after you clean them.
▶ Connect the tubing to the catheter.
▶ Discard the wipes into a biohazard bag.
▶ Remove the gloves. Practice hand hygiene.

DELEGATION GUIDELINES: Drainage Systems

Your delegated tasks may involve urinary drainage systems. If so, you need this information from the nurse and the care plan:

• When to empty the drainage bag
• If the person uses a leg bag
• When to switch drainage bags and leg bags
• If you should clean or discard the drainage bag
• What observations to report and record:
  • The amount of urine measured
  • The color, clarity, and odor of urine
  • Particles in the urine
  • Complaints of pain, burning, irritation, or the need to urinate
  • Drainage system leaks
• When to report observations
• What specific patient or resident concerns to report at once

Leg bags are changed to drainage bags when the person is in bed. This drainage bag stays lower than bladder level. You will have to open the closed drainage system. You must prevent microbes from entering the system.

Drainage bags are emptied and urine is measured:

▶ At the end of every shift
▶ When changing from a leg bag to a drainage bag
▶ When changing from a drainage bag to a leg bag
▶ When the bag is becoming full
  See *Delegation Guidelines: Drainage Systems.*
  See *Promoting Safety and Comfort: Drainage Systems.*

Text continued on p. 372

PROMOTING SAFETY AND COMFORT: Drainage Systems

SAFETY
Urine may contain microbes and blood. Follow Standard Precautions and the Bloodborne Pathogen Standard.

For the procedure: *Changing a Leg Bag to a Drainage Bag,* you will open sterile packages. You must keep sterile items free from contamination. Review "Surgical Asepsis," in Chapter 14.

Leg bags hold less than 1000 mL of urine. Most standard drainage bags hold at least 2000 mL of urine. Therefore leg bags fill faster than standard drainage bags. Check leg bags often. Empty the leg bag if it is becoming half full. Measure the contents.

COMFORT
Having urine in a drainage bag embarrasses some people. Visitors can see the urine when they are with the person. To promote mental comfort, have visitors sit on the side away from the drainage bag. Sometimes you can empty the bag before visitors arrive. Make sure you measure, report, and record the amount of urine.

Some agencies provide drainage bag holders. The drainage bag is placed inside the holder. Urine cannot be seen.

CHANGING A LEG BAG TO A DRAINAGE BAG

✔ Quality of Life *Remember to:*

• Knock before entering the person's room.
• Address the person by name.
• Introduce yourself by name and title.
• Explain the procedure to the person before beginning and during the procedure.

• Protect the person's rights during the procedure.
• Handle the person gently during the procedure.

PRE-PROCEDURE

1 Follow *Delegation Guidelines: Drainage Systems.* See *Promoting Safety and Comfort: Drainage Systems.*
2 Practice hand hygiene.
3 Collect the following:
  • Gloves
  • Drainage bag and tubing
  • Antiseptic wipes
  • Waterproof pad
  • Sterile cap and plug

  • Catheter clamp
  • Paper towels
  • Bedpan
  • Bath blanket
4 Arrange paper towels and equipment on the overbed table.
5 Identify the person. Check the ID bracelet against the assignment sheet. Also call the person by name.
6 Provide for privacy.

CHANGING A LEG BAG TO A DRAINAGE BAG—cont'd

PROCEDURE

7 Have the person sit on the side of the bed.
8 Decontaminate your hands. Put on the gloves.
9 Expose the catheter and leg bag.
10 Clamp the catheter (Fig. 21-15). This prevents urine from draining from the catheter into the drainage tubing.
11 Let urine drain from below the clamp into the drainage tubing. This empties the lower end of the catheter.
12 Help the person lie down.
13 Raise the bed rails if used. Raise the bed for good body mechanics.
14 Lower the bed rail near you if up.
15 Cover the person with a bath blanket. Fan-fold top linens to the foot of the bed. Expose the catheter and leg bag.
16 Place the waterproof pad under the person's leg.
17 Open the antiseptic wipes. Set them on the paper towels.
18 Open the package with the sterile cap and plug. Set the package on the paper towels. Do not let anything touch the sterile cap or plug (Fig. 21-16).
19 Open the package with the drainage bag and tubing.
20 Attach the drainage bag to the bed frame.

21 Disconnect the catheter from the drainage tubing. Do not let anything touch the ends.
22 Insert the sterile plug into the catheter end (Fig. 21-17). Touch only the end of the plug. Do not touch the part that goes inside the catheter. (If you contaminate the end of the catheter, wipe the end with an antiseptic wipe. Do so before you insert the sterile plug.)
23 Place the sterile cap on the end of the leg bag drainage tube (see Fig. 21-17). (If you contaminate the tubing end, wipe the end with an antiseptic wipe. Do so before you put on the sterile cap.)
24 Remove the cap from the new drainage tubing.
25 Remove the sterile plug from the catheter.
26 Insert the end of the drainage tubing into the catheter.
27 Remove the clamp from the catheter.
28 Loop the drainage tubing on the bed. Secure the tubing to the bottom linens.
29 Remove the leg bag. Place it in the bedpan.
30 Remove and discard the waterproof pad.
31 Cover the person. Remove the bath blanket.
32 Take the bedpan to the bathroom.
33 Remove the gloves. Practice hand hygiene.

POST-PROCEDURE

34 Provide for comfort. (See the inside of the front book cover.)
35 Place the signal light within reach.
36 Lower the bed to its lowest position.
37 Raise or lower bed rails. Follow the care plan.
38 Unscreen the person.
39 Put on clean gloves. Discard disposable items.
40 Empty the drainage bag. See procedure: *Emptying a Urinary Drainage Bag.*
41 Discard the drainage tubing and bag following agency policy. Or clean the bag following agency policy.

42 Clean and disinfect the bedpan. Place it in a clean cover.
43 Return the bedpan and other supplies to their proper place.
44 Remove the gloves. Practice hand hygiene.
45 Complete a safety check of the room. (See the inside of the front book cover.)
46 Follow agency policy for soiled linen.
47 Practice hand hygiene.
48 Report and record your observations.

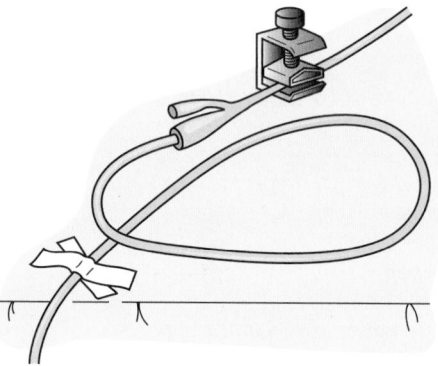

FIGURE 21-15 The clamped catheter prevents urine from draining out of the bladder. The clamp is applied *directly to the catheter*—not to the drainage tube.

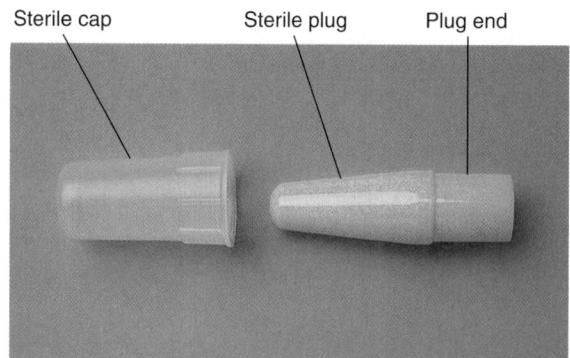

FIGURE 21-16 Sterile cap and catheter plug. The inside of the cap is sterile. Touch only the end of the plug.

EMPTYING A URINARY DRAINAGE BAG

✓ Quality of Life *Remember to:*

- Knock before entering the person's room.
- Address the person by name.
- Introduce yourself by name and title.
- Explain the procedure to the person before beginning and during the procedure.

- Protect the person's rights during the procedure.
- Handle the person gently during the procedure.

PRE-PROCEDURE

1 Follow *Delegation Guidelines: Drainage Systems,* p. 369. See *Promoting Safety and Comfort: Drainage Systems,* p. 369.
2 Collect the following:
   - Graduate (measuring container)
   - Gloves
   - Paper towels

3 Practice hand hygiene.
4 Identify the person. Check the ID bracelet against the assignment sheet. Call the person by name.
5 Provide for privacy.

PROCEDURE

6 Put on the gloves.
7 Place a paper towel on the floor. Place the graduate on top of it.
8 Position the graduate under the collection bag.
9 Open the clamp on the drain.
10 Let all urine drain into the graduate. Do not let the drain touch the graduate (Fig. 21-18).
11 Close and position the clamp (see Fig. 21-11).
12 Measure urine.
13 Remove and discard the paper towel.

14 Empty the contents of the graduate into the toilet and flush.
15 Rinse the graduate. Empty the rinse into the toilet and flush.
16 Clean and disinfect the graduate.
17 Return the graduate to its proper place.
18 Remove the gloves. Practice hand hygiene.
19 Record the time and amount on the intake and output (I&O) record (Chapter 23).

POST-PROCEDURE

20 Provide for comfort. (See the inside of the front cover.)
21 Place the signal light within reach.
22 Unscreen the person.

23 Complete a safety check of the room. (See the inside of the front book cover.)
24 Report and record the amount and other observations.

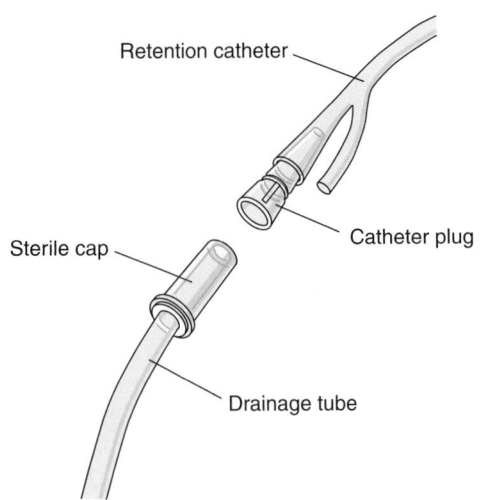

FIGURE 21-17 Sterile plug inserted into the end of the catheter. The sterile cap is on the end of the drainage tube.

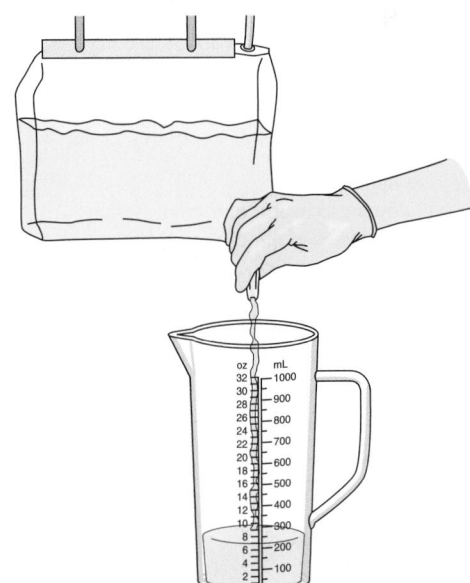

FIGURE 21-18 The clamp on the drainage bag is opened. The drain is directed into the graduate. The drain must not touch the inside of the graduate.

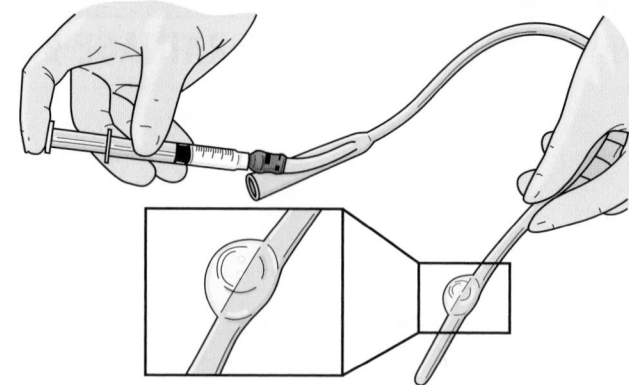

FIGURE 21-19 The balloon of an indwelling catheter is inflated with water. A syringe is used to inject the water.

◆ Removing Indwelling Catheters

An indwelling catheter has two lumens (passage-ways). Sterile water is injected through one lumen to inflate the balloon (Fig. 21-19). A syringe is used to inject the water. Urine drains from the bladder through the other lumen.

To remove the catheter, the balloon is deflated. You need a syringe large enough to hold all of the water in the balloon. Balloon size is marked at the end of the catheter.

A doctor's order is needed to remove a catheter. Most people need bladder training first (p. 374). Dysuria and frequency are common after removing catheters.

See *Delegation Guidelines: Removing Indwelling Catheters.*
See *Promoting Safety and Comfort: Removing Indwelling Catheters.*

DELEGATION GUIDELINES: Removing Indwelling Catheters

Before removing a catheter, make sure that:
- Your state allows you to perform the procedure
- The procedure is in your job description
- You know how to use the agency's supplies and equipment
- You review the procedure with the nurse
- A nurse is available to answer questions and to supervise you

If the above conditions are met, you need this information from the nurse:
- When to remove the catheter
- Balloon size
- Syringe size needed
- What observations to report and record:
  - The amount of urine in the drainage bag
  - Color, clarity, and odor of urine
  - Any particles in the urine
  - How the person tolerated the procedure
  - Complaints of pain, burning, irritation, or the need to urinate
  - Any other observations
- When to report observations
- What specific patient or resident concerns to report at once

---

PROMOTING SAFETY AND COMFORT: Removing Indwelling Catheters

SAFETY
All water must be removed from the balloon. If the balloon size is 5 mL, you should withdraw 5 mL of water into the syringe. Otherwise injury to the urethra is likely as the catheter is removed. Do not remove the catheter if water remains in the balloon.

Urine may contain microbes and blood. Follow Standard Precautions and the Bloodborne Pathogen Standard.

REMOVING AN INDWELLING CATHETER

✔ **Quality of Life** *Remember to:*

- Knock before entering the person's room.
- Address the person by name.
- Introduce yourself by name and title.
- Explain the procedure to the person before beginning and during the procedure.

- Protect the person's rights during the procedure.
- Handle the person gently during the procedure.

PRE-PROCEDURE

1 Follow *Delegation Guidelines: Removing Indwelling Catheters*. See *Promoting Safety and Comfort: Removing Indwelling Catheters.*
2 Practice hand hygiene.
3 Collect the following:
  - Disposable towel
  - Syringe as directed by the nurse
  - Disposable bag
  - Gloves
  - Bath blanket
4 Identify the person. Check the ID bracelet against the assignment sheet. Also call the person by name.
5 Provide for privacy.
6 Raise the bed for good body mechanics. Bed rails are up if used.

PROCEDURE

7 Lower the bed rail near you if up.
8 Decontaminate your hands. Put on the gloves.
9 Position and drape the person as for perineal care (Chapter 19).
10 Cover the person with a bath blanket.
11 Remove the tape or tube holder securing the catheter to the person.
12 Position the towel:
  a Female—between her legs
  b Male—over his thighs
13 Attach the syringe to the balloon port on the catheter.
14 Pull back on the syringe slowly. Withdraw all water from the balloon. Call for the nurse if you cannot remove all of the water.
15 Pull the catheter straight out. Remove the catheter gently. Do not remove the catheter if there is water in the balloon.
16 Discard the catheter into the bag.
17 Dry the perineal area with the towel. Discard the towel in the bag.
18 Remove the gloves. Practice hand hygiene.
19 Cover the person. Remove the bath blanket.

POST-PROCEDURE

20 Provide for comfort. (See the inside of the front book cover.)
21 Place the signal light within reach.
22 Lower the bed to its lowest position.
23 Raise or lower bed rails. Follow the care plan.
24 Unscreen the person.
25 Put on clean gloves. Discard disposable items.
26 Empty the drainage bag. See procedure: *Emptying a Urinary Drainage Bag*, p. 371. Note the amount of urine.
27 Discard the drainage tubing and bag following agency policy.
28 Remove the gloves. Practice hand hygiene.
29 Complete a safety check of the room. (See the inside of the front book cover.)
30 Decontaminate your hands.
31 Report and record your observations.

◆ Condom Catheters

Condom catheters are often used for incontinent men. They also are called *external catheters, Texas catheters,* and *urinary sheaths*. A condom catheter is a soft sheath that slides over the penis. Tubing connects the condom catheter and the drainage bag. Many men prefer leg bags (Fig. 21-20, p. 374).

Condom catheters are changed daily after perineal care. To apply a condom catheter, follow the manufacturer's instructions. Thoroughly wash the penis with soap and water. Then dry it before applying the catheter.

Some condom catheters are self-adhering. Adhesive inside the catheter adheres to the penis. Other catheters are secured in place with elastic tape. Use the elastic tape packaged with the catheter. Elastic tape expands when the penis changes size. This allows blood flow to the penis. *Never use adhesive tape to secure catheters. It does not expand. Blood flow to the penis is cut off, injuring the penis.*

See *Delegation Guidelines: Condom Catheters.*
See *Promoting Safety and Comfort: Condom Catheters.*

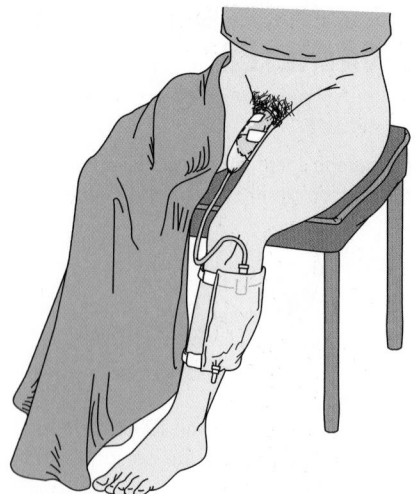

FIGURE 21-20 Condom catheter attached to a leg bag.

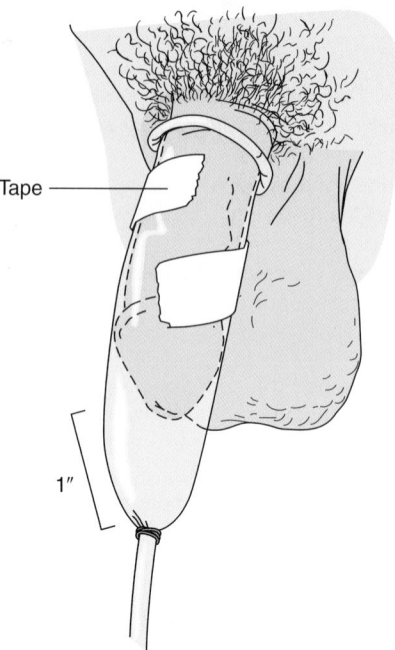

Tape

1"

FIGURE 21-21 A condom catheter applied to the penis. A 1-inch space is between the penis and the end of the catheter. Elastic tape is applied in a spiral fashion to secure the condom catheter to the penis.

DELEGATION GUIDELINES: Condom Catheters

Before removing or applying a condom catheter, you need this information from the nurse and the care plan:

• What size to use—small, medium, or large
• When to remove the catheter and apply a new one
• If a leg bag or standard drainage system is used
• What observations to report and record:
  • Reddened or open areas on the penis
  • Swelling of the penis
  • Color, clarity, and odor of urine
  • Particles in the urine
• When to report observations
• What specific patient or resident concerns to report at once

---

PROMOTING SAFETY AND COMFORT: Condom Catheters

SAFETY

Do not apply a condom catheter if the penis is red, irritated, or shows signs of skin breakdown. Report your observations to the nurse at once.

If you do not know how to use the condom catheters used at your agency, ask the nurse to show you the correct application. Then ask the nurse to observe you applying the catheter.

Blood must flow to the penis. If tape is needed, use elastic tape packaged with the catheter. Apply it in a spiral.

Urine may contain microbes and blood. Follow Standard Precautions and the Bloodborne Pathogen Standard.

COMFORT

To apply a condom catheter, you need to touch and handle the penis. This can embarrass the man. Some men become sexually aroused. Always act in a professional manner. If necessary, allow the man some privacy. Provide for his safety and place the urinal within reach. Tell him when you will return, and then leave the room. Knock before entering the room again.

BLADDER TRAINING

Bladder training helps some persons with urinary incontinence. Some persons need bladder training after indwelling catheter removal. Control of urination is the goal. Bladder control promotes comfort and quality of life. It also increases self-esteem. You assist with bladder training as directed by the nurse and the care plan.

There are two basic methods for bladder training:

▶ The person uses the toilet, commode, bedpan, or urinal at certain times. The person is given 15 or 20 minutes to start voiding. The rules for normal elimination are followed. The normal position for urination is assumed if possible. Privacy is important.

▶ The person has a catheter. The catheter is clamped to prevent urine flow from the bladder (see Fig. 21-15). It is usually clamped for 1 hour at first. Over time, it is clamped for 3 to 4 hours. Urine drains when the catheter is unclamped. When the catheter is removed, voiding is encouraged every 3 to 4 hours or as directed by the nurse and the care plan.

APPLYING A CONDOM CATHETER

✓ Quality of Life *Remember to:*

- Knock before entering the person's room.
- Address the person by name.
- Introduce yourself by name and title.
- Explain the procedure to the person before beginning and during the procedure.

- Protect the person's rights during the procedure.
- Handle the person gently during the procedure.

PRE-PROCEDURE

1 Follow *Delegation Guidelines: Condom Catheters.* See *Promoting Safety and Comfort: Condom Catheters.*
2 Practice hand hygiene.
3 Collect the following:
   - Condom catheter
   - Elastic tape
   - Drainage bag or leg bag
   - Cap for the drainage bag
   - Basin of warm water
   - Soap
   - Towel and washcloths
   - Bath blanket
   - Gloves
   - Waterproof pad
   - Paper towels
4 Arrange paper towels and equipment on the overbed table.
5 Identify the person. Check the ID bracelet against the assignment sheet. Also call the person by name.
6 Provide for privacy.
7 Raise the bed for good body mechanics. Bed rails are up if used.

PROCEDURE

8 Lower the bed rail near you if up.
9 Decontaminate your hands. Put on the gloves.
10 Cover the person with a bath blanket. Lower top linens to the knees.
11 Ask the person to raise his buttocks off the bed. Or turn him onto his side away from you.
12 Slide the waterproof pad under his buttocks.
13 Have the person lower his buttocks. Or turn him onto his back.
14 Secure the drainage bag to the bed frame. Or have a leg bag ready. Close the drain.
15 Expose the genital area.
16 Remove the condom catheter.
   a Remove the tape. Roll the sheath off the penis.
   b Disconnect the drainage tubing from the condom. Cap the drainage tube.
   c Discard the tape and condom.
17 Provide perineal care (Chapter 19). Observe the penis for reddened areas, skin breakdown, and irritation. Remove the gloves. Practice hand hygiene. Put on clean gloves.

18 Remove the protective backing from the condom. This exposes the adhesive strip.
19 Hold the penis firmly. Roll the condom onto the penis. Leave a 1-inch space between the penis and the end of the catheter (Fig. 21-21).
20 Secure the condom.
   a For a self-adhering condom: press the condom to the penis.
   b For a condom secured with elastic tape: apply elastic tape in a spiral (see Figure 21-21). Do not apply tape completely around the penis.
21 Make sure the penis tip does not touch the condom. Make sure the condom is not twisted.
22 Connect the condom to the drainage tubing. Coil and secure excess tubing on the bed. Or attach a leg bag.
23 Remove the waterproof pad and gloves. Discard them. Practice hand hygiene.
24 Cover the person. Remove the bath blanket.

POST-PROCEDURE

25 Provide comfort. (See the inside of the front book cover.)
26 Place the signal light within reach.
27 Lower the bed to its lowest position.
28 Raise or lower bed rails. Follow the care plan.
29 Unscreen the person.
30 Decontaminate your hands. Put on clean gloves.
31 Measure and record the amount of urine in the bag. Clean or discard the collection bag.

32 Clean and return the wash basin and other equipment. Return items to their proper place.
33 Remove the gloves. Practice hand hygiene.
34 Complete a safety check of the room. (See the inside of the front book cover.)
35 Report and record your observations.

REVIEW QUESTIONS

Circle the BEST answer.

1 Which is *false*?
 a Urine is normally clear and yellow or amber in color.
 b Urine normally has an ammonia odor.
 c Micturition usually occurs before going to bed and after sleep.
 d A person normally voids 1500 mL a day.

2 Which is *not* a rule for normal elimination?
 a Help the person assume a normal position for voiding.
 b Provide for privacy.
 c Help the person to the bathroom or commode. Or provide the bedpan or urinal as soon as requested.
 d Stay with the person who uses the bedpan.

3 The person using a standard bedpan is in
 a Fowler's position
 b The supine position
 c The prone position
 d The side-lying position

4 After using the urinal, the man should
 a Put it on the bedside stand
 b Use the signal light
 c Put it on the overbed table
 d Empty it

5 After a person uses a commode you should
 a Clean and disinfect the container, seat, and commode parts
 b Return the commode to the supply area
 c Get a new container
 d Get a new commode

6 Urinary incontinence
 a Is always permanent
 b Requires good skin care
 c Is treated with a catheter
 d Requires bladder training

7 Which is *not* a cause of functional incontinence?
 a Unanswered signal light
 b No signal light within reach
 c Problems removing clothing
 d Urinary tract infection

8 A person has an indwelling catheter. Which is *not* correct?
 a Keep the drainage bag above the level of the bladder.
 b Keep drainage tubing free of kinks.
 c Coil the drainage tubing on the bed.
 d Secure the catheter according to agency policy.

9 A person has an indwelling catheter. Which is *not* correct?
 a Tape any leaks at the connection site.
 b Follow Standard Precautions and the Bloodborne Pathogen Standard.
 c Empty the drainage bag at the end of your shift.
 d Report complaints of pain, burning, the need to void, or irritation at once.

10 A person has an indwelling catheter. You are going to turn the person from the left side to the right side. What should you do with the drainage bag?
 a Move it to the right side.
 b Keep it on the left side.
 c Hang it from an IV pole.
 d Remove the catheter and the drainage bag.

11 When giving catheter care, you clean the catheter
 a From the meatus down the catheter about 4 inches
 b From the meatus down the entire catheter
 c From the drainage tube connection up the catheter to the meatus
 d From the drainage tube connection up the catheter about 4 inches

12 You are going to remove an indwelling catheter. You
 a Attach a needle to the syringe
 b Check the balloon size
 c Tug on the catheter to see if it will come out
 d Use an antiseptic swab to clean the meatus

13 You are going to remove an indwelling catheter. It has a 5-mL balloon. You withdraw 3 mL. What should you do?
 a Call for the nurse.
 b Inject the fluid.
 c Pull the catheter out gently.
 d Cut the catheter.

14 Mr. Cooper has a condom catheter. You apply elastic tape
 a Completely around the penis
 b To the inner thigh
 c To the abdomen
 d In a spiral fashion

15 The goal of bladder training is to
 a Remove the catheter
 b Allow the person to walk to the bathroom
 c Gain control of urination
 d Heal the stoma

Answers to these questions are on p. 780.

Bowel Elimination

OBJECTIVES

- Define the key terms and key abbreviations listed in this chapter
- Describe normal defecation
- List the observations to make about defecation
- Identify the factors that affect bowel elimination
- Describe the common bowel elimination problems
- Explain how to promote comfort and safety during defecation
- Describe bowel training
- Explain why enemas are given
- Describe the common enema solutions
- Describe the rules for giving enemas
- Describe how to care for a person with an ostomy
- Perform the procedures described in this chapter

PROCEDURES

- Checking For a Fecal Impaction
- Removing a Fecal Impaction
- Giving a Cleansing Enema
- Giving a Small-Volume Enema
- Giving an Oil-Retention Enema
- Changing an Ostomy Pouch

KEY TERMS

colostomy A surgically created opening (stomy) between the colon (colo) and abdominal wall

constipation The passage of a hard, dry stool

defecation The process of excreting feces from the rectum through the anus; a bowel movement

dehydration The excessive loss of water from tissues

diarrhea The frequent passage of liquid stools

enema The introduction of fluid into the rectum and lower colon

fecal impaction The prolonged retention and buildup of feces in the rectum

fecal incontinence The inability to control the passage of feces and gas through the anus

feces The semi-solid mass of waste products in the colon that is expelled through the anus

flatulence The excessive formation of gas or air in the stomach and intestines

flatus Gas or air passed through the anus

ileostomy A surgically created opening (stomy) between the ileum (small intestine [ileo]) and the abdominal wall

ostomy A surgically created opening; see colostomy and ileostomy

peristalsis The alternating contraction and relaxation of intestinal muscles

stoma An opening

stool Excreted feces

suppository A cone-shaped, solid drug that is inserted into a body opening; it melts at body temperature

KEY ABBREVIATIONS

F Fahrenheit

GI Gastrointestinal

IV Intravenous

mL Milliliter

oz Ounce

SSE Soapsuds enema

Bowel elimination is a basic physical need. It is the excretion of wastes from the gastrointestinal system (Chapter 8). Many factors affect bowel elimination. They include privacy, habits, age, diet, exercise and activity, fluids, and drugs. Problems easily occur. Promoting normal bowel elimination is important. You assist patients and residents in meeting their elimination needs. See Box 22-1 for a review of the gastrointestinal tract.

NORMAL BOWEL ELIMINATION

Some people have a bowel movement every day. Others have one every 2 to 3 days. Some people have 2 or 3 bowel movements a day. Many people defecate after breakfast. Others do so in the evening.

Stools are normally brown. Bleeding in the stomach and small intestine causes black or tarry stools. Bleeding in the lower colon and rectum causes red-colored stools. So do beets, tomato juice or soup, red Jell-O, and foods with red food coloring. A diet high in green vegetables can cause green stools. Diseases and infection can cause clay-colored or white, pale, orange-colored, or green-colored stools.

Stools are normally soft, formed, moist, and shaped like the rectum. They have a normal odor caused by bacterial action in the intestines. Certain foods and drugs also cause odors.

See *Focus on Children and Older Persons: Normal Bowel Elimination.*

Observations

Your observations are used for the nursing process. Carefully observe stools before disposing of them. Ask the nurse to observe abnormal stools. Observe and report the following to the nurse. If allowed to chart, also record the following:

▶ Color
▶ Amount
▶ Consistency
▶ Presence of blood or mucus
▶ Odor
▶ Shape
▶ Frequency of defecation
▶ Complaints of pain or discomfort
See *Focus on Communication: Observations.*

FOCUS ON **CHILDREN** AND **OLDER PERSONS**

Normal Bowel Elimination

CHILDREN
Breast-fed infants have yellow stools. Stools range from thick liquid to very soft. Bottle-fed infants have liquid-like stools that are yellowish brown or greenish brown, pasty stools. Stool color and consistency change with solid foods.

Newborns usually have a bowel movement with every feeding. Frequency changes as they grow older. Some infants have 2 or 3 bowel movements a day. Others have just one.

BOX 22-1 The Gastrointestinal Tract: Body Structure and Function

The gastrointestinal (GI) tract is part of the digestive system (Chapter 8). Bowel elimination is the excretion of wastes through the GI tract. Foods and fluids are normally taken through the mouth. They are partially digested in the stomach. The partially digested food and fluids are called *chyme*.

Chyme passes from the stomach into the small intestine. Further digestion and absorption of nutrients occur as the chyme passes through the small bowel. Then chyme enters the large intestine (large bowel or colon) where fluid is absorbed. Chyme becomes less fluid and more solid in consistency. **Feces** refer to the semi-solid mass of waste products in the colon that are expelled through the anus.

Feces move through the intestines by peristalsis. **Peristalsis** is the alternating contraction and relaxation of intestinal muscles. The feces move through the large intestine to the rectum. Feces are stored in the rectum until excreted from the body (Fig. 22-1). **Defecation** (bowel movement) is the process of excreting feces from the rectum through the anus. **Stool** refers to excreted feces.

See Chapter 8 for more information.

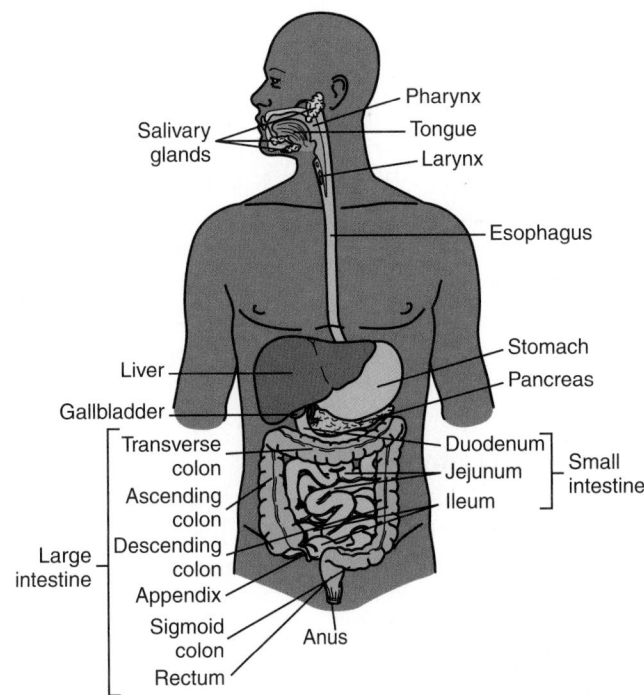

FIGURE 22-1 The gastrointestinal tract.

FOCUS ON COMMUNICATION

Observations

Many patients and residents tend to their own bowel elimination needs. However, information is still needed for the person's record and the nursing process. You many need to ask these questions:

- "Did you have a bowel movement today?"
- "Please tell me about your bowel movement."
- "When did you have a bowel movement?"
- "What was the amount?"
- "Were the stools formed or loose?"
- "What was the color?"
- "Did you have any bleeding, pain, or problems having a bowel movement?"
- "Did you pass any gas?"
- "How much gas did you pass?"
- "Do you need to pass more gas?"
- "Do you need help cleaning yourself?"

FACTORS AFFECTING BOWEL ELIMINATION

These factors affect stool frequency, consistency, color, and odor. The nurse considers them when using the nursing process to meet the person's elimination needs. Normal, regular elimination is the goal.

- *Privacy.* Bowel elimination is a private act. Odors and sounds are embarrassing. Lack of privacy can prevent defecation despite having the urge. Some people ignore the urge when others are present.
- *Habits.* Many people have a bowel movement after breakfast. Some drink a hot beverage, read, or take a walk. These activities are relaxing. Defecation is easier when a person is relaxed, not tense.

- *Diet—high-fiber foods.* High-fiber foods leave a residue for needed bulk. Fruits, vegetables, and whole grain cereals and breads are high in fiber. Many people do not eat enough fruits and vegetables. Some cannot chew these foods. They may not have teeth, or dentures fit poorly. Some people think that they cannot digest fruits and vegetables. So they refuse to eat them. In nursing centers, bran is added to cereal, prunes, or prune juice. These foods provide fiber and prevent constipation.
- *Diet—other foods.* Milk and milk products cause constipation in some people. They cause diarrhea in others. Chocolate and other foods cause similar reactions. Spicy foods can irritate the intestines. Frequent stools or diarrhea can result. Gas-forming foods stimulate peristalsis, which aids defecation. Such foods include onions, beans, cabbage, cauliflower, radishes, and cucumbers.
- *Fluids.* Feces contain water. Stool consistency depends on the amount of water absorbed in the colon. The amount of fluid intake, urine output, and vomiting are factors. Feces harden and dry when large amounts of water are absorbed or when fluid intake is poor. Hard, dry feces move slowly through the colon. Constipation can occur. Drinking 6 to 8 glasses of water daily promotes normal bowel elimination. Warm fluids—coffee, tea, hot cider, warm water—increase peristalsis.
- *Activity.* Exercise and activity maintain muscle tone and stimulate peristalsis. Irregular elimination and constipation often occur from inactivity and bedrest. Inactivity may result from disease, surgery, injury, and aging.

▶ *Drugs.* Drugs can prevent constipation or control diarrhea. Other drugs have diarrhea or constipation as side effects. Drugs for pain relief often cause constipation. Antibiotics (used to fight or prevent infections) often cause diarrhea. Diarrhea occurs when the antibiotics kill normal flora in the colon. Normal flora is needed to form feces.

▶ *Disability.* Some people cannot control bowel movements. They defecate whenever feces enter the rectum. A bowel training program is needed (p. 384).

▶ *Aging.* Age affects bowel elimination. See *Focus on Children and Older Persons: Factors Affecting Bowel Elimination.*

Safety and Comfort

The care plan includes measures to meet the person's elimination needs. It may involve diet, fluids, and exercise. Follow the measures in Box 22-2 to promote safety and comfort.

See *Teamwork and Time Management: Safety and Comfort.*

BOX 22-2 Safety and Comfort During Bowel Elimination

- Provide for privacy. Ask visitors to leave the room. Close doors and privacy curtains. Also close window coverings.
- Help the person to the toilet or commode. Or provide the bedpan as soon as requested.
- Wheel the person into the bathroom on the commode if possible. Place the commode over the toilet. This provides privacy. Remember to lock the commode wheels.
- Make sure the bedpan is warm.
- Position the person in a normal sitting or squatting position.
- Cover the person for warmth and privacy.
- Allow enough time for defecation.
- Place the signal light and toilet tissue within reach.
- Leave the room if the person can be alone. Check on the person every 5 minutes.
- Stay nearby if the person is weak or unsteady.
- Provide perineal care.
- Dispose of stools promptly. This reduces odors and prevents the spread of microbes.
- Assist the person with hand washing after elimination.
- Follow the care plan if the person has fecal incontinence. The care plan tells you when to assist with elimination.
- Follow Standard Precautions and the Bloodborne Pathogen Standard.

COMMON PROBLEMS

Common problems include constipation, fecal impaction, diarrhea, fecal incontinence, and flatulence.

Constipation

Constipation is the passage of a hard, dry stool. The person usually strains to have a bowel movement. Stools are large or marble-size. Large stools cause pain as they pass through the anus. Constipation occurs when feces move slowly through the bowel. This allows more time for water absorption. Common causes of constipation include:

▶ A low-fiber diet
▶ Ignoring the urge to defecate
▶ Decreased fluid intake
▶ Inactivity
▶ Drugs
▶ Aging
▶ Certain diseases

Dietary changes, fluids, and activity prevent or relieve constipation. So do drugs and enemas.

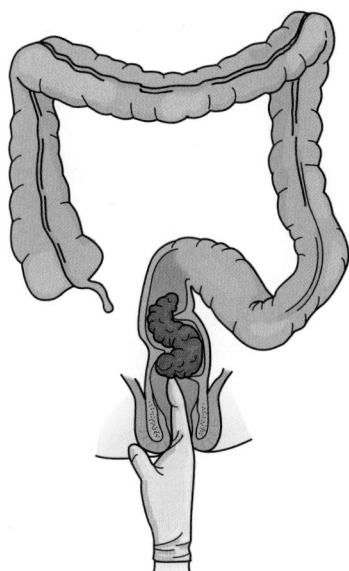

FIGURE 22-2 An index finger is used to check for an impaction.

◆ Fecal Impaction

A **fecal impaction** is the prolonged retention and buildup of feces in the rectum. Feces are hard or putty-like. Fecal impaction results if constipation is not relieved. The person cannot defecate. More water is absorbed from the already hard feces. Liquid feces pass around the hardened fecal mass in the rectum. The liquid feces seep from the anus.

The person tries many times to have a bowel movement. Abdominal discomfort, abdominal distention (swelling), nausea, cramping, and rectal pain are common. Older persons may have poor appetite or confusion. Some persons may have a fever. Report these signs and symptoms to the nurse.

A digital (finger) exam is done to check for an impaction. A lubricated, gloved finger is inserted into the rectum to feel for a hard mass (Fig. 22-2). The mass is felt in the lower rectum. Sometimes it is higher in the colon and out of reach. The digital exam often causes the urge to defecate. The doctor may order drugs and enemas to remove the impaction.

DELEGATION GUIDELINES: Fecal Impactions

Before you check for and remove fecal impactions, make sure that:
- Your state allows you to perform such procedures
- The procedures are in your job description
- You have the necessary education and training
- You review the procedures with a nurse
- A nurse is available to answer questions and to supervise you

If the above conditions are met, you need the following information from the nurse:
- What the doctor's order says
- If you should remove the impaction if one is felt
- When to take the person's pulse
- What pulse rates to report at once
- If the nurse needs to observe removed feces or the person's bowel movement
- What observations to report and record:
  - Color amount, consistency, and odor of feces
  - Signs of bleeding
  - Complaints of pain or discomfort
  - How the person tolerated the procedure
- When to report observations
- What specific patient or resident concerns to report at once

---

PROMOTING SAFETY AND COMFORT: Fecal Impactions

Safety
You must be very careful and gentle. Rectal bleeding can occur. Contact with feces is likely. They may contain microbes or blood. Follow Standard Precautions and the Bloodborne Pathogen Standard.

Sometimes the fecal mass is removed with a gloved finger. This is called *digital removal of an impaction*. A finger is hooked around a piece of feces. Then the finger and feces are removed. The stool is dropped into the bedpan. The process is repeated as needed. Most people find the procedure uncomfortable and embarrassing.

Checking for and removing impactions are very dangerous. The vagus nerve in the rectum can be stimulated. This nerve also affects the heart. Stimulation of the vagus nerve slows the heart rate. The heart rate can slow to dangerous levels in some persons.

See *Delegation Guidelines: Fecal Impactions.*
See *Promoting Safety and Comfort: Fecal Impactions.*

CHECKING FOR A FECAL IMPACTION

✔ Quality of Life *Remember to:*

- Knock before entering the person's room.
- Address the person by name.
- Introduce yourself by name and title.
- Explain the procedure to the person before beginning and during the procedure.

- Protect the person's rights during the procedure.
- Handle the person gently during the procedure.

PRE-PROCEDURE

1 Follow *Delegation Guidelines: Fecal Impactions,* p. 381. See *Promoting Safety and Comfort: Fecal Impactions,* p. 381.
2 Practice hand hygiene.
3 Collect the following:
- Bedpan and cover
- Bath blanket
- Toilet tissue
- Gloves
- Lubricant
- Waterproof pad

- Basin of warm water
- Soap
- Washcloth
- Bath towel
4 Decontaminate your hands.
5 Identify the person. Check the ID bracelet against the assignment sheet. Also call the person by name.
6 Provide for privacy.
7 Raise the bed for good body mechanics. Bed rails are up if used.

PROCEDURE

8 Lower the bed rail near you if up.
9 Cover the person with a bath blanket. Fan-fold top linens to the foot of the bed.
10 Position the person in Sims' position or in a left side-lying position.
11 Put on the gloves.
12 Place the waterproof pad under the buttocks.
13 Expose the anal area.
14 Lubricate your gloved index finger.
15 Ask the person to take a deep breath through his or her mouth.
16 Insert the gloved finger while the person is taking a deep breath.
17 Check for a fecal mass.
18 Remove your finger.
19 Remove the gloves, and practice hand hygiene. Put on clean gloves.
20 Help the person onto the bedpan. Raise the head of the bed, and raise the bed rail if used. Or assist the person to the bathroom or commode. The person wears a robe and non-skid footwear when up. The bed is in the lowest position.

21 Place the signal light and toilet tissue within reach. Remind the person not to flush the toilet.
22 Discard disposable items.
23 Remove the gloves. Practice hand hygiene.
24 Leave the room if the person can be left alone.
25 Return when the person signals. Or check on the person every 5 minutes. Knock before entering.
26 Decontaminate your hands, and put on gloves. Lower the bed rail if up.
27 Observe stools for amount, color, consistency, shape, and odor.
28 Provide perineal care as needed.
29 Remove the waterproof pad.
30 Empty, clean, and disinfect equipment. Flush the toilet after the nurse observes the bowel movement.
31 Return equipment to its proper place.
32 Remove the gloves, and practice hand hygiene.
33 Assist with hand washing. Wear gloves for this step.
34 Cover the person. Remove the bath blanket.

POST-PROCEDURE

35 Provide for comfort. (See the inside of the front book cover.)
36 Place the signal light within reach.
37 Lower the bed to its lowest position.
38 Raise or lower bed rails. Follow the care plan.
39 Unscreen the person.

40 Complete a safety check of the room. (See the inside of the front book cover.)
41 Follow agency policy for dirty linen and used supplies.
42 Practice hand hygiene.
43 Report and record your observations.

REMOVING A FECAL IMPACTION

✔ Quality of Life *Remember to:*

- Knock before entering the person's room.
- Address the person by name.
- Introduce yourself by name and title.
- Explain the procedure to the person before beginning and during the procedure.

- Protect the person's rights during the procedure.
- Handle the person gently during the procedure.

PROCEDURE

1 Follow steps 1 through 10 in procedure: *Checking for a Fecal Impaction.*
2 Check the person's pulse. Note the rate and rhythm.
3 Decontaminate your hands. Put on the gloves.
4 Place the waterproof pad under the buttocks.
5 Expose the anal area.
6 Lubricate your gloved index finger.
7 Ask the person to take a deep breath through the mouth.
8 Insert your lubricated, gloved index finger.
9 Hook your index finger around a small piece of feces.
10 Remove your finger and the feces.
11 Drop the stool into the bedpan.
12 Clean your finger with toilet tissue. Place the toilet tissue in the bedpan.
13 Repeat steps 7 through 12 until you no longer feel feces.
14 *Check the person's pulse at intervals. Use your clean gloved hand. Note the rate and rhythm. Stop the procedure if the pulse rate has slowed or if the rhythm is irregular.*

15 Wipe the anal area with toilet tissue.
16 Cover the person with a bath blanket.
17 Cover the bedpan.
18 Remove and discard the gloves. Practice hand hygiene, and put on clean gloves.
19 Raise the bed rail if used. Take the bedpan to the bathroom.
20 Empty, clean, and disinfect the bedpan.
21 Return the bedpan to the bedside stand.
22 Remove and discard the gloves. Practice hand hygiene.
23 Put on clean gloves.
24 Provide perineal care.
25 Remove the waterproof pad and your gloves. Practice hand hygiene.
26 Cover the person. Remove the bath blanket.

POST-PROCEDURE

27 Provide for comfort. (See the inside of the front book cover.)
28 Place the signal light within reach.
29 Lower the bed to its lowest position.
30 Raise or lower bed rails. Follow the care plan.
31 Unscreen the person.
32 Clean and return equipment to its proper place. Discard disposable items. (Wear gloves for this step.)

33 Complete a safety check of the room. (See the inside of the front book cover.)
34 Follow agency policy for dirty linen.
35 Practice hand hygiene.
36 Report and record your observations.

Diarrhea

Diarrhea is the frequent passage of liquid stools. Feces move through the intestines rapidly. This reduces the time for fluid absorption. The need to defecate is urgent. Some people cannot get to a bathroom in time. Abdominal cramping, nausea, and vomiting may occur.

Causes of diarrhea include infections, some drugs, irritating foods, and microbes in food and water. Diet and drugs are ordered to reduce peristalsis. You need to:

▶ Assist with elimination needs promptly.
▶ Dispose of stools promptly. This prevents odors and the spread of microbes.
▶ Give good skin care. Liquid stools irritate the skin. So does frequent wiping with toilet tissue. Skin breakdown and pressure ulcers are risks.

Fluid lost through diarrhea is replaced. Otherwise dehydration occurs. **Dehydration** is the excessive loss of water from tissues. The person has pale or flushed skin, dry skin, and a coated tongue. The urine is dark and scant in amount (oliguria). Thirst, weakness, dizziness, and confusion also occur. Falling blood pressure and increased pulse and respirations are serious signs. Death can occur. The nursing process is used to meet the person's fluid needs. The doctor may order IV (intravenous) fluids in severe cases (Chapter 24).

Diarrhea

CHILDREN

Infants and young children have large amounts of body water. They are at risk for dehydration. Death can be rapid. Report any liquid or watery stool at once. Ask the nurse to observe the stool. Note the number of wet diapers. Infants wet less when dehydrated.

OLDER PERSONS

Older persons are at risk for dehydration. The amount of body water decreases with aging. Many diseases common in older persons affect body fluids. So do many drugs. Report signs of diarrhea at once. Ask the nurse to observe the stool. Death is a risk when dehydration is not recognized and treated.

Fecal Incontinence

CHILDREN

Infants and toddlers normally have fecal incontinence until toilet trained.

OLDER PERSONS

Persons with dementia may smear stools on themselves, furniture, and walls. Some are not aware of having bowel movements. Some resist care. Follow the person's care plan. The measures for urinary incontinence (Chapter 21) may be part of the care plan. Be patient. Ask for help from co-workers. Talk to the nurse if you have problems keeping the person clean.

Microbes can cause diarrhea. Preventing the spread of infection is important. Always follow Standard Precautions and the Bloodborne Pathogen Standard when in contact with stools.

See *Focus on Children and Older Persons: Diarrhea.*

Fecal Incontinence

Fecal incontinence is the inability to control the passage of feces and gas through the anus. Causes include:

▶ Intestinal diseases
▶ Nervous system diseases and injuries
▶ Fecal impaction
▶ Diarrhea
▶ Some drugs
▶ Chronic illness
▶ Aging
▶ Mental health problems or dementia (Chapters 43 and 44)—the person may not recognize the need for or act of defecating
▶ Not answering signal lights when help is needed with elimination
▶ Not getting to the bathroom in time
▶ Not finding the bathroom when in a new setting

Fecal incontinence affects the person emotionally. Frustration, embarrassment, anger, and humiliation are common. The person may need:

▶ Bowel training
▶ Help with elimination after meals and every 2 to 3 hours
▶ Incontinence products to keep garments and linens clean
▶ Good skin care

See *Focus on Children and Older Persons: Fecal Incontinence.*

Flatulence

Gas and air are normally in the stomach and intestines. They are expelled through the mouth (burping, belching, eructating) and anus. Gas or air passed through the anus is called **flatus. Flatulence** is the excessive formation of gas or air in the stomach and intestines. Causes include:

▶ Swallowing air while eating and drinking (This includes chewing gum, eating fast, drinking through a straw, and drinking carbonated beverages. Tense or anxious people may swallow large amounts of air when drinking.)
▶ Bacterial action in the intestines
▶ Gas-forming foods (onions, beans, cabbage, cauliflower, radishes, and cucumbers)
▶ Constipation
▶ Bowel and abdominal surgeries
▶ Drugs that decrease peristalsis

If flatus is not expelled, the intestines distend. That is, they swell or enlarge from the pressure of gases. Abdominal cramping or pain, shortness of breath, and a swollen abdomen occur. "Bloating" is a common complaint. Exercise, walking, moving in bed, and the left side-lying position often produce flatus. Doctors may order enemas and drugs to relieve flatulence.

BOWEL TRAINING

Bowel training has two goals:

▶ To gain control of bowel movements.
▶ To develop a regular pattern of elimination. Fecal impaction, constipation, and fecal incontinence are prevented.

Meals, especially breakfast, stimulate the urge to defecate. The person's usual time of day for defecation is noted on the care plan. So is toilet, commode, or bedpan use. Offer help with elimination at the times noted. Factors that promote elimination are part of the care plan and bowel training program. These include a high-fiber diet, increased fluids, warm fluids, activity, and privacy. The nurse tells you about a person's bowel training program.

The doctor may order a suppository to stimulate defecation. A **suppository** is a cone-shaped, solid drug that is inserted into a body opening. It melts at body temperature. A nurse inserts a rectal suppository into the rectum (Fig. 22-3). A bowel movement occurs about 30 minutes later.

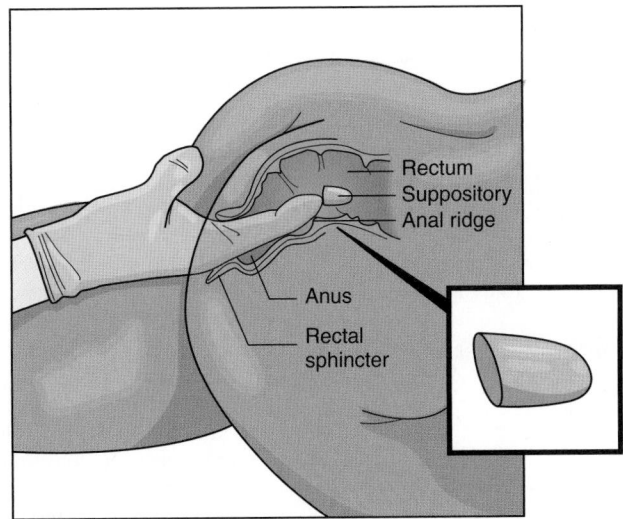

FIGURE 22-3 The suppository *(inset)* is inserted into the rectum.

ENEMAS

An **enema** is the introduction of fluid into the rectum and lower colon. Doctors order enemas:

▶ To remove feces
▶ To relieve constipation, fecal impaction, or flatulence
▶ To clean the bowel of feces before certain surgeries and diagnostic procedures

Safety and comfort measures for bowel elimination are practiced when giving an enema (see Box 22-2). So are the rules in Box 22-3.

The doctor orders the enema solution. The solution depends on the enema's purpose:

▶ *Tap-water enema*—obtained from a faucet.
▶ *Saline enema*—a solution of salt and water. For adults, add 1 to 2 teaspoons of table salt to 500 to 1000 mL (milliliters) of tap water.
▶ *Soapsuds enema (SSE)*—for adults, add 3 to 5 mL (milliliters) of castile soap to 500 to 1000 mL of tap water.
▶ *Small-volume enema*—the adult size contains about 120 mL (4 ounces [4 oz]) of solution. The child size contains 60 mL (2 ounces [2 oz]). The commercially prepared enema is ready to use.
▶ *Oil-retention enema*—mineral, olive, or cottonseed oil. The adult size contains about 120 mL (4 ounces [4 oz]) of solution. Children receive half the bottle—60 mL (2 ounces [2 oz]). The commercially prepared enema is ready to use.

Other enema solutions may be ordered. Consult with the nurse and use the agency's procedure manual to safely prepare and give enemas. You do not give enemas that contain drugs. Nurses give them.

See *Delegation Guidelines: Enemas,* p. 386.
See *Promoting Safety and Comfort: Enemas,* p. 386.

BOX 22-3 Safety and Comfort Measures for Giving Enemas

• Have the person void first. This increases the person's comfort during the enema procedure.
• Measure solution temperature with a bath thermometer. See *Delegation Guidelines: Enemas,* p. 386.
• Give the amount of solution ordered.
• Position the person as the nurse directs. The Sims' position or the left side-lying position is preferred.
• Ask the nurse and check the procedure manual for how far to insert the enema tubing. It is usually inserted 2 to 4 inches in adults.
• Lubricate the enema tip before inserting it.
• Stop tube insertion if you feel resistance, the person complains of pain, or bleeding occurs.
• Ask the nurse how high to raise the enema bag. For adults, it is usually held 12 inches above the anus.
• Give the solution slowly. Usually it takes 10 to 15 minutes to give 750 to 1000 mL.
• Hold the enema tube in place while giving the solution.
• Ask the nurse how long the person should retain the solution. The length of time depends on the amount and type of solution.
• Make sure the bathroom will be vacant when the person needs to defecate. Make sure that another person will not use the bathroom. If the person uses the commode, have the commode ready.
• Ask the nurse to observe the enema results.

DELEGATION GUIDELINES: Enemas

Some states and agencies let nursing assistants give enemas. Others do not. Before giving an enema, make sure that:
* Your state allows you to perform the procedure
* The procedure is in your job description
* You have the necessary education and training
* You review the procedure with the nurse
* A nurse is available to answer questions and to supervise you
  If the above conditions are met, you need this information from the nurse:
* What type of enema to give—cleansing, small-volume, or oil-retention
* What size enema tube to use
* When to give the enema
* How many times to repeat the enema
* The amount of solution ordered by the doctor—usually 500 to 1000 mL for a cleansing enema (for adults)
* How much castile soap to use for an SSE
* How much salt to use for a saline enema
* What the solution temperature should be—usually body temperature (98.6° F); sometimes warmer temperatures are used (105° F for adults; 100° F for children)

* How to position the person—Sims' or the left side-lying position
* How far to insert the enema tubing—usually 2 to 4 inches for adults
* How high to hold the solution container—usually 12 inches above the anus
* How fast to give the solution—750 to 1000 mL are usually given over 10 to 15 minutes
* How long the person should try to retain the solution
* What to report and record:
  * The amount of solution given
  * If you noted bleeding or resistance when inserting the tube
  * How long the person retained the enema solution
  * Color, amount, consistency, shape, and odor of stools
  * Complaints of cramping, pain, or discomfort
  * Complaints of nausea or weakness
  * How the person tolerated the procedure
* When to report observations
* What specific patient or resident concerns to report at once

PROMOTING SAFETY AND COMFORT: Enemas

SAFETY
Enemas are usually safe procedures. Many people give themselves enemas at home. However, enemas are dangerous for older persons and those with certain heart and kidney diseases.

Contact with stools is likely when giving enemas. They may contain microbes and blood. Follow Standard Precautions and the Bloodborne Pathogen Standard.

COMFORT
Before starting the procedure, make sure that the bathroom will be available for the person's use. If the person will use the commode or bedpan, make sure the device is ready. Always keep a bedpan nearby in case the person starts to expel the enema solution and stools. Mental comfort is promoted when the person knows that the bathroom, commode, or bedpan is ready for his or her use.

Make sure the person is comfortable in the Sims' or left side-lying position. When comfortable, it is easier for the person to tolerate the procedure.

Prevent cramping by:
* Using the correct water temperature. Cool water causes cramping.
* Giving the solution slowly.

◆ The Cleansing Enema

Cleansing enemas clean the bowel of feces and flatus. They relieve constipation and fecal impaction. They are needed before certain surgeries and diagnostic procedures. Cleansing enemas take effect in 10 to 20 minutes.

The doctor orders a tap water, saline, or soapsuds enema. The doctor may order *enemas until clear.* This means that enemas are given until the return solution is clear and free of stools. Ask the nurse how many enemas to give. Agency policy may allow repeating enemas 2 or 3 times.

Tap-water enemas can be dangerous. The colon may absorb some of the water into the bloodstream. This creates a fluid imbalance. *Only one tap-water enema is given. Do not repeat the enema.* Repeated enemas increase the risk of excessive fluid absorption.

The *saline enema* solution is similar to body fluid. However, some of the salt solution may be absorbed. This too can cause a fluid imbalance. When excess salt is in the body, the body retains water.

Soapsuds enemas irritate the bowel's mucous lining. Repeated enemas can damage the bowel. So can using more than 3 to 5 mL of castile soap or stronger soaps.

See *Focus on Children and Older Persons: The Cleansing Enema.*

FOCUS ON **CHILDREN** AND **OLDER PERSONS**

The Cleansing Enema

CHILDREN

Saline enemas are used for cleansing enemas in children. Check with the nurse for the amount of solution to give. These are guidelines:

- Infants—50 to 200 mL
- Toddlers—200 to 300 mL
- School-age children—300 to 500 mL
- 12 years and older—500 to 1000 mL

The nurse tells you how far to insert the enema tube. These are guidelines:

- Infants—1 to 1½ inches
- Toddlers and older children—2 to 3 inches, but never more than 4 inches

Infants cannot tell you they hurt. If cramping occurs, the child will draw up the knees. The child's cry is higher-pitched than normal.

In children, cleansing enemas take effect in about 2 to 5 minutes.

GIVING A CLEANSING ENEMA

✔ Quality of Life *Remember to:*

- Knock before entering the person's room.
- Address the person by name.
- Introduce yourself by name and title.
- Explain the procedure to the person before beginning and during the procedure.
- Protect the person's rights during the procedure.
- Handle the person gently during the procedure.

PRE-PROCEDURE

1. Follow *Delegation Guidelines: Enemas.* See *Promoting Safety and Comfort: Enemas.*
2. Practice hand hygiene.
3. Collect the following before going to the person's room:
   - Disposable enema kit as directed by the nurse (enema bag, tube, clamp, and waterproof pad)
   - Bath thermometer
   - Waterproof pad (if not part of the enema kit)
   - Water-soluble lubricant
   - 3 to 5 mL (1 teaspoon) of castile soap or 1 to 2 teaspoons of salt
   - IV pole
4. Arrange collected items in the person's room and bathroom.
5. Decontaminate your hands.
6. Identify the person. Check the ID bracelet against the assignment sheet. Also call the person by name.
7. Put on gloves.
8. Collect the following:
   - Commode or bedpan and cover
   - Gloves
   - Toilet tissue
   - Bath blanket
   - Robe and non-skid footwear
   - Paper towels
9. Provide for privacy.
10. Raise the bed for good body mechanics. Bed rails are up if used.

PROCEDURE

11. Lower the bed rail near you if up.
12. Remove the gloves, and practice hand hygiene. Put on clean gloves.
13. Cover the person with a bath blanket. Fan-fold top linens to the foot of the bed.
14. Position the IV pole so the enema bag is 12 inches above the anus. Or it is at the height directed by the nurse.
15. Raise the bed rail if used.

Continued

GIVING A CLEANSING ENEMA—cont'd

PROCEDURE—cont'd

16 Prepare the enema:
  a Close the clamp on the tube.
  b Adjust water flow until it is lukewarm.
  c Fill the enema bag for the amount ordered.
  d Measure water temperature with the bath thermometer. The nurse tells you what temperature to use.
  e Prepare the solution as directed by the nurse:
    (1) Tap water: add nothing
    (2) Saline enema: add salt as directed
    (3) Soapsuds enema: add castile soap as directed
  f Stir the solution with the bath thermometer. Scoop off any suds (SSE).
  g Seal the bag.
  h Hang the bag on the IV pole.
17 Lower the bed rail near you if up.
18 Position the person in Sims' position or in a left side-lying position.
19 Place a waterproof pad under the buttocks.
20 Expose the anal area.
21 Place the bedpan behind the person.
22 Position the enema tube in the bedpan. Remove the cap from the tubing.
23 Open the clamp. Let solution flow through the tube to remove air. Clamp the tube.
24 Lubricate the tube 2 to 4 inches from the tip.
25 Separate the buttocks to see the anus.
26 Ask the person to take a deep breath through the mouth.
27 Insert the tube gently 2 to 4 inches into the adult's rectum (Fig. 22-4). Do this when the person is exhaling. Stop if the person complains of pain, you feel resistance, or bleeding occurs.
28 Check the amount of solution in the bag.
29 Unclamp the tube. Give the solution slowly (Fig. 22-5).
30 Ask the person to take slow deep breaths. This helps the person relax.
31 Clamp the tube if the person needs to defecate, has cramping, or starts to expel solution. Also clamp the tube if the person is sweating or complains of nausea or weakness. Unclamp when symptoms subside.

32 Give the amount of solution ordered. Stop if the person cannot tolerate the procedure.
33 Clamp the tube before it is empty. This prevents air from entering the bowel.
34 Hold toilet tissue around the tube and against the anus. Remove the tube.
35 Discard toilet tissue into the bedpan.
36 Wrap the tubing tip with paper towels. Place it inside the enema bag.
37 Assist the person to the bathroom or commode. The person wears a robe and non-skid footwear when up. The bed is in the lowest position. Or help the person onto the bedpan. Raise the head of the bed. Raise or lower bed rails according to the care plan.
38 Place the signal light and toilet tissue within reach. Remind the person not to flush the toilet.
39 Discard disposable items.
40 Remove the gloves. Decontaminate your hands.
41 Leave the room if the person can be left alone.
42 Return when the person signals. Or check on the person every 5 minutes. Knock before entering the room or bathroom.
43 Decontaminate your hands, and put on gloves. Lower the bed rail if up.
44 Observe enema results for amount, color, consistency, shape, and odor. Call the nurse to observe the results.
45 Provide perineal care as needed.
46 Remove the waterproof pad.
47 Empty, clean, and disinfect equipment. Flush the toilet after the nurse observes the results.
48 Return equipment to its proper place.
49 Remove the gloves, and practice hand hygiene.
50 Assist with hand washing. Wear gloves for this step.
51 Cover the person. Remove the bath blanket.

POST-PROCEDURE

52 Provide for comfort. (See the inside of the front book cover.)
53 Place the signal light within reach.
54 Lower the bed to its lowest position.
55 Raise or lower bed rails. Follow the care plan.
56 Unscreen the person.

57 Complete a safety check of the room. (See the inside of the front book cover.)
58 Follow agency policy for dirty linen and used supplies.
59 Practice hand hygiene.
60 Report and record your observations.

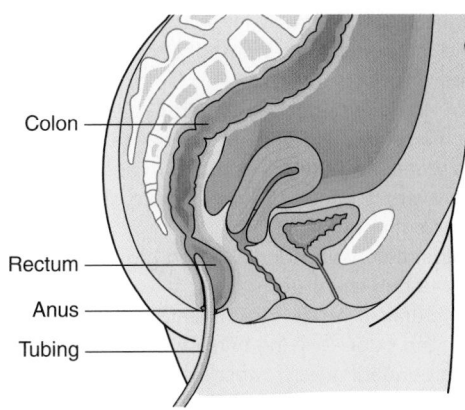

FIGURE 22-4 Enema tubing inserted into the adult rectum.

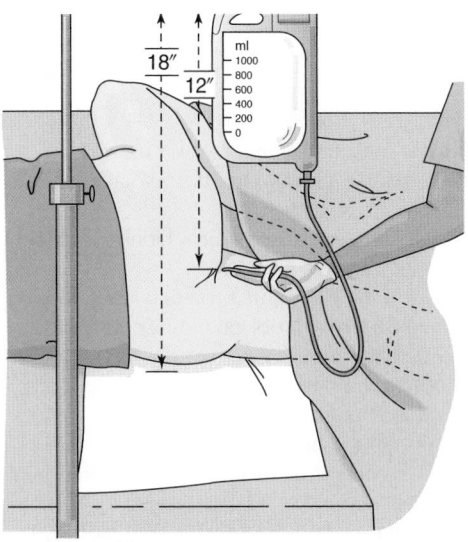

FIGURE 22-5 Giving an enema. The person is in Sims' position. The enema bag hangs from an IV pole. The bag is 12 inches above the anus and 18 inches above the mattress.

 The Small-Volume Enema

Small-volume enemas irritate and distend the rectum. This causes defecation. They are often ordered for constipation or when the bowel does not need complete cleansing.

These enemas are ready to give. The solution is usually given at room temperature. To give the enema, squeeze and roll up the plastic bottle from the bottom. Do not release pressure on the bottle. Otherwise, solution is drawn from the rectum back into the bottle.

Urge the person to retain the solution until there is a need to defecate. This usually takes about 5 to 10 minutes. Staying in the Sims' or left side-lying position helps to retain the enema.

GIVING A SMALL-VOLUME ENEMA

✔ Quality of Life *Remember to:*

- Knock before entering the person's room.
- Address the person by name.
- Introduce yourself by name and title.
- Explain the procedure to the person before beginning and during the procedure.
- Protect the person's rights during the procedure.
- Handle the person gently during the procedure.

PRE-PROCEDURE

1 Follow *Delegation Guidelines: Enemas*, p. 386. See *Promoting Safety and Comfort: Enemas*, p. 386.
2 Practice hand hygiene.
3 Collect the following before going to the person's room:
   - Small-volume enema
   - Waterproof pad
4 Arrange items in the person's room.
5 Decontaminate your hands.
6 Identify the person. Check the ID bracelet against the assignment sheet. Also call the person by name.
7 Put on gloves.

8 Collect the following:
   - Commode or bedpan
   - Waterproof pad
   - Toilet tissue
   - Gloves
   - Robe and non-skid footwear
   - Bath blanket
9 Provide for privacy.
10 Raise the bed for good body mechanics. Bed rails are up if used.

Continued

Bowel Elimination **Chapter 22** **389**

GIVING A SMALL-VOLUME ENEMA — cont'd

PROCEDURE

11 Lower the bed rail near you if up.
12 Remove the gloves, and decontaminate your hands. Put on clean gloves.
13 Cover the person with a bath blanket. Fan-fold top linens to the foot of the bed.
14 Position the person in Sims' or a left side-lying position.
15 Place the waterproof pad under the buttocks.
16 Expose the anal area.
17 Position the bedpan near the person.
18 Remove the cap from the enema tip.
19 Separate the buttocks to see the anus.
20 Ask the person to take a deep breath through the mouth.
21 Insert the enema tip 2 inches into the adult's rectum (Fig. 22-6). Do this when the person is exhaling. Insert the tip gently. Stop if the person complains of pain, you feel resistance, or bleeding occurs.
22 Squeeze and roll the bottle gently. Release pressure on the bottle after you remove the tip from the rectum.
23 Put the bottle into the box, tip first.
24 Assist the person to the bathroom or commode. The person wears a robe and non-skid footwear when up. The bed is in the lowest position. Or help the person onto the bedpan, and raise the head of the bed. Raise or lower bed rails according to the care plan.

25 Place the signal light and toilet tissue within reach. Remind the person not to flush the toilet.
26 Discard disposable items.
27 Remove the gloves. Practice hand hygiene.
28 Leave the room if the person can be left alone.
29 Return when the person signals. Or check on the person every 5 minutes. Knock before entering the room or bathroom.
30 Decontaminate your hands. Put on gloves.
31 Lower the bed rail if up.
32 Observe enema results for amount, color, consistency, shape, and odor. Call the nurse to observe the results.
33 Provide perineal care as needed.
34 Remove the waterproof pad.
35 Empty, clean, and disinfect equipment. Flush the toilet after the nurse observes the results.
36 Return equipment to its proper place.
37 Remove the gloves, and practice hand hygiene.
38 Assist with hand washing. Wear gloves for this step.
39 Cover the person. Remove the bath blanket.

POST-PROCEDURE

40 Provide for comfort. (See the inside of the front book cover.)
41 Place the signal light within reach.
42 Lower the bed to its lowest position.
43 Raise or lower bed rails. Follow the care plan.
44 Unscreen the person.

45 Complete a safety check of the room. (See the inside of the front book cover.)
46 Follow agency policy for dirty linen and used supplies.
47 Practice hand hygiene.
48 Report and record your observations.

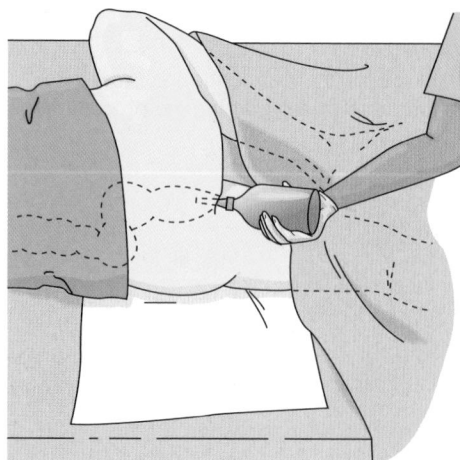

FIGURE 22-6 The small-volume enema tip is inserted 2 inches into the rectum.

◆ The Oil-Retention Enema

Oil-retention enemas relieve constipation and fecal impactions. The oil is retained for 30 to 60 minutes or longer (1 to 3 hours). Retaining oil softens feces and lubricates the rectum. This lets feces pass with ease. Most oil-retention enemas are commercially prepared.

See *Promoting Safety and Comfort: The Oil-Retention Enema.*

PROMOTING SAFETY AND COMFORT: The Oil-Retention Enema

SAFETY

The oil-retention enema is retained for at least 30 to 60 minutes. You will leave the room after giving the enema. Make sure you check on the person often. After checking on the person, tell him or her when you will return. Remind the person to signal for you if he or she needs help.

GIVING AN OIL-RETENTION ENEMA

✔ Quality of Life *Remember to:*

- Knock before entering the person's room.
- Address the person by name.
- Introduce yourself by name and title.
- Explain the procedure to the person before beginning and during the procedure.

- Protect the person's rights during the procedure.
- Handle the person gently during the procedure.

PRE-PROCEDURE

1 Follow *Delegation Guidelines: Enemas,* p. 386. See *Promoting Safety and Comfort:*
   - *Enemas,* p. 386
   - *Oil-Retention Enemas*
2 Practice hand hygiene.
3 Collect the following before going to the person's room:
   - Oil-retention enema
   - Waterproof pads
4 Arrange items in the person's room.

5 Decontaminate your hands.
6 Identify the person. Check the ID bracelet against the assignment sheet. Also call the person by name.
7 Put on gloves.
8 Collect the following:
   - Gloves
   - Bath blanket
9 Provide for privacy.
10 Raise the bed for good body mechanics. Bed rails are up if used.

PROCEDURE

11 Follow steps 11 through 23 in procedure: *Giving a Small-Volume Enema.*
12 Cover the person. Leave him or her in the Sims' or left side-lying position.

13 Encourage him or her to retain the enema for the time ordered.
14 Place more waterproof pads on the bed if needed.
15 Remove the gloves. Practice hand hygiene.

POST-PROCEDURE

16 Provide for comfort. (See the inside of the front book cover.)
17 Place the signal light within reach.
18 Lower the bed to its lowest position.
19 Raise or lower bed rails. Follow the care plan.
20 Unscreen the person.
21 Complete a safety check of the room. (See the inside of the front book cover.)

22 Follow agency policy for dirty linen and used supplies.
23 Practice hand hygiene.
24 Report and record your observations.
25 Check the person often.

THE PERSON WITH AN OSTOMY

Sometimes part of the intestines is removed surgically. Cancer, bowel disease, and trauma (stab or bullet wounds) are common reasons. An ostomy is sometimes necessary. An **ostomy** is a surgically created opening. The opening is called a **stoma.** The person wears a pouch over the stoma to collect stools and flatus.

Colostomy

A **colostomy** is a surgically created opening *(stomy)* between the colon *(colo)* and abdominal wall. Part of the colon is brought out onto the abdominal wall and a stoma made. Feces and flatus pass through the stoma instead of through the anus.

Colostomies are temporary or permanent. If permanent, the diseased part of the colon is removed. A temporary colostomy gives the diseased or injured bowel time to heal. After healing, surgery is done to reconnect the bowel.

The colostomy site depends on the site of disease or injury (Fig. 22-7, p. 392). Stool consistency depends on the colostomy site. Consistency ranges from liquid to formed. The more colon remaining to absorb water, the more solid and formed the stool. If the colostomy is near the start of the colon, stools are liquid. A colostomy near the end of the colon results in formed stools.

Stools irritate the skin. Skin care prevents skin breakdown around the stoma. The skin is washed and dried. Then a skin barrier is applied around the stoma. It prevents stools from having contact with the skin. The skin barrier is part of the pouch or a separate device.

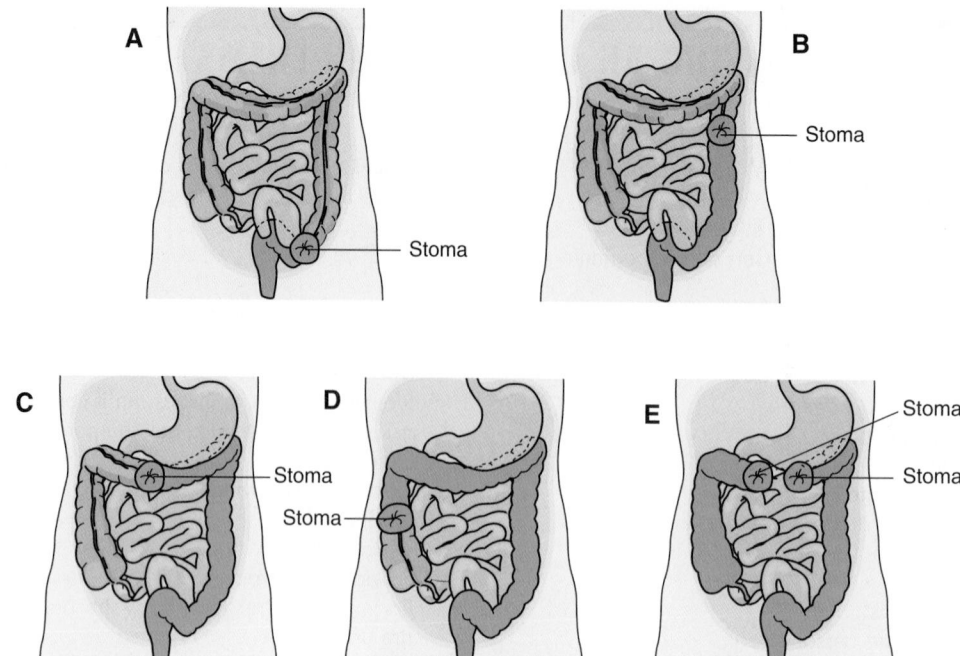

FIGURE 22-7 Colostomy sites. *Shading* shows the part of the bowel surgically removed. **A,** Sigmoid colostomy. **B,** Descending colostomy. **C,** Transverse colostomy. **D,** Ascending colostomy. **E,** Double-barrel colostomy has two stomas. One allows for the excretion of feces. The other is for the introduction of drugs to help the bowel heal. This type of colostomy is usually temporary.

Ileostomy

An **ileostomy** is a surgically created opening *(stomy)* between the ileum *(small intestine [ileo])* and the abdominal wall. Part of the ileum is brought out onto the abdominal wall, and a stoma is made. The entire colon is removed (Fig. 22-8).

Liquid stools drain constantly from an ileostomy. Water is not absorbed because the colon was removed. Feces in the small intestine contain digestive juices that are very irritating to the skin. The ileostomy pouch must fit well. Stools must not touch the skin. Good skin care is required.

◆ Ostomy Pouches

The pouch has an adhesive backing that is applied to the skin. Sometimes pouches are secured to ostomy belts (Fig. 22-9).

Many pouches have a drain at the bottom that close with a clip, clamp, or wire closure. The drain is opened to empty the pouch. The pouch is emptied when stools are present. It is opened when it balloons or bulges with flatus. The drain is wiped with toilet tissue before it is closed.

The pouch is changed every 3 to 7 days and when it leaks. Frequent pouch changes can damage the skin.

Odors are prevented by:
▶ Good hygiene
▶ Emptying the pouch
▶ Avoiding gas-forming foods
▶ Putting deodorants into the pouch (The nurse tells you what to use.)

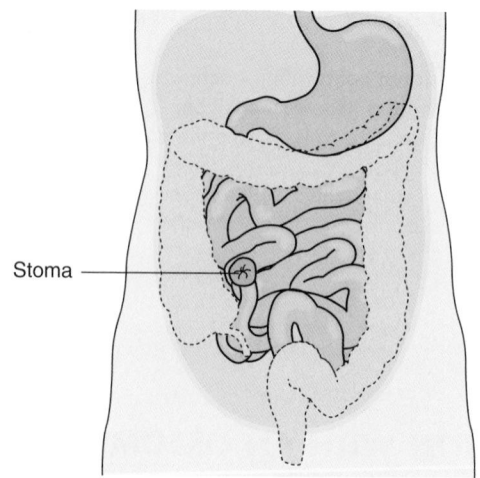

FIGURE 22-8 An ileostomy. The entire large intestine is surgically removed.

The person can wear normal clothes. However, tight garments can prevent feces from entering the pouch. Also, bulging from stools and flatus can be seen with tight clothes.

Peristalsis increases after eating and drinking. Therefore stomas are usually quiet after sleep. That is, expelling feces is less likely at this time. If the person showers or

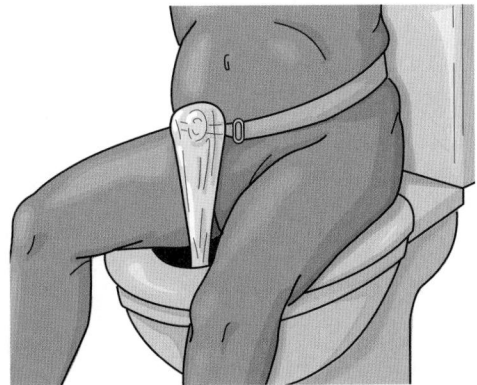

FIGURE 22-9 The ostomy pouch is secured to an ostomy belt. The pouch is emptied by directing it into the toilet and opening the end.

bathes with the pouch off, it is best done before breakfast. Showers and baths are delayed for 1 to 2 hours after applying a new pouch. This gives adhesive time to seal to the skin.

Do not flush pouches down the toilet. Follow agency policy for disposing of them.

See *Focus on Children and Older Persons: Ostomy Pouches.*
See *Delegation Guidelines: Ostomy Pouches.*
See *Promoting Safety and Comfort: Ostomy Pouches.*

FOCUS ON **CHILDREN** AND **OLDER PERSONS**

Ostomy Pouches

CHILDREN
Children of all ages can have ostomies, even premature infants. If changing or emptying a child's ostomy pouch is delegated to you, the nurse gives you the necessary instructions.

DELEGATION GUIDELINES: Ostomy Pouches

Many people manage their own ostomies. Others need help. When the nurse delegates changing an ostomy pouch to you, make sure that:
- Your state allows you to perform the procedure
- The procedure is in your job description
- You have the necessary education and training
- You review the procedure with the nurse
- The nurse is available to answer questions and to supervise you

If the above conditions are met, you need this information from the nurse and the care plan:
- What kind of ostomy the person has—colostomy or ileostomy
- When to change the pouch
- What equipment and supplies to use
- What soap or cleaning agent to use
- How long the skin barrier takes to dry (usually 1 to 2 minutes)
- What pouch deodorant to use
- What observations to report and record:
  - Signs of skin breakdown (the normal stoma is red like a mucous membrane)
  - Color, amount, consistency, and odor of stools
  - Complaints of pain or discomfort
- When to report observations
- What specific patient or resident concerns to report at once

PROMOTING SAFETY AND COMFORT: Ostomy Pouches

SAFETY
When changing an ostomy pouch, contact with stools and the stoma is likely. Stools contain microbes and may contain blood. The stoma may bleed slightly when washed. Follow Standard Precautions and the Bloodborne Pathogen Standard.

COMFORT
The stoma does not have sensation. Touching the stoma does not cause pain or discomfort.

CHANGING AN OSTOMY POUCH

✔ Quality of Life *Remember to:*

- Knock before entering the person's room.
- Address the person by name.
- Introduce yourself by name and title.
- Explain the procedure to the person before beginning and during the procedure.

- Protect the person's rights during the procedure.
- Handle the person gently during the procedure.

PRE-PROCEDURE

1 Follow *Delegation Guidelines: Ostomy Pouches.* See *Promoting Safety and Comfort: Ostomy Pouches.*
2 Practice hand hygiene.
3 Collect the following before going to the person's room:
  - Clean pouch with skin barrier
  - Pouch clamp, clip, or wire closure
  - Clean ostomy belt (if used)
  - Gauze pads or washcloths
  - Adhesive remover wipes
  - Skin paste (optional)
  - Pouch deodorant
  - Disposable bag
4 Arrange your work area.
5 Decontaminate your hands.
6 Identify the person. Check the ID bracelet against the assignment sheet. Also call the person by name.

Continued

CHANGING AN OSTOMY POUCH—cont'd

PRE-PROCEDURE—cont'd

7 Put on gloves.
8 Collect the following:
  • Bedpan with cover
  • Waterproof pad
  • Bath blanket
  • Wash basin with warm water
  • Paper towels
  • Gloves
9 Provide for privacy.
10 Raise the bed for good body mechanics. Bed rails are up if used.

PROCEDURE

11 Lower the bed rail near you if up.
12 Remove the gloves, and decontaminate your hands. Put on clean gloves.
13 Cover the person with a bath blanket. Fan-fold linens to the foot of the bed.
14 Place the waterproof pad under the buttocks.
15 Disconnect the pouch from the belt if one is worn. Remove the belt.
16 Remove the pouch and skin barrier. Gently push the skin down and lift up on the barrier. Use the adhesive remover wipes if necessary.
17 Wipe the stoma and around it with a gauze pad. This removes excess stool and mucus. Discard the gauze pad into the disposable bag.
18 Wet the gauze pads or the washcloth.
19 Wash the stoma and the skin around it with a gauze pad or washcloth. Wash gently. Do not scrub or rub the skin.
20 Pat dry with a gauze pad or the towel.
21 Observe the stoma and the skin around the stoma. Report bleeding, skin irritation, or skin breakdown to the nurse.
22 Remove the backing from the new pouch.
23 Apply a thin layer of paste around the pouch opening. Let it dry following the manufacturer's instructions.
24 Pull the skin around the stoma taut. The skin must be wrinkle-free.
25 Center the pouch over the stoma. The drain points downward.
26 Press around the pouch and skin barrier so it seals to the skin. Apply gentle pressure with your fingers. Start at the bottom and work up around the sides to the top.
27 Maintain the pressure for 1 to 2 minutes. Follow the manufacturer's instructions.
28 Tug downward on the pouch gently. Make sure the pouch is secure.
29 Add deodorant to the pouch.
30 Close the pouch at the bottom. Use a clamp, clip, or wire closure.
31 Attach the ostomy belt if used. The belt should not be too tight. You should be able to slide 2 fingers under the belt.
32 Remove the waterproof pad.
33 Discard disposable supplies into the disposable bag.
34 Remove the gloves. Practice hand hygiene.
35 Cover the person. Remove the bath blanket.

POST-PROCEDURE

36 Provide for comfort. (See the inside of the front book cover.)
37 Place the signal light within reach.
38 Lower the bed to its lowest position.
39 Raise or lower bed rails. Follow the care plan.
40 Unscreen the person.
41 Decontaminate your hands. Put on gloves.
42 Take the bedpan and disposable bag into the bathroom.
43 Empty the pouch and bedpan into the toilet. Observe the color, amount, consistency, and odor of stools. Flush the toilet.
44 Discard the pouch into the disposable bag. Discard the disposable bag.
45 Empty, clean, and disinfect equipment. Return the equipment to its proper place.
46 Remove the gloves. Practice hand hygiene.
47 Complete a safety check of the room. (See the inside of the front book cover.)
48 Follow agency policy for dirty linens.
49 Practice hand hygiene.
50 Report and record your observations.

Circle the BEST answer.

1 Which is *false*?
   a A person must have a bowel movement every day.
   b Stools are normally brown, soft, and formed.
   c Diarrhea occurs when feces move rapidly through the bowels.
   d Constipation results when feces move slowly through the colon.

2 The prolonged retention and accumulation of feces in the rectum is called
   a Constipation
   b Fecal impaction
   c Diarrhea
   d Fecal incontinence

3 Which does *not* promote comfort and safety for bowel elimination?
   a Asking visitors to leave the room
   b Helping the person to a sitting position
   c Offering the bedpan after meals
   d Telling the person that you will return very soon

4 Bowel training is aimed at
   a Bowel control and regular elimination
   b Ostomy control
   c Preventing fecal impaction, constipation, and fecal incontinence
   d Preventing bleeding

5 Which is *not* used for a cleansing enema?
   a Castile soap
   b Salt
   c Oil
   d Tap water

6 These statements are about enemas. Which is *false*?
   a The solution should be cool.
   b The Sims' position is used.
   c The enema bag is held 12 inches above the anus.
   d The solution is given slowly.

7 In adults, the enema tube is inserted
   a 2 to 4 inches
   b 4 to 6 inches
   c 6 to 8 inches
   d 8 to 10 inches

8 The oil-retention enema is retained for at least
   a 10 to 15 minutes
   b 15 to 30 minutes
   c 30 to 60 minutes
   d 60 to 90 minutes

9 These statements are about ostomies. Which is *false*?
   a Good skin care around the stoma is needed.
   b Deodorants can control odors.
   c The person wears a pouch.
   d Stools are liquid.

10 An ostomy pouch is usually emptied
   a Every 4 to 6 hours
   b Every shift
   c Every 3 to 7 days
   d When stools are present

Answers to these questions are on p. 780.

OBJECTIVES

- Define the key terms and key abbreviations listed in this chapter
- Explain the purpose and use of the MyPyramid food guidance system
- Explain how to use the *Dietary Guidelines for Americans*
- Describe the functions and sources of nutrients
- Explain how to read and use food labels
- Describe the factors that affect eating and nutrition
- Describe the OBRA requirements for serving food
- Describe the special diets and between-meal nourishments
- Identify the signs, symptoms, and precautions for aspiration
- Describe fluid requirements and the causes of dehydration

- Explain what to do when the person has special fluid orders
- Explain the purpose of intake and output records
- Identify what is counted as fluid intake
- Explain how to assist with food and fluid needs
- Explain how to assist with calorie counts
- Explain how to safely providing drinking water
- Explain how to prevent foodborne illnesses
- Perform the procedures described in this chapter

PROCEDURES

  Measuring Intake and Output
- Preparing the Person For a Meal
- Serving Meal Trays

  Feeding the Person
- Providing Drinking Water

Procedures with this icon are on the CDCompanion in this book; those with this icon ![View Video] are on the Evolve Student Resources Website.

KEY TERMS

anorexia The loss of appetite

aspiration Breathing fluid, food, vomitus, or an object into the lungs

calorie The amount of energy produced when the body burns food

Daily Value (DV) How a serving fits into the daily diet; expressed in a percent (%) based on a daily diet of 2000 calories

dehydration A decrease in the amount of water in body tissues

dysphagia Difficulty *(dys)* swallowing *(phagia)*

edema The swelling of body tissues with water

graduate A measuring container for fluid

intake The amount of fluid taken in

nutrient A substance that is ingested, digested, absorbed, and used by the body

nutrition The processes involved in the ingestion, digestion, absorption, and use of foods and fluids by the body

output The amount of fluid lost

KEY ABBREVIATIONS

ADEAR Alzheimer's Disease Education and Referral Center

DASH Dietary Approaches to Stop Hypertension

DV Daily Value

F Fahrenheit

FDA Food and Drug Administration

GI Gastrointestinal

I&O Intake and output

IV Intravenous

mg Milligrams

mL Milliliter

NPO Non per os; nothing by mouth

OBRA Omnibus Budget Reconciliation Act of 1987

oz Ounce

USDA United States Department of Agriculture

Food and water are physical needs. They are necessary for life. The person's diet affects physical and mental well-being. A poor diet and poor eating habits:

▶ Increase the risk for infection
▶ Increase the risk of acute and chronic diseases
▶ Cause chronic illnesses to become worse
▶ Cause healing problems
▶ Affect physical and mental function, increasing the risk for accidents and injuries

Eating and drinking provide pleasure. They often are part of social times with family and friends. A friendly, social setting for meals is important. Otherwise, the person may eat poorly.

Many factors affect dietary practices. They include culture, finances, and personal choice. Dietary practices also include selecting, preparing, and serving food. The health team considers these factors when planning to meet the person's nutrition needs.

See Box 23-1, p. 398 for a review of the structure and function of the digestive system.

See *Caring About Culture: Mealtime Practices*, p. 398.

BASIC NUTRITION

Nutrition is the processes involved in the ingestion, digestion, absorption, and use of foods and fluids by the body. Good nutrition is needed for growth, healing, and body functions. A well-balanced diet and correct calorie intake are needed. A high-fat and high-calorie diet causes weight gain and obesity. Weight loss occurs with a low-calorie diet.

Foods and fluids contain nutrients. A **nutrient** is a substance that is ingested, digested, absorbed, and used by the body. Nutrients are grouped into fats, proteins, carbohydrates, vitamins, minerals, and water.

Fats, proteins, and carbohydrates give the body fuel for energy. The amount of energy provided by a nutrient is measured in calories. A **calorie** is the amount of energy produced when the body burns food:

▶ 1 gram of fat—9 calories
▶ 1 gram of protein—4 calories
▶ 1 gram of carbohydrate—4 calories

Dietary Guidelines

The *Dietary Guidelines for Americans 2005* are for persons 2 years of age and older (Box 23-2, p. 399). Through diet and physical activity, the guidelines serve to:

▶ Promote health.
▶ Reduce the risk of chronic diseases.

Certain diseases are linked to poor diet and the lack of physical activity. They include cardiovascular diseases, hypertension (high blood pressure), diabetes, overweight and obesity, osteoporosis, and some cancers.

The Guidelines describe a healthy diet as one that:

▶ Is high in fruits, vegetables, whole grains, and fat-free or low-fat milk and milk products
▶ Includes lean meats, poultry, fish, beans, eggs, and nuts
▶ Is low in fats, cholesterol, salt (sodium), and added sugars

See *Focus on Children and Older Persons: Dietary Guidelines*, p. 401.

Text continued on p. 401

BOX 23-1 Digestive System: Review of Body Structure and Function

The digestive system breaks down food physically and chemically so it can be absorbed for use by the cells. This process is called *digestion*. The digestive system is also called the *gastrointestinal (GI) system*. The system also removes solid wastes from the body.

The digestive system involves the *alimentary canal (GI tract)* and the accessory organs of digestion (Fig. 23-1). The alimentary canal extends from the mouth to the anus. Its major parts are the mouth, pharynx, esophagus, stomach, small intestine, and large intestine. Accessory organs are the teeth, tongue, salivary glands, liver, gallbladder, and pancreas.

Digestion begins in the *mouth (oral cavity)*. It receives food and prepares it for digestion. Using chewing motions, the *teeth* cut, chop, and grind food into small particles for digestion and swallowing. The *tongue* aids in chewing and swallowing. *Taste buds* on the tongue's surface contain nerve endings. Taste buds allow sweet, sour, bitter, and salty tastes to be sensed. *Salivary glands* in the mouth secrete *saliva*. Saliva moistens food particles to ease swallowing and begin digestion. During swallowing, the tongue pushes food into the pharynx.

The *pharynx* (throat) is a muscular tube. Swallowing continues as the pharynx contracts. Contraction of the pharynx pushes food into the esophagus. The *esophagus* is a muscular tube about 10 inches long. It extends from the pharynx to the stomach. Involuntary muscle contractions called *peristalsis* move food down the esophagus through the alimentary canal.

The *stomach* is a muscular, pouch-like sac. It is in the upper left part of the abdominal cavity. Strong stomach muscles stir and churn food to break it up into even smaller particles. A mucous membrane lines the stomach. It contains glands that secrete *gastric juices*. Food is mixed and churned with the gastric juices to form a semi-liquid substance called *chyme*. Through peristalsis, the chyme is pushed from the stomach into the small intestine.

The *small intestine* is about 20 feet long. It has three parts. The first part is the *duodenum*. There, more digestive juices are added to the chyme. One is called *bile*. Bile is a greenish liquid made in the *liver*. Bile is stored in the *gallbladder*. Juices from the *pancreas* and small intestine are added to the chyme. Digestive juices chemically break down food so it can be absorbed.

Peristalsis moves the chyme through the two other parts of the small intestine: the *jejunum* and the *ileum*. Tiny projections called *villi* line the small intestine. Villi absorb the digested food into the capillaries. Most food absorption takes place in the jejunum and the ileum.

Some chyme is not digested. Undigested chyme passes from the small intestine into the *large intestine (large bowel* or *colon)*. Chyme eventually enters the large intestine. More fluid is absorbed. The solid waste that remains is eliminated through the anus. See Chapters 8 and 22.

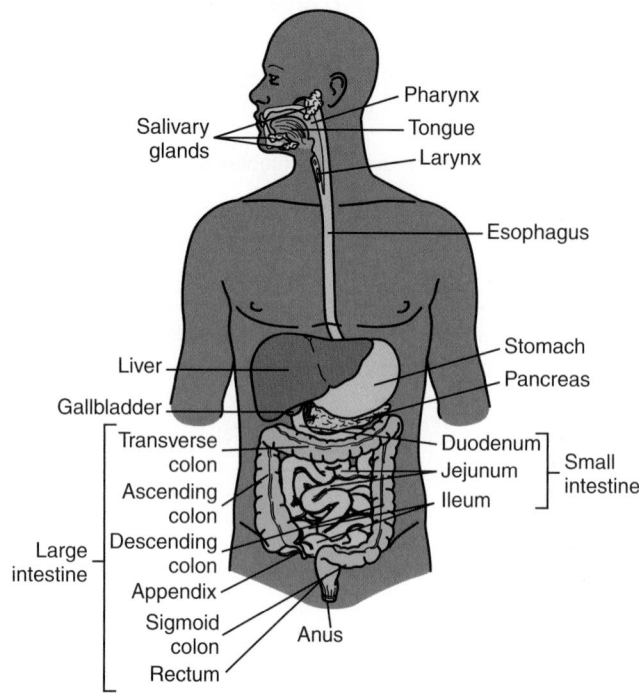

FIGURE 23-1 The digestive system.

CARING ABOUT CULTURE

Mealtime Practices

Many cultural groups have their main meal at mid-day. The *Austrians* do so. They eat light meals in the early evening and at the end of the day. Persons from *Brazil* also eat their main meal at noon. They have a light meal in the evening. A main meal at noon also is common in *Finland, Germany, Greece,* and *Iran.*

(Modified from D'Avanzo CE, Geissler EM: *Pocket guide to cultural health assessment,* ed 3, St Louis, 2003, Mosby.)

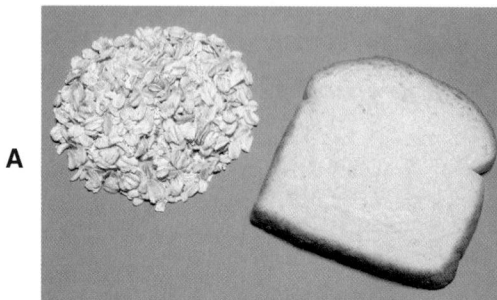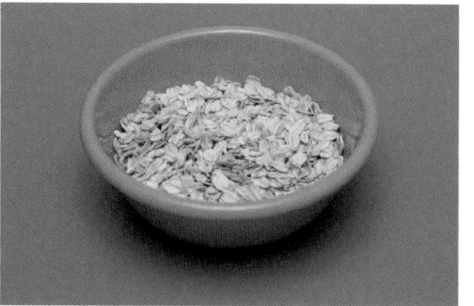

FIGURE 23-2 A, The amount of whole grain that equals a 1-ounce slice of bread. **B,** A 3 ounce-equivalent serving of whole grain.

BOX 23-2 Dietary Guidelines for Americans 2005

CONSUME AN ADEQUATE AMOUNT OF NUTRIENTS WITHIN YOUR DAILY CALORIE NEEDS
- Consume a variety of nutrient-dense foods and beverages from the basic food groups. Nutrient-dense foods have little or no solid fats or added sugar.
- Limit the intake of fats, cholesterol, added sugars, salt, and alcohol.
- Use the MyPyramid Food Guidance System (p. 401) or the DASH Eating Plan (Dietary Approaches to Stop Hypertension p. 411). Use the plans to determine energy needs (calories needed) for your gender (male or female), age, and activity level.

WEIGHT MANAGEMENT
- To maintain a healthy body weight—balance your calorie intake with the calories used for energy.
- To prevent gradual weight gain over time—make small decreases in calorie intake and increase physical activity.

PHYSICAL ACTIVITY
- Engage in regular physical activity to promote health, mental well-being, and a healthy body weight. Avoid a sedentary life-style. *Sedentary* means a life-style with little or no physical activity.
  - To reduce the risk of chronic disease in adulthood—engage in at least 30 minutes of moderate to vigorous activity on most days of the week. This activity is in addition to your usual activity at work or at home.
  - For greater health benefits—engage in physical activity that is more vigorous or longer in duration.
  - To manage body weight and prevent gradual, unhealthy weight gain—engage in up to 60 minutes of moderate to vigorous activity on most days of the week. Do not exceed calorie needs.
  - To maintain weight loss in adulthood—engage in 60 to 90 minutes of moderate activity daily. Do not exceed calorie needs.
- To achieve physical fitness include the following physical activities:
  - Cardiovascular conditioning
  - Stretching exercises for flexibility
  - Resistance exercise or calisthenics for muscle strength and endurance

FOOD GROUPS TO ENCOURAGE
- Eat enough fruits and vegetables but stay within energy (calorie) needs.
  - For a daily intake of 2000 calories—2 cups of fruit and 2½ cups of vegetables are recommended.
  - For a daily intake of more than 2000 calories—more than 2 cups of fruit and 2½ cups of vegetables are recommended.
  - For daily intake of less than 2000 calories—less than 2 cups of fruit and 2½ cups of vegetables are recommended.
- Choose a variety of fruits and vegetables each day. Select from all five vegetable subgroups—dark green, orange, legumes, starchy vegetables, and others. Do so several times a week.

- Eat at least 3 ounces of whole-grain products a day. An ounce-equivalent of whole grain is the amount of whole grain that equals a 1-ounce slice of bread (Fig. 23-2).
  - At least half of the daily grain requirement should come from whole grains. Examples include brown rice, buckwheat, bulgur, oatmeal, and wild rice. Whole wheat bran, crackers, pasta, and tortillas are other examples.
  - The rest of the daily grain requirement comes from enriched or whole-grain products.
- Consume 3 cups per day of fat-free or low-fat milk or equivalent milk products:
  - 1 cup of yogurt = 1 cup of fat-free or low-fat milk
  - 1½ ounce of natural cheese = 1 cup of fat-free or low-fat milk
  - 2 ounces of processed cheese = 1 cup of fat-free or low-fat milk

FATS
- Limit intake of fats and oils high in:
  - Saturated fats—fat from animal products such as meat and dairy products (milk, cheese). Many of these fats are solid at room temperature—butter, lard, and shortening.
  - Trans fats—fats found in shortening and commercially prepared baked goods, snack foods, fried foods, and margarine. Trans fats also are found in dairy products, beef, and lamb.
  - Cholesterol—a fat-related substance that is found in all animal foods. It is not found in plants. Main sources are egg yolks and organ meats (liver, kidneys). Other sources include meat, poultry, fish, and shellfish.
- Keep total fat intake between 20 and 30 percent of calories. Most fat should come from fish, nuts, and vegetable oils.
- Select and prepare meat, poultry, dry beans, milk, and milk products that are lean, low-fat, or fat-free.

CARBOHYDRATES
- Choose fiber-rich fruits, vegetables, and whole grains often.
- Choose and prepare foods and beverages with little added sugars or caloric sweeteners.
- Consume sugar- and starch-containing foods and beverages less frequently. Along with good oral hygiene, this helps prevents dental caries (cavities).

SODIUM AND POTASSIUM
- Consume less than 2300 mg (milligrams) (about 2 teaspoon of salt) of sodium per day.
- Choose and prepare foods with little salt.
- Consume potassium-rich foods. Fruits and vegetables are examples.

ALCOHOLIC BEVERAGES
- Persons who drink alcohol should do so sensibly and in moderation. Moderation means 12 ounces of regular beer, 5 ounces of wine, or 1½ ounces of 80-proof distilled spirits.
  - Women—up to 1 drink per day
  - Men—up to 2 drinks per day

Modified from *Dietary Guidelines for Americans 2005* and *Finding Your Way to a Healthier You: based on the Dietary Guidelines for Americans,* U.S. Department of Health and Human Services and U.S. Department of Agriculture.

Continued

BOX 23-2 Dietary Guidelines for Americans 2005—cont'd

ALCOHOLIC BEVERAGES—cont'd
- Alcohol should not be consumed by:
  - Persons who cannot restrict their alcohol intake
  - Women of child-bearing age who may become pregnant
  - Pregnant and breast-feeding women
  - Children and adolescents
  - Persons taking drugs that interact with alcohol
  - Persons with certain medical conditions
- Alcohol should not be consumed by persons who engage in activities that require attention, skill, or coordination. Driving and operating machinery are examples.

FOOD SAFETY
- To avoid foodborne illnesses:
  - Wash your hands.
  - Clean food contact surfaces.
  - Clean fruits and vegetables.

- Do not wash or rinse meat and poultry.
- Separate raw, cooked, and ready-to-eat foods while shopping, preparing, or storing foods.
- Cook foods to a safe temperature to kill microorganisms (Fig. 23-3).
- Chill perishable foods promptly.
- Defrost foods properly.
- Avoid the following foods:
  - Raw (unpasteurized) milk or any products made from unpasteurized milk
  - Raw or partially cooked eggs or food containing raw eggs
  - Raw or undercooked meat and poultry
  - Unpasteurized juices
  - Raw sprouts
- See "Foodborne Illnesses" on p. 422.

Modified from *Dietary Guidelines for Americans 2005* and *Finding Your Way to a Healthier You: based on the Dietary Guidelines for Americans,* U.S. Department of Health and Human Services and U.S. Department of Agriculture.

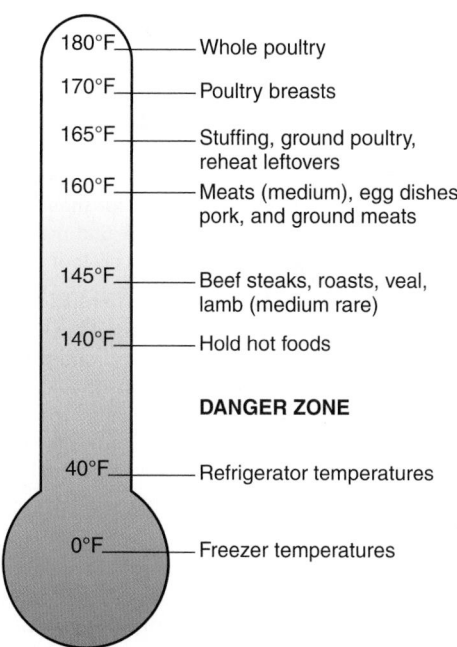

FIGURE 23-3 Food temperature guide. (Redrawn from U.S. Department of Health and Human Services and U.S. Department of Agriculture: *Finding Your Way to a Healthier You: based on the Dietary Guidelines for Americans,* updated April 5, 2005.)

Dietary Guidelines

CHILDREN

The *Dietary Guidelines for Americans 2005* include these key recommendations for children:

- Engage in at least 60 minutes of physical activity on most days of the week. Every day is preferred.
- Eat whole-grain products often. At least half of the grains consumed should be whole-grains.
- Consume fat-free or low-fat milk or equivalent milk products as follows:
  - Children 2 to 8 years of age—2 cups per day
  - Children 9 years of age and older—3 cups per day
- Keep total fat intake as follows:
  - Children 2 to 3 years of age—30 to 35 percent of calories
  - Children 4 to 18 years of age—25 to 35 percent of calories
- Have most fat intake from fish, nuts, and vegetable oils.
- Do not drink alcoholic beverages.
- Do not eat or drink:
  - Raw (unpasteurized) milk or any products made from unpasteurized milk
  - Raw or partially cooked eggs or foods containing raw eggs
  - Raw or undercooked meat and poultry
  - Raw or undercooked fish or shellfish
  - Unpasteurized juices
  - Raw sprouts

OLDER PERSONS

The *Dietary Guidelines for Americans 2005* include these key recommendations for older persons:

- Consume vitamin B_{12} through fortified foods or supplements.
- Consume extra vitamin D from vitamin D-fortified foods and/or supplements.
- Participate in regular physical activity to:
  - Reduce functional declines associated with aging
  - Achieve the other benefits of physical activity identified for all adults
- Aim to consume no more than 1500 mg of sodium per day.
- Meet the potassium recommendation (4700 mg/day) with food.
- Eat certain deli meats and frankfurters that have been reheated to steaming hot.
- Do not eat or drink:
  - Raw (unpasteurized) milk or any products made from unpasteurized milk
  - Raw or partially cooked eggs or foods containing raw eggs
  - Raw or undercooked meat and poultry
  - Raw or undercooked fish or shellfish
  - Unpasteurized juices
  - Raw sprouts

MyPyramid

The MyPyramid food guidance system (Fig. 23-4, p. 402) is based on the *Dietary Guidelines for Americans 2005*. Smart and healthy food choices and daily activity are encouraged.

The MyPyramid symbol shows the "Steps To a Healthier You."

▶ *The kind and amounts of food to eat daily.* This depends on the person's age, gender (male or female), and activity level. There are 12 different calorie levels. (See Appendix D, p. 812.)

▶ *Gradual improvement.* People can take small steps each day to improve their diet and life-style.

▶ *Physical activity.* This is shown by the steps and the person climbing them. They are a reminder of the importance of physical activity. For health benefits, at least 30 minutes of physical activity are needed on most days of the week. It is best to do so every day. Activity should be moderate or vigorous (Box 23-3, p. 403). The activity can be done in one 30-minute period. Or it can be done in 2 or 3 parts as long as the total time is at least 30 minutes a day.

▶ *Variety.* The six color bands stand for the 5 food groups and oils. Food from the 5 groups are needed each day for good health.

▶ *Moderation.* This means to avoid extremes. The bands narrow as they go from the bottom to the top of the pyramid. Foods near the base have the most nutritional value and the fewest calories. They have little or no solid fats, added sugars, or caloric sweeteners. Foods lower in the band should be chosen more often than those higher in the band.

▶ *The right amount from each food group band.* The bands differ in width. The widths suggest how much food to choose from each group. The wider the band, the more foods the person should choose from that group.

Grains

The orange band is for grains. Any food made from wheat, rice, oats, cornmeal, barley, or other cereal grain is a grain product. Bread, pasta, oatmeal, breakfast cereals, tortillas, and grits are examples. There are two types of grains:

▶ *Whole grains* contain the entire grain kernel. Whole-wheat flour, bulgur (cracked wheat), oatmeal, whole cornmeal, and brown rice are examples.

▶ *Refined grains* have been processed to remove the grain kernel. These grains have a finer texture. White flour, white bread, and white rice are examples. They have less dietary fiber than whole grains.

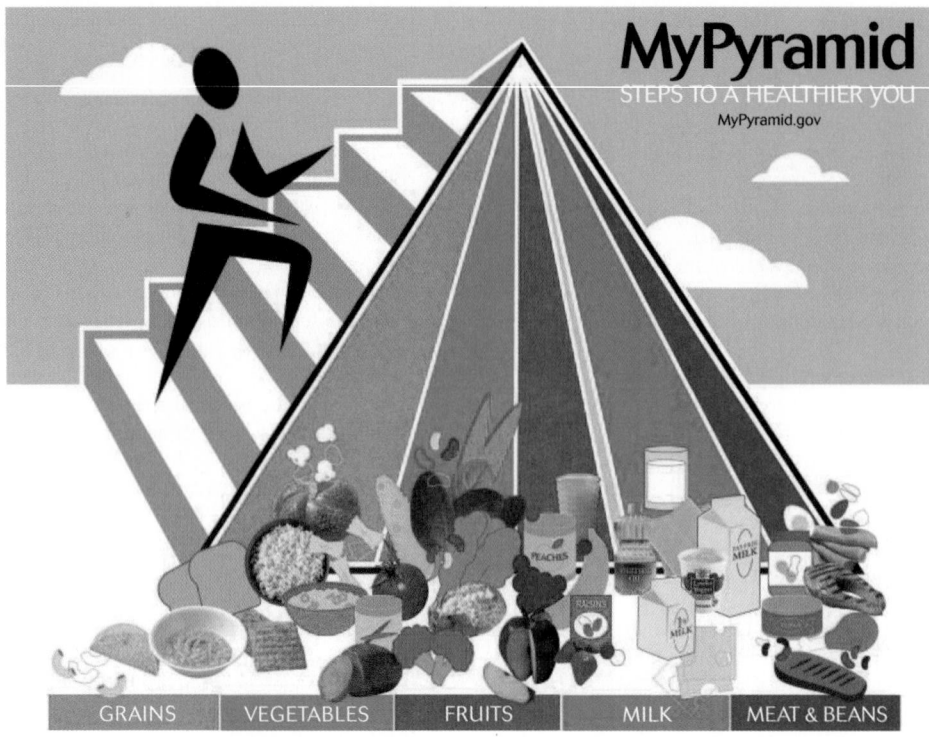

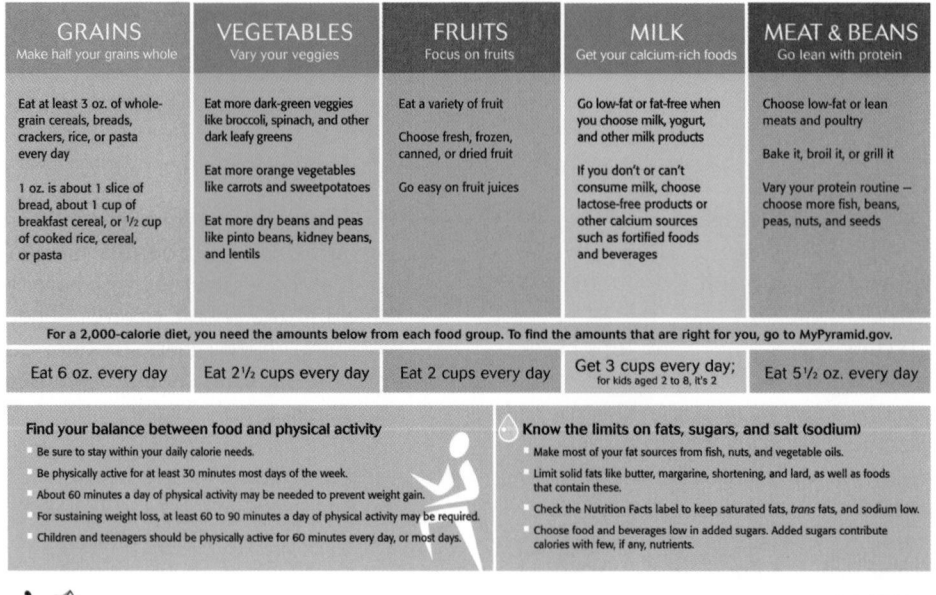

FIGURE 23-4 *MyPyramid: Steps to a Healthier You.* (Courtesy U.S. Department of Agriculture, Center for Nutrition and Policy Promotion, April 2005, CNPP-15.)

A person needs at least 3 ounces of whole-grain cereals, breads, crackers, rice, or pasta every day. For a 2000 calorie diet, 6 ounces are needed daily. See Figure 23-4 and Table 23-1.

Grains have the following health benefits:

▶ Reduce the risk of coronary artery disease.
▶ May prevent constipation.
▶ May help with weight management.
▶ May prevent certain birth defects.
▶ Contain these nutrients—dietary fiber, several B vitamins (thiamine, riboflavin, niacin, folate), and minerals (iron, magnesium, and selenium).

TABLE 23-1 MyPyramid Serving Sizes for a 2000-Calorie Diet

GROUP (COLOR BAND)	SERVINGS	SERVING SIZES
Grains (orange band)	At least 6 ounces (6 oz) of whole-grain cereals, breads, crackers, rice, or pasta daily	1 ounce = 1 slice of bread 1 ounce = 1 cup of breakfast cereal 1 ounce = ½ cup of cooked rice, cereal, or pasta
Vegetables (green band)	At least 2½ cups per day Vegetable subgroups, amounts per week: *Dark green*—3 cups *Orange*—2 cups *Dry beans and peas*—3 cups *Starchy*—3 cups *Other*—6½ cups	1 cup = 1 cup of raw or cooked vegetables or vegetable juice 1 cup = 2 cups of raw leafy greens
Fruits (red band)	At least 2 cups per day	1 cup = 1 cup of fruit 1 cup = 1 cup of fruit juice 1 cup = ½ cup of dried fruit
Milk (blue band)	At least 3 cups per day	1 cup = 1 cup of milk or yogurt 1 cup = 1½ ounces of natural cheese 1 cup = 2 ounces of processed cheese
Meat and beans (purple band)	At least 5½ ounces per day	1 ounce = 1 ounce of lean meat, poultry, or fish 1 ounce = 1 egg 1 ounce = 1 tablespoon of peanut butter 1 ounce = ¼ cup of cooked dry beans 1 ounce = ½ ounce of nuts or seeds
Oils (yellow band)	At least 6 teaspoons daily	1 teaspoon = 1 teaspoon

Modified from *MyPyramid: Food Intake Patterns*, U.S. Department of Agriculture, Center for Nutrition and Policy Promotion, April 2005.

BOX 23-3 MyPyramid: Physical Activity

MODERATE PHYSICAL ACTIVITIES
- Walking briskly (about 3½ miles per hour)
- Hiking
- Gardening and yard work
- Dancing
- Golf (walking and carrying clubs)
- Bicycling (less than 10 miles per hour)
- Weight training (general light workout)

VIGOROUS PHYSICAL ACTIVITIES
- Running and jogging (5 miles per hour)
- Bicycling (more than 10 miles per hour)
- Swimming (freestyle laps)
- Aerobics
- Walking very fast (4½ miles per hour)
- Heavy yard work (chopping wood)
- Weight lifting (vigorous effort)
- Basketball (competitive)

Vegetables

The green band is for vegetables. A person should vary the kinds of vegetables eaten. Most should come from the dark green, orange, and dry peas and beans subgroups:

- *Dark green vegetables*—bok choy, collard greens, dark green leafy lettuce, kale, mesclun, mustard greens, romaine lettuce, spinach, turnips, watercress
- *Orange vegetables*—acorn squash, butternut squash, carrots, hubbard squash, pumpkin, sweet potatoes

- *Dry beans and peas (legumes)*—black beans, black-eyed peas, garbanzo peas (chickpeas), kidney beans, lentils, lima beans (mature), navy beans, pinto beans, soy beans, split peas, tofu, white beans
- *Starchy vegetables*—corn, green peas, lima beans (green), potatoes
- *Other vegetables*—artichokes, asparagus, bean sprouts, beets, Brussels sprouts, cabbage, cauliflower, celery, cucumbers, eggplant, green beans, green or red peppers, iceberg (head) lettuce, mushrooms, okra, onions, parsnips, tomatoes, tomato juice, vegetable juice, turnips, wax beans, zucchini

At least 1 cup of vegetables is needed daily on a 1000 calorie diet. For a 2000 calorie diet, 2½ cups are needed daily. See Figure 23-4 and Table 23-1. A person can choose fresh, frozen, canned, and dried vegetables as well as vegetable juices.

Vegetables have these health benefits:

- May reduce the risk for stroke, coronary artery disease, other cardiovascular diseases, and type 2 diabetes.
- Protect against certain cancers. Cancers of the mouth, stomach, and colon-rectum are examples.
- May reduce the risk of developing kidney stones.
- May reduce the risk of bone loss.
- May help lower calorie intake. Most vegetables are naturally low in fat and calories.
- Contain no cholesterol.
- Contain these nutrients—potassium, dietary fiber, folate (folic acid), vitamins A, E, and C.

Fruits

The red band is for fruits. Any fruit or 100% fruit juice counts as part of the fruit group. Fruit choices should vary. Fresh, frozen, canned, or dried fruits are best. Avoid fruits canned in syrup. Syrup contains added sugar. Choose fruits canned in 100% fruit juice or water.

For a 1000 calorie diet, at least 1 cup of fruit is needed daily. For a 2000 calorie diet, 2 cups are needed daily. See Figure 23-4 and Table 23-1.

Fruits have these health benefits:
▶ May reduce the risk for stroke, coronary artery disease, other cardiovascular diseases, and type 2 diabetes.
▶ Protect against certain cancers. Cancers of the mouth, stomach, and colon-rectum are examples.
▶ May reduce the risk of developing kidney stones.
▶ May reduce the risk of bone loss.
▶ May help lower calorie intake. Most fruits are naturally low in fat and calories.
▶ Contain no cholesterol.
▶ Are naturally low in sodium.
▶ Contain these nutrients—potassium, dietary fiber, vitamin C, and folate (folic acid).

Milk

The blue band is for milk and milk products. Low-fat or fat-free choices are best. The milk group includes all fluid milk. It also includes yogurt and cheese. (Cream, cream cheese, and butter are not part of the group.)

On a 1000 calorie diet, 2 cups are needed daily. A 2000 calorie diet requires 3 cups daily. See Figure 23-4 and Table 23-1.

Milk has these health benefits:
▶ Helps build and maintain bone mass throughout the life span. This may reduce the risk of osteoporosis.
▶ Improves the overall quality of the diet.
▶ Contains these nutrients—calcium, potassium, and vitamin D.

Meat and Beans

The purple band is for meats and beans. This group includes all foods made from meat, poultry, fish, dry beans or peas, eggs, nuts, and seeds. Most meat and poultry choices should be lean or low-fat. Fish, nuts, and seeds contain healthy oils. They should be chosen often instead of meat or poultry.

Remember the following when selecting foods from this group:
▶ Choose lean or low-fat meat and poultry. Higher fat choices include regular ground beef (75 to 80% lean) and chicken with skin.
▶ Using fat for cooking increases the caloric value of the food. Fried chicken and eggs fried in butter are examples.
▶ Salmon, trout, and herring are rich in substances that may reduce the risk of heart disease.

▶ Liver and other organ meats are high in cholesterol.
▶ Egg yolks are high in cholesterol. Egg whites are cholesterol-free.
▶ Processed meats have added sodium (salt). They include ham, sausage, frankfurters, and luncheon and deli meats.
▶ Sunflower seeds, almonds, and hazelnuts are rich sources of vitamin E.

A 1000 calorie diet allows 2 ounces daily from the meat and beans group. A 2000 calorie diet allows 5½ ounces daily. See Figure 23-4 and Table 23-1.

Foods in this group are high in fat and cholesterol. Heart disease is a major risk. However, the meat and beans group provides these nutrients needed for health and body maintenance:
▶ Protein
▶ B vitamins (niacin, thiamine, riboflavin, and vitamin B_6) and vitamin E
▶ Iron, zinc, and magnesium

Oils

The yellow band is for oils. Oils are fats that are liquid at room temperature. Vegetable oils used in cooking are examples. They include canola oil, corn oil, and olive oil. Some foods are naturally high in oil—nuts, olives, some fish, and avocados.

Remember the following when making oil choices:
▶ Oils are high in calories.
▶ The best oil choices come from fish, nuts, and vegetable oils.
▶ Some foods are mainly oil. Mayonnaise, certain salad dressings, and soft margarine (tub or squeeze) are examples.
▶ Oils from plant sources do not contain cholesterol.
▶ Solid fats are those that are solid at room temperature. Common solid fats include butter, beef fat (tallow, suet), chicken fat, pork fat (lard), stick margarine, and shortening.

Oils contain some fatty acids that are essential for health. Oils also are a major source of vitamin E.

Enough oil is usually consumed daily from nuts, fish, cooking oil, and salad dressings. On a 1000 calorie diet, 3 teaspoons of oils are allowed. On a 2000 calorie diet, 6 teaspoons of oils are allowed. See Figure 23-4 and Table 23-1.

See *Focus on Children and Older Persons: MyPyramid.*

Nutrients

No food or food group has every essential nutrient. A well-balanced diet assures an adequate intake of essential nutrients.
▶ *Protein*—is the most important nutrient. It is needed for tissue growth and repair. Sources include meat, fish, poultry, eggs, milk and milk products, cereals, beans, peas, and nuts.

MyPyramid

CHILDREN

The U.S. Department of Agriculture (USDA) offers these tips to help children eat vegetables and fruits. Some of the measures depend on the child's age.

- Serve vegetables and fruits with meals and as snacks.
- Let children choose vegetables and fruits and what goes in salads.
- Let children help shop for vegetables and fruits. Let them choose new ones to try.
- Let children clean, peel, or cut up vegetables and fruits.
- Do not mix vegetables. Serve them separately. For example, do not combine peas and carrots.
- Decorate plates and serving dishes with fruit slices.
- Top cereal with berries.
- Make a "smiley face" with fruit. You can use banana slices for the eyes, raisins for the nose, and an orange slice for the mouth.
- Offer dried fruits and raisins in place of candy and chewy fruit snacks.
- Make fruit kabobs. Use pineapple chunks, bananas, grapes, and berries.
- Offer 100% fruit juices instead of soda or other drinks with sugar.

- *Carbohydrates*—provide energy and fiber for bowel elimination. They are found in fruits, vegetables, breads, cereals, and sugar. Carbohydrates break down into sugars during digestion. The sugars are absorbed into the bloodstream. Fiber is not digested. It provides the bulky part of chyme for elimination.
- *Fats*—provide energy. They add flavor to food and help the body use certain vitamins. Sources include meats, lard, butter, shortening, oils, milk, cheese, egg yolks, and nuts. Dietary fat not needed by the body is stored as body fat *(adipose tissue)*.
- *Vitamins*—are needed for certain body functions. They do not provide calories. The body stores vitamins A, D, E, and K. Vitamin C and the B complex vitamins are not stored. They must be ingested daily. The lack of a certain vitamin results in signs and symptoms of an illness. Table 23-2 lists the sources and major functions of common vitamins.
- *Minerals*—are used for many body processes. They are needed for bone and tooth formation, nerve and muscle function, fluid balance, and other body processes. Table 23-3 (p. 406) lists the major functions and dietary sources of common minerals.
- *Water*—is needed for all body processes (p. 412).

TABLE 23-2 Functions and Sources of Common Vitamins

VITAMIN	MAJOR FUNCTIONS	SOURCES
Vitamin A	Growth; vision; healthy hair, skin, and mucous membranes; resistance to infection	Liver, spinach, green leafy and yellow vegetables, yellow fruits, fish liver oils, egg yolks, butter, cream, whole milk
Vitamin B_1 (thiamine)	Muscle tone, nerve function, digestion, appetite, normal elimination, carbohydrate use	Pork, fish, poultry, eggs, liver, breads, pastas, cereals, oatmeal, potatoes, peas, beans, soybeans, peanuts
Vitamin B_2 (riboflavin)	Growth, healthy eyes, protein and carbohydrate metabolism, healthy skin and mucous membranes	Milk and milk products, liver, green leafy vegetables, eggs, breads, cereals
Vitamin B_3 (niacin)	Protein, fat, and carbohydrate metabolism; nervous system function; appetite; digestive system function	Meat, pork, liver, fish, peanuts, breads and cereals, green vegetables, dairy products
Vitamin B_{12}	Formation of red blood cells, protein metabolism, nervous system function	Liver, meats, poultry, fish, eggs, milk, cheese
Folate (folic acid)	Formation of red blood cells, intestinal function, protein metabolism	Liver, meats, fish, poultry, green leafy vegetables, whole grains
Vitamin C (ascorbic acid)	Formation of substances that hold tissue together; healthy blood vessels, skin, gums, bones, and teeth; wound healing; prevention of bleeding; resistance to infection	Citrus fruits, tomatoes, potatoes, cabbage, strawberries, green vegetables, melons
Vitamin D	Absorption and metabolism of calcium and phosphorus, healthy bones	Fish liver oils, milk, butter, liver, exposure to sunlight
Vitamin E	Normal reproduction, formation of red blood cells, muscle function	Vegetable oils, milk, eggs, meats, cereals, green leafy vegetables
Vitamin K	Blood clotting	Liver, green leafy vegetables, egg yolks, cheese

TABLE 23-3 Functions and Sources of Common Minerals

MINERAL	MAJOR FUNCTIONS	SOURCES
Calcium	Formation of teeth and bones, blood clotting, muscle contraction, heart function, nerve function	Milk and milk products, green leafy vegetables, whole grains, egg yolks, dried peas and beans, nuts
Phosphorus	Formation of bones and teeth; use of proteins, fats, and carbohydrates; nerve and muscle function	Meat, fish, poultry, milk and milk products, nuts, egg yolks, dried peas and beans
Iron	Allows red blood cells to carry oxygen	Liver, meat, eggs, green leafy vegetables, breads and cereals, dried peas and beans, nuts
Iodine	Thyroid gland function, growth, metabolism	Iodized salt, seafood, shellfish
Sodium	Fluid balance, nerve and muscle function	Almost all foods
Potassium	Nerve function, muscle contraction, heart function	Fruits, vegetables, cereals, meats, dried peas and beans

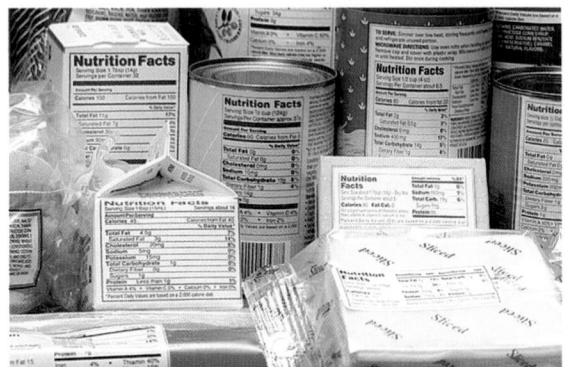

FIGURE 23-5 Food labels. The labels are required by the Nutrition Labeling and Education Act of 1990.

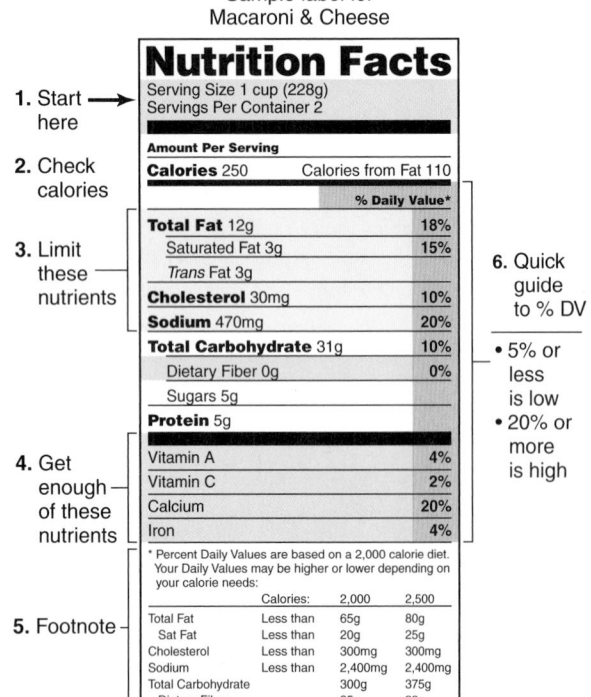

Sample label for Macaroni & Cheese

Nutrition Facts

Serving Size 1 cup (228g)
Servings Per Container 2

1. Start here

Amount Per Serving

Calories 250   Calories from Fat 110

2. Check calories

	% Daily Value*
Total Fat 12g	18%
Saturated Fat 3g	15%
Trans Fat 3g	
Cholesterol 30mg	10%
Sodium 470mg	20%
Total Carbohydrate 31g	10%
Dietary Fiber 0g	0%
Sugars 5g	
Protein 5g	

3. Limit these nutrients

6. Quick guide to % DV

• 5% or less is low
• 20% or more is high

Vitamin A	4%
Vitamin C	2%
Calcium	20%
Iron	4%

4. Get enough of these nutrients

* Percent Daily Values are based on a 2,000 calorie diet. Your Daily Values may be higher or lower depending on your calorie needs:

	Calories:	2,000	2,500
Total Fat	Less than	65g	80g
Sat Fat	Less than	20g	25g
Cholesterol	Less than	300mg	300mg
Sodium	Less than	2,400mg	2,400mg
Total Carbohydrate		300g	375g
Dietary Fiber		25g	30g

5. Footnote

FIGURE 23-6 Nutrition Facts Label. (From U.S. Food and Drug Administration, November 2004.)

Food Labels

Most foods have labels (Fig. 23-5). They are used to make informed food choices for a healthy diet. Figure 23-6 shows how to use a food label. Food labels contain information about:

▶ Serving size and the number of servings in each package.

▶ Calories and calories from fat. The number of servings consumed determines the number of calories eaten of that food. For example: 1 cup of macaroni and cheese contains 250 calories with 110 of them from fat. If you eat 2 cups, you consume 500 calories—220 from fat.

▶ Nutrients—total fat (saturated fat and trans fat), cholesterol, sodium, carbohydrate (dietary fibers and sugar), protein, vitamins A and C, calcium, and iron.

How a serving fits into the daily diet is called the **Daily Value (DV)**. The DV is expressed in a percent (%). The percent is based on a daily diet of 2000 calories. The % DV helps you decide if a food is high or low in a nutrient. According to the Food and Drug Administration (FDA), a 5% DV is low. A DV of 20% or more is high. In Figure 23-6, a serving of macaroni and cheese is low in dietary fiber, vitamins A and C, and iron. It is high in sodium and calcium.

FACTORS AFFECTING EATING AND NUTRITION

Meeting a person's nutritional needs requires a team approach. The nursing team, doctor, dietitian, speech-language pathologist, and occupational therapist are involved. The person is involved. So is the family if necessary. The person's likes, dislikes, and life-long habits are part of his or her nutritional care plan.

Some of the following factors begin during infancy and continue throughout life. Others develop later.

See *Focus on Long-Term Care and Home Care: Factors Affecting Eating and Nutrition.*

▶ *Age.* Age affects nutrition. See *Focus on Children and Older Persons: Factors Affecting Eating and Nutrition—Age*, p. 408.

FOCUS ON LONG-TERM CARE AND HOME CARE

Factors Affecting Eating and Nutrition

LONG-TERM CARE

The Omnibus Budget Reconciliation Act of 1987 (OBRA) has requirements for food served in nursing centers:

- Each person's nutritional and dietary needs are met.
- The person's diet is well-balanced. It is nourishing and tastes good. Food is well-seasoned. It is not too salty or too sweet.
- Food is appetizing. It has an appealing aroma and is attractive.
- Hot food is served hot. Cold food is served cold. Food servers keep food at the correct temperature.
- Food is served promptly. Otherwise, hot food cools and cold food warms.
- Food is prepared to meet each person's needs. Some people need food cut, ground, or chopped. Others have special diets ordered by the doctor.
- Other foods are offered to residents who refuse the food served. The substituted food must have a similar nutritional value to the first foods served.
- Each person receives at least 3 meals a day. A bedtime snack is offered.
- The center provides needed adaptive equipment and utensils (Fig. 23-7).

HOME CARE

You may be assigned to shop for groceries, plan meals, and cook. You need to understand the MyPyramid, basic nutrition, and food labels. You also need to know the person's food likes and dislikes and eating habits. For example, some people have the same breakfast every day. Some people have their large meal in the evening, others at noon.

Review the foods allowed on the person's diet (p. 408). Consider eating, digestive, and other problems when preparing and serving meals. The nurse and dietitian advise you about what to prepare. Use a good cookbook to plan and prepare meals.

Plan menus for a full week. Check recipe ingredients. If not on hand, place needed items on your shopping list. To save money, check newspapers for sales. Also check them and the Internet for coupons. Give all receipts to the person or family member.

Properly store foods. Refrigerate dairy products and most fresh fruits and vegetables right away. Do the same for the meat, fish, or poultry that you will use that day. Freeze the rest and frozen foods. Dried, packaged, canned, and bottled foods keep well in cabinets. See p. 422 for preventing "Foodborne Illnesses."

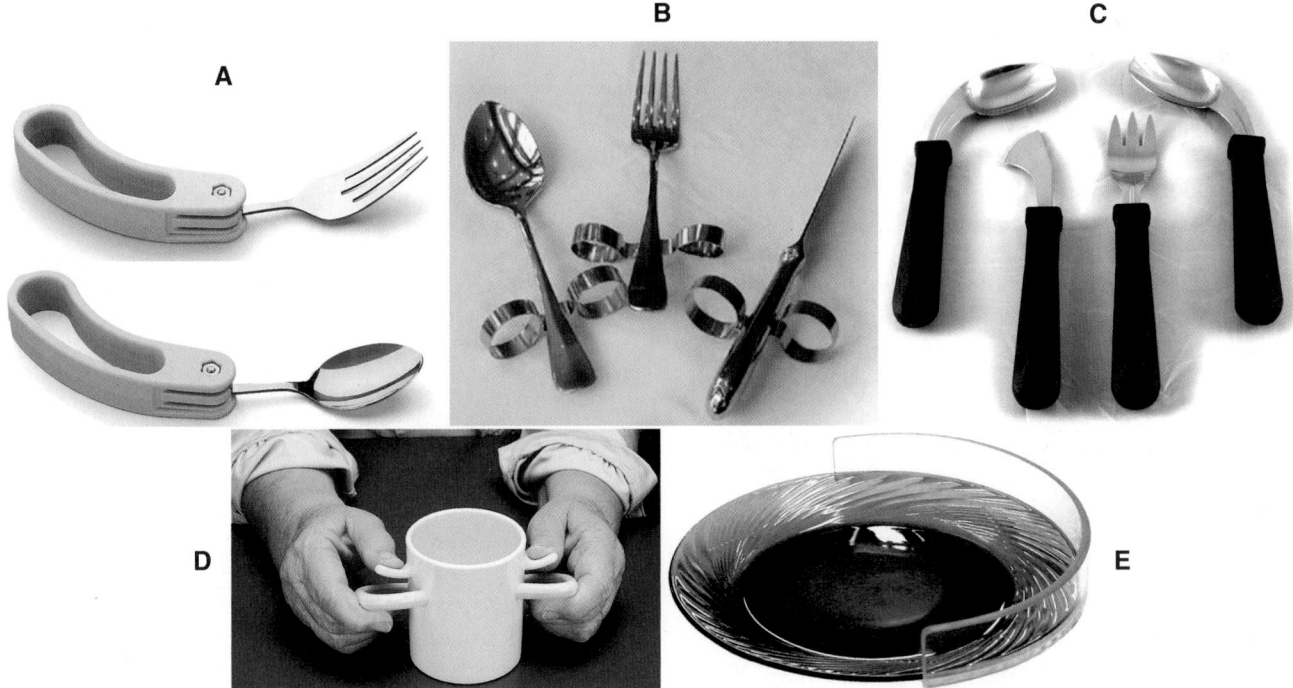

FIGURE 23-7 Eating utensils for persons with special needs. **A,** The fork and spoon are angled. Fingers are inserted through the opening or wrapped around the handle. **B,** The utensils can be adjusted for the person's grip strength. **C,** Eating utensils have tapered and angled handles. The knife cuts with slicing and rocking motions. **D,** The thumb grips on the cup help prevent spilling. **E,** The plate guard helps keep food on the plate. (Courtesy ElderStore, Alpharetta, Georgia.)

► *Culture.* Culture influences dietary practices, food choices, and food preparation. Frying, baking, smoking, or roasting food and eating raw food are cultural practices. So is the use of sauces, herbs, and spices. See *Caring About Culture: Food Practices.*

► *Religion.* Selecting, preparing, and eating food often involve religious practices (Box 23-4). A person may follow all, some, or none of the dietary practices of his or her faith. You must respect the person's religious practices.

► *Finances.* People with limited incomes often buy the cheaper carbohydrate foods. Their diets often lack protein and certain vitamins and minerals.

► *Appetite.* Appetite relates to the desire for food. When hungry, a person seeks food. He or she eats until the appetite is satisfied. Aromas and thoughts of food can stimulate the appetite. However, loss of appetite (**anorexia**) can occur. Causes include illness, drugs, anxiety, pain, and depression. Unpleasant sights, thoughts, and smells are other causes.

► *Personal choice.* Food likes and dislikes are personal. They begin in childhood. They are influenced by foods served in the home. As children grow older, they try new foods at school and social events. Food choices depend on how food looks, how it is prepared, its smell, and its ingredients. Usually food likes expand with age and social experiences. Patients and residents make food choices from menus.

► *Body reactions.* People usually avoid foods that cause allergic reactions. They also avoid foods that cause nausea, vomiting, diarrhea, indigestion, gas, or headaches.

► *Illness.* Appetite usually decreases during illness and recovery from injuries. However, nutritional needs are increased. The body must fight infection, heal tissue, and replace lost blood cells. Nutrients lost through vomiting and diarrhea need replacement. Some diseases and drugs cause a sore mouth. This makes eating painful. Tooth loss affects chewing, especially protein foods (the meat group). Poor nutrition is common in persons needing long-term care. They need good nutrition to correct or prevent health problems.

► *Disability.* Disease or injury can affect the hands, wrists, and arms. Adaptive equipment lets the person eat independently. The speech-language pathologist and occupational therapist teach the person how to use them. Make sure each person has needed equipment.

SPECIAL DIETS

Doctors may order special diets for a nutritional deficiency or a disease (Table 23-4). They also order them for weight control or to eliminate or decrease certain substances in the diet. The doctor, nurses, and dietitian work together to meet the person's nutritional needs. They consider the need for dietary changes, personal choices, religion, culture, and eating problems. They also consider food allergies and sensitivities. The nurse and dietitian teach the person and family about the diet.

FOCUS ON **CHILDREN** AND **OLDER PERSONS**

Factors Affecting Eating and Nutrition—Age

CHILDREN
Infants are breast-fed or bottle-fed. For bottle-fed babies, the doctor orders the formula to use. Solid foods are introduced at 4 to 6 months. Usually baby rice cereal is the first solid food given. The cereal is mixed with breast milk or formula to a thin consistency. Other solid foods are added as the baby grows. The nurse tells you what foods the baby can have.

The MyPyramid applies to children 2 years of age and older. The nurse tells you about the child's needs.

OLDER PERSONS
With aging, changes occur in the gastrointestinal system:
• Taste and smell dull.
• Appetite decreases.
• Secretion of digestive juices decreases. Therefore fried and fatty foods are hard to digest. They may cause indigestion.

Dry, fried, and fatty foods are avoided. This helps digestion and swallowing problems (p. 412). Good oral hygiene and denture care improve taste.

Some people have to avoid high-fiber foods needed for bowel elimination. High-fiber foods are hard to chew and can irritate the intestines. Such foods include apricots, celery, and fruits and vegetables with skins and seeds.

Foods providing soft bulk are often ordered for persons with chewing problems or constipation. These foods include whole-grain cereals and cooked fruits and vegetables.

Older persons need fewer calories than younger people do. Energy and activity levels are lower. Foods that contain calcium help prevent musculoskeletal changes. Protein is needed for tissue growth and repair. The diets of some older persons may lack protein. High-protein foods are costly.

CARING ABOUT CULTURE

Food Practices

Food practices vary among cultural groups. Rice and beans are protein sources in *Mexico.* In the *Philippines,* rice is preferred with every meal. A diet high in starch and fat is common in *Poland.* Potatoes, rye, and wheat are common. The diet in *China* is low in fat and high in sodium. The sodium content is from the use of soy sauce and dried and preserved foods.

Eating beef is common in the *United States.* In *India,* Hindus do not eat beef.

(Modified from D'Avanzo CE, Geissler EM: *Pocket guide to cultural health assessment,* ed 3, St Louis, 2003, Mosby.)

Regular diet, general diet, and *house diet* mean no dietary limits or restrictions. Persons with diseases of the heart, kidneys, gallbladder, liver, stomach, or intestines often need special diets. Persons with wounds or pressure ulcers need high-protein diets for healing. Older and disabled persons may have bran added to their food. It provides fiber for bowel elimination. Allergies, excess weight, and other disorders also require special diets.

BOX 23-4 Religion and Dietary Practices

ADVENTIST (SEVENTH DAY ADVENTIST)
- Coffee, tea, and alcohol are not allowed.
- Beverages with caffeine (colas) are not allowed.
- Some groups have restrictions about beef, pork, lamb, chicken, seafood, and fish.

BAPTIST
- Some groups forbid coffee, tea, and alcohol.

CHRISTIAN SCIENTIST
- Alcohol and coffee are not allowed.

CHURCH OF JESUS CHRIST OF LATTER DAY SAINTS (MORMON)
- Alcohol, coffee, and tea are not allowed.
- Meat is not forbidden. Members are encouraged to eat meat infrequently.

GREEK ORTHODOX
- Fasting is required during the Great Lent and before other holy days.
- Meat, fish, and dairy products are not eaten during a fast.

ISLAM
- All pork and pork products are forbidden.
- Alcohol is not allowed.
- Fasting (no food or fluids) is required from dawn to sunset during Ramadan.

JUDAISM (JEWISH FAITH)
- Foods must be kosher. (*Kosher* means fit or proper.) Food must be prepared according to Jewish law.
- Meat of kosher animals can be eaten—cows, goats, and lambs.
- Chickens, ducks, and geese are kosher fowl.
- Kosher fish have scales and fins—tuna, sardines, carp, salmon, herring, whitefish, and so on.
- Milk, milk products, and eggs from kosher animals and fowl are allowed.
- Meat and milk cannot be cooked together.
- Meat and milk products cannot be eaten together.
- Meat and milk products are not prepared or served with the same utensils and dishes. Two sets of utensils and dishes are needed. They are washed and stored separately.
- Fermented grain products are not consumed during Passover—cookies, noodles, alcohol, and so on.

ROMAN CATHOLIC
- Fasting is required for 1 hour before receiving Holy Communion.
- Fasting from meat is required on Ash Wednesday, Good Friday, and all Fridays during Lent.

TABLE 23-4 Special Diets

DIET	USE	FOODS ALLOWED
Clear-liquid—foods liquid at body temperature and that leave small amounts of residue; non-irritating and non-gas forming	Post-operatively, acute illness, infection, nausea and vomiting, and to prepare for GI exams	Water, tea, and coffee (without milk or cream); carbonated drinks; gelatin; clear fruit juices (apple, grape, cranberry); fat-free clear broth; hard candy, sugar, and Popsicles
Full-liquid—foods liquid at room temperature or melt at body temperature	Advance from clear-liquid diet post-operatively; for stomach irritation, fever, nausea, and vomiting; for persons unable to chew, swallow, or digest solid foods	Foods on the clear-liquid diet; custard; eggnog; strained soups; strained fruit and vegetable juices; milk and milk shakes; strained, cooked cereals; plain ice cream and sherbet; pudding; yogurt
Mechanical soft—semi-solid foods that are easily digested	Advance from full-liquid diet, chewing problems, GI disorders, and infections	All liquids; eggs (not fried); broiled, baked, or roasted meat, fish, or poultry that is chopped or shredded; mild cheeses (American, Swiss, cheddar, cream, cottage); strained fruit juices; refined bread (no crust) and crackers; cooked cereal; cooked or pureed vegetables; cooked or canned fruit without skin or seeds; pudding; plain cakes and soft cookies without fruit or nuts
Fiber- and residue-restricted—food that leaves a small amount of residue in the colon	Diseases of the colon and diarrhea	Coffee, tea, milk, carbonated drinks, strained fruit juices; refined bread and crackers; creamed and refined cereal; rice; cottage and cream cheese; eggs (not fried); plain puddings and cakes; gelatin; custard; sherbet and ice cream; strained vegetable juices; canned or cooked fruit without skin or seeds; potatoes (not fried); strained cooked vegetables; plain pasta; *no raw fruits or vegetables*
High-fiber—foods that increase the amount of residue and fiber in the colon to stimulate peristalsis	Constipation and GI disorders	All fruits and vegetables; whole wheat bread; whole-grain cereals; fried foods; whole-grain rice; milk, cream, butter, and cheese; meats

Continued

TABLE 23-4 Special Diets—cont'd

DIET	USE	FOODS ALLOWED
Bland—foods that are mechanically and chemically non-irritating and low in roughage; foods served at moderate temperatures; no strong spices or condiments	Ulcers, gallbladder disorders, and some intestinal disorders; after abdominal surgery	Lean meats; white bread; creamed and refined cereals; cream or cottage cheese; gelatin; plain puddings, cakes, and cookies; eggs (not fried); butter and cream; canned fruits and vegetables without skin and seeds; strained fruit juices; potatoes (not fried); pastas and rice; strained or soft cooked carrots, peas, beets, spinach, squash, and asparagus tips; creamed soups from allowed vegetables; no fried foods
High-calorie—calorie intake is increased to about 3000 to 4000 daily; includes 3 full meals and between-meal snacks	Weight gain and some thyroid imbalances	Dietary increases in all foods; large portions of regular diet with 3 between-meal snacks
Calorie-controlled—provides adequate nutrients while controlling calories to promote weight loss and reduce body fat	Weight reduction	Foods low in fats and carbohydrates and lean meats; avoid butter, cream, rice, gravies, salad oils, noodles, cakes, pastries, carbonated and alcoholic drinks, candy, potato chips, and similar foods
High-iron—foods that are high in iron	Anemia, following blood loss, for women during the reproductive years	Liver and other organ meats, lean meats, egg yolks, shellfish, dried fruits, dried beans, green leafy vegetables, lima beans, peanut butter, enriched breads and cereals
Fat-controlled (low cholesterol)—foods low in fat and prepared without adding fat	Heart disease, gallbladder disease, disorders of fat digestion, liver disease, diseases of the pancreas	Skim milk (fat free) or buttermilk; cottage cheese (no other cheeses allowed); gelatin; sherbet; fruit; lean meat, poultry, and fish (baked, broiled, or roasted); fat-free broth; soups made with skim milk (fat free); margarine; rice, pasta, breads, and cereals; vegetables; potatoes
High-protein—aids and promotes tissue healing	For burns, high fever, infection, and some liver diseases	Meat, milk, eggs, cheese, fish, poultry; breads and cereals; green leafy vegetables
Sodium-controlled—a certain amount of sodium is allowed	Heart disease, fluid retention, liver disease, and some kidney diseases	Fruits and vegetables and unsalted butter are allowed; adding salt at the table is not allowed; highly salted foods and foods high in sodium are not allowed; the use of salt during cooking may be restricted
Diabetes meal plan—the same amounts of carbohydrates, protein, and fat are eaten at the same time each day	Diabetes	Determined by nutritional and energy requirements

The sodium-controlled diet is often ordered. So is a diabetes meal plan. Persons with difficulty swallowing may need a dysphagia diet.

The Sodium-Controlled Diet

The average amount of sodium in the daily diet is 3000 to 5000 mg. The body needs no more than 2400 mg a day. Healthy people excrete excess sodium in the urine.

Heart, liver, and kidney diseases and certain drugs cause the body to retain extra sodium. A sodium-controlled diet is often needed. Sodium causes the body to retain water. If there is too much sodium, the body retains more water. Tissues swell with water. There is excess fluid in the blood vessels. The heart has to work

harder. That is, the workload of the heart increases. With heart disease, the extra workload can cause serious problems or death.

Sodium control decreases the amount of sodium in the body. The body retains less water. Less water in the tissues and blood vessels reduces the heart's workload.

The doctor orders the amount of sodium allowed. Sodium-controlled diets involve:

▶ Omitting high-sodium foods (Box 23-5)
▶ Not adding salt to food at the table
▶ Limiting the amount of salt used in cooking
▶ Diet planning

See *Focus on Long-Term Care and Home Care: The Sodium-Controlled Diet.*

BOX 23-5 High-Sodium Foods

GRAINS (ORANGE BAND)
- Baked goods—biscuits, muffins, cakes, cookies, pies, pastries, sweet rolls, donuts, and so on
- Breads and rolls
- Cereals—cold, instant hot
- Noodle mixes
- Pancakes
- Salted snack foods—pretzels, corn chips, popcorn, crackers, chips, and so on
- Stuffing mixes
- Waffles

VEGETABLES (GREEN BAND)
- Canned vegetables
- Olives
- Pickles and other pickled vegetables
- Relish
- Sauerkraut
- Tomato sauce or paste
- Vegetable juices—tomato, V-8, bloody Mary mixes
- Vegetables with sauces, creams, or seasonings

FRUITS (RED BAND)
- None—fruits are not high in sodium

MILK (BLUE BAND)
- Buttermilk
- Cheese
- Commercial dips made with sour cream

MEAT AND BEANS (PURPLE BAND)
- Bacon
- Canadian bacon
- Canned meats and fish—chicken, tuna, salmon, anchovies, sardines
- Caviar
- Chipped and corned beef
- Dried beef and other meats
- Dried fish
- Ham

- Herring
- Hot dogs (frankfurters)
- Liverwurst
- Lox
- Luncheon meats—turkey, ham, bologna, salami
- Mackerel
- Pastrami
- Pepperoni
- Salt pork
- Sausages
- Scrapple
- Shellfish—shrimp, crab, clams, oysters, scallops, lobster
- Smoked salmon

OILS (YELLOW BAND)
- Mayonnaise
- Salad dressings

OTHER
- Asian foods—Chinese, Japanese, East Indian, Thai, Vietnamese
- Baking soda and baking powder
- Catsup (ketchup)
- Cocoa mixes
- Commercially prepared dinners—frozen, canned, boxed, and so on
- Mexican foods
- Mustard
- Pasta dishes—lasagna, manicotti, ravioli
- Peanut butter
- Pizzas
- Pot pies
- Salted nuts or seeds
- Sauces—soy, teriyaki, Worcestershire, steak, barbecue, pasta, chili, cocktail
- Seasoning salts—garlic, onion, celery, meat tenderizers, monosodium glutamate (MSG), and so on
- Soups—canned, packaged, instant, dried, bouillon

FOCUS ON LONG-TERM CARE AND HOME CARE

The Sodium-Controlled Diet

HOME CARE

Eating too much sodium is a factor in high blood pressure. (See "Hypertension" in Chapter 40.) Blood pressure can be lowered by reducing the amount of sodium consumed. Your home care patients, with and without high blood pressure, may follow the DASH Eating Plan. The plan:
- Is low in fat.
- Encourages healthy foods—fruits, vegetables, low-fat dairy foods, whole-grain products, fish, poultry, and nuts.
- Reduces the amount of red meat, sweets, and sugar-containing beverages in the diet.
- Is rich in magnesium, potassium, and calcium.
- Is rich in protein and fiber.
  Some people follow the 2400 mg of daily sodium plan. Others follow the 1500 mg of daily sodium plan.
- 1 teaspoon of table salt equals about 2400 mg of sodium
- 2/3 teaspoon of table salt equals about 1500 mg of sodium
  The following measures reduce salt and sodium in the diet. Always follow the nurse's directions and the care plan.

- Use reduced sodium or no-salt-added products.
- Use fresh, plain frozen, or canned with "no-salt-added" vegetables.
- Use fresh poultry, fish, and lean meat. Avoid canned, smoked, and processed types.
- Choose ready-to-eat breakfast cereals that are low in sodium.
- Limit the foods listed in Box 23-5.
- Flavor foods with herbs, spices, lemon, lime, vinegar, or salt-free seasonings. Do so in cooking and at the table.
- Cook rice, pasta, and hot cereals without salt.
- Cut back on instant or flavored rice, pasta, and cereal mixes. These usually have added salt.
- Choose convenience foods that are lower in sodium.
- Cut back on frozen dinners and mixed dishes. They often are high in sodium. Examples include pizza, packaged mixes, canned soups or broths, and salad dressings.
- Rinse canned foods to remove sodium.

(From the U.S. Department of Health and Human Services: *Facts about the DASH eating plan.*)

Diabetes Meal Plan

Diabetes meal planning is for people with diabetes. Diabetes is a chronic illness in which the body cannot use sugar for energy (Chapter 41). The pancreas produces and secretes insulin. Insulin lets the body use sugar. Without enough insulin, sugar builds up in the bloodstream. It is not used by cells for energy. Diabetes is usually treated with insulin or other drugs, diet, and exercise.

The dietitian and person develop a meal plan for healthy eating. Consistency is key. It involves:

▶ The person's food preferences (likes, eating habits, meal times, culture, and life-style). It may be necessary to limit the amount of food or change how it is prepared.
▶ Calories needed. The same amounts of carbohydrates, protein, and fat are eaten each day.
▶ Eating meals and snacks at regular times. The person should eat at the same time every day.

Serve the person's meals and snacks on time. The person eats at regular times to maintain a certain blood sugar level.

Always check the tray to see what was eaten. Tell the nurse what the person did and did not eat. If all food was not eaten, a between-meal nourishment is needed (p. 422). The nurse tells you what to give the person. It makes up for what was not eaten at the meal. The amount of insulin given also depends on daily food intake. Tell the nurse about changes in the person's eating habits.

The Dysphagia Diet

Dysphagia means difficulty (*dys*) swallowing (*phagia*). Food thickness is changed to meet the person's needs (Box 23-6). The doctor, speech-language pathologist, occupational therapist, dietitian, and nurse choose the right food thickness.

A *slow swallow* means the person has difficulty getting enough food and fluids for good nutrition and fluid balance. An *unsafe swallow* means that food enters the airway (aspiration). **Aspiration** is breathing fluid, food, vomitus, or an object into the lungs (Chapter 24).

BOX 23-6 Dysphagia Diet

CONSISTENCY	DESCRIPTION
Thickened liquid	No lumps. Pureed with milk, gravy, or broth to thickness of baby food. Thickener is added to some pureed foods as needed. Does not mound on a plate. May be called creamy or a sauce. Stir before serving if the food settles. Use a spoon.
Medium thick	The thickness of nectar or V-8 juice (does not hold its shape). Stir right before serving.
Extra thick	Thick like honey. Mounds a bit on a spoon. Drinkable from a cup. Stir before serving.
Yogurt-like	Thick like yogurt or pudding. Holds its shape. Served with a spoon.
Puree	No lumps; mounds on a plate. May be thick like mashed potatoes.

BOX 23-7 Signs and Symptoms of Dysphagia

- The person avoids food that needs chewing.
- The person avoids food with certain textures and temperatures.
- The person tires during a meal.
- Food spills out of the person's mouth while eating.
- Food "pockets" or is "squirreled" in the person's cheeks.
- The person eats slowly, especially solid foods.
- The person complains that food will not go down or that the food is stuck.
- The person frequently coughs or chokes before, during, or after swallowing.
- The person regurgitates food after eating (Chapter 24).
- The person spits out food suddenly and almost violently.
- Food comes up through the person's nose.
- The person is hoarse—especially after eating.
- After swallowing, the person makes gargling sounds while talking or breathing.
- The person has a runny nose, sneezes, or has excessive drooling of saliva.
- The person complains of frequent heartburn.
- Appetite is decreased.

BOX 23-8 Aspiration Precautions

- Help the person with meals and snacks. Follow the care plan.
- Position the person in Fowler's position or upright in a chair for meals and snacks.
- Support the upper back, shoulders, and neck with a pillow. Follow the care plan.
- Observe for signs and symptoms of aspiration during meals and snacks (Chapter 24).
- Check the person's mouth after eating for pocketing. Check inside the cheeks, under the tongue, and on the roof of the mouth. Remove any food.
- Position the person in a chair or in semi-Fowler's position after eating. The person maintains this position for at least 1 hour after eating. Follow the care plan.
- Provide mouth care after eating.
- Report and record your observations.

You may need to feed a person with dysphagia. To promote the person's safety and comfort, you must:
▶ Know the signs and symptoms of dysphagia (Box 23-7).
▶ Feed the person according to the care plan.
▶ Follow aspiration precautions (Box 23-8).
▶ Report changes in how the person eats.
▶ Report choking, coughing, or difficulty breathing during or after meals. Also report abnormal breathing or respiratory sounds. Report these observations at once.

FLUID BALANCE

Water is needed to live. Death can result from too much or too little water. Water is ingested through fluids and foods. Water is lost through urine, feces, and vomit. It is also lost through the skin (perspiration) and the lungs (expiration).

Fluid balance is needed for health. The amount of fluid taken in (intake) and the amount of fluid lost (output) must be equal. If fluid intake exceeds fluid output, body tissues swell with water. This is called **edema**. Edema is common in people with heart and kidney diseases. **Dehydration** is a decrease in the amount of water in body tissues. Fluid output exceeds intake. Common causes are poor fluid intake, vomiting, diarrhea, bleeding, excess sweating, and increased urine production.

Normal Fluid Requirements

An adult needs 1500 mL (milliliters) of water daily to survive. About 2000 to 2500 mL of fluid per day are needed for normal fluid balance. The water requirement increases with hot weather, exercise, fever, illness, and excess fluid losses.

See *Focus on Children and Older Persons: Normal Fluid Requirements.*

See *Focus on Ethics and Laws: Normal Fluid Requirements.*

Special Fluid Orders

The doctor may order the amount of fluid a person can have during a 24-hour period. This is done to maintain fluid balance. Found in the care plan and in the Kardex, common orders are:

- *Encourage fluids.* The person drinks an increased amount of fluid. The order states the amount to ingest. Intake records are kept. The person is given a variety of fluids allowed on the diet. They are kept within the person's reach. They are served at the correct temperature. Fluids are offered regularly to persons who cannot feed themselves.
- *Restrict fluids.* Fluids are limited to a certain amount. They are offered in small amounts and in small containers. The water pitcher is removed from the room or kept out of sight. Intake records are kept. The person needs frequent oral hygiene. It helps keep mucous membranes of the mouth moist.
- *Nothing by mouth.* The person cannot eat or drink anything. *NPO* is the abbreviation for *non per os.* It means nothing *(non)* by *(per)* mouth *(os)*. NPO often is ordered before and after surgery, before some laboratory tests and diagnostic procedures, and in treating certain illnesses. An NPO sign is posted above the bed. The water pitcher and glass are removed. Frequent oral hygiene is needed, but the person must not swallow any fluid. The person is NPO for 6 to 8 hours before surgery and before some laboratory tests and diagnostic procedures.
- *Thickened liquids.* All fluids are thickened, including water. The thickness depends on the person's ability to swallow (see Box 23-6). Thickener is added before fluids are served. Or commercial fluids are used. They are already thickened.

FOCUS ON **CHILDREN** AND **OLDER PERSONS**

Normal Fluid Requirements

CHILDREN
Fluid requirements vary with age. Infants and young children have more body water. They need more fluids than adults do. Excess fluid losses cannot be tolerated. They quickly cause death in an infant or child.

OLDER PERSONS
The amount of body water decreases with age. Older persons also are at risk for diseases that affect fluid balance. Examples include heart disease, kidney disease, cancer, and diabetes. Some drugs cause the body to lose fluids. Others cause the body to retain water. The older person is at risk for dehydration and edema.

Older persons may have a decreased sense of thirst. Their bodies need water, but they may not feel thirsty. You need to offer water often. Some persons have special fluid orders.

FOCUS ON **ETHICS** AND **LAWS**

Normal Fluid Requirements

Mr. Phillip Caruso was admitted to a nursing center on January 22 after needing hospital care for about 5 weeks. He had nervous and urinary system disorders. A doctor examined him on January 23. The doctor found him to be in stable condition. He showed signs of adequate hydration and responded to the doctor's commands.

The nursing center "did not keep a chart of Phillip's intake or output of fluids." According to the center nurses, Mr. Caruso received the following:
- Three meals a day.
- Three snacks [a day] with juice or milk.
- Drugs four times a day. He was given 4 ounces of water with the drugs.
- Offers of something to drink every two hours during the night.

Seven days after being admitted to the nursing center (January 29), Mr. Caruso was taken to the hospital. The emergency room doctor diagnosed severe dehydration. He was weak and confused, had tremors, and had dry skin with poor turgor. (Author note: *poor skin turgor* means that the skin slowly returns to its normal position after being grasped between two fingers.) In the hospital Mr. Caruso was treated with IV (intravenous) fluids and a catheter. He was also treated for a urinary tract infection caused by the catheter.

Mr. Caruso returned to the nursing center on February 19. He died on May 14.

His family sued the nursing center. They charged the nursing center with negligence and with abuse and neglect because of failing to give Mr. Caruso enough water. They claimed that the dehydration led to declines in his physical and mental condition.

The jury found in favor of Mr. Caruso's family. The jury awarded the family $195,000 and attorney fees. The nursing home appealed the case. Because of a legal technicality, a judge ordered a new trial.

(I. Caruso v Pine Manor Nursing Center, Ill, 1989.)

Intake and Output Records

The doctor or nurse may order intake and output (I&O) measurements. I&O records are kept. They are used to evaluate fluid balance and kidney function. They help in evaluating and planning medical treatment. They also are kept when the person has special fluid orders.

All fluids taken by mouth are measured and recorded—water, milk, coffee, tea, juices, soups, and soft drinks. So are foods that melt at room temperature—ice cream, sherbet, custard, pudding, gelatin, and Popsicles. The nurse measures and records IV fluids and tube feedings (Chapter 24). Output includes urine, vomitus, diarrhea, and wound drainage.

◆ *Measuring Intake and Output*

Intake and output are measured in milliliters (mL). You need to know these amounts:

▶ 1 ounce (oz) equals 30 mL
▶ 1 pint is about 500 mL
▶ 1 quart is about 1000 mL

You also need to know the serving sizes of bowls, dishes, cups, pitchers, glasses, and other containers. This information may be on the I&O record (Fig. 23-8).

A measuring container for fluid is called a **graduate.** It is used to measure left-over fluids, urine, vomitus, and drainage from suction. Like a measuring cup, the graduate is marked in ounces and milliliters (Fig. 23-9). Plastic

---

OSF
ST. JOSEPH MEDICAL CENTER
Bloomington, Illinois

FLUID BALANCE CHART

Water Glass	250mL	Ice Cream	120mL
Styrofoam Cup	180mL	Ice Chips	1/2 amt. of mL's in cup
Cup (coffee)	250mL		
Milk Carton	240mL	Pitcher	
Pop (1 can)	360mL	(Yellow)	1000mL
Broth-Soup	175mL		
Juice Carton	120mL		
Juice Glass	120mL		
Jello	120mL		

DATE __6/15__

	INTAKE				OUTPUT					
		Parenteral	Amt. mL Absbd.		URINE		OTHER		CONT. IRRIGATION	
TIME	ORAL				Method Collected	Amt. (mL)	Method Collected	Amt. (mL)	In	Out
2400-0100		mL from previous shift			V	150				
0100-0200							Vom.	150		
0200-0300										
0300-0400										
0400-0500										
0500-0600	125				V	200				
0600-0700										
0700-0800										
	125	8 - hour Sub-total			8-hr T	350	8-hr T	150		
0800-0900	400	mL from previous shift			V	250				
0900-1000	100									
1000-1100										
1100-1200										
1200-1300	400				V	250				
1300-1400										
1400-1500	200									
1500-1600										
	1100	8 - hour Sub-total			8-hr T	500	8-hr T			
1600-1700		mL from previous shift			V	270				
1700-1800	350									
1800-1900	50									
1900-2000	200									
2000-2100					V	400				
2100-2200										
2200-2300										
2300-2400										
	600	8 - hour Sub-total			8-hr T	670	8-hr T			
	1825	24 - hour Sub-total			24-hr T	1520	24-hr T	150		

Source Key:
URINE
V - Voided
C - Catheter
INC - Incontinent
U.C. - Ureteral Catheter

Source Key:
OTHER
G.I.T. - Gastric Intestinal Tube
T.T. - T. Tube
Vom. - Vomitus
Liq S. - Liquid Stool
H.V. - Hemovac

310¹ Marie Mills

Form No. MF36722 (Rev. 5/97) **MFI**

FIGURE 23-8 An intake and output record. (Modified from OSF St. Joseph Medical Center, Bloomington, Ill.)

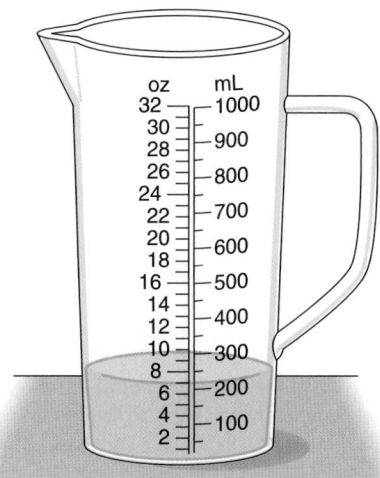

FIGURE 23-9 A graduate marked in ounces and milliliters.

urinals and kidney basins also have amounts marked. The measuring device is held at eye level to read the amount.

An I&O record is kept at the bedside. When intake or output is measured, the amount is recorded in the correct column (see Fig. 23-8). Amounts are totaled at the end of the shift. The totals are recorded in the person's chart. They also are shared during the end-of-shift report.

The purpose of measuring I&O and how to help are explained to the person. Some persons measure and record their intake. Family members may help. The urinal, commode, bedpan, or specimen pan is used for voiding. Remind the person not to void in the toilet. Also remind the person not to put toilet tissue into the receptacle.

See *Delegation Guidelines: Intake and Output*.
See *Promoting Safety and Comfort: Intake and Output*.

DELEGATION GUIDELINES: Intake and Output

When measuring I&O, you need this information from the nurse and the care plan:

- If the person has a special fluid order—encourage fluids, restrict fluids, NPO, or thickened fluids
- When to report measurements—hourly or end-of-shift
- What the person uses for voiding—urinal, bedpan, commode, or specimen pan
- If the person has a catheter
- What specific patient or resident concerns to report at once

---

PROMOTING SAFETY AND COMFORT: Intake and Output

SAFETY

Urine may contain microbes or blood. Microbes can grow in urinals, commodes, bedpans, specimen pans, and drainage systems. Follow Standard Precautions and the Bloodborne Pathogen Standard when handling such equipment. Thoroughly clean the item after it is used. Use a disinfectant for cleaning.

COMFORT

Promptly measure the contents of urinals, bedpans, commodes, and specimen pans. This helps prevent or reduce odors. Odors can disturb the person.

 NNAAP™ Skill

MEASURING INTAKE AND OUTPUT

✔**Quality of Life** *Remember to:*

- Knock before entering the person's room.
- Address the person by name.
- Introduce yourself by name and title.
- Explain the procedure to the person before beginning and during the procedure.

- Protect the person's rights during the procedure.
- Handle the person gently during the procedure.

PRE-PROCEDURE

1 Follow *Delegation Guidelines: Intake and Output*. See *Promoting Safety and Comfort: Intake and Output*.
2 Practice hand hygiene.

3 Collect the following:
  - Intake and output (I&O) record
  - Graduates
  - Gloves

Continued

MEASURING INTAKE AND OUTPUT—cont'd

PROCEDURE

4 Put on gloves.
5 Measure intake as follows:
  a Pour liquid remaining in the container into the graduate.
  b Measure the amount at eye level. Keep the container level.
  c Check the serving amount on the I&O record.
  d Subtract the remaining amount from the full serving amount. Note the amount.
  e Pour fluid in the graduate back into the container.
  f Repeat steps 5a through 5e for each liquid.
  g Add the amounts from each liquid together.
  h Record the time and amount on the I&O record.

6 Measure output as follows:
  a Pour the fluid into the graduate used to measure output.
  b Measure the amount at eye level. Keep the container level.
  c Dispose of fluid in the toilet. Avoid splashes.
7 Clean and rinse the graduates. Dispose of rinse into the toilet. Return the graduates to their proper place.
8 Clean and rinse the bedpan, urinal, commode container, specimen pan, kidney basin, or other drainage container. Dispose of the rinse into the toilet. Return the item to its proper place.
9 Remove the gloves. Practice hand hygiene.
10 Record the output amount on the I&O record.

POST-PROCEDURE

11 Provide for comfort. (See the inside of the front book cover.)
12 Make sure the signal light is within reach.

13 Complete a safety check of the room. (See the inside of the front book cover.)
14 Report and record your observations.

MEETING FOOD AND FLUID NEEDS

Weakness, illness, and confusion can affect appetite and ability to eat. So can unpleasant odors, sights, and sounds. An uncomfortable position, the need for oral hygiene, the need to eliminate, and pain also affect appetite.

See *Focus on Communication: Meeting Food and Fluid Needs.*

◆ Preparing For Meals

Preparing patients and residents for meals promotes their comfort. To promote comfort:
▶ Assist with elimination needs.
▶ Provide oral hygiene. Make sure dentures are in place.
▶ Make sure eyeglasses and hearing aids are in place.
▶ Make sure incontinent persons are clean and dry.
▶ Position the person in a comfortable position. Assist the person with hand washing.
  See *Delegation Guidelines: Preparing for Meals.*
  See *Promoting Safety and Comfort: Preparing for Meals.*

DELEGATION GUIDELINES: Preparing for Meals

To prepare a person for a meal, you need this information from the nurse and the care plan:
• How much help the person needs
• Where the person will eat—room or dining room
• What the person uses for elimination—bathroom, commode, bedpan, urinal, or specimen pan
• What type of oral hygiene the person needs
• If the person wears dentures
• How to position the person—in bed or in a chair or wheelchair
• If the person wears eyeglasses or hearing aids
• How the person gets to the dining room—by self or with help
• If the person uses a wheelchair, walker, or cane

FOCUS ON COMMUNICATION

Meeting Food and Fluid Needs

The person may not eat or drink all the food and fluids served. You need to find out why and tell the nurse. You can ask these questions. Then ask the person to explain his or her answer.
• "Please tell me why you didn't eat everything."
• "Was there something wrong with your food?"
• "Did your food taste okay?"
• "Was your food too hot or too cold?"
• "Would you like something else?"
• "Weren't you hungry?"

PROMOTING SAFETY AND COMFORT: Preparing for Meals

SAFETY

Before meals, the person needs to eliminate and have oral hygiene. Follow Standard Precautions and the Bloodborne Pathogen Standard. Also follow them when cleaning equipment and the room.

COMFORT

The meal setting must be free of unpleasant sights, sounds, and odors. Remove unpleasant equipment from the room.

PREPARING THE PERSON FOR A MEAL

✔ Quality of Life *Remember to:*

- Knock before entering the person's room.
- Address the person by name.
- Introduce yourself by name and title.
- Explain the procedure to the person before beginning and during the procedure.

- Protect the person's rights during the procedure.
- Handle the person gently during the procedure.

PRE-PROCEDURE

1 Follow *Delegation Guidelines: Preparing for Meals.* See *Promoting Safety and Comfort: Preparing for Meals.*
2 Practice hand hygiene.
3 Collect the following:
- Equipment for oral hygiene
- Bedpan and cover, urinal, commode, or specimen pan

- Toilet tissue
- Wash basin
- Soap
- Washcloth
- Towel
- Gloves
4 Provide for privacy.

PROCEDURE

5 Make sure eyeglasses and hearing aids are in place.
6 Assist with oral hygiene. Make sure dentures are in place. Wear gloves, and decontaminate your hands after removing gloves.
7 Assist with elimination. Make sure the incontinent person is clean and dry. Wear gloves, and practice hand hygiene after removing them.
8 Assist with hand washing. Wear gloves and practice hand hygiene after removing gloves.
9 Do the following if the person will eat in bed:
  a Raise the head of the bed to a comfortable position. Usually Fowler's position is preferred.

  b Remove items from the overbed table. Clean the overbed table.
  c Adjust the overbed table in front of the person.
10 Do the following if the person will sit in a chair:
  a Position the person in a chair or wheelchair.
  b Remove items from the overbed table. Clean the table.
  c Adjust the overbed table in front of the person.
11 Assist the person to the dining area. (This step is for the person who eats in a dining area.)

POST-PROCEDURE

12 Provide for comfort. (See the inside of the front book cover.)
13 Place the signal light within reach.
14 Empty, clean, and disinfect equipment. Return equipment to its proper place. Wear gloves, and practice hand hygiene after removing gloves.

15 Straighten the room. Eliminate unpleasant noise, odors, or equipment.
16 Unscreen the person.
17 Complete a safety check of the room. (See the inside of the front book cover.)
18 Practice hand hygiene.

◆ Serving Meal Trays

Food is served in containers that keep foods at the correct temperature. Hot food is kept hot. Cold food is kept cold.

You serve meal trays after preparing patients and residents for meals. You can serve trays promptly if they are ready to eat. Prompt serving keeps food at the correct temperature.

Some agencies have "room service" meal programs. A full menu (breakfast, lunch, dinner) is in the person's room. When ready to eat, the person calls the dietary department to order what he or she wants. Food is served a short while later. This program allows the person to eat when hungry. For a fee, visitors can also order food so they can dine with the person.

Serve trays in the order assigned by the health team. In nursing centers, some residents are seated at tables. Everyone at a table is served at the same time.

If food is not served within 15 minutes, recheck food temperatures. Follow agency policy. If not at the correct temperature, get a fresh tray. Some agencies allow reheating in microwave ovens.

See *Focus on Long-Term Care and Home Care: Serving Meal Trays,* p. 418.

See *Delegation Guidelines: Serving Meal Trays,* p. 418.

See *Promoting Safety and Comfort: Serving Meal Trays,* p. 418.

See *Teamwork and Time Management: Serving Meal Trays,* p. 418.

Text continued on p. 420

FOCUS ON **LONG-TERM CARE** AND **HOME CARE**

Serving Meal Trays

LONG-TERM CARE

OBRA requires that food be served at the correct temperature. Temperature guides and food thermometers are in dining rooms. They also are in the kitchen on each nursing unit.

The following dining programs are common in nursing centers:

- *Social dining.* Four to six residents are seated at a dining room table (Fig. 23-10). Tables have tablecloths or placemats. Food is served as in a restaurant. This program is for persons who are oriented and can feed themselves. Sometimes quietly confused persons are included. They must be able to feed themselves and not disrupt others.
- *Family dining.* This is like social dining. However, food is served in bowls and on platters. Residents serve themselves as at home.
- *Assistive dining.* Horse-shoe shaped tables are in the dining room. A nursing assistant sits at the center of the table and feeds up to four persons (Fig. 23-11). Very confused persons are with others for meals. Food is served at the correct temperature. And residents are fed in a timely manner.
- *Low-stimulation dining.* Mealtime distractions are prevented. The health team decides on the best place for each person to sit.
- *Restaurant-style menus.* The person selects food from a menu. This program allows more food choices. The person is served as in a restaurant.
- *Open-dining.* A buffet is open for several hours. A breakfast buffet is an example. Residents can eat any time while the buffet is open.

Some centers have dining areas where residents can dine privately with guests. The person can have a meal with a partner, children, and other family or friends. They can celebrate holidays, birthdays, anniversaries, or other events. Food is provided by guests or the dietary department.

DELEGATION GUIDELINES: Serving Meal Trays

Before serving meal trays, you need this information from the nurse and the care plan:
- What adaptive equipment the person uses
- How much help the person needs opening cartons, cutting food, buttering bread, and so on
- If the person's I&O are measured
- If calorie counts are done (p. 422)

PROMOTING SAFETY AND COMFORT: Serving Meal Trays

SAFETY

Always check food temperature after reheating. Food that is too hot can burn the person.

COMFORT

Check the person's position when serving meal trays. The position may have changed after the person was prepared to eat. Provide other comfort measures as needed. See the inside of the front book cover for comfort measures.

TEAMWORK AND TIME MANAGEMENT

Serving Meal Trays

Trays are served in the order set by the health team. You will serve trays to your patients and residents and to those assigned to other nursing assistants. Your co-workers will do the same. The goal is to serve trays as fast as possible. This keeps food at the desired temperature.

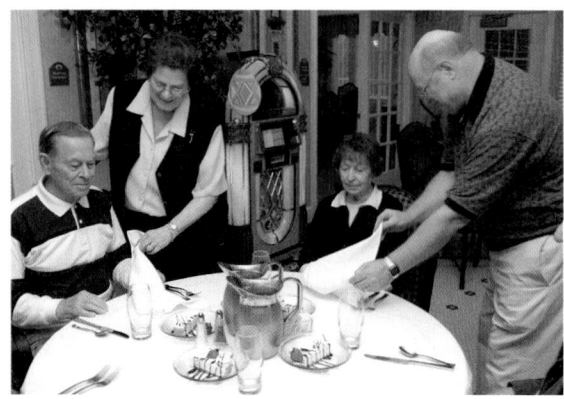

FIGURE 23-10 These residents are eating in the dining room.

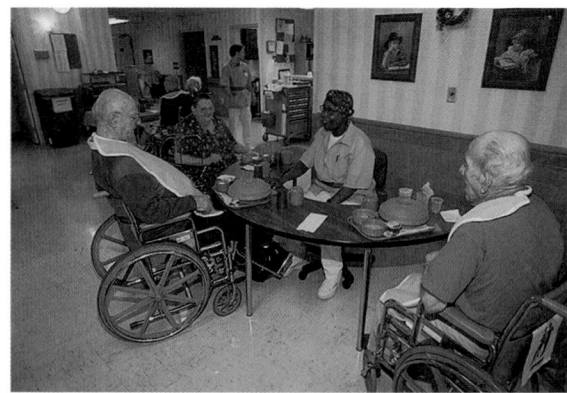

FIGURE 23-11 A horse-shoe shaped table is used for assistive dining. The nursing assistant feeds three residents at one time. Residents are in the company of others.

SERVING MEAL TRAYS

✔ Quality of Life *Remember to:*

- Knock before entering the person's room.
- Address the person by name.
- Introduce yourself by name and title.
- Explain the procedure to the person before beginning and during the procedure.

- Protect the person's rights during the procedure.
- Handle the person gently during the procedure.

PRE-PROCEDURE

1 Follow *Delegation Guidelines: Serving Meal Trays.* See *Promoting Safety and Comfort: Serving Meal Trays.*
2 Practice hand hygiene.

PROCEDURE

3 Make sure the tray is complete. Check items on the tray with the dietary card. Make sure adaptive equipment is included.
4 Identify the person. Check the ID bracelet against the dietary card. Also call the person by name.
5 Place the tray within the person's reach. Adjust the overbed table as needed.
6 Remove food covers. Open cartons, cut food into bite-size pieces, butter bread, and so on as needed (Fig. 23-12).
7 Place the napkin, clothes protector, adaptive equipment, and eating utensils within reach.
8 Place the signal light within reach.

9 Do the following when the person is done eating:
  a Measure and record intake if ordered.
  b Note the amount and type of foods eaten. (See "Calorie Counts" on p. 422.)
  c Check for and remove any food in the mouth (pocketing). Wear gloves. Decontaminate your hands after removing gloves.
  d Remove the tray.
  e Clean spills. Change soiled linen and clothing.
  f Help the person return to bed if needed.
  g Assist with oral hygiene and hand washing. Wear gloves. Decontaminate your hands after removing the gloves.

POST-PROCEDURE

10 Provide for comfort. (See the inside of the front book cover.)
11 Place the signal light within reach.
12 Raise or lower bed rails. Follow the care plan.
13 Complete a safety check of the room. (See the inside of the front book cover.)

14 Follow agency policy for soiled linen.
15 Decontaminate your hands.
16 Report and record your observations.

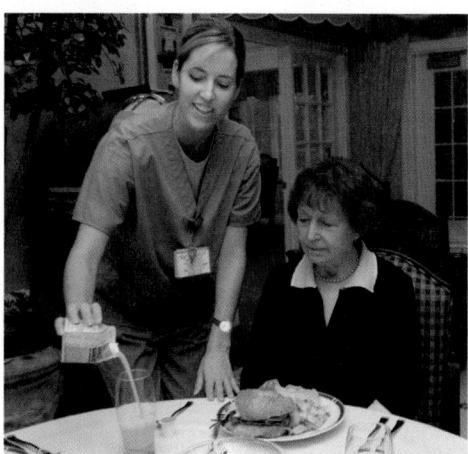

FIGURE 23-12 Cartons and containers are opened for the person.

◆ Feeding the Person

Weakness, paralysis, casts, confusion, and other limits may make self-feeding impossible. These persons are fed.

Serve food and fluids in the order the person prefers. Offer fluids during the meal. Fluids help the person chew and swallow.

Use teaspoons to feed the person. They are less likely to cause injury than forks. The teaspoon should only be one-third full. This portion is chewed and swallowed easily. Some people need smaller portions. Follow the care plan.

Persons who need to be fed are often angry, humiliated, and embarrassed. Some are depressed or resentful or refuse to eat. Let them do as much as possible. Some can manage "finger foods" (bread, cookies, crackers). If strong enough, let them hold milk or juice glasses (never hot drinks). Do not exceed ordered activity limits. Provide support. Encourage them to try, even if food is spilled.

Visually impaired persons are often very aware of food aromas. They may know the food served. Always tell the person what is on the tray. When feeding visually impaired persons, describe what you are offering. For persons who feed themselves, describe foods and fluids and their place on the tray. Use the numbers on a clock for the location of foods (Fig. 23-13).

Many people pray before eating. Allow time and privacy for prayer. This shows respect and care about the person.

Meals provide social contact with others. Engage the person in pleasant conversation. However, allow time for chewing and swallowing. Also, sit facing the person. Sitting is more relaxing. It shows that you have time for the person. By facing the person, you can see how well the person is eating. You can also see if the person has problems swallowing.

See *Focus on Children and Older Persons: Feeding the Person.*

See *Delegation Guidelines: Feeding the Person.*

See *Promoting Safety and Comfort: Feeding the Person.*

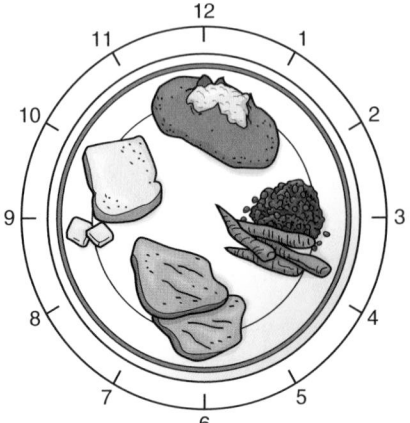

FIGURE 23-13 The numbers on a clock are used to help a visually impaired person locate food.

Feeding the Person

OLDER PERSONS

Some older persons have dementia. They may become distracted during meals. Some persons cannot sit long enough for a meal. Others forget how to use eating utensils. Some persons resist your efforts to assist them with eating. A confused person may throw or spit food.

The Alzheimer's Disease Education and Referral Center (ADEAR) recommends the following. The measures may be part of the person's care plan.

- Provide a calm, quiet setting for eating. Limit noise and other distractions. This helps the person focus on the meal.
- Limit the number of food choices.
- Offer several small meals throughout the day instead of larger ones.
- Use straws or cups with lids. These make drinking easier.
- Provide finger foods if the person has problems with utensils. A bowl may be easier to use than a plate.
- Provide healthy snacks. Keep snacks where the person can see them.

You must be patient. Talk to the nurse if you feel upset or impatient. Remember, the person has the right to be treated with dignity and respect.

DELEGATION GUIDELINES: Feeding the Person

Before feeding a person, you need this information from the nurse and the care plan:
- Why the person needs help
- How much help the person needs
- If the person can manage finger foods
- What the person's activity limits are
- What the person's dietary restrictions are
- What size portion to feed the person—⅓ teaspoonful or less
- What safety measures are needed if the person has dysphagia
- If the person can use a straw
- What observations to report and record:
  - The amount and kind of food eaten
  - Complaints of nausea or dysphagia
  - Signs and symptoms of dysphagia
  - Signs and symptoms of aspiration
- When to report observations
- What specific patient or resident concerns to report at once

---

PROMOTING SAFETY AND COMFORT: Feeding the Person

SAFETY

Check food temperature. Very hot foods can burn the person.

Prevent aspiration. Check the person's mouth before offering more food or fluids. The person's mouth must be empty between bites and swallows.

COMFORT

The person will eat better if not rushed. Sit to show the person that you have time for him or her. Standing communicates that you are in a hurry.

Wipe the person's hands, face, and mouth as needed during the meal. Use the napkin. If necessary, use a wet washcloth. Then dry the person with a towel.

FEEDING THE PERSON

✔ Quality of Life *Remember to:*

- Knock before entering the person's room.
- Address the person by name.
- Introduce yourself by name and title.
- Explain the procedure to the person before beginning and during the procedure.

- Protect the person's rights during the procedure.
- Handle the person gently during the procedure.

PRE-PROCEDURE

1 Follow *Delegation Guidelines: Feeding the Person.* See *Promoting Safety and Comfort: Feeding the Person.*
2 Practice hand hygiene.

3 Position the person in a comfortable position for eating—usually sitting or Fowler's.
4 Get the tray. Place it on the overbed table or dining table.

PROCEDURE

5 Identify the person. Check the ID bracelet against the dietary card. Also call the person by name.
6 Drape a napkin across the person's chest and underneath the chin.
7 Tell the person what foods and fluids are on the tray.
8 Prepare food for eating. Cut food into bite-size pieces. Season foods as the person prefers and is allowed on the care plan.
9 Serve foods in the order the person prefers. Identify foods as you serve them. Alternate between solid and liquid foods. Use a spoon for safety (Fig. 23-14). Allow enough time for chewing and swallowing. Do not rush the person.
10 Check the person's mouth before offering more food or fluids. Make sure the person's mouth is empty between bites and swallows.
11 Use straws for liquids if the person cannot drink out of a glass or cup. Have one straw for each liquid. Provide short straws for weak persons.

12 Wipe the person's hands, face, and mouth as needed during the meal. Use the napkin.
13 Follow the care plan if the person has dysphagia. (Some persons with dysphagia do not use straws.) Give thickened liquid with a spoon.
14 Converse with the person in a pleasant manner.
15 Encourage him or her to eat as much as possible.
16 Wipe the person's mouth with a napkin. Discard the napkin.
17 Note how much and which foods were eaten. See "Calorie Counts," p. 422.
18 Measure and record intake if ordered (p. 414).
19 Remove the tray.
20 Take the person back to his or her room (if in a dining area).
21 Assist with oral hygiene and hand washing. Provide for privacy, and put on gloves. Decontaminate your hands after removing the gloves.

POST-PROCEDURE

22 Provide for comfort. (See the inside of the front book cover.)
23 Place the signal light within reach.
24 Raise or lower bed rails. Follow the care plan.
25 Complete a safety check of the room. (See the inside of the front book cover.)

26 Return the food tray to the food cart.
27 Decontaminate your hands.
28 Report and record your observations.

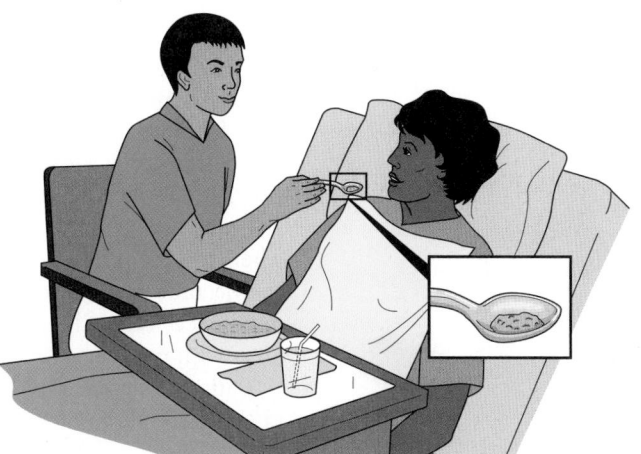

FIGURE 23-14 A spoon is used to feed the person. The spoon is one-third full.

Between-Meal Nourishments

Many special diets involve between-meal nourishments. Common nourishments are crackers, milk, juice, a milkshake, cake, wafers, a sandwich, gelatin, and custard.

These nourishments are served upon arrival on the nursing unit. Provide needed utensils, a straw, and a napkin. Follow the same considerations and procedures for serving meal trays and feeding persons.

Calorie Counts

Calorie records are kept for some people. On a flow sheet, note what the person ate and how much. For example, a chicken breast, rice, beans, a roll, pudding, and two pats of butter were served. The person ate all the chicken, half the rice, and the roll. One pat of butter was used. The beans and pudding were not eaten. You note these on the flow sheet. A nurse or dietitian converts these portions into calories. The nurse tells you which persons need calorie counts.

◆ Providing Drinking Water

Patients and residents need fresh drinking water each shift. They also need water whenever the pitcher is empty.

Some agencies do not use the procedure that follows. Each person's water pitcher is filled as needed. The pitcher is taken to an ice and water dispenser. If so, fill the water pitcher with ice first. Then add water to the pitcher. Follow the center's procedure for providing fresh drinking water.

See *Delegation Guidelines: Providing Drinking Water.*

See *Promoting Safety and Comfort: Providing Drinking Water.*

DELEGATION GUIDELINES: Providing Drinking Water

Before providing water, you need this information from the nurse and the care plan:
- The person's fluid orders
- If the person can have ice
- If the person uses a straw

PROMOTING SAFETY AND COMFORT: Providing Drinking Water

SAFETY

Water glasses and pitchers can spread microbes. To prevent the spread of microbes:
- Make sure the water pitcher is labeled with the person's name and room and bed number.
- Do not touch the rim or inside of the water glass or pitcher.
- Do not let the ice scoop touch the rim or inside of the water cup or pitcher.
- Do not put the ice scoop in the ice container or dispenser. Place it in the scoop holder or on a towel for the scoop.
- Make sure the person's water pitcher and cup are clean. Also check for cracks and chips. Provide a new water pitcher or cup as needed.

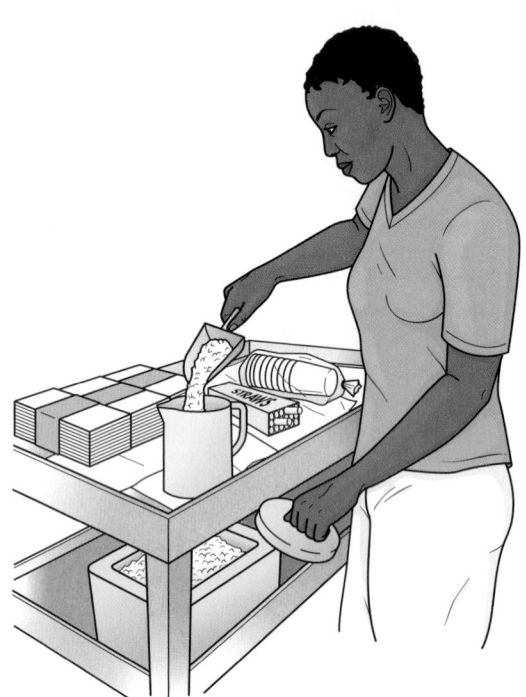

FIGURE 23-15 Providing drinking water.

FOODBORNE ILLNESSES

A foodborne illness (food poisoning) is caused by pathogens in food and fluids. Signs and symptoms depend on the pathogen. Report the signs and symptoms listed in Box 23-9 to the nurse at once.

Food is not sterile. Therefore pathogens are present when food is purchased. Cooked and ready-to-eat foods can become contaminated from other food. For example, meat juices can spill or splash onto other food. Food handlers with poor hygiene can contaminate the food.

Pathogens grow rapidly between 40° and 140° F. This range is called the "danger zone" by the USDA. You must keep food out of the "danger zone." To do so, keep cold food cold and hot food hot.

PROVIDING DRINKING WATER

✔ Quality of Life *Remember to:*

- Knock before entering the person's room.
- Address the person by name.
- Introduce yourself by name and title.
- Explain the procedure to the person before beginning and during the procedure.

- Protect the person's rights during the procedure.
- Handle the person gently during the procedure.

PRE-PROCEDURE

1 Follow *Delegation Guidelines: Providing Drinking Water.* See *Promoting Safety and Comfort: Providing Drinking Water.*
2 Obtain a list of persons who have special fluid orders from the nurse. Or use your assignment sheet.
3 Practice hand hygiene.
4 Collect the following:
- Cart
- Ice chest filled with ice
- Cover for the ice chest

- Scoop
- Disposable cups
- Straws
- Paper towels
- Water pitchers for the patient and resident use
- Large water pitcher filled with cold water (optional, depending on center procedure)
- Towel for the scoop
5 Cover the cart with paper towels. Arrange equipment on top of the paper towels.

PROCEDURE

6 Take the cart to the person's room door. Do not take the cart into the room.
7 Check the person's fluid orders. Use the list obtained from the nurse.
8 Identify the person. Check the ID bracelet against the fluid orders sheet or your assignment sheet. Also call the person by name.
9 Take the pitcher from the person's overbed table. Empty it into the bathroom sink.
10 Determine if a new water pitcher is needed.
11 Use the scoop to fill the pitcher with ice (Fig. 23-15). Do not let the scoop touch the rim or inside of the pitcher.

12 Place the ice scoop on the towel.
13 Fill the water pitcher with water. Get water from the bathroom or use the larger water pitcher on the cart.
14 Place the pitcher, disposable cup, and straw (if used) on the overbed table. Fill the cup with water. Do not let the water pitcher touch the rim or inside of the cup.
15 Make sure the water pitcher, cup, and straw (if used) are within the person's reach.

POST-PROCEDURE

16 Provide for comfort. (See the inside of the front book cover.)
17 Place the signal light within reach.
18 Complete a safety check of the room. (See the inside of the front book cover.)

19 Decontaminate your hands.
20 Repeat steps 6 through 19 for each person.

To keep food safe, the USDA recommends these 4 safety tips:

▸ *Clean.* Wash hands, utensils, and counter tops often.
▸ *Separate.* Avoid cross-contamination. Do not let raw meat, poultry, or their juices touch other foods that will not be cooked.
▸ *Cook.* Cook food to a safe internal temperature (see Fig. 23-3). Use a food thermometer to check the internal temperature. When re-heating cooked food, re-heat to 165° F.
▸ *Chill.* Refrigerate or freeze food within 2 hours. If the air is 90° F or above, chill food within 1 hour.

See *Focus on Long-Term Care and Home Care: Foodborne Illnesses,* p. 424.

BOX 23-9 Signs and Symptoms of Foodborne Illnesses

- Abdominal cramps or pain
- Backache
- Breathing problems
- Chills
- Double vision
- Diarrhea (may be bloody)
- Droopy eyelids

- Fever
- Headache
- Muscle pain
- Nausea
- Speaking problems
- Swallowing problems
- Vomiting

FOCUS ON LONG-TERM CARE AND HOME CARE

Foodborne Illnesses

HOME CARE

You need to protect the patient and family from foodborne illnesses. Follow the *clean*, *separate*, *cook*, and *chill* safety tips. Other aspects of clean, separate, cook, and chill listed by the USDA include:

Vegetables and Fruits

- Wash vegetables and fruits before preparing or eating them.
- Rub vegetables and fruits under clean running water. Rub briskly with your hands to remove dirt and microbes.
- Dry vegetables and fruits after washing them.
- Keep vegetables and fruits separate from raw meat, poultry, and seafood. Do this while shopping, preparing, and storing food.

Milk

- Avoid raw (unpasteurized) milk or any products made from unpasteurized milk.
- Refrigerate promptly milk and milk products that can perish.
- Defrost foods properly.
- Refrigerate or freeze prepared food and left-overs as soon as possible.
- Discard food that has been left at temperatures between 40° and 140° F for more than 2 hours.
- Separate raw, cooked, and ready-to-eat foods.

Beef, Poultry, and Seafood

- Select meat, poultry, and seafood just before checking out at the grocery store. Place each item in a disposable plastic bag to prevent juices from leaking onto other foods.
- Separate beef, poultry, and seafood from other foods in the grocery cart, at check-out, and in grocery bags.
- Follow safe handling instructions on the package.
- Do the following for fully cooked, take-out, or fast food:
  - Make sure the food is hot at the time of purchase.
  - Use the food within 2 hours or refrigerate it in shallow, covered containers. Use within 1 hour if the air temperature is above 90° F.
  - Eat refrigerated food within 3 to 4 days.
  - Eat the food cold or reheated to 165° F. The food is hot, but not steaming.
  - Use frozen ready-prepared dishes within 4 months.
- Separate raw, cooked, and ready-to-eat foods.
- Refrigerate or freeze beef, poultry, and seafood at once.
- Do not wash or rinse beef, poultry, or seafood.
- Use or freeze beef products with a "Sell-By" date within 3 to 5 days of purchase.
- Use or freeze poultry within 1 to 2 days of purchase.
- Observe the "Use-By" date on the package unless the food is properly frozen.
- Wash cutting boards, knives, utensils, and counter tops with hot soapy water. Do so:
  - After preparing each food item
  - Before going to the next food item
- Store raw meat, poultry, and seafood on the bottom shelf of the refrigerator. This prevents juices from dripping onto other foods.
- Cook foods to a safe temperature to kill microbes. Use a meat thermometer to measure the internal temperature.
- Chill promptly food that can perish.

Beef, Poultry, and Seafood—cont'd

- Defrost foods properly. To thaw food:
  - Place it in the refrigerator. Thawing can take 1 to 2 days depending on the size.
  - Submerge air-tight packaged food in cold tap water. Change the water every 30 minutes. Thawing can take 30 minutes to 3 hours depending on the size.
  - Place on a plate and thaw in a microwave oven. Cook at once after thawing.
- Do not defrost food on a counter at room temperature.
- Refrigerate or freeze prepared food and left-overs within 2 hours. Place the food in clean, shallow, covered containers.
- Boil used marinade before brushing on cooked food. Discard any uncooked, left-over marinade.

Eggs

- Do not eat or serve raw eggs. This includes milk shakes, Caesar salad dressing, Hollandaise sauce, homemade mayonnaise, and other foods in which the raw egg ingredients are not cooked.
- Buy eggs with clean, uncracked shells.
- Do not wash eggs.
- Store eggs in the grocery carton.
- Refrigerate eggs at once. Store them in the coldest part of the refrigerator. Do not store them on the door.
- Do not keep eggs (including Easter eggs) out of the refrigerator for more than 2 hours.
- Use raw eggs in the shell within 3 to 5 weeks.
- Use left-over yolks and whites within 4 days.
- Use refrigerated, hard-cooked eggs within 1 week.
- Wash hands, utensils, equipment, and work areas with warm, soapy water. Do so before and after contact with eggs and dishes containing eggs.
- Serve cooked eggs and dishes containing eggs at once after cooking. Or place them in shallow containers for quick cooling and refrigerate. Use within 3 to 4 days.
- Cook eggs until the yolks are firm. Scrambled eggs should not be runny. Casseroles and dishes containing eggs should be cooked to 160° F.

Other

- Wash your hands with soap and hot water before and after:
  - Handling food
  - Using the bathroom
  - Giving care (including changing diapers)
  - Handling pets
- Use hot, soapy water and paper towels or clean cloths to wipe up kitchen surfaces or spills.
- Use the hot cycle of the washing machine to wash dish towels and washcloths.
- Wash cutting boards, dishes, and counter tops with hot soapy water before and after preparing each food item.
- Use a solution of 1 teaspoon of bleach in 1 quart of water to sanitize surfaces and utensils.
- Use a clean cutting board.
- Use one cutting board for fresh produce. Use a separate one for raw meat, poultry, and seafood.
- Marinate food in the refrigerator, not on the counter.
- Use a clean plate to serve food.
- Do not place cooked food back on the same plate or cutting board that held raw food.

REVIEW QUESTIONS

Circle the BEST answer.

1 Nutrition is
   a Fats, proteins, carbohydrates, vitamins, and minerals
   b The many processes involved in the ingestion, digestion, absorption, and use of food and fluids by the body
   c The MyPyramid food guidance system
   d The balance between calories taken in and used by the body

2 The MyPyramid food guidance system encourages the following *except*
   a The same diet for everyone
   b Smart food choices
   c Physical activity
   d Small steps to improve diet and life-style

3 On a 2000-calorie a day diet, what is the amount of grains needed?
   a 6 ounces
   b 4 to 5 ounces
   c 3 to 4 ounces
   d 2 ounces

4 On a 2000-calorie a day diet, what is the amount of meat and beans needed?
   a 2½ ounces
   b 3 to 4 ounces
   c 4 to 5 ounces
   d 5½ ounces

5 Which food group contains the *most* fat?
   a Grains
   b Vegetables
   c Milk
   d Meat and beans

6 These statements are about oils. Which is *false?*
   a Oils are high in calories.
   b The best oil choices come from fish, nuts, and vegetable oils.
   c Oils from plant sources contain cholesterol.
   d Mayonnaise, certain salad dressings, and soft margarine are mainly oil.

7 Protein is needed for
   a Tissue growth and repair
   b Energy and the fiber for bowel elimination
   c Body heat and to protect organs from injury
   d Improving the taste of food

8 Which foods provide the *most* protein?
   a Butter and cream
   b Tomatoes and potatoes
   c Meats and fish
   d Corn and lettuce

9 The sodium-controlled diet involves
   a Omitting high-sodium foods
   b Adding salt to food at the table
   c Using 2400 mg of salt in cooking
   d A sodium-intake flow sheet

10 A person on a sodium-controlled diet wants a salt shaker. You should
   a Provide the salt
   b Tell the nurse
   c Explain that added salt is not allowed on the diet
   d Ignore the request

11 Diabetes meal planning involves the following *except*
   a Food the person likes
   b Eating the same amount of carbohydrates, protein, and fat each day
   c Eating at regular times
   d Sodium control

12 OBRA requires the following *except*
   a Offering 24-hour meal service
   b Serving hot food hot; serving cold food cold
   c Providing needed eating equipment
   d Serving food promptly

13 OBRA requires
   a 2 regular meals
   b 3 regular meals
   c 3 regular meals and a bedtime snack
   d Meals every 6 hours

14 Adult fluid requirements for normal fluid balance are about
   a 1000 to 1500 mL daily
   b 1500 to 2000 mL daily
   c 2000 to 2500 mL daily
   d 2500 to 3000 mL daily

15 A person is NPO. You should
   a Provide a variety of fluids
   b Offer fluids in small amounts and in small containers
   c Remove the water pitcher and cup from the room
   d Remove oral hygiene equipment from the room

16 Which are *not* counted as liquid foods?
   a Coffee, tea, juices, and soft drinks
   b Butter, sauces, and melted cheese
   c Ice cream, sherbet, custard, pudding
   d Jell-O, Popsicles, and creamed cereals

17 Nursing center residents are eating in the dining room. They serve themselves from bowls and platters on their tables. This is
   a A social dining program
   b A family dining program
   c A low-stimulation feeding program
   d An open-dining program

18 Persons with dysphagia
   a Use straws for all liquids
   b Have a regular diet
   c Are fed according to the care plan
   d Eat alone in their rooms

19 Which is *not* a sign of a swallowing problem?
   a Drooling
   b Coughing while eating
   c Pocketing
   d Edema

Continued

425

20 You are feeding a person. Which action is *not correct?*
 a Ask if he or she wants to pray before eating.
 b Use a fork to feed the person.
 c Ask the person the order in which to serve food and fluids.
 d Engage the person in a pleasant conversation.

21 Before providing fresh drinking water, you need to know the person's
 a I&O
 b Diet
 c Fluid orders
 d Preferred beverages

22 You are re-heating cooked food. The food temperature should be
 a 40° F
 b 90° F
 c 140° F
 d 165° F

Circle T if the statement is true and F if it is false.

23 T F Vegetables and fruits should be washed before serving them.

24 T F Unpasteurized milk is safe to drink.

25 T F Raw meat can touch other foods.

26 T F Fully cooked refrigerated foods should be eaten within 3 to 4 days.

27 T F Poultry is washed and rinsed before cooking.

28 T F A cutting board can be used for all foods. Then the board is washed.

29 T F Raw meat, poultry, and seafood are stored on the top shelf of the refrigerator.

30 T F Ground beef can be placed on a counter top to thaw.

31 T F Left-over foods should be refrigerated or frozen within 2 hours.

32 T F Eggs are washed before using them.

33 T F Eggs are stored in the egg tray on the refrigerator door.

34 T F Hot, soapy water and paper towels are used to clean kitchen surfaces.

35 T F Poultry is used or frozen within 1 to 2 days of purchase.

Answers to these questions are on p. 780.

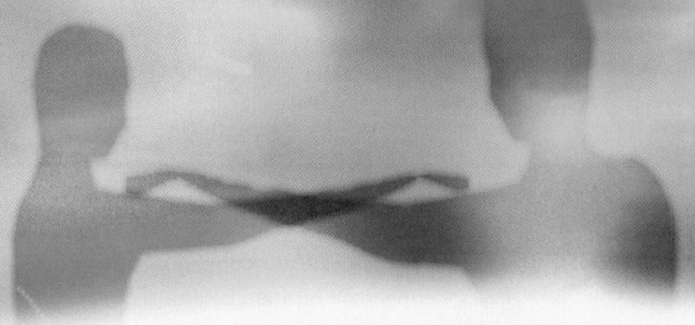

Nutritional Support and IV Therapy

OBJECTIVES

- Define the key terms and key abbreviations listed in this chapter
- Identify the reasons for nutritional support and IV therapy
- Explain how tube feedings are given
- Describe scheduled and continuous feedings
- Explain how to prevent aspiration
- Describe the comfort measures for the person with a feeding tube
- Describe parenteral nutrition
- Describe the IV therapy sites
- Identify the equipment used in IV therapy
- Describe how to assist with the IV flow rate
- Identify the safety measures for IV therapy
- Identify the observations to report when a person has nutritional support or IV therapy
- Explain how to assist with nutritional support and IV therapy

KEY TERMS

aspiration Breathing fluid, food, vomitus, or an object into the lungs

enteral nutrition Giving nutrients into the gastrointestinal (GI) tract *(enteral)* through a feeding tube

flow rate The number of drops per minute *(gtt/min)*

gastrostomy tube A tube inserted through a surgically created opening *(stomy)* in the stomach *(gastro)*; stomach tube

gavage The process of giving a tube feeding

intravenous (IV) therapy Giving fluids through a needle or catheter inserted into a vein; IV and IV infusion

jejunostomy tube A feeding tube inserted into a surgically created opening *(stomy)* in the *jejunum* of the small intestine

nasogastric (NG) tube A feeding tube inserted through the nose *(naso)* into the stomach *(gastro)*

nasoduodenal tube A feeding tube inserted through the nose *(naso)* into the *duodenum* of the small intestine

nasointestinal tube A feeding tube inserted through the nose *(naso)* into the small intestine *(intestinal)*

nasojejunal tube A feeding tube inserted through the nose *(naso)* into the *jejunum* of the small intestine

parenteral nutrition Giving nutrients through a catheter inserted into a vein; *para* means beyond; *enteral* relates to the bowel

percutaneous endoscopic gastrostomy (PEG) tube A feeding tube inserted into the stomach *(gastro)* through a small incision *(stomy)* made through *(per)* the skin *(cutaneous)*; a lighted instrument *(scope)* used to see inside a body cavity or organ *(endo)*

regurgitation The backward flow of stomach contents into the mouth

KEY ABBREVIATIONS

AIDS Acquired immunodeficiency syndrome

GI Gastrointestinal

gtt Drops

gtt/min Drops per minute

IV Intravenous

mL Milliliter

NG Nasogastric

NPO Nothing by mouth

PEG Percutaneous endoscopic gastrostomy

PICC Peripherally inserted central catheter

TPN Total parenteral nutrition

Many persons cannot eat or drink because of illness, surgery, or injury. They may have chewing or swallowing problems. Aspiration is a risk. **Aspiration** is breathing fluid, food, vomitus, or an object into the lungs. Some persons have problems eating or refuse to eat or drink. Others cannot eat enough to meet their nutritional needs. The doctor may order nutritional support or IV (intravenous) therapy to meet food and fluid needs.

ENTERAL NUTRITION

Some persons cannot or will not ingest, chew, or swallow food. Or food cannot pass from the mouth into the esophagus and into the stomach or small intestine. Poor nutrition results. Common causes are:

▶ Cancer, especially cancers of the head, neck, and esophagus
▶ Trauma to the face, mouth, head, or neck
▶ Coma
▶ Dysphagia
▶ Dementia
▶ Eating disorders
▶ Nervous system disorders (Chapter 39)
▶ Prolonged vomiting
▶ Major trauma or surgery
▶ Acquired immunodeficiency syndrome (AIDS)
▶ Illnesses and disorders affecting eating and nutrition

Enteral nutrition is giving nutrients into the gastrointestinal (GI) tract *(enteral)* through a feeding tube. **Gavage** is the process of giving a tube feeding. Tube feedings replace or supplement normal nutrition.

Types of Feeding Tubes

These feeding tubes are common:

▶ **Nasogastric (NG) tube.** A feeding tube is inserted through the nose *(naso)* into the stomach *(gastro)*. See Figure 24-1. A doctor or an RN inserts the tube.
▶ **Nasointestinal tube.** A feeding tube is inserted through the nose *(naso)* into the small intestine *(intestinal)*. See Figure 24-2. A nasoduodenal tube is inserted into the *duodenum*. A nasojejunal tube is inserted into *the jejunum*. A doctor or RN inserts the tube.
▶ **Gastrostomy tube.** Also called a *stomach tube*, it is inserted into the stomach. A doctor surgically creates an opening *(stomy)* in the stomach *(gastro)*. See Figure 24-3.
▶ **Jejunostomy tube.** A feeding tube is inserted into a surgically created opening *(stomy)* in the *jejunum* of the small intestine. See Figure 24-4.
▶ **Percutaneous endoscopic gastrostomy (PEG) tube.** The doctor inserts the feeding tube with an endoscope. An endoscope is a lighted instrument *(scope)* used to see inside a body cavity or organ *(endo)*. The tube is

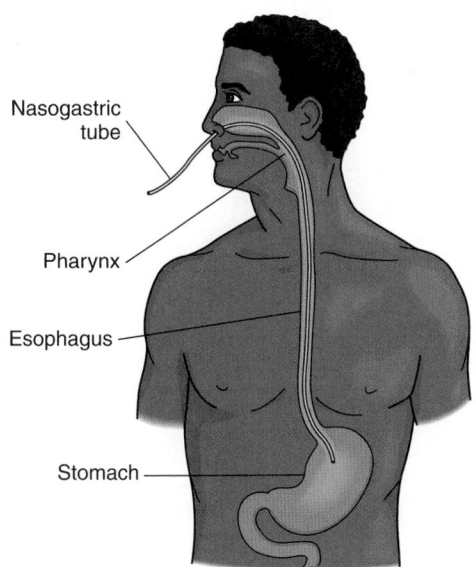

FIGURE 24-1 A nasogastric (NG) tube is inserted through the nose and esophagus and into the stomach.

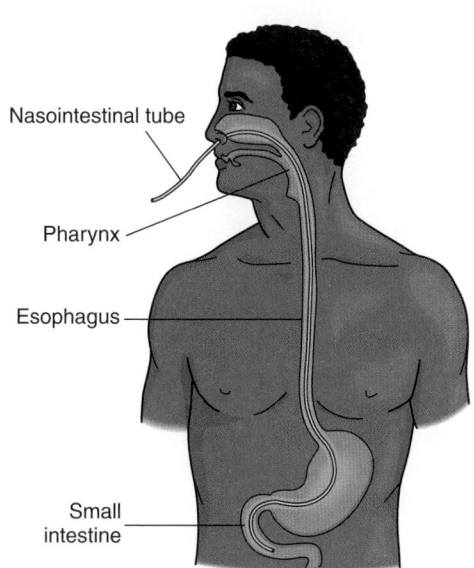

FIGURE 24-2 A nasointestinal tube is inserted through the nose and into the duodenum or jejunum of the small intestine.

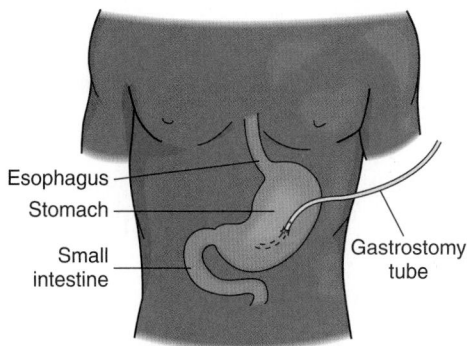

FIGURE 24-3 A gastrostomy tube.

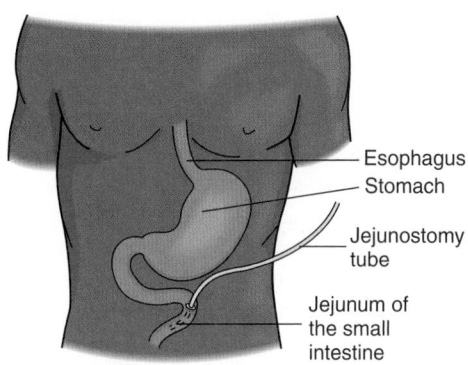

FIGURE 24-4 A jejunostomy tube.

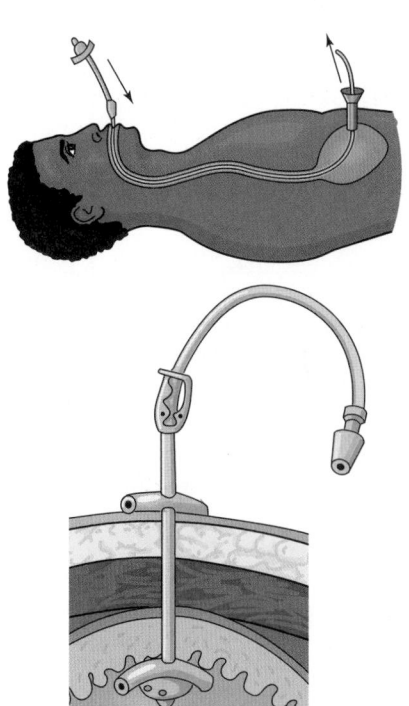

FIGURE 24-5 A percutaneous endoscopic gastrostomy (PEG) tube.

inserted through the mouth and esophagus and into the stomach. The doctor makes a small incision *(stomy)* through *(per)* the skin *(cutaneous)* and into the stomach *(gastro)*. A tube is inserted into the stomach through the incision (Fig. 24-5). The endoscope allows the doctor to see correct tube placement in the stomach.

Nasogastric and nasointestinal tubes are used for short-term nutritional support. Short-term support is usually less than 6 weeks. Gastrostomy, jejunostomy, and PEG tubes are used for long-term nutritional support. Long-term support is usually longer than 6 weeks.

Formulas

The doctor orders the type of formula, the amount to give, and when to give tube feedings. Most formulas contain protein, carbohydrates, fat, vitamins, and minerals. Commercial formulas are common.

A nurse gives formula through the feeding tube. Formula is given at room temperature. Cold fluids can cause cramping.

Opened formula can remain at room temperature for about 4 hours. Microbes can grow in warm formula. Sometimes formula is kept cold with ice chips around the container. The chilled formula warms as it passes through the connecting tubing and feeding tube.

See *Teamwork and Time Management: Formulas.*

Feeding Times

Tube feedings are given at certain times (scheduled feedings). Or they are given over a 24-hour period (continuous feedings).

Scheduled Feedings

Such feedings also are called intermittent feedings. (*Intermittent* means to start, stop, and then start again.) Feeding times are scheduled. Four or more feedings are given each day. Usually 8 to 12 ounces (240 to 360 milliliters [mL]) are given over about 30 minutes. The frequency, amount, and time are like a normal eating pattern.

The nurse uses a syringe or a feeding bag (Fig. 24-6). The syringe attaches to the feeding tube. Connecting tubing connects the feeding bag to the tube. Formula is added to the syringe or to the feeding bag. Then it slowly flows through the feeding tube into the stomach.

The nurse removes the syringe or connecting tubing after the feeding. Then the nurse clamps and covers the

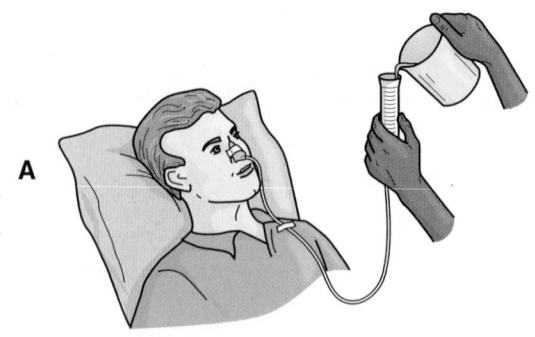

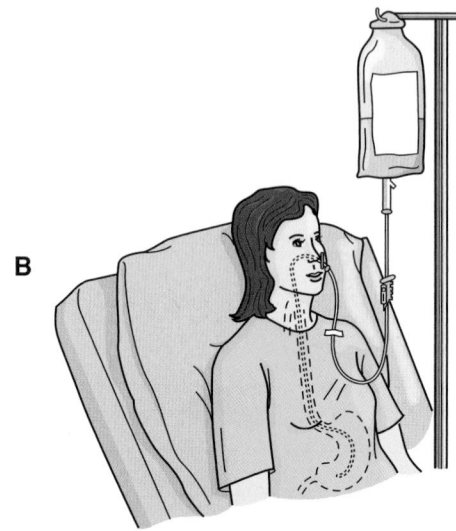

FIGURE 24-6 A, A tube feeding given with a syringe. **B,** Formula drips from a feeding bag into the feeding tube.

end of the feeding tube with a cap or gauze. Gauze is secured in place with a rubber band. Clamping prevents air from entering the tube. It also prevents fluid from leaking out of the tube. Covering the end of the tube also prevents leaking.

Continuous Feedings

These feedings are usually given over 24 hours. A feeding pump is used (Fig. 24-7). Formula drips into the feeding tube at a certain rate per minute. The person receives a certain amount every hour.

An alarm on the pump sounds if something is wrong. When you hear an alarm, tell the nurse.

Observations

Diarrhea, constipation, delayed stomach emptying, and aspiration are risks. Report the following at once:
- Nausea
- Discomfort during the feeding
- Vomiting
- Distended (enlarged and swollen) abdomen
- Coughing
- Complaints of indigestion or heartburn

TEAMWORK AND TIME MANAGEMENT

Formulas

Refrigerated formula needs to warm to room temperature. The nurse may ask you to warm the formula. To do so, place the container in a wash basin filled with warm water. If warmed in the sink, other staff cannot use the sink. They need to go elsewhere. This wastes their time and energy. Or someone may remove the container to use the sink. The container does not warm in a timely manner. That affects you, the nurse, and the patient or resident.

You can help keep hanging formula cool. Add ice chips following the nurse's directions.

The manufacturer's instructions tell how long formula can hang. This is usually 4 hours; 6 hours if chilled with ice. Check the instructions. Also check the time that the feeding started. Remind the nurse when the time limit is near. For example, the feeding started at 0800. The formula can hang for 4 hours. At 1130 or 1145, tell the nurse how much time is left. Also report the amount of formula left.

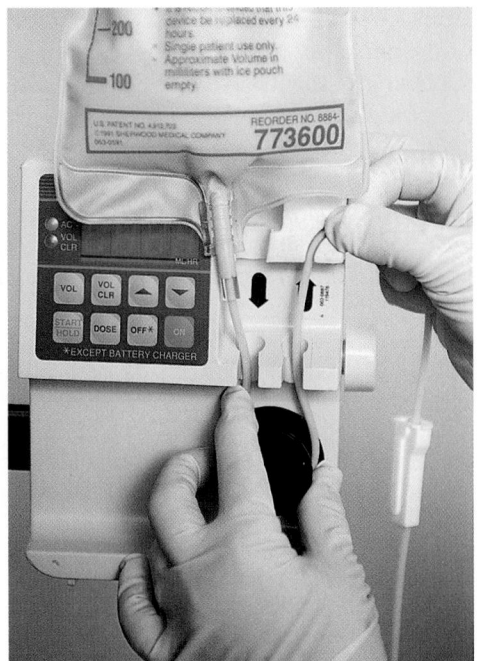

FIGURE 24-7 Feeding pump. (From Potter PA, Perry AG: *Fundamentals of nursing*, ed 6, St Louis, 2005, Mosby.)

- Redness, swelling, drainage, odor, or pain at the ostomy site
- Fever
- Signs and symptoms of respiratory distress (Chapter 34)
- Increased pulse rate
- Complaints of flatulence (Chapter 22)
- Diarrhea (Chapter 22)

Preventing Aspiration

Aspiration is a major risk from tube feedings. It can cause pneumonia and death. Aspiration can occur:

- *During insertion.* NG tubes and nasointestinal tubes are passed through the esophagus and then into the stomach or small intestine. The tube can slip into the airway. An x-ray is taken after insertion to check tube placement.
- *From tube movement out of place.* Coughing, sneezing, vomiting, suctioning, and poor positioning are common causes. A tube can move from the stomach or intestines into the esophagus and then into the airway. The RN checks tube placement before every scheduled tube feeding. With continuous feedings, the RN checks tube placement every 4 hours. To do so, the RN attaches a syringe to the tube. Gastrointestinal secretions are withdrawn through the syringe. Then the pH of the secretions is measured (Chapter 30). *You are never responsible for checking feeding tube placement.*
- *From regurgitation.* **Regurgitation** is the backward flow of stomach contents into the mouth. Delayed stomach emptying and over-feeding are common causes.

To assist the nurse in preventing regurgitation and aspiration:

- Position the person in Fowler's or semi-Fowler's position before the feeding. Follow the care plan and the nurse's directions.
- Maintain Fowler's or semi-Fowler's position after the feeding. This position may be required for 1 to 2 hours after the feeding or at all times. The position allows formula to move through the GI tract. Follow the care plan and the nurse's directions.
- Avoid the left side-lying position. When the person lays on the left side, the stomach cannot empty into the small intestine.

Persons with NG or gastrostomy tubes are at great risk for regurgitation. The risk is less with intestinal tubes. Formula passes directly into the small intestine. Also, formula is given at a slow rate. During digestion, food slowly passes from the stomach into the small intestine. The stomach handles larger amounts of food at one time than does the small intestine.

See *Focus on Children and Older Persons: Preventing Aspiration.*

Comfort Measures

Persons with feeding tubes usually are not allowed to eat or drink. They are NPO—nothing by mouth. (See Chapter 23.) Dry mouth, dry lips, and sore throat can cause discomfort. Sometimes hard candy or gum is allowed. The following measures are common:

- Oral hygiene every 2 hours while the person is awake
- Lubricant for the lips every 2 hours while the person is awake
- Mouth rinses every 2 hours while the person is awake

Feeding tubes can irritate and cause pressure on the nose. They can change the shape of the nostrils or cause pressure ulcers. The following measures are common:

- Clean the nose and nostrils every 4 to 8 hours.
- Secure the tube to the nose (Fig. 24-8, p. 432). Use tape or a tube holder. (Tube holders have foam cushions that prevent pressure on the nose. Re-taping is not needed. Re-taping irritates the nose.)
- Secure the tube to the person's garment at the shoulder area. This prevents the tube from pulling or dangling. Both can cause pressure on the nose. The following methods are common. Follow agency policy.
    - Loop a rubber band around the tube. Then pin the rubber band to the garment with a safety pin.
    - Tape the tube to the garment.

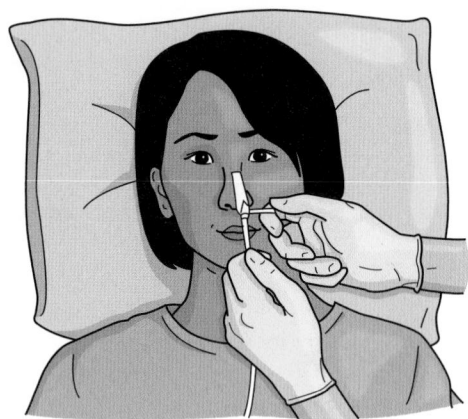

FIGURE 24-8 The feeding tube is secured to the nose.

Giving Tube Feedings

You assist the nurse with tube feedings. In some states and agencies, nursing assistants give tube feedings and remove NG tubes. *Remember, you are never responsible for inserting feeding tubes or checking their placement. This is the RN's responsibility.*

See *Delegation Guidelines: Giving Tube Feedings.*
See *Promoting Safety and Comfort: Giving Tube Feedings.*
See *Focus on Ethics and Laws: Giving Tube Feedings.*

PROMOTING SAFETY AND COMFORT: Giving Tube Feedings

SAFETY

The person may have an IV, a breathing tube (Chapter 34), and drainage tubes (Chapter 32). You must know the purpose of each tube. Ask the nurse to label each tube to identify its purpose. Formula must enter only the feeding tube. Otherwise, the person can die.

Before giving a tube feeding always:
- Turn on the light if the room is dark. Do so even if the person is sleeping.
- Check and inspect the feeding tube and label with the nurse.
- Make sure an RN checks for tube placement.
- Make sure every tube, catheter, and needle is labeled.
- Trace the feeding tube back to the insertion site. Start at the end of the tube into which you will give the feeding. Trace the tube backward. For example, if the person has an NG tube, you will end at the nose. If the person has a gastrostomy tube, you will end at the abdomen. *If you do not end at the correct place, do not give the tube feeding. Call for the nurse.*

Nasal secretions may contain blood or microbes. So can drainage at an ostomy site. Wear gloves. Follow Standard Precautions and the Bloodborne Pathogen Standard.

Remind visitors to call for a nurse if a any tube becomes disconnected or needs to be reconnected. They could connect the wrong tubes together.

DELEGATION GUIDELINES: Giving Tube Feedings

Before giving tube feedings or removing an NG tube make sure that:
- Your state allows you to perform the procedure
- The procedure is in your job description
- You have had the necessary education and training
- You know how to use the agency's equipment and supplies
- You review the procedure in the agency's procedure manual
- You review the procedure with the nurse
- A nurse is available to answer questions and to supervise you
- An RN has identified and labeled all other tubes, catheters, and needles
- An RN checks tube placement

If the above conditions are met, you need this information from the nurse and the care plan:
- The type of tube—NG, nasointestinal, PEG, or jejunostomy
- What feeding method to use—syringe, feeding bag, or feeding pump
- What size syringe to use—usually 30 or 60 mL for an adult
- How to position the person for the feeding—Fowler's or semi-Fowler's
- How to position the person after the feeding—Fowler's or semi-Fowler's
- What formula to use
- How much formula to give
- How high to raise the syringe or hang the feeding bag (usually 18 inches above the stomach or intestines)
- The amount of flushing solution to use—usually 30 to 60 mL (1 to 2 ounces) of water for an adult
- How fast to give the feeding if using a syringe—usually over 30 minutes
- The flow rate if a feeding bag is used (Flow rate is the number of drops per minute. See p. 434.)
- The flow rate if a feeding pump is used
- If ice is kept around the bag for a continuous feeding
- If you are to remove an NG tube, when to remove the tube
- What observations to report and record—see p. 430
- When to report observations
- What specific patient or resident concerns to report at once

FOCUS ON ETHICS AND LAWS

Feeding Tubes

After a kidney transplant, a 62-year-old male patient had another surgery for a stomach problem. A feeding tube was placed on the left side of his abdomen. A drainage tube was placed on the right side. The feeding tube was marked with tape.

Five days after the tubes were placed, a nurse gave the feeding through the drainage tube. Four hours later, a doctor found the error. Surgery was done to clean the abdomen of the feeding material. Laboratory tests showed an infection.

The patient developed many complications. The abdominal wound did not heal. The transplanted kidney was rejected, which required surgery to remove it. Shortly after the surgery, the patient developed serious respiratory complications and died.

His wife sued. She claimed that there was negligence for not knowing the feeding tube from the drainage tube. The case settled for $1,450,000.

(M. Weinberg as Executrix of the Estate of J. Weinberg, etc. v Westchester County Healthcare Corp., Westchester Medical Center, Ratik El-Sabrout, MD, and Eric Presser, MD, New York, 2005.)

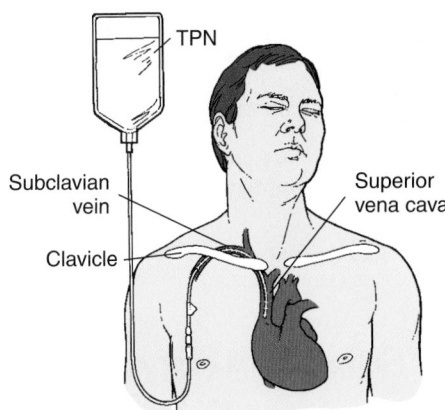

FIGURE 24-9 Parenteral nutrition. (From *Mosby's dictionary of medicine, nursing, and health professions*, ed 7, St Louis, 2006, Mosby.)

PARENTERAL NUTRITION

Parenteral nutrition is giving nutrients through a catheter inserted into a vein (Fig. 24-9). (*Para* means beyond; *enteral* relates to the bowel). A nutrient solution is given directly into the bloodstream. Nutrients do not enter the GI tract for absorption. Parenteral nutrition is often called *total parenteral nutrition (TPN)* or *hyperalimentation*. (*Hyper* means high or *excessive*. *Alimentation* means *nourishment*.)

The nutrient solution contains water, proteins, carbohydrates, vitamins, and minerals. The solution drips through a catheter inserted into a large vein (p. 434). This method is used when the person cannot receive oral feedings or enteral feedings. Or it is used when oral or enteral feedings are not enough to meet the person's needs.

Common reasons for TPN include:

▶ Disease, injury, or surgery to the GI tract
▶ Severe trauma, infection, or burns
▶ Being NPO for more than 5 to 7 days
▶ GI side effects from cancer treatments (Chapter 38)
▶ Prolonged coma
▶ Prolonged anorexia (loss of appetite)

Observations

TPN has many risks. They include infection, fluid imbalances, and blood sugar imbalances. Report the following signs and symptoms to the nurse at once:

▶ Fever, chills, and other signs and symptoms of infection (Chapter 14)
▶ Signs and symptoms of sugar imbalances (see "Diabetes" in Chapter 41)
▶ Chest pain
▶ Difficulty breathing or shortness of breath
▶ Cough
▶ Nausea and vomiting
▶ Diarrhea
▶ Thirst
▶ Rapid heart rate or an irregular heartbeat
▶ Weakness or fatigue
▶ Sweating
▶ Pallor (pale skin)
▶ Trembling
▶ Confusion or changes in behavior

Assisting With TPN

The nurse is responsible for all aspects of TPN. You assist the nurse by carefully observing the person. You also assist with the person's basic needs and activities of daily living. Persons receiving TPN may be NPO. Provide frequent oral hygiene, lubricant to the lips, and mouth rinses as the nurse and care plan direct (p. 431). Also follow other aspects of the person's care plan.

Many aspects of IV therapy apply to TPN.

IV THERAPY

Intravenous (IV) therapy is giving fluids through a needle or catheter inserted into a vein (Fig. 24-10). Fluid flows directly into the bloodstream. *IV* and *IV infusion* also refer to IV therapy. Doctors order IV therapy to:

▶ Provide fluids when they cannot be taken by mouth
▶ Replace minerals and vitamins lost because of illness or injury
▶ Provide sugar for energy
▶ Give drugs and blood

RNs are responsible for IV therapy. They start and maintain the infusion according to the doctor's orders. RNs also give IV drugs and administer blood. State laws vary regarding the role of LPNs/LVNs and nursing assistants in IV therapy.

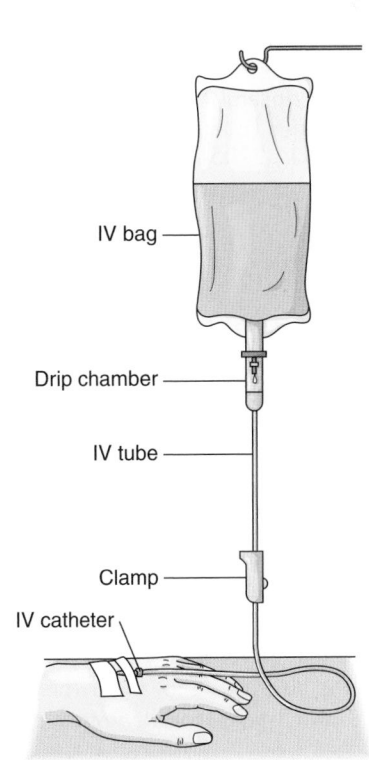

FIGURE 24-10 Equipment for IV therapy.

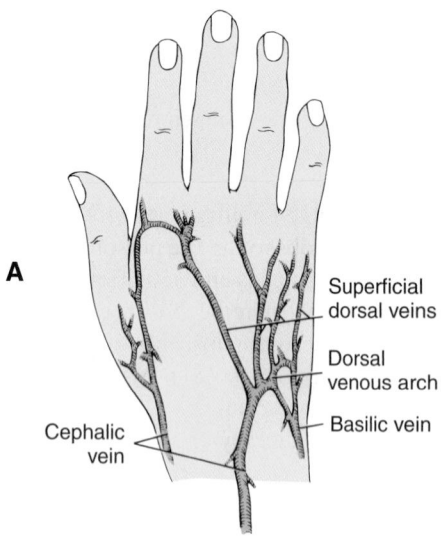

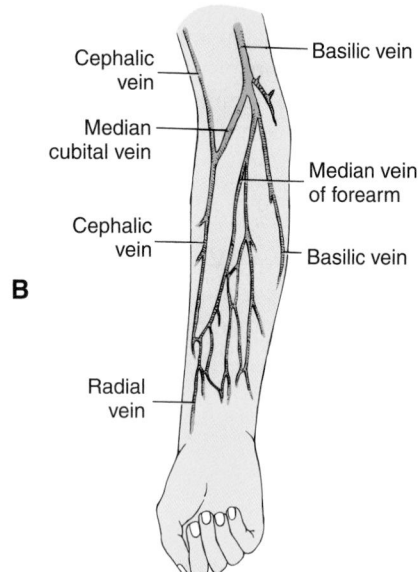

FIGURE 24-11 Peripheral IV sites, **A,** Back of the hand. **B,** Inner forearm. (From Potter PA, Perry AG: *Fundamentals of nursing,* ed 6, St Louis, 2005, Mosby.)

IV Sites

Peripheral and central venous sites are used. Peripheral means around *(peri)* a boundary *(pheral)*. The boundary is the center of the body near the heart. *Peripheral IV sites* are away from the center of the body. For adults, the back of the hand and inner forearm provide useful sites (Fig. 24-11).

The subclavian vein and the internal jugular vein are *central venous sites.* They are close to the heart. A catheter is threaded into the superior vena cava or right atrium (Fig. 24-12, *A* and *B*). The catheter is called a *central venous catheter* or a *central line.* The cephalic and basilic veins in the arm also are used. Catheters inserted into these sites are called *peripherally inserted central catheters*

(PICCs). The catheter is threaded into the subclavian vein or the superior vena cava (Fig. 24-12, *C*).

Central venous sites are used:
▶ For parenteral nutrition
▶ To give large amounts of fluid
▶ For long-term IV therapy
▶ To give drugs that irritate peripheral veins
  See *Focus on Children and Older Persons: IV Sites.*
  See *Focus on Long-Term Care and Home Care: IV Sites.*

IV Equipment

The basic equipment used in IV therapy is shown in Figure 24-10:
▶ The solution container is a plastic bag. It is called the *IV bag.*
▶ A *catheter* or *needle* is inserted into a vein (Fig. 24-13).
▶ The *IV tube* or *infusion tubing* connects the IV bag to the catheter or needle. Fluid drips from the bag into the *drip chamber.* The *clamp* is used to regulate the flow rate.
▶ The IV bag hangs from an IV pole or ceiling hook. *IV standard* is another name for an IV pole.

Flow Rate

The doctor orders the amount of fluid to give (infuse) and the amount of time to give it in. With this information, the RN figures the flow rate. The **flow rate** is the number of drops per minute *(gtt/min).* The abbreviation *gtt* means drops. The Latin word *guttae* means drops.

The RN sets the clamp for the flow rate. Or an electronic pump is used to control the flow rate (Fig. 24-14). An alarm sounds if something is wrong. Tell the nurse at once if you hear an alarm. *Never change the position of the clamp or adjust any controls on IV pumps.*

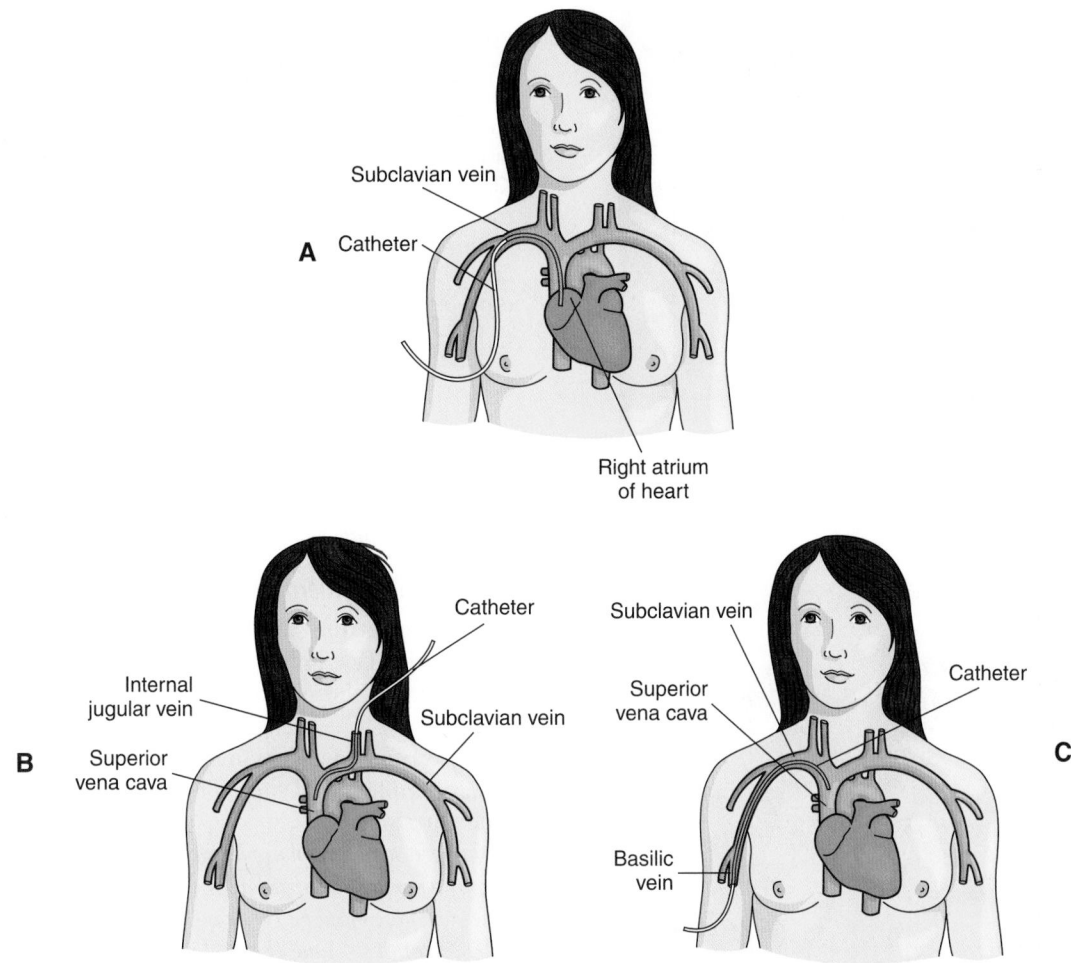

FIGURE 24-12 Central venous sites. **A,** Subclavian vein. The catheter tip is in the right atrium. **B,** Internal jugular vein. The catheter tip is in the superior vena cava. **C,** Basilic vein. This is a peripherally inserted central catheter (PICC).

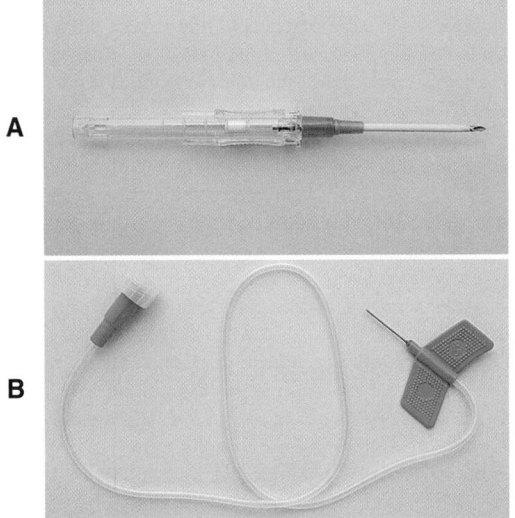

FIGURE 24-13 A, Intravenous catheter. **B,** Butterfly needle.

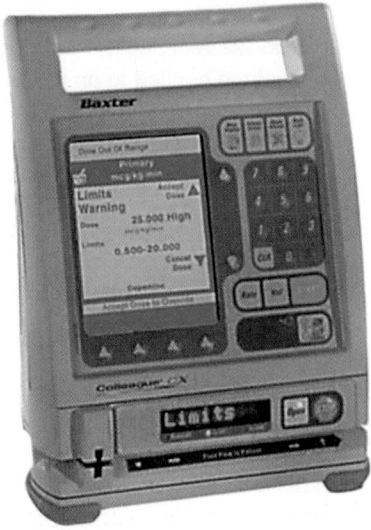

FIGURE 24-14 Electronic IV pump. (Courtesy Baxter Healthcare Corp., Round Lake, Ill.)

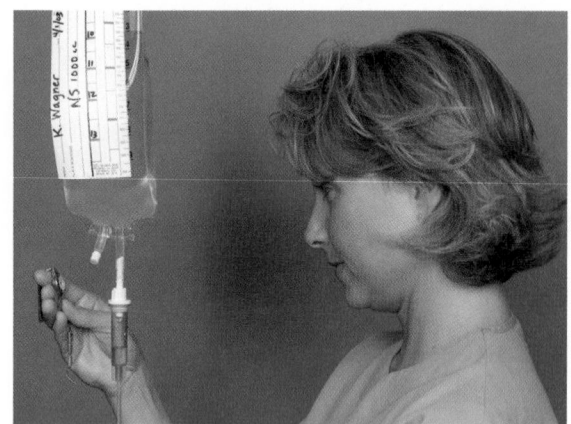

FIGURE 24-15 The flow rate is checked by counting the number of drops per minute.

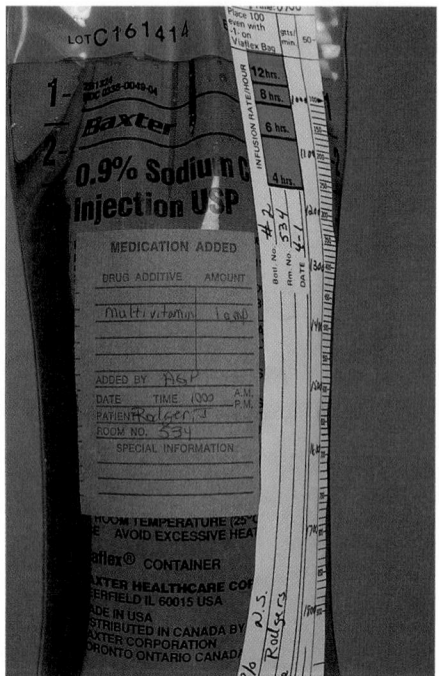

FIGURE 24-16 Time tape applied to an IV bag. (From Elkin MK, Perry AG, Potter PA: *Nursing interventions & clinical skills*, ed 4, St Louis, 2007, Mosby.)

You can check the flow rate. The RN tells you the number of drops per minute. To check the flow rate, count the number of drops in 1 minute (Fig. 24-15). Tell the RN at once if:

▶ No fluid is dripping
▶ The rate is too fast
▶ The rate is too slow

The time tape shows how much fluid to give over a period of time (Fig. 24-16). For example, the doctor orders 1000 mL of fluid over 8 hours. The RN marks the tape in 8 one-hour intervals. To check if the fluid is being given on time, compare the fluid line with the time line on the tape. If the fluid line is above or below the time line, the flow rate is too slow or too fast. Tell the RN at once if too much or too little fluid was given.

See *Promoting Safety and Comfort: Flow Rate.*

Assisting With IV Therapy

You help meet the safety, hygiene, and activity needs of persons with IVs. Follow the safety measures in Box 24-1. Report any of the signs and symptoms listed in Box 24-2 at once.

Your state and agency may allow you to change dressings at peripheral IV sites. They also may let you discontinue a peripheral IV.

You are never responsible for starting or maintaining IV therapy. Nor do you regulate the flow rate or change IV bags. You never give blood or IV drugs.

See *Teamwork and Time Management: Assisting With IV Therapy.*

See *Delegation Guidelines: Assisting With IV Therapy.*

PROMOTING SAFETY AND COMFORT: Flow Rate

SAFETY

The person can suffer serious harm if the flow rate is too fast or too slow. The flow rate can change from position changes. Kinked tubes and lying on the tube also affect the flow rate.

Never change the position of the clamp or adjust any controls on infusion pumps. Tell the nurse at once if there is a problem with the flow rate.

BOX 24-1 Safety Measures for IV Therapy

- Follow Standard Precautions and the Bloodborne Pathogen Standard.
- Do not move the needle or catheter. Needle or catheter position must be maintained. If the needle or catheter is moved, it may come out of the vein. Then fluid flows into tissues (infiltration). Or the flow stops.
- Follow the safety measures for restraints (Chapter 13). The nurse may splint or restrain the extremity to prevent movement (Fig. 24-17). Or the nurse may apply a protective device (Fig. 24-18). This helps prevent the needle or catheter from moving.
- Protect the IV bag, tubing, and needle or catheter when the person walks. Portable IV standards are rolled along next to the person (Fig. 24-19).
- Assist the person with turning and repositioning. Move the IV bag to the side of the bed on which the person is lying. Always allow enough slack in the tubing. The needle or catheter can move from pressure on the tube.
- Tell the nurse at once if bleeding occurs from the insertion site. Follow Standard Precautions and the Bloodborne Pathogen Standard.
- Tell the nurse at once of any signs and symptoms listed in Box 24-2.

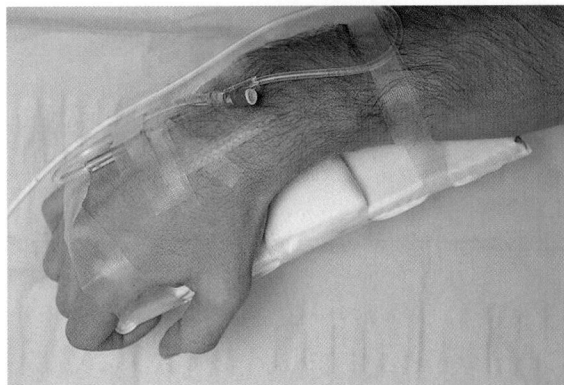

FIGURE 24-17 An armboard prevents movement at an IV site. (From Elkin MK, Perry AG, Potter PA: *Nursing interventions & clinical skills,* ed 4, St Louis, 2007, Mosby.)

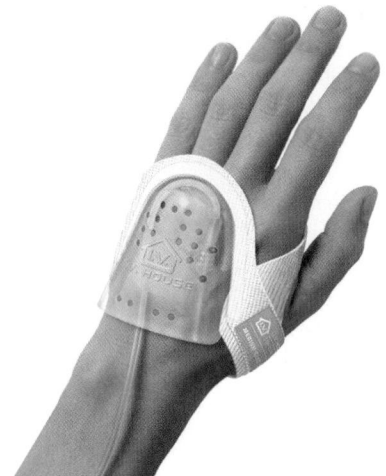

FIGURE 24-18 I.V. House Protective Device. (Courtesy I.V. House, St. Louis, Mo.)

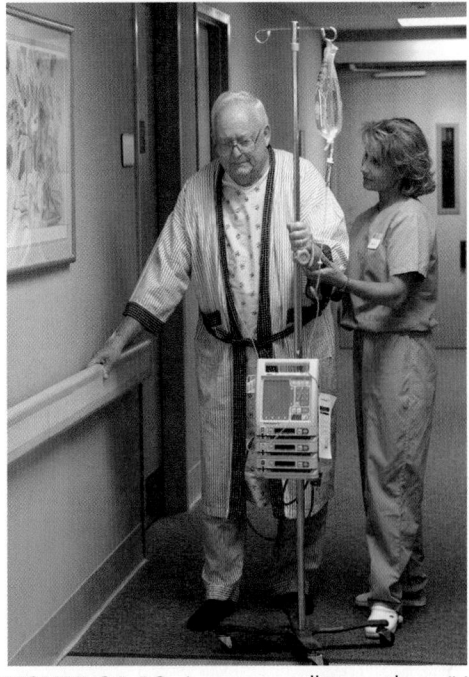

FIGURE 24-19 A person walking with an IV.

TEAMWORK AND TIME MANAGEMENT

Assisting With IV Therapy

If a person's care is part of your assignment, you must know the IV flow rate. When you are with the person, check the flow rate. Report any problems to the nurse at once.

Also check the amount of fluid in the bag. Tell the nurse at once if the bag is empty or almost empty.

Patients and residents cared for by other staff may have IVs. When you are near the person or walking past the person's room, make sure the IV is dripping. Also check the amount of fluid in the bag. Report any problems to a nurse at once.

DELEGATION GUIDELINES: Assisting With IV Therapy

Before changing a peripheral IV dressing or discontinuing a peripheral IV, make sure that:

- Your state lets nursing assistants perform the procedure
- The procedure is in your job description
- You have the necessary education and training
- You know how to use the agency's supplies and equipment
- You review the procedure in the agency's procedure manual
- You review the procedure with the nurse
- A nurse is available to answer questions and to supervise you
- An RN has identified and labeled all other tubes, catheters, and needles

If the above conditions are met, you need this information from the nurse and the care plan:

- When to change the IV dressing
- If the person has an IV needle or catheter
- When to discontinue the IV
- If the person has more than one IV, which IV to discontinue
- What supplies to use
- What observations to report and record (see Box 24-2)
- When to report observations
- What specific patient and resident concerns to report at once

---

BOX 24-2 Signs and Symptoms of IV Therapy Complications

LOCAL—AT THE IV SITE
- Bleeding
- Puffiness or swelling
- Pale or reddened skin
- Complaints of pain at or above the IV site
- Hot or cold skin near the site

SYSTEMIC—INVOLVING THE WHOLE BODY
- Fever
- Itching
- Drop in blood pressure
- Pulse rate greater than 100 beats per minute
- Irregular pulse
- Cyanosis
- Confusion or changes in mental function
- Loss of consciousness
- Difficulty breathing
- Shortness of breath
- Decreasing or no urine output
- Chest pain
- Nausea

Circle the BEST answer.

1 Enteral nutrition
   a Requires an NG tube
   b Is given into a central venous site
   c Is given into the GI tract
   d Requires an IV

2 The process of giving a tube feeding is called
   a Gavage
   b Parenteral nutrition
   c Aspiration
   d Regurgitation

3 For a tube feeding the person is positioned in
   a Fowler's or semi-Fowler's position
   b The left side-lying position
   c The right side-lying position
   d The supine position

4 Formula for a tube feeding is given
   a At body temperature
   b At room temperature
   c Hot
   d Cold

5 Continuous feedings are given with a
   a Syringe
   b Feeding bag
   c PEG tube
   d Feeding pump

6 The nurse checks feeding tube placement to prevent
   a Aspiration
   b Regurgitation
   c Over-feeding
   d Cramping

7 Which position prevents regurgitation after a tube feeding?
   a Fowler's or semi-Fowler's position
   b The supine position
   c The left or right side-lying position
   d The prone position

8 The risk of regurgitation is the greatest with
   a NG and gastrostomy tubes
   b A PEG tube
   c Nasointestinal tubes
   d A jejunostomy tube

9 A person with a feeding tube is NPO. You should do the following *except*
   a Give the person hard candy or gum
   b Provide oral hygiene
   c Provide mouth rinses
   d Apply lubricant to the lips

10 A person has an NG tube. The care plan includes the following measures to prevent nasal irritation. Which measure should you question?
   a Clean the nose and nostrils every 4 hours.
   b Tape the tube to the nose.
   c Remove the tube every 4 hours.
   d Secure the tube to the person's gown.

11 A nurse asks you to give a tube feeding. The procedure is not in your job description. What should you do?
   a Refuse to perform the task.
   b Give the tube feeding.
   c Tell the director of nursing.
   d Ask another nurse what you should do.

12 A person is receiving TPN. The person complains of chest pain and difficulty breathing. What should you do?
   a Position the person in Fowler's position.
   b Call for the nurse.
   c Stop the TPN.
   d Provide oral hygiene.

13 A person is receiving TPN. You know that TPN
   a Involves a nutrient solution
   b Is given through a feeding tube
   c Can cause pressure ulcers on the nose
   d Requires that the person be NPO

14 Which is a peripheral IV site?
   a Subclavian vein
   b Superior vena cava
   c Jugular vein
   d A vein on the back of the hand

15 A nurse asks you to check an IV flow rate. What should you do?
   a Count the drops in 30 seconds; multiply the number by 2.
   b Count the drops for 1 minute.
   c Check if the fluid is dripping too fast or slow.
   d Measure the amount of fluid.

16 The IV flow rate is
   a The number of gtt/mL
   b The number of gtt/min
   c The amount of fluid given in 1 hour
   d The amount of fluid in the IV bag

17 You note that an IV bag is almost empty. What should you do?
   a Clamp the IV tubing.
   b Tell the nurse.
   c Discontinue the IV.
   d Adjust the flow rate.

18 You note bleeding from an IV insertion site. What should you do?
   a Tell the nurse.
   b Move the needle or catheter.
   c Discontinue the IV.
   d Clamp the IV tubing.

Answers to these questions are on p. 780.

Measuring Vital Signs

OBJECTIVES

- ■ Define the key terms and key abbreviations listed in this chapter
- ■ Explain why vital signs are measured
- ■ List the factors affecting vital signs
- ■ Identify the normal ranges for each temperature site
- ■ Explain when to use each temperature site
- ■ Identify the pulse sites
- ■ Describe a normal pulse and normal respirations
- ■ Describe the practices to follow when measuring blood pressure
- ■ Know the normal vital signs for different age-groups
- ■ Perform the procedures described in this chapter

PROCEDURES

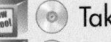 Taking a Temperature With a Glass Thermometer

 Taking a Temperature With an Electronic Thermometer

 Taking a Radial Pulse

 Taking an Apical Pulse

■ Taking an Apical-Radial Pulse

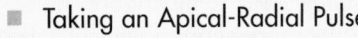 Counting Respirations

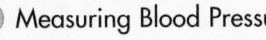 Measuring Blood Pressure

---

Procedures with this icon are on the CDCompanion in this book; those with this icon are on the Evolve Student Resources Website.

KEY TERMS

apical-radial pulse Taking the apical and radial pulses at the same time

blood pressure The amount of force exerted against the walls of an artery by the blood

body temperature The amount of heat in the body that is a balance between the amount of heat produced and the amount lost by the body

bradycardia A slow *(brady)* heart rate *(cardia)*; less than 60 beats per minute

diastole The period of heart muscle relaxation; the period when the heart is at rest

diastolic pressure The pressure in the arteries when the heart is at rest

fever Elevated body temperature

hypertension Blood pressure measurements that remain above *(hyper)* a systolic pressure of 140 mm Hg or a diastolic pressure of 90 mm Hg

hypotension When the systolic blood pressure is below *(hypo)* 90 mm Hg and the diastolic pressure is below 60 mm Hg

pulse The beat of the heart felt at an artery as a wave of blood passes through the artery

pulse deficit The difference between the apical and radial pulse rates

pulse rate The number of heartbeats or pulses felt in 1 minute

respiration Breathing air into *(inhalation)* and out of *(exhalation)* the lungs

sphygmomanometer A cuff and measuring device used to measure blood pressure

stethoscope An instrument used to listen to sounds produced by the heart, lungs, and other body organs

systole The period of heart muscle contraction; the period when the heart is pumping blood

systolic pressure The amount of force needed to pump blood out of the heart into the arterial circulation

tachycardia A rapid *(tachy)* heart rate *(cardia)*; more than 100 beats per minute

vital signs Temperature, pulse, respirations, and blood pressure

KEY ABBREVIATIONS

A Axillary

Ap Apical

BP Blood pressure

C Centigrade; Celsius

CPR Cardiopulmonary resuscitation

F Fahrenheit

Hg Mercury

IV Intravenous

mm Millimeters

mm Hg Millimeters of mercury

R Rectal

TPR Temperature, pulse, and respirations

Vital signs reflect the function of three body processes essential for life: regulation of body temperature, breathing, and heart function. The four **vital signs** of body function are:

▶ Temperature
▶ Pulse
▶ Respirations
▶ Blood pressure

Vital signs are often called TPR (temperature, pulse, and respiration) and BP (blood pressure). Some agencies consider "pain" to be a vital sign. See Chapter 27 for how to assist the nurse with pain assessment.

MEASURING AND REPORTING VITAL SIGNS

A person's vital signs vary within certain limits. They are affected by sleep, activity, eating, weather, noise, exercise, drugs, anger, fear, anxiety, pain, and illness.

Vital signs are measured to detect changes in normal body function. They tell about responses to treatment. They often signal life-threatening events. Vital signs are

part of the assessment step in the nursing process. Vital signs are measured:

▶ During physical exams
▶ When the person is admitted to a health care agency
▶ As often as required by the person's condition
▶ Before and after surgery
▶ Before and after complex procedures or diagnostic tests
▶ After some care measures, such as ambulation
▶ After a fall or other injury
▶ When drugs affect the respiratory or circulatory system
▶ When there are complaints of pain, dizziness, light-headedness, feeling faint, shortness of breath, a rapid heart rate, or not feeling well
▶ As stated on the care plan (usually daily or weekly in nursing centers)

Vital signs show even minor changes in the person's condition. Accuracy is essential when you measure, record, and report vital signs. If unsure of your measurements,

---

FOCUS ON CHILDREN AND OLDER PERSONS

Measuring and Reporting Vital Signs

OLDER PERSONS

Measuring vital signs on persons with dementia may be difficult. The person may move about, hit at you, and grab equipment. This is not safe for the person or for you. Two workers may be needed. One uses touch and a soothing voice to calm and distract the person. The other measures the vital signs.

You may need to try the procedure when the person is calmer. Or take the pulse and respirations at one time. Then take the temperature and blood pressure at another time.

Always approach the person calmly. Use a soothing voice. Tell the person what you are going to do. Do not rush the person. Follow the care plan. If you cannot measure vital signs, tell the nurse right away.

FOCUS ON COMMUNICATION

Measuring and Reporting Vital Signs

Patients and residents like to know their measurements. If agency policy allows, you can tell the person the measurements. Remember, this information is private and confidential. Roommates and visitors must not hear what you are saying.

A measurement may be abnormal. Or you may not be able to feel a pulse or hear a blood pressure. Do not alarm the person. You can say:

- "I'm not sure that I counted your pulse correctly. I want the nurse to take it too."
- "I'm not sure that I heard your blood pressure correctly. I'll ask the nurse to take it again."
- "Your pulse is a little slow (or fast). I'll ask the nurse to check it."
- "Your temperature is higher than normal. I'm going to check it with another thermometer. I'll also ask the nurse to check you."

BOX 25-1 Temperature Sites

ORAL SITE
Oral temperatures are *not* taken if the person:
- Is under 4 or 5 years of age
- Is unconscious
- Has had surgery or an injury to the face, neck, nose, or mouth
- Is receiving oxygen
- Breathes through the mouth
- Has a nasogastric tube
- Is delirious, restless, confused, or disoriented
- Is paralyzed on one side of the body
- Has a sore mouth
- Has a convulsive (seizure) disorder

RECTAL SITE
The rectal site is used for infants and children under 3 years old. Rectal temperatures are taken when the oral site cannot be used. Rectal temperatures are *not* taken if the person:
- Has diarrhea
- Has a rectal disorder or injury
- Has heart disease
- Had rectal surgery
- Is confused or agitated

TYMPANIC MEMBRANE SITE
The site has fewer microbes than the mouth or rectum. Therefore the risk of spreading infection is reduced. This site is *not* used if the person has:
- An ear disorder
- Ear drainage

TEMPORAL ARTERY SITE
Measures body temperature at the temporal artery in the forehead. The site is non-invasive.

AXILLARY SITE
Less reliable than the other sites. It is used when the other sites cannot be used.

---

promptly ask the nurse to take them again. Unless otherwise ordered, take vital signs with the person lying or sitting. The person is at rest when vital signs are measured. Report the following at once:

► Any vital sign that is changed from a prior measurement
► Vital signs above the normal range
► Vital signs below the normal range

Vital signs are recorded in the person's medical record. If they are measured often, a flow sheet is used. The doctor or nurse compares current and previous measurements.

See *Focus on Children and Older Persons: Measuring and Reporting Vital Signs.*

See *Focus on Communication: Measuring and Reporting Vital Signs.*

BODY TEMPERATURE

Body temperature is the amount of heat in the body. It is a balance between the amount of heat produced and the amount lost by the body. Heat is produced as cells use food for energy. It is lost through the skin, breathing, urine, and feces. Body temperature stays fairly stable. It is lower in the morning and higher in the afternoon and evening. Body temperature is affected by age, weather, exercise, emotions, stress, and illness. Pregnancy and the menstrual cycle are other factors.

Thermometers are used to measure temperature. It is measured using the Fahrenheit (F) and centigrade or Celsius (C) scales.

Temperature Sites

Temperature sites are the mouth, rectum, axilla (underarm), tympanic membrane (ear), and temporal artery (forehead) (Box 25-1). Each site has a normal range (Table 25-1, p. 442). **Fever** means an elevated body temperature. Always report temperatures that are above or below the normal range.

See *Focus on Children and Older Persons: Temperature Sites,* p. 442.

See *Promoting Safety and Comfort: Temperature Sites,* p. 442.

TABLE 25-1 Normal Body Temperatures

Site	Baseline	Normal Range
Oral	98.6° F (37° C)	97.6° to 99.6° F (36.5° to 37.5° C)
Rectal	99.6° F (37.5° C)	98.6° to 100.6° F (37.0° to 38.1° C)
Axillary	97.6° F (36.5° C)	96.6° to 98.6° F (35.9° to 37.0° C)
Tympanic membrane	98.6° F (37° C)	98.6° F (37°C)
Temporal artery	99.6° F (37.5° C)	99.6° F (37.5° C)

FOCUS ON CHILDREN AND OLDER PERSONS

Temperature Sites

CHILDREN

The oral site is not used for infants and children younger than 4 to 5 years. Other routes are used as directed by the nurse and the care plan. See Box 25-1.

OLDER PERSONS

Older persons have lower body temperatures than younger persons. An oral temperature of 98.6° F may signal fever in an older person.

PROMOTING SAFETY AND COMFORT: Temperature Sites

SAFETY

Rectal temperatures are dangerous for persons with heart disease. The thermometer can stimulate the vagus nerve in the rectum. This nerve also affects the heart. Stimulation of the vagus nerve slows the heart rate. The heart rate can slow to dangerous levels in some persons.

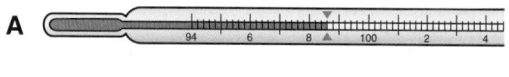

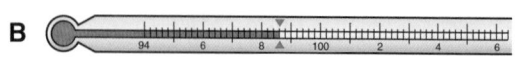

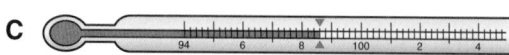

FIGURE 25-1 Types of glass thermometers. **A,** The long or slender tip. **B,** The stubby tip (rectal thermometer). **C,** The pear-shaped tip.

Glass Thermometers

The glass thermometer is a hollow glass tube (Fig. 25-1) with a bulb (tip) at the end. The device is filled with a substance—a mercury-free mixture or mercury. When heated, the substance texpands and rises in the tube. When cooled, the substance contracts and moves down the tube.

Long- or slender-tip thermometers are used for oral and axillary temperatures. So are thermometers with stubby and pear-shaped tips. Rectal thermometers have stubby tips. Thermometers are color-coded:

▶ Blue—oral and axillary thermometers
▶ Red—rectal thermometers

Glass thermometers are reusable. However, the following are problems:

▶ They take a long time to register—3 to 10 minutes depending on the site (p. 444).
▶ They break easily. Broken thermometers can injure the rectum and colon.
▶ The person may bite down and break an oral thermometer. Cuts in the mouth are risks. Swallowed mercury can cause mercury poisoning.

See *Focus on Long-Term Care and Home Care: Glass Thermometers.*

See *Promoting Safety and Comfort: Glass Thermometers.*

Reading a Glass Thermometer

Fahrenheit thermometers have long and short lines. Every other long line is an even degree from 94° to 108° F. The short lines mean 0.2 (two tenths) of a degree (Fig. 25-2, *A*).

On a centigrade thermometer, each long line means 1 degree. Degrees range from 34° to 42° C. Each short line means 0.1 (one tenth) of a degree (Fig. 25-2, *B*).

To read a glass thermometer:

▶ Hold it at the stem (Fig. 25-3). Bring it to eye level.
▶ Turn it until you can see the numbers and the long and short lines.
▶ Turn it back and forth slowly until you can see the silver or red line.
▶ Read the nearest degree (long line).
▶ Read the nearest tenth of a degree (short line)—an even number on a Fahrenheit thermometer.

FOCUS ON LONG-TERM CARE AND HOME CARE

Glass Thermometers

HOME CARE

Patients in home settings may have mercury-glass thermometers. If so, tell the nurse. Do not use a mercury-glass thermometer to measure a child's temperature.

PROMOTING SAFETY AND COMFORT: Glass Thermometers

SAFETY

If a mercury-glass thermometer breaks, tell the nurse at once. Mercury is a hazardous substance. Do not touch the mercury. Do not let the person do so. The agency must follow special procedures for handling all hazardous materials. See Chapter 11.

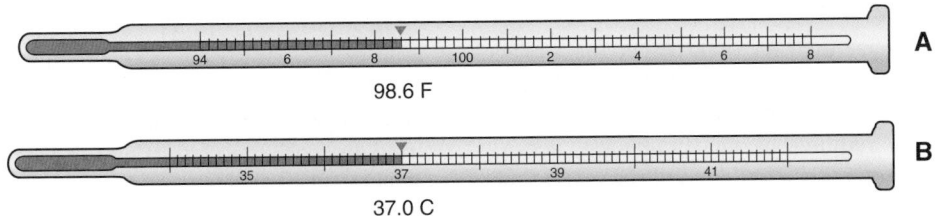

FIGURE 25-2 A, A Fahrenheit thermometer. The temperature measurement is 98.6° F. **B,** Centigrade thermometer. The temperature measurement is 37.0° C.

Using a Glass Thermometer

Do the following to prevent infection, promote safety, and obtain an accurate measurement:

▶ Use the person's thermometer.
▶ Use a rectal thermometer only for rectal temperatures.
▶ Rinse the thermometer under cold, running water if it was soaking in a disinfectant. Dry it from the stem to the bulb end with tissues.
▶ Check the thermometer for breaks, cracks, and chips. Discard it following agency policy if it is broken, cracked, or chipped.
▶ Shake down the thermometer to move the substance down in the tube. Hold it at the stem; stand away from walls, tables, or other hard surfaces. Flex and snap your wrist until the substance is below 94° F or 34° C. See Figure 25-4.
▶ Use plastic covers following agency policy (Fig. 25-5). To take a temperature, insert the thermometer into a cover. Remove the cover to read the thermometer. Discard the cover after use.
▶ Clean and store the thermometer following agency policy. Wipe it with tissues first to remove mucus, feces, or sweat. Do not use hot water. It causes the mercury or mercury-free mixture to expand so much that the thermometer could break. After cleaning, rinse the thermometer under cold, running water. Then store it in a container with a disinfectant solution.
▶ Practice medical asepsis.
▶ Follow Standard Precautions and the Bloodborne Pathogen Standard.

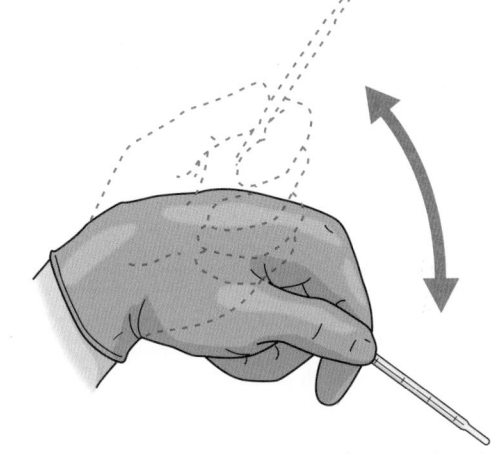

FIGURE 25-4 The wrist is snapped to shake down the thermometer.

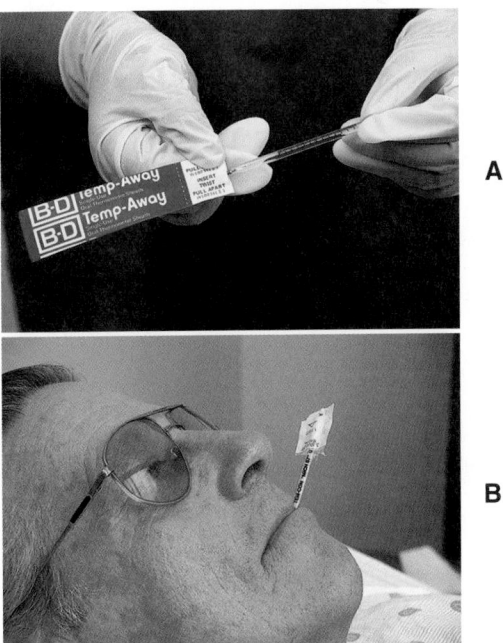

FIGURE 25-5 A, Thermometer inserted in a plastic cover. **B,** The person's temperature is taken with thermometer in a plastic cover.

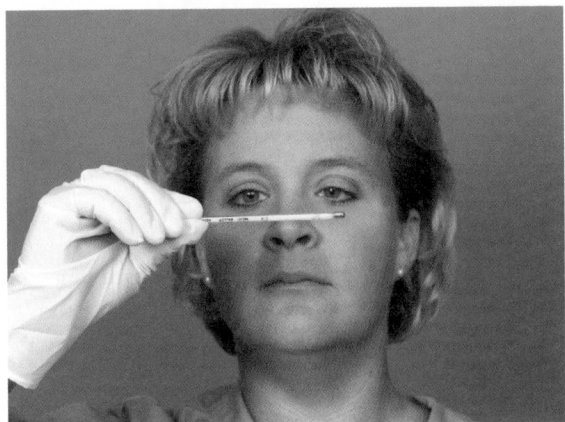

FIGURE 25-3 The thermometer is held at the stem. It is read at eye level.

◆ Taking Temperatures

Glass thermometers are used for oral, rectal, and axillary temperatures. Special measures are needed for each site.

▶ *The oral site.* The glass thermometer remains in place 2 to 3 minutes or as required by agency policy.

▶ *The rectal site.* Lubricate the bulb end of the rectal thermometer for easy insertion and to prevent tissue injury. Hold the thermometer in place so it is not lost into the rectum or broken. A glass thermometer remains in the rectum for 2 minutes or as required by agency policy. Privacy is important. The buttocks and anus are exposed. The procedure embarrasses many people.

▶ *The axillary site.* The axilla (underarm) must be dry. Do not use this site right after bathing. The glass thermometer stays in place for 5 to 10 minutes or as required by agency policy.

See *Delegation Guidelines: Taking Temperatures.*
See *Promoting Safety and Comfort: Taking Temperatures.*

PROMOTING SAFETY AND COMFORT: Taking Temperatures

SAFETY

Thermometers are inserted into the mouth, rectum, axilla, and ear. Each area has many microbes. The area may contain blood. Therefore each person has his or her own glass thermometer. This prevents the spread of microbes and infection. Follow Standard Precautions and the Bloodborne Pathogen Standard when taking temperatures.

When taking a rectal temperature, your gloved hands may come in contact with feces. If so, remove the gloves and decontaminate your hands. Then note the temperature on your notepad or assignment sheet. Put on clean gloves to complete the procedure.

COMFORT

Remove the thermometer in a timely manner. Do not leave it in place longer than needed. This affects the person's comfort. For example, an oral thermometer is left in place for 2 to 3 minutes. Do not leave it in place longer than that.

DELEGATION GUIDELINES: Taking Temperatures

The nurse may ask you to take temperatures. If so, you need this information from the nurse and the care plan:

- What site to use for each person—oral, rectal, axillary, tympanic membrane, or temporal artery
- What thermometer to use for each person—glass, electronic, or other type
- How long to leave a glass thermometer in place
- When to take temperatures
- Which persons are at risk for elevated temperatures
- What observations to report and record
  - A temperature that is changed from a prior measurement
  - A temperature above or below the normal range for the site used
- When to report observations
- What specific patient or resident concerns to report at once

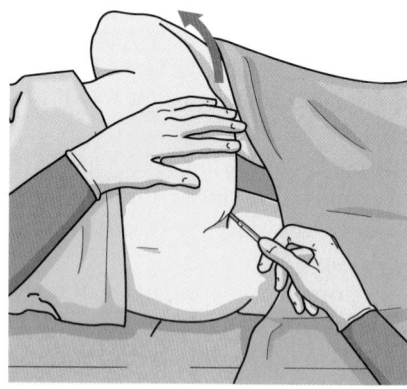

FIGURE 25-7 The rectal temperature is taken with the person in Sims' position. The buttock is raised to expose the anus.

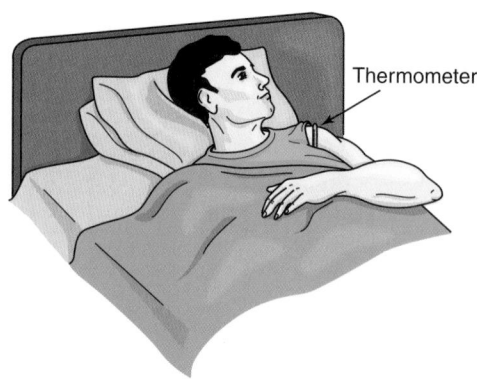

FIGURE 25-8 The thermometer is held in place in the axilla by bringing the person's arm over the chest.

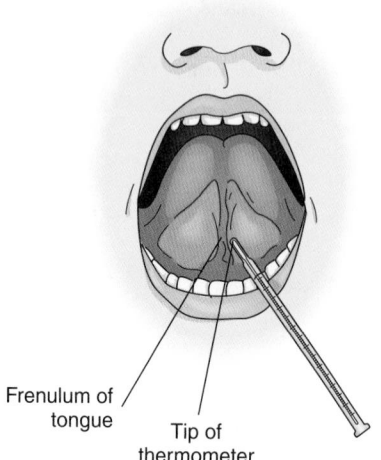

Frenulum of tongue

Tip of thermometer

FIGURE 25-6 The thermometer is placed at the base of the tongue and to one side.

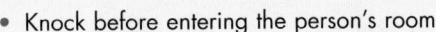

TAKING A TEMPERATURE WITH A GLASS THERMOMETER

✔ Quality of Life *Remember to:*

- Knock before entering the person's room.
- Address the person by name.
- Introduce yourself by name and title.

- Explain the procedure to the person before beginning and during the procedure.
- Protect the person's rights during the procedure.
- Handle the person gently during the procedure.

PRE-PROCEDURE

1 Follow *Delegation Guidelines: Taking Temperatures.* See *Promoting Safety and Comfort:*
   - *Glass Thermometers,* p. 442
   - *Taking Temperatures*
2 For an *oral temperature,* ask the person not to eat, drink, smoke, or chew gum for at least 15 to 20 minutes before the measurement or as required by agency policy.
3 Practice hand hygiene.
4 Collect the following:
   - Oral or rectal thermometer and holder

- Tissues
- Plastic covers if used
- Gloves
- Toilet tissue (rectal temperature)
- Water-soluble lubricant (rectal temperature)
- Towel (axillary temperature)
5 Decontaminate your hands.
6 Identify the person. Check the ID bracelet against the assignment sheet. Also call the person by name.
7 Provide for privacy.

PROCEDURE

8 Put on the gloves.
9 Rinse the thermometer in cold water if it was soaking in a disinfectant. Dry it with tissues.
10 Check for breaks, cracks, or chips.
11 Shake down the thermometer below the lowest number. Hold the thermometer by the stem.
12 Insert it into a plastic cover if used.
13 *For an oral temperature:*
   a Ask the person to moisten his or her lips.
   b Place the bulb end of the thermometer under the tongue and to one side (Fig. 25-6).
   c Ask the person to close the lips around the thermometer to hold it in place.
   d Ask the person not to talk. Remind the person not to bite down on the thermometer.
   e Leave it in place for 2 to 3 minutes or as required by agency policy. (*NOTE:* Some state competency tests require leaving the thermometer in place for 3 minutes.)
14 *For a rectal temperature:*
   a Position the person in Sims' position.
   b Put a small amount of lubricant on a tissue.
   c Lubricate the bulb end of the thermometer.
   d Fold back top linens to expose the anal area.
   e Raise the upper buttock to expose the anus (Fig. 25-7).
   f Insert the thermometer 1 inch into the rectum. Do not force the thermometer. Remember, glass thermometers can break.
   g Hold the thermometer in place for 2 minutes or as required by agency policy. Do not let go of it while it is in the rectum.

15 *For an axillary temperature:*
   a Help the person remove an arm from the gown. Do not expose the person.
   b Dry the axilla with the towel.
   c Place the bulb end of the thermometer in the center of the axilla.
   d Ask the person to place the arm over the chest to hold the thermometer in place (Fig. 25-8). Hold it and the arm in place if he or she cannot help.
   e Leave the thermometer in place for 5 to 10 minutes or as required by agency policy.
16 Remove the thermometer.
17 Use tissues to remove the plastic cover. Discard the cover and tissues. Wipe the thermometer with a tissue if no cover was used. Wipe from the stem to the bulb end. Discard the tissue.
18 Read the thermometer.
19 Note the person's name and temperature on your notepad or assignment sheet. Write *R* for a rectal temperature. Write *A* for an axillary temperature.
20 *For a rectal temperature:*
   a Place used toilet tissue on several thicknesses of clean toilet tissue.
   b Place the thermometer on clean toilet tissue.
   c Wipe the anal area to remove lubricant and feces.
   d Cover the person.
21 *For an axillary temperature:* Help the person put the gown back on.
22 Shake down the thermometer.
23 Clean the thermometer according to agency policy. Return it to the holder.
24 Discard tissues and dispose of toilet tissue.
25 Remove the gloves. Decontaminate your hands.

POST-PROCEDURE

26 Provide for comfort. (See the inside of the front book cover.)
27 Place the signal light within reach.
28 Unscreen the person.
29 Complete a safety check of the room. (See the inside of the front book cover.)

30 Decontaminate your hands.
31 Report and record the temperature. Note the temperature site when reporting and recording. Report an abnormal temperature at once.

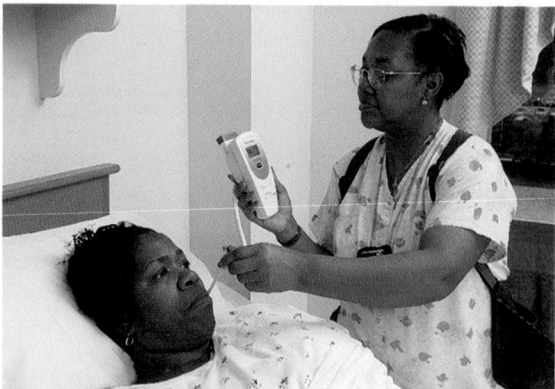

FIGURE 25-9 The covered probe of the electronic thermometer is inserted under the tongue.

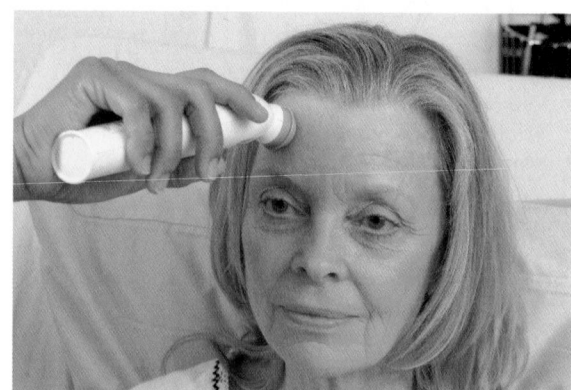

FIGURE 25-11 Temporal artery thermometer.

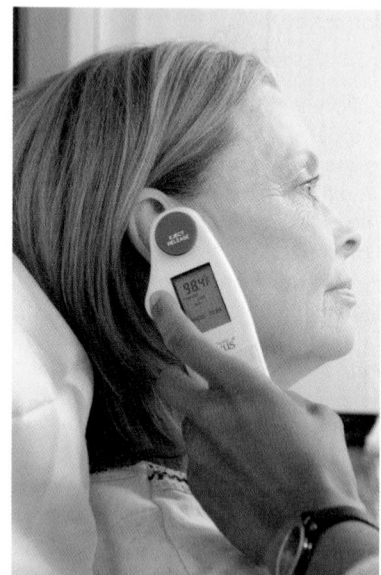

FIGURE 25-10 Tympanic membrane thermometer.

Electronic Thermometers

Electronic thermometers are battery-operated (Fig. 25-9). They measure temperature in a few seconds. The temperature is shown on the front of the device. Some contain batteries. Others are kept in battery chargers when not in use.

Some electronic thermometers have oral and rectal probes. A disposable cover (sheath) protects the probe. The probe cover is discarded after use. This helps prevent the spread of infection.

Tympanic Membrane Thermometers

Tympanic membrane thermometers measure temperature at the tympanic membrane in the ear (Fig. 25-10). The covered probe is gently inserted into the ear. The temperature is measured in 1 to 3 seconds.

Tympanic membrane thermometers are comfortable. They are not invasive like rectal thermometers and probes. There are fewer microbes in the ear than in the mouth or rectum. Therefore the risk of spreading infection is reduced. These thermometers are not used if there is ear drainage.

Temporal Artery Thermometers

Body temperature is measured at the temporal artery in the forehead (Fig. 25-11). The device is gently stroked across the forehead and across the temporal artery. It measures the temperature of the blood in the temporal artery—the same temperature of the blood coming from the heart.

These thermometers measure body temperature in 3 to 4 seconds. They are non-invasive. Nothing is inserted into the mouth, ear, or rectum. Follow the manufacturer's instructions for using, cleaning, and storing the device. Some devices have probe covers. To measure temperature:

▶ Choose the side of the head that is exposed. Do not use the side covered by hair, a dressing, hat, or other covering. If the person was in the side-lying position, do not use the side that was on a pillow.
▶ Place the thermometer at the side of forehead between the hairline and eyebrows.
▶ Slide the thermometer across the forehead.
▶ Read the temperature display.

See *Focus on Children and Older Persons: Electronic Thermometers.*

See *Teamwork and Time Management: Electronic Thermometers.*

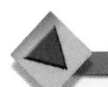

TAKING A TEMPERATURE WITH AN ELECTRONIC THERMOMETER

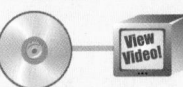

✔ **Quality of Life** *Remember to:*

- Knock before entering the person's room.
- Address the person by name.
- Introduce yourself by name and title.
- Explain the procedure to the person before beginning and during the procedure.

- Protect the person's rights during the procedure.
- Handle the person gently during the procedure.

PRE-PROCEDURE

1 Follow *Delegation Guidelines: Taking Temperatures,* p. 444. See *Promoting Safety and Comfort: Taking Temperatures,* p. 444.

2 For an oral temperature, ask the person not to eat, drink, smoke, or chew gum for at least 15 to 20 minutes before the measurement or as required by agency policy.

3 Practice hand hygiene.

4 Collect the following:
- Thermometer—electronic, tympanic membrane, temporal artery
- Probe (Blue for an oral or axillary temperature. Red for a rectal temperature.)

- Probe covers
- Toilet tissue (rectal temperature)
- Water-soluble lubricant (rectal temperature)
- Gloves
- Towel (axillary temperature)

5 Plug the probe into the thermometer. (This is not done for a tympanic membrane or temporal artery thermometer.)

6 Decontaminate your hands.

7 Identify the person. Check the ID bracelet against the assignment sheet. Also call the person by name.

PROCEDURE

8 Provide for privacy. Position the person for an oral, rectal, axillary, or tympanic membrane temperature.

9 Put on gloves if contact with blood, body fluids, secretions, or excretions is likely.

10 Insert the probe into a probe cover.

11 *For an oral temperature:*
- a Ask the person to open the mouth and raise the tongue.
- b Place the covered probe at the base of the tongue and to one side (see Fig. 25-9).
- c Ask the person to lower the tongue and close the mouth.

12 *For a rectal temperature:*
- a Place some lubricant on toilet tissue.
- b Lubricate the end of the covered probe.
- c Expose the anal area.
- d Raise the upper buttock.
- e Insert the probe ½ inch into the rectum.
- f Hold the probe in place.

13 *For an axillary temperature:*
- a Help the person remove an arm from the gown. Do not expose the person.
- b Dry the axilla with the towel.
- c Place the covered probe in the center of the axilla.
- d Place the person's arm over the chest.
- e Hold the probe in place.

Continued

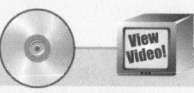

TAKING A TEMPERATURE WITH AN ELECTRONIC THERMOMETER—cont'd

PROCEDURE—cont'd

14 For a tympanic membrane temperature:
  a Ask the person to turn his or her head so the ear is in front of you.
  b Pull up and back on the adult's ear to straighten the ear canal (Fig. 25-12).
  c Insert the covered probe gently.
15 Start the thermometer.
16 Hold the probe in place until you hear a tone or see a flashing or steady light.
17 Read the temperature on the display.
18 Remove the probe. Press the eject button to discard the cover.

19 Note the person's name and temperature on your notepad or assignment sheet. Note the temperature site. Write R for a rectal temperature. Write A for an axillary temperature.
20 Return the probe to the holder.
21 Help the person put the gown back on (axillary temperature). For a rectal temperature:
  a Wipe the anal area with toilet tissue to remove lubricant.
  b Cover the person.
  c Dispose of used toilet tissue.
  d Remove the gloves. Decontaminate your hands.

POST-PROCEDURE

22 Provide for comfort. (See the inside of the front book cover.)
23 Place the signal light within reach.
24 Unscreen the person.
25 Complete a safety check of the room. (See the inside of the front book cover.)

26 Return the thermometer to the charging unit.
27 Decontaminate your hands.
28 Report and record the temperature. Note the temperature site when reporting and recording. Report an abnormal temperature at once.

Other Thermometers

Other thermometers are used. Follow the manufacturer's instructions.

▶ *Digital thermometers*—show the temperature on the front of the thermometer (Fig. 25-13). Depending on the type, they measure temperature in 6 to 60 seconds.
▶ *Disposable oral thermometers*—have small chemical dots (Fig. 25-14). The dots change color when heated. Each dot is heated to a certain temperature before it changes color. These thermometers are used once. They measure temperatures in 45 to 60 seconds.
▶ *Temperature-sensitive tape*—changes color in response to body heat (Fig. 25-15). The tape is applied to the forehead or abdomen. The measurement takes about 15 seconds.

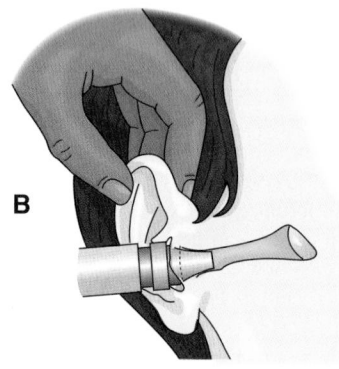

FIGURE 25-12 Using a tympanic membrane thermometer. **A,** The ear is pulled up and back. **B,** The probe is inserted into the ear canal.

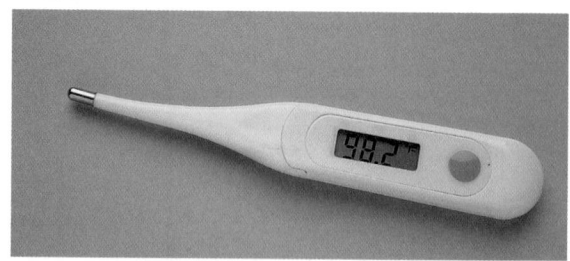

FIGURE 25-13 Digital thermometer.

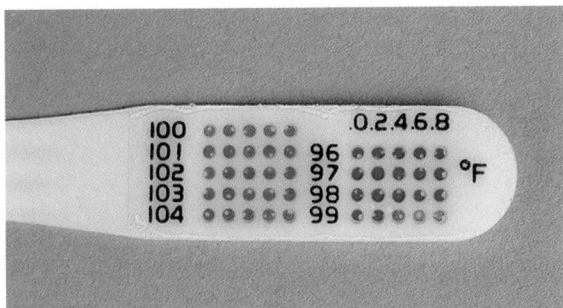

FIGURE 25-14 Disposable oral thermometer with chemical dots. The dots change color when heated by the body.

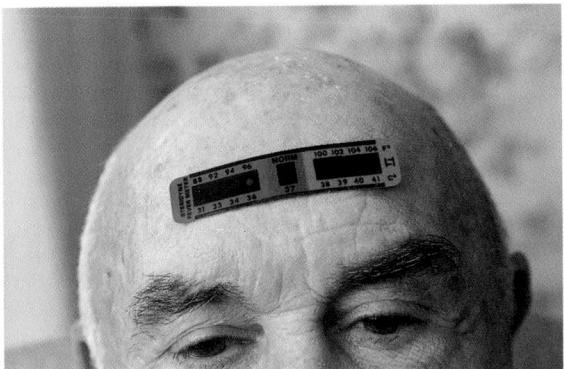

FIGURE 25-15 Temperature sensitive tape.

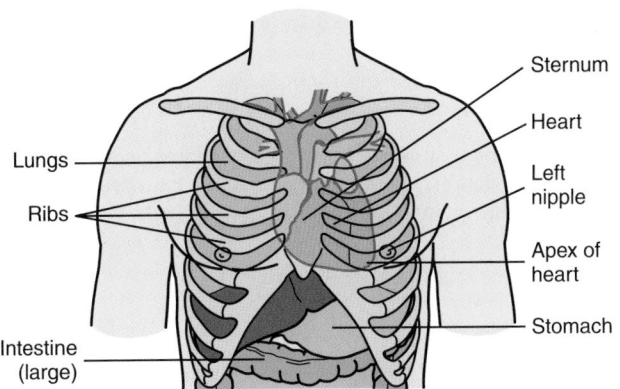

FIGURE 25-16 Location of the heart.

PULSE

Arteries carry blood from the heart to all body parts (Box 25-2). The **pulse** is the beat of the heart felt at an artery as a wave of blood passes through the artery. A pulse is felt every time the heart beats.

BOX 25-2 The Heart and Blood Vessels: Body Structure and Function

The heart is a muscle. It pumps blood through the blood vessels to the tissues and cells. The heart lies in the middle to lower part of the chest cavity toward the left side (Fig. 25-16).

The heart has four chambers (Chapter 8). Upper chambers receive blood and are called the *atria*. The *right atrium* receives blood from body tissues. The *left atrium* receives blood from the lungs. Lower chambers are called ventricles. Ventricles pump blood. The *right ventricle* pumps blood to the lungs for oxygen. The *left ventricle* pumps blood to all parts of the body.

There are two phases of heart action. *Diastole* is the resting phase. Heart chambers fill with blood. *Systole* is the working phase. The heart contracts. Blood is pumped through the blood vessels when the heart contracts.

Blood flows to body tissues and cells through the blood vessels. *Arteries* carry blood away from the heart. Arterial blood is rich in oxygen. The *aorta* is the largest artery. The aorta receives blood directly from the left ventricle. The aorta branches into other arteries that carry blood to all parts of the body (Fig. 25-17). *Veins* return blood to the heart.

See Chapter 8 for more detailed information.

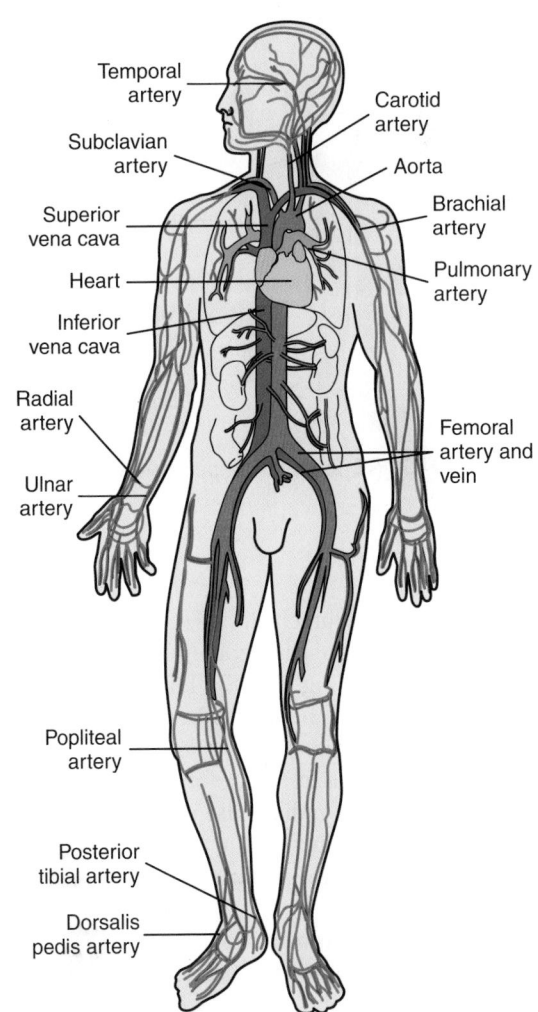

FIGURE 25-17 The arterial system.

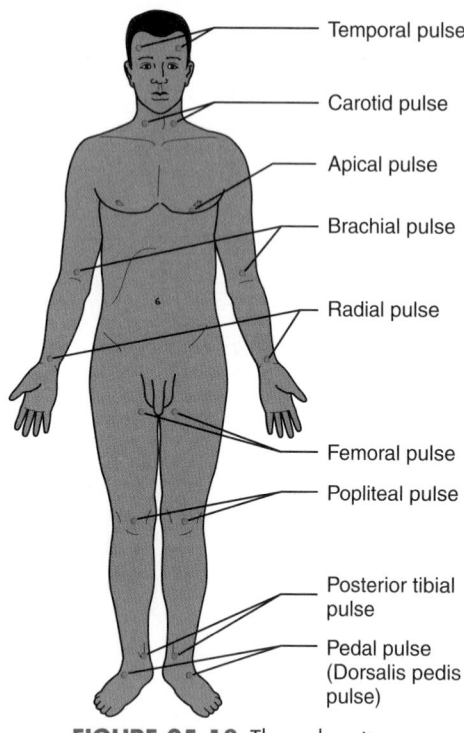

FIGURE 25-18 The pulse sites.

Temporal pulse
Carotid pulse
Apical pulse
Brachial pulse
Radial pulse
Femoral pulse
Popliteal pulse
Posterior tibial pulse
Pedal pulse (Dorsalis pedis pulse)

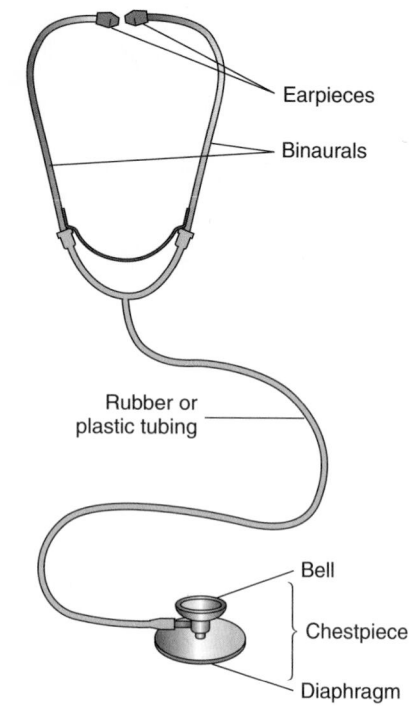

Earpieces
Binaurals
Rubber or plastic tubing
Bell
Chestpiece
Diaphragm

FIGURE 25-19 Parts of a stethoscope.

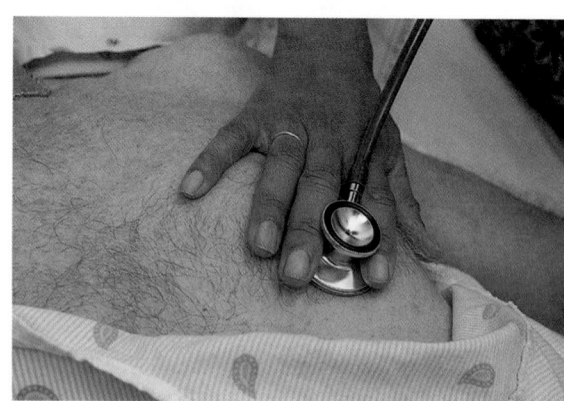

FIGURE 25-20 The stethoscope is held in place with the fingertips of the index and middle fingers.

Pulse Sites

The temporal, carotid, brachial, radial, femoral, popliteal, posterior tibial, and dorsalis pedis (pedal) pulses are on each side of the body (Fig. 25-18). The arteries are close to the body surface and lie over a bone. Therefore they are easy to feel.

The radial pulse is used most often. It is easy to reach and find. You can take a radial pulse without disturbing or exposing the person. The carotid pulse is taken during CPR (cardiopulmonary resuscitation) and other emergencies (Chapter 49).

The apical pulse is felt over the heart. The apex *(apical)* of the heart is at the tip of the heart, just below the left nipple (p. 453). This pulse is taken with a stethoscope.

See *Focus on Children and Older Persons: Pulse Sites.*

Using a Stethoscope

A **stethoscope** is an instrument used to listen to the sounds produced by the heart, lungs, and other body organs (Fig. 25-19). It is used to take apical pulses and blood pressures. The device makes sounds louder for easy hearing.

To use a stethoscope:
▶ Wipe the earpieces and diaphragm with antiseptic wipes before and after use.
▶ Place the earpiece tips in your ears. The bend of the tips points forward. Earpieces should fit snugly to block out noises. They should not cause pain or ear discomfort.
▶ Tap the diaphragm gently. You should hear the tapping. If not, turn the chest piece at the tubing. Gently tap the diaphragm again. Proceed if you hear the tapping sound. Check with the nurse if you do not hear the tapping.
▶ Place the diaphragm over the artery. Hold it in place as in Figure 25-20.
▶ Prevent noise. Do not let anything touch the tubing. Ask the person to be silent.
See *Promoting Safety and Comfort: Using a Stethoscope.*

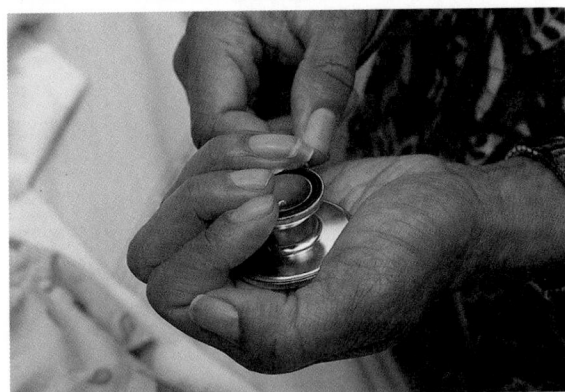

FIGURE 25-21 The diaphragm of the stethoscope is warmed in the palm of the hand.

TABLE 25-2 Pulse Ranges by Age

Age	Pulse Rate (beats per minute)
Birth to 1 year	80-190
2 years	80-160
6 years	75-120
10 years	70-110
12 years and older	60-100

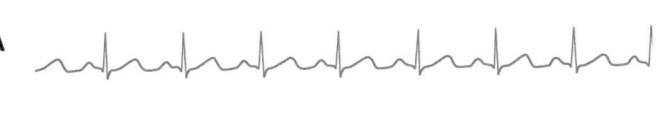

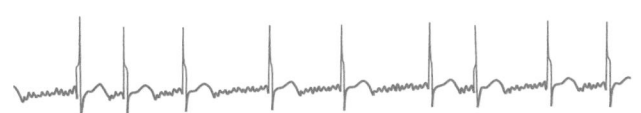

FIGURE 25-22 A, The electrocardiogram shows a regular pulse. The beats occur at regular intervals. **B,** These beats are at irregular intervals.

Pulse Rate

The **pulse rate** is the number of heartbeats or pulses felt in 1 minute. The rate varies for each age-group (Table 25-2). The pulse rate is affected by many factors. They include fever, exercise, fear, anger, anxiety, excitement, heat, position, and pain. These and other factors cause the heart to beat faster. Some drugs also increase the pulse rate. Other drugs slow down the pulse.

The adult pulse rate is between 60 and 100 beats per minute. A rate of less than 60 or more than 100 is considered abnormal. Report abnormal pulses to the nurse at once.

▶ **Tachycardia** is a rapid (*tachy*) heart rate (*cardia*). The heart rate is more than 100 beats per minute.
▶ **Bradycardia** is a slow (*brady*) heart rate (*cardia*). The heart rate is less than 60 beats per minute.

Rhythm and Force of the Pulse

The *rhythm* of the pulse should be regular. That is, pulses are felt in a pattern. The same time interval occurs between beats. An irregular pulse occurs when the beats are not evenly spaced or beats are skipped (Fig. 25-22).

Force relates to pulse strength. A forceful pulse is easy to feel. It is described as *strong, full,* or *bounding.* Hard-to-feel pulses are described as *weak, thready,* or *feeble.*

Electronic blood pressure equipment (p. 458) can also count pulses. The pulse rate and blood pressures are shown. Information is not given about pulse rhythm and force. You need to feel the pulse to determine rhythm and force.

Taking Pulses

You will take radial, apical, and apical-radial pulses. You must count accurately. And you must report and record the pulse rate accurately.

See *Delegation Guidelines: Taking Pulses.*
See *Promoting Safety and Comfort: Taking Pulses,* p. 452.

PROMOTING SAFETY AND COMFORT: Taking Pulses

SAFETY

Do not use your thumb to take a pulse. The thumb has a pulse. You could mistake the pulse in your thumb for the person's pulse. Reporting and recording the wrong pulse rate can harm the person.

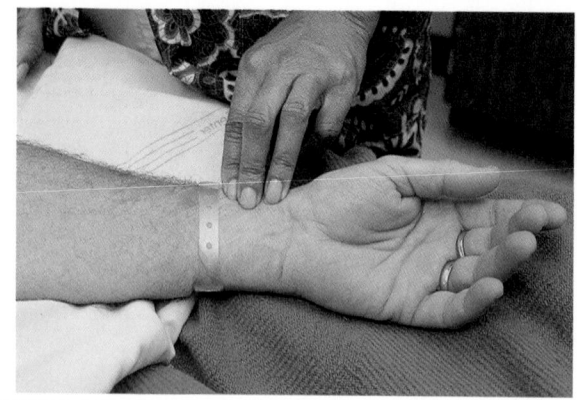

FIGURE 25-23 The middle three fingertips are used to take the radial pulse.

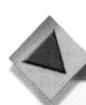 *Taking a Radial Pulse*

The radial pulse is used for routine vital signs. Place the first 2 or 3 fingertips of one hand against the radial artery. The radial artery is on the thumb side of the wrist (Fig. 25-23). Count the pulse for 30 seconds. Then multiply the number by 2. This gives the number of beats per minute. If the pulse is irregular, count it for 1 minute.

In some agencies, all radial pulses are taken for 1 minute. Follow agency policy.

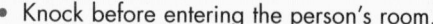

NNAAP™ Skill

TAKING A RADIAL PULSE

✔ **Quality of Life** *Remember to:*

- Knock before entering the person's room.
- Address the person by name.
- Introduce yourself by name and title.
- Explain the procedure to the person before beginning and during the procedure.

- Protect the person's rights during the procedure.
- Handle the person gently during the procedure.

PRE-PROCEDURE

1 Follow *Delegation Guidelines: Taking Pulses.* See *Promoting Safety and Comfort: Taking Pulses.*
2 Practice hand hygiene.

3 Identify the person. Check the ID bracelet against the assignment sheet. Also call the person by name.
4 Provide for privacy.

PROCEDURE

5 Have the person sit or lie down.
6 Locate the radial pulse. Use your first 2 or 3 middle fingertips (see Fig. 25-23).
7 Note if the pulse is strong or weak, and regular or irregular.
8 Count the pulse for 30 seconds. Multiply the number of beats by 2. Or count the pulse for 1 minute if:
  • Directed by the nurse and care plan
  • Required by agency policy

  • The pulse was irregular
  • Required for your state competency test
9 Note the person's name and pulse on your notepad or assignment sheet. Note the strength of the pulse. Note if it was regular or irregular.

POST-PROCEDURE

10 Provide for comfort. (See the inside of the front book cover.)
11 Place the signal light within reach.
12 Unscreen the person.

13 Complete a safety check of the room. (See the inside of the front book cover.)
14 Decontaminate your hands.
15 Report and record pulse rate and your observations. Report an abnormal pulse at once.

◆ *Taking an Apical Pulse*

The apical pulse is on the left side of the chest slightly below the nipple (Fig. 25-24). It is taken with a stethoscope. Apical pulses are taken on:

▶ Infants and children up to about 2 years of age
▶ Persons who have heart disease
▶ Persons who have irregular heart rhythms
▶ Persons who take drugs that affect the heart

Count the apical pulse for 1 minute. The heartbeat normally sounds like a *lub-dub*. Count each *lub-dub* as one beat. Do not count the *lub* as one beat and the *dub* as another.

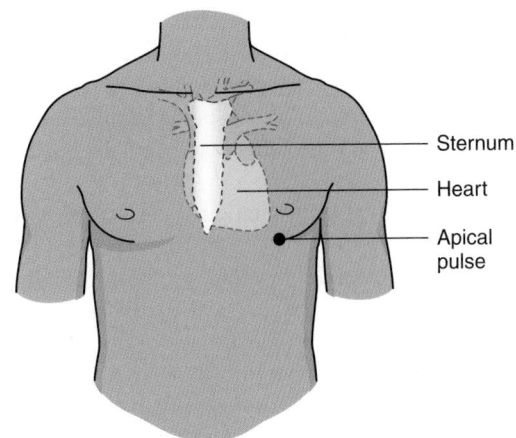

FIGURE 25-24 The apical pulse is located 2 to 3 inches to the left of the sternum (breastbone) and below the left nipple.

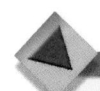

TAKING AN APICAL PULSE

✔ Quality of Life *Remember to:*

- Knock before entering the person's room.
- Address the person by name.
- Introduce yourself by name and title.
- Explain the procedure to the person before beginning and during the procedure.

- Protect the person's rights during the procedure.
- Handle the person gently during the procedure.

PRE-PROCEDURE

1 Follow *Delegation Guidelines: Taking Pulses.* See *Promoting Safety and Comfort: Using a Stethoscope,* p. 451.
2 Practice hand hygiene.
3 Collect a stethoscope and antiseptic wipes.

4 Decontaminate your hands.
5 Identify the person. Check the ID bracelet against the assignment sheet. Also call the person by name.
6 Provide for privacy.

PROCEDURE

7 Clean the earpieces and diaphragm with the wipes.
8 Have the person sit or lie down.
9 Expose the nipple area of the left chest. Limit exposure of a woman's breasts to the extent necessary.
10 Warm the diaphragm in your palm.
11 Place the earpieces in your ears.
12 Find the apical pulse. Place the diaphragm 2 to 3 inches to the left of the breastbone and below the left nipple (see Fig. 25-24).

13 Count the pulse for 1 minute. Note if it was regular or irregular.
14 Cover the person. Remove the earpieces.
15 Note the person's name and pulse on your notepad or assignment sheet. Note if the pulse was regular or irregular.

POST-PROCEDURE

16 Provide for comfort. (See the inside of the front book cover.)
17 Place the signal light within reach.
18 Unscreen the person.
19 Complete a safety check of the room. (See the inside of the front book cover.)

20 Clean the earpieces and diaphragm with the wipes.
21 Return the stethoscope to its proper place.
22 Decontaminate your hands.
23 Report and record your observations. Record the pulse rate with *Ap* for apical. Report an abnormal pulse rate at once.

Taking an Apical-Radial Pulse

The apical pulse and radial pulse should be equal. Sometimes heart contractions are not strong enough to create pulses in the radial artery. Then the radial pulse rate is less than the apical pulse rate. This may occur in people with heart disease.

To see if the apical and radial pulses are equal, two staff members are needed. One takes the radial pulse; the other takes the apical pulse. Taking the apical and radial pulses at the same time is called the **apical-radial pulse**.

The **pulse deficit** is the difference between the apical and radial pulse rates. To obtain the pulse deficit, subtract the radial rate from the apical rate. (The apical pulse rate is never less than the radial pulse rate.) For example:

▶ The apical pulse rate is 84 beats per minute. The radial pulse rate is 84 beats per minute. The pulse deficit is zero (0).
▶ The apical pulse rate is 90 beats per minute. The radial pulse rate is 86 beats per minute. The pulse deficit is 4.

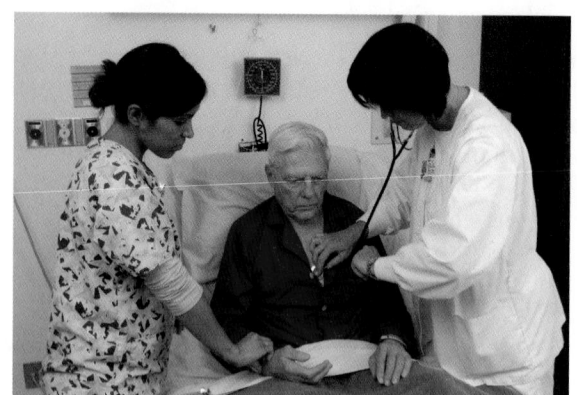

FIGURE 25-25 Taking an apical-radial pulse. One worker takes the apical pulse. The other takes the radial pulse.

TAKING AN APICAL-RADIAL PULSE

✔ Quality of Life *Remember to:*

- Knock before entering the person's room.
- Address the person by name.
- Introduce yourself by name and title.
- Explain the procedure to the person before beginning and during the procedure.

- Protect the person's rights during the procedure.
- Handle the person gently during the procedure.

PRE-PROCEDURE

1 Follow *Delegation Guidelines: Taking Pulses*, p. 452. See *Promoting Safety and Comfort:*
  a *Using a Stethoscope*, p. 451
  b *Taking Pulses*, p. 452
2 Ask a nursing team member to help you.
3 Practice hand hygiene.

4 Collect a stethoscope and antiseptic wipes.
5 Decontaminate your hands.
6 Identify the person. Check the ID bracelet against the assignment sheet. Also call the person by name.
7 Provide for privacy.

PROCEDURE

8 Clean the earpieces and diaphragm with the wipes.
9 Have the person sit or lie down.
10 Expose the nipple area of the left chest. Limit exposure of a woman's breasts to the extent necessary.
11 Warm the diaphragm in your palm.
12 Place the earpieces in your ears.
13 Find the apical pulse. Your helper finds the radial pulse (Fig. 25-25).
14 Give the signal to begin counting.

15 Count the pulse for 1 minute.
16 Give the signal to stop counting.
17 Cover the person. Remove the stethoscope earpieces.
18 Note the person's name and the apical and radial pulses on your notepad or assignment sheet. Subtract the radial pulse from the apical pulse for the pulse deficit. Note whether the pulse was regular or irregular.

POST-PROCEDURE

19 Provide for comfort. (See the inside of the front book cover.)
20 Place the signal light within reach.
21 Unscreen the person.
22 Complete a safety check of the room. (See the inside of the front book cover.)
23 Clean the earpieces and diaphragm with the wipes.

24 Return the stethoscope to its proper place.
25 Decontaminate your hands.
26 Report and record your observations. (Report an abnormal pulse at once.) Include:
- The apical and radial pulse rates
- The pulse deficit

◆ RESPIRATIONS

Respiration means breathing air into *(inhalation)* and out of *(exhalation)* the lungs. Oxygen enters the lungs during inhalation. Carbon dioxide leaves the lungs during exhalation. Each respiration involves one inhalation and one exhalation. The chest rises during inhalation. It falls during exhalation. See Box 25-3 for a review of the respiratory system.

The healthy adult has 12 to 20 respirations per minute. The respiratory rate is affected by the factors that affect temperature and pulse. Heart and respiratory diseases usually increase the respiratory rate.

Respirations are normally quiet, effortless, and regular. Both sides of the chest rise and fall equally. See Chapter 34 for abnormal respiratory patterns.

Count respirations when the person is at rest. Position the person so you can see the chest rise and fall. To a certain extent, a person can control the rate and depth of breathing. People tend to change their breathing patterns when they know their respirations are being counted. Therefore the person should not know that you are counting them.

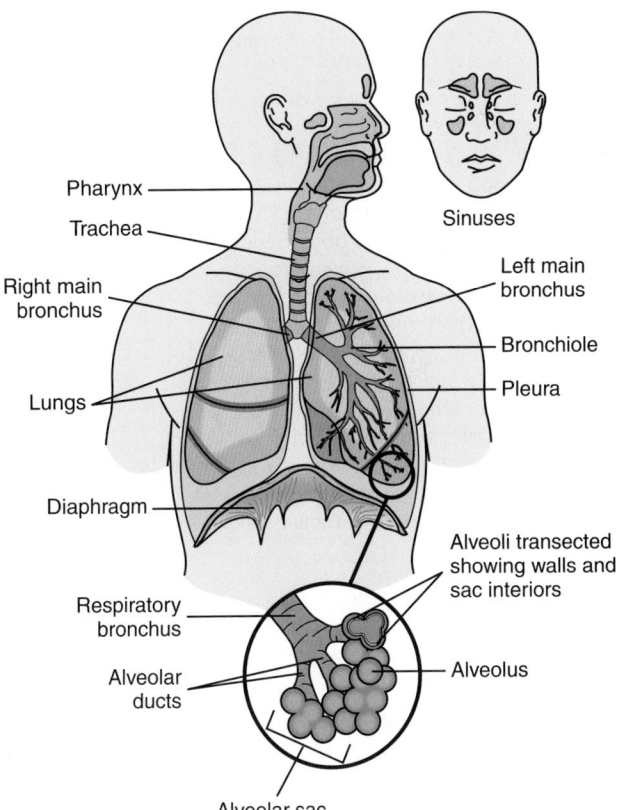

FIGURE 25-26 The respiratory system.

Count respirations right after taking a pulse. Keep your fingers or stethoscope over the pulse site. (The person assumes you are taking the pulse). To count respirations, watch the chest rise and fall. Count them for 30 seconds. Multiply the number by 2 for the number of respirations in 1 minute. If an abnormal pattern is noted, count the respirations for 1 minute.

In some agencies, respirations are counted for 1 minute. Follow agency policy.

See *Focus on Children and Older Persons: Respirations.*
See *Delegation Guidelines: Respirations,* p. 456.

BOX 25-3 The Respiratory System: Body Structure and Function

Oxygen is needed for life. Every cell needs oxygen. The respiratory system (Fig. 25-26) brings oxygen into the lungs and rids the body of carbon dioxide. *Respiration* is the process of supplying the cells with oxygen and removing carbon dioxide from them. Respiration involves *inhalation* (breathing in) and *exhalation* (breathing out). The terms *inspiration* (breathing in) and *expiration* (breathing out) are also used.

Air enters the body through the *nose.* The air then passes into the *pharynx* (throat), a tube-shaped passageway for both air and food. Air passes from the pharynx into the *larynx* (the voice box). Air passes from the larynx into the *trachea* (the windpipe). The trachea divides at its lower end into the *right bronchus* and *left bronchus.* Each bronchus enters a lung.

On entering the lungs, the bronchi divide many times into smaller branches called *bronchioles.* Eventually the bronchioles further divide. They end in tiny one-celled air sacs called *alveoli.* They are supplied by capillaries.

Oxygen and carbon dioxide are exchanged between the alveoli and capillaries. Blood in the capillaries picks up oxygen from the alveoli. Then the blood returns to the left side of the heart and is pumped to the rest of the body. Alveoli pick up carbon dioxide from the capillaries for exhalation.

Each lung is divided into lobes. The right lung has three lobes; the left lung has two. The lungs are separated from the abdominal cavity by a muscle called the *diaphragm.* A bony framework made up of the ribs, sternum, and vertebrae protects the lungs.

See Chapter 8 for more detailed information.

FOCUS ON **CHILDREN** AND **OLDER PERSONS**

Respirations

CHILDREN
Infants and children have higher respiratory rates than adults (Table 25-3, p. 456). Count an infant's respirations for 1 minute.

DELEGATION GUIDELINES: Respirations

Before counting respirations, you need this information from the nurse and the care plan:

- How long to count respirations for each person—30 seconds or 1 minute
- When to count respirations
- If the nurse has concerns about certain patients or residents
- What other vital signs to measure
- What observations to report and record:
  - The respiratory rate
  - Equality and depth of respirations
  - If the respirations were regular or irregular
  - If the person has pain or difficulty breathing
  - Any respiratory noises
  - An abnormal respiratory pattern (Chapter 34)
- When to report observations
- What specific patient or resident concerns to report at once

TABLE 25-3 Normal Respiratory Rates for Children

Age	Respirations per Minute
Newborn	35
1 year	30
2 years	25
4 years	23
6 years	21
8 years	20
10 years	19
12 years	19
14 years	18
16 years	17
18 years	16-18

Modified from Hockenberry MJ and Wilson D: *Wong's nursing care of infants and children*, ed 8, St Louis, 2007, Mosby.

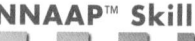

NNAAP™ Skill

COUNTING RESPIRATIONS

PROCEDURE

1 Follow *Delegation Guidelines: Respirations.*
2 Keep your fingers or stethoscope over the pulse site.
3 Do not tell the person you are counting respirations.
4 Begin counting when the chest rises. Count each rise and fall of the chest as 1 respiration.
5 Note the following:
  - If respirations are regular
  - If both sides of the chest rise equally
  - The depth of respirations
  - If the person has any pain or difficulty breathing
  - An abnormal respiratory pattern

6 Count respirations for 30 seconds. Multiply the number by 2. Count respirations for 1 minute if:
  - Directed by the nurse and care plan
  - Required by agency policy
  - They are abnormal or irregular
  - Required for your state competency test
7 Note the person's name, respiratory rate, and other observations on your notepad or assignment sheet.

POST-PROCEDURE

8 Provide for comfort. (See the inside of the front book cover.)
9 Place the signal light within reach.
10 Unscreen the person.
11 Complete a safety check of the room. (See the inside of the front book cover.)

12 Decontaminate your hands.
13 Report and record the respiratory rate and your observations. Report abnormal respirations at once.

BLOOD PRESSURE

Blood pressure is the amount of force exerted against the walls of an artery by the blood. Blood pressure is controlled by:

▶ The force of heart contractions

▶ The amount of blood pumped with each heartbeat

▶ How easily the blood flows through the blood vessels

The period of heart muscle contraction is called **systole.** The heart is pumping blood. The period of heart muscle relaxation is called **diastole.** The heart is at rest.

Systolic and diastolic pressures are measured. The **systolic pressure** is the amount of force needed to pump blood out of the heart into the arterial circulation. It is the higher pressure. The **diastolic pressure** is the pressure in the arteries when the heart is at rest. It is the lower pressure.

Blood pressure is measured in millimeters (mm) of mercury (Hg). The systolic pressure is recorded over the diastolic pressure. A systolic pressure of 120 mm Hg (millimeters of mercury) and a diastolic pressure of 80 mm Hg is written as 120/80 mm Hg.

Normal and Abnormal Blood Pressures

Blood pressure can change from minute to minute. Factors affecting blood pressure are listed in Box 25-4.

Because it can vary so easily, blood pressure has normal ranges:

▶ *Systolic pressure*—less than 120 mm Hg

▶ *Diastolic pressure*—less than 80 mm Hg

Treatment is indicated for:

▶ **Hypertension**—blood pressure measurements that remain above *(hyper)* a systolic pressure of 140 mm Hg or a diastolic pressure of 90 mm Hg. Report any systolic measurement at or above 120 mm Hg. Also report a diastolic pressure at or above 80 mm Hg.

▶ **Hypotension**—when the systolic blood pressure is below *(hypo)* 90 mm Hg and the diastolic pressure is below 60 mm Hg. Report a systolic pressure below 90 mm Hg. Also report a diastolic pressure below 60 mm Hg. Some people normally have low blood pressures. However, hypotension can signal a life-threatening problem.

See *Focus on Children and Older Persons: Normal and Abnormal Blood Pressures.*

BOX 25-4 Factors Affecting Blood Pressure

- *Age.* Blood pressure increases with age. It is lowest in infancy and childhood. It is highest in adulthood.
- *Gender (male or female).* Women usually have lower blood pressures than men do. Blood pressures rise in women after menopause.
- *Blood volume.* This is the amount of blood in the system. Severe bleeding lowers the blood volume. Therefore blood pressure lowers. Giving IV (intravenous) fluids rapidly increases the blood volume. The blood pressure rises.
- *Stress.* Stress includes anxiety, fear, and emotions. Blood pressure increases as the body responds to stress.
- *Pain.* Pain generally increases blood pressure. However, severe pain can cause shock. Blood pressure is seriously low in the state of shock (Chapter 49).
- *Exercise.* Blood pressure increases. Do not measure blood pressure right after exercise.
- *Weight.* Blood pressure is higher in overweight persons. It lowers with weight loss.
- *Race.* Black persons generally have higher blood pressures than white persons do.
- *Diet.* A high-sodium diet increases the amount of water in the body. The extra fluid volume increases blood pressure.
- *Drugs.* Drugs can be given to raise or lower blood pressure. Other drugs have the side effects of high or low blood pressure.
- *Position.* Blood pressure is lower when lying down. It is higher in the standing position. Sudden changes in position can cause a sudden drop in blood pressure (orthostatic hypotension). When standing suddenly, the person may have a sudden drop in blood pressure. Dizziness and fainting can occur (Chapter 26).
- *Smoking.* Blood pressure increases. Nicotine in cigarettes causes blood vessels to narrow. The heart must work harder to pump blood through narrowed vessels.
- *Alcohol.* Excessive alcohol intake can raise blood pressure.

FOCUS ON CHILDREN AND OLDER PERSONS

Normal and Abnormal Blood Pressures

CHILDREN

Age, sex, and height are used to determine what a child's normal blood pressure should be. Young children can have high blood pressure. Overweight children usually have higher blood pressures than do children with a normal weight. Children 3 years of age and older are screened for high blood pressure.

OLDER PERSONS

Older persons also are at risk for orthostatic hypotension (Chapter 26).

Equipment

A stethoscope and a sphygmomanometer are used to measure blood pressure. The **sphygmomanometer** has a cuff and a measuring device.

▶ The *aneroid type* has a round dial and a needle that points to the numbers (Fig. 25-27, *A*).
▶ The *mercury type* has a column of mercury within a calibrated tube (Fig. 25-27, *B*).
▶ The *electronic type* shows the systolic and diastolic blood pressures on the front of the device (Fig. 25-27, *C*). It also shows the pulse rate. To use the device, follow the manufacturer's instructions.

The blood pressure cuff is wrapped around the upper arm. Tubing connects the cuff to the manometer. Another tube connects the cuff to a small, hand-held bulb. A valve on the bulb is turned clockwise to close the valve so the cuff inflates as the bulb is squeezed. The inflated cuff causes pressure over the brachial artery. The valve is turned counter-clockwise to open the valve to deflate the cuff. Blood pressure is measured as the cuff is deflated.

Sounds are produced as the blood flows through the arteries. The stethoscope is used to listen to the sounds in the brachial artery as the cuff is deflated. Stethoscopes are not needed with electronic manometers.

See *Focus on Children and Older Persons: Equipment.*
See *Promoting Safety and Comfort: Equipment.*

FOCUS ON CHILDREN AND OLDER PERSONS

Equipment

CHILDREN

Pediatric blood pressure cuffs are used for children. Infant and child sizes are available. The nurse tells you what size to use.

PROMOTING SAFETY AND COMFORT: Equipment

SAFETY

Mercury is a hazardous substance. Mercury thermometers are being phased out of health care although some agencies may still use them. Handle mercury thermometers carefully. If one breaks, call for the nurse at once. Do not touch the mercury. Do not let the person touch it. The agency must follow special procedures for handling all hazardous substances. See Chapter 11.

COMFORT

Inflate the cuff only to the extent necessary (see procedure: *Measuring Blood Pressure*). The inflated cuff causes discomfort. The higher the inflation, the greater the discomfort.

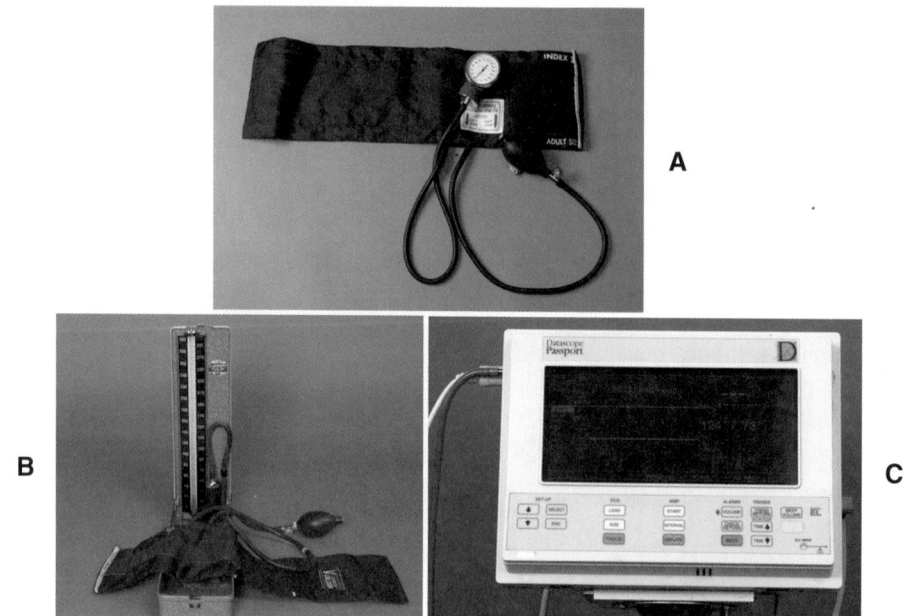

FIGURE 25-27 Blood pressure equipment. **A,** Aneroid manometer and cuff. **B,** Mercury manometer and cuff. **C,** Electronic sphygmomanometer.

Measuring Blood Pressure

Blood pressure is normally measured in the brachial artery. Box 25-5 lists the guidelines for measuring blood pressure.

See *Delegation Guidelines: Measuring Blood Pressure.*

DELEGATION GUIDELINES: Measuring Blood Pressure

Before measuring blood pressure, you need this information from the nurse and the care plan:
- When to measure blood pressure
- What arm to use
- The person's normal blood pressure range
- If the nurse has concerns about certain patients or residents
- If the person needs to be lying down, sitting, or standing
- What size cuff to use—regular, child-size, or extra large
- What observations to report and record
- When to report the blood pressure measurement
- What specific patient or resident concerns to report at once

---

BOX 25-5 Guidelines For Measuring Blood Pressure

- Do not take blood pressure on an arm with an IV infusion, a cast, or a dialysis access site. If a person had breast surgery, do not take blood pressure on that side. Avoid taking blood pressure on an injured arm.
- Let the person rest for 10 to 20 minutes before measuring blood pressure.
- Measure blood pressure with the person sitting or lying. Sometimes the doctor orders blood pressure measured in the standing position.
- Apply the cuff to the bare upper arm. Clothing can affect the measurement.
- Make sure the cuff is snug. Loose cuffs can cause inaccurate readings.
- Use a larger cuff if the person is obese or has a large arm. Use a small cuff if the person has a very small arm. Ask the nurse what size to use. Also check the care plan.
- Place the diaphragm of the stethoscope firmly over the brachial artery. The entire diaphragm must have contact with the skin.
- Make sure the room is quiet. Talking, TV, radio, and sounds from the hallway can affect an accurate measurement.
- Have the sphygmomanometer where you can clearly see it.
- Measure the systolic and diastolic pressures.
  - Expect to hear the first blood pressure sound at the point where you last felt the radial or brachial pulse. The first sound is the systolic pressure.
  - The point where the sound disappears is the diastolic pressure.
- Take the blood pressure again if you are not sure of an accurate measurement. Wait 30 to 60 seconds before repeating the measurement. Ask the nurse to take the blood pressure if you are unsure of the measurement.
- Tell the nurse at once if you cannot hear the blood pressure.

NNAAP™ Skill

MEASURING BLOOD PRESSURE

✔ Quality of Life *Remember to:*

- Knock before entering the person's room.
- Address the person by name.
- Introduce yourself by name and title.
- Explain the procedure to the person before beginning and during the procedure.

- Protect the person's rights during the procedure.
- Handle the person gently during the procedure.

PRE-PROCEDURE

1 Follow *Delegation Guidelines: Measuring Blood Pressure.* See *Promoting Safety and Comfort:*
  - *Using a Stethoscope,* p. 451
  - *Equipment*
2 Practice hand hygiene.
3 Collect the following:
  - Sphygmomanometer
  - Stethoscope
  - Antiseptic wipes

4 Decontaminate your hands.
5 Identify the person. Check the ID bracelet against the assignment sheet. Also call the person by name.
6 Provide for privacy.

Continued

MEASURING BLOOD PRESSURE—cont'd

PROCEDURE

7 Wipe the stethoscope earpieces and diaphragm with the wipes. Warm the diaphragm in your palm.
8 Have the person sit or lie down.
9 Position the person's arm level with the heart. The palm is up.
10 Stand no more than 3 feet away from the manometer. The mercury type is vertical, on a flat surface, and at eye level. The aneroid type is directly in front of you.
11 Expose the upper arm.
12 Squeeze the cuff to expel any remaining air. Close the valve on the bulb.
13 Find the brachial artery at the inner aspect of the elbow. (The brachial artery is on the little finger side of the arm.) Use your fingertips.
14 Place the arrow on the cuff over the brachial artery (Fig. 25-28, A). Wrap the cuff around the upper arm at least 1 inch above the elbow. It is even and snug.
15 *Method one:*
   a Place the stethoscope earpieces in your ears.
   b Find the radial or brachial artery.
   c Inflate the cuff until you can no longer feel the pulse. Note this point.
   d Inflate the cuff 30 mm Hg beyond the point where you last felt the pulse.
16 *Method two:*
   a Find the radial or brachial artery.
   b Inflate the cuff until you can no longer feel the pulse. Note this point.

c Inflate the cuff 30 mm Hg beyond the point where you last felt the pulse.
d Deflate the cuff slowly. Note the point when you feel the pulse.
e Wait 30 seconds.
f Place the stethoscope earpieces in your ears.
g Inflate the cuff again, 30 mm Hg beyond the point where you felt the pulse return.
17 Place the diaphragm of the stethoscope over the brachial artery (Fig. 25-28, B). Do not place it under the cuff.
18 Deflate the cuff at an even rate of 2 to 4 millimeters per second. Turn the valve counter-clockwise to deflate the cuff.
19 Note the point where you hear the first sound. This is the systolic reading. It is near the point where the radial pulse disappeared.
20 Continue to deflate the cuff. Note the point where the sound disappears. This is the diastolic reading.
21 Deflate the cuff completely. Remove it from the person's arm. Remove the stethoscope earpieces from your ears.
22 Note the person's name and blood pressure on your notepad or assignment sheet.
23 Return the cuff to the case or wall holder.

POST-PROCEDURE

24 Provide for comfort. (See the inside of the front book cover.)
25 Place the signal light within reach.
26 Unscreen the person.
27 Complete a safety check of the room. (See the inside of the front book cover.)

28 Clean the earpieces and diaphragm with the wipes.
29 Return the equipment to its proper place.
30 Decontaminate your hands.
31 Report and record the blood pressure (Fig. 25-29). Report an abnormal blood pressure at once.

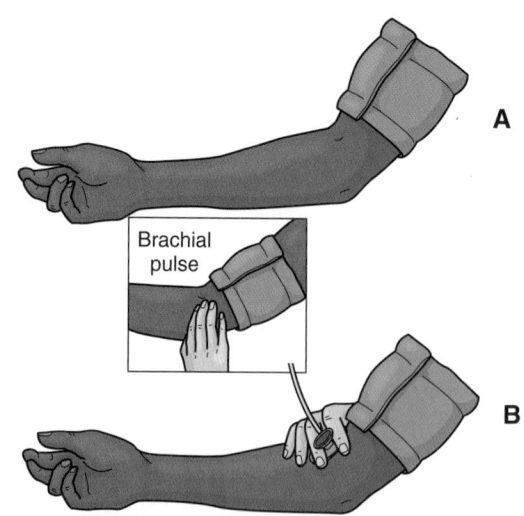

FIGURE 25-28 Measuring blood pressure. **A,** The cuff is over the brachial artery. **B,** The diaphragm of the stethoscope is over the brachial artery.

Date	Time	Weight	T	P	R	BP				Signatures	
10/19	0700	126	98.4	72	20	142/84				*Mary Smith CNA*	
10/26	0715	125	98.6	72	18	140/84				Jane Doe CNA	
11/2	0715	126	98.6	70	18	144/82				*Mary Smith CNA*	

FIGURE 25-29 Charting sample.

REVIEW QUESTIONS

Circle the BEST answer.

1 Which statement is *false*?
   a The vital signs are temperature, pulse, respirations, and blood pressure.
   b Vital signs detect changes in body function.
   c Vital signs change only during illness.
   d Sleep, exercise, drugs, emotions, and noise affect vital signs.

2 Which should you report at once?
   a An oral temperature of 98.4° F
   b A rectal temperature of 101.6° F
   c An axillary temperature of 97.6° F
   d An oral temperature of 99.0° F

3 A rectal temperature is taken when the person
   a Is unconscious
   b Has heart disease
   c Is confused
   d Has diarrhea

4 Which gives the *least* accurate measurement of body temperature?
   a Oral site
   b Rectal site
   c Axillary site
   d Tympanic membrane site

5 Which site is used to take an infant's temperature?
   a Oral site
   b Rectal site
   c Axillary site
   d Tympanic membrane site

6 Which is usually used to take an adult's pulse?
   a The radial pulse
   b The apical pulse
   c The apical-radial pulse
   d The brachial pulse

7 Which is reported to the nurse at once?
   a An adult has a pulse of 120 beats per minute.
   b An infant has a pulse of 130 beats per minute.
   c An adult has a pulse of 80 beats per minute.
   d An adult has a pulse of 64 beats per minute.

8 Which statement about the apical-radial pulse is *true*?
   a The radial pulse can be greater than the apical pulse.
   b The apical pulse can be greater than the radial pulse.
   c The apical and radial pulses are always equal.
   d The pulse deficit is 0.

9 In an adult, normal respirations are
   a 10 to 18 per minute
   b 12 to 20 per minute
   c Less than 20 per minute
   d More than 20 per minute

10 Normal respirations
   a Are heard as the person inhales
   b Are heard as the person exhales
   c Are quiet
   d Sound like wheezing with inhalation and exhalation

11 Respirations are usually counted
   a After taking the temperature
   b After taking the pulse
   c Before taking the pulse
   d After taking the blood pressure

12 Which blood pressure is normal for an adult?
   a 88/54 mm Hg
   b 140/90 mm Hg
   c 100/60 mm Hg
   d 112/78 mm Hg

13 When measuring blood pressure, you should do the following *except*
   a Use the arm with an IV infusion
   b Apply the cuff to a bare upper arm
   c Turn off the TV
   d Locate the brachial artery

14 The systolic pressure is the point
   a Where the pulse is no longer felt
   b Where the first sound is heard
   c Where the last sound is heard
   d 30 mm Hg above where the pulse was felt

Answers for these questions are on p. 781.

Exercise and Activity

OBJECTIVES

- Define the key terms and key abbreviations listed in this chapter
- Describe bedrest
- Explain how to prevent the complications from bedrest
- Describe the devices used to support and maintain body alignment
- Explain the purpose of a trapeze
- Describe range-of-motion exercises
- Describe four walking aids
- Perform the procedures described in this chapter

PROCEDURES

 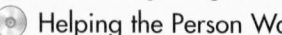 Performing Range-of-Motion Exercises

Helping the Person Walk

Procedures with this icon ⊙ are on the CDCompanion in this book; those with this icon 📹 are on the Evolve Student Resources Website.

KEY TERMS

abduction Moving a body part away from the midline of the body

adduction Moving a body part toward the midline of the body

ambulation The act of walking

atrophy The decrease in size or the wasting away of tissue

contracture The lack of joint mobility caused by abnormal shortening of a muscle

deconditioning The loss of muscle strength from inactivity

dorsiflexion Bending the toes and foot up at the ankle

extension Straightening a body part

external rotation Turning the joint outward

flexion Bending a body part

footdrop The foot falls down at the ankle; permanent plantar flexion

hyperextension Excessive straightening of a body part

internal rotation Turning the joint inward

orthostatic hypotension Abnormally low (hypo) blood pressure when the person suddenly stands up (ortho and static); postural hypotension

plantar flexion The foot (plantar) is bent (flexion); bending the foot down at the ankle

postural hypotension Orthostatic hypotension

pronation Turning the joint downward

range of motion (ROM) The movement of a joint to the extent possible without causing pain

rotation Turning the joint

supination Turning the joint upward

syncope A brief loss of consciousness; fainting

KEY ABBREVIATIONS

ADL Activities of daily living

AFO Ankle-foot orthosis

BRP Bathroom privileges

LNA Licensed nursing assistant

OBRA Omnibus Budget Reconciliation Act of 1987

ROM Range of motion

Being active is important for physical and mental well-being. Most people move about and function without help. Illness, surgery, injury, pain, and aging cause weakness and some activity limits. Some people are in bed for a long time. Some are paralyzed. Some disorders worsen over time. They cause decreases in activity. Examples include arthritis and nervous system and muscular disorders (Chapter 39). Inactivity, whether mild or severe, affects every body system. It also affects mental well-being.

Nurses use the nursing process to promote exercise and activity in all persons to the extent possible. The care plan and your assignment sheet include the person's activity level and needed exercises.

To help promote exercise and activity, you need to understand:

- Bedrest
- How to prevent complications from bedrest
- How to help with exercise

See *Focus on Children and Older Persons: Exercise and Activity.*

BEDREST

The doctor orders bedrest to treat a health problem. It may be a nursing measure if the person's condition changes. Generally bedrest is ordered to:

- Reduce physical activity
- Reduce pain
- Encourage rest
- Regain strength
- Promote healing

These types of bedrest are common:

- *Strict bedrest.* Everything is done for the person. No activities of daily living (ADL) are allowed.
- *Bedrest.* Some ADL are allowed. Self-feeding, oral hygiene, bathing, shaving, and hair care are often allowed.
- *Bedrest with commode privileges.* The person uses the commode for elimination.
- *Bedrest with bathroom privileges (bedrest with BRP).* The person uses the bathroom for elimination.

The person's care plan and your assignment sheet tell you the activities allowed. Always ask the nurse what bedrest means for each person. Check with the nurse if you have questions about a person's activity limits.

FOCUS ON **CHILDREN** AND **OLDER PERSONS**

Exercise and Activity

OLDER PERSONS

Deconditioning is the loss of muscle strength from inactivity. When not active, older persons become deconditioned quickly.

Persons with dementia may resist exercise and activity. They do not understand what is happening and may fear harm. They may become agitated and combative. Some cry out for help. Do not force the person to exercise or take part in activities. Stay calm, and ask the nurse for help. Follow the care plan.

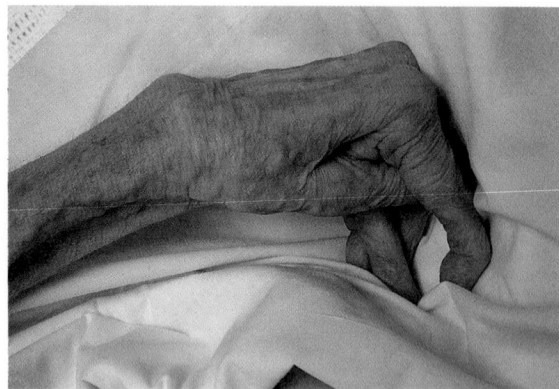

FIGURE 26-1 A contracture.

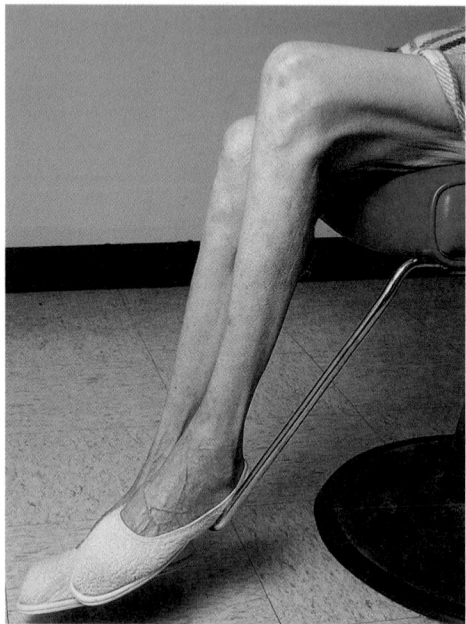

FIGURE 26-2 Muscle atrophy.

Complications of Bedrest

Bedrest and lack of exercise and activity can cause serious complications. Every system is affected. Pressure ulcers, constipation, and fecal impaction can result. Urinary tract infections and renal calculi (kidney stones) can occur. So can blood clots (thrombi) and pneumonia (inflammation and infection of the lung).

The musculoskeletal system is affected by lack of exercise and activity. These complications must be prevented to maintain normal movement:

▶ A **contracture** is the lack of joint mobility caused by abnormal shortening of a muscle. The contracted muscle is fixed into position, is deformed, and cannot stretch (Fig. 26-1). Common sites are the fingers, wrists, elbows, toes, ankles, knees, and hips. They can also occur in the neck and spine. The person is permanently deformed and disabled.

▶ **Atrophy** is the decrease in size or the wasting away of tissue. Tissues shrink in size. Muscle atrophy is a decrease in size or a wasting away of muscle (Fig. 26-2).

BOX 26-1 Preventing Orthostatic Hypotension

- Measure blood pressure, pulse, and respirations with the person supine.
- Position the person in Fowler's position. Raise the head of the bed slowly.
  - Ask the person about weakness, dizziness, or spots before the eyes. Lower the head of the bed if symptoms occur.
  - Measure blood pressure, pulse, and respirations.
  - Keep the person in Fowler's position for a short while. Ask about weakness, dizziness, or spots before the eyes.
- Help the person sit on the side of the bed (Chapter 16).
  - Ask about weakness, dizziness, or spots before the eyes. Help the person to Fowler's position if symptoms occur.
  - Measure blood pressure, pulse, and respirations.
  - Have the person sit on the side of the bed for a short while.
- Help the person stand.
  - Ask about weakness, dizziness, or spots before the eyes. Help the person sit on the side of the bed if any symptoms occur.
  - Measure blood pressure, pulse, and respirations.
- Help the person sit in a chair or walk as directed by the nurse.
  - Ask about weakness, dizziness, or spots before the eyes. If the person is walking, help the person to sit if symptoms occur.
  - Measure blood pressure, pulse, and respirations.
- Report blood pressure, pulse, and respirations to the nurse. Also report other symptoms or complaints.

FOCUS ON COMMUNICATION

Complications of Bedrest

Orthostatic hypotension can occur when the person moves from lying to sitting or standing. Fainting is a risk. To check for orthostatic hypotension, ask the person these questions:
- "Do you feel weak?"
- "Do you feel dizzy?"
- "Do you see spots before your eyes?"
- "Do you feel like fainting?"

Orthostatic hypotension and blood clots (Chapter 31) occur in the circulatory system. **Orthostatic hypotension** is abnormally low (*hypo*) blood pressure when the person suddenly stands up (*ortho* and *static*). When a person moves from lying or sitting to a standing position, the blood pressure drops. The person is dizzy and weak and has spots before the eyes. Syncope can occur. **Syncope** (fainting) is a brief loss of consciousness. (Syncope comes from the Greek word *synkoptein*. It means to cut short.) Orthostatic hypotension also is called **postural hypotension**. (*Postural* relates to posture or standing.) Box 26-1 lists the measures that prevent orthostatic hypotension. Slowly changing positions is key.

Good nursing care prevents complications from bedrest. Good alignment, range-of-motion exercises, and frequent position changes are important measures. These are part of the care plan.

See *Focus on Communication: Complications of Bedrest.*

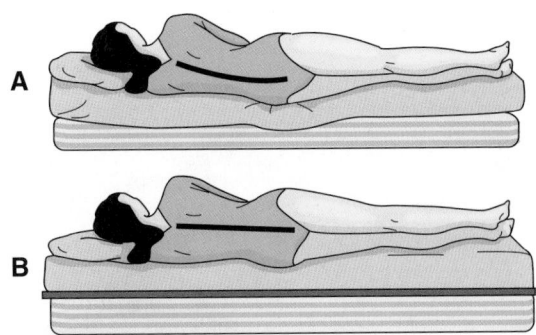

FIGURE 26-3 Bed boards. **A,** Mattress sagging without bed boards. **B,** Bed boards are under the mattress. No sagging occurs.

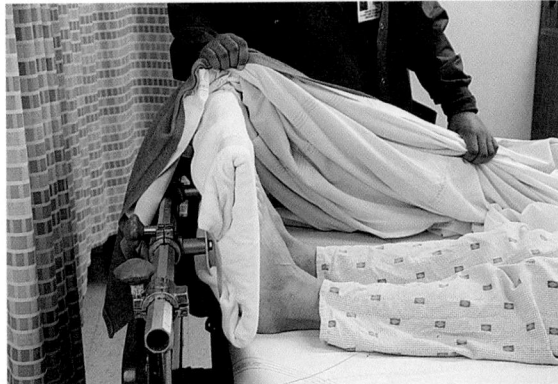

FIGURE 26-4 A foot board. Feet are flush with the board to keep them in normal alignment.

Positioning

Body alignment and positioning were discussed in Chapter 15. Supportive devices are often used to support and maintain the person in a certain position:

▶ *Bed boards*—are placed under the mattress. They prevent the mattress from sagging (Fig. 26-3). Usually made of plywood, they are covered with canvas or other material. There are two sections so the head of the bed can be raised. One section is for the head of the bed. The other is for the foot of the bed.

▶ *Foot boards*—are placed at the foot of mattresses (Fig. 26-4). They prevent plantar flexion that can lead to footdrop. In **plantar flexion,** the foot (*plantar*) is bent (*flexion*). **Footdrop** is when the foot falls down at the ankle (permanent plantar flexion). The foot board is placed so the soles of the feet are flush against it. The feet are in good alignment as when standing. Foot boards also serve as bed cradles. They prevent pressure ulcers by keeping top linens off the feet and toes.

▶ *Trochanter rolls*—prevent the hips and legs from turning outward (external rotation) (Fig. 26-5). A bath blanket is folded to the desired length and rolled up. The loose end is placed under the person from the hip to the knee. Then the roll is tucked alongside the body. Pillows or sandbags also keep the hips and knees in alignment.

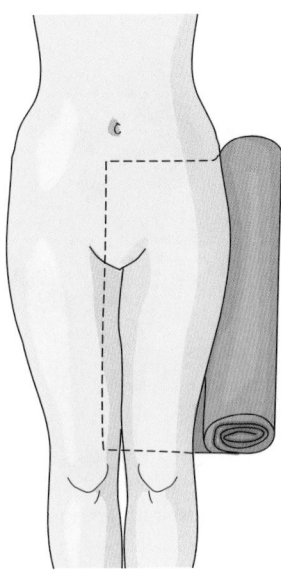

FIGURE 26-5 A trochanter roll is made from a bath blanket. It extends from the hip to the knee.

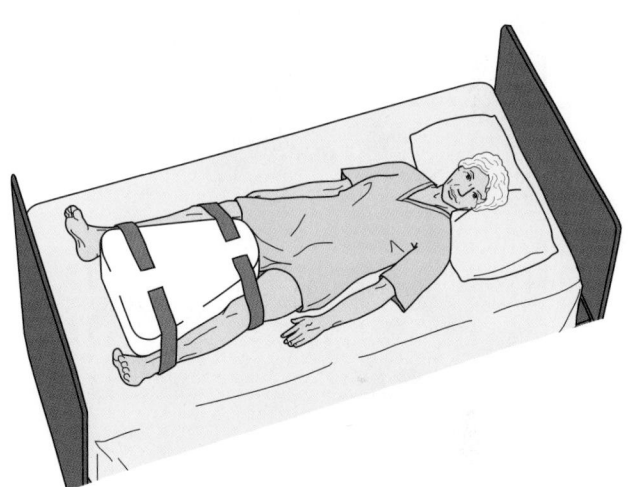

FIGURE 26-6 Hip abduction wedge.

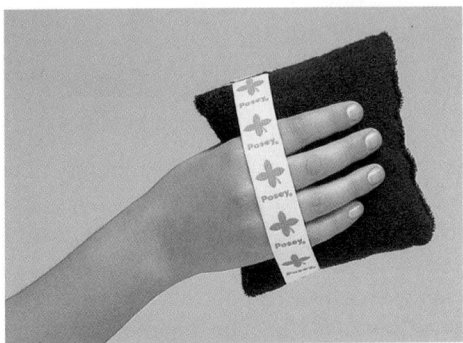

FIGURE 26-7 Handgrip. (Image courtesy J.T. Posey Co., Arcadia, Calif.)

▶ *Hip abduction wedges*—keep the hips abducted (Fig. 26-6). The wedge is placed between the person's legs. These are common after hip replacement surgery.

▶ *Handrolls or handgrips*—prevent contractures of the thumb, fingers, and wrist (Fig. 26-7). Foam rubber sponges, rubber balls, and finger cushions (Fig. 26-8, p. 466) also are used.

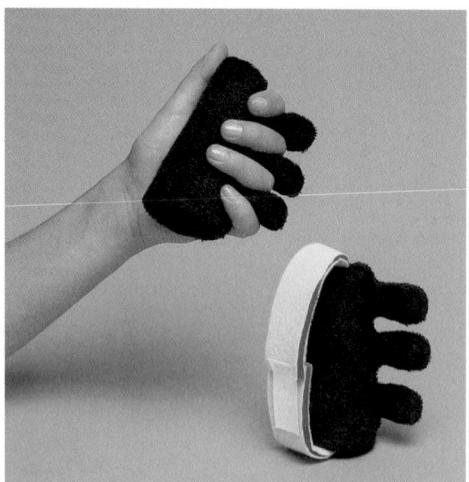

FIGURE 26-8 Finger cushion. (Image courtesy J.T. Posey Co., Arcadia, Calif.)

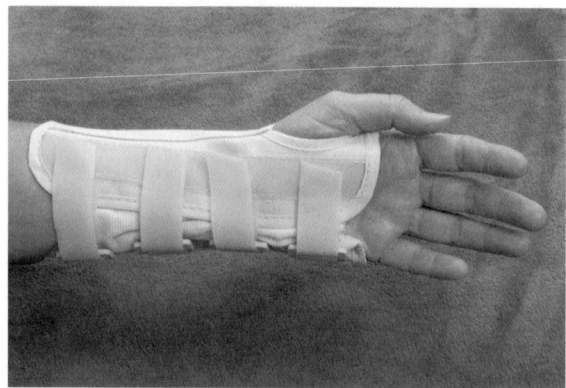

FIGURE 26-9 A splint.

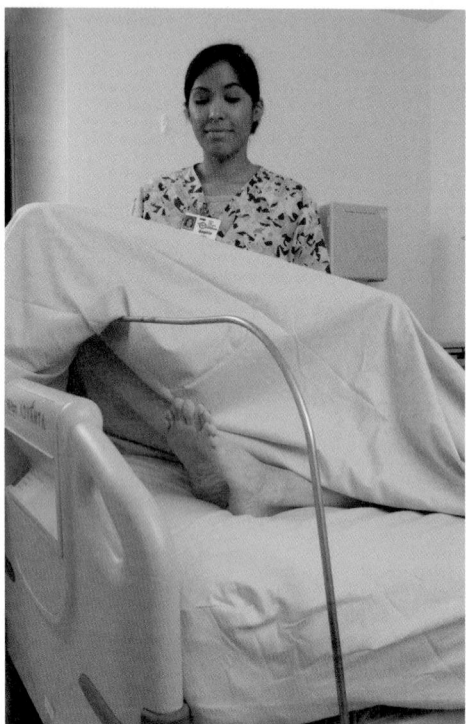

FIGURE 26-10 A bed cradle.

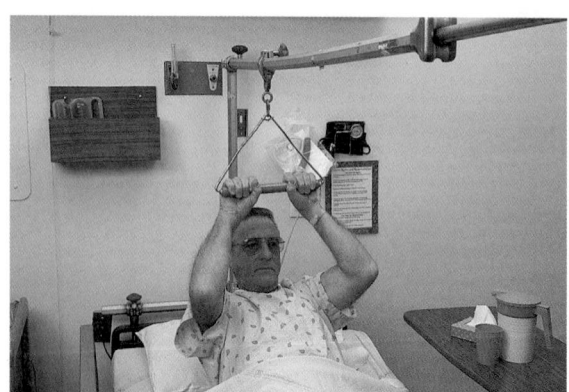

FIGURE 26-11 A trapeze is used to strengthen arm muscles.

- *Splints*—keep the elbows, wrists, thumbs, fingers, ankles, and knees in normal position. They are usually secured in place with Velcro. Some have foam padding (Fig. 26-9).
- *Bed cradles*—keep the weight of top linens off the feet and toes (Fig. 26-10). The weight of top linens can cause footdrop and pressure ulcers.

Exercise

Exercise helps prevent contractures, muscle atrophy, and other complications of bedrest. Some exercise occurs with ADL and when turning and moving in bed without help. Other exercises are needed for muscles and joints. (See "Range-of-Motion Exercises," and "Ambulation," p. 472.)

A trapeze is used for exercises to strengthen arm muscles. The trapeze hangs from an overbed frame (Fig. 26-11). The person grasps the bar with both hands to lift the trunk off the bed. The trapeze is also used to move up and turn in bed.

◆ RANGE-OF-MOTION EXERCISES

The movement of a joint to the extent possible without causing pain is the **range of motion (ROM)** of that joint. Range-of-motion exercises involve moving the joints through their complete range of motion (Box 26-2). They are usually done at least 2 times a day.

- *Active* range-of-motion exercises—are done by the person.
- *Passive* range-of-motion exercises—someone moves the joints through their range of motion.
- *Active-assistive* range-of-motion exercises—the person does the exercises with some help.

BOX 26-2 Joint Movements

Abduction—moving a body part away from the midline of the body

Adduction—moving a body part toward the midline of the body

Extension—straightening a body part

Flexion—bending a body part

Hyperextension—excessive straightening of a body part

Dorsiflexion—bending the toes and foot up at the ankle

Rotation—turning the joint

Internal rotation—turning the joint inward

External rotation—turning the joint outward

Plantar flexion—bending the foot down at the ankle

Pronation—turning the joint downward

Supination—turning the joint upward

FOCUS ON CHILDREN AND OLDER PERSONS

Range-of-Motion Exercises

CHILDREN

Depending on the child's activity limits, most play activities promote active range-of-motion exercises. For example:

- Kicking a Mylar balloon or foam ball.
- Touching a Mylar balloon that is held or hung in different places. For example, for the child in traction you can hang a Mylar balloon from the trapeze.
- Playing basketball with bean-bags, wadded paper, or foam balls. Use a hoop or wastebasket as the target.
- Playing "pat-a-cake" or "Simon Says" (clap, kick, jump, and other motions).
- Having the child act like a bird, butterfly, spider, monkey, horse, and other animals.
- Playing video or computer games for finger and hand movements.
- Playing with finger paints, clay, or play dough.
- Having tricycle or wheelchair races.
- Playing "hide and seek." Hide a toy in the bed or room.

Always check with the nurse for the child's activity limits. Make sure the nurse approves of the play activity.

OLDER PERSONS

The Omnibus Budget Reconciliation Act of 1987 (OBRA) requires an assessment and care planning process to prevent unnecessary loss in a person's range of motion. Prevention may involve range-of-motion exercises. Sometimes splints and braces are used (p. 477).

Modified from Hockenberry MJ and others: *Wong's nursing care of infants and children*, ed 8, St Louis, 2007, Mosby.

Bathing, hair care, eating, reaching, dressing and undressing, and walking all involve joint movements. Persons on bedrest need more frequent range-of-motion exercises. So do those who cannot walk, turn, or transfer themselves because of illness or injury. The doctor or nurse may order range-of-motion exercises.

See *Focus on Children and Older Persons: Range-of-Motion Exercises.*

See *Focus on Communication: Range-of-Motion Exercises.*

See *Delegation Guidelines: Range-of-Motion Exercises.*

See *Promoting Safety and Comfort: Range-of-Motion Exercises.*

See *Focus on Ethics and Laws: Range-of-Motion Exercises*, p. 468.

FOCUS ON COMMUNICATION

Range-of-Motion Exercises

You must not force a joint beyond its present range of motion or to the point of pain. Ask the person to tell you if he or she:

- Feels that the joint cannot move any farther
- Feels pain or discomfort in the joint

DELEGATION GUIDELINES: Range-of-Motion Exercises

When delegated range-of-motion exercises, you need this information from the nurse and the care plan:

- The kind of range-of-motion exercises ordered—active, passive, active-assistive
- Which joints to exercise
- How often the exercises are done
- How many times to repeat each exercise
- What observations to report and record:
  - The time the exercises were performed
  - The joints exercised
  - The number of times the exercises were performed on each joint
  - Complaints of pain or signs of stiffness or spasm
  - The degree to which the person took part in the exercises
- When to report observations
- What specific patient or resident concerns to report at once

---

PROMOTING SAFETY AND COMFORT: Range-of-Motion Exercises

SAFETY

Range-of-motion exercises can cause injury if not done properly. Muscle strain, joint injury, and pain are possible. Practice the rules in Box 26-3 when performing or assisting with range-of-motion exercises.

Range-of-motion exercises to the neck can cause serious injury if not done properly. Some agencies require that nursing assistants have special training before doing such exercises. Other agencies do not let nursing assistants do them. Know your agency's policy. *Perform range-of-motion exercises to the neck only if allowed by your agency and if the nurse instructs you to do so.*

COMFORT

To promote physical comfort during range-of-motion exercises, follow the rules in Box 26-3. Also cover the person with a bath blanket. Expose only the part being exercised. Providing for privacy promotes mental comfort.

FOCUS ON **ETHICS** AND **LAWS**

Range-of-Motion Exercises

A licensed nursing assistant (LNA) cared for a person with Alzheimer's disease. The resident was severely contracted. Her ability to communicate was poor. And she could not make decisions. The LNA admitted to:

- Being observed pulling the resident's arms away from her body and allowing them to snap back
- Being observed pulling the resident's legs upward from the bed and allowing them to fall back down
- Failing to remove a bowel movement while cleaning the resident

The Board found that the LNA abused and improperly cared for the resident. The unprofessional conduct violated the Administrative Rules of the Board of Nursing because of:

- Abusing or improperly caring for a patient
- Performing unsafe or unacceptable patient care
- Failing to conform to acceptable standards of practice
- Engaging in conduct likely to harm the public

The LNA's license was suspended indefinitely.

Author note: "Suspend indefinitely" means that the LNA:

- *Had to give her license to the Board*
- *Could ask the Board to re-instate her license but had to prove that:*
  - *She posed no danger to the public or practice of nursing*
  - *She would safely and competently perform an LNA's duties*
  - *She meets the requirements for license renewal and re-instatement*

(State of Vermont Board of Nursing in regard to A. Willard, 2000.)

BOX 26-3 **Performing Range-Of-Motion Exercises**

- Exercise only the joints the nurse tells you to exercise.
- Expose only the body part being exercised.
- Use good body mechanics.
- Support the part being exercised.
- Move the joint slowly, smoothly, and gently.
- Do not force a joint beyond its present range of motion.
- Do not force a joint to the point of pain.
- Ask the person if he or she has pain or discomfort.
- *Perform range-of-motion exercises to the neck only if allowed by agency policy.* In some agencies, only physical or occupational therapists do neck exercises. This is because of the danger of neck injuries.

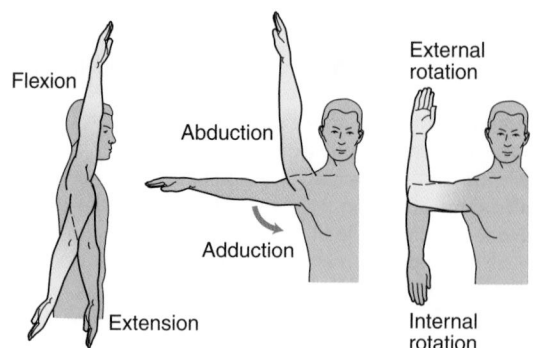

FIGURE 26-13 Range-of-motion exercises for the shoulder.

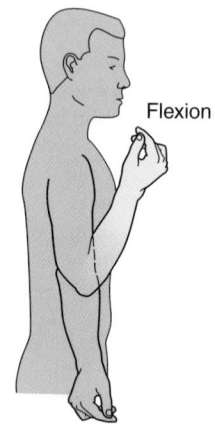

FIGURE 26-14 Range-of-motion exercises for the elbow.

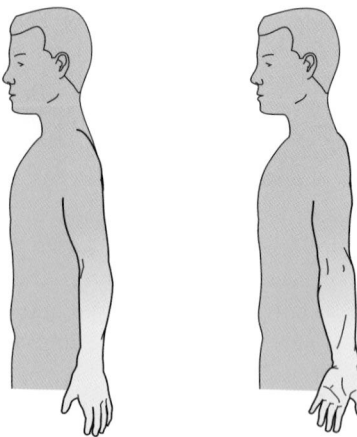

FIGURE 26-15 Range-of-motion exercises for the forearm.

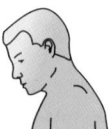 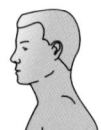 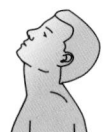 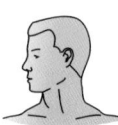 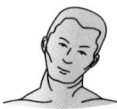

Flexion　Extension　Hyperextension　Rotation　Lateral flexion

FIGURE 26-12 Range-of-motion exercises for the neck.

PERFORMING RANGE-OF-MOTION EXERCISES

✔ Quality of Life *Remember to:*

- Knock before entering the person's room.
- Address the person by name.
- Introduce yourself by name and title.
- Explain the procedure to the person before beginning and during the procedure.
- Protect the person's rights during the procedure.
- Handle the person gently during the procedure.

PRE-PROCEDURE

1 Follow *Delegation Guidelines: Range-of-Motion Exercises*, p. 467. See *Promoting Safety and Comfort: Range-of-Motion Exercises*, p. 467.
2 Practice hand hygiene.

3 Identify the person. Check the ID bracelet against the assignment sheet. Also call the person by name.
4 Obtain a bath blanket.
5 Provide for privacy.
6 Raise the bed for good body mechanics. Bed rails are up if used.

PROCEDURE

7 Lower the bed rail near you if up.
8 Position the person supine.
9 Cover the person with a bath blanket. Fan-fold top linens to the foot of the bed.
10 Exercise the neck *if allowed by your agency and if the RN instructs you to do so* (Fig. 26-12, p. 468):
   a Place your hands over the person's ears to support the head. Support the jaws with your fingers.
   b Flexion—bring the head forward. The chin touches the chest.
   c Extension—straighten the head.
   d Hyperextension—bring the head backward until the chin points up.
   e Rotation—turn the head from side to side.
   f Lateral flexion—move the head to the right and to the left.
   g Repeat flexion, extension, hyperextension, rotation, and lateral flexion 5 times—or the number of times stated on the care plan.
11 Exercise the shoulder (Fig. 26-13, p. 468):
   a Grasp the wrist with one hand. Grasp the elbow with the other hand.
   b Flexion—raise the arm straight in front and over the head.
   c Extension—bring the arm down to the side.
   d Hyperextension—move the arm behind the body. (Do this if the person sits in a straight-backed chair or is standing.)
   e Abduction—move the straight arm away from the side of the body.
   f Adduction—move the straight arm to the side of the body.
   g Internal rotation—bend the elbow. Place it at the same level as the shoulder. Move the forearm down toward the body.
   h External rotation—move the forearm toward the head.
   i Repeat flexion, extension, hyperextension, abduction, adduction, and internal and external rotation 5 times—or the number of times stated on the care plan.

12 Exercise the elbow (Fig. 26-14, p. 468):
   a Grasp the person's wrist with one hand. Grasp the elbow with your other hand.
   b Flexion—bend the arm so the same-side shoulder is touched.
   c Extension—straighten the arm.
   d Repeat flexion and extension 5 times—or the number of times stated on the care plan.
13 Exercise the forearm (Fig. 26-15, p. 468):
   a Continue to support the wrist and elbow.
   b Pronation—turn the hand so the palm is down.
   c Supination—turn the hand so the palm is up.
   d Repeat pronation and supination 5 times—or the number of times stated on the care plan.
14 Exercise the wrist (Fig. 26-16, p. 470):
   a Hold the wrist with both of your hands.
   b Flexion—bend the hand down.
   c Extension—straighten the hand.
   d Hyperextension—bend the hand back.
   e Radial flexion—turn the hand toward the thumb.
   f Ulnar flexion—turn the hand toward the little finger.
   g Repeat flexion, extension, hyperextension, and radial flexion and ulnar flexion 5 times—or the number of times stated on the care plan.
15 Exercise the thumb (Fig. 26-17, p. 470):
   a Hold the person's hand with one hand. Hold the thumb with your other hand.
   b Abduction—move the thumb out from the inner part of the index finger.
   c Adduction—move the thumb back next to the index finger.
   d Opposition—touch each fingertip with the thumb.
   e Flexion—bend the thumb into the hand.
   f Extension—move the thumb out to the side of the fingers.
   g Repeat abduction, adduction, opposition, flexion, and extension 5 times—or the number of times stated on the care plan.
16 Exercise the fingers (Fig. 26-18, p. 470):
   a Abduction—spread the fingers and the thumb apart.
   b Adduction—bring the fingers and thumb together.

Continued

PERFORMING RANGE-OF-MOTION EXERCISES—cont'd

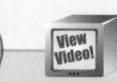

PROCEDURE—cont'd

c Extension—straighten the fingers so the fingers, hand, and arm are straight.

d Flexion—make a fist.

e Repeat abduction, adduction, extension, and flexion 5 times—or the number of times stated on the care plan.

17 Exercise the hip (Fig. 26-19):

  a Support the leg. Place one hand under the knee. Place your other hand under the ankle.

  b Flexion—raise the leg.

  c Extension—straighten the leg.

  d Abduction—move the leg away from the body.

  e Adduction—move the leg toward the other leg.

  f Internal rotation—turn the leg inward.

  g External rotation—turn the leg outward.

  h Repeat flexion, extension, abduction, adduction, and internal and external rotation 5 times—or the number of times stated on the care plan.

18 Exercise the knee (Fig. 26-20):

  a Support the knee. Place one hand under the knee. Place your other hand under the ankle.

  b Flexion—bend the knee.

  c Extension—straighten the knee.

  d Repeat flexion and extension of the knee 5 times—or the number of times stated on the care plan.

19 Exercise the ankle (Fig. 26-21):

  a Support the foot and ankle. Place one hand under the foot. Place your other hand under the ankle.

  b Dorsiflexion—pull the foot forward. Push down on the heel at the same time.

  c Plantar flexion—turn the foot down. Or point the toes.

  d Repeat dorsiflexion and plantar flexion 5 times—or the number of times stated on the care plan.

20 Exercise the foot (Fig. 26-22):

  a Continue to support the foot and ankle.

  b Pronation—turn the outside of the foot up and the inside down.

  c Supination—turn the inside of the foot up and the outside down.

  d Repeat pronation and supination 5 times—or the number of times stated on the care plan.

21 Exercise the toes (Fig. 26-23):

  a Flexion—curl the toes.

  b Extension—straighten the toes.

  c Abduction—spread the toes apart.

  d Adduction—pull the toes together.

  e Repeat flexion, extension, abduction, and adduction 5 times—or the number of times stated on the care plan.

22 Cover the leg. Raise the bed rail if used.

23 Go to the other side. Lower the bed rail near you if up.

24 Repeat steps 11 through 21.

POST-PROCEDURE

25 Provide for comfort. (See the inside of the front book cover.)

26 Remove the bath blanket.

27 Place the signal light within reach.

28 Lower the bed to its lowest level.

29 Raise or lower bed rails. Follow the care plan.

30 Return the bath blanket to its proper place.

31 Unscreen the person.

32 Complete a safety check of the room. (See the inside of the front book cover.)

33 Decontaminate your hands.

34 Report and record your observations.

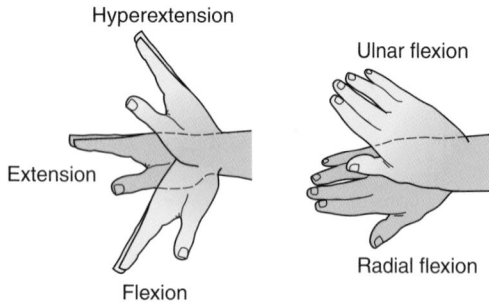

FIGURE 26-16 Range-of-motion exercises for the wrist.

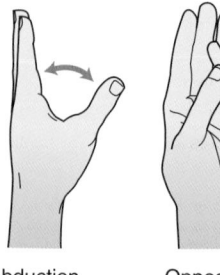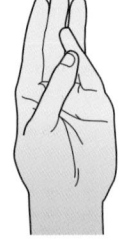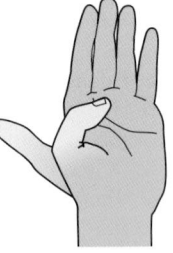

FIGURE 26-17 Range-of-motion exercises for the thumb.

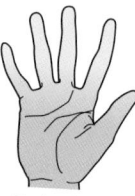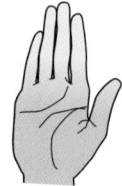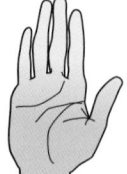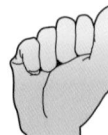

FIGURE 26-18 Range-of-motion exercises for the fingers.

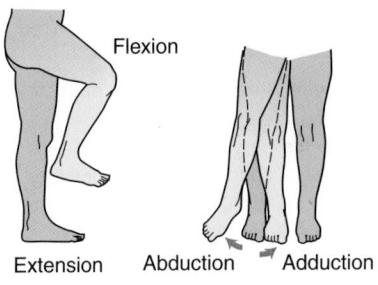

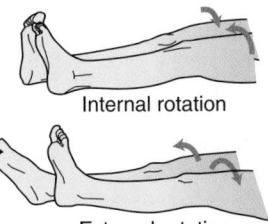

FIGURE 26-19 Range-of-motion exercises for the hip.

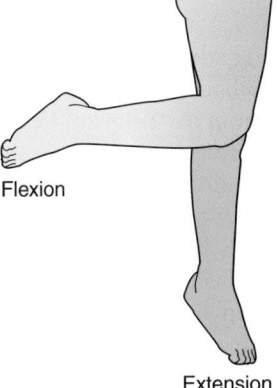

FIGURE 26-20 Range-of-motion exercises for the knee.

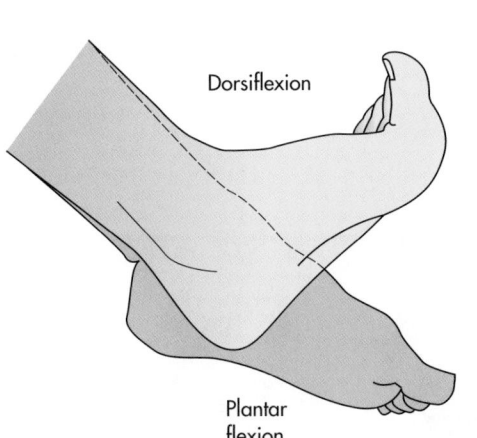

FIGURE 26-21 Range-of-motion exercises for the ankle.

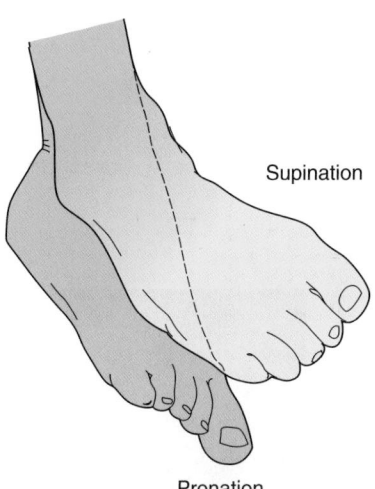

FIGURE 26-22 Range-of-motion exercises for the foot.

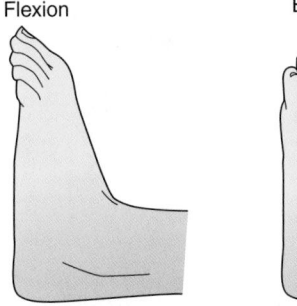 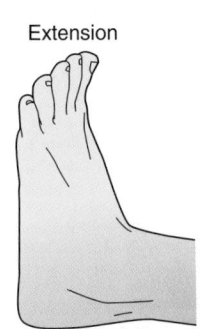 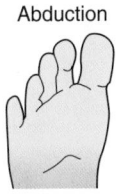 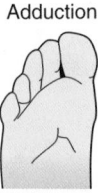

FIGURE 26-23 Range-of-motion exercises for the toes.

◆ AMBULATION

Ambulation is the act of walking. Some people are weak and unsteady from bedrest, illness, surgery, or injury. They may need help walking. Some become strong enough to walk alone. Others will always need help.

After bedrest, activity increases slowly and in steps. First the person dangles (sits on the side of the bed). Sitting in a bedside chair follows. Next the person walks in the room and then in the hallway. To achieve the goal of walking, contractures and muscle atrophy must be prevented. Proper positioning and exercises are needed during bedrest.

Walking regularly helps prevent deconditioning. Some persons who use wheelchairs can walk with help. Follow the care plan when helping a person walk. Use a gait (transfer) belt if the person is weak or unsteady. The person also uses hand rails along the wall. Always check the person for orthostatic hypotension (p. 464).

See *Delegation Guidelines: Ambulation.*
See *Promoting Safety and Comfort: Ambulation.*

DELEGATION GUIDELINES: Ambulation

Before helping with ambulation, you need this information from the nurse and the care plan:
• How much help the person needs
• If the person uses a cane, walker, crutches, or a brace
• Areas of weakness—right arm or leg, left arm or leg
• How far to walk the person
• What observations to report and record:
  • How well the person tolerated the activity
  • Shuffling, sliding, limping, or walking on tip-toes
  • Complaints of pain or discomfort
  • Complaints of orthostatic hypotension—weakness, dizziness, spots before the eyes, feeling faint
  • The distance walked
• When to report observations
• What specific patient or resident concerns to report at once

---

PROMOTING SAFETY AND COMFORT: Ambulation

SAFETY
Practice the safety measures to prevent falls (Chapter 12). Use a gait belt to help the person stand. Also use it during ambulation.

COMFORT
The fear of falling affects the person's mental comfort. Explain the purpose of the gait belt. Also explain how you will help the person if he or she starts to fall (Chapter 12).

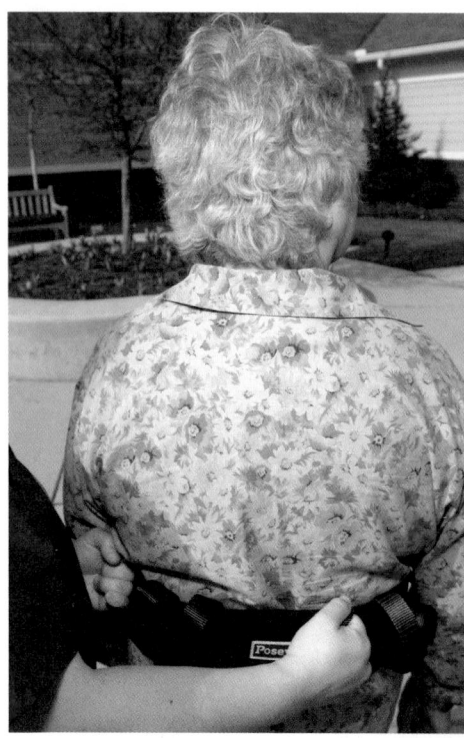
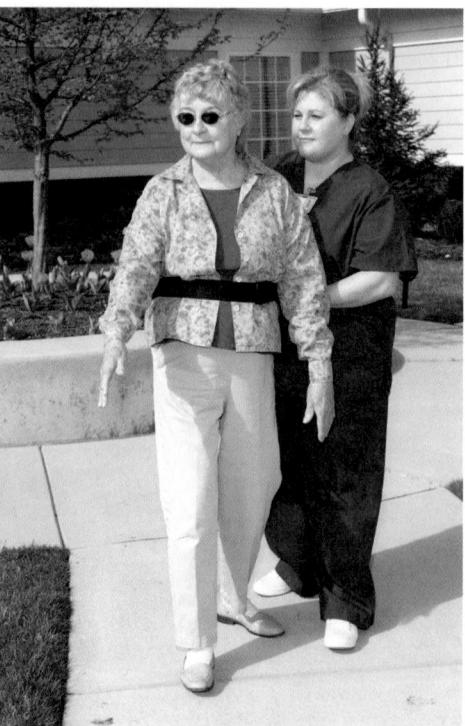

FIGURE 26-24 Assist with ambulation. **A,** The nursing assistant uses a gait belt for the person's safety. **B,** The nursing assistant walks at the person's side and slightly behind her.

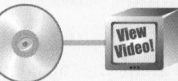

HELPING THE PERSON WALK

✔ Quality of Life *Remember to:*

- Knock before entering the person's room.
- Address the person by name.
- Introduce yourself by name and title.
- Explain the procedure to the person before beginning and during the procedure.

- Protect the person's rights during the procedure.
- Handle the person gently during the procedure.

PRE-PROCEDURE

1 Follow *Delegation Guidelines: Ambulation*. See *Promoting Safety and Comfort: Ambulation*.
2 Practice hand hygiene.
3 Collect the following:
 - Robe and non-skid shoes
 - Paper or sheet to protect bottom linens
 - Gait (transfer) belt

4 Identify the person. Check the ID bracelet against the assignment sheet. Also call the person by name.
5 Provide for privacy.

PROCEDURE

6 Lower the bed to its lowest position. Lock the bed wheels. Lower the bed rail if up.
7 Fan-fold top linens to the foot of the bed.
8 Place the paper or sheet under the person's feet. Put the shoes on the person. Fasten the shoes.
9 Help the person dangle. (See procedure: *Sitting on the Side of the Bed [Dangling]*, Chapter 16.)
10 Help the person put on the robe.
11 Apply the gait belt. (See procedure: *Applying a Transfer Belt*, Chapter 12.)
12 Help the person stand. (See procedure: *Transferring the Person to a Chair or Wheelchair*, Chapter 16.) Grasp the gait belt at each side. If not using a gait belt, place your arms under the person's arms around to the shoulder blades.
13 Stand at the person's weak side while he or she gains balance. Hold the belt at the side and back. If not using a gait belt, have one arm around the back and the other at the elbow to support the person.
14 Encourage the person to stand erect with the head up and back straight.

15 Help the person walk. Walk to the side and slightly behind the person on the person's weak side. Provide support with the gait belt (Fig. 26-24). If not using a gait belt, have one arm around the back and the other at the elbow to support the person. Encourage the person to use the hand rail on his or her strong side.
16 Encourage the person to walk normally. The heel strikes the floor first. Discourage shuffling, sliding, or walking on tip-toes.
17 Walk the required distance if the person tolerates the activity. Do not rush the person.
18 Help the person return to bed. Remove the gait belt. (See procedure: *Transferring the Person From a Chair or Wheelchair to a Bed*, Chapter 16.)
19 Lower the head of the bed. Help the person to the center of the bed.
20 Remove the shoes. Remove the paper or sheet over the bottom sheet.

POST-PROCEDURE

21 Provide for comfort. (See the inside of the front book cover.)
22 Place the signal light within reach.
23 Raise or lower bed rails. Follow the care plan.
24 Return the robe and shoes to their proper place.

25 Unscreen the person.
26 Complete a safety check of the room. (See the inside of the front book cover.)
27 Decontaminate your hands.
28 Report and record your observations (Fig. 26-25).

	Date	Time	Nursing Margin	Other Depts Margin
	10/10	1400	Ambulated 25 feet in the hallway c̄ assist of one and use of a gait belt.	
			Reminded not to shuffle her feet. Showed no signes of distress or discomfort.	
			Denied feeling dizzy, lightheaded, or weak. No c/o pain. Assisted to her recliner	
			chair and elevated her feet after ambulating. BP-132/84 L arm sitting. P-76	
			regular rate and rhythm. R-20 and unlabored. Overbed table c̄ water pitcher	
			and glass within reach. Signal light within reach. Adam Aims, CNA ———	

FIGURE 26-25 Charting sample.

Walking Aids

Walking aids support the body. The doctor, RN, or physical therapist orders them. The need may be temporary or permanent. The type ordered depends on the person's condition, the amount of support needed, and the type of disability. Older persons often need walkers or canes for safety. The physical therapist or RN measures and teaches the person to use the device.

Crutches

Crutches are used when the person cannot use one leg or when one or both legs need to gain strength. Some persons with permanent leg weakness can use crutches. They usually use forearm crutches (Fig. 26-26). Underarm crutches extend from the underarm to the ground (Fig. 26-27).

The person learns to crutch walk, use stairs, and sit and stand. Safety is important. The person on crutches is at risk for falls. Follow these safety measures:

▶ Check the crutch tips. They must not be worn down, torn, or wet. Replace worn or torn crutch tips. Dry wet tips with a towel or paper towels.
▶ Check crutches for flaws. Check wooden crutches for cracks and metal crutches for bends.
▶ Tighten all bolts.
▶ Street shoes are worn. They must be flat and have non-skid soles.
▶ Clothes must fit well. Loose clothes may get caught between the crutches and underarms. Loose clothes and long skirts can hang forward and block the person's view of the feet and crutch tips.

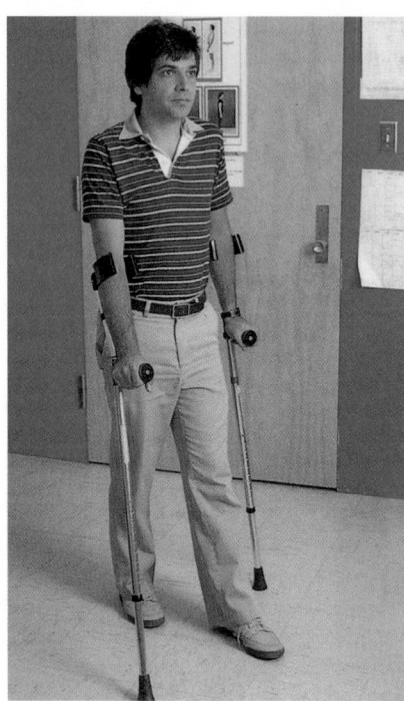

FIGURE 26-26 Forearm crutches. (From Elkin MK, Perry AG, Potter PA: *Nursing interventions & clinical skills*, ed 2, St Louis, 2000, Mosby.)

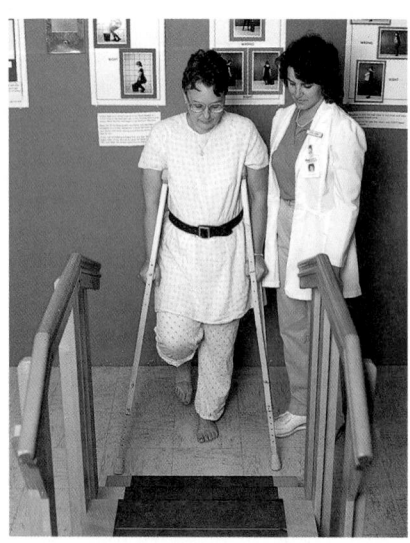

FIGURE 26-27 Underarm crutches. (From Elkin MK, Perry AG, Potter PA: *Nursing interventions & clinical skills*, ed 4, St Louis, 2007, Mosby.)

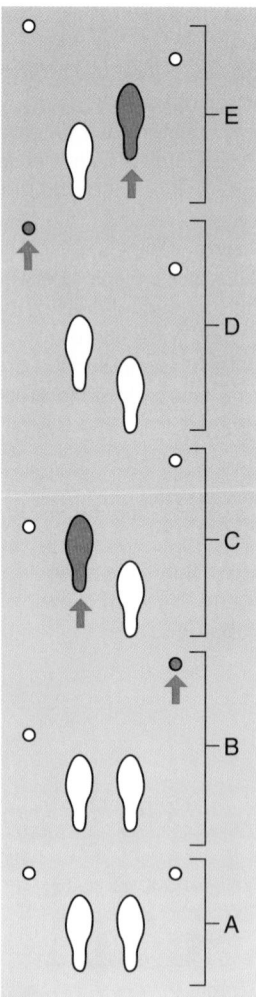

FIGURE 26-28 The four-point gait. The person uses both legs. The right crutch is moved forward and then the left foot. Then the left crutch is moved forward followed by the right foot.

▶ Practice safety rules to prevent falls (Chapter 12).
▶ Keep crutches within the person's reach. Put them by the person's chair or against a wall.
▶ Know which crutch gait the person uses:
  ▶ Four-point gait (Fig. 26-28)
  ▶ Three-point gait (Fig. 26-29)
  ▶ Two-point gait (Fig. 26-30)
  ▶ Swing-to gait (Fig. 26-31)
  ▶ Swing-through gait (Fig. 26-32)

Canes

Canes are used for weakness on one side of the body. They help provide balance and support. Single-tip and four-point (quad) canes are common (Fig. 26-33, p. 476).

A cane is held on the *strong side* of the body. (If the left leg is weak, the cane is held in the right hand.) Four-point canes give more support than single-tip canes. However, they are harder to move.

The cane tip is about 6 to 10 inches to the side of the foot. It is about 6 to 10 inches in front of the foot on the strong side. The grip is level with the hip. The person walks as follows:

▶ *Step A:* The cane is moved forward 6 to 10 inches (Fig. 26-34, *A*, p. 476).
▶ *Step B:* The weak leg (opposite the cane) is moved forward even with the cane (Fig. 26-34, *B*, p. 476).
▶ *Step C:* The strong leg is moved forward and ahead of the cane and the weak leg (Fig. 26-34, *C*, p. 476).

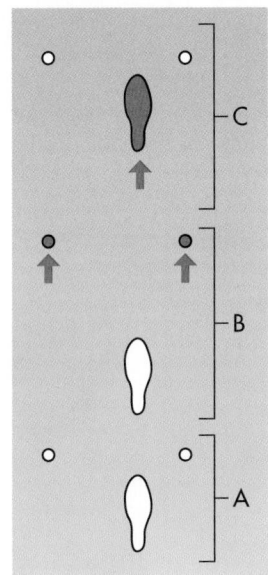

FIGURE 26-29 The three-point gait. One leg is used. Both crutches are moved forward. Then the good foot is moved forward.

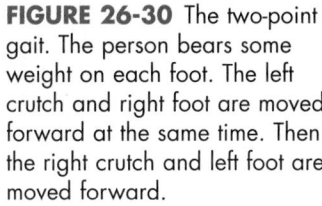

FIGURE 26-30 The two-point gait. The person bears some weight on each foot. The left crutch and right foot are moved forward at the same time. Then the right crutch and left foot are moved forward.

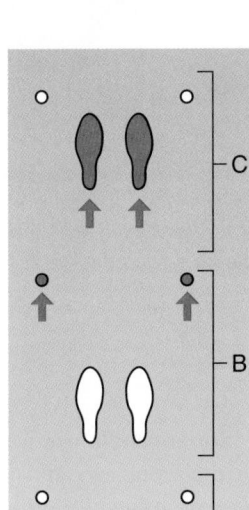

FIGURE 26-31 Swing-to gait. The person bears some weight on each leg. Both crutches are moved forward. Then the person lifts both legs and *swings to* the crutches.

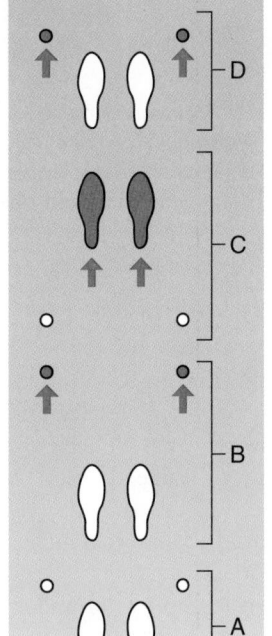

FIGURE 26-32 Swing-through gait. The person bears some weight on each leg. Both crutches are moved forward. Then the person lifts both legs and *swings through* the crutches.

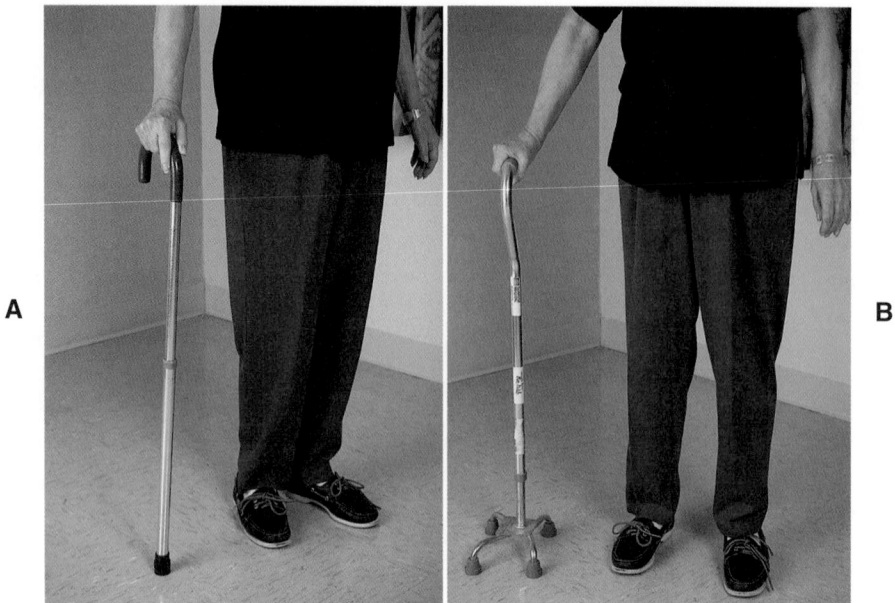

FIGURE 26-33 A, Single-tip cane. **B,** Four-point cane.

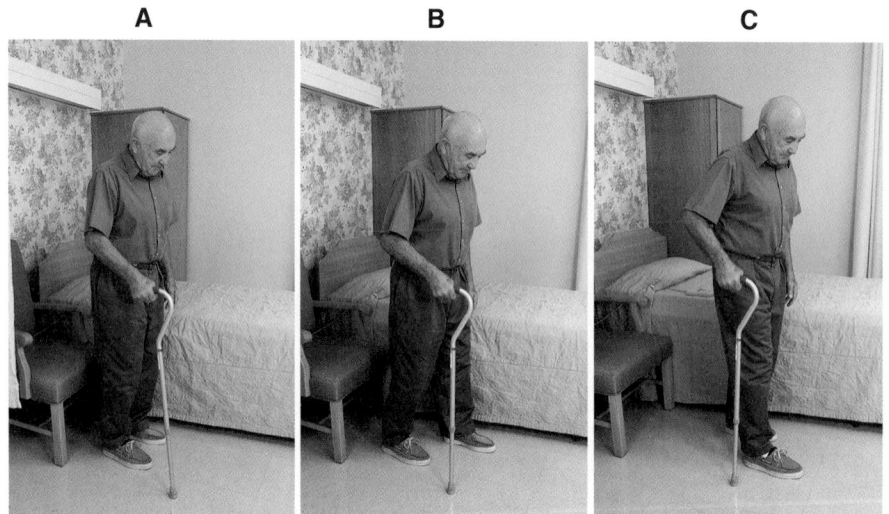

FIGURE 26-34 Walking with a cane. **A,** The cane is moved forward about 6 to 10 inches. **B,** The leg opposite the cane (weak leg) is brought forward even with the cane. **C,** The leg on the cane side (strong side) is moved ahead of the cane and the weak leg.

Walkers

A walker is a four-point walking aid (Fig. 26-35). It gives more support than a cane. Many people feel safer and more secure with walkers than with canes. There are many kinds of walkers. The standard walker is used as follows:

▶ The walker is picked up and moved about 6 to 8 inches in front of the person (Fig. 26-36, *A*).
▶ The person moves one foot and leg up to the walker (Fig. 26-36, *B*).
▶ The person moves the other foot and leg up to the walker.

Some people use wheeled walkers. They have wheels on the front legs and rubber tips on the back legs. The person pushes the walker about 6 to 8 inches in front of his or her feet. Rubber tips on the back legs prevent the walker from moving while the person is walking or standing. Some have a braking action when weight is applied to the walker's back legs.

Baskets, pouches, and trays attach to the walker (see Fig. 26-35). They are used for needed items. This allows more independence. They also free the hands to grip the walker.

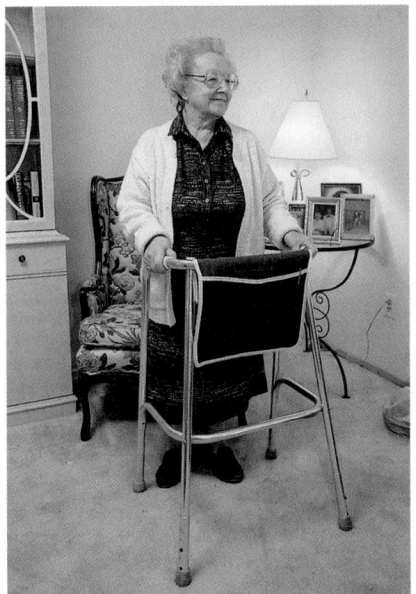

FIGURE 26-35 A walker.

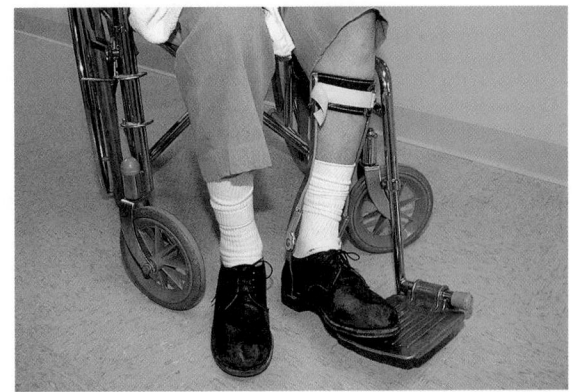

FIGURE 26-37 Leg brace.

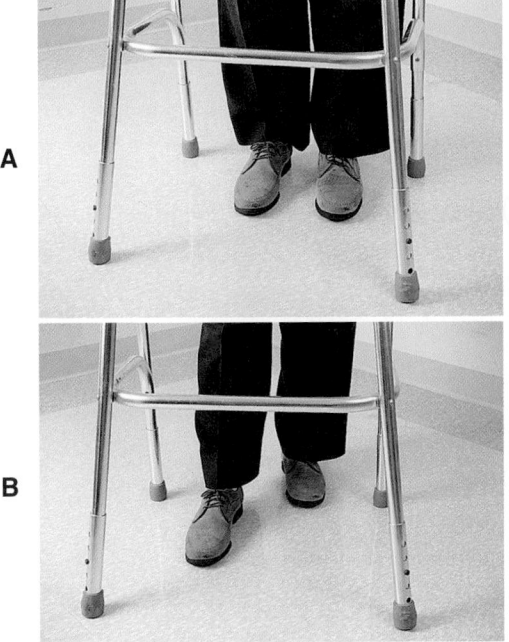

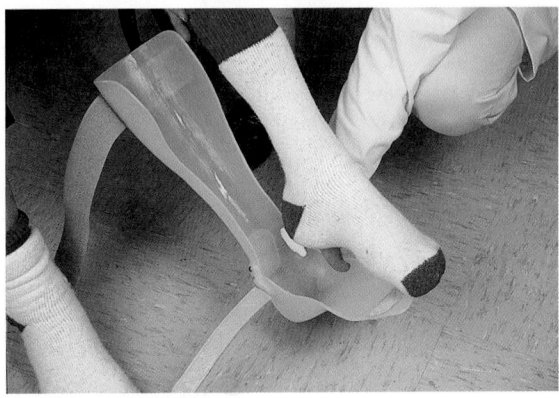

FIGURE 26-38 Ankle-foot orthosis (AFO).

FIGURE 26-36 Walking with a walker. **A,** The walker is moved about 6 to 8 inches in front of the person. **B,** The person moves one foot and leg up to the walker. Then the other foot and leg are moved up to the walker.

Braces

Braces support weak body parts. They also prevent or correct deformities or prevent joint movement. Metal, plastic, or leather is used for braces. A brace is applied over the ankle, knee, or back (Fig. 26-37). An ankle-foot orthosis (AFO) is placed in the shoe (Fig. 26-38). Then the foot is inserted. The AFO is secured in place with a Velcro strap. This type of brace is common after a stroke.

Skin and bony points under braces are kept clean and dry. This prevents skin breakdown. Report redness or signs of skin breakdown at once. Also report complaints of pain or discomfort. The nurse assesses the skin under braces every shift. The care plan tells you when to apply and remove a brace.

RECREATIONAL ACTIVITIES

OBRA requires activity programs for residents. Recreational activities are important for an older person's physical and mental well-being. Joints and muscles are exercised. Circulation is stimulated. Recreational activities also are social events and are mentally stimulating. A good activity program improves a person's quality of life.

According to OBRA, activities must meet each person's interests and physical, mental, and psychosocial needs. Bingo, movies, dances, exercise groups, shopping trips, museum trips, concerts, guest speakers, and gardening activities are common.

The right to personal choice is protected. Well-being is promoted when the person attends activities of personal choice. The person is not forced to do things that do not interest him or her.

Some persons need help getting to an activity. Some also need help taking part in them. You must assist as needed.

See *Teamwork and Time Management: Recreational Activities.*

TEAMWORK AND TIME MANAGEMENT

Recreational Activities

Some persons need help getting to activity programs. Some also need help with activities. When you can, help co-workers assist patients and residents to and from and with activity programs. For example, you have 1 or 2 people who need help. A co-worker may have 4 to 5 persons needing help.

REVIEW QUESTIONS

Circle the BEST answer.

1 The purpose of bedrest is to
   a Prevent orthostatic hypotension
   b Reduce pain and promote healing
   c Prevent pressure ulcers, constipation, and blood clots
   d Cause contractures and muscle atrophy

2 Which helps prevent plantar flexion?
   a Bed boards   c A trochanter roll
   b A foot board   d Handrolls

3 Which prevents the hip from turning outward?
   a Bed boards   **c** Trochanter roll
   b A foot board   d A leg brace

4 A contracture is
   a The loss of muscle strength from inactivity
   b The lack of joint mobility from shortening of a muscle
   c A decrease in the size of a muscle
   d A blood clot in the muscle

5 A trapeze is used to
   a Prevent footdrop   **c** Strengthen arm muscles
   b Prevent contractures   d Strengthen leg muscles

6 Passive range-of-motion exercises are performed by
   a The person
   b Someone else
   c The person with the help of another
   d The person with the use of a trapeze

7 ROM exercises are ordered. You do the following *except*
   a Support the part being exercised
   b Move the joint slowly, smoothly, and gently
   c Force the joint though its full range of motion
   d Exercise only the joints indicated by the nurse

8 Flexion involves
   a Bending the body part
   b Straightening the body part
   c Moving the body part toward the body
   d Moving the body part away from the body

9 When ambulating a person
   a A gait belt is used if the person is weak or unsteady
   b The person can shuffle or slide when walking after bedrest
   c Walking aids are needed
   d You walk on the person's strong side

10 You are getting a person ready to crutch walk. You should do the following *except*
   a Check the crutch tips
   b Have the person wear non-skid shoes
   c Get a pair of crutches from physical therapy
   d Tighten the bolts on the crutches

11 A single-tip cane is used
   a At waist level
   b On the strong side
   c On the weak side
   d On either side

Circle T if the statement is true and F if it is false.

12 T **F** A single-tip cane and a four-point cane give the same support.

13 T **F** When using a cane, the feet are moved first.

14 **T** F When using a walker, the feet are moved first.

15 **T** F A person has a brace. Bony areas need protection from skin breakdown.

Answers to these questions are on p. 781.

Comfort, Rest, and Sleep

OBJECTIVES

- Define the key terms and key abbreviations listed in this chapter
- Explain why comfort, rest, and sleep are important
- List the OBRA room requirements for comfort, rest, and sleep
- Describe four types of pain and the factors affecting pain
- Explain why pain is personal
- List the signs and symptoms of pain
- List the nursing measures that relieve pain
- Explain why meeting basic needs is important for rest
- Identify when rest is needed
- Explain how circadian rhythm affects sleep
- Describe the stages of sleep
- Know the sleep requirements for each age-group
- Describe the factors that affect sleep
- Describe the common sleep disorders
- List the nursing measures that promote rest and sleep
- Explain how dementia affects sleep

KEY TERMS

acute pain Pain that is felt suddenly from injury, disease, trauma, or surgery

chronic pain Pain lasting longer than 6 months; it is constant or occurs off and on

circadian rhythm Daily rhythm based on a 24-hour cycle; the day-night cycle or body rhythm

comfort A state of well-being; the person has no physical or emotional pain and is calm and at peace

discomfort Pain

distraction To change the person's center of attention

enuresis Urinary incontinence in bed at night

guided imagery Creating and focusing on an image

insomnia A chronic condition in which the person cannot sleep or stay asleep all night

NREM sleep The phase of sleep when there is *no rapid eye movement*; non-REM sleep

pain To ache, hurt, or be sore; discomfort

phantom pain Pain felt in a body part that is no longer there

radiating pain Pain felt at the site of tissue damage and in nearby areas

relaxation To be free from mental and physical stress

REM sleep The phase of sleep when there is *rapid eye movement*

rest To be calm, at ease, and relaxed; no anxiety or stress

sleep A state of unconsciousness, reduced voluntary muscle activity, and lowered metabolism

KEY ABBREVIATIONS

F Fahrenheit
ICU Intensive care unit
NREM No rapid eye movement

OBRA Omnibus Budget Reconciliation Act of 1987
REM Rapid eye movement

Comfort, rest, and sleep are needed for well-being. The total person—the physical, emotional, social, and spiritual—is affected by comfort, rest, and sleep problems. Discomfort and pain can be physical or emotional. Whatever the cause, they affect rest and sleep. They also decrease function and quality of life.

Rest and sleep restore energy and well-being. Illness and injury increase the need for rest and sleep. The body needs more energy for healing and repair. During illness or injury, more energy is needed to perform daily functions.

See *Focus on Long-Term Care and Home Care: Comfort, Rest, and Sleep.*

COMFORT

Comfort is a state of well-being. The person has no physical or emotional pain. He or she is calm and at peace. Age, illness, and activity affect comfort. So do temperature, ventilation, noise, odors, and lighting. Those factors are controlled to meet the person's needs (Chapter 17).

See *Focus on Communication: Comfort.*

PAIN

Pain or **discomfort** means to ache, hurt, or be sore. It is unpleasant. Comfort and discomfort are subjective (Chapter 6). That is, you cannot see, hear, touch, or smell pain or discomfort. You must rely on what the person says. Report complaints to the nurse. The information is used for the nursing process.

Pain is personal. It differs for each person. What *hurts* to one person may *ache* to another. What one person calls *sore*, another may call *aching*. If a person complains of pain

---

FOCUS ON **LONG-TERM CARE** AND **HOME CARE**

Comfort, Rest, and Sleep

LONG-TERM CARE

The Omnibus Budget Reconciliation Act of 1987 (OBRA) requires that persons receive care that promotes well-being. Comfort, rest, and sleep are needed for physical, emotional, and mental well-being. Rooms are designed and equipped for comfort.

These OBRA room requirements promote comfort:
- No more than four persons in a room
- A suspended curtain that goes around the bed for privacy
- A bed of proper height and size for the person
- A clean, comfortable mattress
- Linens (sheets, blankets, spreads) that suit the weather and climate
- A clean and orderly room
- An odor-free room
- A room temperature between 71° and 81° F
- An acceptable noise level
- Adequate ventilation and room humidity
- Appropriate lighting

FOCUS ON **COMMUNICATION**

Comfort

Do not assume that a person is comfortable. You can ask the following:
- "Are you comfortable?"
- "What can I do to help you be more comfortable?"
- "Are you warm enough?"
- "Do you need another blanket?"
- "Do you need another pillow?"
- "Do you want me to adjust your pillow?"

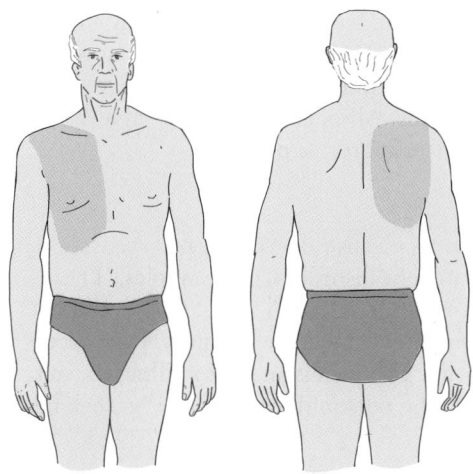

FIGURE 27-1 Gallbladder pain radiates to the right upper abdomen, the back, and the right shoulder.

or discomfort, the person *has* pain or discomfort. You must believe the person. You cannot see, hear, feel, or smell the pain.

Pain is a warning from the body. It means there is tissue damage. Pain often causes the person to seek health care.

Types of Pain

There are different types of pain. The doctor uses the type of pain when diagnosing. The nurse uses it for the nursing process.

▶ **Acute pain** is felt suddenly from injury, disease, trauma, or surgery. There is tissue damage. Acute pain lasts a short time, usually less than 6 months. It lessens with healing.

▶ **Chronic pain** lasts longer than 6 months. Pain is constant or occurs off and on. There is no longer tissue damage. Chronic pain remains long after healing. Arthritis and cancer are common causes.

▶ **Radiating pain** is felt at the site of tissue damage and in nearby areas. Pain from a heart attack is often felt in the left chest, left jaw, left shoulder, and left arm. Gallbladder disease can cause pain in the right upper abdomen, the back, and the right shoulder (Fig. 27-1).

▶ **Phantom pain** is felt in a body part that is no longer there. A person with an amputated leg may still sense leg pain.

Factors Affecting Pain

A person may handle pain well one time and poorly the next time. Many factors affect reactions to pain.

Past Experience

We learn from past experiences. They help us know what to do or what to expect. Whether it is going to school, driving, taking a test, shopping, having a baby, or caring for children, the past prepares us for similar events at another time. We also learn from the experiences of family and friends.

A person may have had pain before. The severity of pain, its cause, how long it lasted, and if relief occurred all affect the person's current response to pain. Knowing what to expect can help or hinder how the person handles pain.

Some people have not had pain. When it occurs, pain can cause fear and anxiety. They can make pain worse.

Anxiety

Anxiety relates to feelings of fear, dread, worry, and concern. The person is uneasy and tense. The person may feel troubled or threatened. Or the person may sense danger. Something is wrong but the person does not know what or why.

Pain and anxiety are related. Pain can cause anxiety. Anxiety increases how much pain the person feels. Reducing anxiety helps lessen pain. For example, the nurse explains to Mr. Smith that he will have pain after surgery. The nurse also explains that he will receive drugs for pain relief. Mr. Smith knows the cause of the pain. And he knows what to expect. This helps reduce his anxiety and therefore the amount of pain felt.

Rest and Sleep

Rest and sleep restore energy. They reduce body demands, and the body repairs itself. Lack of needed rest and sleep affects thinking and coping with daily life. Sleep and rest needs increase with illness and injury. Pain seems worse when tired or restless. Also, the person tends to focus on pain when tired and unable to rest or sleep.

Attention

The more a person thinks about the pain, the worse it seems. Sometimes severe pain is all the person thinks about. However, even mild pain can seem worse if the person thinks about it all the time.

Pain often seems worse at night. Activity is less, and it is quiet. There are no visitors. The radio or TV is off. Others are asleep. When unable to sleep, the person has time to think about the pain.

Personal and Family Duties

Personal and family duties affect pain responses. Often pain is ignored when there are children to care for. Some people go to work with pain. Others deny pain if a serious illness is feared. The illness can interfere with a job, going to school, or caring for children, a partner, or ill parents.

The Value or Meaning of Pain

To some people, pain is a sign of weakness. It may mean a serious illness and the need for painful tests and treatments. Therefore pain is ignored or denied. Sometimes pain gives pleasure. The pain of childbirth is one example.

For some persons, pain means not having to work or assume daily routines. Pain is used to avoid certain people or things. The pain is useful. Some people like doting and pampering by others. The person values and wants such attention.

Support From Others

Dealing with pain is often easier when family and friends offer comfort and support. The pain of childbirth is easier when a loving father gives support and encouragement. A child bears pain much better when comforted by a caring parent or family member. The use of touch by a valued person is very comforting. Just being nearby also helps.

Some people do not have caring family or friends. They deal with pain alone. Being alone can increase anxiety. The person has more time to think about the pain. Facing pain alone is hard for everyone, especially children and older persons.

Culture

Culture affects pain responses. In some cultures, the person in pain is *stoic*. To be stoic means to show no reaction to joy, sorrow, pleasure, or pain. Strong verbal and nonverbal reactions to pain are seen in other cultures. See *Caring About Culture: Pain Reactions.*

CARING ABOUT CULTURE

Pain Reactions

People of *Mexico* and the *Philippines* may appear stoic in reaction to pain. In the *Philippines,* pain is viewed as the will of God. It is believed that God will give strength to bear the pain.

In *Vietnam,* pain may be severe before pain relief measures are requested. The people of *India* accept pain quietly. They will accept some pain relief measures.

In *China,* showing emotion is a weakness of character. Therefore pain is often suppressed.

From D'Avanzo CE, Geissler EM: *Pocket guide to cultural health assessment,* ed 3, St Louis, 2003, Mosby.

Non-English speaking persons may have problems describing pain. The agency must know who these persons are. Someone must be available to interpret the person's needs. All persons have the right to be comfortable and as pain-free as possible.

Illness

Some diseases cause decreased pain sensations. Central nervous system disorders are examples. The person may not feel pain. Or it may not feel severe. The person is at risk for undetected disease or injury. Pain occurs with tissue damage. The pain is an alert to illness or injury. If pain is not felt, the person does not know to seek health care.

Age

See *Focus on Children and Older Persons: Factors Affecting Pain.*

Signs and Symptoms

You cannot see, hear, feel, or smell the person's pain. You must rely on what the person tells you. Promptly report any information you collect about pain. Write down what the person says. Use the person's exact words when reporting and recording. The nurse needs this information to assess the person's pain:

▶ *Location.* Where is the pain? Ask the person to point to the area of pain (Fig. 27-2). Pain can radiate. Ask the person if the pain is anywhere else and to point to those areas.
▶ *Onset and duration.* When did the pain start? How long has it lasted?

FOCUS ON CHILDREN AND OLDER PERSONS

Factors Affecting Pain

CHILDREN

Children may not understand pain. They know it feels bad. They have fewer pain experiences. They do not know what to expect.

Children do not have many ways to deal with pain. They may restrict play, school, and sports activities to lessen pain. Adults can buy some pain drugs. They can go to a doctor. They know that heat or cold applications help relieve pain. They can distract attention away from the pain with music, working, reading, and hobbies. Children do not know how to relieve their own pain. They rely on adults for help.

Adults must be alert to behaviors and situations that signal a child's pain. Infants cry, fuss, and are restless. Such behaviors also mean hunger and needing a diaper changed. Toddlers and preschoolers may not have the words to express pain.

OLDER PERSONS

Older persons may have decreased pain sensations. They may not feel pain. Or it may not feel severe. The person is at risk for undetected disease or injury. Pain occurs with tissue damage. The pain signals illness or injury. If pain is not felt, the person does not know to seek health care.

Some older persons have many painful health problems. Chronic pain may mask new pain. Older persons may ignore or deny new pain. They may think it relates to a known health problem. Older persons often deny or ignore pain because of what it may mean.

Thinking and reasoning are affected in some older persons. Some cannot verbally communicate pain. Changes in usual behavior may signal pain. A person who normally moans and groans may become quiet and withdrawn. A person who is friendly and outgoing may become agitated and aggressive. One who is nonverbal and quiet may become restless and cry easily. Loss of appetite also signals pain.

Report any changes in a person's usual behavior to the nurse. All persons have the right to correct pain management. The nurse needs to do a pain assessment when the person's behavior changes.

▶ *Intensity.* Does the person complain of mild, moderate, or severe pain? Ask the person to rate the pain on a scale of 0 to 10, with 10 as the most severe (Fig. 27-3). Or use the Wong-Baker Faces Pain Rating Scale (Fig. 27-4). Designed for children, the scale is useful for persons of all ages. To use the scale, tell the person that each face shows how a person is feeling. Read the description for each face. Then ask the person to choose the face that best describes how he or she feels.

▶ *Description.* Ask the person to describe the pain. If the person cannot describe the pain, offer some of the words listed in Box 27-1.

▶ *Factors causing pain.* These are called *precipitating* factors. To precipitate means to cause. Such factors include moving or turning in bed, coughing or deep breathing, and exercise. Ask what the person was doing before the pain started and when it started.

▶ *Factors affecting pain.* Ask the person what makes the pain better. Also ask what makes it worse.

▶ *Vital signs.* Measure the person's pulse, respirations, and blood pressure. Increases in these vital signs often occur with acute pain. Vital signs may be normal with chronic pain.

▶ *Other signs and symptoms.* Does the person have other symptoms—dizziness, nausea, vomiting, weakness, numbness or tingling, or others? Box 27-2, p. 484 lists the signs and symptoms that often occur with pain. See *Focus on Communication: Signs and Symptoms.*

FOCUS ON COMMUNICATION

Signs and Symptoms

A person may use the word "hurt" instead of "pain." Children may use "owie" or "boo boo" when referring to pain. Use words that the person uses.

BOX 27-1 Words Used to Describe Pain

- Aching
- Burning
- Cramping
- Crushing
- Dull
- Gnawing
- Knife-like
- Piercing
- Pressure
- Sharp
- Sore
- Squeezing
- Stabbing
- Throbbing
- Vise-like

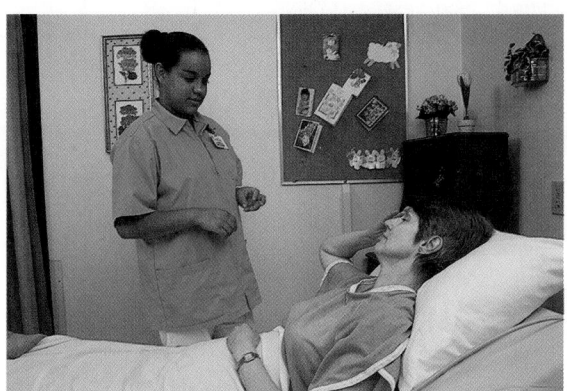

FIGURE 27-2 The person points to the area of pain.

PAIN: Ask patient to rate pain on scale of 0-10										
No pain										Worst pain imaginable
0	1	2	3	4	5	6	7	8	9	10

FIGURE 27-3 Pain rating scale. (From deWit SC: *Fundamental concepts and skills for nursing,* ed 2, Philadelphia, 2005, Saunders.)

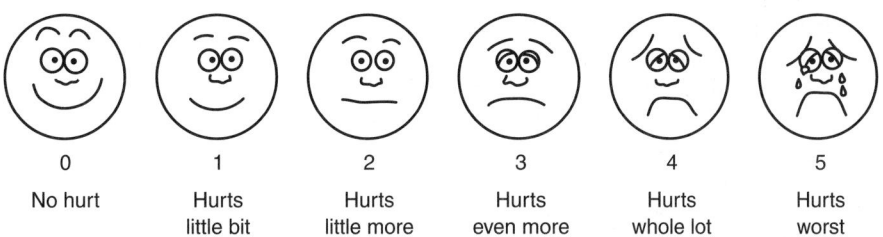

0	1	2	3	4	5
No hurt	Hurts little bit	Hurts little more	Hurts even more	Hurts whole lot	Hurts worst

FIGURE 27-4 Wong-Baker Faces Pain Rating Scale. (From Hockenberry MJ and Wilson D: *Wong's nursing care of infants and children,* ed 8, St Louis, 2007, Mosby.)

BOX 27-2 Signs and Symptoms of Pain

BODY RESPONSES
- Appetite: changes in
- Dizziness
- Nausea
- Numbness
- Pulse, respirations, and blood pressure: increased
- Skin: pale (pallor)
- Sleep: difficulty with
- Sweating (diaphoresis)
- Tingling
- Vomiting
- Weakness

BEHAVIORS
- Crying
- Gasping
- Grimacing
- Groaning
- Grunting
- Holding the affected body part (splinting; guarding)
- Irritability
- Moaning
- Mood: changes in
- Positioning: maintaining one position; refusing to move
- Quietness
- Restlessness
- Rubbing
- Screaming
- Speech: slow or rapid; loud or quiet

BOX 27-3 Nursing Measures to Promote Comfort and Relieve Pain

- Position the person in good alignment. Use pillows for support.
- Keep bed linens tight and wrinkle-free.
- Make sure the person is not lying on drainage tubes.
- Assist with elimination needs.
- Provide blankets for warmth and to prevent chilling.
- Use correct handling, moving, and turning procedures.
- Wait 30 minutes after pain drugs are given before giving care or starting activities.
- Give a back massage.
- Provide soft music to distract the person.
- Talk softly and gently.
- Use touch to provide comfort.
- Allow family and friends at the bedside as requested by the person.
- Avoid sudden or jarring movements of the bed or chair.
- Handle the person gently.
- Practice safety measures if the person takes strong pain drugs or sedatives:
  - Keep the bed in the low position.
  - Raise bed rails as directed. Follow the care plan.
  - Check on the person every 10 to 15 minutes.
  - Provide help when the person needs to get up and when he or she is up and about.
- Apply warm or cold applications as directed by the nurse (Chapter 33).
- Provide a calm, quiet, darkened setting.

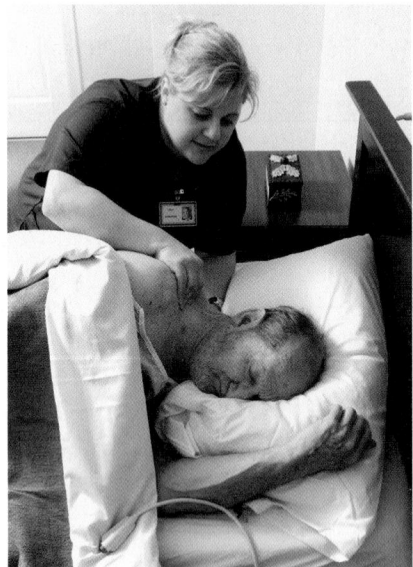

FIGURE 27-5 Measures are implemented to relieve pain. The person is positioned in good alignment with pillows used for comfort. The room is darkened. Blankets provide warmth. A back massage provides touch and promotes relaxation.

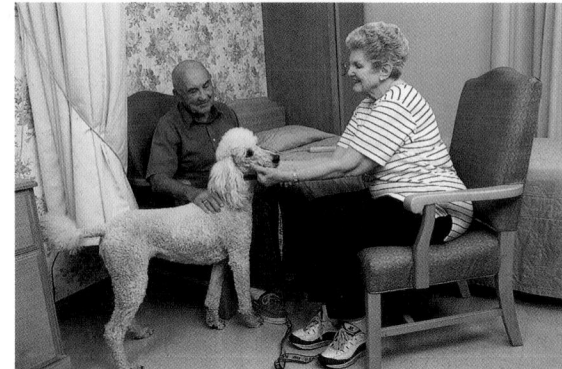

FIGURE 27-6 A comforting pet can distract attention away from pain.

Nursing Measures

The nurse uses the nursing process to promote comfort and relieve pain. The care plan may include the measures in Box 27-3. See Figure 27-5.

Other measures are often needed. They include distraction, relaxation, and guided imagery. Nurses and physical, occupational, and recreational therapists may assist with these measures. If asked to assist, they tell you what to do.

Distraction means to change the person's center of attention. Attention is moved away from the pain. Music, games, singing, praying, TV, and needlework can distract attention (Fig. 27-6).

Relaxation means to be free from mental and physical stress. This state reduces pain and anxiety. The person is taught relaxation methods. The person is taught to breathe deeply and slowly and to contract and relax muscle groups. A comfortable position is important. So is a quiet room.

Guided imagery is creating and focusing on an image. The person is asked to create a pleasant scene. This is noted on the care plan so all staff members use the same image with the person. A calm, soft voice is used to help the person focus on the image. Soft music, a blanket for warmth, and a darkened room may help. The person is coached to focus on the image and then to practice relaxation exercises.

Doctors often order drugs to control or relieve pain. Nurses give these drugs. Such drugs can cause orthostatic hypotension (Chapter 26). They also can cause drowsiness, dizziness, and coordination problems. Therefore the person is protected from injury, falls, and fractures. The nurse and care plan alert you to needed safety measures.

See *Focus on Children and Older Persons: Nursing Measures.*

REST

Rest means to be calm, at ease, and relaxed. The person has no anxiety or stress. Rest may involve inactivity. Or the person does things that are calming and relaxing. Examples include reading, music, TV, needlework, and prayer. Some people garden, bake, golf, walk, or do woodworking.

You can promote rest by meeting physical needs. Thirst, hunger, and elimination needs can affect rest. So can pain or discomfort. A comfortable position and good alignment are important. A quiet setting promotes rest. So does a clean, dry, and wrinkle-free bed. Some people rest easier in a clean, neat, and uncluttered room.

Meet safety and security needs. The person must feel safe from falling or other injuries. The person is secure with the signal light within reach. Understanding the reasons for care also helps the person feel safe. So does knowing how care is given. That is why you always explain procedures before doing them.

Many people have rituals or routines before resting. These may include going to the bathroom, brushing teeth, and washing the face and hands. Some people pray. Some have a snack or beverage, lock doors, or make sure loved ones are safe at home. The person may want a certain blanket or afghan. Follow routines and rituals whenever possible.

Love and belonging promote rest. Visits or calls from family and friends may relax the person. The person knows that others care and are concerned. Reading cards and letters may also help the person relax and rest (Fig. 27-7).

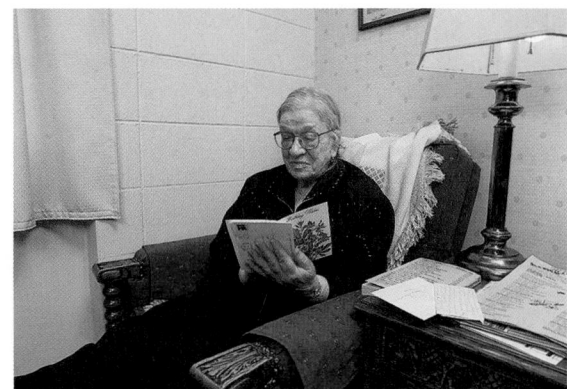

FIGURE 27-7 The resident reads cards and letters from family and friends.

Self-esteem needs relate to feeling good about oneself. Some people find patient gowns embarrassing. Others fear exposure. Many persons rest better in their own sleepwear. Hygiene and grooming also affect self-esteem. This includes hair care and being clean and odor-free. Hygiene and grooming measures help people feel good about themselves. If esteem needs are met, the person may rest easier.

Some people are refreshed after a 15- or 20-minute rest. Others need more time. Health care routines usually allow time for afternoon rest.

Ill or injured persons need to rest more often. Some rest during or after a procedure. For example, a bath tires a person. So does getting dressed. The person needs to rest before you make the bed. Some people need a few hours for hygiene and grooming. Others need to rest after meals. Do not push the person beyond his or her limits. Allow rest when needed. Do not rush the person.

Distraction, relaxation, and guided imagery also promote rest. So does a back massage. Plan and organize care to allow uninterrupted rest.

The doctor may order bedrest for a person. Bedrest is presented in Chapter 26.

SLEEP

Sleep is a state of unconsciousness, reduced voluntary muscle activity, and lowered metabolism. An unconscious person is unaware of the environment. He or she cannot respond to people and things in the environment. There are no voluntary arm or leg movements. *Metabolism* is the burning of food to produce energy for the body. Less energy is needed during sleep. Thus metabolism is reduced during sleep. The sleep state is temporary. People wake up from sleep.

Sleep is a basic need. It lets the mind and body rest. The body saves energy. Body functions slow. Vital signs are lower than when awake. Tissue healing and repair occur. Sleep lowers stress, tension, and anxiety. It refreshes and renews the person. The person regains energy and mental alertness. The person thinks and functions better after sleep.

BOX 27-4 Sleep Cycle

STAGE 1: NREM SLEEP
- Lightest sleep level
- Lasts a few minutes
- Gradual decrease in vital signs
- Gradual lowering of metabolism
- Person feels drowsy and relaxed
- Person is easily aroused
- Daydreaming feeling after being aroused

STAGE 2: NREM SLEEP
- Sound sleep
- Relaxation increases
- Still easy to arouse
- Lasts 10 to 20 minutes
- Body functions continue to slow

STAGE 3: NREM SLEEP
- First stage of deep sleep
- Hard to arouse the person
- Person rarely moves
- Muscles relax completely
- Vital signs decrease
- Lasts 15 to 30 minutes

STAGE 4: NREM SLEEP
- Deepest stage of sleep
- Hard to arouse the person
- Body rests and is restored
- Vital signs much lower than when awake
- Lasts about 15 to 30 minutes
- Sleepwalking may occur
- **Enuresis** (urinary incontinence in bed at night) may occur

REM SLEEP
- Vivid, full-color dreaming
- Usually starts 50 to 90 minutes after sleep has begun
- Rapid eye movements
- Blood pressure, pulse, and respirations may fluctuate
- Voluntary muscles are relaxed
- Mental restoration occurs
- Hard to arouse the person
- Lasts about 20 minutes

Modified from Potter PA, Perry AG: *Fundamentals of nursing*, ed 6, St Louis, 2005, Mosby.

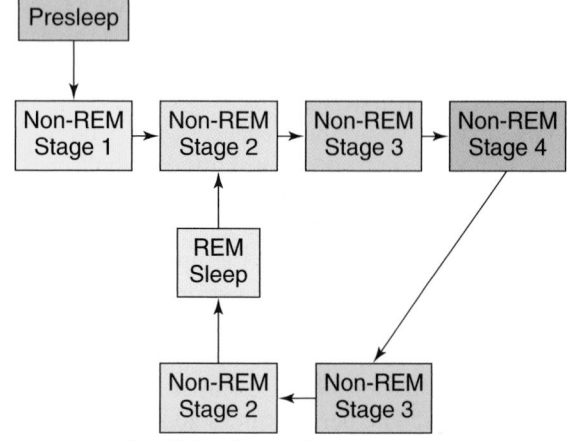

FIGURE 27-8 Adult sleep cycle.

Circadian Rhythm

Sleep is part of circadian rhythm. (*Circa* means *about. Dies* means *day.*) **Circadian rhythm** is a daily rhythm based on a 24-hour cycle. It is called the *day-night cycle* or *body rhythm*. It affects functioning. Some people function better in the morning. They are more alert and active. They think and react better. Others do better in the evening.

Circadian rhythm includes a sleep-wake cycle. The person's *biological clock* signals when to sleep and when to wake up. You sleep and wake up at certain times. You may awaken before the alarm clock goes off. That is part of your biological clock. Health care often interferes with a person's circadian rhythm and the sleep-wake cycle. Sleep problems easily occur.

Many people work evening and night shifts. Their bodies must adjust to changes in the sleep-wake cycle.

Sleep Cycle

There are two phases of sleep (Box 27-4). **NREM sleep** *(non-REM sleep)* is the phase of sleep where there is *no rapid eye movement*. NREM sleep has 4 stages. Sleep goes from light to deep as the person moves through the four stages.

The *rapid eye movement* phase is called **REM sleep**. The person is hard to arouse. Mental restoration occurs. Events and problems of the day are thought to be reviewed. The person prepares for the next day.

There are usually 4 to 6 cycles of NREM and REM sleep during 7 to 8 hours of sleep. Stage 1 of NREM is usually not repeated (Fig. 27-8).

Sleep Requirements

Sleep needs vary for each age-group. The amount needed decreases with age (Table 27-1). Infants need more sleep than toddlers. Toddlers need more than preschool children. School-age children need more than teenagers. Older persons need less sleep than middle-age adults.

Factors Affecting Sleep

Many factors affect the amount and quality of sleep. Quality relates to how well the person slept. It also involves getting needed amounts of NREM and REM sleep.

▶ *Illness.* Illness increases the need for sleep. However, signs and symptoms of illness can interfere with sleep. They include pain, nausea, vomiting, coughing, difficulty breathing, diarrhea, frequent voiding, and itching. Treatments and therapies can also interfere with sleep. Often patients and residents are awakened for treatments or drugs. Care devices can cause uncomfortable positions. The emotional effects of illness can affect sleep. These include fear, anxiety, and worry.

▶ *Nutrition.* Sleep needs increase with weight gain. They decrease with weight loss. Some foods affect sleep. Those with caffeine (chocolate, coffee, tea, or colas) prevent sleep. The protein tryptophan tends to help sleep. It is found in protein sources—milk, cheese, red meat, fish, poultry, and peanuts.

TABLE 27-1 Average Sleep Requirements

AGE-GROUP	HOURS PER DAY
Newborns (birth to 4 weeks)	14 to 18
Infants (4 weeks to 1 year)	12 to 14
Toddlers (1 to 3 years)	11 to 12
Preschoolers (3 to 6 years)	11 to 12
Middle and late childhood (6 to 12 years)	10 to 11
Adolescents (12 to 18 years)	8 to 9
Young adults (18 to 40 years)	7 to 8
Middle-age adults (40 to 65 years)	7 to 8
Older adults (65 years and older)	5 to 7

▶ *Exercise.* Exercise improves health and fitness. Exercise requires energy. People usually feel good after exercising. Eventually they tire. Being tired helps them sleep well. Exercise before bedtime interferes with sleep. Exercise causes the release of substances into the bloodstream that stimulate the body. Exercise is avoided 2 hours before bedtime.

▶ *Environment.* People adjust to their usual sleep settings. They get used to such things as the bed, pillows, noises, lighting, and a sleeping partner. Any change in the usual setting can affect the amount and quality of sleep.

▶ *Drugs and other substances.* Sleeping pills promote sleep. Drugs for anxiety, depression, and pain may cause the person to sleep. However, these drugs and sleeping pills reduce the length of REM sleep. Mental restoration occurs during REM sleep. Behavior problems and sleep deprivation can occur. Alcohol is a drug. It causes drowsiness and sleep. However, it interferes with REM sleep. Those under the influence of alcohol may awaken during sleep. Difficulty returning to sleep is common. Some drugs contain caffeine. Caffeine is a stimulant and prevents sleep. Besides in drugs, caffeine is found in coffee, tea, chocolate, and colas. The side effects of some drugs cause frequent voiding and nightmares.

▶ *Life-style changes.* Life-style relates to a person's daily routines and way of living. Work, school, play, and social events are all part of life-style. Life-style changes can affect sleep. Travel, vacation, and social events often affect usual sleep and wake times. Children usually stay up later during school holidays. They may sleep later, too. If work hours change, sleep hours may change. Such changes affect normal sleep-wake cycles and the circadian rhythm.

▶ *Emotional problems.* Fear, worry, depression, and anxiety affect sleep. Causes include work, personal, or family problems. Loss of a loved one or friend is another cause. Money problems are stressful. People may have problems falling asleep, or they awaken often. Some have problems getting back to sleep.

BOX 27-5 Signs and Symptoms of Sleep Disorders

- Agitation
- Attention: decreased
- Coordination: problems with
- Disorientation
- Eyes: red, puffy, dark circles under the eyes
- Fatigue
- Hallucinations (Chapters 43 and 44)
- Irritability
- Memory: reduced word memory; problems finding the right word
- Mood: moodiness; mood swings
- Pulse: irregular
- Reasoning and judgment: decreased
- Responses to questions, conversations, or situations: slowed
- Restlessness
- Sleepiness
- Speech: slurred
- Tremors: in the hands

Sleep Disorders

Sleep disorders involve repeated sleep problems. The amount and quality of sleep are affected. Sleep disorders affect life-style. Box 27-5 lists the signs and symptoms that occur.

Insomnia

Insomnia is a chronic condition in which the person cannot sleep or stay asleep all night. There are three forms of insomnia:

▶ Cannot fall asleep
▶ Cannot stay asleep
▶ Early awakening and cannot fall back asleep

Emotional problems are common causes of insomnia. The fear of dying during sleep is another cause. Some people are afraid of not waking up. This may occur with heart disease or when told of a terminal illness. The fear of not being able to sleep is another cause. The physical and emotional discomforts of illness can also cause insomnia.

The nurse plans measures to promote sleep. However, the emotional or physical problems causing the insomnia also are treated.

Sleep Deprivation

With sleep deprivation, the amount and quality of sleep are decreased. Sleep is interrupted. NREM and REM sleep stages are not completed. Illness, pain, and hospital care are common causes. Patients in hospital intensive care units (ICUs) are at great risk. ICU lights, the many care measures, and equipment sounds interfere with sleep. Factors that affect sleep can also lead to sleep deprivation. The signs and symptoms in Box 27-5 may occur.

Sleepwalking

The person leaves the bed and walks about. The person is not aware of sleepwalking. He or she has no memory of the event on awakening. Children sleepwalk more than adults. The event may last 3 to 4 minutes or longer.

Stress, fatigue, and some drugs are common causes. Protect the person from injury. Falling is a risk. Intravenous therapy, catheters, nasogastric tubes, and other tubing can cause injury. The tubes or catheters can be pulled out of the body when the person gets out of bed. Guide sleepwalkers back to bed. They startle easily. Awaken them gently.

See *Teamwork and Time Management: Sleepwalking.*

TEAMWORK AND TIME MANAGEMENT

Sleepwalking

You may find a person sleepwalking. Help him or her back to bed even if you are not assigned to provide the person's care. Provide for the person's comfort. Then tell the nurse what happened and what you did.

BOX 27-6 Nursing Measures to Promote Sleep

- Plan care for uninterrupted rest.
- Avoid physical activity before bedtime.
- Encourage the person to avoid business or family matters before bedtime.
- Allow a flexible bedtime. Bedtime is when the person is tired, not a certain time.
- Provide a comfortable room temperature.
- Let the person take a warm bath or shower.
- Provide a bedtime snack.
- Avoid caffeine (coffee, tea, colas, chocolate).
- Avoid alcoholic beverages.
- Have the person void before going to bed.
- Make sure incontinent persons are clean and dry. Change a baby's diaper.
- Follow bedtime routines.
- Have the person wear loose-fitting sleepwear.
- Provide for warmth (blankets, socks) for those who tend to be cold.
- Reduce noise.
- Darken the room—close window coverings and the privacy curtain. Shut off or dim lights.
- Dim lights in hallways and the nursing unit.
- Make sure linens are clean, dry, and wrinkle-free.
- Position the person in good alignment and in a comfortable position.
- Support body parts as ordered.
- Give a back massage.
- Provide measures to relieve pain.
- Let the person read. Read to children.
- Let the person listen to music or watch TV.
- Assist with relaxation exercises as ordered.
- Sit and talk with the person.

Promoting Sleep

The nurse assesses the person's sleep patterns. Report any of the signs and symptoms listed in Box 27-5. Measures are planned to promote sleep (Box 27-6). Follow the care plan. Also report your observations about how the person slept. This helps the nurse evaluate if the person develops a regular sleep pattern.

Many people have rituals and routines before bedtime. They are important to the person. They are allowed if safe. The person may perform personal hygiene in a certain order. A bedtime snack may be important. Some watch certain TV shows in bed. Others read religious writings, pray, or say a rosary before going to sleep.

See *Focus on Children and Older Persons: Promoting Sleep.*

See *Focus on Long-Term Care and Home Care: Promoting Sleep.*

FOCUS ON CHILDREN AND OLDER PERSONS

Promoting Sleep

OLDER PERSONS

Older persons have less energy than younger people. They may nap during the day. You need to let the person sleep. Plan the person's care to allow uninterrupted naps.

Sleep problems are common in persons with Alzheimer's disease and other dementias. Night wandering is common. Restlessness and confusion often increase at night. This increases the risk of falls. It often helps to quietly and calmly direct the person to his or her room. Allowing night-time wandering in a safe and supervised setting is the best approach for some persons. The measures listed in Box 27-6 are tried. Follow the care plan.

FOCUS ON LONG-TERM CARE AND HOME CARE

Promoting Sleep

LONG-TERM CARE

Some persons like to check on other residents before going to bed. Some have the duty of turning off the lights at bedtime. These actions promote the person's dignity and mental comfort.

The person is involved in planning care. The person chooses when to nap or go to bed. The person chooses the measures that promote comfort, rest, and sleep. Follow the care plan and the person's wishes.

REVIEW QUESTIONS

Circle the BEST answer.

1 These statements are about pain. Which is *false*?
  a Pain can be seen, heard, smelled, or felt.
  b Pain is a warning from the body.
  c Pain is personal. It is different for each person.
  d Pain is used to make diagnoses.

2 A person has pain in the left chest, the left jaw, and the left shoulder and arm. This is
  a Acute pain
  b Chronic pain
  c Radiating pain
  d Phantom pain

3 A person complains of pain. You should ask the person to do the following *except*
  a Point to where the pain is felt
  b Tell you when the pain started
  c Describe the pain
  d Let you look at the pain

4 The nurse gives a person a drug for pain relief. Care is scheduled for this time. You should
  a Give the care before the drug is given
  b Give care right after the drug is given
  c Wait 30 minutes to let the drug take effect
  d Omit the care for the day

5 A person was given a drug for pain relief. To promote safety, you should do the following *except*
  a Keep the bed in the high position
  b Raise bed rails as directed
  c Check on the person every 10 to 15 minutes
  d Provide help if the person needs to get up

6 Which measure will *not* help relieve pain?
  a Providing blankets as needed
  b Keeping the room well lighted
  c Providing soft music
  d Giving a back massage

7 A person's care plan has these measures. Which will *not* promote rest or sleep?
  a Voiding before rest or sleep
  b Positioning in a comfortable position
  c Having the person walk before rest or sleep
  d Letting the person choose sleepwear

8 A person tires easily. Morning care includes a bath, hair care, and getting dressed. The bed is made after the person is dressed. When should the person rest?
  a After you complete morning care
  b After the bath and before hair care
  c After you make the bed
  d When the person needs to

9 These statements are about sleep. Which is *false*?
  a Tissue healing and repair occur during sleep.
  b Voluntary muscle activity increases during sleep.
  c Sleep refreshes and renews the person.
  d Sleep lowers stress, tension, and anxiety.

10 A person was awake several nights. Which is *false*?
  a Circadian rhythm may be affected.
  b NREM and REM sleep are affected.
  c The person's biological clock still tells when to sleep and wake up.
  d Functioning may be affected.

11 A healthy 70-year-old person probably needs about
  a 12 to 14 hours of sleep
  b 8 to 9 hours of sleep
  c 7 to 8 hours of sleep
  d 5 to 7 hours of sleep

12 Which prevents sleep?
  a Chocolate
  b Cheese
  c Milk
  d Beef

13 These measures to promote sleep are part of a person's care plan. Which should you question?
  a Let the person choose the bedtime.
  b Provide hot tea and a cheese sandwich at bedtime.
  c Position the person in good alignment.
  d Follow the person's bedtime rituals.

Circle T if the statement is true and F if the statement is false.

14 **T** **F** Changes in a person's usual behavior may signal pain.

15 **T** **F** Persons with dementia usually sleep well at night.

16 **T** **F** A person's culture may affect how he or she reacts to pain.

Answers to these questions are on p. 781.

CHAPTER
28 Admissions, Transfers, and Discharges

OBJECTIVES

- Define the key terms listed in this chapter
- Describe your role during admissions, transfers, and discharges
- Explain how you can help new residents feel comfortable in the nursing center
- Identify the rules for measuring weight and height
- Explain the reasons for transfers to another nursing unit
- Perform the procedures described in this chapter

PROCEDURES

- Preparing the Person's Room
- Admitting the Person
- Measuring Weight and Height
- Measuring Height—The Person Is in Bed
- Transferring the Person to Another Nursing Unit
- Discharging the Person

KEY TERMS

admission Official entry of a person into an agency

discharge Official departure of a person from an agency

transfer Moving a person from one room or nursing unit to another

Procedures with this icon are on the CDCompanion in this book; those with this icon are on the Evolve Student Resources Website.

Admission to a hospital or nursing center causes anxiety and fear in patients, residents, and families. They may worry about treatments and surgeries and their outcomes. They may fear serious health problems. The fear of pain is common.

Patients, residents, and their families are in new, strange settings. They may have concerns and fears about:
▶ Where to go, what to do, and what to expect
▶ Never returning home
▶ Who gives care, how care is given, and if the correct care is given
▶ Getting meals
▶ Finding the bathroom
▶ How to get help
▶ Being abused
▶ Strange sights and sounds
▶ Being apart from family and friends
▶ Making new friends
▶ Leaving homes and possessions behind

Discharge is usually a happy time. However, the person may need home care or long-term care.

Admission, transfer, and discharge are critical events. They involve:
▶ Privacy and confidentiality
▶ Reporting and recording
▶ Understanding and communicating with the person
▶ Communicating with the health team
▶ Respect for the person and the person's property
▶ Being kind, courteous, and respectful

See *Focus on Long-Term Care and Home Care: Admissions, Transfers, and Discharges.*

See *Teamwork and Time Management: Admissions, Transfers, and Discharges.*

See *Delegation Guidelines: Admissions, Transfers, and Discharges.*

See *Promoting Safety and Comfort: Admissions, Transfers, and Discharges.*

ADMISSIONS

The admission process usually starts in the admitting office. **Admission** is the official entry of a person into an agency. Admitting staff or a nurse obtains information for the admission record. This includes the person's:
▶ Full name
▶ Age and birth date
▶ Doctor's name
▶ Religion

The person is given an identification number and an ID bracelet (Chapter 11). Admitting papers and a general consent for treatment are signed at this time.

The admitting office tells the nursing unit when there is a new patient or resident. The person's room and bed number are given. In some agencies, the person can walk to the room if able. Most persons require transport by wheelchair or stretcher.

See *Focus on Long-Term Care and Home Care: Admissions,* p. 492.

FOCUS ON LONG-TERM CARE AND HOME CARE
Admissions, Transfers, and Discharges

LONG-TERM CARE
The Omnibus Budget Reconciliation Act of 1987 (OBRA) has standards for transfers and discharges. The person's rights must be protected. Therefore reasons for a transfer or discharge are part of the person's medical record. The person and family are told of the transfer or discharge plans. A procedure is followed if the person objects. An ombudsman makes sure the person's best interests are considered.

TEAMWORK AND TIME MANAGEMENT
Admissions, Transfers, and Discharges

Transfers and discharges are easier if a co-worker helps you. When asking for help, politely tell your co-worker:
• The procedure you need help with
• When you plan to do the procedure
• What you need the person to do
• How much time it will take
  Remember to thank the person for helping you.

DELEGATION GUIDELINES: Admissions, Transfers, and Discharges

When admitting, transferring, or discharging a person, you need this information from the nurse:
• If you need to admit, transfer, or discharge the person
• The person's method of transportation to or from the agency—car, ambulance, or wheelchair van
• How the person will move about within the agency—walking, wheelchair, stretcher, or bed
• The person's room and bed number
• What special equipment and supplies are needed
• If the person can stay dressed or needs to wear a gown or sleepwear
• If the person stays in bed or can be in a chair
• When to report observations
• What specific patient or resident concerns to report at once

---

PROMOTING SAFETY AND COMFORT: Admissions, Transfers, and Discharges

SAFETY
The person may develop pain or become distressed during admission, a transfer, or discharge. If so, call for the nurse at once. Stay with the person. When the nurse arrives, assist as needed.

COMFORT
Admission, transfer, or discharge may be stressful for the person. Some persons are happy. Others are sad and fearful. Some anxiety is expected. To provide for the person's mental comfort:
• Explain what you are doing and why
• Do not rush the person
• Be sensitive to the person's needs and feelings

FOCUS ON LONG-TERM CARE AND HOME CARE

Admissions

LONG-TERM CARE

Nursing centers have admission coordinators. They make the person's admission simple and easy. Often admission procedures are done 2 or 3 days before the person enters the center. Needed information is obtained from the person or family member.

The room assignment is made before the person arrives. Some residents arrive by ambulance or wheelchair van. The attendants take them to their rooms. Some arrive by car. Nurses or nursing assistants take them to their rooms. Often a family member is present.

A nurse or social worker explains the resident's rights to the person and family. They also get a booklet explaining the rights.

The person's photo is taken. Then the person receives an ID bracelet. The photo and ID bracelet are used to identify the person (Chapter 11).

Persons with dementia and their families may need extra help during the admission process. Often confusion increases in a new setting. Fear, agitation, and wanting to leave are common. The family also is fearful. Many feel guilty about the need for nursing center care. The health team helps the person and family feel safe and welcome.

Admission is often a hard time for the person and family. They do not part until ready to do so. Remember, the center is now the person's home.

◆ Preparing the Room

You prepare the room before the person arrives. Figure 28-1 shows a room ready for a new resident.

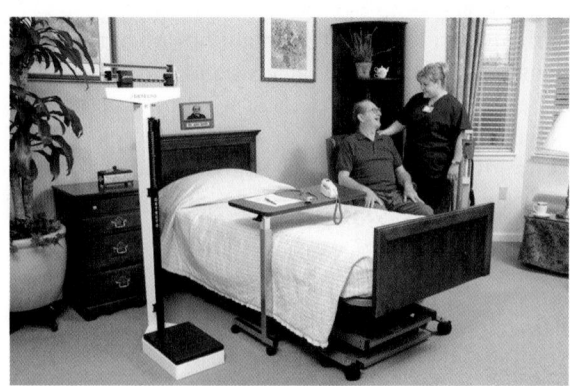

FIGURE 28-1 The room is ready for a new resident.

PREPARING THE PERSON'S ROOM

PROCEDURE

1 Follow *Delegation Guidelines: Admissions, Transfers, and Discharges*, p. 491.
2 Practice hand hygiene.
3 Collect the following:
   - Admission kit—wash basin, soap, toothpaste, toothbrush, water pitcher and cup, and so on
   - Bedpan and urinal (for a man)
   - Admission form (Fig. 28-2)
   - Urine specimen container (if a urine specimen is ordered)
   - Thermometer
   - Sphygmomanometer
   - Stethoscope
   - Gown or pajamas (if needed)
   - Towels and washcloth
   - IV pole (if needed)
   - Other items requested by the nurse
4 Place the following on the overbed table:
   - Thermometer
   - Sphygmomanometer
   - Stethoscope
   - Admission form
5 Place the water pitcher and cup and the urine specimen container on the bedside stand or overbed table.
6 Place the following in the bedside stand:
   - Admission kit
   - Bedpan and urinal
   - Gown or pajamas
   - Towels and washcloth
7 If the person arrives by stretcher:
   a Make a surgical bed (Chapter 18).
   b Raise the bed to its highest level.
8 If the person is ambulatory or arrives by wheelchair:
   a Open the bed for a hospital patient. Leave the bed closed for a nursing center resident.
   b Lower the bed to its lowest position.
9 Attach the signal light to the bed linens.
10 Decontaminate your hands.

ADMISSION NURSING ASSESSMENT
STATUS UPON ADMISSION

Admission Notes

Date of admission ____/____/____   Time _____ a.m. p.m.

Transported by _____

Accompanied by _____

Age _____ Sex _____ Weight _____ Height: _____ Ft. _____ In.

Vitals: T _____ P _____ (❑ Reg ❑ Irreg) R _____ B/P _____/_____

Attending physician notified? ❑ No ❑ Yes, date/time ____/____/____ _____ a.m. p.m.

Diagnosis: _____ Date last chest x-ray or PPD ____/____/____

Allergies

Meds _____

Food _____

Other _____

Skin Condition

Using the diagrams provided, indicate all body marks such as old/recent scars (surgical and other), bruises, discolorations, abrasions, pressure ulcers, or questionable markings. Indicate size, depth (in cms), color and drainage.

COMMENTS: _____

SPECIAL TREATMENTS & PROCEDURES: _____

PAIN
(As described by resident/representative)

Frequency:
❑ No pain   ❑ Daily, but not constant
❑ Less than daily   ❑ Constant

Location: _____

Intensity:
❑ No pain   ❑ Severe pain
❑ Mild pain   ❑ Horrible pain
❑ Distressing pain   ❑ Excruciating pain

Pain on admission:
❑ No   ❑ Yes, describe _____

RIGHT   LEFT

CURRENT STATUS

General Skin Condition

Check all that apply.
❑ Reddened   ❑ Pale   ❑ Jaundiced
❑ Cyanotic   ❑ Ashen
❑ Dry   ❑ Moist   ❑ Oily   ❑ Warm   ❑ Cold
❑ Edema, site _____

Physical Status (describe if applicable otherwise indicate NA)

Paralysis/paresis-site, degree _____
Contracture(s)-site, degree _____
Congenital anomalies _____
Prosthesis: _____
Other _____

Functional Status

TRANSFERS-ABLE TO TRANSFER
❑ Independently
❑ 1 person assist
❑ 2 person assist
❑ Total assist

WEIGHT BEARING-ABLE TO BEAR
❑ Full weight
❑ Partial weight
❑ Non-weight bearing

AMBULATION-ABLE TO AMBULATE
❑ Independently
❑ 1 person assist
❑ 2 person assist
❑ With device
Type _____
❑ Wheelchair only
❑ Wheelchair/propels self
❑ Bedrest

SUPPORTIVE DEVICES USED:
❑ Elastic hose   ❑ Footboard
❑ Bed cradle   ❑ Air mattress
❑ Sheepskin   ❑ Eggcrate
❑ Hand rolls   ❑ Sling   ❑ Trapeze
❑ Other _____
❑ Other _____

Drug Therapy

DRUG	DOSE/FREQUENCY	DRUG	DOSE/FREQUENCY
1		6	
2		7	
3		8	
4		9	
5		10	

NAME–Last	First	Middle	Attending Physician	Record No.	Room/Bed

CFS 5-3HH R1001 © 1992 Briggs Corporation, Des Moines, IA 50306 (800) 247-2343 PRINTED IN U.S.A.

ADMISSION NURSING ASSESSMENT
❑ Continued on Reverse

FIGURE 28-2 Admission form. (Courtesy Briggs Corp., Des Moines, Iowa.)
Continued

CURRENT STATUS - CONTINUED

Hearing	Right	Left	R & L	Vision	Right	Left	R & L	Communication
Adequate				Adequate				❏ Clear
Adequate w/aid				Adequate w/glasses				❏ Aphasic ❏ Dysphasic
Poor				Poor				Language(s) Spoken:
Deaf				Blind				

Oral Assessment | **Eating/Nutrition**

Complete oral cavity exam: ❏ Yes ❏ No
  If yes, condition _____
_____

Own teeth: ❏ Yes ❏ No
  If yes, condition _____

Dentures: Upper ❏ Comp ❏ Part
  Lower ❏ Comp ❏ Part
Do dentures fit? ❏ Yes ❏ No

❏ Dependent ❏ Independent ❏ Needs assist

❏ Dysphagic; reason _____

❏ Adaptive equipment (specify) _____

Type/consistency of diet _____
_____

Food likes _____

Food dislikes _____

Bev. preference _____

HS snack preferred: ❏ Yes ❏ No

Sleep Patterns	Bathing/Oral Hyg.	Indep.	Assist	Dep.	General Grooming	Indep.	Assist	Dep.
Usual bed time _____ a.m./p.m.	Tub				Shave			
Usual arising time _____ a.m./p.m.	Shower				Grooming			
Usual nap time _____ a.m./p.m.	Bed bath				Dressing			
Other _____	Oral hygiene				Shampoo			

Psychosocial Functioning

FAMILY RELATIONSHIPS:

Members visit (frequency) _____
_____

Closest relationship with _____
_____
_____

ORIENTED: ❏ Yes ❏ No, if No,
DISORIENTED TO: ❏ Time ❏ Place
  ❏ Person
RESIDENT GIVEN EXPLANATION OF/OR INVOLVED IN PLAN OF CARE? ❏ Yes ❏ No
RESIDENT ORIENTED TO FACILITY? ❏ Call light ❏ Bathroom ❏ Mealtime ❏ Activities

WHICH WORDS BEST DESCRIBE RESIDENT? ❏ Alert ❏ Angry ❏ Fearful
  ❏ Noisy ❏ Friendly ❏ Cooperative ❏ Lethargic ❏ _____
  ❏ Non-questioning ❏ Combative
ANSWERS QUESTIONS: ❏ Readily ❏ Reluctantly ❏ Inappropriately
MOOD: ❏ Passive ❏ Depressed ❏ Elated ❏ Quiet ❏ Secure
  ❏ Questioning ❏ Talkative ❏ Homesick ❏ Wanders mentally
  ❏ Hyperactive ❏ _____
COMPREHENSION: ❏ Slow ❏ Quick ❏ Unable to understand
MOTIVATION: ❏ Good ❏ Fair ❏ Poor
PERSONAL HABITS: Smokes? ❏ Yes ❏ No Uses alcohol? ❏ Yes ❏ No

Bowel and Bladder Evaluation

Uses: ❏ Toilet ❏ Urinal ❏ Bedpan ❏ Bedside commode
BOWEL HABITS: Continent? ❏ Yes ❏ No Constipated? ❏ Yes ❏ No Laxative used? ❏ Yes ❏ No
  Enemas used? ❏ Yes ❏ No Last bowel movement _____ a.m./p.m.
BLADDER HABITS: Continent? ❏ Yes ❏ No Dribbles? ❏ Yes ❏ No Catheter? ❏ Yes, type _____ ❏ No
  Urine color _____ Consistency _____ Time last voiding _____ a.m./p.m.

Restorative Programs Indicated | Therapy Indicated

Based on the foregoing assessment, check all that apply.

❏ ROM

❏ Splint or brace assistance

❏ Bed mobility training & skill practice

❏ Transfer training & skill practice

❏ Walking training & skill practice

❏ Dressing/grooming training & skill practice

❏ Eating/swallowing training & skill practice

❏ Appliance/prosthesis training & skill practice

❏ Communication training & skill practice

❏ Scheduled tolieting

❏ Bladder retraining

Comments: _____
_____

❏ Physical

❏ Occupational

❏ Speech

Comments: _____
_____
_____
_____
_____

Completed by:
Signature/Title _____ Date _____

NAME–Last	First	Middle	Attending Physician	Record No.	Room/Bed

ADMISSION NURSING ASSESSMENT

FIGURE 28-2, cont'd Admission form. (Courtesy Briggs Corp., Des Moines, Iowa.)

Admitting the Person

A nurse usually greets and escorts the person to the room. The nurse may ask you to do so if the person has no discomfort or distress.

Admission is your first chance to make a good impression. You must:

▶ Greet the person by name and title. Use the admission form to find out the person's name.

▶ Introduce yourself by name and title (Fig. 28-3). Do so to the person, family, and friends.

▶ Make roommate introductions.

▶ Act in a professional manner.

▶ Treat the person with dignity and respect.

See *Focus on Long-Term Care and Home Care: Admitting the Person.*

FOCUS ON **LONG-TERM CARE** AND **HOME CARE**

Admitting the Person

LONG-TERM CARE

Physical and mental comfort are important. So is feeling safe and secure. Do not rush to complete the admission procedures. Rather, treat the person and family as guests in your home. Offer them a beverage. Visit with them. Tell them some of the good things about the center.

Besides the roommate, introduce residents in nearby rooms. This way the person knows other residents. They can provide comfort and support. They understand, better than anyone else, what a nursing center is like.

The center is the person's home. Help make the room as home-like as possible. Also help the person unpack. Perhaps the person needs help putting clothes away. The person may want to hang pictures or display photos. Show caring and compassion. Help the person feel safe, comfortable, and secure. When the person is comfortable, complete the admission.

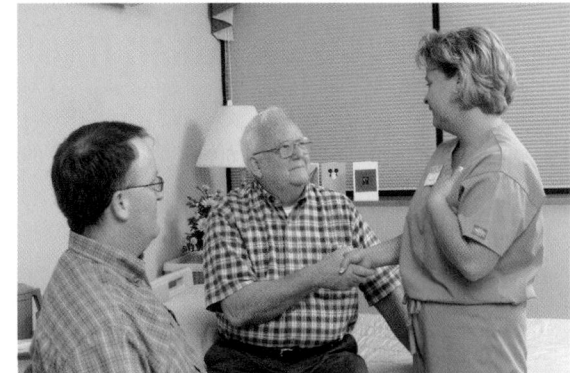

FIGURE 28-3 The nursing assistant introduces herself to the person and family member.

◄ The Admission Procedure

During the admission procedure you will:

- ► Collect some information for the admission form
- ► Measure the person's weight and height
- ► Measure the person's vital signs
- ► Obtain a urine specimen if one is ordered (Chapter 30)
- ► Complete a clothing and personal belongings list
- ► Orient the person to the room, the nursing unit, and the center

ADMITTING THE PERSON

■ ■ ■ ■ ■

✔ Quality of Life *Remember to:*

- Knock before entering the person's room.
- Address the person by name.
- Introduce yourself by name and title.
- Explain the procedure to the person before beginning and during the procedure.

- Protect the person's rights during the procedure.
- Handle the person gently during the procedure.

PRE-PROCEDURE

1 Follow *Delegation Guidelines: Admissions, Transfers, and Discharges*, p. 491. See *Promoting Safety and Comfort: Admissions, Transfers, and Discharges*, p. 491.

2 Practice hand hygiene.
3 Prepare the room. See procedure: *Preparing the Person's Room*, p. 492.

PROCEDURE

4 Check the person's name on the admission form.
5 Greet the person by name. Ask if he or she prefers a certain name.
6 Introduce yourself to the person and others present. Give your name and title. Explain that you assist the nurses in giving care.
7 Introduce the roommate.
8 Provide for privacy. Ask family or friends to leave the room. Tell them how much time you need, and direct them to the waiting area. Let a family member or friend stay if the person prefers.

9 Let the person stay dressed if his or her condition permits. Or help the person change into a gown or pajamas.
10 Provide for comfort. The person is in bed or in a chair as directed by the nurse.
11 Assist the nurse with assessment:
   a Measure vital signs (Chapter 25).
   b Measure weight and height (p. 496).
   c Collect information for the admission form as requested by the nurse.
12 Complete a clothing and personal belongings list (Chapter 11).

Continued

ADMITTING THE PERSON—cont'd

PROCEDURE—cont'd

13 Help the person put away clothes and personal items. Put them in the closet, drawers, and bedside stand. (The family may wish to help with this step.)

14 Explain ordered activity limits.

15 Obtain a urine specimen if ordered. Take the specimen to the storage area or laboratory. Clean equipment, and decontaminate your hands.

16 Orient the person to the area:
- Give names of the nurses.
- Identify items in the bedside stand. Explain the purpose of each.
- Explain how to use the overbed table.
- Show how to use the signal light.
- Show how to use the bed, TV, and light controls.
- Explain how to make phone calls. Place the phone within reach.
- Show the person the bathroom. Also show how to use the signal light in the bathroom.

- Explain visiting hours and policies.
- Explain where to find the nurses' station, lounge, chapel, dining room, and other areas.
- Identify staff—housekeeping, dietary, physical therapy, and others. Also identify students who are in the agency.
- Explain when meals and nourishments are served.

17 Fill the water pitcher and cup if oral fluids are allowed.

18 Place the signal light within reach.

19 Place other controls and needed items within reach.

20 Provide a denture container if needed. Label it with the person's name and room and bed number.

21 Label the person's property and personal care items for the nursing center resident. Items are labeled with the person's name.

POST-PROCEDURE

22 Provide for comfort. (See the inside of the front book cover.)

23 Lower the bed to its lowest position.

24 Raise or lower bed rails. Follow the care plan.

25 Complete a safety check of the room. (See the inside of the front book cover.)

26 Decontaminate your hands.

27 Report and record your observations.

◆ Measuring Weight and Height

Weight and height are measured on admission to the agency. Then the person is weighed daily, weekly, or monthly. This is done to measure weight gain or loss.

Standing, chair, bed, and lift scales are used (Fig. 28-4). Chair, bed, and lift scales are used for persons who cannot stand. Follow the manufacturer's instructions and agency procedures.

When measuring weight and height, follow these guidelines:

▶ The person only wears a gown or pajamas. Clothes add weight. No footwear is worn. Footwear adds to the weight and height measurement.

▶ The person voids before being weighed. A full bladder adds weight. If a urine specimen is needed, collect it at this time.

▶ Weigh the person at the same time of day. Before breakfast is the best time. Food and fluids add weight.

▶ Use the same scale for daily, weekly, and monthly weights. Scales weigh differently.

▶ Balance the scale at zero (0) before weighing the person. For balance scales, move the weights to zero. A digital scale should read at zero.

See *Teamwork and Time Management: Measuring Weight and Height.*

See *Delegation Guidelines: Measuring Weight and Height.*

See *Promoting Safety and Comfort: Measuring Weight and Height.*

TEAMWORK AND TIME MANAGEMENT

Measuring Weight and Height

Nursing units usually have just one standing scale. In some agencies, chair and lift scales are shared with other nursing units. Return the device to the storage area as quickly as possible. Do not have your co-workers wait or look for the scale.

DELEGATION GUIDELINES: Measuring Weight and Height

Before measuring weight and height, you need this information from the nurse and the care plan:
- When to measure weight and height
- What scale to use
- If height is measured with the person in bed (p. 499)
- When to report the measurements
- What specific patient and resident concerns to report at once

PROMOTING SAFETY AND COMFORT: Measuring Weight and Height

SAFETY

Follow the manufacturer's instructions when using chair, bed, or lift scales. Also follow the agency's procedures. Practice safety measures to prevent falls.

COMFORT

The person wears only a gown or pajamas for the weight measurement. Prevent chilling and drafts (Chapter 17).

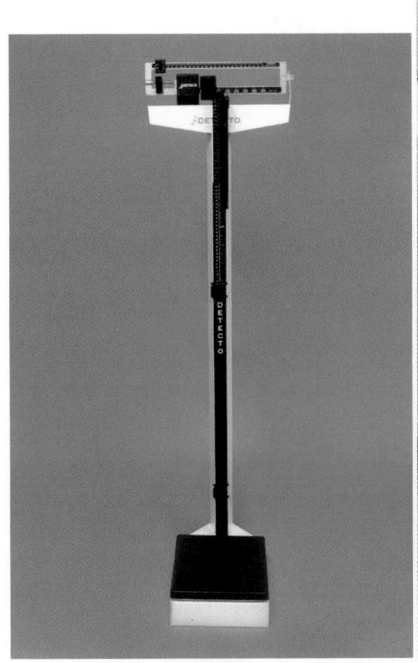
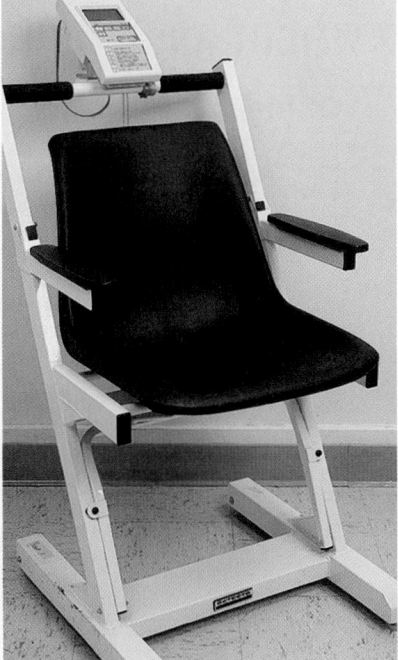
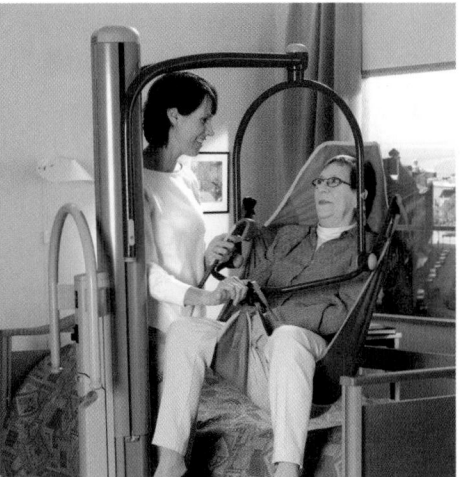

A   B   C

FIGURE 28-4 Types of scales. **A,** Standing scale. **B,** Chair scale. **C,** Lift scale. (**C,** Courtesy ARJO, Roselle, Ill., (800)323-1245.)

MEASURING WEIGHT AND HEIGHT

✔ Quality of Life *Remember to:*

- Knock before entering the person's room.
- Address the person by name.
- Introduce yourself by name and title.
- Explain the procedure to the person before beginning and during the procedure.

- Protect the person's rights during the procedure.
- Handle the person gently during the procedure.

PRE-PROCEDURE

1 Follow *Delegation Guidelines: Measuring Weight and Height.* See *Promoting Safety and Comfort: Measuring Weight and Height.*
2 Ask the person to void.
3 Practice hand hygiene.
4 Bring the scale and paper towels (for a standing scale) to the person's room.

5 Decontaminate your hands.
6 Identify the person. Check the ID bracelet against the assignment sheet. Also call the person by name.
7 Provide for privacy.

PROCEDURE

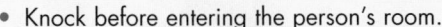

8 Place the paper towels on the scale platform.
9 Raise the height rod.
10 Move the weights to zero (0). The pointer is in the middle.
11 Have the person remove the robe and footwear. Assist as needed.
12 Help the person stand on the scale. The person stands in the center of the scale. Arms are at the sides.
13 Move the weights until the balance pointer is in the middle (Fig. 28-5, p. 498).
14 Note the weight on your notepad or assignment sheet.

15 Ask the person to stand very straight.
16 Lower the height rod until it rests on the person's head (Fig. 28-6, p. 498).
17 Note the height on your notepad or assignment sheet.
18 Raise the height rod. Help the person step off of the scale.
19 Help the person put on a robe and non-skid footwear if he or she will be up. Or help the person back to bed.
20 Lower the height rod. Adjust the weights to zero (0) if this is your agency's policy.

Continued

MEASURING WEIGHT AND HEIGHT—cont'd

POST-PROCEDURE

21 Provide for comfort. (See the inside of the front book cover.)
22 Place the signal light within reach.
23 Raise or lower bed rails. Follow the care plan.
24 Unscreen the person.
25 Complete a safety check of the room. (See the inside of the front book cover.)
26 Discard the paper towels.
27 Return the scale to its proper place.
28 Decontaminate your hands.
29 Report and record the measurements.

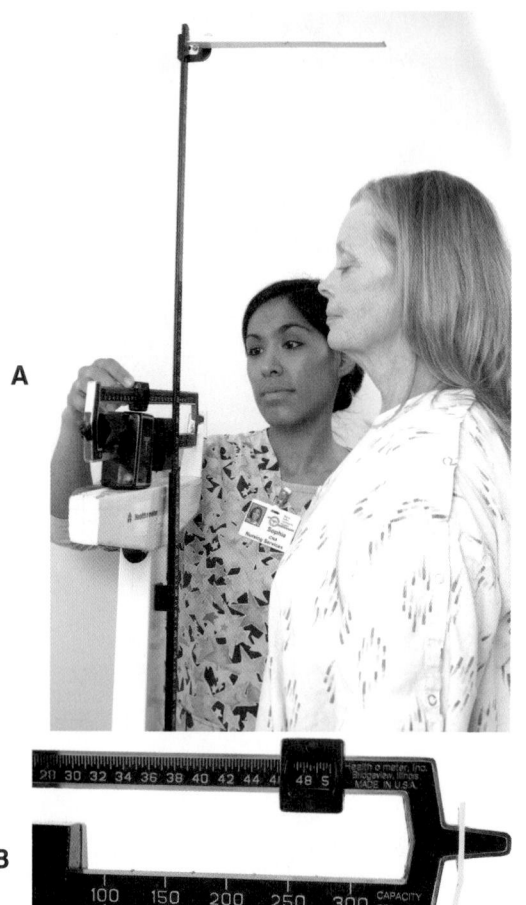

A

B

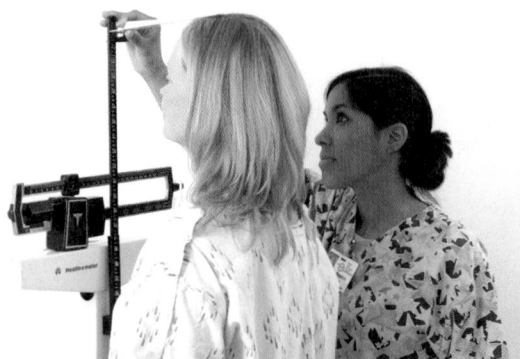

FIGURE 28-5 A, The person is weighed. **B,** The weight is read when the balance pointer is in the middle.

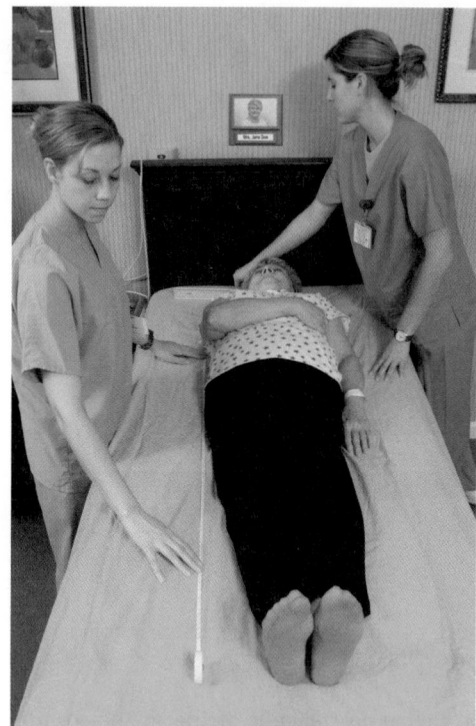

FIGURE 28-7 The person's height is measured in bed. The tape measure extends from the top of the head to the heel. The ruler is flat across the top of the person's head.

◆ TRANSFERS

A **transfer** is moving a person from one room or nursing unit to another. Reasons for transfers include:
► A change in condition
► The person requests a room change
► Roommates do not get along
► Changes in care needs

The doctor, nurse, or social worker explains the reasons for the transfer. The family and business office are told. You assist with the transfer or perform the entire procedure. The person is transported by wheelchair, stretcher, or the bed.

Support and reassure the person. The person does not know staff on the new unit. Use good communication skills.
► Avoid pat answers. "It will be OK" is an example.
► Use touch to provide comfort.
► Introduce the person to the staff and roommate.
► Wish the person well as you leave him or her.

FIGURE 28-6 Height is measured.

MEASURING HEIGHT—THE PERSON IS IN BED

✔ Quality of Life *Remember to:*

- Knock before entering the person's room.
- Address the person by name.
- Introduce yourself by name and title.
- Explain the procedure to the person before beginning and during the procedure.

- Protect the person's rights during the procedure.
- Handle the person gently during the procedure.

PRE-PROCEDURE

1 Follow *Delegation Guidelines: Measuring Weight and Height*, p. 496. See *Promoting Safety and Comfort: Measuring Weight and Height*, p. 496.
2 Practice hand hygiene.
3 Ask a co-worker to help you.
4 Collect a measuring tape and ruler.

5 Decontaminate your hands.
6 Identify the person. Check the ID bracelet against the assignment sheet. Also call the person by name.
7 Provide for privacy.
8 Raise the bed for good body mechanics. Bed rails are up if used.

PROCEDURE

9 Lower the bed rails if up.
10 Position the person supine if the position is allowed.
11 Have your co-worker hold the end of the measuring tape at the person's heel.
12 Pull the measuring tape along the person's body. Pull until it extends past the head (Fig. 28-7).

13 Place the ruler flat across the top of the person's head. It extends from the person's head to the measuring tape. Make sure the ruler is level.
14 Note the height on your notepad or assignment sheet.

POST-PROCEDURE

15 Provide for comfort. (See the inside of the front book cover.)
16 Place the signal light within reach.
17 Lower the bed to its lowest position.
18 Raise or lower bed rails. Follow the care plan.

19 Complete a safety check of the room. (See the inside of the front book cover.)
20 Return equipment to its proper place.
21 Decontaminate your hands.
22 Report and record the height.

TRANSFERRING THE PERSON TO ANOTHER NURSING UNIT

✔ Quality of Life *Remember to:*

- Knock before entering the person's room.
- Address the person by name.
- Introduce yourself by name and title.
- Explain the procedure to the person before beginning and during the procedure.

- Protect the person's rights during the procedure.
- Handle the person gently during the procedure.

PRE-PROCEDURE

1 Follow *Delegation Guidelines: Admissions, Transfers, and Discharges*, p. 491. See *Promoting Safety and Comfort: Admissions, Transfers, and Discharges*, p. 491.
2 Ask a co-worker to help you.
3 Practice hand hygiene.
4 Collect the following:
 - Wheelchair or stretcher
 - Utility cart
 - Bath blanket

5 Decontaminate your hands.
6 Identify the person. Check the ID bracelet against the assignment sheet. Call the person by name.
7 Provide for privacy.

Continued

TRANSFERRING THE PERSON TO ANOTHER NURSING UNIT—cont'd

PROCEDURE

8 Collect the person's belongings and care equipment. Place them on the utility cart.
9 Transfer the person to a wheelchair or stretcher (Chapter 16). Cover him or her with the bath blanket.
10 Transport the person to the new room. Your co-worker brings the utility cart.
11 Help transfer the person to the bed or chair. Help position the person (Chapter 15).

12 Help arrange the person's belongings and equipment.
13 Report the following to the receiving nurse:
- How the person tolerated the transfer
- Any observations made during the transfer
- That the nurse will bring the medical record, care plan, Kardex, and drugs

POST-PROCEDURE

14 Return the wheelchair or stretcher and the utility cart to the storage area.
15 Decontaminate your hands.
16 Report and record the following:
- The time of the transfer
- Who helped you with the transfer
- Where the person was taken
- How the person was transferred (bed, wheelchair, or stretcher)
- How the person tolerated the transfer

- Who received the person
- Any other observations
17 Strip the bed, and clean the unit. Decontaminate your hands, and put on gloves for this step. (The housekeeping staff may do this step.)
18 Remove the gloves. Decontaminate your hands.
19 Follow agency policy for dirty linen.
20 Make a closed bed.
21 Decontaminate your hands.

◀ DISCHARGES

Discharges are usually planned in advance. **Discharge** is the official departure of a person from an agency. This is a happy time if the person is going home. Some persons go to another hospital or nursing center. Others need home care.

The health team plans the discharge. They teach the person and family about diet, exercise, and drugs. They also teach them about procedures and treatments. They arrange for home care, equipment, and therapies as needed. A doctor's appointment is given.

The nurse tells you when to start the discharge procedure. The doctor must write a discharge order before the person can leave. The nurse tells you when the person may leave and how to transport him or her. Usually a wheelchair is used. Some agencies let the person walk if able. If leaving by ambulance, a stretcher is used.

Use good communication skills when assisting with a discharge. Wish the person and family well as they leave the agency.

A person may want to leave the agency without the doctor's permission. Tell the nurse at once of the wish or intent to leave. The nurse or social worker handles the matter.

DISCHARGING THE PERSON

✔ Quality of Life *Remember to:*

- Knock before entering the person's room.
- Address the person by name.
- Introduce yourself by name and title.
- Explain the procedure to the person before beginning and during the procedure.

- Protect the person's rights during the procedure.
- Handle the person gently during the procedure.

PRE-PROCEDURE

1 Follow *Delegation Guidelines: Admissions, Transfers, and Discharges,* p. 491. See *Promoting Safety and Comfort: Admissions, Transfers, and Discharges,* p. 491.
2 Ask a co-worker to help you.
3 Practice hand hygiene.

4 Identify the person. Check the ID bracelet against the assignment sheet. Also call the person by name.
5 Provide for privacy.

DISCHARGING THE PERSON—cont'd

PROCEDURE

6 Help the person dress as needed.

7 Help the person pack. Check all drawers and closets. Make sure all items are collected.

8 Check off the clothing list and personal belongings list. Give the lists to the nurse.

9 Tell the nurse that the person is ready for the final visit. The nurse:
- Gives prescriptions written by the doctor
- Provides discharge instructions
- Gets valuables from the safe
- Has the person sign the clothing and personal belongings lists

10 Get a wheelchair and a utility cart for the person's items. Ask a co-worker to help you.

11 Help the person into the wheelchair.

12 Take the person to the exit area.

13 Lock the wheelchair wheels.

14 Help the person out of the wheelchair and into the car.

15 Help put the person's items into the car.

POST-PROCEDURE

16 Return the wheelchair and cart to the storage area.

17 Decontaminate your hands.

18 Report and record the following:
- The time of the discharge
- Who helped you with the discharge
- How the person was transported
- Who was with the person
- The person's destination
- Any other observations

19 Strip the bed, and clean the unit. Decontaminate your hands, and put on gloves for this step. (The housekeeping staff may do this step.)

20 Remove the gloves. Decontaminate your hands.

21 Follow agency policy for dirty linen.

22 Make a closed bed.

23 Decontaminate your hands.

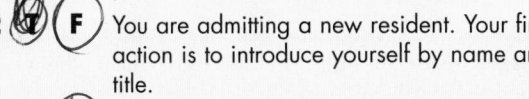

REVIEW QUESTIONS

Circle T if the statement is true and F if it is false.

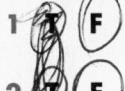

1 T **F** Identifying information is obtained when the person arrives on the nursing unit.

2 T **F** You are admitting a new resident. Your first action is to introduce yourself by name and title.

3 T **F** A person arrives at the agency by ambulance. You transport the person to his or her room.

4 **T** F The person is greeted by name and title during the admission process.

5 **T** F Vital signs are measured during the admission procedure.

6 T **F** You explain the resident's rights to the person and family.

7 T **F** A person complains of pain. Report the complaint after the admission form is complete.

8 T **F** The person arrives by stretcher. You make an occupied bed.

9 **T** F You help orient the person to the new setting.

10 T **F** A robe and footwear are worn when measuring weight.

11 T **F** A robe and footwear are worn when measuring height.

12 **T** F Clothing and personal belongings lists are made during the admission process.

13 **T** F A person's condition may require a transfer to another nursing unit.

14 **T** F A doctor's order is required for discharge from the agency.

15 T **F** You teach the person about diet and drugs.

16 **T** F Starting with admission, the person's rights are protected.

17 **T** F A person with dementia may become more confused in a new setting.

18 **T** F A person objects to a transfer. An ombudsman makes sure the person's rights are protected.

Answers to these questions are on p. 781.

Assisting With the Physical Examination

OBJECTIVES

- Define the key terms listed in this chapter
- Explain what to do before, during, and after an examination (exam)
- Identify the equipment used for an exam
- Describe how to prepare and drape a person for an exam
- Explain the rules for assisting with an exam
- Perform the procedure described in this chapter

PROCEDURES

- Preparing the Person For an Examination

KEY TERMS

dorsal recumbent position The supine position with the legs together; horizontal recumbent position

horizontal recumbent position The dorsal recumbent position

knee-chest position The person kneels and rests the body on the knees and chest; the head is turned to one side, the arms are above the head or flexed at the elbows, the back is straight, and the body is flexed about 90 degrees at the hips

laryngeal mirror An instrument used to examine the mouth, teeth, and throat

lithotomy position The woman lies on her back with her hips at the edge of the exam table, her knees are flexed, her hips are externally rotated, and her feet are in stirrups

nasal speculum An instrument used to examine the inside of the nose

ophthalmoscope A lighted instrument used to examine the internal structures of the eye

otoscope A lighted instrument used to examine the external ear and the eardrum (tympanic membrane)

percussion hammer An instrument used to tap body parts to test reflexes; reflex hammer

tuning fork An instrument vibrated to test hearing

vaginal speculum An instrument used to open the vagina so it and the cervix can be examined

Doctors and many RNs perform physical exams. You may need to assist them. Exams are done to:
- Promote health
- Determine fitness for work
- Diagnose disease

YOUR ROLE

What you do depends on agency policies and procedures. It also depends on the examiner's preferences. You may do some or all of the following:
- Collect linens to drape the person for the procedure.
- Collect exam equipment and supplies.
- Prepare the room for the exam.
- Provide lighting.
- Transport the person to and from the exam room.
- Measure vital signs, weight, and height.
- Position and drape the person.
- Hand equipment and supplies to the examiner.
- Label specimen containers.
- Discard used supplies.
- Clean equipment.
- Help the person dress or to a comfortable position after the exam.
- Follow agency policy for soiled linens.

EQUIPMENT

Some items needed for an exam are used to give care. You need to know the instruments in Figure 29-1:
- **Laryngeal mirror**—used to examine the mouth, teeth, and throat.
- **Nasal speculum**—used to examine the inside of the nose.
- **Ophthalmoscope**—a lighted instrument used to examine the internal structures of the eye.
- **Otoscope**—a lighted instrument used to examine the external ear and the eardrum (tympanic membrane). Some scopes have parts for examining eyes and ears. They are changed into an ophthalmoscope or otoscope.
- **Percussion hammer**—used to tap body parts to test reflexes. It is also called a *reflex hammer*.
- **Tuning fork**—vibrated to test hearing.
- **Vaginal speculum**—used to open the vagina so it and the cervix can be examined.

Some agencies have exam trays in the supply department. If not, collect the items listed in the procedure: *Preparing the Person for an Examination*, p. 504. Arrange them on a tray or table.

◆ PREPARING THE PERSON

The physical exam concerns many people. They worry about possible findings. Some are confused or fearful about what the examiner will do. Discomfort, embarrassment, fearing exposure, and not knowing the procedure cause anxiety. You must be sensitive to the person's feelings and concerns. The person is prepared physically and

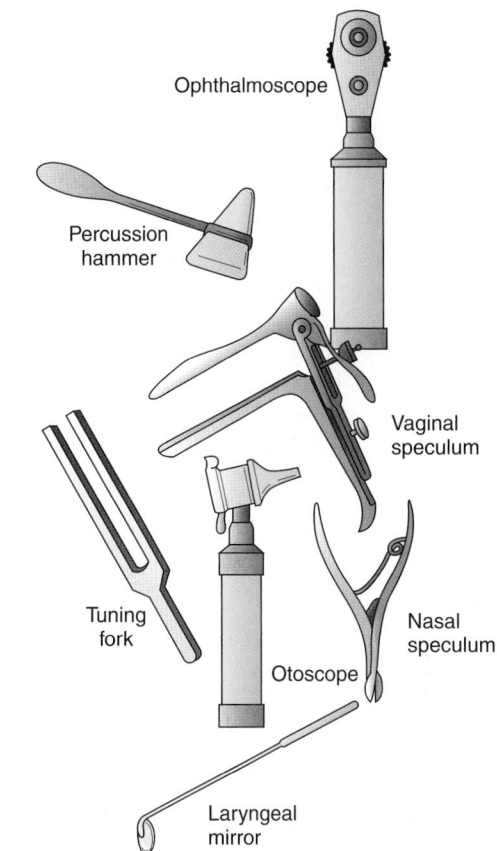

FIGURE 29-1 Instruments used for a physical exam.

mentally for the exam. The nurse explains its purpose and what to expect.

Privacy is protected. The person is screened and the room door is closed. All clothes are removed for a complete exam. Usually a patient gown is worn. It reduces the naked feeling and the fear of exposure. So does covering the person with a drape—paper drape, bath blanket, sheet, or drawsheet. Explain that there is little exposure during the exam. Only the part being examined is exposed.

The person voids before the exam. An empty bladder lets the examiner feel the abdominal organs. A full bladder can change the normal position and shape of organs. It also causes discomfort, especially when the abdominal organs are felt. If a urine specimen is needed, obtain it at this time. Explain how to collect the specimen (Chapter 30). Label the container.

Measure weight and height (Chapter 28) and vital signs (Chapter 25) before the exam starts. Record the measurements on the exam form. Then drape and position the person for the exam.

See *Focus on Children and Older Persons: Preparing the Person*, p. 504.

See *Delegation Guidelines: Preparing the Person*, p. 504.

See *Promoting Safety and Comfort: Preparing the Person*, p. 504.

FOCUS ON **CHILDREN** AND **OLDER PERSONS**

Preparing the Person

CHILDREN

Babies are undressed for a physical exam. Leave diapers on baby boys to prevent urine sprays. Toddlers, preschool children, and school-age children can wear underpants. The pants are lowered or removed as needed during the exam.

OLDER PERSONS

In nursing centers, residents have an exam at least once a year. The resident has the right to personal choice. The doctor or nurse tells the person about the exam. Reasons for it are given. The person is told who will do the exam and when it will be done. The procedure is explained. The exam is done only with the person's consent. The person may want a different examiner. Or the person may want a family member present during the exam and when the results are explained.

DELEGATION GUIDELINES: Preparing the Person

To prepare a person for an exam, you need this information from the nurse and the care plan:
- When to prepare the person
- Where the exam will be done—an exam room or the person's room
- How to position the person
- What equipment and supplies are needed
- If a urine specimen is needed
- What specific patient or resident concerns to report at once

PROMOTING SAFETY AND COMFORT: Preparing the Person

SAFETY

Protect the person from falls and injury. Do not leave the person unattended.

COMFORT

Warmth is a major concern during an exam. Protect the person from chilling. Have an extra bath blanket nearby. Also, take measures to prevent drafts.

PREPARING THE PERSON FOR AN EXAMINATION

✔ Quality of Life *Remember to:*

- Knock before entering the person's room.
- Address the person by name.
- Introduce yourself by name and title.
- Explain the procedure to the person before beginning and during the procedure.

- Protect the person's rights during the procedure.
- Handle the person gently during the procedure.

PRE-PROCEDURE

1 Follow *Delegation Guidelines: Preparing the Person.* See *Promoting Safety and Comfort: Preparing the Person.*
2 Practice hand hygiene.
3 Collect the following:
- Flashlight
- Sphygmomanometer
- Stethoscope
- Thermometer
- Tongue depressors (blades)
- Laryngeal mirror
- Ophthalmoscope
- Otoscope
- Nasal speculum
- Percussion (reflex) hammer
- Tuning fork
- Tape measure
- Gloves
- Water-soluble lubricant
- Vaginal speculum
- Cotton-tipped applicators
- Specimen containers and labels

- Disposable bag
- Kidney basin
- Towel
- Bath blanket
- Tissues
- Drape (sheet, bath blanket, drawsheet, or paper drape)
- Paper towels
- Cotton balls
- Waterproof pad
- Eye chart (Snellen chart)
- Slides
- Gown
- Alcohol wipes
- Wastebasket
- Container for soiled instruments
- Marking pencils or pens
4 Decontaminate your hands.
5 Identify the person. Check the ID bracelet against the assignment sheet. Also call the person by name.
6 Provide for privacy.

PREPARING THE PERSON FOR AN EXAMINATION—cont'd

PROCEDURE

7 Have the person put on the gown. Tell the person to remove all clothes. Assist as needed.

8 Ask the person to void. Offer the bedpan, commode, or urinal if necessary. Provide for privacy.

9 Transport the person to the exam room. (This is not done for an exam in the person's room.)

10 Measure weight and height (Chapter 28). Record the measurements on the exam form.

11 Help the person onto the exam table. Provide a step stool if necessary. (Omit this step for an exam in the person's room.)

12 Raise the far bed rail (if used). Raise the bed to its highest level. (This step is not done if an exam table is used.)

13 Measure vital signs. Record them on the exam form.

14 Position the person as directed.

15 Drape the person.

16 Place a waterproof pad under the buttocks.

17 Raise the bed rail near you (if used).

18 Provide adequate lighting.

19 Put the signal light on for the examiner. Do not leave the person alone.

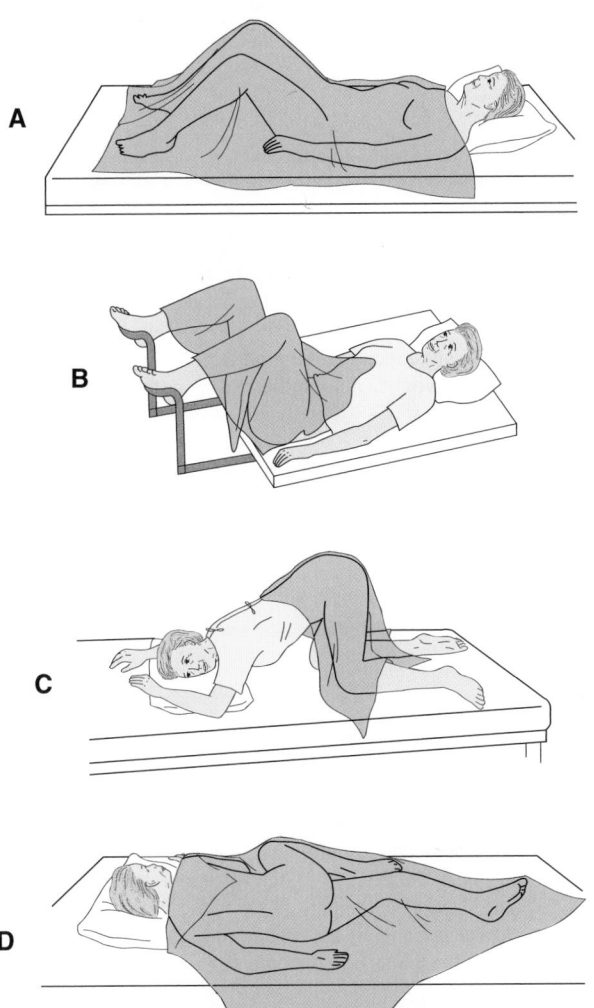

FIGURE 29-2 Positioning and draping for the physical exam. **A,** Dorsal recumbent position. **B,** Lithotomy position. **C,** Knee-chest position. **D,** Sims' position.

POSITIONING AND DRAPING

Sometimes a special position is needed for the exam. Some positions are uncomfortable and embarrassing. The examiner tells you how to position the person. Before helping the person assume and maintain the position, explain the following:

▶ Why the position is needed
▶ How to assume the position
▶ How the body is draped for warmth and privacy
▶ How long to expect to stay in the position

The **dorsal recumbent position** is used to examine the abdomen, chest, and breasts. It is also called the **horizontal recumbent position**. The person is supine with the legs together. To examine the perineal area, the knees are flexed and hips externally rotated. Drape the person as in Figure 29-2, A.

The **lithotomy position** (Fig. 29-2, B) is used to examine the vagina. The woman lies on her back. Her hips are at the edge of the exam table. Her knees are flexed and her hips externally rotated. Her feet are in stirrups. Drape the person as for perineal care (Chapter 19). Some agencies provide socks to cover the feet and calves. Some women cannot assume this position. If so, the examiner tells you how to position the woman.

The **knee-chest position** (Fig. 29-2, C) is used to examine the rectum. Sometimes it is used to examine the vagina. The person kneels and rests the body on the knees and chest. The head is turned to one side. The arms are above the head or flexed at the elbows. The back is straight. The body is flexed about 90 degrees at the hips. Apply the drape in a diamond shape to cover the back, buttocks, and thighs. The person wears a gown and sometimes socks.

The Sims' position (Fig. 29-2, D) is sometimes used to examine the rectum or vagina (Chapter 15). Apply the drape in a diamond shape. The examiner folds back the near corner to expose the rectum or vagina.

See *Focus on Children and Older Persons: Positioning and Draping*, p. 506.

ASSISTING WITH THE EXAM

You may be asked to prepare, position, and drape the person. And you might assist the doctor or RN during the exam. To assist with the exam, follow the rules in Box 29-1.

See *Focus on Children and Older Persons: Assisting With the Exam.*

See *Focus on Communication: Assisting With the Exam.*

After the Exam

After the exam, the person dresses or returns to bed. Lubricant is used to examine the vagina or rectum. The area is wiped or cleaned before the person dresses or returns to the room. Assist as needed. You also need to:

- Discard disposable items—waterproof pad, drape, tongue blades, cotton balls, and so on.
- Replace supplies so the tray is ready for the next exam.
- Clean reusable items according to agency policy. Return them to the tray or storage area. This includes the otoscope and ophthalmoscope tips and stethoscope.
- Send the speculum to the supply area for sterilization.
- Cover the exam table with a clean drawsheet or paper.

- Label specimens. Take them to the designated area with a requisition slip.
- Clean and straighten the person's unit or exam room.
- Follow agency policy for soiled linens.

See *Teamwork and Time Management: After the Exam.*

REVIEW QUESTIONS

Circle the BEST answer.

1 The otoscope is used to examine
  a Internal structures of the eye
  b The external ear and the eardrum
  c Reflexes
  d The vagina

2 You are preparing a person for an exam. You should do the following *except*
  a Ask the person to void
  b Ask the person to undress
  c Drape the person
  d Go tell the nurse when the person is ready

3 Which part of an exam can you do?
  a Test reflexes
  b Inspect the mouth, teeth, and throat
  c Measure weight, height, and vital signs
  d Observe the perineum and rectum

4 A person is supine. The hips are flexed and externally rotated. The feet are supported in stirrups. The person is in the
  a Dorsal recumbent position
  b Lithotomy position
  c Knee-chest position
  d Sims' position

5 You will assist with Mrs. Janz's exam. Which is *false?*
  a Hand hygiene is practiced before and after the exam.
  b Instruments are placed near the examiner.
  c A male nursing team member stays in the room.
  d Provide for privacy by screening, closing the door, and proper draping.

Answers to these questions are on p. 781.

Collecting and Testing Specimens

OBJECTIVES

- Define the key terms and key abbreviations listed in this chapter
- Explain why urine, stool, sputum, and blood specimens are collected
- Explain the rules for collecting specimens
- Describe the different types of urine specimens
- Describe the equipment used for blood glucose testing
- Identify the sites used for skin punctures
- Perform the procedures described in this chapter

PROCEDURES

- Collecting a Random Urine Specimen
- Collecting a Midstream Specimen
- Collecting a 24-Hour Urine Specimen
- Collecting a Double-Voided Specimen
- Collecting a Urine Specimen From the Infant or Child
- Testing Urine With Reagent Strips

- Straining Urine
- Collecting a Stool Specimen
- Testing a Stool Specimen For Blood
- Collecting a Sputum Specimen
- Measuring Blood Glucose

KEY TERMS

acetone A substance that appears in urine from the rapid breakdown of fat for energy; ketone body or ketone

glucosuria Sugar *(glucos)* in the urine *(uria)*; glycosuria

glycosuria Sugar *(glycos)* in the urine *(uria)*; glucosuria

hematoma A swelling *(oma)* that contains blood *(hemat)*

hematuria Blood *(hemat)* in the urine *(uria)*

hemoptysis Bloody *(hemo)* sputum *(ptysis* means to *spit)*

ketone Acetone, ketone body

ketone body Acetone; ketone

melena A black, tarry stool

sputum Mucus from the respiratory system that is expectorated *(expelled)* through the mouth

KEY ABBREVIATIONS

I&O Intake and output

mL Milliliter

MSDS Material safety data sheet

oz Ounce

TB Tuberculosis

Specimens *(samples)* are collected and tested to prevent, detect, and treat disease. The doctor orders what specimen to collect and the test needed. Most specimens are tested in the laboratory. All specimens sent to the laboratory require requisition slips. The slip has the person's identifying information and the test ordered. And the specimen container is labeled according to agency policy. Some tests are done at the bedside. When collecting specimens, follow the rules in Box 30-1.

See *Teamwork and Time Management: Collecting and Testing Specimens.*

BOX 30-1 Rules For Collecting Specimens

- Follow the rules of medical asepsis.
- Follow Standard Precautions and the Bloodborne Pathogen Standard.
- Use a clean container for each specimen.
- Use the correct container.
- Do not touch the inside of the container or lid.
- Identify the person. Check the ID bracelet against the laboratory requisition slip or assignment sheet. Compare *all* information.
- Label the container in the person's presence. Provide accurate information.
- Collect the specimen at the correct time.
- Ask the person not to have a bowel movement when collecting a urine specimen. The specimen must not contain stools.
- Ask the person to void before collecting a stool specimen. The specimen must not contain urine.
- Ask the person to put toilet tissue in the toilet or wastebasket. Urine and stool specimens must not contain tissue.
- Place the specimen container in a plastic bag. Do not let the container touch the outside of the bag. Apply a BIOHAZARD label according to agency policy.
- Take the specimen and requisition slip to the laboratory. Or take it to the storage area.

URINE SPECIMENS

Urine specimens are collected for urine tests. Follow the rules in Box 30-1.

See *Focus on Children and Older Persons: Urine Specimens,* p. 510.

See *Delegation Guidelines: Urine Specimens,* p. 510.

See *Promoting Safety and Comfort: Urine Specimens,* p. 510.

◆ The Random Urine Specimen

The random urine specimen is collected for a routine urinalysis. It is collected any time during a 24-hour period. Many people can collect the specimen themselves. Weak and very ill persons need help.

TEAMWORK AND TIME MANAGEMENT

Collecting and Testing Specimens

Nursing centers do not have laboratories on-site. A nursing center contracts with a laboratory for its services. Specimens are sent to that laboratory for study or analysis.

The nursing center has a storage area for specimens. A driver picks up specimens at a certain time and transports them to the laboratory.

You need to have ordered specimens collected and in the storage area by the pick-up time. If the specimen is not yet collected, the results are delayed at least one day. This can cause the person harm. If the specimen was not collected in time, it may need to be discarded. If discarded, another is collected the next day. This also causes a delay in the results and can cause the person harm. And more supplies and equipment are needed. This costs the person more money.

FOCUS ON **CHILDREN** AND **OLDER PERSONS**

Urine Specimens

CHILDREN

For infants and toddlers who are not toilet-trained, a collection is bag is applied to the genital area (p. 515). It is hard for toilet-trained toddlers and young children to void on request and into a collection device. Potty chairs and specimen pans are useful. Remember to use terms the child understands. "Pee pee," "wee, wee," "potty," and "tinkle" are examples.

The nurse may ask you to give the child water or other fluids when a urine specimen is needed. Usually the child needs to void about 30 minutes after drinking fluids.

Urine specimens may embarrass older children and teenagers. They do not like clear specimen containers that show urine. Placing the urine specimen container in a paper bag is often helpful.

DELEGATION GUIDELINES: Urine Specimens

Before collecting a urine specimen, you need this information from the nurse:
- If the person uses the toilet, bedpan, urinal, or commode for voiding
- The type of specimen needed
- What time to collect the specimen
- What special measures are needed
- If you need to test the specimen (p. 517)
- If measuring intake and output (I&O) is ordered
- What observations to report and record:
  - Problems obtaining the specimen
  - Color, clarity, and odor of urine
  - Particles in the urine
  - Complaints of pain, burning, urgency, dysuria, or other problems
  - The time the specimen was collected or when the 24-hour urine specimen was started
- When to report observations
- What specific patient or resident concerns to report at once

PROMOTING SAFETY AND COMFORT: Urine Specimens

SAFETY

Microbes can grow in urine. Urine also may contain blood. Follow Standard Precautions and the Bloodborne Pathogen Standard.

COMFORT

Urine specimens may embarrass some people. They do not like clear specimen containers that show urine. Placing the urine specimen container in a paper bag is often helpful.

COLLECTING A RANDOM URINE SPECIMEN

✔ Quality of Life *Remember to:*

- Knock before entering the person's room.
- Address the person by name.
- Introduce yourself by name and title.
- Explain the procedure to the person before beginning and during the procedure.

- Protect the person's rights during the procedure.
- Handle the person gently during the procedure.

PRE-PROCEDURE

1 Follow *Delegation Guidelines: Urine Specimens.* See *Promoting Safety and Comfort: Urine Specimens.*
2 Practice hand hygiene.
3 Collect the following before going to the person's room:
   - Laboratory requisition slip
   - Specimen container and lid
   - Specimen label
   - Plastic bag
   - BIOHAZARD label (if needed)
4 Arrange collected items in the person's bathroom.

5 Decontaminate your hands.
6 Identify the person. Check the ID bracelet against the requisition slip. Also call the person by name.
7 Label the container in the person's presence.
8 Put on gloves.
9 Collect the following:
   - Voiding receptacle—bedpan and cover, urinal, commode, or specimen pan (Fig. 30-1)
   - Graduate to measure output
   - Gloves
10 Provide for privacy.

COLLECTING A RANDOM URINE SPECIMEN—cont'd

PROCEDURE

11 Ask the person to void into the receptacle. Remind him or her to put toilet tissue into the wastebasket or toilet. Toilet tissue is not put in the bedpan or specimen pan.
12 Take the receptacle to the bathroom.
13 Pour about 120 mL (milliliters) (4 ounces [oz]) into the specimen container.
14 Place the lid on the specimen container. Put the container in the plastic bag. Do not let the container touch the outside of the bag. Apply a BIOHAZARD label according to agency policy.

15 Measure urine if I&O are ordered. Include the amount in the specimen container.
16 Empty, clean, and disinfect equipment. Return equipment to its proper place.
17 Remove the gloves, and practice hand hygiene. Put on clean gloves.
18 Assist with hand washing.
19 Remove the gloves. Practice hand hygiene.

POST-PROCEDURE

20 Provide for comfort. (See the inside of the front book cover.)
21 Place the signal light within reach.
22 Raise or lower bed rails. Follow the care plan.
23 Unscreen the person.
24 Complete a safety check of the room. (See the inside of the front book cover.)

25 Decontaminate your hands.
26 Take the specimen and the requisition slip to the laboratory or storage area. Wear gloves.
27 Report and record your observations.

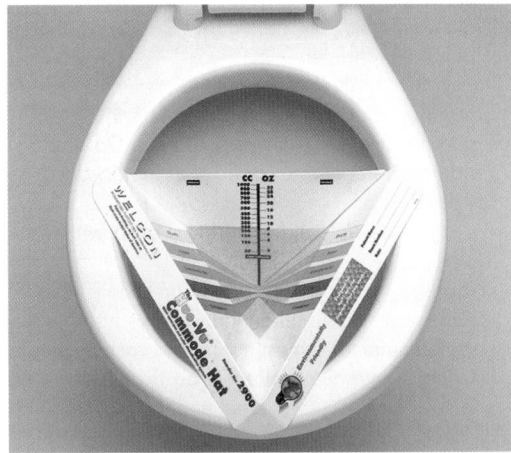

FIGURE 30-1 The specimen pan is placed at the front of the toilet on the toilet rim. It has a color chart for urine. (Courtesy Welcon, Inc., Forth Worth, Tex.)

◆ The Midstream Specimen

The midstream specimen is also called a *clean-voided specimen* or *clean-catch specimen*. The perineal area is cleaned before collecting the specimen. This reduces the number of microbes in the urethral area. The person starts to void into a receptacle. Then the persons stops the stream of urine, and a sterile specimen container is positioned. The person voids into the container until the specimen is obtained.

Stopping the stream of urine is hard for many people. You may need to position and hold the specimen container in place after the person starts to void (Fig. 30-2).

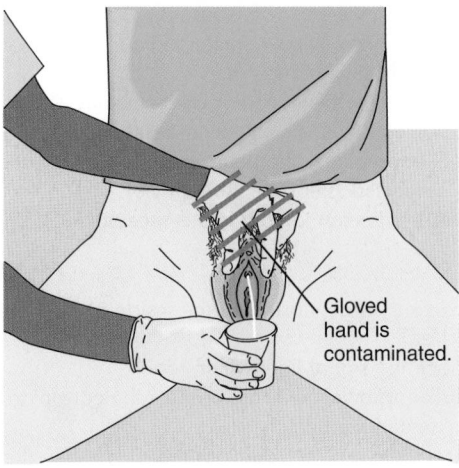

Gloved hand is contaminated.

FIGURE 30-2 The labia are separated to collect a midstream specimen.

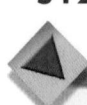

COLLECTING A MIDSTREAM SPECIMEN

✔ Quality of Life *Remember to:*

- Knock before entering the person's room.
- Address the person by name.
- Introduce yourself by name and title.
- Explain the procedure to the person before beginning and during the procedure.

- Protect the person's rights during the procedure.
- Handle the person gently during the procedure.

PRE-PROCEDURE

1 Follow *Delegation Guidelines: Urine Specimens,* p. 510. See *Promoting Safety and Comfort: Urine Specimens,* p. 510.
2 Practice hand hygiene.
3 Collect the following before going to the person's room:
   - Laboratory requisition slip
   - Midstream specimen kit—includes specimen container, label, and towelettes and may include sterile gloves
   - Plastic bag
   - Sterile gloves (if not part of the kit)
   - BIOHAZARD label (if needed)

4 Arrange your work area.
5 Decontaminate your hands.
6 Identify the person. Check the ID bracelet against the requisition slip. Also call the person by name.
7 Put on disposable gloves.
8 Collect the following:
   - Voiding receptacle—bedpan and cover, urinal, commode, or specimen pan if needed
   - Supplies for perineal care
   - Graduate to measure output
   - Disposable gloves
   - Paper towel
9 Provide for privacy.

PROCEDURE

10 Provide perineal care. (Wear gloves for this step. Decontaminate your hands after removing them.)
11 Open the sterile kit.
12 Put on the sterile gloves.
13 Open the packet of towelettes inside the kit.
14 Open the sterile specimen container. Do not touch the inside of the container or lid. Set the lid down so the inside is up.
15 *For a female*—clean the perineal area with the towelettes.
   a Spread the labia with your thumb and index finger. Use your non-dominant hand. (This hand is now contaminated. It must not touch anything sterile.)
   b Clean down the urethral area from front to back. Use a clean towelette for each stroke.
   c Keep the labia separated to collect the urine specimen (steps 17 through 20).
16 *For a male*—clean the penis with the towelettes.
   a Hold the penis with your non-dominant hand. (This hand is now contaminated. It must not touch anything sterile.)
   b Clean the penis starting at the meatus. Clean in a circular motion. Start at the center and work outward.
   c Keep holding the penis until the specimen is collected (steps 17 through 20).
17 Ask the person to void into a receptacle.

18 Pass the specimen container into the stream of urine. Keep the labia separated (see Fig. 30-2).
19 Collect about 30 to 60 mL (1 to 2 ounces [oz]) of urine.
20 Remove the specimen container before the person stops voiding.
21 Release the labia or penis. Let the person finish voiding into the receptacle.
22 Put the lid on the specimen container. Touch only the outside of the container and lid. Wipe the outside of the container. Set the container on a paper towel.
23 Provide toilet tissue after the person is done voiding.
24 Take the receptacle to the bathroom.
25 Measure urine if I&O are ordered. Include the amount in the specimen container.
26 Empty, clean, and disinfect equipment. Return equipment to its proper place.
27 Remove the gloves, and practice hand hygiene. Put on clean disposable gloves.
28 Label the specimen container in the person's presence. Place the container in the plastic bag. Do not let the container touch the outside of the bag. Apply a BIOHAZARD label according to agency policy.
29 Assist with hand washing.
30 Remove the gloves. Practice hand hygiene.

POST-PROCEDURE

31 Provide for comfort. (See the inside of the front book cover.)
32 Place the signal light within reach.
33 Raise or lower bed rails. Follow the care plan.
34 Unscreen the person.
35 Complete a safety check of the room. (See the inside of the front book cover.)

36 Decontaminate your hands.
37 Take the specimen and the requisition slip to the laboratory or storage area. Wear gloves.
38 Report and record your observations.

The 24-Hour Urine Specimen

All urine voided during a 24-hour period is collected for a 24-hour urine specimen. Urine is chilled on ice or refrigerated during this time. This prevents the growth of microbes. A preservative is added to the collection container for some tests.

The person voids to begin the test with an empty bladder. Discard this voiding. Save *all voidings* for the next 24 hours. The person and nursing staff must clearly understand the procedure and the test period. The test is restarted if:

▶ A voiding was not saved
▶ Toilet tissue was discarded into the specimen
▶ The specimen contains feces

See *Promoting Safety and Comfort: The 24-Hour Urine Specimen.*

PROMOTING SAFETY AND COMFORT: The 24-Hour Urine Specimen

SAFETY

The collection container or preservative may contain an acid. Do not get the preservative or urine from the container on your skin or in your eyes. If you do, flush your skin or eyes with a large amount of water. Tell the nurse what happened and check the material safety data sheet (MSDS) (Chapter 11). Also complete an incident report.

The specimen is kept chilled to prevent the growth of microbes. If not refrigerated, the urine collection container is placed in a bucket with ice. Add ice to the bucket as needed.

Assist the person with hand washing after every voiding. This prevents the spread of microbes that may be in the urine.

COLLECTING A 24-HOUR URINE SPECIMEN

✔ Quality of Life *Remember to:*

- Knock before entering the person's room.
- Address the person by name.
- Introduce yourself by name and title.
- Explain the procedure to the person before beginning and during the procedure.

- Protect the person's rights during the procedure.
- Handle the person gently during the procedure.

PRE-PROCEDURE

1 Follow *Delegation Guidelines: Urine Specimens,* p. 510. See *Promoting Safety and Comfort:*
   a *Urine Specimens,* p. 510
   b *The 24-Hour Urine Specimen*
2 Practice hand hygiene.
3 Collect the following before going to the person's room:
   - Laboratory requisition slip
   - Urine container for a 24-hour collection
   - Specimen label
   - Preservative if needed
   - Bucket with ice if needed
   - Two "24-hour Urine" labels
   - Funnel
   - BIOHAZARD label

4 Arrange collected items in the person's bathroom.
5 Place one "24-hour Urine" label in the bathroom. Place the other near the bed.
6 Decontaminate your hands.
7 Identify the person. Check the ID bracelet against the requisition slip. Also call the person by name.
8 Label the specimen container in the person's presence. Apply the BIOHAZARD label.
9 Put on gloves.
10 Collect the following:
   - Voiding receptacle—bedpan and cover, urinal, commode, or specimen pan
   - Gloves
   - Graduate to measure output
11 Provide for privacy.

PROCEDURE

12 Ask the person to void. Provide a voiding receptacle.
13 Measure and discard the urine. Note the time. This starts the 24-hour collection period.
14 Mark the time on the collection container.
15 Empty, clean, and disinfect equipment. Return equipment to its proper place.
16 Remove the gloves, and practice hand hygiene. Put on clean gloves.
17 Assist with hand washing.
18 Remove the gloves. Practice hand hygiene.

19 Mark the time the test began and the time it ends on the room and bathroom labels.
20 Remind the person to:
   a Use the voiding receptacle when voiding during the next 24 hours.
   b Not to have a bowel movement when voiding.
   c Put toilet tissue in the toilet or wastebasket.
   c Put on the signal light after voiding.
21 Return to the room when the person signals for you. Knock before entering the room.

Continued

COLLECTING A 24-HOUR URINE SPECIMEN—cont'd

PROCEDURE—cont'd

22 Do the following after every voiding:
   a Decontaminate your hands. Put on gloves.
   b Measure urine if I&O is ordered.
   c Pour urine into the container using the funnel. Do not spill any urine. Restart the test if you spill or discard the urine.
   c Empty, clean, and disinfect equipment. Return equipment to its proper place.

   e Remove the gloves, and practice hand hygiene. Put on clean gloves.
   f Assisting with hand washing.
   g Remove the gloves. Practice hand hygiene.
   h Follow "Post-Procedure" steps except for steps 28 and 33.
23 Ask the person to void at the end of the 24-hour period. Follow step 22.

POST-PROCEDURE

24 Provide for comfort. (See the inside of the front book cover.)
25 Place the signal light within reach.
26 Raise or lower bed rails. Follow the care plan.
27 Put on gloves.
28 Remove the labels from the room and bathroom.
29 Clean and return equipment to its proper place. Discard disposable items.

30 Remove the gloves. Practice hand hygiene.
31 Unscreen the person.
32 Complete a safety check of the room. (See the inside of the front book cover.)
33 Take the specimen and requisition slip to the laboratory or storage area. Wear gloves.
34 Report and record your observations.

◆ The Double-Voided Specimen

Fresh-fractional urine specimen is another term for double-voided specimen. The person voids twice. The first time the bladder is emptied of "stale" urine. "Fresh" urine collects in the bladder after the first voiding. In 30 minutes the person voids again. The second voiding is usually a small or "fractional" amount of urine.

Fresh-fractional urine specimens are used to test urine for glucose and ketones (p. 517). Specimen containers and urine testing equipment are usually kept in the person's bathroom.

COLLECTING A DOUBLE-VOIDED SPECIMEN

✔ Quality of Life *Remember to:*

- Knock before entering the person's room.
- Address the person by name.
- Introduce yourself by name and title.
- Explain the procedure to the person before beginning and during the procedure.

- Protect the person's rights during the procedure.
- Handle the person gently during the procedure.

PRE-PROCEDURE

1 Follow *Delegation Guidelines: Urine Specimens,* p. 510. See *Promoting Safety and Comfort: Urine Specimens,* p. 510.
2 Practice hand hygiene. Put on gloves.
3 Collect the following:
   • Voiding receptacle—bedpan and cover, urinal, commode, or specimen pan
   • Two specimen containers

   • Urine testing equipment
   • Graduate to measure output
   • Gloves
4 Remove the gloves. Decontaminate your hands.
5 Identify the person. Check the ID bracelet against the assignment sheet. Also call the person by name.
6 Provide for privacy.

COLLECTING A DOUBLE-VOIDED SPECIMEN—cont'd

PROCEDURE

7 Put on gloves.

8 Ask the person to void into the receptacle. Remind the person not to put toilet tissue in the receptacle.

9 Take the receptacle to the bathroom.

10 Measure urine if I&O is ordered.

11 Pour some urine into a specimen container.

12 Test the specimen in case the person cannot provide a second specimen (p. 517). Discard the urine. Note the result on your assignment sheet.

13 Empty, clean, and disinfect equipment. Return equipment to its proper place.

14 Remove the gloves, and practice hand hygiene. Put on clean gloves.

15 Assist with hand washing.

16 Remove the gloves. Practice hand hygiene.

17 Ask the person to drink an 8-ounce glass of water.

18 Do the following before leaving the room:

 a Provide for comfort. (See the inside of the front book cover.)

 b Place the signal light within reach.

 c Raise or lower the bed rails. Follow the care plan.

 c Unscreen the person.

 e Complete a safety check of the room. (See the inside of the front book cover.)

 f Decontaminate your hands.

19 Return to the room in 20 to 30 minutes. Decontaminate your hands.

20 Repeat steps 2 through 16.

POST-PROCEDURE

21 Provide for comfort. (See the inside of the front book cover.)

22 Place the signal light within reach.

23 Raise or lower the bed rails. Follow the care plan.

24 Unscreen the person.

25 Complete a safety check of the room. (See the inside of the front book cover.)

26 Decontaminate your hands.

27 Report and record the results of the second test and any other observations.

◆ Collecting a Urine Specimen From an Infant or Child

Sometimes specimens are needed from infants and children who are not toilet-trained. A collection bag ("wee bag") is applied over the urethra (Fig. 30-3). A parent or another staff member assists if the child is upset.

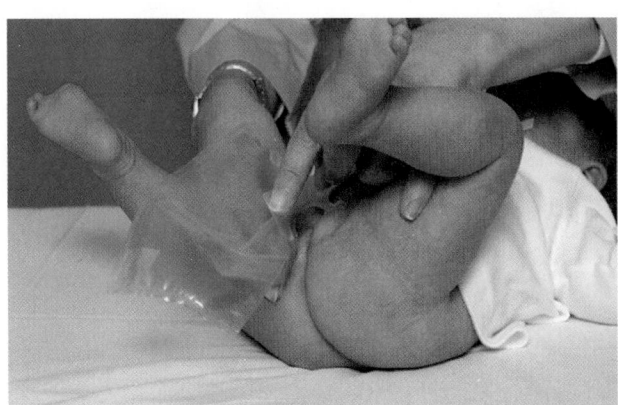 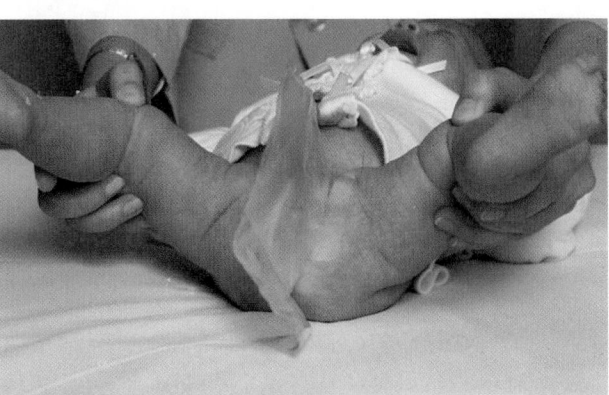

A   B

FIGURE 30-3 A urine collection bag is applied to the female infant's perineum. (From Hockenberry MJ and Wilson D: *Wong's nursing care of infants and children,* ed 8, St Louis, 2007, Mosby.)

COLLECTING A URINE SPECIMEN FROM THE INFANT OR CHILD

✔ **Quality of Life** *Remember to:*

- Knock before entering the child's room.
- Address the child by name.
- Introduce yourself by name and title.
- Explain the procedure to the child and parents before beginning and during the procedure.

- Protect the child's rights during the procedure.
- Handle the child gently during the procedure.

PRE-PROCEDURE

1 Follow *Delegation Guidelines: Urine Specimens,* p. 510. See *Promoting Safety and Comfort: Urine Specimens,* p. 510.
2 Practice hand hygiene.
3 Collect the following:
  - Collection bag ("wee" bag)
  - BIOHAZARD label (if needed)
  - Cotton balls
  - Specimen container
  - Plastic bag

- Scissors
- Wash basin
- Bath towel
- Two diapers
- Gloves

4 Arrange your work area.
5 Decontaminate your hands.
6 Identify the child. Check the ID bracelet against the requisition slip. Also call the child by name.
7 Provide for privacy.

PROCEDURE

8 Decontaminate your hands. Put on gloves.
9 Position the child on his or her back.
10 Remove the diaper, and set it aside.
11 Clean the perineal area with cotton balls. Use a new cotton ball for each stroke. Rinse and dry the area.
12 Remove the gloves. Practice hand hygiene.
13 Put on clean gloves.
14 Flex the child's knees. Spread the legs.
15 Remove the adhesive backing from the collection bag.
16 Apply the bag to the perineum (see Fig. 30-3).
17 Cut a slit in the bottom of a new diaper.
18 Diaper the child.
19 Pull the collection bag through the slit in the diaper.
20 Remove the gloves. Practice hand hygiene.
21 Raise the head of the crib if allowed. This helps urine collect in the bottom of the bag.
22 Raise the crib rails before leaving the bedside.
23 Unscreen the child.
24 Dispose of the removed diaper. Follow agency policy. (Wear gloves for this step.)

25 Practice hand hygiene.
26 Check the child often. Check the bag for urine. (Provide for privacy and wear gloves for this step.)
27 Do the following if the child has voided:
  a Provide for privacy.
  b Decontaminate your hands. Put on clean gloves.
  c Remove the diaper.
  c Remove the collection bag gently.
  e Press the adhesive surfaces of the bag together. Make sure the seal is tight and there are no leaks. Or transfer the urine to the specimen container using the drainage tab.
  f Clean the perineal area. Rinse and dry well.
  g Diaper the child.
  h Remove the gloves. Practice hand hygiene.
28 Put on clean gloves.
29 Label the collection bag or specimen container in the child's presence. Then place it in the plastic bag. Apply the BIOHAZARD label (if needed).

POST-PROCEDURE

30 Provide for comfort. (See the inside of the front book cover.)
31 Raise the crib rail.
32 Unscreen the child.
33 Clean and return equipment to its proper place. Discard disposable items. (Wear gloves for this step.)

34 Complete a safety check of the room. (See the inside of the front book cover.)
35 Decontaminate your hands.
36 Take the specimen and requisition slip to the laboratory or storage area. Wear gloves.
37 Report and record your observations.

Testing Urine

The nurse may ask you to do simple urine tests. You can test for pH, glucose, and blood using reagent strips. The doctor orders the type and frequency of urine tests.

▶ *Testing for pH*—Urine pH measures if urine is acidic or alkaline. Changes in normal pH (4.6 to 8.0) occur from illness, food, and drugs. A routine urine specimen is needed.

▶ *Testing for glucose and ketones*—In diabetes, the pancreas does not secrete enough insulin (Chapter 41). The body needs insulin to use sugar for energy. If not used, sugar builds up in the blood. Some sugar appears in the urine. **Glucosuria** or **glycosuria** means sugar (*glucos*, *glycos*) in the urine (*uria*). The diabetic person may also have **acetone (ketone bodies, ketones)** in the urine. These substances appear in urine from the rapid breakdown of fat for energy. The body uses fat for energy if it cannot use sugar. Urine is also tested for ketones. These tests are usually done four times a day—30 minutes before each meal and at bedtime. The doctor uses the test to make drug and diet decisions. Double-voided specimens are best for these tests.

▶ *Testing for blood*—Injury and disease can cause **hematuria**. It means blood (*hemat*) in the urine (*uria*). Sometimes blood is seen in the urine. At other times it is unseen (*occult*). A routine urine specimen is needed.

See *Teamwork and Time Management: Testing Urine.*
See *Delegation Guidelines: Testing Urine.*
See *Promoting Safety and Comfort: Testing Urine.*

◀ Using Reagent Strips

Reagent strips have sections that change color when they react with urine. To use a reagent strip:

▶ Do not touch the test area on the strip.
▶ Dip the strip into urine.
▶ Compare the strip with the color chart on the bottle (Fig. 30-4).

See *Promoting Safety and Comfort: Using Reagent Strips.*

TEAMWORK AND TIME MANAGEMENT

Testing Urine

Test urine for glucose and ketones at times directed by the nurse and the care plan. The nurse uses the test results to make decisions about giving the person his or her drugs for diabetes. The drugs are given at a certain time. Therefore the nurse needs the test results before giving the drugs.

DELEGATION GUIDELINES: Testing Urine

When testing urine is delegated to you, you need this information from the nurse and the care plan:
• What test is needed
• What urine specimen to collect
• What equipment to use
• When to test urine
• Instructions for the test ordered
• If the nurse wants to observe the results of each test
• What observations to report and record:
  • The time you collected and tested the specimen
  • Test results
  • Problems obtaining the specimen
  • Color, clarity, and odor of urine
  • Particles in the urine
  • Complaints of pain, burning, urgency, dysuria, or other problems
• When to report test results and observations
• What specific patient or resident concerns to report at once

---

PROMOTING SAFETY AND COMFORT: Testing Urine

SAFETY
You must be accurate when testing urine. Promptly report the results to the nurse. Ordered drugs may depend on the results.

Urine may contain microbes and blood. Follow Standard Precautions and the Bloodborne Pathogen Standard.

COMFORT
The person may want to know the test results. If allowed by agency policy, you can tell the person the results. Remember, this information is private and confidential. Make sure only the person hears what you are saying.

PROMOTING SAFETY AND COMFORT: Using Reagent Strips

SAFETY
When using reagent strips, follow the manufacturer's instructions. Otherwise you could get the wrong result. The doctor uses the test results in diagnosing and treating the person. A wrong result could lead to serious harm.

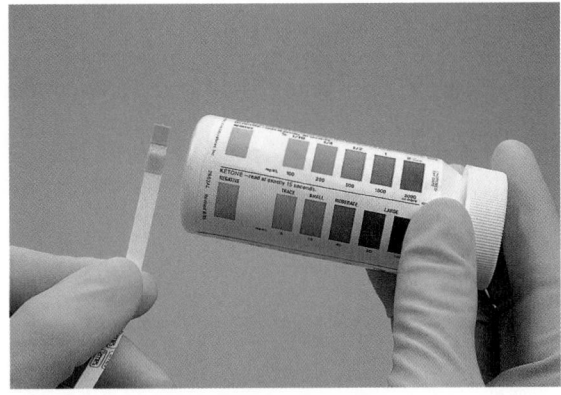

FIGURE 30-4 Reagent strip for sugar and ketones.

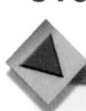

TESTING URINE WITH REAGENT STRIPS

✔ **Quality of Life** *Remember to:*

- Knock before entering the person's room.
- Address the person by name.
- Introduce yourself by name and title.
- Explain the procedure to the person before beginning and during the procedure.

- Protect the person's rights during the procedure.
- Handle the person gently during the procedure.

PRE-PROCEDURE

1 Follow *Delegation Guidelines: Testing Urine*, p. 517. See *Promoting Safety and Comfort:*
   a *Testing Urine*, p. 517
   b *Using Reagent Strips*, p. 517
2 Practice hand hygiene.
3 Collect the reagent strips ordered.
4 Decontaminate your hands.
5 Identify the person. Check the ID bracelet against the assignment sheet. Also call the person by name.

6 Put on gloves.
7 Collect the following:
   - Equipment for collecting the urine specimen needed (See procedure: *Collecting a Random Urine Specimen*, p. 510, or *Collecting a Double-Voided Specimen*, p. 514.)
   - Gloves
8 Provide for privacy.

PROCEDURE

9 Collect the urine specimen. (See procedure: *Collecting a Random Urine Specimen*, p. 510, or *Collecting a Double-Voided Specimen*, p. 514.)
10 Remove the strip from the bottle. Put the cap on the bottle at once. It must be on tight.
11 Dip the strip test areas into the urine.
12 Remove the strip after the correct amount of time. See the manufacturer's instructions.
13 Tap the strip gently against the container. This removes excess urine.

14 Wait the required amount of time. See the manufacturer's instructions.
15 Compare the strip with the color chart on the bottle (see Fig. 30-4). Read the results.
16 Discard disposable items and the specimen.
17 Empty, clean, and disinfect equipment. Return equipment to its proper place.
18 Remove the gloves. Practice hand hygiene.

POST-PROCEDURE

19 Provide for comfort. (See the inside of the front book cover.)
20 Place the signal light within reach.
21 Raise or lower bed rails. Follow the care plan.
22 Unscreen the person.

23 Complete a safety check of the room. (See the inside of the front book cover.)
24 Decontaminate your hands.
25 Report and record the test results and other observations.

◀ Straining Urine

A stone *(calculus)* can develop in the kidney, ureter, or bladder. Stones *(calculi)* vary in size (Chapter 42). Some are as small as grains of sand. They also can be pearl-size or the size of golf balls. Stones causing severe pain and urinary system damage may require surgical removal. Some stones are passed through urine. Therefore all of the person's urine is strained. Passed stones are sent to the laboratory.

The person drinks 2 to 3 quarts (8 to 12 glasses) of water a day to help pass the stone. Expect the person to void in large amounts.

STRAINING URINE

✔ **Quality of Life** *Remember to:*

- Knock before entering the person's room.
- Address the person by name.
- Introduce yourself by name and title.
- Explain the procedure to the person before beginning and during the procedure.

- Protect the person's rights during the procedure.
- Handle the person gently during the procedure.

PRE-PROCEDURE

1 Follow *Delegation Guidelines: Testing Urine*, p. 517. See *Promoting Safety and Comfort: Testing Urine*, p. 517.
2 Practice hand hygiene.
3 Collect the following before going to the person's room:
- Laboratory requisition slip
- Gauze or strainer
- Specimen container
- Specimen label
- Two "Strain All Urine" labels
- Plastic bag
- BIOHAZARD label (if needed)
4 Arrange collected items in the person's bathroom.

5 Place one "Strain All Urine" label in the bathroom. Place the other near the bed.
6 Decontaminate your hands.
7 Identify the person. Check the ID bracelet against the assignment sheet. Call the person by name.
8 Label the specimen container in the person's presence.
9 Put on gloves.
10 Collect the following:
- Voiding receptacle—bedpan and cover, urinal, commode, or specimen pan
- Graduate
- Gloves
11 Provide for privacy.

PROCEDURE

12 Ask the person to use the voiding receptacle for urinating. Ask the person to put on the signal light after voiding.
13 Remove the gloves. Practice hand hygiene.
14 Return to the room when the person signals for you. Knock before entering the room.
15 Decontaminate your hands. Put on clean gloves.
16 Place the gauze or strainer into the graduate.
17 Pour urine into the graduate. Urine passes through the gauze or strainer (Fig. 30-5, p. 520).
18 Place the gauze or strainer in the specimen container if any crystals, stones, or particles appear.

19 Place the specimen container in the plastic bag. Do not let the container touch the outside of the bag. Apply a BIOHAZARD label according to agency policy.
20 Measure urine if I&O were ordered.
21 Empty, clean, and disinfect equipment. Return equipment to its proper place.
22 Remove the gloves, and practice hand hygiene. Put on clean gloves.
23 Assist with hand washing.
24 Remove the gloves. Practice hand hygiene.

POST-PROCEDURE

25 Provide for comfort. (See the inside of the front book cover.)
26 Place the signal light within reach.
27 Raise or lower bed rails. Follow the care plan.
28 Unscreen the person.
29 Complete a safety check of the room. (See the inside of the front book cover.)

30 Decontaminate your hands.
31 Take the specimen container and requisition slip to the laboratory or storage area. Wear gloves.
32 Report and record your observations.

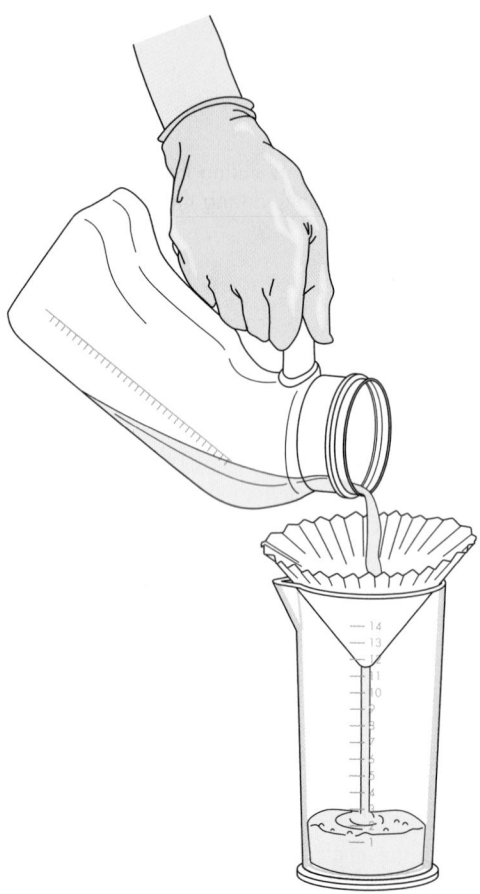

FIGURE 30-5 A strainer is placed in the graduate. Urine is poured through the strainer into the graduate.

◆ STOOL SPECIMENS

When internal bleeding is suspected, stools are checked for blood. Stools also are studied for fat, microbes, worms, and other abnormal contents.

The stool specimen must not be contaminated with urine. The person uses one receptacle for voiding and another for a bowel movement. Some tests require a warm stool. The specimen is taken at once to the laboratory or to the storage area for transport to the laboratory. Follow the rules in Box 30-1.

See *Focus on Children and Older Persons. Stool Specimens.*
See *Focus on Communication: Stool Specimens.*
See *Delegation Guidelines: Stool Specimens.*
See *Promoting Safety and Comfort: Stool Specimens.*

FOCUS ON **CHILDREN** AND **OLDER PERSONS**

Stool Specimens

CHILDREN
If the child wears a diaper, you can obtain stool from the diaper. You may need to scrape the diaper with a tongue blade.

FOCUS ON **COMMUNICATION**

Stool Specimens

Always explain the procedure before you begin. Explain what the person needs to do and what you will do. Also show what equipment and supplies you will use. For example:

"The doctor wants your stools tested. Meaning, we need a specimen from a bowel movement. I'm going to place this specimen pan (show the specimen pan) at the back of the toilet seat. You will urinate into the toilet. Your stools will collect in the specimen pan rather than in the toilet. Please put toilet tissue in the toilet, not in the specimen pan. After you have a bowel movement, put your signal light on right away. I'll use a tongue blade (show the tongue blade) to take some stool from the specimen pan to put in this specimen container (show the specimen container)."

After explaining the procedure, ask the person if he or she has any questions. If you do not know the answer, refer questions to the nurse.

Also make sure the person understands what to do. You can say:

"Mrs Clark, please help me make sure that you understand what I said. To collect a stool specimen, please tell me what you're going to do and what I need to do."

PROMOTING SAFETY AND COMFORT: **Stool Specimens**

SAFETY
Stools contain microbes. And they may contain blood. Follow Standard Precautions and the Bloodborne Pathogen Standard.

COMFORT
Stools normally have an odor. A person may be embarrassed that you need to collect a specimen. Complete the task quickly and carefully. Also act in a professional manner.

DELEGATION GUIDELINES: **Stool Specimens**

Before collecting a stool specimen, you need this information from the nurse:
- What time to collect the specimen
- What special measures are needed
- What observations to report and record:
  - Problems obtaining the specimen
  - Color, amount, consistency, and odor of stools
  - Complaints of pain or discomfort
  - The time when the specimen was collected
- When to report observations
- What specific patient or resident concerns to report at once

COLLECTING A STOOL SPECIMEN

✔ **Quality of Life** *Remember to:*

- Knock before entering the person's room.
- Address the person by name.
- Introduce yourself by name and title.
- Explain the procedure to the person before beginning and during the procedure.

- Protect the person's rights during the procedure.
- Handle the person gently during the procedure.

PRE-PROCEDURE

1 Follow *Delegation Guidelines: Stool Specimens.* See *Promoting Safety and Comfort: Stool Specimens.*
2 Practice hand hygiene.
3 Collect the following before going to the person's room:
   - Laboratory requisition slip
   - Specimen pan for the toilet
   - Specimen container and lid
   - Specimen label
   - Tongue blade
   - Disposable bag
   - Plastic bag
   - BIOHAZARD label (if needed)

4 Arrange collected items in the person's bathroom.
5 Decontaminate your hands.
6 Identify the person. Check the ID bracelet against the requisition slip. Also call the person by name.
7 Label the specimen container in the person's presence.
8 Put on gloves.
9 Collect the following:
   - Receptacle for voiding—bedpan and cover, urinal, commode, or specimen pan
   - Gloves
   - Toilet tissue
10 Provide for privacy.

PROCEDURE

11 Ask the person to void. Provide the receptacle for voiding if the person does not use the bathroom. Empty, clean, and disinfect the device. Return it to its proper place.
12 Put the specimen pan on the toilet if the person will use the bathroom. Place it at the back of the toilet (Fig. 30-6, p. 522). Or provide a bedpan or commode.
13 Ask the person not to put toilet tissue into the bedpan, commode, or specimen pan. Provide a bag for toilet tissue.
14 Place the signal light and toilet tissue within reach. Raise or lower bed rails. Follow the care plan.
15 Remove the gloves. Decontaminate your hands. Leave the room.
16 Return when the person signals. Or check on the person every 5 minutes. Knock before entering.
17 Decontaminate your hands. Put on clean gloves.
18 Lower the bed rail near you if up.
19 Remove the bedpan. Note the color, amount, consistency, and odor of stools.

20 Provide perineal care if needed.
21 Collect the specimen:
   a Use a tongue blade to take about 2 tablespoons of formed or liquid stool to the specimen container (Fig. 30-7, p. 522). Take the sample from the middle of a formed stool.
   b Include pus, mucus, or blood present in the stool.
   c Take stool from 2 different places in the bowel movement if required by agency policy.
   c Put the lid on the specimen container.
   e Place the container in the plastic bag. Do not let the container touch the outside of the bag. Apply a BIOHAZARD label according to agency policy.
22 Wrap the tongue blade in toilet tissue. Discard it into the disposable bag.
23 Empty, clean, and disinfect equipment. Return equipment to its proper place.
24 Remove the gloves, and practice hand hygiene. Put on clean gloves.
25 Assist with hand washing.
26 Remove the gloves. Practice hand hygiene.

POST-PROCEDURE

27 Provide for comfort. (See the inside of the front book cover.)
28 Place the signal light within reach.
29 Raise or lower bed rails. Follow the care plan.
30 Unscreen the person.

31 Complete a safety check of the room. (See the inside of the front book cover.)
32 Take the specimen and requisition slip to the laboratory or storage area. Wear gloves.
33 Report and record your observations.

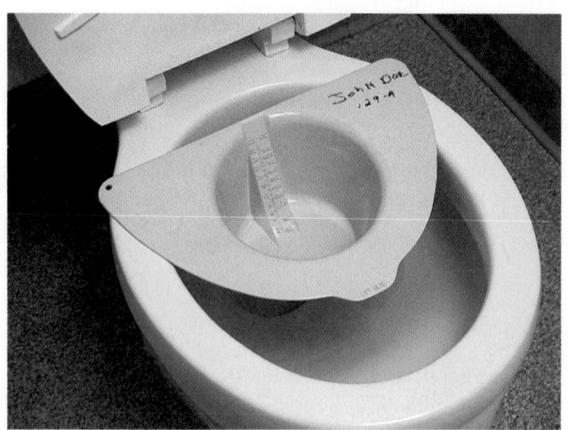

FIGURE 30-6 The specimen pan is placed at the back of the toilet for a stool specimen.

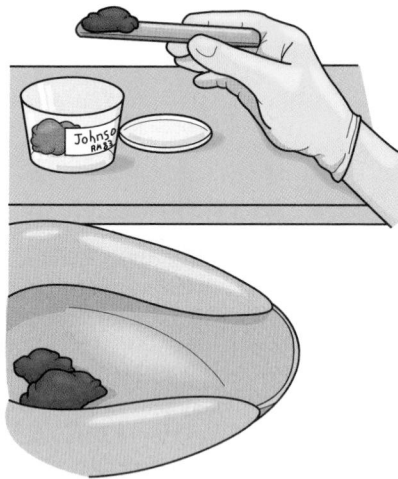

FIGURE 30-7 A tongue blade is used to transfer a small amount of stool from the bedpan to the specimen container.

◆ Testing Stools For Blood

Stools may contain blood for many reasons. Ulcers, colon cancer, and hemorrhoids are common causes. Often blood is seen if it is low in the bowels. Stools are black and tarry if there is bleeding in the stomach or upper gastrointestinal tract. **Melena** is a black, tarry stool.

Sometimes bleeding occurs in very small amounts. Such bleeding is hard to see. Therefore stools are often tested for *occult blood. Occult* means "hidden" or "not seen." The test is often done to screen for colon cancer.

Occult blood test kits vary. Follow the manufacturer's instructions. The following procedure is presented as a guide.

See *Delegation Guidelines: Testing Stools for Blood.*

See *Promoting Safety and Comfort: Testing Stools for Blood.*

DELEGATION GUIDELINES: Testing Stools For Blood

Before testing a stool specimen for blood, you need this information from the nurse:
- What test is needed
- What equipment to use
- When to test the stool
- Instructions for the test ordered
- If the nurse wants to observe the results of each test
- What observations to report and record:
  - The time you collected and tested the specimen
  - Test results
  - Problems obtaining the specimen
  - Color, amount, consistency, and odor of feces
  - Complaints of pain or discomfort
- When to report observations
- What specific patient or resident concerns to report at once

---

PROMOTING SAFETY AND COMFORT: Testing Stools for Blood

SAFETY

You must be accurate when testing stools. Follow the manufacturer's instructions for the test used. Promptly report the results to the nurse.

Stools contain microbes. They may contain blood. Follow Standard Precautions and the Bloodborne Pathogen Standard.

TESTING A STOOL SPECIMEN FOR BLOOD

✓ Quality of Life *Remember to:*

- Knock before entering the person's room.
- Address the person by name.
- Introduce yourself by name and title.
- Explain the procedure to the person before beginning and during the procedure.

- Protect the person's rights during the procedure.
- Handle the person gently during the procedure.

PRE-PROCEDURE

1 Follow *Delegation Guidelines: Testing Stools for Blood.* See *Promoting Safety and Comfort:*
   a *Stool Specimens,* p. 520
   b *Testing Stools for Blood*
2 Practice hand hygiene.
3 Collect the following before going to the person's room:
   - Hemoccult test kit
   - Tongue blades (if needed)
4 Arrange collected items in the person's bathroom.

5 Decontaminate your hands.
6 Identify the person. Check the ID bracelet against the assignment sheet. Also call the person by name.
7 Put on gloves.
8 Collect the following:
   - Equipment for collecting a stool specimen. (See procedure: *Collecting a Stool Specimen,* p. 521.)
   - Paper towels
   - Gloves
9 Provide for privacy.

PROCEDURE

10 Collect a stool specimen. (See procedure: *Collecting a Stool Specimen,* p. 521.)
11 Practice hand hygiene. Put on clean gloves.
12 Open the test kit.
13 Use a tongue blade to obtain a small amount of stool.
14 Apply a thin smear of stool on *box A* on the test paper (Fig. 30-8, *A*).
15 Use another tongue blade to obtain stool from another part of the specimen.
16 Apply a thin smear of stool on *box B* on the test paper (Fig. 30-8, *B*).
17 Close the packet.
18 Turn the test packet to the other side. Open the flap. Apply developer (from the kit) to *boxes A* and *B.* Follow the manufacturer's instructions (Fig. 30-8, *C*).

19 Wait the amount of time noted in the manufacturer's instructions. Time varies from 10 to 60 seconds.
20 Note the color changes on your assignment sheet (Fig. 30-8, *D*).
21 Dispose of the test packet.
22 Wrap the tongue blades with toilet tissue. Then discard them.
23 Empty, clean, and disinfect equipment. Return equipment to its proper place.
24 Remove the gloves. Practice hand hygiene.

POST-PROCEDURE

25 Provide for comfort. (See the inside of the front book cover.)
26 Place the signal light within reach.
27 Raise or lower bed rails. Follow the care plan.
28 Complete a safety check of the room. (See the inside of the front book cover.)

29 Decontaminate your hands.
30 Report and record the test results and your observations.

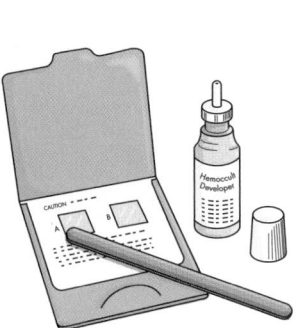
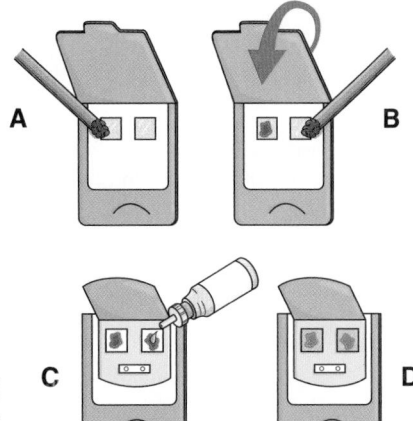

FIGURE 30-8 Testing for occult blood. **A,** Stool is smeared on *box A.* **B,** Stool is smeared on *box B* and then the flap is closed. **C,** Developer is applied to *boxes A* and *B.* **D,** Color changes are noted.

◆ SPUTUM SPECIMENS

Respiratory disorders cause the lungs, bronchi, and trachea to secrete mucus. Mucus from the respiratory system is called **sputum** when expectorated *(expelled)* through the mouth. Sputum is not saliva. Saliva ("spit") is a thin, clear liquid. It is produced by the salivary glands in the mouth.

Sputum specimens are studied for blood, microbes, and abnormal cells. The person coughs up sputum from the bronchi and trachea. This is often painful and hard to do. It is easier to collect a specimen in the morning. Secretions collect in the trachea and bronchi during sleep. They are coughed up on awakening.

To collect a specimen, follow the rules in Box 30-1. Also have the person rinse the mouth with water. Rinsing decreases saliva and removes food particles. Mouthwash is not used. It destroys some of the microbes in the mouth.

See *Focus on Children and Older Persons: Sputum Specimens.*

See *Delegation Guidelines: Sputum Specimens.*

See *Promoting Safety and Comfort: Sputum Specimens.*

DELEGATION GUIDELINES: Sputum Specimens

Before collecting a sputum specimen, you need this information from the nurse:
- When to collect the specimen
- How much sputum is needed—usually 1 to 2 tablespoons
- If the person uses the bathroom
- If the person can hold the specimen container
- What observations to report and record:
  - The time the specimen was collected
  - The amount of sputum collected
  - How easily the person raised the sputum
  - Sputum color—clear, white, yellow, green, brown, or red
  - Sputum odor—none or foul odor
  - Sputum consistency—thick, watery, or frothy (with bubbles or foam)
  - **Hemoptysis**—bloody *(hemo)* sputum *(ptysis*, meaning *to spit)*
  - If the person was not able to produce sputum
  - Any other observations
- When to report observations
- What specific patient or resident concerns to report at once

---

FOCUS ON **CHILDREN** AND **OLDER PERSONS**

Sputum Specimens

CHILDREN

Breathing treatments and suctioning are often needed to produce sputum specimens in infants and small children. The RN or respiratory therapist gives the breathing treatment. The nurse suctions the trachea for the specimen. The infant or child is likely to be uncooperative during suctioning. You can assist by holding the child's head and arms still.

OLDER PERSONS

Older persons may lack the strength to cough up sputum. Coughing is easier after postural drainage. It drains secretions by gravity. Gravity causes fluids to flow down. The person is positioned so a lung part is higher than the airway (Fig. 30-9). The nurse or respiratory therapist does postural drainage.

PROMOTING SAFETY AND COMFORT: Sputum Specimens

SAFETY

Follow Standard Precautions and the Bloodborne Pathogen Standard to prevent contact with mucus. It may contain blood or microbes.

The doctor may order Isolation Precautions if the person has or may have tuberculosis (TB) (Chapter 40). Protect yourself by wearing a tuberculosis respirator (Chapter 14).

COMFORT

The procedure can embarrass the person. Coughing and expectorating sounds can disturb those nearby. Also, sputum is not pleasant to look at. For these reasons, privacy is important. Cover the specimen container and place it in a bag. Some sputum specimen containers are cloudy in color to hide the contents.

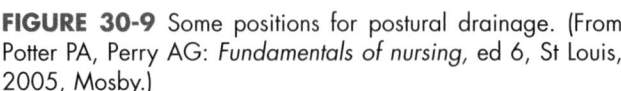
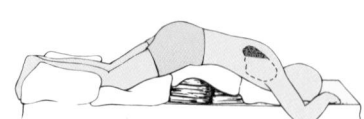
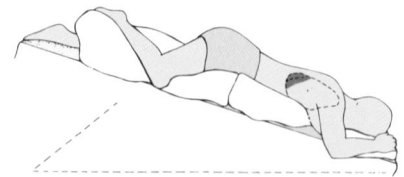

FIGURE 30-9 Some positions for postural drainage. (From Potter PA, Perry AG: *Fundamentals of nursing,* ed 6, St Louis, 2005, Mosby.)

COLLECTING A SPUTUM SPECIMEN

✔ **Quality of Life** *Remember to:*

- Knock before entering the person's room.
- Address the person by name.
- Introduce yourself by name and title.
- Explain the procedure to the person before beginning and during the procedure.

- Protect the person's rights during the procedure.
- Handle the person gently during the procedure.

PRE-PROCEDURE

1 Follow *Delegation Guidelines: Sputum Specimens.* See *Promoting Safety and Comfort: Sputum Specimens.*
2 Practice hand hygiene.
3 Collect the following before going to the person's room:
   - Laboratory requisition slip
   - Sputum specimen container and lid
   - Specimen label
   - Plastic bag
   - BIOHAZARD label (if needed)

4 Arrange collected items in the person's bathroom.
5 Decontaminate your hands.
6 Identify the person. Check the ID bracelet against the requisition slip. Also call the person by name.
7 Label the container in the person's presence.
8 Collect gloves and tissues.
9 Provide for privacy. If able, the person uses the bathroom for the procedure.

PROCEDURE

10 Put on gloves.
11 Ask the person to rinse the mouth out with clear water.
12 Have the person hold the container. Only the outside is touched.
13 Ask the person to cover the mouth and nose with tissues when coughing. Follow agency policy for used tissues.
14 Ask him or her to take 2 or 3 deep breaths and cough up the sputum.
15 Have the person expectorate directly into the container (Fig. 30-10). Sputum should not touch the outside of the container.

16 Collect 1 to 2 tablespoons of sputum unless told to collect more.
17 Put the lid on the container.
18 Place the container in the plastic bag. Do not let the container touch the outside of the bag. Apply a BIOHAZARD label according to agency policy.
19 Remove the gloves, and decontaminate your hands. Put on clean gloves.
20 Assist with hand washing.
21 Remove the gloves. Decontaminate your hands.

POST-PROCEDURE

22 Provide for comfort. (See the inside of the front book cover.)
23 Place the signal light within reach.
24 Raise or lower bed rails. Follow the care plan.
25 Unscreen the person.

26 Complete a safety check of the room. (See the inside of the front book cover.)
27 Decontaminate your hands.
28 Take the specimen and the requisition slip to the laboratory or storage area. Wear gloves.
29 Report and record your observations.

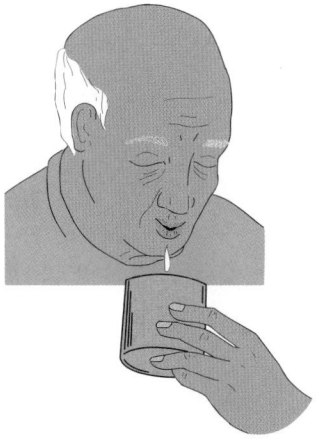

Figure 30-10 The person expectorates into the center of the specimen container.

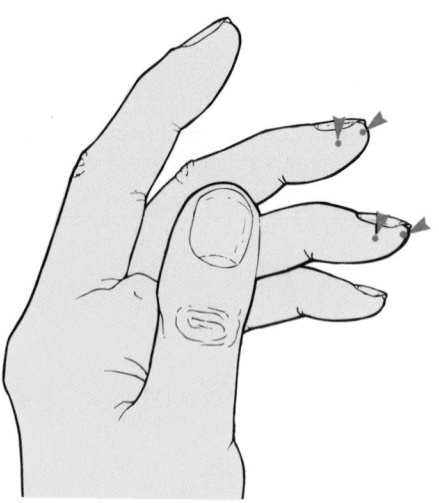

FIGURE 30-11 Site for skin punctures. (From Bonewit-West K: *Clinical procedures for medical assistants,* ed 5, Philadelphia, 2000, Saunders.)

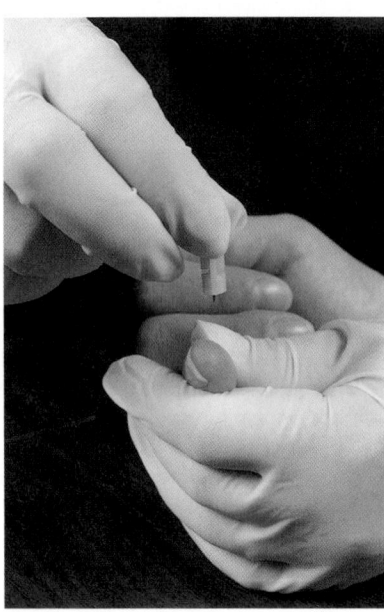

FIGURE 30-12 A lancet. (From Bonewit-West K: *Clinical procedures for medical assistants,* ed 5, Philadelphia, 2000, Saunders.)

◆ BLOOD GLUCOSE TESTING

Blood glucose testing is used for persons with diabetes. The doctor uses the results to regulate the person's drugs and diet. For the test, capillary blood is obtained through a skin puncture.

With skin punctures, a few drops of capillary blood are obtained. A fingertip is the most common site for skin punctures. The earlobe also is a site. These sites provide easy access and do not require clothing removal. The person feels a sharp pinch. Discomfort is brief.

Inspect the site carefully. Look for signs of trauma and skin breaks. Avoid sites that are swollen, bruised, cyanotic (bluish color), scarred, or calloused. Blood flow to these areas is poor. A *callus* is a thick, hardened area on the skin. Calluses often form over frequently used areas, such as the tips of the thumbs and index fingers. Therefore the thumbs and index fingers are not good sites for skin punctures.

Do not use the center, fleshy part of the fingertip. The site has many nerve endings. A puncture at the site is painful. Use the side toward the tip of the fingertip on the middle or ring finger (Fig. 30-11).

A sterile lancet is used to puncture the skin (Fig. 30-12). A *lancet* is a short, pointed blade. The short blade punctures but does not cut the skin. The lancet is inside a protective cover. You do not touch the actual blade. All types of lancets are disposable. A lancet is discarded into the sharps container after use.

A *glucose meter (glucometer)* is used to measure blood glucose. With a drop of blood applied to the reagent strip, the strip is inserted into the glucose meter. The blood glucose level is shown on the monitor. Many different glucose meters are available. The speed with which results are displayed varies with the manufacturer. Some take 1 minute. Others take 15 seconds or less.

Before inserting the reagent strip into the device, follow the manufacturer's instructions. One of the following is usually required:

▶ *Dry-wipe.* Blood is wiped off the reagent strip with a cotton ball.
▶ *Wet-wash.* The reagent strip is flushed with water to rinse blood off.
▶ *No-wipe.* No wiping or rinsing. The reagent strip is inserted directly into the device.

In agencies, glucose meters are tested daily for accuracy. The manufacturer has instructions for testing the device.

There are many different kinds of glucometers. You will learn to use the device used in your agency. Always follow the manufacturer's instructions.

See *Teamwork and Time Management: Blood Glucose Testing.*

See *Delegation Guidelines: Blood Glucose Testing.*

See *Promoting Safety and Comfort: Blood Glucose Testing.*

TEAMWORK AND TIME MANAGEMENT

Blood Glucose Testing

Perform blood glucose testing at times directed by the nurse and the care plan. The nurse uses the test results to make decisions about giving the person his or her drugs for diabetes. The drugs are given at a certain time. Therefore the nurse needs the blood glucose results before giving the drugs.

Glucose meters are shared with other nursing team members. When using the device, tell your co-workers that you have a glucose meter. Work quickly, but carefully. Return the device to the storage area in a timely manner.

Delegation Guidelines: Blood Glucose Testing

Many states and agencies allow nursing assistive personnel to test blood glucose. If the task is delegated to you, make sure that:

- Your state allows nursing assistive personnel to perform the procedure
- The procedure is in your job description
- You have the necessary training
- You know how to use the agency's equipment
- You review the procedure with a nurse
- The nurse is available to answer questions and to supervise you

If the above conditions are met, you need the following information from the nurse:

- What sites to avoid for a skin puncture
- When to collect and test the specimen—usually before meals
- If the person is receiving drugs that affect blood clotting (*NOTE:* If yes, it may take a longer time to stop bleeding. Apply pressure until bleeding stops.)
- What to report and record:
  - The time the specimen was collected
  - The blood glucose test result
  - The site used for the skin puncture
  - The amount of bleeding at the skin puncture site
  - Any signs of a **hematoma** (a swelling [*oma*] that contains blood [*hemat*])
  - How the person tolerated the procedure
  - Complaints of the pain at the skin puncture site
  - Other observations or patient or resident complaints
- When to report observations and the blood glucose measurement
- What specific patient or resident concerns to report at once

PROMOTING SAFETY AND COMFORT: Blood Glucose Testing

SAFETY

Accurate results are important. Inaccurate results can harm the person. Follow the rules in Box 30-2 when testing blood specimens for glucose.

Make sure you know how to use the equipment before testing blood. Also check the manufacturer's instructions for the reagent strip to use. Use only the type of reagent strip specified by the manufacturer. Otherwise you will get inaccurate results.

Contact with blood is likely. Follow Standard Precautions and the Bloodborne Pathogen Standard.

COMFORT

The heel is used for skin punctures in infants who are not yet walking. The third finger (ring finger) is used for children. See Figure 30-13.

Older persons often have poor circulation in their fingers. To increase blood flow, apply a warm wash cloth or wash the hands in warm water.

BOX 30-2 Rules For Blood Glucose Testing

- Follow the manufacturer's instructions for the glucose meter.
- Know how to use the equipment. Request any necessary training.
- Make sure the glucose meter was tested for accuracy. Check the testing log.
- Check the color of reagent strips. Do not use discolored strips.
- Check the expiration date of the reagent strips. Do not use them if the date has passed.
- Use a watch with a sweep hand to time the test. Follow the manufacturer's instructions for test times.
- Report the results to the nurse at once.
- Record the results following agency policy.

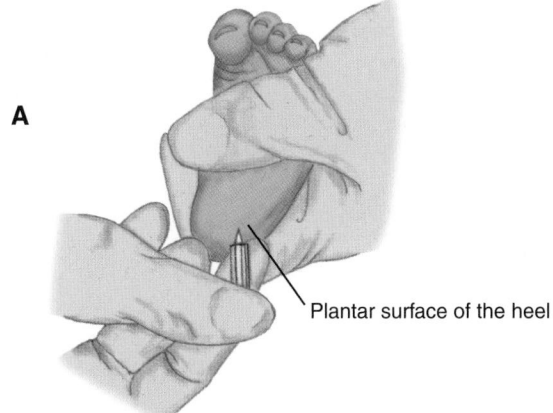

A

Plantar surface of the heel

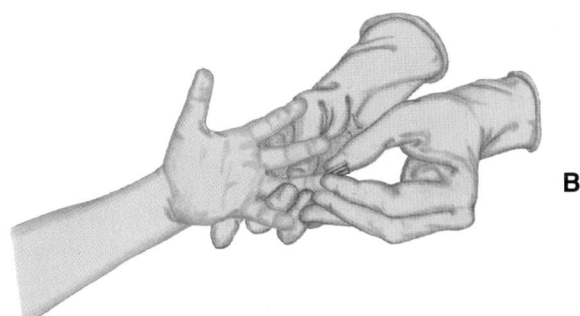

B

FIGURE 30-13 A, Heel site is used for skin punctures in infants. **B,** The third finger (ring finger) is used for skin punctures in children. (From James SR, Ashwill JW, Droske SC: *Nursing care of children: principles and practice,* ed 3, Philadelphia, 2007, Saunders.)

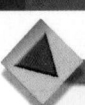

MEASURING BLOOD GLUCOSE

- Knock before entering the person's room.
- Address the person by name.
- Introduce yourself by name and title.
- Explain the procedure to the person before beginning and during the procedure.

- Protect the person's rights during the procedure.
- Handle the person gently during the procedure.

PRE-PROCEDURE

1 Follow *Delegation Guidelines: Blood Glucose Testing,* p. 527. See *Promoting Safety and Comfort: Blood Glucose Testing,* p. 527.
2 Practice hand hygiene.
3 Collect the following:
- Sterile lancet
- Antiseptic wipes
- Gloves
- Cotton balls
- Glucose meter
- Reagent strips (Use the correct ones for the meter. Check the expiration date.)

- Paper towels
- Washcloth
- Soap, towel, and wash basin
4 Read the manufacturer's instructions for the lancet and glucose meter.
5 Arrange your work area.
6 Identify the person. Check the ID bracelet against the assignment sheet. Also call the person by name.
7 Provide for privacy.
8 Raise the bed for good body mechanics. The far bed rail is up if used.

PROCEDURE

9 Help the person to a comfortable position.
10 Assist with hand washing.
11 Put on the gloves.
12 Prepare the supplies:
 a Open the antiseptic wipes.
 b Remove a reagent strip from the bottle. Place it on the paper towel. Place the cap securely on the bottle.
 c Prepare the lancet.
 d Turn on the glucose meter.
 e Insert a reagent strip into the glucose meter (Fig. 30-14).
13 Perform a skin puncture to obtain a drop of blood:
 a Inspect the person's fingers. Select a skin puncture site.
 b Warm the finger. Rub it gently or apply a warm washcloth.
 c Massage the hand and finger toward the puncture site. This brings more blood to the site.
 c Lower the finger below the person's waist. This increases blood flow to the site.
 e Hold the finger with your thumb and forefinger. Use your non-dominant hand. Hold the finger until step 13-k.
 f Clean the site with an antiseptic wipe. *Do not touch the site after cleaning.*
 g Let the site dry.
 h Pick up the sterile lancet.

 i Place the lancet against the side of the finger or the top of the finger tip.
 j Push the button on the lancet to puncture the skin. (Follow the manufacturer's instructions.)
 k Wipe away the first blood drop. Use a cotton ball.
 l Apply gentle pressure below the puncture site.
 m Let a large drop of blood form.
14 Collect and test the specimen. Follow the manufacturer's instructions and agency procedures for the glucose meter used.
 a Hold the test area of the reagent strip close to the drop of blood.
 b Lightly touch the reagent strip to the blood drop (Fig. 30-15). Do not smear the blood.
 c Set the timer on the glucose meter.
 d Wait the length of time required by the manufacturer.
 e Apply pressure to the puncture site until bleeding stops. Use a cotton ball. If able, let the person apply pressure to the site.
 f Read the result on the display (Fig. 30-16). Note the result, and tell the person the result.
 g Turn off the glucose meter.
15 Discard the lancet into the sharps container.
16 Discard the cotton balls following agency policy.
17 Remove and discard the gloves. Decontaminate your hands.

POST-PROCEDURE

18 Provide for comfort. (See the inside of the front book cover.)
19 Place the signal light within reach.
20 Lower the bed to its lowest position.
21 Raise or lower bed rails. Follow the care plan.
22 Unscreen the person.
23 Discard used supplies. Clean and return the bath basin to its proper place.

24 Complete a safety check of the room. (See the inside of the front book cover.)
25 Follow agency policy for soiled linen.
26 Decontaminate your hands.
27 Report and record the test result and your observations.

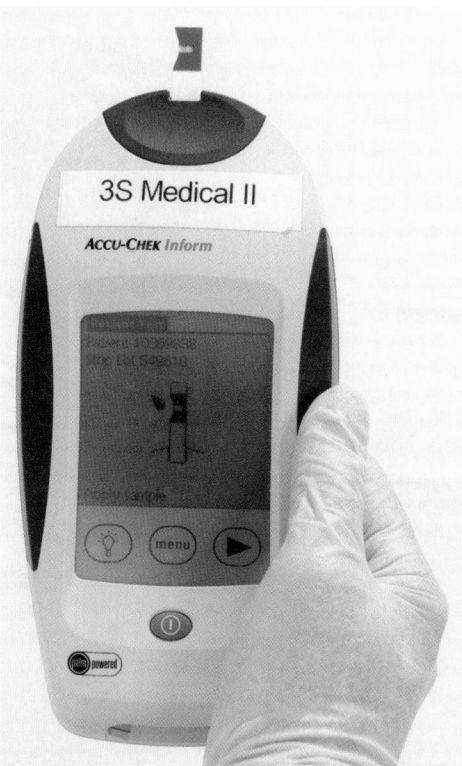

FIGURE 30-14 A reagent strip is in the glucose meter.

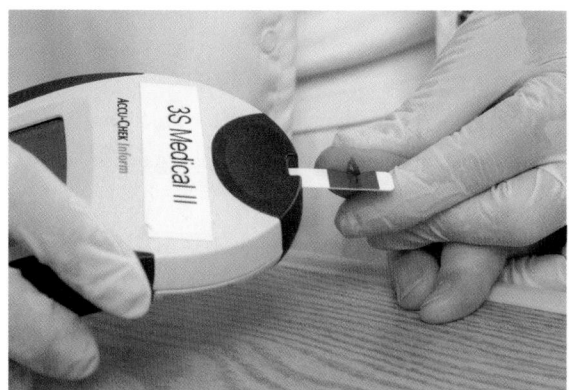

FIGURE 30-15 A drop of blood is applied to the reagent strip.

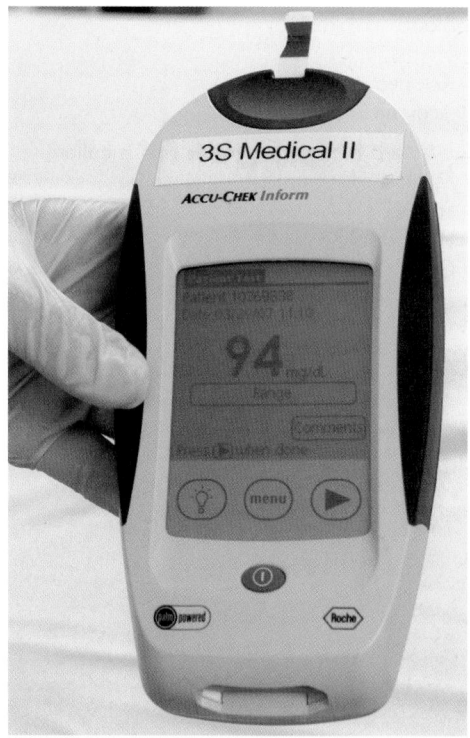

FIGURE 30-16 The result is displayed on the glucose meter.

REVIEW QUESTIONS

Circle the BEST answer.

1 A random urine specimen is collected
   a Upon awakening
   b Before meals
   c After meals
   d Any time

2 Perineal care is given before collecting a
   a Random specimen
   b Midstream specimen
   c Stool specimen
   d Double-voided specimen

3 A 24-hour urine specimen involves
   a Collecting all urine voided during a 24-hour period
   b Collecting a random specimen every hour for 24 hours
   c Testing urine for sugar and ketones every day
   d Measuring output every hour for 24 hours

4 Urine is tested for sugar and ketones
   a At bedtime
   b 30 minutes after meals and at bedtime
   c 30 minutes before meals and at bedtime
   d Before breakfast

5 Which specimen is best for sugar and ketone testing?
   a A random specimen
   b A clean-voided specimen
   c A reagent specimen
   d A double-voided specimen

6 You need to strain a person's urine. Straining is done to find
   a Blood
   b Stones
   c Ketones
   d Acetone

7 You note a black, tarry stool. This is called
   a Melena
   b Feces
   c Hemostool
   d Occult blood

8 A stool specimen must be kept warm. After collecting the specimen
   a Put it in an oven
   b Put it in a paper bag
   c Cover it with a towel
   d Take it to the laboratory

9 The best time to collect a sputum specimen is
   a On awakening
   b After meals
   c At bedtime
   d After oral hygiene

10 A sputum specimen is needed. You should ask the person to
   a Use mouthwash
   b Rinse the mouth with clear water
   c Brush the teeth
   d Remove dentures

11 Which is the best site for a skin puncture?
   a The thumb
   b The index finger
   c The ring finger
   d The little finger

12 Which is used to measure blood glucose?
   a Glucose meter
   b Lancet
   c Reagent strip
   d Sphygmomanometer

13 You are measuring blood glucose. How long should you time the test?
   a 30 seconds
   b 1 minute
   c 2 minutes
   d As stated in the manufacturer's instructions

14 Before using reagent strips for blood glucose testing, you need to
   a Check the expiration date
   b Make sure they are discolored
   c Label each strip with the person's name
   d Check the size of the test area

Answers to these questions are on p. 781.

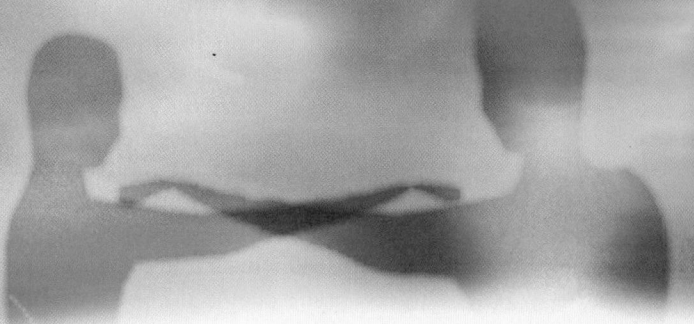

The Person Having Surgery

OBJECTIVES

- Define the key terms and key abbreviations listed in this chapter
- Describe the common fears and concerns of surgical patients
- Explain how people are prepared for surgery
- Describe how to prepare a room for the post-operative patient
- List the signs and symptoms to report after surgery
- Explain how to meet the person's needs after surgery
- Perform the procedures described in this chapter

PROCEDURES

- The Surgical Skin Prep—Shaving the Skin
- Applying Elastic Stockings
- Applying Elastic Bandages

KEY TERMS

anesthesia The loss of feeling or sensation produced by a drug

elective surgery Surgery done by choice to improve the person's life or well-being

embolus A blood clot that travels through the vascular system until it lodges in a blood vessel

emergency surgery Surgery done at once to save life or function

general anesthesia The loss of consciousness and all feeling or sensation

local anesthesia The loss of feeling or sensation in a small area

post-operative After surgery

pre-operative Before surgery

regional anesthesia The loss of feeling or sensation in a large area of the body

thrombus A blood clot

urgent surgery Surgery needed for the person's health; it is done soon to prevent further damage or disease

Procedures with this icon are on the CDCompanion in this book; those with this icon [View Video!] are on the Evolve Student Resources Website.

KEY ABBREVIATIONS

AE Anti-embolism, anti-embolic
CBC Complete blood count
ECG Electrocardiogram
EKG Electrocardiogram
I&O Intake and output
IV Intravenous

NG Nasogastric
NPO Non per os; nothing by mouth
OR Operating room
PACU Post anesthesia care unit
SCD Sequential compression device
TED Thrombo-embolic disease

Doctors perform surgery for many reasons. Surgeries are done to:

▶ Remove a diseased or injured body part
▶ Remove a tumor
▶ Repair an injured body part
▶ Make a diagnoses
▶ Improve appearance
▶ Relieve symptoms
▶ Restore or improve function
▶ Replace a body part

Surgery often requires a hospital stay. Patients are admitted to the hospital before surgery. Patients are admitted the morning of surgery or 1 or 2 days before surgery. Some patients go directly to surgery from the emergency department.

Patients stay for 1, 2, or more days after surgery. Same-day surgery (out-patient, one-day, or ambulatory surgery) is common. The person is admitted in the morning and discharged later in the day. Many same-day surgeries are done in clinics or surgical centers that are part of hospitals or doctors' offices.

Surgeries are elective, urgent, or an emergency:

▶ **Elective surgery** is done by choice to improve the person's life or well-being. It is not life-saving. Joint replacement surgery and cosmetic surgery are examples. The surgery is scheduled in advance.
▶ **Urgent surgery** is needed for the person's health. It is done to prevent further damage or disease. Cancer surgery and coronary artery bypass surgery are examples.
▶ **Emergency surgery** is done at once to save life or function. The need is sudden and not expected. Vehicle crashes, stabbings, and bullet wounds often require emergency surgery.

The person is prepared for what happens before, during, and after surgery. This is done by doctors, nurses, and other health team members. You assist as the nurse and care plan direct.

In hospitals, you will care for patients before and after surgery. **Pre-operative** refers to before surgery. **Post-operative** refers to after surgery. In nursing centers, many residents are recovering from surgery. Some patients need home care after surgery.

PSYCHOLOGICAL CARE

Surgery causes many fears and concerns (Box 31-1). The person's deepest and worst fears are often felt. What if you needed surgery today or tomorrow? Would you fear cancer or losing a body part? Would you worry about pain or death? Who will care for your children and home? Will you have an income to support your family? Imagine having an accident. You wake up hours later. You are told that your right leg was amputated.

Past experiences affect feelings. Some persons have had surgery. Others have not. Patients are affected when family and friends talk about their own surgeries. Most people know about tragic events—surgery on the wrong person or body part, instruments left in the body, death during or after surgery. Some people do not share their fears and concerns. They may cry, be quiet or withdrawn, or talk about other things. Some pace or are very cheerful.

Mental preparation is important. Respect the person's fears and concerns. Show the person warmth, sensitivity, and caring.

BOX 31-1 Common Fears and Concerns of Surgical Patients

THE FEAR OF . . .
- Anesthesia and its effects
- Cancer
- Complications from surgery
- Disfigurement and scarring
- Disability
- Dying during or after surgery
- Exposure
- Not waking up after surgery
- Pain during surgery
- Pain after surgery
- Prolonged recovery
- Separation from family and friends
- Surgery on the wrong body part
- Tubes, needles, and other care equipment
- Waking up during surgery
- What happens after surgery—more surgery, treatments, care, and so on

CONCERN ABOUT . . .
- Caring for children and other family members
- Finances—monthly bills, loan payments, mortgages, hospital bills, doctor bills
- House, lawn, and garden
- Pets
- Plants

Patient Information

The doctor explains the need for surgery to the patient and family. They are told about:

▶ The surgical procedure, its risk, and possible complications

▶ The risks from not having surgery

▶ Who will do the surgery

▶ The date and time of the surgery

▶ How long the surgery will take

Questions from the patient and family are answered. Misunderstandings are cleared up. Instructions about care are given. The doctor and nurse give all the information before surgery.

After surgery the doctor talks to the patient and family. The doctor decides what and when to tell them. Often the health team knows the results before the person.

See *Focus on Communication: Patient Information.*

Your Role

You can assist in the person's psychological care. Do the following if you assist in pre-operative and post-operative care:

▶ Listen to the person. He or she may talk about fears and concerns.

▶ Refer questions about the surgery or its results to the nurse.

▶ Explain the care you will give. Also explain why the care is needed.

▶ Follow communication rules (Chapters 5 and 7).

▶ Use verbal and nonverbal communication (Chapter 7).

▶ Perform procedures and tasks with skill and ease.

▶ Report signs (verbal and nonverbal) of fear or anxiety.

▶ Report a request to see a member of the clergy.

PRE-OPERATIVE CARE

The pre-operative period may be many days or a few minutes. If time permits, the person is prepared mentally and physically for the effects of anesthesia and surgery. The goal is to prevent complications before, during, and after surgery.

See *Teamwork and Time Management: Pre-Operative Care.*

Pre-Operative Teaching

A nurse does the pre-operative teaching. The nurse explains what to expect before, during, and after surgery. Teaching includes:

▶ *Pre-operative activities.* This includes tests and their purpose, skin preparation, and personal care. The person learns about the purpose and effects of pre-operative drugs.

▶ *Deep breathing, coughing, and incentive spirometry.* These are taught and practiced. After surgery, they are done every 1 or 2 hours when the person is awake.

▶ *Leg exercises.* These are taught and practiced. After surgery, they are done every 1 or 2 hours when the person is awake.

▶ *Post anesthesia care unit (PACU).* This is where the person is taken after surgery (Fig. 31-1, p. 534). He or she wakes up in the PACU. Care given in the PACU is explained.

▶ *Vital signs.* These are taken often until they are stable.

▶ *Food and fluids.* The person is NPO and has intravenous (IV) therapy after surgery. The doctor orders food and oral fluids when the person's condition is stable.

▶ *Turning and repositioning.* These are done at least every 1 to 2 hours after surgery.

▶ *Early ambulation.* The person walks as soon as possible after surgery.

▶ *Pain.* The person is told about the type and amount of pain to expect. The nurse explain about pain relief drugs and how they given.

▶ *Treatments and equipment.* The person may need a urinary catheter, NG (nasogastric) tube, oxygen, wound suction, a cast, or traction.

▶ *Position restrictions.* Some surgeries require certain positions. For example, the hip is abducted after hip replacement surgery (Chapter 39).

See *Focus on Children and Older Persons: Pre-Operative Care,* p.534.

Pre-Operative Care

CHILDREN
The child and parents are prepared for the surgery. Often play is used to help the child understand what will happen. For example, dolls are used to show the surgery site. A tour of the operating room and PACU is common. The child and parents meet the nursing staff who will care for the child.

Special Tests

Before surgery, the doctor evaluates the person's health status. The following tests are commonly ordered:
- Chest x-ray.
- Complete blood count (CBC).
- Urinalysis.
- Electrocardiogram (ECG; EKG). See Figure 31-2.

Other tests depend on the person's condition and surgery. If blood loss is expected, the person's blood is tested for blood type and compatible blood. This is called *type and cross-match*.

The person is prepared for the tests as needed. Tests results must be on the chart by the time of surgery.

Nutrition and Fluids

A light meal usually is allowed. Then the person is NPO for 6 to 8 hours before surgery. These measures reduce the risk of vomiting and aspiration during anesthesia and after surgery. An NPO sign is placed in the person's room. The water pitcher and glass are removed.

Bowel Elimination

Bowel surgeries may require cleansing the bowel of feces. This is called a *bowel prep*. Feces contain microbes. When the intestine is opened, feces can spill into the sterile abdominal cavity. The bowel prep prevents this contamination.

For the bowel prep, the person drinks special fluids ordered by the doctor. Or cleansing enemas are ordered. Sometimes enemas are given to prevent constipation after surgery. The doctor orders what enema to give and when.

SAFETY
Check all persons for loose teeth. Loose teeth are common in children. Adults may have loose teeth from periodontal disease (Chapter 19). Report loose teeth to the nurse. The nurse notes this on the pre-operative checklist and tells the surgery staff. A loose tooth can fall out during anesthesia. The person can aspirate on the tooth.

Urinary Elimination

Some surgeries require catheters. For pelvic and abdominal surgeries, the bladder must be empty. A full bladder is easily injured during surgery. Catheters also allow accurate output measurements during and after surgery.

The person without a catheter needs to void before the nurse gives pre-operative drugs.

Personal Care

Personal care before surgery involves:
- *A complete bath, shower, or tub bath.* A special soap or cleanser may be ordered. A shampoo is included. The bath and shampoo reduce the number of microbes on the body. This reduces the risk of a wound infection. A gown is put on after the bath.
- *Removing makeup, nail polish, and fake nails.* The skin, lips, and nail beds are observed for color and circulation. Observations are made during and after surgery.
- *Hair care.* All hairpins, clips, combs, and other items are removed. So are wigs and hairpieces. Some agencies have the patient wear a surgical cap. A cap keeps hair out of the face and the operative site.
- *Oral hygiene for comfort.* Being NPO causes thirst and a dry mouth. The person must not swallow any water during oral hygiene.
- *Removing dentures.* Provide denture care. Then store dentures following agency policy. Some people do not like being seen without their dentures. Let them wear dentures as long as possible. This promotes dignity and self-esteem.
- *Removing prostheses.* Eyeglasses, contact lenses, hearing aids, artificial eyes, and artificial limbs are examples. Follow agency policy for storage and safekeeeping. See *Promoting Safety and Comfort: Personal Care.*

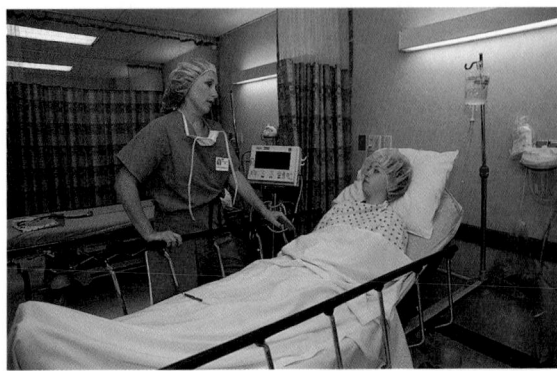

FIGURE 31-1 The post anesthesia care unit (PACU).

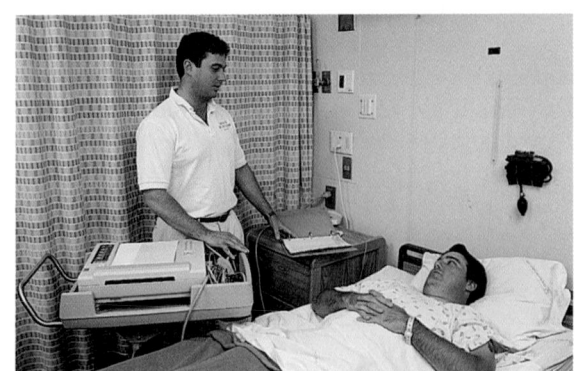

FIGURE 31-2 An electrocardiogram is taken.

Jewelry

Jewelry is easily lost or broken during surgery and during care in the PACU. Transfers to and from the operating room (OR), PACU, and the person's room also present safety risks. Therefore all jewelry is removed and stored for safekeeping. Record its removal and storage according to agency policy.

The person may want to wear a wedding ring or religious medal. The item is secured in place with gauze and tape according to agency policy. Hand, arm, shoulder, and breast surgeries can cause swelling of the fingers. Wedding rings are removed for such surgeries.

◆ Skin Preparation

The skin and hair contain microbes that can enter the body through the surgical incision. Infection is a risk. To reduce the risk of infection, a *skin prep* is done. The doctor orders one or more of the following for the skin prep:

▸ Cleansing the operative area with an anti-microbial soap. (*Anti* means against.)
▸ Clipping the hair at and around the operative site.
▸ Shaving the skin to remove hair at and around the operative site.

The incision site and a large area around it are *prepped* (Fig. 31-3). This is done right before the surgery. The prep is done in the person's room or in the OR. To remove hair, a hair cream remover is used. Or the skin is shaved.

For shaving, a skin prep kit is used. The kit has a razor, a sponge filled with soap, a basin, a drape, and a towel (Fig. 31-4, p. 537). Lather the skin with soap. Then shave in the direction of hair growth (Fig. 31-5, p. 537).

See *Delegation Guidelines: Skin Preparation*, p. 537.
See *Promoting Safety and Comfort: Skin Preparation*, p. 537.

Text continued on p. 538

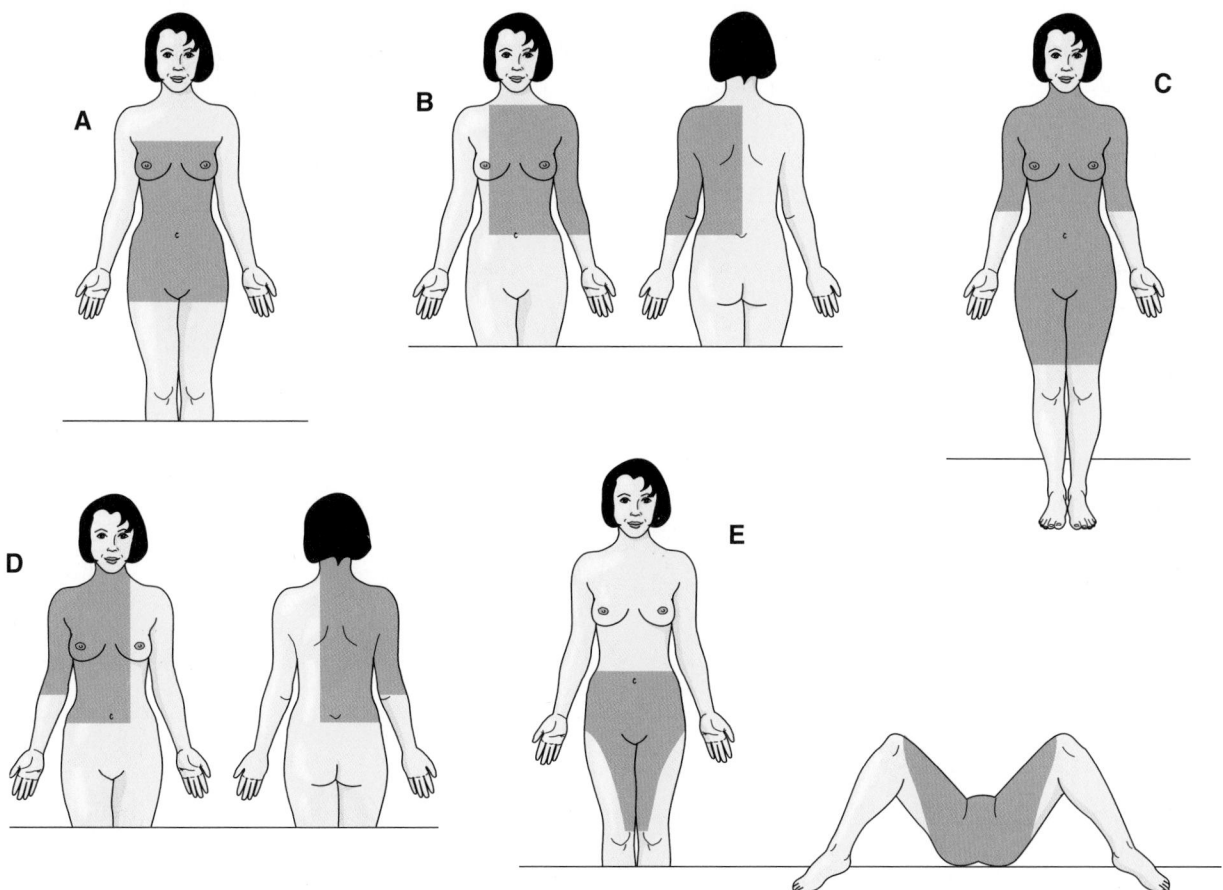

FIGURE 31-3 Skin prep sites. The *shaded area* shows the area to prep. **A,** Abdominal surgery. **B,** Chest or thoracic surgery. **C,** Open-heart surgery. **D,** Breast surgery. **E,** Perineal surgery. *Continued*

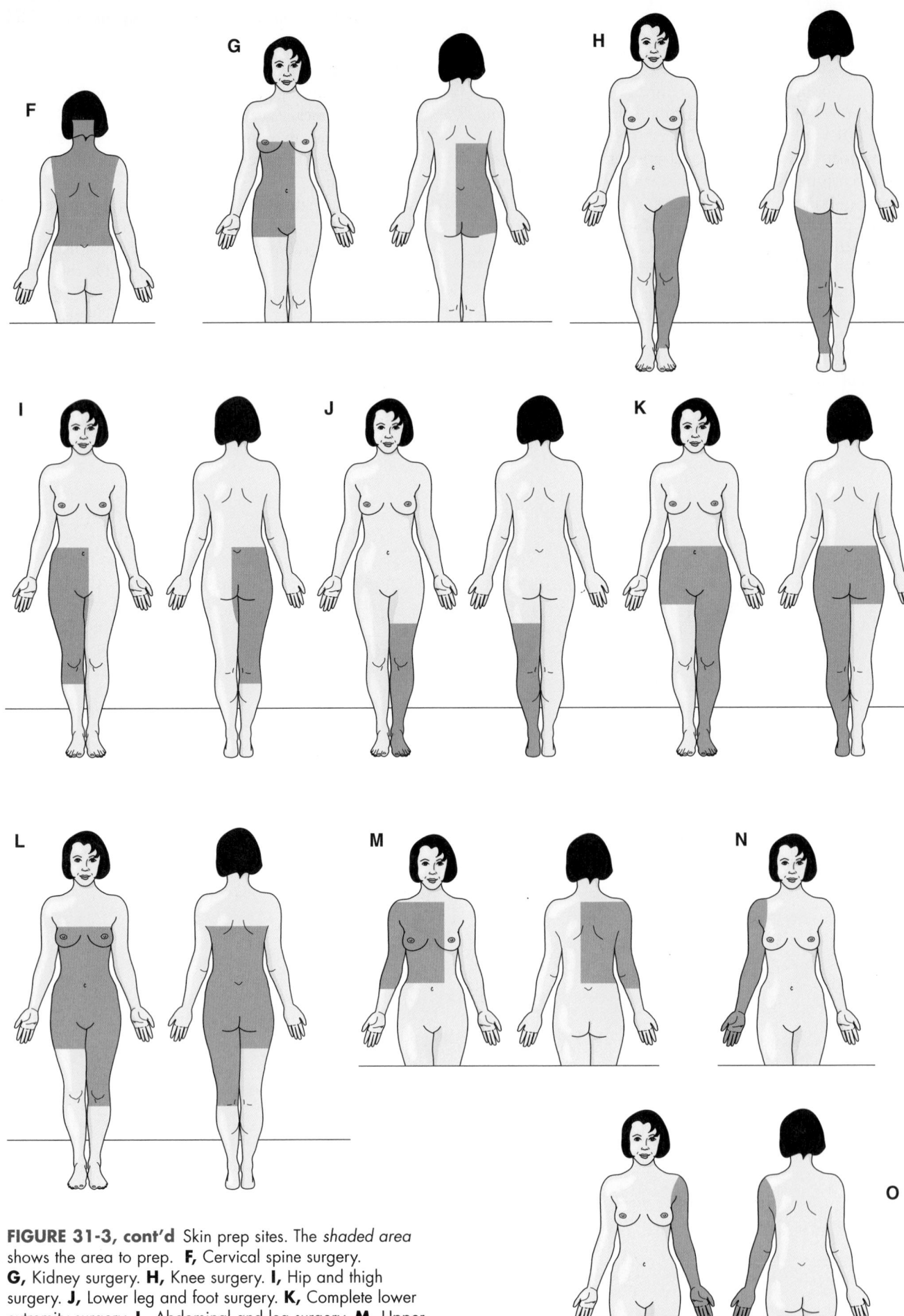

FIGURE 31-3, cont'd Skin prep sites. The *shaded area* shows the area to prep. **F,** Cervical spine surgery. **G,** Kidney surgery. **H,** Knee surgery. **I,** Hip and thigh surgery. **J,** Lower leg and foot surgery. **K,** Complete lower extremity surgery. **L,** Abdominal and leg surgery. **M,** Upper arm surgery. **N,** Lower arm surgery. **O,** Elbow surgery.

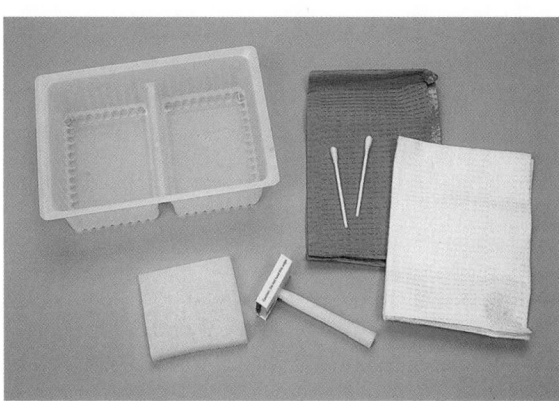

FIGURE 31-4 Skin prep kit.

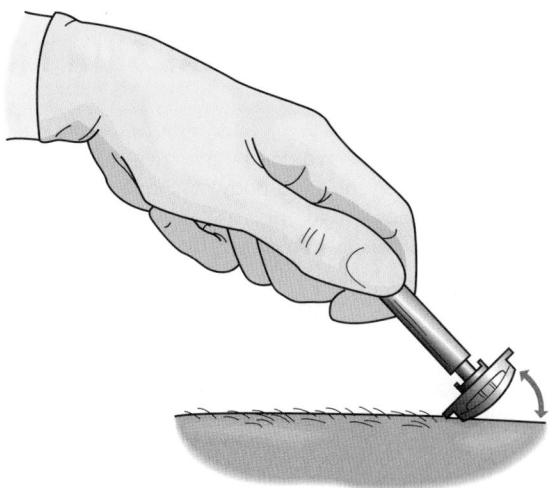

FIGURE 31-5 Shave in the direction of hair growth.

DELEGATION GUIDELINES: Skin Preparation

The nurse may delegate a skin prep to you. When reviewing the procedure with the nurse, you need this information:
- What type of skin prep to do—cleanse the skin, clip hair, shave the skin
- What site to prep
- What observations to report and record
  - The area prepped
  - Any cuts, nicks, or scratches
  - Bleeding
  - Sites of non-intact skin
- When to report observations
- What specific patient or resident concerns to report at once

PROMOTING SAFETY AND COMFORT: Skin Preparation

SAFETY

Any break in the skin is a possible infection site. Be very careful not to cut, scratch, or nick the skin. Follow Standard Precautions and the Bloodborne Pathogen Standard.

THE SURGICAL SKIN PREP—SHAVING THE SKIN

✔ **Quality of Life** *Remember to:*

- Knock before entering the person's room.
- Address the person by name.
- Introduce yourself by name and title.
- Explain the procedure to the person before beginning and during the procedure.
- Protect the person's rights during the procedure.
- Handle the person gently during the procedure.

PRE-PROCEDURE

1 Follow *Delegation Guidelines: Skin Preparation.* See *Promoting Safety and Comfort: Skin Preparation.*
2 Practice hand hygiene.
3 Collect the following:
  - Skin prep kit
  - Bath blanket
  - Warm water
  - Gloves
  - Waterproof pad
  - Bath towel
4 Identify the person. Check the ID bracelet against the assignment sheet. Also call the person by name.
5 Provide for privacy.

Continued

THE SURGICAL SKIN PREP—SHAVING THE SKIN—cont'd

PROCEDURE

6 Make sure you have good lighting.
7 Raise the bed for good body mechanics. Lower the bed rail near you (if up).
8 Cover the person with a bath blanket. Fan-fold top linens to the foot of the bed.
9 Place the waterproof pad under the area you will shave.
10 Open the skin prep kit.
11 Position the person for the skin prep.
12 Drape him or her with the drape.
13 Add warm water to the basin. Bed rails (if used) are up before you leave the bedside.

14 Put on the gloves.
15 Lather the skin with the sponge.
16 Hold the skin taut. Shave in the direction of hair growth (see Fig. 31-5).
17 Shave outward from the center using short strokes.
18 Rinse the razor often.
19 Make sure the entire area is free of hair. Check for cuts, scratches, or nicks.
20 Rinse the skin thoroughly. Pat dry.
21 Remove the drape and waterproof pad.
22 Remove the gloves. Decontaminate your hands.
23 Return top linens. Remove the bath blanket.

POST-PROCEDURE

24 Provide for comfort. (See the inside of the front book cover.)
25 Place the signal light within reach.
26 Lower the bed to its lowest position. Lock the bed wheels.
27 Raise or lower bed rails. Follow the care plan.
28 Unscreen the person.

29 Return equipment to its proper place.
30 Discard supplies.
31 Complete a safety check of the room. (See the inside of the front book cover.)
32 Follow agency policy for dirty linen.
33 Decontaminate your hands.

The Surgery Consent

The person's consent is needed before surgery is done. An operative permit or surgical consent is signed when the person understands the information given by the doctor. The person's spouse or nearest relative may be required to sign the consent. A parent or legal representative signs for a minor child. The legal representative signs for a person who is not mentally competent to sign.

The doctor is reponsible for securing the written consent. Often this is delegated to an RN. *You do not obtain the person's written consent for surgery.*

The Pre-Operative Checklist

A pre-operative checklist (Fig. 31-6) is placed on the front of the person's chart. When the list is complete, the person is ready for surgery. The nurse may ask you to do some of the things on the list. Promptly report when you complete each task. Also report any observations. Except for bed rails, the entire checklist is completed before the nurse gives pre-operative drugs.

Marking the Surgical Site

The surgical site is marked before the surgery. Sometimes the person marks the surgical site. Marking the site prevents surgery on the wrong body part or area.

Marking the site may be part of the pre-operative checklist. It is done before the pre-operative drugs are given.

Pre-Operative Drugs

About 45 to 60 minutes before surgery, the nurse gives pre-operative drugs. They are given to:
▶ Help the person relax and feel drowsy.
▶ Reduce respiratory secretions to prevent aspiration. A dry mouth also results.
▶ Prevent nausea and vomiting.

The person feels sleepy and light-headed. Falls and accidents are prevented after the drugs are given. Bed rails are raised. The person is not allowed out of bed. Therefore the person voids before the drugs are given. After they are given, the person uses the bedpan or urinal for voiding.

After the drugs are given, move furniture to make room for the stretcher. Also clean off the overbed table and the bedside stand. This prevents damage to equipment and valuables. Raise the bed to its highest level to transfer the patient from the bed to a stretcher.

Transport to the Operating Room

An OR staff member brings a stretcher to the room. The patient is transferred to the stretcher and covered with a bath blanket. The blanket provides warmth and prevents exposure. Falls are prevented. Safety straps are secured and the side rails are raised. A pillow is placed under the person's head for comfort.

Identification checks are made. Then the person's chart is given to the OR staff member. The person is transported to the OR. The family may be allowed to go as far as the OR entrance.

See *Focus on Children and Older Persons: Transport to the Operating Room*, p. 540.

SURGICAL CHECK LIST

Patient's Name   Room

PATIENT STICKER ⬆

I.D. Band on	
Surgical Permit Signed	
History & Physical	
Allergies	
Operative Area Prepped	
Pre-op Enema (if ordered)	
NPO after midnight	
Blood Work Done	
Urinalysis	
UCG on females age 12-50	
BP and TRP taken	
Voided and catheterized	
Jewelry removed and secured	
Hairpins, make up and nail polish removed	
Contact lenses and glasses removed	
Dentures removed	
Head cap and gown	
Premedication of _____	
Time given _____	

Date _____   Nurse _____

IV20064   ©2005 133090 LKCS • www.lk-cs.com

FIGURE 31-6 Pre-operative checklist. (Courtesy Illinois Valley Community Hospital, Peru, Ill.)

ANESTHESIA

Anesthesia is the loss of feeling or sensation produced by a drug. These types of anesthesia are common:

▶ **General anesthesia** is the loss of consciousness and all feeling or sensation. A drug is given IV, or a gas is inhaled.

▶ **Regional anesthesia** is the loss of feeling or sensation in a large area of the body. The person is awake. A drug is injected into a body part.

▶ **Local anesthesia** is the loss of feeling or sensation in a small area. A drug is injected at the site.

Anesthetics are given by specially educated doctors and nurses. An *anesthesiologist* is a doctor who specializes in giving anesthetics. An *anesthetist* is an RN with advanced study in giving anesthetics.

POST-OPERATIVE CARE

After surgery the person is taken to the PACU. It is near the OR. There the person recovers from the anesthesia. This takes 1 to 2 hours. The person is watched very closely. Vital signs are taken and observations are made often. The doctor gives the transfer order and the person is transported to his or her room when:

▶ Vital signs are stable.

▶ Respiratory function is good.

▶ The person can respond and call for help.

Preparing the Person's Room

The room must be ready for the person. This is done after the person is taken to the OR. You can do the following:

▶ Make a surgical bed (lower the bed rails; raise the bed to its highest position)

▶ Place equipment and supplies in the room:
  ▶ Thermometer
  ▶ Stethoscope
  ▶ Sphygmomanometer
  ▶ Kidney basin
  ▶ Tissues
  ▶ Waterproof bed protector
  ▶ Vital signs flow sheet
  ▶ I&O (intake and output) record
  ▶ IV pole
  ▶ Other items as directed by the nurse

▶ Move furniture out of the way for the stretcher

Return From the PACU

The PACU staff calls the nursing unit when the person is ready for transfer. The transport is done by PACU nurses. A nurse meets them and the patient in the person's room. Then the person is transferred from the stretcher to bed. Assist as needed. Also help position the person.

Vital signs are measured and observations made. They are compared with those taken in the PACU. The nurse checks the incision for bleeding. Catheter, IV, and other tube placements and functions are checked. Bed rails are raised. The signal light is placed within the person's reach. Necessary care and treatments are given. Then the family can be with the person.

Measurements and Observations

Your role in the person's post-operative care depends on his or her condition. Often you will measure vital signs and observe the person's condition. Vital signs are usually measured:

▶ Every 15 minutes for the first hour

▶ Every 30 minutes for 1 to 2 hours

▶ Every hour for 4 hours

▶ Then every 4 hours

The nurse tells you how often to check the person. This is an important function. Be alert for the signs and symptoms in Box 31-2. Report them to the nurse at once.

Positioning

The person is positioned for comfort and to prevent complications. The type of surgery affects positioning. Position restrictions may be ordered. The person is usually positioned:

▶ For easy and comfortable breathing

▶ To prevent stress on the incision

▶ To prevent aspiration

When the person is supine, the head of the bed is usually raised slightly. His or her head may be turned to the side.

Repositioning is done at least every 1 to 2 hours. This prevents respiratory and circulatory complications. Turning may be painful. Provide support. Use smooth, gentle motions. Pillows and other positioning devices are used as the nurse directs (Chapters 15 and 26).

The nurse tells you when to reposition the person and the positions allowed. Usually you assist the nurse. Sometimes you turn and reposition the person yourself. This occurs when the person's condition is stable and care is simple.

See *Focus on Children and Older Persons: Positioning.*

BOX 31-2 Post-Operative Observations

- Bleeding: from the incision, drainage tubes, suction tubes, or other sites
- Blood pressure: a drop or rise
- Condition: any change in
- Choking
- Confusion
- Cough: weak
- Disorientation
- Drainage:
  - On or under dressings
  - On bed linens (including bottom linens and pillowcases)
  - Appearance from urinary catheter, NG tube, wound suction, and other tubes
- Hypoxia (Chapter 34)
- Intake and output
- IV flow rate
- Nausea
- Pain

- Pulse:
  - More than 100 beats per minute
  - Less than 60 beats per minute
  - Weak
  - Irregular
- Respirations:
  - Shallow, slow breathing
  - Rapid
  - Gasping
  - Difficult
  - Rapid
  - Moist-sounding
  - Gurgling
- Restlessness
- Skin:
  - Moist or clammy
  - Pale
  - Cyanosis (bluish color)
- Temperature: a drop or rise
- Thirst
- Urine: amount, character, and time of first voiding after surgery
- Vomiting

Preventing Respiratory Complications

Respiratory complications are prevented. They include:

▶ *Pneumonia*—an inflammation and infection of the lung
▶ *Atelectasis*—the collapse of a portion of the lung

Coughing and deep-breathing exercises help prevent these complications. So does incentive spirometry. See Chapter 34.

See *Focus on Children and Older Persons: Preventing Respiratory Complications.*

See *Promoting Safety and Comfort: Preventing Respiratory Complications.*

FOCUS ON CHILDREN AND OLDER PERSONS

Positioning

OLDER PERSONS

Many older persons have stiff and painful joints. Sore muscles, bones, and joints occur from being on the OR table. Turn and reposition older persons slowly and gently.

FOCUS ON CHILDREN AND OLDER PERSONS

Preventing Respiratory Complications

OLDER PERSONS

Older persons are at risk for respiratory complications. Respiratory muscles are weaker. Lung tissue is less elastic. The person has less strength for coughing. Coughing, deep breathing, and incentive spirometry are very important.

PROMOTING SAFETY AND COMFORT: Preventing Respiratory Complications

COMFORT

For coughing exercises, comfort is promoted if the person "splints" the incision. To splint means to support or brace. To splint the incision, the person holds a pillow or his or her hands over the incision. See Chapter 34.

Stimulating Circulation

Circulation must be stimulated. This is important for blood flow in the legs. If blood flow is sluggish, blood clots may form. They can form in the deep leg veins in the lower leg or thigh (Fig. 31-7, *A*, p. 542). Many people do not have signs or symptoms. Signs and symptoms to report at once include:

▶ Swollen area of a leg.
▶ Pain or tenderness in a leg. This may occur only when standing or walking.
▶ Warmth in the part of the leg that is swollen or painful.
▶ Red or discolored skin.

A blood clot (**thrombus**) can break loose and travel through the bloodstream. It then becomes an embolus. An **embolus** is a blood clot that travels through the vascular system until it lodges in a vessel (Fig. 31-7, *B*, p. 542). An embolus from a vein lodges in the lungs (pulmonary embolism). A pulmonary embolus can cause severe respiratory problems and death. Report chest pain or shortness of breath at once.

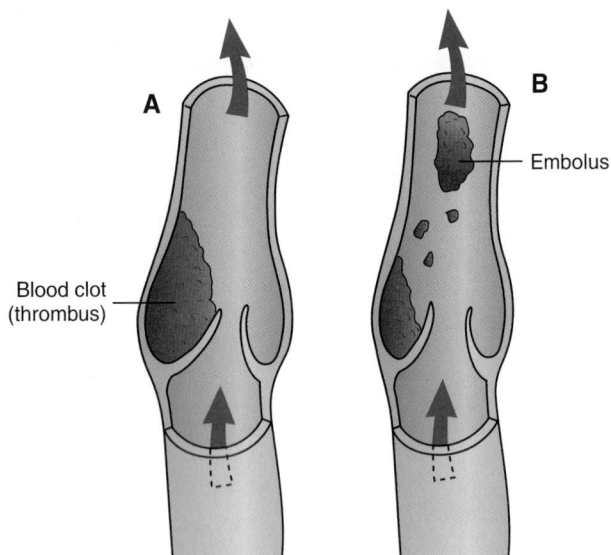

FIGURE 31-7 A, A blood clot is attached to the wall of a vein. The arrow shows the direction of blood flow. **B,** Part of the thrombus breaks off and becomes an embolus. The embolus travels in the bloodstream until it lodges in a distant vessel.

FOCUS ON CHILDREN AND OLDER PERSONS

Stimulating Circulation

OLDER PERSONS
Older persons are at risk for thrombi (blood clots) and emboli (more than one embolus). Blood is pumped through the body with less force. Circulation is already sluggish.

After surgery, circulation is stimulated and thrombi prevented by:

► Leg exercises
► Ambulation as soon as possible
► Elastic stockings
► Elastic bandages
► Sequential compression devices
► No prolonged standing or sitting

See *Focus on Children and Older Persons: Stimulating Circulation.*

Leg Exercises

Leg exercises increase venous blood flow and help prevent thrombi. If the person has had leg surgery, a doctor's order is needed for the exercises.

The nurse tells you when to do the exercises. They are done at least every 1 or 2 hours while the person is awake. Assist if the person is weak. These exercises are done 5 times:

► Making circles with the toes. This rotates the ankles.
► Dorsiflexing and plantar flexing the feet (Chapter 26).
► Flexing and extending one knee and then the other (Fig. 31-8, *A*).
► Raising and lowering the leg off the bed (Fig. 31-8, *B*). Repeat with the other leg.

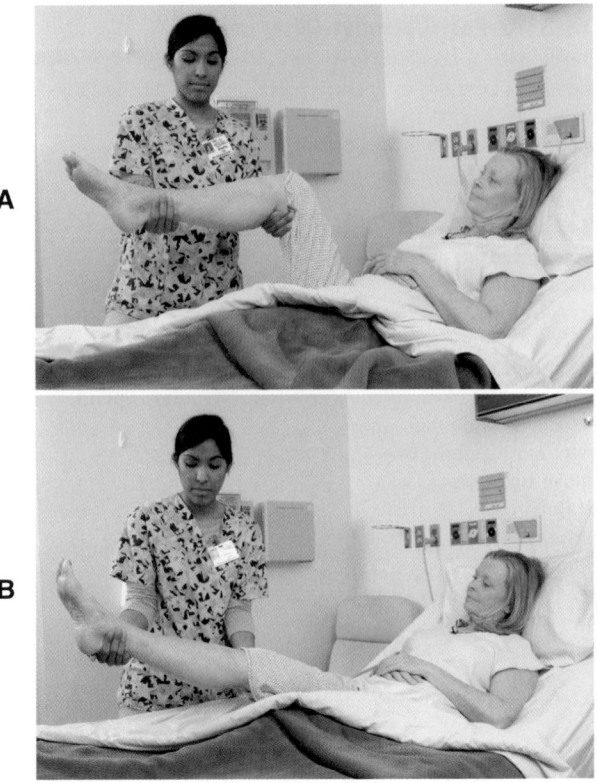

FIGURE 31-8 Leg exercises to stimulate circulation. **A,** The knee is flexed and then extended. **B,** The leg is raised and lowered.

Elastic Stockings

Elastic stockings exert pressure on the veins. The pressure promotes venous blood return to the heart. Elastic stockings also are called AE stockings (AE means *anti-embolism* or *anti-embolic*). They also are called TED hose (TED means *thrombo-embolic disease*). Persons at risk for thrombi include those who:

► Have heart and circulatory disorders
► Are on bedrest
► Have had surgery
► Are older
► Are pregnant

Stockings come in thigh-high and knee-high lengths. The nurse measures the person for the correct size. Most stockings have an opening near the toes. Others have an opening in the top or bottom of the foot. The opening is used to check circulation, skin color, and skin temperature.

The person usually has two pairs of stockings. One pair is washed while the other pair is worn. Wash the stockings by hand with a mild soap. Hang them to dry.

See *Delegation Guidelines: Elastic Stockings.*
See *Promoting Safety and Comfort: Elastic Stockings.*

DELEGATION GUIDELINES: Elastic Stockings

Before applying elastic stockings, you need this information from the nurse and the care plan:
- What size to use—small, medium, or large
- What length to use—thigh-high or knee-high
- When to remove them and for how long—usually every 8 hours for 30 minutes
- What observations to report and record:
  - The size and length of stockings applied
  - When you applied the stockings
  - Skin color and temperature
  - Leg and foot swelling
  - Skin tears, wounds, or signs of skin breakdown
  - Complaints of pain tingling or numbness
  - When you removed the stockings and for how long
  - When you re-applied the stockings
  - When you washed the stockings
- When to report observations
- What specific patient or resident concerns to report at once

PROMOTING SAFETY AND COMFORT: Elastic Stockings

SAFETY
Apply the stocking so the opening in the toe area is over the top of the toes. The opening is used to check circulation to the toes.

Stockings should not have twists, creases, or wrinkles after you apply them. Twists can affect circulation. Creases and wrinkles can cause skin breakdown.

COMFORT
Stockings are applied before the person gets out of bed. Otherwise the person's legs can swell from sitting or standing. Stockings are hard to put on when the legs are swollen. The person lies in bed while they are off. This prevents the legs from swelling.

Gently handle and move the person's foot and leg. Do not force the joints (toes, foot, ankle, knee, and hip) beyond their range of motion or to the point of pain.

NNAAP™ Skill

APPLYING ELASTIC STOCKINGS

✔ **Quality of Life** *Remember to:*

- Knock before entering the person's room.
- Address the person by name.
- Introduce yourself by name and title.
- Explain the procedure to the person before beginning and during the procedure.
- Protect the person's rights during the procedure.
- Handle the person gently during the procedure.

PRE-PROCEDURE

1 Follow *Delegation Guidelines: Elastic Stockings.* See *Promoting Safety and Comfort: Elastic Stockings.*
2 Practice hand hygiene.
3 Obtain elastic stockings in the correct size and length.

4 Identify the person. Check the ID bracelet against the assignment sheet. Also call the person by name.
5 Provide for privacy.
6 Raise the bed for good body mechanics. Bed rails are up if used.

PROCEDURE

7 Lower the bed rail near you if up.
8 Position the person supine.
9 Expose the legs. Fan-fold top linens toward the thighs.
10 Turn the stocking inside out down to the heel.
11 Slip the foot of the stocking over the toes, foot, and heel (Fig. 31-9, A, p. 544).

12 Grasp the stocking top. Pull the stocking up the leg. It turns right side out as it is pulled up. The stocking is even and snug (Fig. 31-9, B, p. 544).
13 Remove twists, creases, or wrinkles.
14 Repeat steps 10 through 13 for the other leg.

POST-PROCEDURE

15 Cover the person.
16 Provide for comfort. (See the inside of the front book cover.)
17 Place the signal light within reach.
18 Lower the bed to its lowest position.
19 Raise or lower bed rails. Follow the care plan.

20 Unscreen the person.
21 Complete a safety check of the room. (See the inside of the front book cover.)
22 Decontaminate your hands.
23 Report and record your observations.

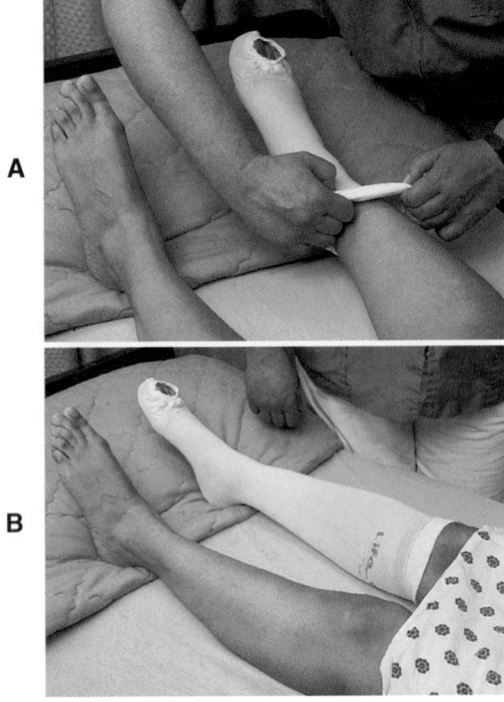

FIGURE 31-9 Applying elastic stockings. **A,** The stocking is slipped over the toes, foot, and heel. **B,** The stocking turns right side out as it is pulled up over the leg.

◆ Elastic Bandages

Elastic bandages have the same purposes as elastic stockings. They also provide support and reduce swelling from injuries. Sometimes they are used to hold dressing in place. They are applied to arms and legs. When applying bandages:

▶ Use the correct size. Use the proper length and width to bandage the extremity.
▶ Position the person in good alignment.
▶ Face the person during the procedure.
▶ Start at the lower (*distal*) part of the extremity. Work upward to the top (*proximal*) part.
▶ Expose fingers or toes if possible. This allows circulation checks.
▶ Apply the bandage with firm, even pressure.
▶ Check the color and temperature of the extremity every hour.
▶ Re-apply a loose or wrinkled bandage.
▶ Replace a moist or soiled bandage.
  See *Focus on Communication: Elastic Bandages.*
  See *Delegation Guidelines: Elastic Bandages.*
  See *Promoting Safety and Comfort: Elastic Bandages.*

FOCUS ON COMMUNICATION

Elastic Bandages

Elastic bandages should promote comfort. To check for comfort, you can ask:
• "Does the bandage feel too tight?"
• "Do you feel pain, itching, tingling, or numbness?" If yes: "What do you feel?" "Where do you feel it?"

DELEGATION GUIDELINES: Elastic Bandages

Before applying elastic bandages, you need this information from the nurse and the care plan:
• Where to apply the bandage
• What width and length to use
• When to remove the bandage and for how long—usually every 8 hours for 30 minutes
• What to do if the bandage is wet or soiled
• What observations to report and record:
  • The width and length applied
  • When you applied the bandage
  • Skin color and temperature
  • Swelling of the part
  • Skin tears, wounds, or signs of skin breakdown
  • Complaints of pain, itching, tingling, or numbness
  • When you removed the bandage and for how long
  • When you re-applied the bandage
• When to report observations
• What specific patient and resident concerns to report at once

---

PROMOTING SAFETY AND COMFORT: Elastic Bandages

SAFETY
Elastic bandages must be firm and snug. However, they must not be tight. A tight bandage can affect circulation.

Elastic bandages are secured in place with clips, tape, or Velcro. Clips are made of metal or plastic. Clips can injure the skin if they become loose or fall off. Use clips only if the nurse tells you to. Check the bandage often to make sure the clips are correctly in place.

Some agencies do not let nursing assistants apply elastic bandages. Know your agency's policy.

COMFORT
A tight bandage can cause pain and discomfort. Apply it with firm, even pressure. If the person complains of pain, tingling, or numbness, remove the bandage and tell the nurse at once.

APPLYING ELASTIC BANDAGES

✔ Quality of Life *Remember to:*

- Knock before entering the person's room.
- Address the person by name.
- Introduce yourself by name and title.
- Explain the procedure to the person before beginning and during the procedure.

- Protect the person's rights during the procedure.
- Handle the person gently during the procedure.

PRE-PROCEDURE

1 Follow *Delegation Guidelines: Elastic Bandages*. See *Promoting Safety and Comfort: Elastic Bandages*.
2 Practice hand hygiene.
3 Collect the following:
   - Elastic bandage as directed by the nurse
   - Tape or clips (unless the bandage has Velcro)

4 Identify the person. Check the ID bracelet against the assignment sheet. Also call the person by name.
5 Provide for privacy.
6 Raise the bed for good body mechanics. Bed rails are up if used.

PROCEDURE

7 Lower the bed rail near you if up.
8 Help the person to a comfortable position. Expose the part you will bandage.
9 Make sure the area is clean and dry.
10 Hold the bandage so the roll is up. The loose end is on the bottom (Fig. 31-10, *A*).
11 Apply the bandage to the smallest part of the wrist, foot, ankle, or knee.
12 Make two circular turns around the part (Fig. 31-10, *B*).
13 Make overlapping spiral turns in an upward direction. Each turn overlaps about ½ to ⅔ of the previous turn (Fig. 31-10, *C*). Make sure each overlap is equal.

14 Apply the bandage smoothly with firm, even pressure. It is not tight.
15 End the bandage with two circular turns.
16 Secure the bandage in place with Velcro, tape, or clips. The clips are not under the body part.
17 Check the fingers or toes for coldness or cyanosis (bluish color). Ask about pain, itching, numbness, or tingling. Remove the bandage if any are noted. Report your observations to the nurse.

POST-PROCEDURE

18 Provide for comfort. (See the inside of the front book cover.)
19 Place the signal light within reach.
20 Lower the bed to its lowest position.
21 Raise or lower bed rails. Follow the care plan.

22 Unscreen the person.
23 Complete a safety check of the room. (See the inside of the front book cover.)
24 Decontaminate your hands.
25 Report and record your observations.

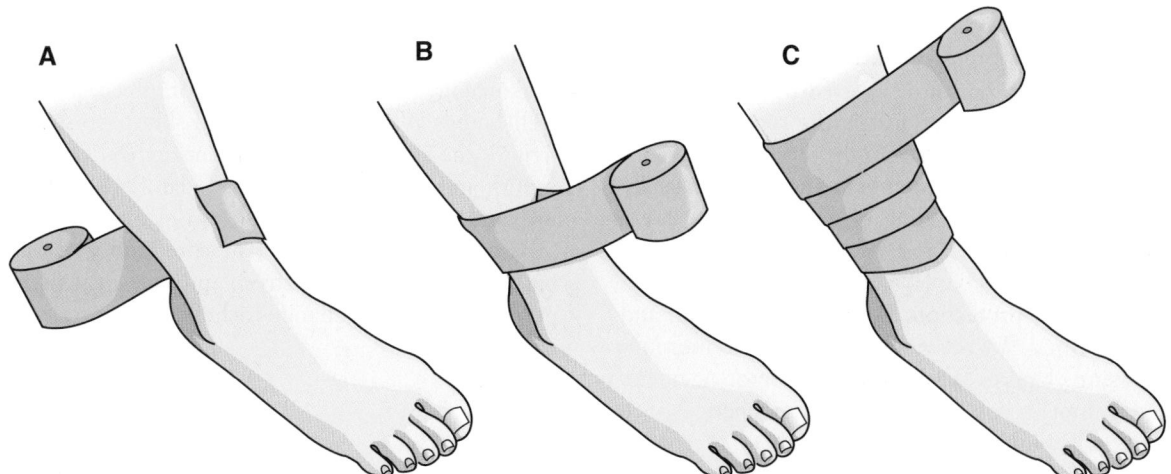

FIGURE 31-10 Applying an elastic bandage. **A,** The roll of the bandage is up. The loose end is at the bottom. **B,** The bandage is applied to the smallest part with two circular turns. **C,** The bandage is applied with spiral turns in an upward direction.

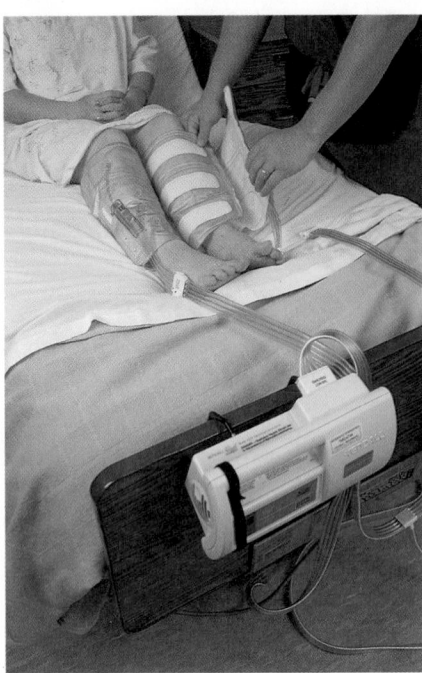

FIGURE 31-11 Sequential compression device. (From deWit SC: *Fundamental concepts and skills for nursing*, ed 2, Philadelphia, 2005, Saunders.)

Sequential Compression Devices

A sequential compression device (SCD) is a sleeve that wraps around the leg (Fig. 31-11). Made of cloth or plastic, the SCD is secured in place with Velcro.

A pump inflates the device with air. This promotes venous blood flow to the heart by causing pressure on the veins. Then the pump deflates the device. After deflation, the device is inflated again. The inflation and deflation sequence is repeated as ordered by the doctor.

Early Ambulation

Early ambulation prevents circulatory complications such as thrombi. It also prevents pneumonia, atelectasis, constipation, and urinary tract infections.

The person usually walks the day of surgery. The person dangles first. Blood pressure and pulse are measured. If they are stable, the person is assisted out of bed. The person does not walk very far, just in the room. Distance increases as the person gains strength.

The nurse tell you when the person can walk. Usually you assist the nurse the first time.

Wound Healing

The incision needs protection. Healing is promoted and infection prevented. A dressing may be over the incision. Sterile dressing changes are done by the doctor or nurse. Your agency may let you do simple dressing changes. See Chapter 32 for wound care.

Nutrition and Fluids

The person returns from the OR with an IV. Continued IV therapy depends on the type of surgery and the person's condition. Anesthesia may cause nausea and vomiting. Diet progresses from NPO to clear liquids, to full liquids, to a regular diet. The doctor orders the diet. Frequent oral hygiene is important when the person is NPO.

Some patients have nasogastric tubes (Chapter 24). Often the NG tube is attached to suction to keep the stomach empty. The person is NPO and has an IV.

Elimination

Anesthesia, the surgery, and being NPO affect normal bowel and urinary elimination. Pain relief drugs can cause constipation. Measures to promote elimination are practiced as directed by the nurse and the care plan (Chapters 21 and 22).

Intake and output are measured. The person must void within 8 hours after surgery. Report the time and amount of the first voiding. If the person does not void within 8 hours, a catheterization usually is ordered. Some patients have a catheter after surgery. See Chapter 21 for the care of a person with a urinary catheter.

Fluid intake and regular diet are needed for bowel elimination. Suppositories or enemas may be ordered for constipation.

Comfort and Rest

Pain is common after surgery. The degree of pain depends on:

▶ The extent of the surgery.
▶ The incision site and size.
▶ If drainage tubes, casts, or other devices are present.
▶ Positioning during surgery. The position can cause muscle strains and discomfort.

The doctor orders drugs for pain relief. The nurse uses the nursing process to promote comfort and rest. Many of the measures listed in Chapter 27 are part of the person's care plan.

Personal Hygiene

Personal hygiene is important for physical and mental well-being. Wound drainage and skin prep solutions can irritate the skin and cause discomfort. NPO causes a dry mouth and breath odors. Moist, clammy skin from blood pressure changes or fever also causes discomfort.

Frequent oral hygiene, hair care, and a complete bed bath after surgery help refresh and renew the person. The gown and lines are changed whenever wet or soiled.

Circle the BEST answer.

1 Which is true of elective surgery?
  a It is done at once.
  b The need is sudden and not expected.
  c It is scheduled at a later date.
  d General anesthesia is always used.

2 A person states "I'm afraid of the surgery." What should you do?
  a Call a member of the clergy.
  b Listen and use touch.
  c Change the subject.
  d Tell the family.

3 You can assist with pre-operative care by explaining
  a The reason for the surgery
  b The procedures you are doing
  c The risks and possible complications of surgery
  d What to expect during and after surgery

4 Before surgery, a person is
  a NPO
  b Allowed only water
  c Given a regular breakfast
  d Given a tube feeding

5 A bowel prep is ordered to
  a Clean the intestines of feces
  b Prevent bleeding
  c Relieve flatus
  d Prevent pain

6 A skin prep is done to
  a Completely bathe the body
  b Sterilize the skin
  c Reduce the amount of microbes on the skin
  d Destroy non-pathogens and pathogens

7 When shaving the skin
  a Shave in the direction opposite of hair growth
  b Shave toward the center of the operative site
  c Do not cut, scratch, or nick the skin
  d Use an electric shaver

8 Pre-operative drugs were given. The patient
  a Must stay in bed
  b Can use the bathroom
  c Can use the commode to void
  d Can have sips of water

9 General anesthesia
  a Is a specially educated nurse
  b Is the loss of consciousness and feeling or sensation
  c Is a specially educated doctor
  d Is the loss of sensation or feeling in a body part

10 Coughing and deep breathing after surgery prevent
  a Bleeding
  b A pulmonary embolus
  c Respiratory complications
  d Pain and discomfort

11 Leg exercises are ordered for a post-operative patient. Which is *false?*
  a They stimulate circulation.
  b They prevent thrombi.
  c They are done 5 times every 1 to 2 hours.
  d They are done only for leg surgery.

12 After surgery, a person's position is changed at least
  a Every 2 hours
  b Every 3 hours
  c Every 4 hours
  d Every shift

13 Elastic stockings
  a Hold dressing in place
  b Prevent blood clots
  c Reduce swelling after injury
  d Prevent pressure ulcers

14 Elastic stockings are applied
  a Before the person gets out of bed
  b When the person is standing
  c After the person's shower or bath
  d For 30 minutes and then removed

15 The purpose of an elastic bandage is to
  a Prevent infection
  b Absorb drainage
  c Provide moisture for wound healing
  d Reduce swelling

16 When applying an elastic bandage
  a Position the part in good alignment
  b Cover the fingers or toes if possible
  c Apply it from the largest to smallest part of the extremity
  d Apply it from the upper to lower part of the extremity

Circle T if the statement is true and F if it is false.

17 T F Hair is kept out of the face for surgery. Pins, clips, or combs are used.

18 T F Nail polish is removed before surgery.

19 T F Makeup can be worn to surgery.

20 T F Pajamas are worn to the OR.

21 T F Contact lenses are removed before surgery.

22 T F A surgical bed is made for the person's return from the PACU.

23 T F A drop in blood pressure is reported at once.

24 T F The person walks for the first time 2 days after surgery.

25 T F Intake and output are measured after surgery.

26 T F The person should void within 8 hours after surgery.

Answers to these questions are on p. 781.

OBJECTIVES

- Define the key terms listed in this chapter
- Describe skin tears, pressure ulcers, circulatory ulcers, and diabetic foot ulcers and their causes
- Identify the pressure points in each body position
- Identify the signs and symptoms of pressure ulcers
- Identify the persons at risk for skin tears, pressure ulcers, circulatory ulcers, and diabetic foot ulcers
- Describe how to prevent skin tears, pressure ulcers, circulatory ulcers, and diabetic foot ulcers
- Describe the process, types, and complications of wound healing
- Describe what to observe about wounds and wound drainage
- Explain how to secure dressings
- Explain the rules for applying dressings
- Explain the purpose of binders and how to apply them
- Describe how to meet the basic needs of persons with wounds
- Perform the procedure described in this chapter

PROCEDURE

- Applying a Dry, Non-Sterile Dressing

KEY TERMS

abrasion A partial-thickness wound caused by the scraping away or rubbing of the skin

arterial ulcer An open wound on the lower legs or feet caused by poor arterial blood flow

chronic wound A wound that does not heal easily

circulatory ulcer An open sore on the lower legs or feet caused by decreased blood flow through the arteries or veins; vascular ulcer

clean-contaminated wound Occurs from the surgical entry of the reproductive, urinary, respiratory, or gastrointestinal system

clean wound A wound that is not infected; microbes have not entered the wound

closed wound Tissues are injured but the skin is not broken

contaminated wound A wound with a high risk of infection

contusion A closed wound caused by a blow to the body; a bruise

dehiscence The separation of wound layers

diabetic foot ulcer An open wound on the foot caused by complications from diabetes

dirty wound An infected wound

edema Swelling caused by fluid collecting in tissues

epidermal stripping Removing the epidermis (outer skin layer) as tape is removed from the skin

evisceration The separation of the wound along with the protrusion of abdominal organs

full-thickness wound The dermis, epidermis, and subcutaneous tissue are penetrated; muscle and bone may be involved

gangrene A condition in which there is death of tissue

hematoma A swelling (oma) that contains blood (hemat)

hemorrhage The excessive loss of blood in a short time

incision An open wound with clean, straight edges; usually intentional from a sharp instrument

infected wound A wound containing large amounts of microbes that shows signs of infection; a dirty wound

intentional wound A wound created for therapy

laceration An open wound with torn tissues and jagged edges

open wound The skin or mucous membrane is broken

partial-thickness wound The dermis and epidermis of the skin are broken

penetrating wound An open wound in which the skin and underlying tissues are pierced

phlebitis Inflammation (itis) of a vein (phleb)

pressure ulcer A localized injury to the skin and/or underlying tissue usually over a bony prominence; the result of pressure or pressure in combination with shear and/or friction

puncture wound An open wound made by a sharp object; entry of the skin and underlying tissues may be intentional or unintentional

purulent drainage Thick green, yellow, or brown drainage

sanguineous drainage Bloody (sanguis) drainage

serosanguineous drainage Thin, watery drainage (sero) that is blood-tinged (sanguineous)

serous drainage Clear, watery fluid (serum)

shock Results when tissues do not get enough blood

skin tear A break or rip in the skin; the epidermis (top skin layer) separates from the underlying tissues

stasis ulcer Venous ulcer

trauma An accident or violent act that injures the skin, mucous membranes, bones, and organs

ulcer A shallow or deep crater-like sore of the skin or a mucous membrane

unintentional wound A wound resulting from trauma

vascular ulcer A circulatory ulcer

venous ulcer An open sore on the lower legs or feet caused by poor blood flow through the veins; stasis ulcer

wound A break in the skin or mucous membrane

The skin is the body's first line of defense. It protects the body from microbes that cause infection. You must prevent skin injury and give good skin care to help prevent skin breakdown.

Box 32-1, p. 550 lists the common causes of skin breakdown. Older and disabled persons are at great risk. Their skin is easily injured.

A **wound** is a break in the skin or mucous membrane. Common causes are:

▶ Surgery.
▶ **Trauma**—an accident or violent act that injures the skin, mucous membranes, bones, and organs. Falls, vehicle crashes, gun shots, stabbings, human and animal bites, burns, and frostbite are examples.

▶ Pressure ulcers from unrelieved pressure.
▶ Decreased blood flow through the arteries or veins.
▶ Nerve damage.

When injury does occur, infection is a major threat. Wound care involves preventing infection and further injury to the wound and nearby tissues. Blood loss and pain also are prevented.

The nurse uses the nursing process to keep the person's skin healthy. Some agencies have a skin care team to manage all skin problems. The team includes an RN, physical therapist, and a dietitian. Your role in wound care depends on state law, your job description, and the person's condition.

BOX 32-1 Skin Breakdown—Common Causes

- Age-related changes in the skin
- Dryness
- Fragile and weak capillaries
- General thinning of the skin
- Loss of the fatty layer under the skin
- Decreased sensation to touch, heat, and cold
- Decreased mobility
- Sitting in a chair or laying in bed most or all of the day
- Chronic diseases (diabetes, high blood pressure)
- Diseases that decrease circulation

- Poor nutrition
- Poor hydration
- Incontinence (urinary, fecal)
- Moisture in dark body areas (skin folds, under breasts, perineal area)
- Pressure on bony parts (Fig. 32-1)
- Poor fingernail and toenail care
- Friction and shearing
- Edema

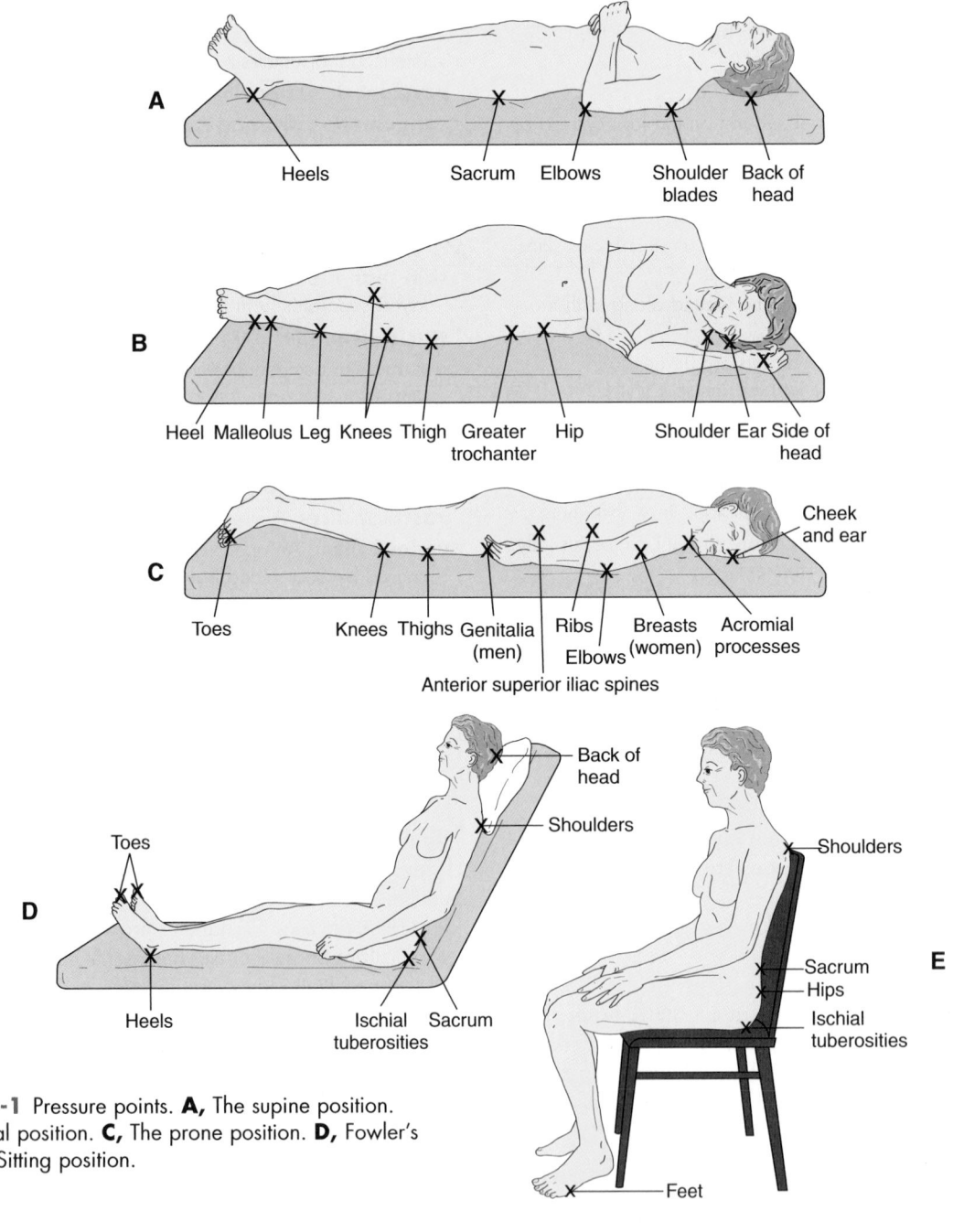

FIGURE 32-1 Pressure points. **A,** The supine position. **B,** The lateral position. **C,** The prone position. **D,** Fowler's position. **E,** Sitting position.

BOX 32-2 Types of Wounds

INTENTIONAL AND UNINTENTIONAL WOUNDS
- **Intentional wound**—is created for therapy. Surgical incisions are examples. So are venipunctures for starting intravenous therapy and for drawing blood specimens.
- **Unintentional wound**—results from trauma (p. 549).

OPEN AND CLOSED WOUNDS
- **Open wound**—when the skin or mucous membrane is broken. Intentional and most unintentional wounds are open.
- **Closed wound**—tissues are injured but the skin is not broken. Bruises, twists, and sprains are examples.

CLEAN AND DIRTY WOUNDS
- **Clean wound**—is not infected. Microbes have not entered the wound. Closed wounds are usually clean. So are intentional wounds created under surgically aseptic conditions. The reproductive, urinary, respiratory, and gastrointestinal systems are not entered.
- **Clean-contaminated wound**—occurs from the surgical entry of the reproductive, urinary, respiratory, or gastrointestinal system. Some or all parts of these systems are not sterile and contain normal flora.

- **Contaminated wound**—has a high risk of infection. Unintentional wounds are generally contaminated. Wound contamination occurs from breaks in surgical asepsis and spillage of intestinal contents. Tissues may show signs of inflammation.
- **Infected wound (dirty wound)**—contains large amounts of microbes and shows signs of infection. Examples include old wounds, surgical incisions into infected areas, and traumatic injuries that rupture the bowel.
- **Chronic wound**—does not heal easily. Pressure ulcers and circulatory ulcers are examples.

PARTIAL- AND FULL-THICKNESS WOUNDS (DESCRIBE WOUND DEPTH)
- **Partial-thickness wound**—the dermis and epidermis of the skin are broken.
- **Full-thickness wound**—the dermis, epidermis, and subcutaneous tissue are penetrated. Muscle and bone may be involved.

TYPES OF WOUNDS

Types of wounds are described in Box 32-2. Wounds also are described by their cause:

- **Abrasion**—a partial-thickness wound caused by the scraping away or rubbing of the skin
- **Contusion**—a closed wound caused by a blow to the body (a bruise)
- **Incision**—an open wound with clean, straight edges; usually intentional from a sharp instrument
- **Laceration**—an open wound with torn tissues and jagged edges
- **Penetrating wound**—an open wound in which the skin and underlying tissues are pierced
- **Puncture wound**—an open wound made by a sharp object; entry of the skin and underlying tissues may be intentional or unintentional

SKIN TEARS

A **skin tear** is a break or rip in the skin. The epidermis (top skin layer) separates from the underlying tissues (Chapter 8). The hands, arms, and lower legs are common sites for skin tears. Very thin and fragile skin is common in older persons. Slight pressure can cause a skin tear.

Causes

Skin tears are caused by friction, shearing (Chapter 16), pulling, or pressure on the skin. Bumping a hand, arm, or leg on any hard surface can cause a skin tear. Beds, bed rails, chairs, wheelchair footplates, and tables are dangers. So is holding the person's arm or leg too tight.

FOCUS ON CHILDREN AND OLDER PERSONS

Persons at Risk (Skin Tears)

OLDER PERSONS

Some persons are confused and may resist care. They often move quickly and without warning. Or they pull away from you during care. Some try to hit or kick. These sudden movements can cause skin tears.

Never force care on a person. Chapter 44 describes how to care for persons who are confused and resist care. Always follow the care plan.

Be careful when moving, repositioning, or transferring the person. Bathing, dressing, and other tasks can cause skin tears. So can pulling buttons and zippers across fragile skin. Jewelry—yours or the person's—also can cause skin tears. Rings, watches, and bracelets are examples.

Skin tears are painful. They are portals of entry for microbes. Wound complications can develop. Tell the nurse at once if you cause or find a skin tear.

Persons at Risk

Persons at risk for skin tears:
- Need moderate to total help in moving
- Have poor nutrition
- Have poor hydration
- Have altered mental awareness (See *Focus on Children and Older Persons: Persons at Risk.*)
- Are very thin

BOX 32-3 Measures to Prevent Skin Tears

- Keep your fingernails short and smoothly filed.
- Keep the person's fingernails short and smoothly filed. Report long and tough toenails.
- Do not wear rings with large or raised stones. Do not wear bracelets.
- Be patient and calm when the person is confused or agitated or resists care.
- Follow the care plan and safety rules to handle, move, turn, position, or transfer the person.
  - Prevent shearing and friction.
  - Use an assist device to move and turn the person in bed.
  - Use pillows to support arms and legs. Follow the care plan.
- Pad bed rails and wheelchair arms, footplates, and leg supports. Follow the care plan.
- Follow the care plan and safety rules to bathe the person.
- Dress and undress the person carefully.
- Dress the person in soft clothes with long sleeves and long pants.
- Provide good lighting so the person can see. The person needs to avoid bumping into furniture, walls, and equipment.
- Provide a safe area for wandering (Chapter 44).
- Keep the skin moisturized. Apply lotion according to the care plan.
- Offer fluids. Follow the care plan.

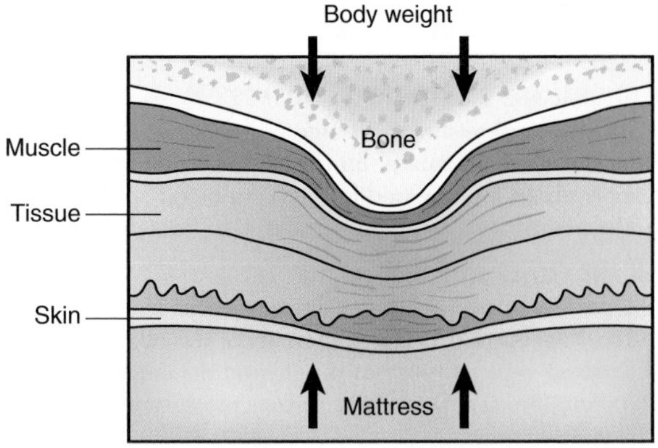

FOCUS ON CHILDREN AND OLDER PERSONS

Pressure Ulcers

OLDER PERSONS
Older and disabled persons are at great risk for pressure ulcers. Their skin is easily injured. Causes include age-related skin changes, chronic disease, and general disability.

Prevention and Treatment

Careful and safe care helps prevent skin tears and further injury. Follow the measures in Box 32-3. Also follow the care plan and the nurse's directions. They may include dressings (p. 565) and elastic bandages (Chapter 31) to protect the skin and promote healing.

PRESSURE ULCERS

The National Pressure Ulcer Advisory Panel defines a **pressure ulcer** as a localized injury to the skin and/or underlying tissue usually over a bony prominence. It is the result of pressure or pressure in combination with shear and/or friction. *Decubitus ulcer, bed sore,* or *pressure sore* are other terms for pressure ulcer.

A pressure ulcer usually occurs over a bony prominence. *Prominence* means to stick out. A *bony prominence* is an area where the bone sticks out or projects from the flat surface of the body. The back of the head, shoulder blades, elbows, hips, spine, sacrum, knees, ankles, heels, and toes are bony prominences.

See *Focus on Children and Older Persons: Pressure Ulcers.*

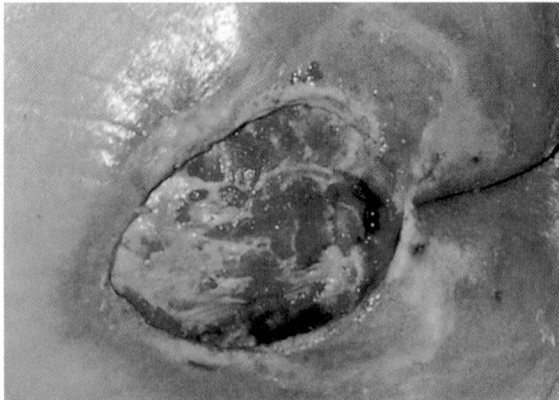

FIGURE 32-2 Tissue under pressure. The skin is squeezed between two hard surfaces: the bone and the mattress. (Redrawn from *Understanding your body: what are pressure ulcers?* August 2001, Life Sciences Education and Health Literacy, Agency for Healthcare Research and Quality, Rockville, Md.)

FIGURE 32-3 A pressure ulcer. (From Proceedings from the November National V.A.C.®, *Ostomy wound management,* Feb 2005, Vol. 51, 2A[suppl]:7S, HMP Communications. Used with permission.)

Causes and Risk Factors

Pressure, shearing, and friction are causes of skin breakdown and pressure ulcers. Risk factors include breaks in the skin, poor circulation to an area, moisture, dry skin, and irritation by urine and feces.

Pressure occurs when the skin over a bony area is squeezed between hard surfaces (Fig. 32-2). The bone is one hard surface. The other is usually the mattress or chair seat. Squeezing or pressure prevents blood flow to the skin and underlying tissues. Lack of blood flow means oxygen and nutrients cannot get to the cells. Therefore involved skin and tissues die (Fig. 32-3).

Friction scrapes the skin, causing an open area. The open area needs to heal. A good blood supply is needed. Infection is prevented so healing occurs. A poor blood supply or an infection can lead to a pressure ulcer.

Shearing is when the skin sticks to a surface (usually the bed or chair) while deeper tissues move downward. This occurs when the person slides down in the bed or chair. Blood vessels and tissues are damaged. Blood flow to the area is reduced.

Persons at Risk

Persons at risk for pressure ulcers are those who:

▶ Are *bedfast* (confined to a bed) or *chairfast* (confined to a chair).
▶ Need some or total help in moving. Coma, paralysis, or a hip fracture increases the risk of pressure ulcers.
▶ Are agitated or have involuntary muscle movements. The person's movements cause rubbing against linens and other surfaces. The rubbing causes friction.
▶ Have loss of bowel or bladder control. Urine and feces are sources of moisture. Moisture irritates the skin.
▶ Are exposed to moisture. Moisture irritates the skin. Wound drainage or heavy perspiration expose the person to moisture.
▶ Have poor nutrition. A balanced diet is needed to properly nourish the skin. The risk of pressure ulcers increases when the skin is not healthy.
▶ Have poor fluid balance. Fluid balance is needed for healthy skin.
▶ Have lowered mental awareness. The person cannot act (move, change positions) to prevent pressure ulcers. Drugs and health problems affect mental awareness.
▶ Have problems sensing pain or pressure. These are symptoms of tissue damage.
▶ Have circulatory problems. Good blood flow is needed to bring oxygen and nutrients to the cells.
▶ Are older. Older persons have thin and fragile skin. Such skin is easily injured. Many older persons also have chronic diseases that affect mobility, nutrition, circulation, and mental awareness.
▶ Are obese. Friction can damage the skin.
▶ Are very thin. Friction can damage the skin. There is less tissue to protect bony areas.

See *Focus on Children and Older Persons: Persons at Risk.*

Pressure Ulcer Stages

In persons with light skin, a reddened bony area is the first sign of a pressure ulcer. In persons with dark skin, skin color may differ from surrounding areas. The area may feel warm or cool. The person may complain of pain, burning, tingling, or itching in the area. Some persons do not feel anything unusual. Box 32-4 describes pressure ulcer stages.

See *Focus on Long-Term Care and Home Care: Signs of Pressure Ulcers*

BOX 32-4 Stages of Pressure Ulcers

Stage 1 The skin is intact. There is usually redness over a bony prominence. The color does not return to normal when the skin is relieved of pressure. In persons with dark skin, skin color may differ from surrounding areas. See Figure 32-4, *A,* p. 554.

Stage 2 Partial-thickness skin loss (Fig. 32-4, *B,* p. 554). The wound may involve a blister or shallow ulcer. An ulcer may appear to be reddish-pink. A blister may be intact or open.

Stage 3 Full-thickness skin loss (Fig. 32-4, *C,* p. 554). The skin is gone. Subcutaneous fat may be exposed. Tissue shedding *(slough)* may be present.

Stage 4 Full-thickness tissue loss with muscle, tendon, and bone exposure (Fig. 32-4, *D,* p. 554). Slough (tissue shedding) or *eschar* (a scab or dry crust) may be present.

Unstageable Full-thickness tissue loss with the ulcer covered by slough and/or eschar. Slough is yellow, tan, gray, green, or brown. Eschar is tan, brown, or black.

Modified from National Pressure Ulcer Advisory Panel, February 2007.

FOCUS ON **LONG-TERM CARE** AND **HOME CARE**

Signs of Pressure Ulcers

HOME CARE

Persons needing home care can develop pressure ulcers. Make sure you check the person's skin during every visit. Report and record your observations.

Remind family members to check the person's skin. They need to call the nurse if signs of a pressure ulcer are noted.

FOCUS ON **CHILDREN** AND **OLDER PERSONS**

Persons at Risk

CHILDREN

Infants and children also are at risk for pressure ulcers. Poor mobility, lack of bowel and bladder control (incontinence), poor nutrition, and infection are risk factors. Pressure, friction, and shearing are causes. Epidermal stripping is another cause. **Epidermal stripping** is removing the epidermis (outer skin layer) as tape is removed from the skin. Newborns are at risk because of their fragile skin.

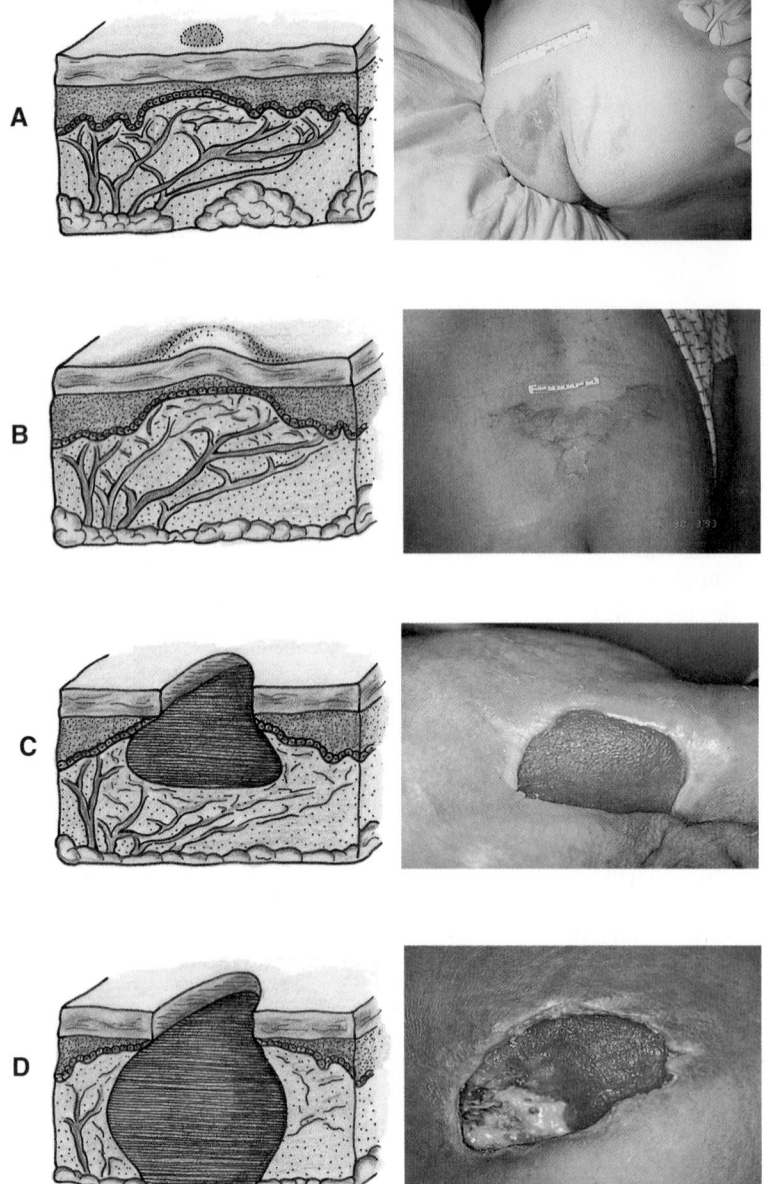

FIGURE 32-4 Stages of pressure ulcers. **A,** Stage 1. **B,** Stage 2. **C,** Stage 3. **D,** Stage 4. (Courtesy Laurel Wiersema-Bryant, RN, MSN, Clinical Nurse Specialist, Barnes-Jewish Hospital, St Louis, Mo.)

Sites

Pressure ulcers usually occur over bony areas. The bony areas are called *pressure points*. This is because they bear the weight of the body in a certain position (see Fig. 32-1). Pressure from body weight can reduce the blood supply to the area.

The ears also are sites for pressure ulcers. This is from pressure of the ear on the mattress when in the side-lying position. Eyeglasses and oxygen tubing (Chapter 34) also can cause pressure on the ears.

In obese people, pressure ulcers can occur in areas where skin has contact with skin. Common sites are between abdominal folds, the legs, the buttocks, the thighs, and under the breasts. Friction occurs in these areas.

Prevention and Treatment

Preventing pressure ulcers is much easier than trying to heal them. Good nursing care, cleanliness, and skin care are essential. The Joint Commission, an accrediting agency, estimates that it costs $500 to $40,000 to treat a pressure ulcer.

The measures in Box 32-5 help prevent skin breakdown and pressure ulcers. The Omnibus Budget Reconciliation Act of 1987 and the Joint Commission require pressure ulcer prevention. The health team must develop a plan of care for each person at risk. You must know and follow the care plan.

The person at risk for pressure ulcers is placed on a surface that reduces or relieves pressure. Such surfaces include foam, air, alternating air, gel, or water mattresses. The health team decides on the best surface for the person.

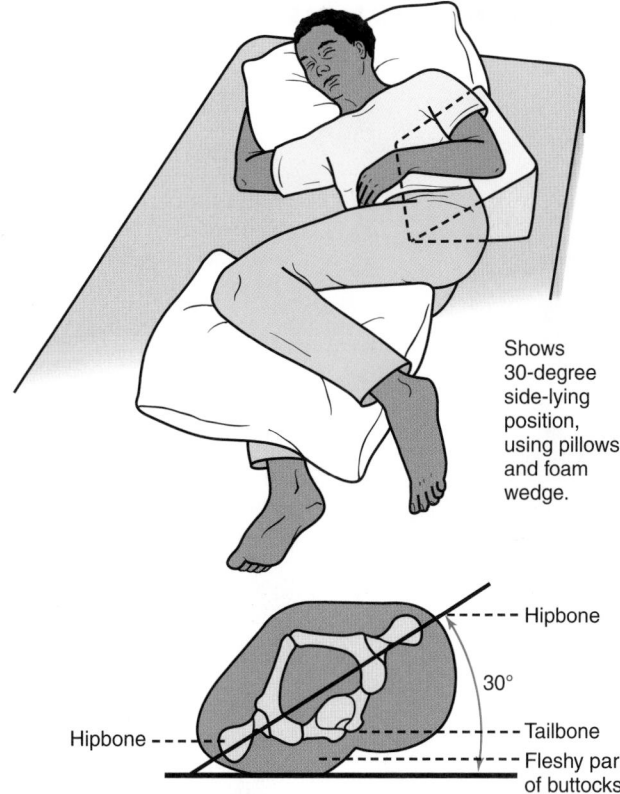

Shows 30-degree side-lying position, using pillows and foam wedge.

Hipbone

30°

Hipbone

Tailbone

Fleshy part of buttocks

FIGURE 32-5 The 30-degree lateral position. Pillows are placed under the head, shoulder, and leg. This position inclines (lifts up) the hip to avoid pressure on the hip. The person does not lie on the hip as in the side-lying position.

BOX 32-5 Measures to Prevent Pressure Ulcers

HANDLING, MOVING, AND POSITIONING
- Follow the repositioning schedule in the person's care plan. Reposition bedfast persons at least every 1 to 2 hours. Reposition chairfast persons every hour. Some persons are repositioned every 15 minutes.
- Position the person according to the care plan. Use pillows for support as instructed by the nurse. The 30-degree lateral position is recommended (Fig. 32-5).
- Prevent shearing and friction during handling, moving, and transfer procedures. Use assist devices as directed by the nurse and the care plan.
- Prevent friction in bed. Powder sheets lightly to prevent friction. Follow the care plan.
- Prevent shearing. Do not raise the head of the bed more than 30 degrees. Follow the care plan. The care plan tells you:
  - When to raise the head of the bed
  - How far to raise the head of the bed
  - How long (in minutes) to raise the head of the bed
- Use pillows, foam wedges, or other devices to prevent bony areas from contact with bony areas. The knees and ankles are examples. Follow the care plan.
- Keep the heels and ankles off the bed. Use pillows or other devices as the nurse directs. Place the pillows or devices under the lower legs from mid-calf to the ankles.
- Use protective devices as the nurse and care plan direct.
- Remind persons sitting in chairs to shift their positions every 15 minutes. This decreases pressure on bony points.

SKIN CARE
- Do not use hot water to bathe or clean the skin. Hot water can irritate the skin.
- Use a cleansing agent as directed by the nurse and the care plan. Soap can dry and irritate the skin.

- Provide good skin care. The skin is clean and dry after bathing. The skin is free of moisture from urine, stools, perspiration, and wound drainage.
- Follow the care plan to prevent incontinence.
- Prevent skin exposure to moisture. Check persons who are incontinent of urine or feces often. Provide good skin care at once and change linens and garments as needed. Use incontinence products as directed by the nurse and the care plan.
- Check persons often who perspire heavily or have wound drainage. Change linens and garments as needed. Provide good skin care.
- Prevent friction by applying a thin layer of cornstarch to the bottom sheets.
- Apply moisturizer to dry areas—hands, elbows, legs, ankles, heels, and so on. The nurse tells you what to use and what areas need attention.
- Give a back massage when repositioning the person. *Do not massage bony areas.*
- Do not massage over pressure points. *Never rub or massage reddened areas.*
- Keep linens clean, dry, and wrinkle-free.
- Apply cornstarch where skin touches skin. Apply it in a thin layer.
- Do not irritate the skin. Avoid scrubbing or vigorous rubbing when bathing or drying the person.
- Use pillows and blankets to prevent skin from being in contact with skin. They also reduce moisture and friction.
- Make sure socks and shoes are in good repair. Socks should not have wrinkles or creases. Make sure there is nothing in the shoes before the person puts them on.

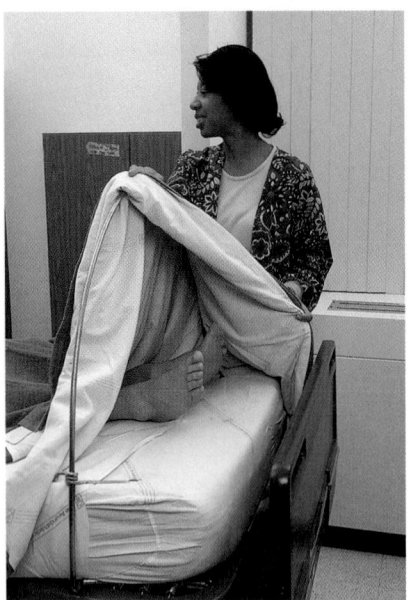

FIGURE 32-6 A bed cradle. Linens are brought over the top of the cradle.

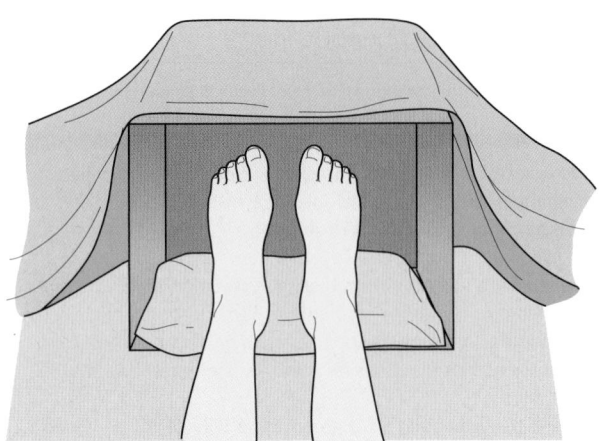

FIGURE 32-7 A box serves as a bed cradle. It keeps the top linens off of the feet.

The doctor orders wound care products, drugs, treatments, and special equipment to promote healing. The nurse and care plan tell you what to do. Protective devices are often used to prevent and treat pressure ulcers and skin breakdown. These devices are common:

▶ *Bed cradle*—A bed cradle is a metal frame placed on the bed and over the person (Chapter 26). Top linens are brought over the cradle to prevent pressure on the legs, feet, and toes (Fig. 32-6). Protect the person from air drafts and chilling. To do so, tuck and miter linens at the bottom of the mattress. Also tuck them in under the mattress sides. See *Focus on Long-Term Care and Home Care: Prevention and Treatment.*

Prevention and Treatment

HOME CARE

A cardboard box is useful as a bed cradle (Fig. 32-7). The nurse tells you how to line the box to prevent pressure on the heels.

TEAMWORK AND TIME MANAGEMENT

Prevention and Treatment

The entire nursing team must prevent pressure ulcers. As you walk down hallways, look into rooms to see if a person has slid down in bed or in a chair. Do the same when people are in dining and lounge areas. Help reposition the person. Ask a co-worker to help you as needed. Report the repositioning to the nurse.

▶ *Heel and elbow protectors*—These devices are made of foam padding, pressure-relieving gel, sheepskin, and other cushion materials. They fit the shape of heels and elbows (Fig. 32-8). Some are inserted inside sleeves or mesh. Others are secured in place with straps. These devices prevent pressure and friction.

▶ *Heel and foot elevators*—These raise the heels and feet off of the bed (Fig. 32-9). They prevent pressure. Some also prevent footdrop (Chapter 26). Many are secured in place with Velcro straps.

▶ *Gel or fluid-filled pads and cushions*—These devices involve a pressure-relieving gel or fluid (Fig. 32-10). They are used for chairs and wheelchairs to prevent pressure. The outer case is vinyl. The pad or cushion is placed in a fabric cover to protect the person's skin. Some covers are two colors (Fig. 32-11). The colors remind the staff to reposition the person.

▶ *Eggcrate-type pads*—These devices are placed on beds or in chairs or wheelchairs (Fig. 32-12). The foam pad looks like an egg carton. Peaks in the pad distribute the person's weight more evenly. The pad is put in a special cover. The cover protects against heat, moisture, and soiling. Only a bottom sheet is used over the eggcrate-type pad and cover. No other bottom linens are used.

▶ *Special beds*—Some beds have air flowing through the mattresses (Fig. 32-13). The person *floats* on the mattress. Body weight is distributed evenly. There is little pressure on body parts. Some beds allow repositioning without moving the person. The person is turned to the prone or supine position or the bed is tilted various degrees. Alignment does not change. Pressure points change as the position changes. There is little friction. Some beds constantly rotate from side to side. They are useful for persons with spinal cord injuries.

▶ *Other equipment*—Pillows, trochanter rolls, foot boards, and other positioning devices are used (Chapter 26). They help keep the person in good alignment.

See *Teamwork and Time Management: Prevention and Treatment.*

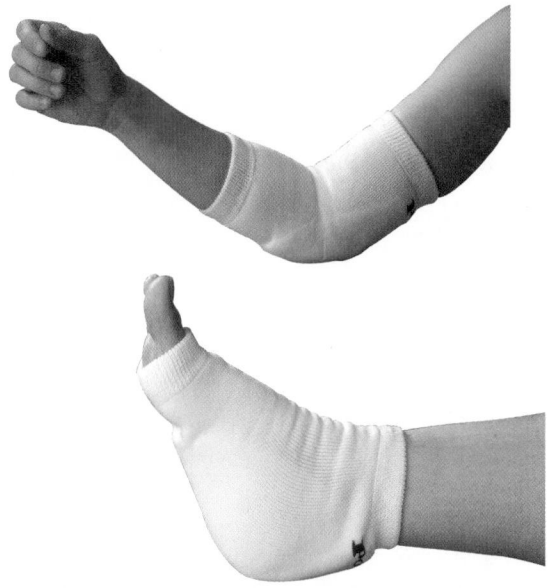

FIGURE 32-8 Heel and elbow protector. (Image courtesy J.T. Posey Company, Arcadia, Calif.)

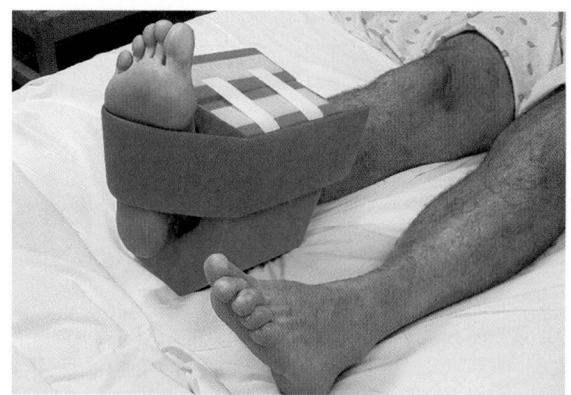

FIGURE 32-9 Heel elevator.

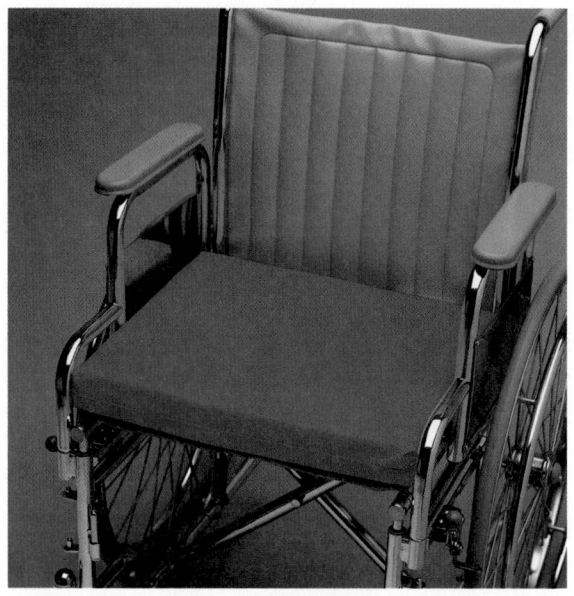

FIGURE 32-10 Gel and foam cushion. (Image courtesy J.T. Posey Company, Arcadia, Calif.)

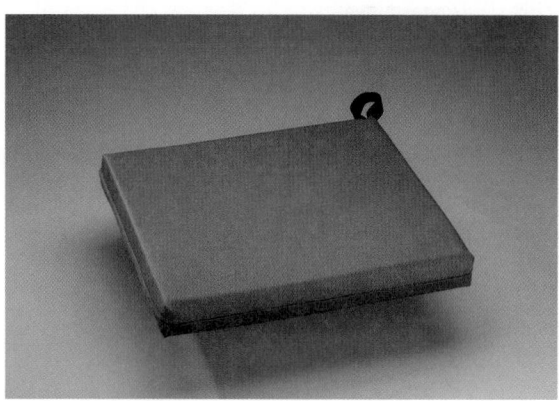

FIGURE 32-11 Gel and foam cushion with a two-color cover. (Image courtesy J.T. Posey Company, Arcadia, Calif.)

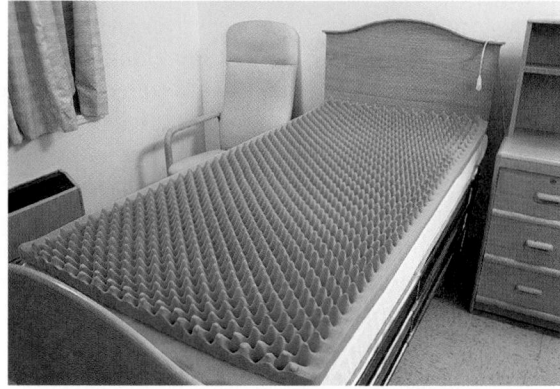

FIGURE 32-12 Eggcrate-type pad on the bed.

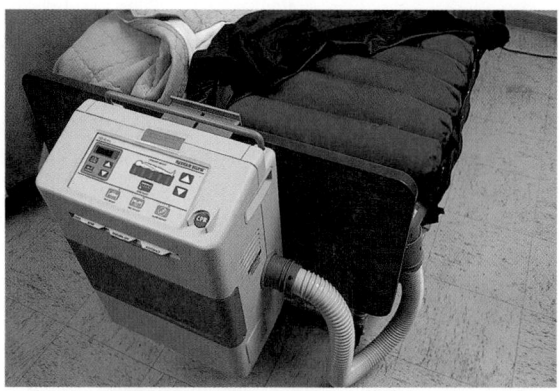

FIGURE 32-13 Air flotation bed.

Date	Time	Nursing Margin	Other Depts Margin
8-27	0830	While assisting resident with a tub bath, a blister the size of a	
		quarter was noted on the outer aspect of the L heel. There is a 1/4	
		inch reddened area around the blister. No drainage noted. Resident	
		states, "It hurts a little." She said she thinks her shoes are rubbing	
		Asked Barabara Lane, RN to observe the area. Jean Hein, CNA	

FIGURE 32-14 Charting sample.

BOX 32-6 Measures to Prevent Circulatory Ulcers

- Remind the person not to sit with the legs crossed.
- Reposition the person according to the care plan. The person is repositioned at least every 2 hours.
- Do not use elastic or rubber band-type garters to hold socks or hose in place.
- Do not dress the person in tight clothes.
- Provide good skin care daily. Keep the feet clean and dry. Clean and dry between the toes.
- Do not scrub or rub the skin during bathing and drying.
- Keep linens clean, dry, and wrinkle-free.
- Avoid injury to the legs and feet.
- Make sure shoes fit well.
- Keep pressure off the heels and other bony areas. Use pillows or other devices as the nurse and care plan direct.
- Check the person's legs and feet. Report skin breaks or changes in skin color.
- Do not massage over pressure points. *Never rub or massage reddened areas.*
- Use protective devices as the nurse directs. Follow the care plan.
- Follow the care plan for walking and exercise.

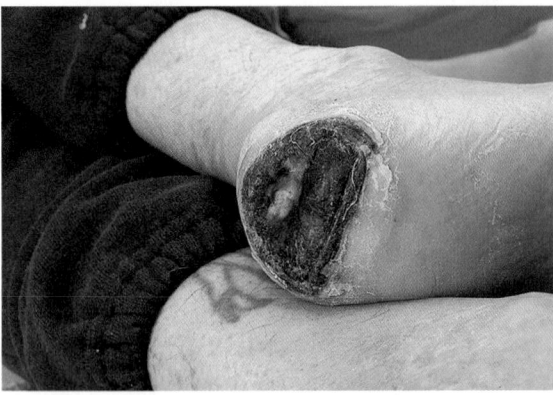

FIGURE 32-15 Venous ulcer.

Reporting and Recording

Report and record any signs of skin breakdown or pressure ulcers at once. See Figure 32-14. See "Wound Appearance" on p. 563.

CIRCULATORY ULCERS

Some diseases affect blood flow to and from the legs and feet. Such poor circulation can lead to pain, open wounds, and edema. **Edema** is swelling caused by fluid collecting in tissues. Infection and gangrene can result from the open wound and poor circulation. **Gangrene** is a condition in which there is death of tissue (Chapter 39).

An **ulcer** is a shallow or deep crater-like sore of the skin or a mucous membrane. **Circulatory ulcers (vascular ulcers)** are open sores on the lower legs or feet. They are caused by decreased blood flow through the arteries or veins. Persons with diseases affecting the blood vessels are at risk. These wounds are painful and hard to heal.

The doctor orders drugs and treatments as needed. The nurse uses the nursing process to meet the person's needs (Box 32-6). You must help prevent skin breakdown on the legs and feet.

Venous Ulcers

Venous ulcers are open sores on the lower legs or feet. They are caused by poor blood flow through the veins (Fig. 32-15). Venous ulcers also are called **stasis ulcers.** Stasis comes from a Greek word that means to *stand still.*

These ulcers can develop when valves in the legs do not close well. The veins cannot pump blood back to the heart in a normal way. Blood and fluid collect in the legs and feet. Small veins in the skin can rupture. Hemoglobin gives blood its red color. When veins rupture, hemoglobin enters the tissues. This causes the skin to turn brown. The skin is dry, leathery, and hard. Itching is common.

The heels and inner aspect of the ankles are common sites for venous ulcers. They can occur from skin injury. Scratching is an example. Or they can occur without trauma.

Venous ulcers are painful and make walking difficult. Fluid may seep from the wound. Infection is a risk. Healing is slow.

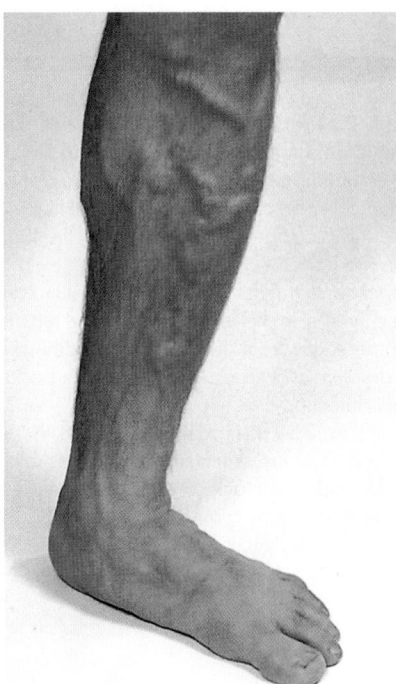

FIGURE 32-16 Varicose veins. Veins under the skin are dilated (wide) and bulging. (From Belch J and others: *Color atlas of peripheral vascular diseases*, ed 2, London, 1996, Wolfe Medical Publishers.)

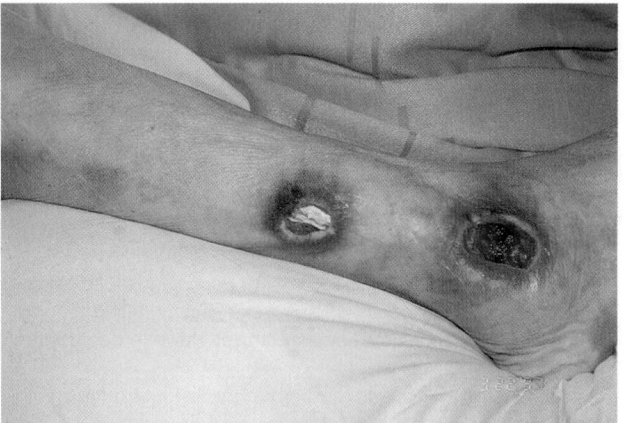

FIGURE 32-17 Arterial ulcer. (From Black JM, Hawks JH: *Medical-surgical nursing: clinical management for positive outcomes*, ed 7, St Louis, 2005, WB Saunders.)

Risk Factors

Risk factors for venous ulcers include:
► History of blood clots
► History of varicose veins (Fig. 32-16)
► Decreased mobility
► Obesity
► Leg or foot surgery
► Advanced age
► Surgery on the bones and joints
► **Phlebitis** (inflammation *[itis]* of a vein *[phleb]*)

Prevention and Treatment

To prevent venous ulcers:
► Follow the person's care plan to prevent skin breakdown. The care plan may include the measures in Box 32-6.
► Prevent injury. Do not bump the legs and feet.
► Handle, move, and transfer the person carefully and gently.

Persons at risk need professional foot care. Attention is given to toenails, corns, calluses, and other toe and foot problems. *You do not cut the toenails of persons with diseases affecting the circulation.*

Venous ulcers are hard to heal. The doctor may order drugs for infection and to decrease swelling. Medicated bandages and other wound care products are often ordered. So are devices used for pressure ulcers. The doctor may order elastic stockings or elastic bandages (Chapter 31).

Arterial Ulcers

Arterial ulcers are open wounds on the lower legs or feet caused by poor arterial blood flow. They are found between the toes, on top of the toes, and on the outer side of the ankle (Fig. 32-17). The leg and foot may feel cold and look blue or shiny. The ulcer is very painful.

These ulcers are caused by diseases or injuries that decrease arterial blood flow to the legs and feet. High blood pressure and diabetes are common causes. So are narrowed arteries from aging. Smoking is a risk factor.

The doctor treats the disease causing the ulcer. Drugs, wound care, and a walking and exercise program are ordered. Professional foot care is important. Follow the care plan (see Box 32-6) and prevent further injury.

Diabetic Foot Ulcers

A **diabetic foot ulcer** is an open wound on the foot caused by complications from diabetes. Diabetes (Chapter 41) can affect the nerves and blood vessels.
► *Nerves.* When nerves are affected, the person can lose sensation in a foot or leg. Loss of sensation can be complete or partial. The person may not feel pain, heat, or cold. Therefore the person may not feel a cut, blister, burn, or other trauma to the foot. Infection and a large sore can develop.
► *Blood vessels.* Diabetes affects the blood vessels. Blood flow decreases. Tissues and cells do not get needed oxygen and nutrients. A sore does not heal properly. Tissue death (gangrene) can occur.

Some persons with diabetes have both nerve and blood vessel damage. Both problems can lead to diabetic foot ulcers. Infection and gangrene are risks. Sometimes amputation of the affected part is needed to prevent the spread of gangrene.

Check the person's feet every day. Look for the foot problems described in Box 32-7, p. 560. Report any sign of a foot problem to the nurse at once. Follow the care plan to prevent and treat diabetic foot ulcers.

BOX 32-7 **Foot Problems Common in Persons With Diabetes**

- *Corns and calluses* (Fig. 32-18, *A*). These are thick layers of the skin caused by too much rubbing or pressure on the same spot. They can occur over bony areas or the soles of the feet. They can become infected.
- *Blisters* (Fig. 32-18, *B*). These form when shoes rub on the same spot. They are caused by shoes that do not fit well and by wearing shoes without socks. They can become infected.
- *Ingrown toenails* (Fig. 32-18, *C*). An edge of a toenail grows into the skin. They occur when the skin is cut while trimming toenails. Tight shoes are another cause. The skin becomes red and infected.
- *Bunions* (Fig. 32-18, *D*). The big toe slants toward the small toes. The space between the bones near the base of the big toe grows larger. Bunions can occur on one or both feet. Heredity is a factor. Shoes that fit poorly and pointy shoes are causes. Bunions are removed by surgery.
- *Plantar warts* (Fig. 32-18, *E*). *Plantar* means sole. Plantar warts occur on the soles (bottoms) of the feet. They are caused by a virus. Plantar warts are painful.

- *Hammer toes* (Fig. 32-18, *F*). One or more toes are permanently flexed. They form when a foot muscle weakens. Diabetic nerve damage can weaken foot muscles. Hammer toe is most common in the second toe. Because the toes are deformed, the person has problems walking. Also, shoes do not fit well. Sores can develop on the tops of the toes and on the bottoms of the feet.
- *Dry and cracked skin* (Fig. 32-18, *G*). Dry skin can occur from nerve damage in the legs and feet. The legs and feet do not receive messages from the brain to keep the skin soft and moist. The dry skin can crack. The cracks are portals of entry for microbes. Infection can occur.
- *Athlete's foot* (Fig. 32-18, *H*). This is a fungus that causes redness and cracking of the skin between the toes and on the bottoms of the feet. The cracks are portals of entry for microbes. The fungus can spread to the toenails. The toenails become thick, yellow, and hard to cut.

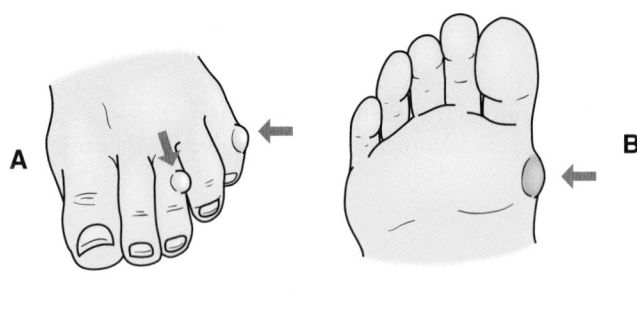
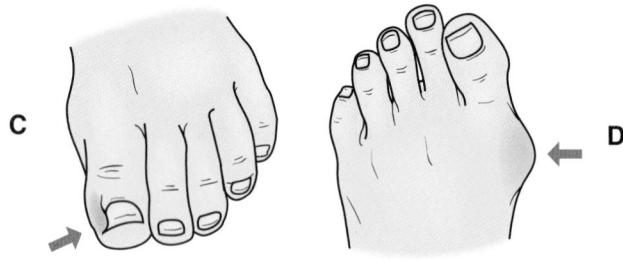
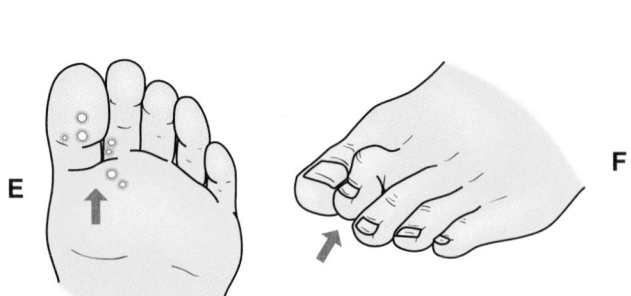
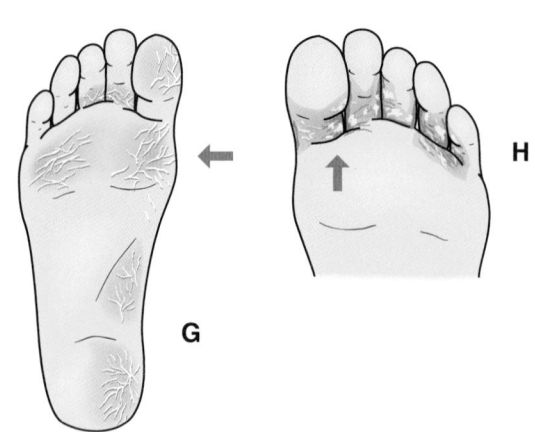

FIGURE 32-18 Diabetic foot problems. **A,** Corns. **B,** A blister. **C,** An in-grown toenail. **D,** A bunion. **E,** Plantar warts. **F,** Hammer toe. **G,** Dry and cracked skin. **H,** Athlete's foot. (Redrawn from *Prevent diabetes problems: keep your feet and skin healthy,* National Diabetes Information Clearinghouse [NDIC], NIH Publication No. 07-4282, February 2007, Bethesda, Md.)

WOUND HEALING

The healing process has three phases:

▶ *Inflammatory phase* (3 days). Bleeding stops. A scab forms over the wound. The scab protects against microbes entering the wound. Blood supply to the wound increases. The blood brings nutrients and healing substances. Because blood supply increases, signs and symptoms of inflammation appear. They are redness, swelling, heat or warmth, and pain. Loss of function may occur.

▶ *Proliferative phase* (day 3 to day 21). Proliferate means to multiply rapidly. Tissue cells multiply to repair the wound.

▶ *Maturation phase* (day 21 to 2 years). The scar gains strength. The red, raised scar becomes thin and pale.

Types of Wound Healing

Healing occurs in three ways:

▶ *First intention (primary intention, primary closure).* Wound edges are brought together to close the wound. Sutures (stitches), staples, clips, special glue, or adhesive strips hold the wound edges together. See Figure 32-19, *A*, p. 562.

▶ *Second intention (secondary intention).* This is used for contaminated and infected wounds. Wounds are cleaned and dead tissue removed. Wound edges are not brought together. The wound gaps. Healing occurs naturally. However, healing takes longer and leaves a larger scar. The threat of infection is great. See Figure 32-19, *B*, p. 562.

▶ *Third intention (delayed intention, tertiary intention).* The wound is left open and closed later. It combines second and first intention. Infection and poor circulation are common reasons for third intention. See Figure 32-19, *C*, p. 562.

Complications of Wound Healing

Many factors affect healing and increase the risk of complications. The type of wound is one factor. Other factors include the person's age, general health, nutrition, and life-style.

Good circulation is important. Age, smoking, circulatory disease, and diabetes all affect circulation. Certain drugs (Coumadin and heparin) prolong bleeding.

Good nutrition is needed. Protein is needed for tissue growth and repair.

Infection is a risk for persons with immune system changes and for those taking antibiotics. Antibiotics kill pathogens. Specific antibiotics kill specific pathogens. In doing so, an environment may be created that allows other pathogens to grow and multiply.

Hemorrhage and Shock

Hemorrhage is the excessive loss of blood in a short time (Chapter 49). If bleeding is not stopped, death results. Hemorrhage may be internal or external.

▶ *Internal hemorrhage.* You cannot see internal hemorrhage. Bleeding occurs inside the body into tissues and body cavities. A hematoma may form. A **hematoma** is a swelling (*oma*) that contains blood (*hemat*). The area is swollen and reddish blue in color. Shock, vomiting blood, coughing up blood, and loss of consciousness signal internal hemorrhage.

▶ *External hemorrhage.* You can see external bleeding. Common signs are bloody drainage and dressings soaked with blood. Gravity causes fluid to flow down. Blood can flow down and collect under a body part. Check under the body part for pooling of blood. Shock can occur with external hemorrhage.

Shock results when tissues and organs do not get enough blood (Chapter 49). Blood pressure falls, the pulse is rapid and weak, and respirations are rapid. The skin is cold, moist, and pale. The person is restless and may complain of thirst. Confusion and loss of consciousness occur as shock worsens.

Hemorrhage and shock are emergencies. Alert the nurse at once. Assist as requested.

See *Promoting Safety and Comfort: Hemorrhage and Shock.*

Infection

Wound contamination can occur during or after the injury. Trauma often causes contaminated wounds. Surgical wounds can be contaminated during or after surgery. An infected wound appears inflamed (reddened) and has drainage (p. 564). The wound is painful and tender. The person has a fever.

Dehiscence and Evisceration

Dehiscence is the separation of wound layers (Fig. 32-20, p. 563). Separation may involve the skin layer or underlying tissues. Abdominal wounds are commonly affected. Coughing, vomiting, and abdominal distention place stress on the wound. The person often describes the sensation of the wound "popping open."

Evisceration is the separation of the wound along with the protrusion of abdominal organs (Fig. 32-21, p. 563). Causes are the same as for dehiscence.

Dehiscence and evisceration are surgical emergencies. The wound is covered with large sterile dressings saturated with saline. You must tell the nurse at once and help prepare the person for surgery.

PROMOTING SAFETY AND COMFORT: Hemorrhage and Shock

SAFETY

Follow Standard Precautions and the Bloodborne Pathogen Standard when in contact with blood. Gloves, gowns, masks, and eye protection are necessary when blood splashes and splatters are likely.

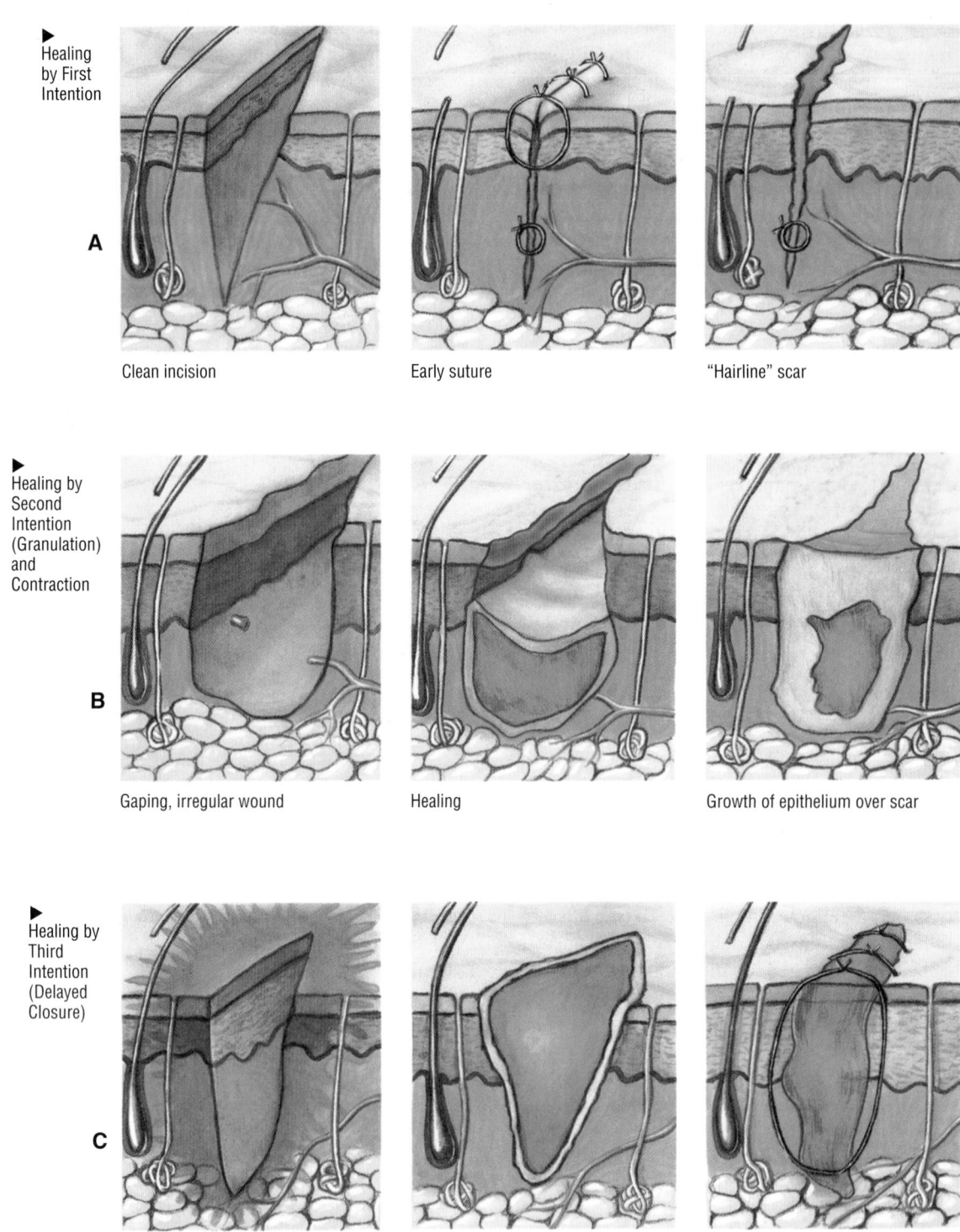

► Healing by First Intention

A

Clean incision   Early suture   "Hairline" scar

► Healing by Second Intention (Granulation) and Contraction

B

Gaping, irregular wound   Healing   Growth of epithelium over scar

► Healing by Third Intention (Delayed Closure)

C

Infected wound   Healing   Closure with wide scar

FIGURE 32-19 Wound healing. **A,** First intention. **B,** Second intentnion. **C,** Third intention. (Modified from Ignatavicius DD, Workman ML: *Medical-surgical nursing: critical thinking for collaborative care,* ed 5, St Louis, 2006, Saunders.)

Wound Appearance

Doctors and nurses observe the wound and its drainage. They observe for healing and complications. You need to make certain observations when assisting with wound care (Box 32-8). Report and record your observations according to agency policy.

See *Focus on Long-Term Care and Home Care: Wound Appearance*.

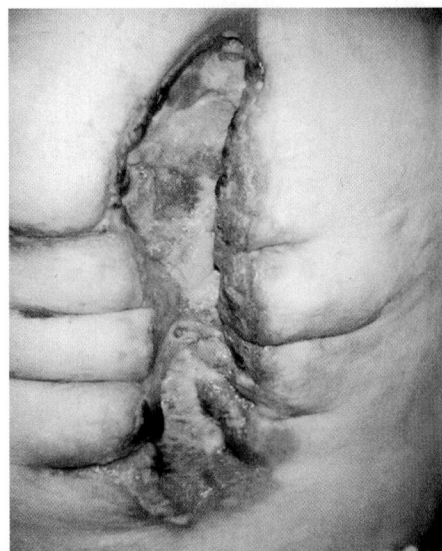

FIGURE 32-20 Wound dehiscence. (Courtesy KCI Licensing, Inc., San Antonio, Tex.)

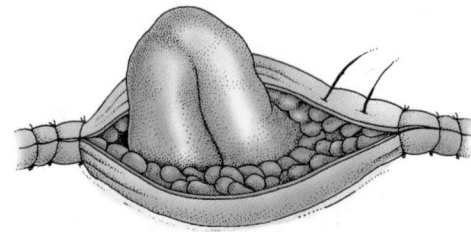

FIGURE 32-21 Wound evisceration. (From Ignatavicius DD, Workman ML: *Medical-surgical nursing: critical thinking for collaborative care,* ed 5, St Louis, 2006, Saunders.)

FOCUS ON **LONG-TERM CARE** AND **HOME CARE**

Wound Appearance

HOME CARE

The nurse may asked you to take photos of wounds. The photos help the nurse assess and evaluate the wound. Before taking a photo, make sure the person has signed a consent for photography. (The nurse obtains the consent.)

If using a Polaroid camera, write the person's name, the date, and the time on the back of the photo. For regular film or a digital camera, note the frame number, the person's name, and the date and time in the person's record.

The photo does not replace making accurate observations. See Box 32-8.

BOX 32-8 **Wound Observations**

- Wound location
  - The person may have multiple wounds from surgery or trauma.
- Wound size and depth (measure in centimeters)
  - Size: Measure from top to bottom and side to side (Fig. 32-22).
  - Depth. The nurse measures depth by:
    —Inserting a swab inside the deepest part of the wound
    —Removing the swab
    —Measuring the distance on the swab
  - Use a disposable ruler.
- Wound appearance
  - Is the wound red and swollen?
  - Is the area around the wound warm to touch?
  - Are sutures, staples, or clips intact or broken?
  - Are wound edges closed or separated?
  - Did the wound break open?
- Drainage (p. 564)
  - Is the drainage serous, sanguineous, serosanguineous, or purulent?
  - What is the amount of drainage?
- Odor
  - Does the wound or drainage have an odor?
- Surrounding skin
  - Is surrounding skin intact?
  - What is the color of surrounding skin?
  - Are surrounding tissues swollen?

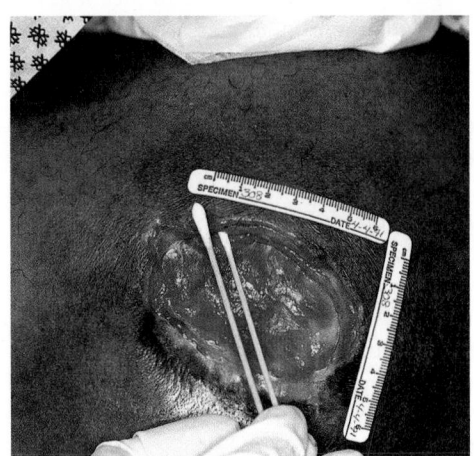

FIGURE 32-22 The size and depth of this pressure ulcer are measured. (From Potter PA, Perry AG: *Fundamentals of nursing,* ed 6, St Louis, 2005, Mosby.)

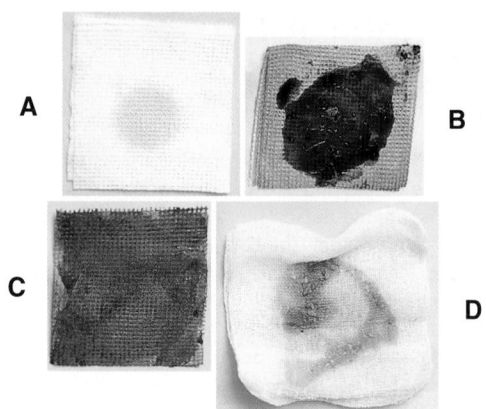

FIGURE 32-23 Wound drainage. **A,** Serous drainage. **B,** Sanguineous drainage. **C,** Serosanguineous drainage. **D,** Purulent drainage. (From Potter PA, Perry AG: *Fundamentals of nursing,* ed 6, St Louis, 2005, Mosby.)

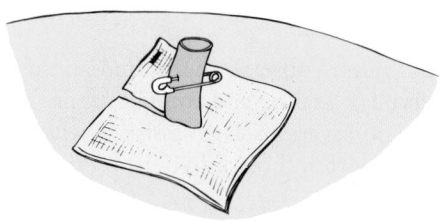

FIGURE 32-24 Penrose drain. (From Potter PA, Perry AG: *Fundamentals of nursing,* ed 6, St Louis, 2005, Mosby.)

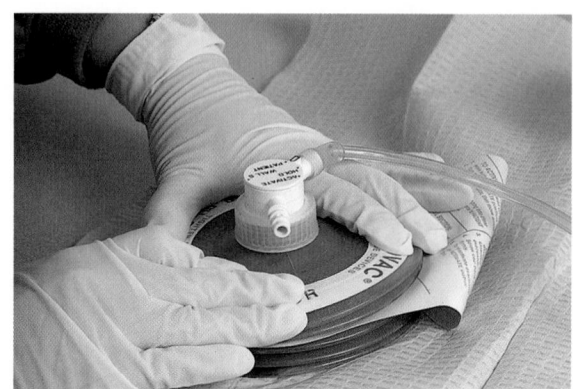

FIGURE 32-25 Hemovac. Drains are sutured to the wound and connected to a reservoir. (From Potter PA, Perry AG: *Fundamentals of nursing,* ed 6, St Louis, 2005, Mosby.)

Wound Drainage

During injury and the inflammatory phase of wound healing, fluid and cells escape from the tissues. The amount of drainage may be small or large. This depends on wound size and location. Bleeding and infection also affect the amount and kind of drainage. Wound drainage is observed and measured.

▶ **Serous drainage**—clear, watery fluid (Fig. 32-23, *A*). *Serous* comes from the word *serum.* The fluid in a blister is serous. Serum is the clear, thin, fluid portion of blood. Serum does not contain blood cells or platelets.

▶ **Sanguineous drainage**—bloody drainage (Fig. 32-23, *B*). The Latin word *sanguis* means blood. The amount and color of sanguineous drainage are important. Hemorrhage is suspected when large amounts are present. Bright drainage means fresh bleeding. Older bleeding is darker.

▶ **Serosanguineous drainage**—thin, watery drainage *(sero)* that is blood-tinged *(sanguineous)* (Fig. 32-23, *C*).

▶ **Purulent drainage**—thick and green, yellow, or brown drainage (Fig. 32-23, *D*).

Drainage must leave the wound for healing. If drainage is trapped inside the wound, underlying tissues swell. The wound may heal at the skin level, but underlying tissues do not close. Infection and complications can occur.

When large amounts of drainage are expected, the doctor inserts a drain. A *Penrose drain* is a rubber tube that drains onto a dressing (Fig. 32-24). It opens onto the dressing. Therefore it is an open drain. Microbes can enter the drain and wound.

Closed drainage systems prevent microbes from entering the wound. A drain is placed in the wound and attached to suction. The Hemovac (Fig. 32-25) and Jackson-Pratt systems are examples (Fig. 32-26). Other systems are used depending on wound type, size, and location.

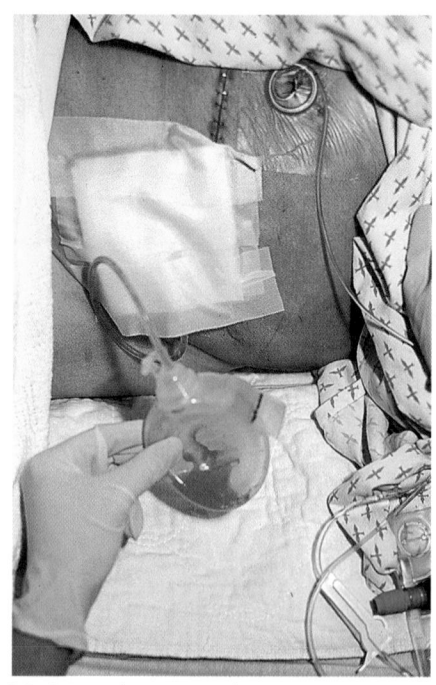

FIGURE 32-26 Jackson-Pratt drainage system. (From Potter PA, Perry AG: *Fundamentals of nursing,* ed 6, St Louis, 2005, Mosby.)

Drainage is measured in three ways:

▶ Weighing dressings before applying them to the wound. The weight of each new dressing is noted. Dressings are weighed after removal. The dry dressing weight is subtracted from the wet dressing weight. (Wet dressings weigh more.)

▶ Noting the number and size of dressings with drainage. What is the amount and kind of drainage? Are dressings saturated? Is drainage on just part of the dressing? If so, which part? Is drainage through some or all layers?

▶ Measuring the amount of drainage in the collection container if closed drainage is used.

DRESSINGS

Wound dressings have many functions. They:

▶ Protect wounds from injury and microbes.
▶ Absorb drainage.
▶ Remove dead tissue.
▶ Promote comfort.
▶ Cover unsightly wounds.
▶ Provide a moist environment for wound healing.
▶ Apply pressure (pressure dressings) to help control bleeding.

Dressing type and size depend on many factors. These include the type of wound, its size and location, and amount of drainage. Infection is a factor. The dressing's function and the frequency of dressing changes are other factors. The doctor and nurse choose the best type of dressing for each wound.

Types of Dressings

Dressings are described by the material used and application method. There are many dressing products (Fig. 32-27). The following are common:

▶ *Gauze.* It comes in squares, rectangles, pads, and rolls. Gauze dressings absorb drainage and moisture.

▶ *Non-adherent gauze.* It is a gauze dressing with a non-stick surface. It does not stick to the wound. It removes easily without injuring tissue.

▶ *Transparent adhesive film.* Air can reach the wound but fluids and microbes cannot. The wound is kept moist. Drainage is not absorbed. The transparent film allows wound observation.

Some dressings contain special agents to promote wound healing. If you assist with a dressing change, the nurse explains its use to you.

Dressings are wet or dry:

▶ *Dry dressing.* A dry gauze dressing is placed over the wound. More dressings are placed on top of the first dressing as needed. The dressings absorb drainage. Therefore drainage is removed with the dressing. A dry dressing can stick to the wound. The dressing is removed carefully to prevent tissue injury and discomfort.

▶ *Wet-to-dry dressing.* This dressing is used to remove dead tissue from the wound. Gauze dressings are saturated with a solution. These "wet" dressings are applied to the wound. The solution softens dead tissue. The dressing absorbs the dead tissue, which is removed when the dressings are dry.

▶ *Wet-to-wet dressing.* Gauze dressings saturated with solution are placed in the wound. The dressing is kept moist. It is not allowed to dry.

Securing Dressings

Dressings must be secured over wounds. Microbes can enter the wound, and drainage can escape if the dressing is dislodged. Tape and Montgomery ties are used to secure dressings. Binders hold dressings in place.

Tape

Adhesive, paper, plastic, cloth, and elastic tapes are common. Adhesive tape sticks well to the skin. Any adhesive remaining on the skin is hard to remove. It can irritate the skin. An abrasion occurs if skin is removed with tape. Many people are allergic to adhesive tape. Paper, plastic, and cloth tapes usually do not cause allergic reactions. Elastic tape allows movement of the body part.

Tape comes in different sizes—½, ¾, 1, 2, and 3 inch widths. Tape is applied to the top, middle, and bottom parts of the dressing. The tape extends several inches beyond each side of the dressing (Fig. 32-28). *Tape is not applied to circle the entire body part. If swelling occurs, circulation to the part is impaired.*

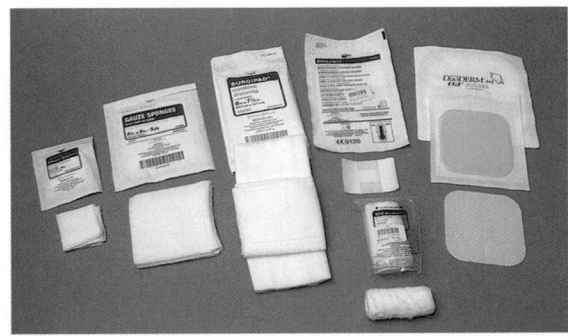

FIGURE 32-27 Types of dressings. (From deWit SC: *Fundamental concepts and skills for nursing,* ed 2, St Louis, 2005, Saunders.)

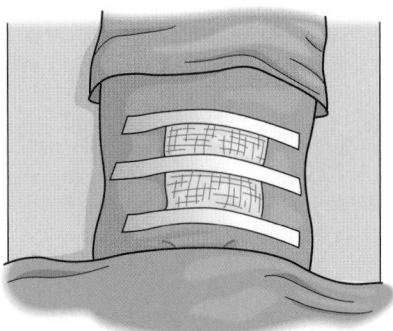

FIGURE 32-28 Tape is applied at the top, middle, and bottom of the dressing. The tape extends several inches beyond both sides of the dressing.

Montgomery Ties

Montgomery ties (Fig. 32-29) are used for large dressings and frequent dressing changes. A Montgomery tie has an adhesive strip and a cloth tie. When the dressing is in place, the adhesive strips are placed on both sides of the dressing. Then the cloth ties are secured over the dressing. Two or three Montgomery ties may be needed on each side. The ties are undone for the dressing change. The adhesive strips stay in place. They are not removed unless soiled. Montgomery ties protect the skin from frequent tape application and removal.

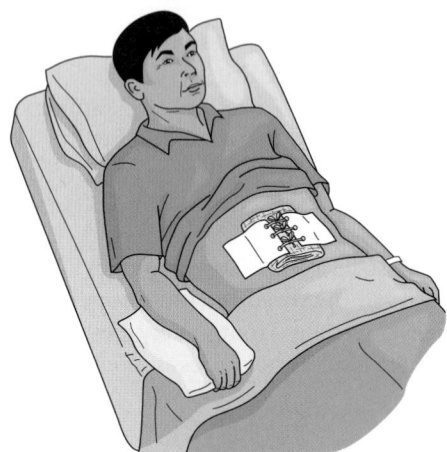

FIGURE 32-29 Montgomery ties.

BOX 32-9 Rules For Applying Dressings

- Allow pain drugs time to take effect, usually 30 minutes. The dressing change may cause discomfort. The nurse gives the drug and tells you how long to wait.
- Meet the person's fluid and elimination needs before you begin.
- Collect needed equipment and supplies before you begin.
- Do not bend or reach over your work area.
- Control your non-verbal communication. Wound odors, appearance, and drainage may be unpleasant. Do not communicate your thoughts or reactions to the person.
- Remove soiled dressings so the person cannot see the soiled side. The drainage and its odor may upset the person.
- Do not force the person to look at the wound. A wound can affect body image and self-esteem. The nurse helps the person deal with the wound.
- Remove tape by pulling it toward the wound.
- Remove dressings gently. They may stick to the wound, drain, or surrounding skin. If the dry dressing sticks, the nurse may have you wet the dressing with a saline solution. A wet dressing is easier to remove.
- Touch only the outer edges of old and new dressings. (See Chapter 14.)
- Report and record your observations. See *Delegation Guidelines: Applying Dressings*.

◆ Applying Dressings

The nurse may ask you to assist with dressing changes. Some agencies let you apply simple, dry, non-sterile dressings to simple wounds. Box 32-9 lists the rules for applying dressings.

See *Focus on Children and Older Persons: Applying Dressings*.

See *Focus on Communication: Applying Dressings*.

See *Teamwork and Time Management: Applying Dressings*.

See *Delegation Guidelines: Applying Dressings*.

See *Promoting Safety and Comfort: Applying Dressings*.

FOCUS ON **CHILDREN** AND **OLDER PERSONS**

Applying Dressings

CHILDREN

Children are often afraid of dressing changes. Tape removal is often painful. Wound appearance can be frightening. A calm, cooperative child helps prevent contamination of the sterile field. A parent or caregiver holds the child so the wound can be reached with ease. Holding or playing with a toy can comfort the child.

OLDER PERSONS

Older persons have thin, fragile skin. Skin tears must be prevented. Extreme care is necessary when removing tape.

FOCUS ON **COMMUNICATION**

Applying Dressings

The person may not report discomfort from a dressing. You should ask:
- "Is the dressing comfortable?"
- "Does the tape cause pain or itching?"

TEAMWORK AND **TIME MANAGEMENT**

Applying Dressings

Collect all needed items before you start the procedure. Have extra dressings, tape, and other supplies on-hand. Leave unused items in the room for the next dressing change. Wound contamination can occur if you need to leave the room during the procedure.

DELEGATION GUIDELINES: Applying Dressings

When applying a dressing is delegated to you, make sure that:

- Your state allows you to perform the procedure
- The procedure is in your job description
- You have the necessary training
- You are familiar with the equipment
- You review the procedure with the nurse
- A nurse is available to answer questions and to supervise you

If the above conditions are met, you need this information from the nurse:

- When to change the dressing
- When the person received a pain-relief drug; when it will take effect
- What to do if the dressing sticks to the wound
- How to clean the wound
- What dressings to use
- How to secure the dressing—tape or Montgomery ties
- What kind of tape to use—adhesive, paper, plastic, cloth, or elastic
- What size tape to use

- What observations to report and record:
  - What you used to dress the wound and secure the dressing
  - A red or swollen wound
  - An area around the wound that is warm to touch
  - If wound edges are closed or separated
  - A wound that has broken open
  - Drainage appearance—clear, bloody, or watery and blood-tinged; thick and green, yellow, or brown
  - The amount of drainage
  - Wound or drainage odor
  - Intactness and color of surrounding tissues
  - Swelling of surrounding tissues
  - Possible dressing contamination—urinary or fecal incontinence; other body fluids, secretions, or excretions; dislodged dressing
  - Pain
  - Fever
- When to report observations
- What specific patient and resident concerns to report at once

PROMOTING SAFETY AND COMFORT: Applying Dressings

SAFETY

Contact with blood, body fluids, secretions, or excretions is likely. Follow Standard Precautions and the Bloodborne Pathogen Standard. Wear personal protective equipment as needed.

Do not apply tape to irritated, injured, or non-intact skin. Tape can further damage the skin.

COMFORT

Wounds and dressing changes can cause discomfort or pain. If so, the nurse gives a pain-relief drug before the dressing change. Allow time for the drug to take effect. Be gentle when applying and removing tape and dressings.

APPLYING A DRY, NON-STERILE DRESSING

✔ Quality of Life *Remember to:*

- Knock before entering the person's room.
- Address the person by name.
- Introduce yourself by name and title.
- Explain the procedure to the person before beginning and during the procedure.

- Protect the person's rights during the procedure.
- Handle the person gently during the procedure.

PRE-PROCEDURE

1 Follow *Delegation Guidelines: Applying Dressings*. See *Promoting Safety and Comfort: Applying Dressings*.
2 Practice hand hygiene.
3 Collect the following:
- Gloves
- Personal protective equipment as needed
- Tape or Montgomery ties
- Dressings as directed by the nurse
- Saline solution as directed by the nurse

- Cleansing solution as directed by the nurse
- Adhesive remover
- Dressing set with scissors and forceps
- Plastic bag
- Bath blanket

Continued

APPLYING A DRY, NON-STERILE DRESSING—cont'd

PRE-PROCEDURE—cont'd

4 Decontaminate your hands.
5 Identify the person. Check the ID bracelet against the assignment sheet. Also call the person by name.
6 Provide for privacy.

7 Arrange your work area. You should not have to reach over or turn your back on your work area.
8 Raise the bed for good body mechanics. Bed rails are up if used.

PROCEDURE

9 Lower the bed rail near you if up.
10 Help the person to a comfortable position.
11 Cover the person with a bath blanket. Fan-fold top linens to the foot of the bed.
12 Expose the affected body part.
13 Make a cuff on the plastic bag. Place it within reach.
14 Decontaminate your hands.
15 Put on needed personal protective equipment. Put on gloves.
16 Remove tape or undo Montgomery ties.
   a *Tape:* hold the skin down. Gently pull the tape toward the wound.
   b *Montgomery ties:* fold ties away from the wound.
17 Remove any adhesive from the skin. Wet a 4 x 4 gauze dressing with adhesive remover. Clean away from the wound.
18 Remove gauze dressings. Start with the top dressing, and remove each layer. Keep the soiled side of each dressing away from the person's sight. Put dressings in the plastic bag. They must not touch the outside of the bag.

19 Remove the dressing over the wound very gently. It may stick to the wound or drain site. Moisten the dressing with saline if it sticks to the wound.
20 Observe the wound, drain site, and wound drainage.
21 Remove the gloves, and put them in the plastic bag. Decontaminate your hands.
22 Open the new dressings.
23 Cut the length of tape needed.
24 Put on clean gloves.
25 Clean the wound with saline as directed by the nurse. See Figure 32-30.
26 Apply dressings as directed by the nurse.
27 Secure the dressings in place. Use tape or Montgomery ties.
28 Remove the gloves. Put them in the bag.
29 Remove and discard personal protective equipment.
30 Decontaminate your hands.
31 Cover the person. Remove the bath blanket.

POST-PROCEDURE

32 Provide for comfort. (See the inside of the front book cover.)
33 Place the signal light within reach.
34 Lower the bed to its lowest position.
35 Raise or lower bed rails. Follow the care plan.
36 Return equipment and supplies to the proper place. Leave extra dressings and tape in the room.
37 Discard used supplies into the bag. Tie the bag closed. Discard the bag following agency policy. (Wear gloves for this step.)

38 Clean your work area. Follow the Bloodborne Pathogen Standard.
39 Unscreen the person.
40 Complete a safety check of the room. (See the inside of the front book cover.)
41 Decontaminate your hands.
42 Report and record your observations.

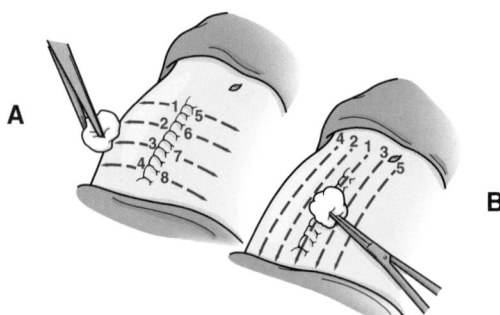

FIGURE 32-30 Cleaning a wound. **A,** Clean starting at the wound and stroking out to the surrounding skin. Use new gauze for each stroke. **B,** Clean the wound from the top to bottom. Start at the wound. Then clean the surrounding areas. Use new gauze for each stroke. (Redrawn from Potter PA, Perry AG: *Fundamentals of nursing*, ed 6, St Louis, 2005, Mosby.)

BOX 32-10 Rules For Applying Binders

- Follow the manufacturer's instructions.
- Apply the binder so there is firm, even pressure over the area.
- Apply the binder so it is snug. It must not interfere with breathing or circulation.
- Position the person in good alignment.
- Re-apply the binder if it is loose or wrinkled.
- Re-apply the binder if it is out of position or causes discomfort.
- Secure safety pins so they point away from the wound.
- Change binders that are moist or soiled. This prevents the growth of microbes.
- Tell the nurse at once if there is a change in the person's breathing.
- Check the person's skin under and around the binder. Tell the nurse at once if there is redness, irritation, or other signs of a skin problem.

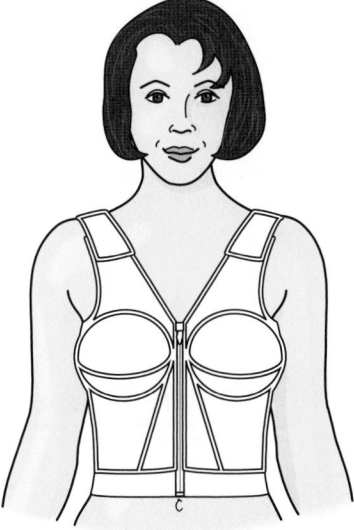

FIGURE 32-32 Breast binder.

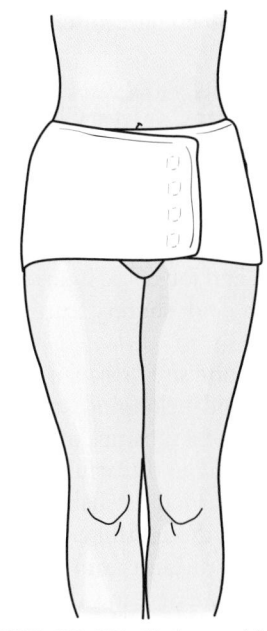

FIGURE 32-31 Abdominal binder.

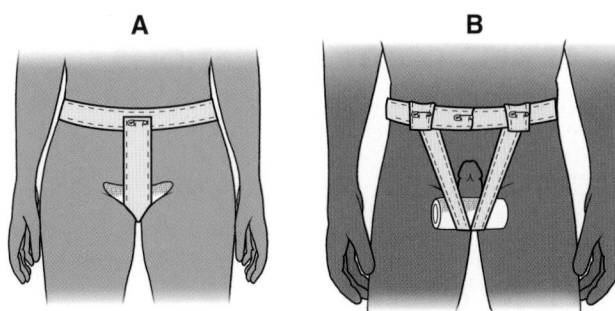

FIGURE 32-33 A, Single T binder. **B,** Double T binder. (From deWit SC: *Fundamental concepts and skills for nursing,* ed 2, St Louis, 2005, Saunders.)

BINDERS

Binders are wide bands of elastic fabric. They are applied to the abdomen, chest, or perineal areas. Binders promote healing by:

▶ Supporting wounds
▶ Holding dressings in place
▶ Preventing or reducing swelling
▶ Promoting comfort
▶ Preventing injury

Box 32-10 lists the rules for applying these binders:

▶ *Abdominal binder*—provides abdominal support and holds dressings in place (Fig. 32-31). The top part is at the person's waist. The lower part is over the hips. Binders are secured in place with Velcro or with hook and loop closures.

▶ *Breast binder*—supports the breasts after surgery (Fig. 32-32). It also applies pressure to the breasts after childbirth in the non-breastfeeding mother. Pressure from the binder helps dry up the milk in the breasts. The binder also promotes comfort and supports swollen breasts after childbirth. Breast binders are secured in place with Velcro or padded zippers.

▶ *T binders*—secure dressings in place after rectal and perineal surgeries. The single T binder is for women (Fig. 32-33, *A*). The double T binder is for men (Fig. 32-33, *B*). If perineal dressings are large, women many need double T binders. The waistbands are brought around the waist and pinned at the front. The tails are brought between the legs and up to the waistband. They are pinned in place at the waistband.

See *Focus on Communication: Binders*, p. 570.
See *Promoting Safety and Comfort: Binders*, p. 570.

Binders

The person may not tell you about pain or discomfort. Therefore you need to ask these questions:
- "Is the binder too tight or too loose?"
- "Does the binder cause pain?"
- "Do you feel pressure from the binder?" If yes: "Where? Please show me."

PROMOTING SAFETY AND COMFORT: Binders

SAFETY

Binders must be applied properly. Otherwise, severe discomfort, skin irritation, and circulatory and respiratory problems can occur. Correct application is needed for the person's safety and for the binder to work effectively.

COMFORT

A binder should promote comfort. Re-apply the binder if it causes pain or discomfort.

HEAT AND COLD APPLICATIONS

Heat and cold applications promote healing and comfort. They also reduce tissue swelling. See Chapter 33.

MEETING BASIC NEEDS

The wound can affect the person's basic needs. However, it is only one part of the person's care. Remember, the *person* has the wound.

The person is recovering from surgery or trauma. The wound causes pain and discomfort. The wound and pain may affect breathing and moving. Turning, repositioning, and walking may be painful. Handle the person gently. Allow pain drugs to take effect before giving care.

Good nutrition is needed for healing. However, pain and discomfort can affect appetite. So can odors from wound drainage. Remove soiled dressings promptly from the room. Use room deodorizers as directed. Also keep drainage containers out of the person's sight. Tell the nurse if the person has a taste for certain foods or drinks.

Infection is always a threat. Follow Standard Precautions and the Bloodborne Pathogen Standard. Carefully observe the wound. Also observe for signs and symptoms of infection.

Delayed healing is a risk for persons who are older or obese or have poor nutrition. Protein is needed for tissue growth and repair. Poor circulation and diabetes also affect healing. These conditions are risk factors for infection.

Many factors affect safety and security needs. The person fears scarring, disfigurement, delayed healing, and infection. Fears about the wound "popping open" are common. Medical bills are other concerns. The person may need care for a long time.

Victims of violence have many other concerns. Future attacks, finding and convicting the attacker, and fear for family members are common concerns. Victims of domestic, child, and elder abuse often hide the source of their injuries.

The wound may be large or small. Others can see wounds on the face, arms, or legs. Clothing can hide some wounds. Wound drainage may have odors. Some wounds are large and disfiguring. They can affect sexual performance or feelings of sexual attraction. Amputation of a finger, hand, arm, toe, foot, or leg can affect function, everyday activities, and jobs. Eye injuries can affect vision. Abdominal trauma and surgery can affect eating and elimination.

Whatever the wound site or size, it affects function and body image. Love and belonging and self-esteem needs are affected. You must be sensitive to the person's feelings. The person may be sad and tearful or angry and hostile. Adjustment may be hard and rehabilitation necessary. Be gentle and kind, give thoughtful care, and practice good communication. Other health team members—therapists, social workers, psychiatrists, and the clergy—may be involved in the person's care.

REVIEW QUESTIONS

Circle the BEST answer.

1. A person has a laceration on the right leg from a fall. The wound is
   a. Open, unintentional, and contaminated
   b. Open, unintentional, and infected
   c. Closed, intentional, and clean
   d. Closed, intentional, and chronic

2. A person had rectal surgery. The person has a
   a. Clean wound
   c. Clean-contaminated wound
   b. Dirty wound
   d. Contaminated wound

3. The skin and underlying tissues are pierced. This is
   a. A penetrating wound
   b. An incision
   c. A contusion
   d. An abrasion

4. Which can cause skin tears?
   a. Keeping your nails trim and smooth
   b. Dressing the person in soft clothing
   c. Wearing rings
   d. Padding wheelchair footplates

5 The first sign of a pressure ulcer is
   a A blister   c Drainage
   b A reddened area   d Gangrene

6 Which can cause pressure ulcers?
   a Repositioning the person every 2 hours
   b Scrubbing and rubbing the skin
   c Applying lotion to dry areas
   d Keeping linens clean, dry, and wrinkle-free

7 Pressure ulcers usually occur
   a On the feet
   b Over a bony area
   c On the buttocks
   d Where skin has contact with skin

8 Which can cause pressure ulcers?
   a Diabetes   c Bed cradles
   b Dressings   d Shearing and friction

9 Which are *not* used to treat pressure ulcers?
   a Special beds
   b Gel or fluid-filled pads and cushions
   c Plastic drawsheets and waterproof pads
   d Heel and elbow protectors

10 What is the preferred position for preventing pressure ulcers?
    a 30-degree lateral position   c Prone position
    b Semi-Fowler's position   d Supine position

11 Persons sitting in chairs should shift their positions every
    a 15 minutes   c Hour
    b 30 minutes   d Two hours

12 A person is at risk for pressure ulcers. Which measure should you question?
    a Apply lotion to the hands, elbows, legs, ankles, and heels.
    b Massage bony areas.
    c Give a back massage when repositioning the person.
    d Apply powder under the breasts.

13 A person has a venous ulcer. Which measure should you question?
    a Hold socks in place with elastic garters.
    b Do not cut or trim toenails.
    c Apply elastic stockings.
    d Reposition the person every hour.

14 Arterial ulcers commonly occur
    a Between the toes   c Over a bony area
    b Behind the ear   d Over an artery

15 Persons with diabetes are at risk for diabetic foot ulcers because of
    a Gangrene
    b Amputation
    c Infection
    d Nerve and blood vessel damage

16 A person has diabetes. You should check the person's feet every
    a 2 hours   c Week
    b Day   d Month

17 A person with diabetes needs to wear socks with shoes to prevent
    a Corns   c Plantar warts
    b Bunions   d Blisters

18 A wound is separating. This is called
    a Primary intention   c Dehiscence
    b Third intention   d Evisceration

19 Clear, watery drainage from a wound is called
    a Purulent drainage
    b Serous drainage
    c Sero-purulent drainage
    d Serosanguineous drainage

20 You note large amounts of sanguineous drainage in a Hemovac. Which is *true*?
    a The person is bleeding.
    b You need to tell the doctor.
    c The person has an infection.
    d The person has a Penrose drain.

21 A dressing does the following *except*
    a Protect the wound from injury
    b Absorb drainage
    c Provide moisture for wound healing
    d Support the wound and reduce swelling

22 To secure a dressing, apply tape
    a Around the entire part
    b Along the sides of the dressing
    c To the top, middle, and bottom of the dressing
    d As the person prefers

23 A person has frequent dressing changes. The nurse will likely have the dressings secured with
    a A binder   c Paper or cloth tape
    b Montgomery ties   d An elastic bandage

24 A person receives a pain-relief drug before a dressing change. How long should you wait for the drug to take effect?
    a 5 minutes   c 15 minutes
    b 10 minutes   d 30 minutes

25 To remove tape
    a Pull it toward the wound
    b Pull it away from the wound
    c Use an adhesive remover
    d Use a saline solution

26 An abdominal binder is used to
    a Prevent blood clots
    b Prevent wound infection
    c Provide support and hold dressings in place
    d Decrease swelling and circulation

Answers to these questions are on p. 781.

OBJECTIVES

- Define the key terms and key abbreviations listed in this chapter
- Identify the purposes, effects, and complications of heat and cold applications
- Identify the persons at risk for complications from heat and cold applications
- Describe moist and dry heat applications
- Describe moist and dry cold applications
- Describe the rules for applying heat and cold
- Explain how cooling and warming blankets are used
- Perform the procedure described in this chapter

PROCEDURE

- Applying Heat and Cold Applications

KEY TERMS

compress A soft pad applied over a body area

constrict To narrow

cyanosis Bluish color

dilate To expand or open wider

hyperthermia A body temperature *(thermia)* that is much higher *(hyper)* than the person's normal range

hypothermia A very low *(hypo)* body temperature *(thermia)*

pack A treatment that involves wrapping a body part with a wet or dry application

KEY ABBREVIATIONS

F Fahrenheit

C Centigrade

eat and cold applications promote healing and comfort. They also reduce tissue swelling. Heat and cold have opposite effects on body function. Severe injuries and changes in body function can occur. The risks are great. You must understand the purposes, effects, and complications of heat and cold applications.

Doctors order heat and cold applications. In some agencies, only nurses apply heat and cold. Other agencies let nursing assistants do so. Before you perform these procedures, make sure that:

▶ Your state allows you to perform the procedure.

▶ The procedure is in your job description.

▶ You have the necessary training.

▶ You know how to use the equipment.

▶ You review the procedure with a nurse.

▶ A nurse is available to answer questions and to supervise you.

See *Focus on Children and Older Persons: Heat and Cold Applications.*

HEAT APPLICATIONS

Heat applications can be applied to almost any body part. They are often used for musculoskeletal injuries or problems (sprains, arthritis). Heat:

▶ Relieves pain

▶ Relaxes muscles

▶ Promotes healing

▶ Reduces tissue swelling

▶ Decreases joint stiffness

When heat is applied to the skin, blood vessels in the area dilate. **Dilate** means to expand or open wider (Fig. 33-1). Blood flow increases. Tissues have more oxygen and nutrients for healing. Excess fluid is removed from the area faster. The skin is red and warm.

Complications

High temperatures can cause burns. Report pain, excessive redness, and blisters at once. Also observe for pale skin. When heat is applied too long, blood vessels **constrict** (narrow) (see Fig. 33-1). Blood flow decreases. Tissues receive less blood. Tissue damage occurs, and the skin is pale.

Older and fair-skinned persons have fragile skin that is easily burned. Persons with problems sensing heat and pain are also at risk. Nervous system damage, loss of consciousness, and circulatory disorders affect sensation. So do confusion and some drugs.

Metal implants pose risks. Metal conducts heat. Deep tissues can be burned. Pacemakers (cardiac devices) and joint replacements are made of metal. Do not apply heat to an implant area.

Heat is not applied to a pregnant woman's abdomen. The heat can affect fetal growth.

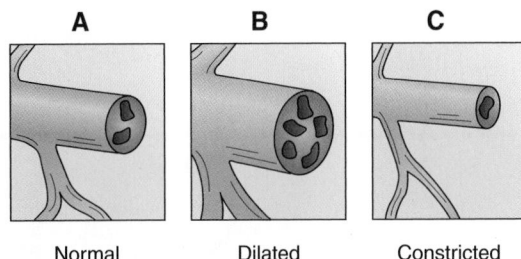

Normal   Dilated   Constricted

FIGURE 33-1 A, Blood vessel under normal conditions. **B,** Dilated blood vessel. **C,** Constricted blood vessel.

Moist and Dry Heat Applications

With a moist heat application, water is in contact with the skin. Water conducts heat. Moist heat has greater and faster effects than dry heat. Heat penetrates deeper with a moist application. To prevent injury, moist heat applications have lower (cooler) temperatures than dry heat applications. Moist heat applications include:

▶ *Hot compresses* (Fig. 33-2, *A*, p. 574)—A **compress** is a soft pad applied over a body area. It is usually made of cloth. Sometimes an aquathermia pad (p. 574) is applied over the compress. It maintains the temperature of the compress.

▶ *Hot soaks* (Fig. 33-2, *B*, p. 574)—A body part is put into water. This is usually used for smaller parts—a hand, lower arm, foot, or lower leg. A tub is used for larger areas.

▶ *Sitz baths* (Fig. 33-2, *C* and *D*, p. 574)—The perineal and rectal areas are immersed in warm water. (*Sitz* means *seat* in German.) Sitz baths are common for hemorrhoids and after rectal or female pelvic surgeries. They are used to:

  ▶ Clean perineal and anal wounds

  ▶ Promote healing

  ▶ Relieve pain and soreness

  ▶ Increase circulation

  ▶ Stimulate voiding

▶ *Hot packs* (Fig. 33-2, *E*)—A **pack** is a treatment that involves wrapping a body part with a wet or dry application. There are single-use (disposable) and re-usable packs. Some can be used for heat or cold. Follow the manufacturer's instructions to activate the heat or cold. Some hot packs are put in boiling water for a few minutes. Or they are warmed in a microwave oven. For other types, you strike, knead, or squeeze the package to activate the heat. Clean re-usable packs after use. Wipe them with alcohol or wash them with soap and water. Follow agency policy and the manufacturer's instructions.

Some *hot packs* and the *aquathermia pad* (Aqua-K, K-Pad) are dry heat applications (Fig. 33-3). With dry heat applications, water is not in contact with the skin. A dry heat application stays at the desired temperature longer. Dry heat does not penetrate as deeply as moist heat. Because water is not used, dry heat needs higher (hotter) temperatures to achieve the desired effect. Therefore burns are still a risk.

The aquathermia pad is an electrical device. Tubes inside the pad are filled with distilled water. Heated water flows to the pad through a hose. Another hose returns water to the heating unit. The water is reheated and

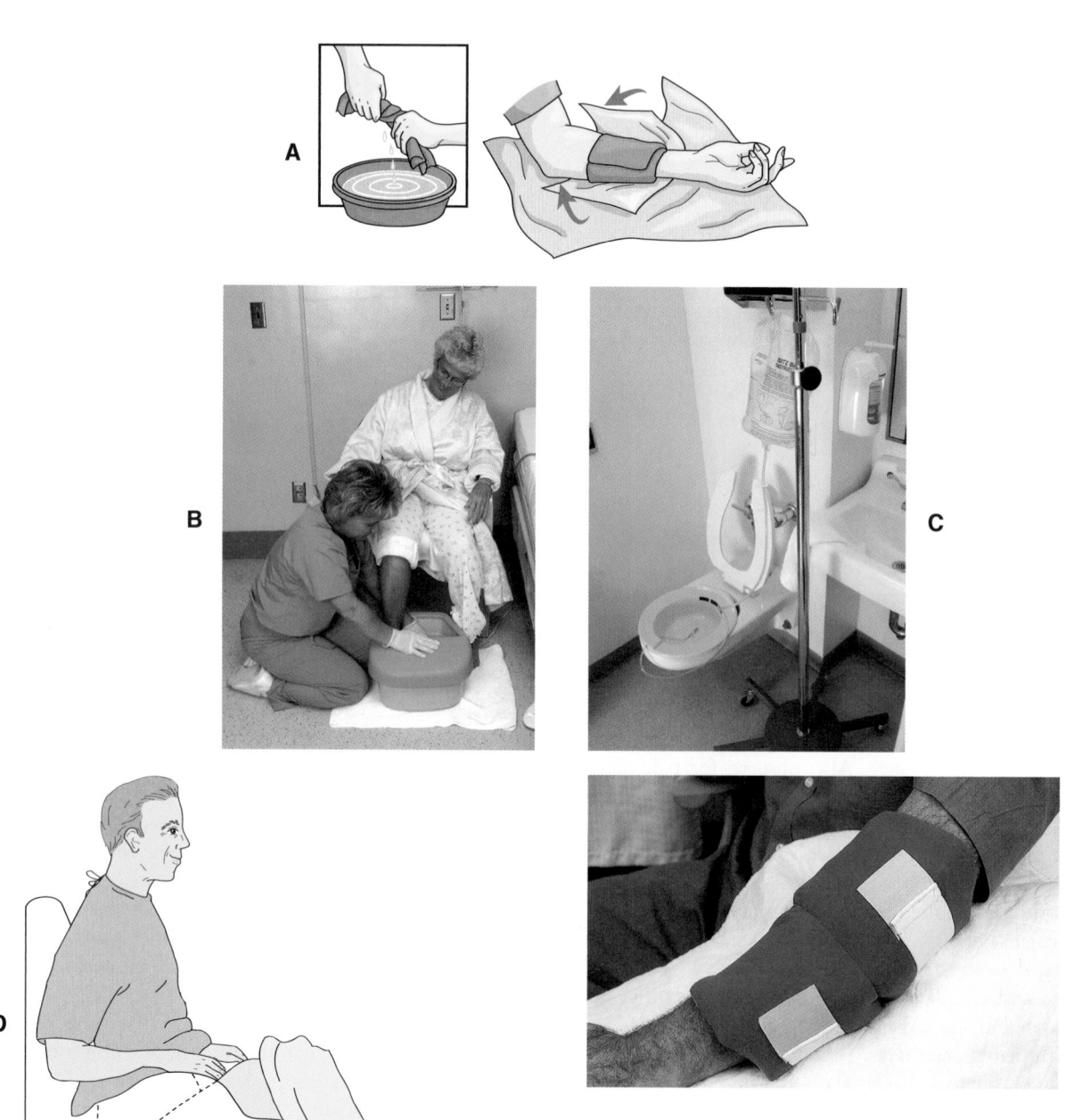

FIGURE 33-2 Wet heat applications. **A,** Compress. **B,** Hot soak. **C,** Disposable sitz bath. **D,** Built-in sitz bath. **E,** Hot pack.

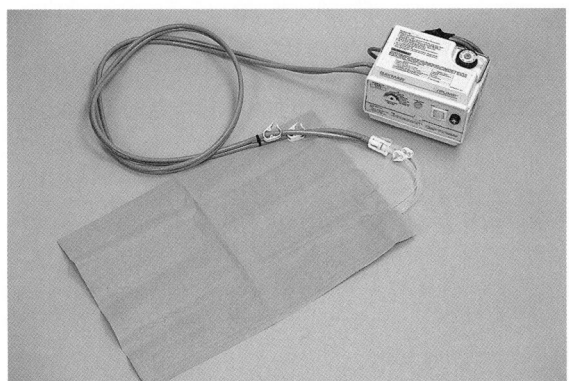

FIGURE 33-3 The aquathermia pad.

Moist and Dry Heat Applications

HOME CARE

Many people have heating pads with electrical coils made of wire. The coils present fire hazards if they break. Always make sure the heating pad is in good repair.

The temperature is easily adjusted. Burns are a great risk. Check the temperature often. Make sure the person has not changed it.

Some devices serve as heating pads and cold applications. They are filled with a special fluid. The pad is kept in the freezer until needed. For a heating pad, heat it following the manufacturer's instructions.

returned back into the pad. Keep the heating unit level with the pad and connecting hoses. Water must flow freely. Hoses must not have kinks and bubbles. The temperature is set at 105° F (Fahrenheit) (40.5° C [centigrade]) with a key. Then the key is removed to prevent anyone from changing the temperature. Often the temperature is set in the supply department. The key is kept there.

See *Focus on Long-Term Care and Home Care: Moist and Dry Heat Applications.*

COLD APPLICATIONS

Cold applications are often used to treat sprains and fractures. They reduce pain, prevent swelling, and decrease circulation and bleeding. Cold cools the body when fever is present.

Cold has the opposite effect of heat. When cold is applied to the skin, blood vessels constrict (see Fig. 33-1). Blood flow decreases. Less oxygen and nutrients are carried to the tissues.

Cold applications are useful right after an injury. Decreased blood flow reduces the amount of bleeding. Less fluid collects in the tissues. Cold has a numbing effect on the skin. This helps reduce or relieve pain in the part.

Complications

Complications include pain, burns, blisters, and poor circulation. Burns and blisters occur from intense cold. They also occur when dry cold is in direct contact with the skin.

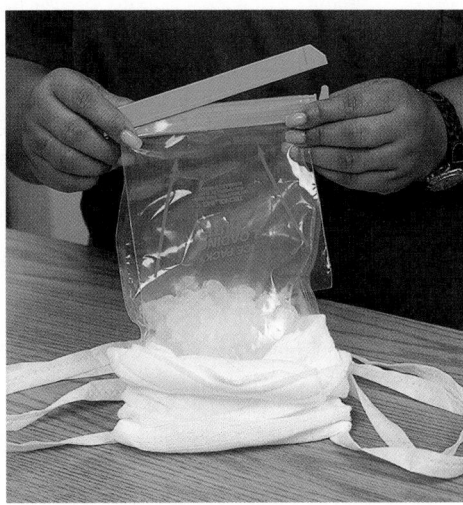

FIGURE 33-4 The ice bag is filled ½ to ⅔ full with ice.

When cold is applied for a long time, blood vessels dilate. Blood flow increases. The prolonged application of cold has the same effect as heat applications.

Older and fair-skinned persons have fragile skin. They are at great risk for complications. So are persons with sensory impairments.

See *Focus on Children and Older Persons: Heat and Cold Applications,* p. 573.

Moist and Dry Cold Applications

Moist cold applications penetrate deeper than dry ones. Therefore moist applications are not as cold as dry applications.

The cold compress is a moist cold application (see Fig. 33-2, *A*). Dry cold applications include ice bags, ice collars, and ice gloves (Fig. 33-4). The device is filled with crushed ice.

Cold packs can be moist or dry applications (see Fig. 33-2, *E*). Commercial cold packs are single-use (disposable) or re-usable. Single-use cold packs are discarded after use. To activate the cold, follow the manufacturer's instructions. You will need to strike, knead, or squeeze the pack. Re-usable cold packs are kept in the freezer. They are cleaned after use (see *Hot packs*).

See *Focus on Long-Term Care and Home Care: Moist and Dry Cold Applications.*

Text continued on p. 579

Moist and Dry Cold Applications

HOME CARE

Disposable ice packs are common in home settings. A bag of frozen peas or corn can serve as an ice bag. So can plastic bags. If using a plastic bag:
- Fill the plastic bag with ice.
- Close the bag securely to prevent leaks.

Wrap the pack, bag of peas or corn, or plastic bag in a towel, dishcloth, or pillowcase.

BOX 33-1 Rules for Applying Heat and Cold

- Know how to use the equipment. Follow the manufacturer's instructions for commercial devices.
- Measure the temperature of moist applications. Use a bath thermometer. Or follow agency policy for measuring temperature.
- Follow agency policies for safe temperature ranges. See Table 33-1.
- Do not apply *very hot* (above 106° F [41.1° C]) applications. Tissue damage can occur. A nurse applies *very hot* applications.
- Ask the nurse what the temperature of the application should be.
  - *Heat*—cooler temperatures are needed for persons at risk.
  - *Cold*—warmer temperatures are needed for persons at risk.
- Know the precise site of the application. Ask the nurse to show you the site.
- Cover dry heat or cold applications before applying them. Use a flannel cover, towel, or other cover as directed by the nurse.
- Provide for privacy. Properly screen and drape the person. Expose only the body part involved. Avoid unnecessary exposure.
- Maintain comfort and body alignment during the procedure.
- Observe the skin every 5 minutes for signs of complications. See *Delegation Guidelines: Applying Heat and Cold.*
- Do not let the person change the temperature of the application.
- Know how long to leave the application in place. See *Delegation Guidelines: Applying Heat and Cold.* Carefully watch the time. Heat and cold are applied no longer than 15 to 20 minutes.
- Follow the rules of electrical safety when using electrical appliances to apply heat.
- Place the signal light within the person's reach.
- Complete a safety check before leaving the room. (See the inside of the front book cover.)

◀ APPLYING HEAT AND COLD

Protect the person from injury during heat and cold applications. Follow the rules listed in Box 33-1, p. 576. Temperature ranges for heat and cold are listed in Table 33-1.

See *Focus on Communication: Applying Heat and Cold.*

See *Teamwork and Time Management: Applying Heat and Cold.*

See *Delegation Guidelines: Applying Heat and Cold.*

See *Promoting Safety and Comfort: Applying Heat and Cold.*

TABLE 33-1 Heat and Cold Temperature Ranges

Temperature	Fahrenheit Range	Centigrade Range
Hot	98° to 106° F	36.6° to 41.1° C
Warm	93° to 98° F	33.8° to 36.6° C
Tepid	80° to 93° F	26.6° to 33.8° C
Cool	65° to 80° F	18.3° to 26.6° C
Cold	50° to 65° F	10.0° to 18.3° C

Modified from Perry AG, Potter PA: *Clinical nursing skills and techniques,* ed 6, St Louis, 2006, Mosby.

FOCUS ON COMMUNICATION

Applying Heat and Cold

The person may not tell you about pain or discomfort. The person may not know what symptoms to report. For heat and cold applications, you need to ask:
- "Does the application feel too hot or too cold?"
- "Do you feel any pain, numbness, or burning?"
- "Are you warm enough?"
- "Do you feel weak, faint, or drowsy?" If yes: "Tell me how you feel?"

TEAMWORK AND TIME MANAGEMENT

Applying Heat and Cold

After applying heat or cold, you need to check the person and the application every 5 minutes. Plan your work so that you can stay in or near the person's room. For example, during the application:
- Make the bed and straighten the person's unit.
- Provide care to the person's roommate if you are assigned to him or her.
- Help the person complete his or her daily or weekly menu.
- Read cards and letters to the person, with his or her consent.
- Address envelopes and other correspondence for the person.
- Take time to visit with the person.

DELEGATION GUIDELINES: Applying Heat and Cold

Before applying heat or cold, you need this information from the nurse and the care plan:
- The type of application—hot compress or pack, commercial compress, hot soak, sitz bath, aquathermia pad; ice bag, ice collar, ice glove, cold pack, or cold compress
- How to cover the application
- What temperature to use (see Table 33-1)
- The application site
- How long to leave the application in place
- What observations to report and record:
  - Complaints of pain or discomfort, numbness, or burning
  - Excessive redness
  - Blisters
  - Pale, white, or gray skin
  - **Cyanosis** (bluish color)
  - Shivering
  - Rapid pulse, weakness, faintness, and drowsiness (sitz bath)
  - Time, site, and length of application
- When to report observations
- What specific patient or resident concerns to report at once

PROMOTING SAFETY AND COMFORT: Applying Heat and Cold

SAFETY

Check the person every 5 minutes. Also follow these safety measures:

- *Sitz bath.* Blood flow increases to the perineum and rectum. Therefore less blood flows to other body parts. The person may become weak or feel faint. Drowsiness can occur from the bath's relaxing effect. Observe for signs of weakness, fainting, or fatigue. Also protect the person from injury. Check the person often. Keep the signal light within reach, and prevent chills and burns.
- *Commercial hot and cold packs.* Read warning labels and follow the manufacturer's instructions.
- *Aquathermia pad:*
  - Follow electrical safety precautions (Chapter 11).
  - Check the device for damage or flaws.
  - Follow the manufacturer's instructions.

- Place the heating unit on an even, uncluttered surface. This prevents it from being knocked over or knocked off of the surface.
- Use a flannel cover to insulate the pad. It absorbs perspiration at the application site. (Some agencies use towels or pillowcases.)
- Secure the pad in place with ties, tape, or rolled gauze. Do not use pins. They can puncture the pad and cause leaks.
- Do not place the pad under the person or under a body part. This prevents the escape of heat. Burns can result if heat cannot escape.

COMFORT

Cold applications can cause chilling and shivering. Provide for warmth. Use bath blankets or other blankets as needed.

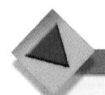

APPLYING HEAT AND COLD APPLICATIONS

✔ **Quality of Life** *Remember to:*

- Knock before entering the person's room.
- Address the person by name.
- Introduce yourself by name and title.
- Explain the procedure to the person before beginning and during the procedure.

- Protect the person's rights during the procedure.
- Handle the person gently during the procedure.

PRE-PROCEDURE

1 Follow *Delegation Guidelines: Applying Heat and Cold.* See *Promoting Safety and Comfort: Applying Heat and Cold.*
2 Practice hand hygiene.
3 Collect needed equipment.
   a *For a hot compress:*
   - Basin
   - Bath thermometer
   - Small towel, washcloth, or gauze squares
   - Plastic wrap or aquathermia pad
   - Ties, tape, or rolled gauze
   - Bath towel
   - Waterproof pad
   b *For a hot soak:*
   - Water basin or arm or foot bath
   - Bath thermometer
   - Waterproof pad
   - Bath blanket
   - Towel
   c *For a sitz bath:*
   - Disposable sitz bath
   - Bath thermometer
   - Two bath blankets, bath towels, and a clean gown
   d *For a hot or cold pack:*
   - Commercial pack

   - Pack cover
   - Ties, tape, or rolled gauze (if needed)
   - Waterproof pad
   e *For an aquathermia pad:*
   - Aquathermia pad and heating unit
   - Distilled water
   - Flannel cover or other cover as directed by the nurse
   - Ties, tape, or rolled gauze
   f *For an ice bag, ice collar, ice glove, or dry cold pack:*
   - Ice bag, collar, or glove or cold pack
   - Crushed ice (except for a cold pack)
   - Flannel cover or other cover as directed by the nurse
   - Paper towels
   g *For a cold compress:*
   - Large basin with ice
   - Small basin with cold water
   - Gauze squares, washcloths, or small towels
   - Waterproof pad
4 Identify the person. Check the ID bracelet against the assignment sheet. Also call the person by name.
5 Provide for privacy.

Continued

APPLYING HEAT AND COLD APPLICATIONS—cont'd

PROCEDURE

6 Position the person for the procedure.

7 Place the waterproof pad (if needed) under the body part.

8 For a hot compress:
   a Fill the basin ½ to ⅔ full with hot water as directed by the nurse. Measure water temperature.
   b Place the compress in the water.
   c Wring out the compress.
   d Apply the compress over the area. Note the time.
   e Cover the compress quickly. Use one of the following as directed by the nurse:
      (1) Apply plastic wrap and then a bath towel. Secure the towel in place with ties, tape, or rolled gauze.
      (2) Apply an aquathermia pad.

9 For a hot soak:
   a Fill the container ½ full with hot water as directed by the nurse. Measure water temperature.
   b Place the part into the water. Pad the edge of the container with a towel. Note the time.
   c Cover the person with a bath blanket for warmth.

10 For a sitz bath:
   a Place the disposable sitz bath on the toilet seat.
   b Fill the sitz bath ⅔ full with water as directed by the nurse. Measure water temperature.
   c Secure the gown above the waist.
   d Help the person sit on the sitz bath. Note the time.
   e Provide for warmth. Place a bath blanket around the shoulders. Place another over the legs.
   f Stay with the person if he or she is weak or is unsteady.

11 For a hot or cold pack:
   a Squeeze, knead, or strike the pack as directed by the manufacturer.
   b Place the pack in the cover.
   c Apply the pack. Note the time.
   d Secure the pack in place with ties, tape, or rolled gauze. Some packs are secured with Velcro straps.

12 For an aquathermia pad:
   a Fill the heating unit to the fill line with distilled water.
   b Remove the bubbles. Place the pad and tubing below the heating unit. Tilt the heating unit from side to side.
   c Set the temperature as the nurse directs (usually 105° F [40.5° C]). Remove the key. (Give the key to the nurse after the procedure.)

d Place the pad in the cover.
e Plug in the unit. Let water warm to the desired temperature.
f Set the heating unit on the bedside stand. Keep the pad and connecting hoses level with the unit. Hoses must not have kinks.
g Apply the pad to the part. Note the time.
h Secure the pad in place with ties, tape, or rolled gauze. Do not use pins.

13 For an ice bag, collar, or glove:
   a Fill the device with water. Put in the stopper. Turn the device upside down to check for leaks.
   b Empty the device.
   c Fill the device ½ to ⅔ full with crushed ice or ice chips.
   d Remove excess air. Bend, twist, or squeeze the device. Or press it against a firm surface.
   e Place the cap or stopper on securely.
   f Dry the device with paper towels.
   g Place the device in the cover.
   h Apply the device. Note the time.
   i Secure the device in place with ties, tape, or rolled gauze.

14 For a cold compress:
   a Place the small basin with cold water into the large basin with ice.
   b Place the compresses into the cold water.
   c Wring out a compress.
   d Apply the compress to the part. Note the time.

15 Place the signal light within reach. Unscreen the person.

16 Raise or lower bed rails. Follow the care plan.

17 Check the person every 5 minutes. Check for signs and symptoms of complications (see *Delegation Guidelines: Applying Heat and Cold*). Remove the application if any complications occur. Tell the nurse at once.

18 Check the application every 5 minutes. Change the application if cooling (hot applications) or warming (cold applications) occurs.

19 Remove the application at the specified time. Heat and cold applications are usually left on for 15 to 20 minutes. (If bed rails are up, lower the near one for this step.)

POST-PROCEDURE

20 Provide for comfort. (See the inside of the front book cover.)

21 Place the signal light within reach.

22 Raise or lower bed rails. Follow the care plan.

23 Unscreen the person.

24 Clean and return re-usable items to their proper place. Follow agency policy for soiled linen. Wear gloves for this step.

25 Complete a safety check of the room. (See the inside of the front book cover.)

26 Remove and discard the gloves. Decontaminate your hands.

27 Report and record your observations (Fig. 33-5).

Date	Time	Nursing Margin	Other Depts Margin
3/6	1000	Aquathermia heating unit set at 105° F. The pad was placed in a flannel	
		cover and applied to the anterior R thigh. Secured in place with tape.	
		Resident positioned in semi-Fowler's position. States she is comfortable.	
		States the pad does not feel too hot. Overbed table with water pitcher and	
		water glass within reach. Bed in the low position. Signal light within	
		reach. Adam Aims, CNA	
3/6	1005	Aquathermia pad checked. Resident states she feels comfortable. States the	
		pad is not too hot. Denies pain or discomfort. There is no redness, swelling,	
		or blistering of the skin under the pad. Pad re-secured with tape. Overbed	
		table with water pitcher and glass within reach. Bed in the low position.	
		Signal light within reach. Adam Aims, CNA	

FIGURE 33-5 Charting sample.

COOLING AND WARMING BLANKET

Hyperthermia is a body temperature *(thermia)* that is much higher *(hyper)* than the person's normal range. With hyperthermia, body temperature is usually greater than 103° F (39.4° C). It is often called *heat stroke* when caused by hot weather. Other causes include illness, dehydration, and not being able to perspire. Lowering the person's body temperature is necessary. Otherwise death can occur. The doctor orders ice packs applied to the head, neck, underarms, and groin. Sometimes cooling blankets are used alone or with ice packs.

A cooling blanket is an electrical device. Made of rubber or plastic, the device has tubes filled with fluid. The fluid flows through the tubes. The blanket is placed on the bed and covered with a sheet. The blanket is turned on the cool setting and allowed to cool. The person lies on the blanket. Vital signs are measured often. Rapid and excess cooling is prevented.

Hypothermia is a very low *(hypo)* body temperature *(thermia)*. Body temperature is less than 95° F (35° C). Cold weather is a common cause. The person is warmed to prevent death. Treatment may include a warming blanket. A warming blanket is like a cooling blanket except warm settings are used. Vital signs are checked often to prevent rapid or excess warming.

When used for cooling, the device is called a *hypothermia blanket*. When used for warming, it is called a *hyperthermia blanket*. The device has warm and cool settings.

See *Focus on Children and Older Persons: Cooling and Warming Blankets.*

FOCUS ON CHILDREN AND OLDER PERSONS

Cooling and Warming Blankets

CHILDREN
Rapid temperature changes can occur in infants and children. Observe them closely. Measure temperature as the nurse directs. Always report the measurement at once. Also report changes in other vital signs or in the child's condition.

REVIEW QUESTIONS

Circle the BEST answer.

1 Heat applications have these effects *except*
  a Pain relief
  b Muscle relaxation
  c Healing
  d Decreased blood flow

2 The *greatest* threat from heat applications is
  a Infection
  b Burns
  c Chilling
  d Pressure ulcers

3 Who has the *greatest* risk of complications from heat applications?
  a An older person with dark skin
  b An older person with nerve damage
  c An adult with a circulatory disorder
  d A child with fair skin

4 These statements are about moist heat applications. Which is *false?*
  a Water is in contact with the skin.
  b The effects from moist heat are less than from a dry heat application.
  c Moist heat penetrates deeper than dry heat.
  d A moist heat application has a lower temperature than a dry heat application.

5 A hot application is usually between
  a 80° and 93° F
  b 93° and 98° F
  c 98° and 106° F
  d 106° and above

6 These statements are about sitz baths. Which is *false?*
  a The perineal and rectal areas are immersed in warm water.
  b Sitz baths last 25 to 30 minutes.
  c They clean the perineum, relieve pain, increase circulation, or stimulate voiding.
  d Weakness and fainting can occur.

7 A person uses an aquathermia pad. Which is *false?*
  a It is a dry heat application.
  b A flannel cover is used.
  c Electrical safety precautions are practiced.
  d Pins secure the pad in place.

8 Cold applications
  a Reduce pain, prevent swelling, and decrease circulation
  b Dilate blood vessels
  c Prevent the spread of microbes
  d Prevent infection

9 Which is *not* a complication of cold applications?
  a Pain
  b Burns
  c Blisters
  d Infection

10 Before applying an ice bag
  a Place the bag in the freezer
  b Measure the temperature of the bag
  c Place the bag in a cover
  d Provide perineal care

11 Moist cold compresses are left in place no longer than
  a 20 minutes
  b 30 minutes
  c 45 minutes
  d 60 minutes

12 A cooling blanket is used for
  a Hypothermia
  b Hyperthermia
  c Cyanosis
  d Shivering

Answers to these questions are on p. 781.

Oxygen Needs

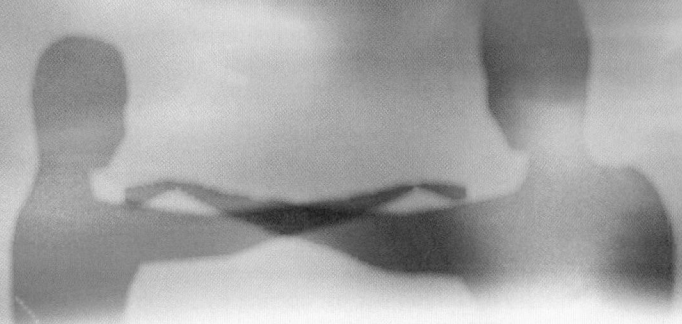

OBJECTIVES

- Define the key terms and key abbreviations listed in this chapter
- Describe the factors affecting oxygen needs
- List the signs and symptoms of hypoxia and altered respiratory function
- Describe the tests used to diagnose respiratory problems
- Explain the measures that promote oxygenation
- Describe the oxygen devices
- Explain how to safely assist with oxygen therapy
- Perform the procedures described in this chapter

PROCEDURES

- Using a Pulse Oximeter
- Assisting With Deep-Breathing and Coughing Exercises
- Setting Up for Oxygen Administration

KEY TERMS

allergy A sensitivity to a substance that causes the body to react with signs and symptoms

apnea The lack or absence *(a)* of breathing *(pnea)*

Biot's respirations Rapid and deep respirations followed by 10 to 30 seconds of apnea

bradypnea Slow *(brady)* breathing *(pnea)*; respirations are fewer than 12 per minute

Cheyne-Stokes respirations Respirations gradually increase in rate and depth and then become shallow and slow; breathing may stop *(apnea)* for 10 to 20 seconds

dyspnea Difficult, labored, or painful *(dys)* breathing *(pnea)*

hemoptysis Bloody *(hemo)* sputum *(ptysis* means *to spit)*

hyperventilation Respirations *(ventilation)* are rapid *(hyper)* and deeper than normal

hypoventilation Respirations *(ventilation)* are slow *(hypo)*, shallow, and sometimes irregular

hypoxemia A reduced amount *(hypo)* of oxygen *(ox)* in the blood *(emia)*

hypoxia Cells do not have enough *(hypo)* oxygen *(oxia)*

Kussmaul respirations Very deep and rapid respirations

orthopnea Breathing *(pnea)* deeply and comfortably only when sitting *(ortho)*

orthopneic position Sitting up *(ortho)* and leaning over a table to breathe *(pneic)*

oxygen concentration The amount (percent) of hemoglobin containing oxygen

pollutant A harmful chemical or substance in the air or water

respiratory arrest When breathing stops

respiratory depression Slow, weak respirations at a rate of fewer than 12 per minute

sputum Mucus from the respiratory system that is expectorated *(expelled)* through the mouth

tachypnea Rapid *(tachy)* breathing *(pnea)*; respirations are more than 20 per minute

KEY ABBREVIATIONS

ABGs Arterial blood gases

CO_2 Carbon dioxide

COPD Chronic obstructive pulmonary disease

CXR Chest x-ray

L/min Liters per minute

O_2 Oxygen

NPO Non per os; nothing by mouth

RBC Red blood cell

SMI Sustained maximal inspiration

SpO_2 Oxygen saturation

Oxygen (O_2) is a gas. It has no taste, odor, or color. It is a basic need required for life. Death occurs within minutes if breathing stops. Brain damage and serious illnesses can occur without enough oxygen. Illness, surgery, and injuries affect the amount of oxygen in the blood and cells.

You assist in the care of persons with oxygen needs. You must give safe and effective care. See Box 34-1 for a review of the respiratory system.

FACTORS AFFECTING OXYGEN NEEDS

The respiratory and circulatory systems must function properly for cells to get enough oxygen. Any disease, injury, or surgery involving these systems affects the intake and use of oxygen. Body systems depend on each other. Altered function of any system (for example, the nervous, musculoskeletal, or urinary system) affects oxygen needs. Oxygen needs are affected by:

▸ *Respiratory system status.* Structures must be intact and function properly. An open *(patent)* airway is needed. Alveoli (air sacs) must exchange O_2 and carbon dioxide (CO_2).

▸ *Circulatory system function.* Blood must flow to and from the heart. Narrowed vessels affect blood flow. Capillaries and cells must exchange O_2 and CO_2.

▸ *Red blood cell count.* Red blood cells (RBCs) contain hemoglobin. Hemoglobin picks up O_2 in the lungs and carries it to the cells. The bone marrow must produce enough RBCs. Poor diet, chemotherapy, and leukemia affect bone marrow function. Blood loss also reduces the number of RBCs.

▸ *Nervous system function.* Nervous system diseases and injuries can affect respiratory muscles. Breathing may be difficult or impossible. Brain damage affects respiratory rate, rhythm, and depth. Narcotics and depressant drugs affect the brain. They slow respirations. O_2 and CO_2 blood levels also affect brain function. Respirations increase when O_2 is lacking. The body tries to bring in more oxygen. Respirations also increase when CO_2 increases. The body tries to get rid of CO_2.

▸ *Aging.* Respiratory muscles weaken. Lung tissue is less elastic. Strength for coughing decreases. The person must cough and remove secretions from the upper airway. Otherwise, *pneumonia* (inflammation and infection of the lung) can develop. Older persons are at risk for respiratory complications after surgery.

- *Exercise.* O_2 needs increase with exercise. Normally, respiratory rate and depth increase to bring enough O_2 into the lungs. Persons with heart and respiratory diseases may have enough oxygen at rest. However, even slight activity can increase O_2 needs. Their bodies may not be able to bring in O_2 and carry it to the cells.
- *Fever.* O_2 needs increase. Respiratory rate and depth increase to meet the body's needs.
- *Pain.* O_2 needs increase. Respirations increase to meet this need. However, chest and abdominal injuries and surgeries often involve respiratory muscles. It hurts to breathe in and out.
- *Drugs.* Some drugs depress the respiratory center in the brain. **Respiratory depression** means slow, weak respirations at a rate of fewer than 12 per minute. Respirations are too shallow to bring enough O_2 into the lungs. **Respiratory arrest** is when breathing stops. Narcotics (morphine, Demerol, and others) can have these effects. (Narcotic comes from the Greek word *narkoun*. It means *stupor* or *to be numb.*) In safe amounts, these drugs relieve severe pain. Substance abusers are at risk for respiratory depression and respiratory arrest. They can overdose on drugs.

- *Smoking.* Smoking causes lung cancer and chronic obstructive pulmonary disease (COPD). It is a risk factor for coronary artery disease.
- *Allergies.* An **allergy** is a sensitivity to a substance that causes the body to react with signs and symptoms. Runny nose, wheezing, and congestion are common. Mucous membranes in the upper airway swell. With severe swelling, the airway closes. Shock and death are risks. Pollens, dust, foods, drugs, insect bites, and cigarette smoke often cause allergies. Chronic bronchitis and asthma are risks.
- *Pollutant exposure.* A **pollutant** is a harmful chemical or substance in the air or water. Examples are dust, fumes, toxins, asbestos, coal dust, and sawdust. They damage the lungs. Pollutant exposure occurs in home, work, and public settings.
- *Nutrition.* Good nutrition is needed to produce blood cells. The body needs iron and vitamins (vitamin B_{12}, vitamin C, and folate) to produce RBCs.
- *Alcohol.* Alcohol depresses the brain. Excessive amounts reduce the cough reflex and increase the risk of aspiration. Obstructed airway and pneumonia are risks from aspiration.

BOX 34-1 The Respiratory System: Body Structure and Function

Oxygen is needed to live. Every cell needs oxygen. The respiratory system (Fig. 34-1) brings oxygen into the lungs and removes carbon dioxide. *Respiration* is the process of supplying the cells with oxygen and removing carbon dioxide from them. Respiration involves *inhalation* (breathing in) and *exhalation* (breathing out). The terms *inspiration* (breathing in) and *expiration* (breathing out) also are used.

Air enters the body through the *nose*. The air then passes into the *pharynx* (throat). It is a tube-shaped passageway for air and food. Air passes from the pharynx into the *larynx* (voice box). Air passes from the larynx into the *trachea* (windpipe).

The trachea divides at its lower end into the *right bronchus* and the *left bronchus*. Each bronchus enters a lung. Upon entering the lungs, the bronchi divide many times into smaller branches *(bronchioles)*. Eventually the bronchioles subdivide. They end up in tiny one-celled air sacs called *alveoli*.

Oxygen and carbon dioxide are exchanged between the alveoli and capillaries. Blood in the capillaries picks up oxygen from the alveoli. Then the blood is returned to the left side of the heart and pumped to the rest of the body. Alveoli pick up carbon dioxide from the capillaries for exhalation.

Each lung is divided into lobes. The right lung has three lobes; the left lung has two. The lungs are separated from the abdominal cavity by a muscle called the *diaphragm*. A bony framework made up of the ribs, sternum, and vertebrae protects the lungs.

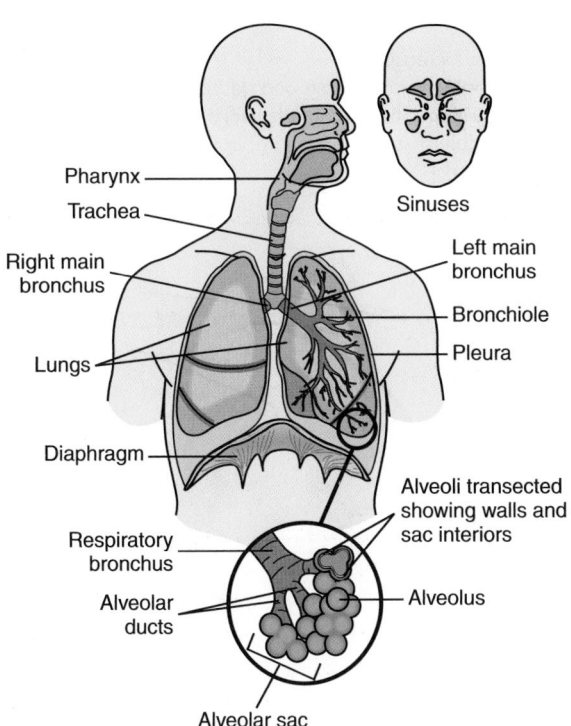

FIGURE 34-1 The respiratory system.

ALTERED RESPIRATORY FUNCTION

Respiratory function involves three processes. Respiratory function is altered if even one process is affected.

▶ Air moves into and out of the lungs.
▶ O_2 and CO_2 are exchanged at the alveoli.
▶ The blood carries O_2 to the cells and removes CO_2 from them.

Hypoxia

Hypoxia means that cells do not have enough *(hypo)* oxygen *(oxia)*. When cells do not have enough oxygen, they cannot function properly. Anything that affects respiratory function can cause hypoxia. The brain is very sensitive to inadequate O_2. Restlessness is an early sign. So are dizziness and disorientation. Report the signs and symptoms in Box 34-2 to the nurse at once.

Hypoxia is life-threatening. All organs need oxygen to function. Oxygen is given. The cause of hypoxia is treated.

BOX 34-2 Signs and Symptoms of Hypoxia

- Restlessness
- Dizziness
- Disorientation
- Confusion
- Behavior and personality changes
- Concentrating and following directions: problems with
- Apprehension
- Anxiety
- Fatigue
- Agitation
- Pulse rate: increased
- Respirations: increased rate and depth
- Sitting position: often leaning forward
- Cyanosis (bluish color to the skin, lips, mucous membranes, and nail beds)
- Dyspnea

Abnormal Respirations

Adults normally have 12 to 20 respirations per minute. Infants and children have faster rates. Normal respirations are quiet, effortless, and regular. Both sides of the chest rise and fall equally. These breathing patterns are abnormal (Fig. 34-2):

▶ **Tachypnea**—rapid *(tachy)* breathing *(pnea)*. Respirations are more than 20 per minute. Fever, exercise, pain, pregnancy, airway obstruction, and hypoxemia are common causes. **Hypoxemia** is a reduced amount *(hypo)* of oxygen *(ox)* in the blood *(emia)*.

▶ **Bradypnea**—slow *(brady)* breathing *(pnea)*. Respirations are fewer than 12 per minute. Drug overdose and central nervous system disorders are common causes.

▶ **Apnea**—lack or absence *(a)* of breathing *(pnea)*. It occurs in sudden cardiac arrest and respiratory arrest. Sleep apnea and periodic apnea of newborns are other types of apnea.

▶ **Hypoventilation**—respirations *(ventilation)* are slow *(hypo)*, shallow, and sometimes irregular. Lung disorders affecting the alveoli are common causes. Pneumonia is an example. Other causes include obesity, airway obstruction, and drug side effects. Nervous system and musculoskeletal disorders affecting the respiratory muscles are other causes.

▶ **Hyperventilation**—respirations *(ventilation)* are rapid *(hyper)* and deeper than normal. Its many causes include asthma, emphysema, infection, fever, nervous system disorders, hypoxia, anxiety, pain, and some drugs.

▶ **Dyspnea**—difficult, labored, or painful *(dys)* breathing *(pnea)*. Heart disease, exercise, and anxiety are common causes.

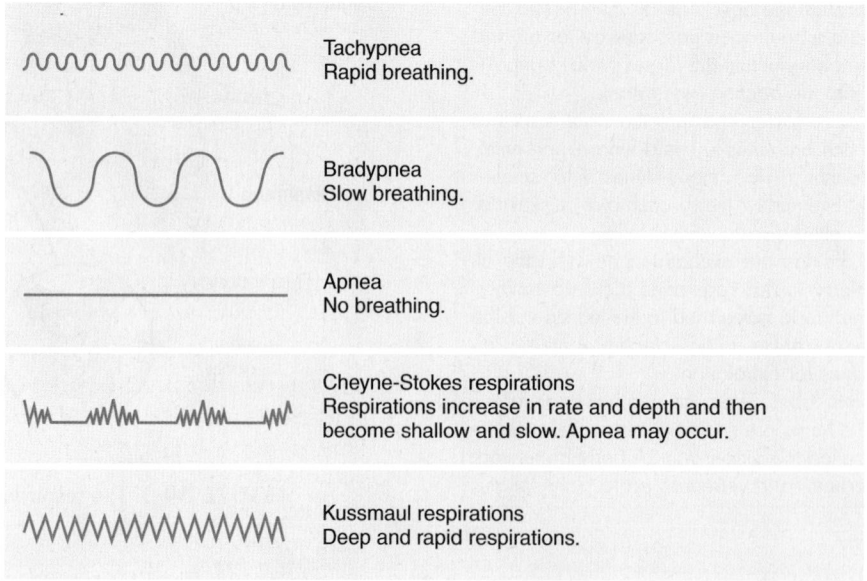

Tachypnea
Rapid breathing.

Bradypnea
Slow breathing.

Apnea
No breathing.

Cheyne-Stokes respirations
Respirations increase in rate and depth and then become shallow and slow. Apnea may occur.

Kussmaul respirations
Deep and rapid respirations.

FIGURE 34-2 Some abnormal breathing patterns. (Modified from Talbot L, Meyers-Marquardt M: *Pocket guide to critical care assessment,* ed 3, St Louis, 1997, Mosby.)

▶ **Cheyne-Stokes respirations**—respirations gradually increase in rate and depth. Then they become shallow and slow. Breathing may stop (*apnea*) for 10 to 20 seconds. Drug overdose, heart failure, renal failure, and brain disorders are common causes. Cheyne-Stokes are common when death is near.

▶ **Orthopnea**—breathing (*pnea*) deeply and comfortably only when sitting (*ortho*). Common causes include emphysema, asthma, pneumonia, angina, and other heart and respiratory disorders.

▶ **Biot's respirations**—rapid and deep respirations followed by 10 to 30 seconds of apnea. They occur with nervous system disorders.

▶ **Kussmaul respirations**—very deep and rapid respirations. They signal diabetic coma.

ASSISTING WITH ASSESSMENT AND DIAGNOSTIC TESTS

Altered respiratory function may be an acute or chronic problem. Report your observations promptly and accurately (Box 34-3). Quick action is needed to meet the

---

BOX 34-3 Signs and Symptoms of Altered Respiratory Function

- Hypoxia: signs and symptoms of (see Box 34-2)
- Breathing pattern: abnormal
- Shortness of breath or complaints of being "winded" or "short-winded"
- Cough (note frequency and time of day)
  - Dry and hacking
  - Harsh and barking
  - Productive (produces sputum) or non-productive
- Sputum (mucus from the respiratory system)
  - Color: clear, white, yellow, green, brown, or red
  - Odor: none or foul odor
  - Consistency: thick, watery, or frothy (with bubbles or foam)
  - **Hemoptysis:** bloody (*hemo*) sputum (*ptysis* means *to spit*); note if the sputum is bright red, dark red, blood-tinged, or streaked with blood
- Respirations: noisy
  - Wheezing
  - Wet-sounding
  - Crowing sounds
- Chest pain (note location)
  - Constant or intermittent (comes and goes)
  - Person's description (stabbing, knife-like, aching)
  - What makes it worse (movement, coughing, yawning, sneezing, sighing, deep breathing)
- Cyanosis (bluish color)
  - Skin
  - Mucous membranes
  - Lips
  - Nail beds
- Vital signs: changes in
- Position
  - Sitting upright
  - Leaning forward or hunched over a table

FOCUS ON COMMUNICATION

Assisting With Assessment and Diagnostic Tests

The questions you ask the person aid the nurse in the assessment step of the nursing process. For example:
- "Do you need more pillows?"
- "Do you want the head of your bed raised more?"
- "How often are you coughing?"
- "Are you coughing anything up?"
- "Please use a tissue when you cough up mucus, then put on your signal light. The nurse needs to observe the mucus."

---

person's oxygen needs. Measures are taken to correct the problem and to prevent it from becoming worse.

See *Focus on Communication: Assisting With Assessment and Diagnostic Tests.*

The doctor orders tests to find the cause of the problem. These tests are common:

▶ *Chest x-ray (CXR).* An x-ray is taken of the chest. Lung changes are studied. All clothing and jewelry from the waist to the neck are removed. A patient gown (without snaps) is worn. A portable x-ray machine is used in the person's room.

▶ *Lung scan.* The lungs are scanned to see what areas are not getting air or blood. The person inhales radioactive gas. *Radioactive* means to give off radiation. A radioisotope is injected into a vein. A *radioisotope* is a substance that gives off radiation. Lung tissue getting air and blood flow "take up" the substance. All clothing from the waist to the neck is removed. An x-ray garment is worn.

▶ *Bronchoscopy.* A scope (*scopy*) is passed into the trachea and bronchi (*broncho*). Airway structures are checked for bleeding and tumors. Tissue samples (*biopsies*) are taken. Or mucous plugs and foreign objects are removed. The person is NPO (non per os; nothing by mouth) for 6 to 8 hours before the procedure. This reduces the risks of vomiting and aspiration. An anesthetic is given. After the procedure, the person is NPO and observed carefully until the gag and swallow reflexes return. This can take about 2 hours. The nurse directs pre-operative and post-operative care.

▶ *Thoracentesis.* The pleura (*thora*) is punctured. Air or fluid is removed (*centesis*) from it. The doctor inserts a needle through the chest wall into the pleural sac (Fig. 34-3, p. 586). Injury or disease can cause the sac to fill with air, blood, or fluid. Sometimes fluid is removed for laboratory study. Anti-cancer drugs can be injected into the pleural sac. A thoracentesis takes a few minutes. Vital signs are taken. Then a local anesthetic is given. The person sits up and leans forward. He or she is asked not to talk, cough, or move suddenly. Afterward a dressing is applied to the puncture site. Vital signs are taken. A chest x-ray is taken to detect lung damage. The person is observed for shortness of breath, dyspnea, cough, sputum, chest pain, cyanosis, vital sign changes, and other respiratory signs and symptoms.

▶ *Pulmonary function tests.* These tests measure the amount of air moving into and out of the lungs *(volume).* They also measure how much air the lungs can hold *(capacity).* The person takes as deep a breath as possible. Using a mouthpiece, the person blows into a machine (Fig. 34-4). The tests help assess the risk for lung diseases or post-operative lung complications. They also measure the progress of lung disease and its treatment. Fatigue is common after the tests. The person needs to rest.

▶ *Arterial blood gases (ABGs).* A radial, femoral, or brachial artery is punctured to obtain arterial blood. Laboratory tests measure the amount of oxygen in the blood. Hemorrhage from the artery must be prevented. Pressure is applied to the artery for at least 5 minutes after the procedure. Pressure is applied longer if there are blood-clotting problems. The procedure is done by a specially trained nurse, respiratory therapist, or laboratory technician.

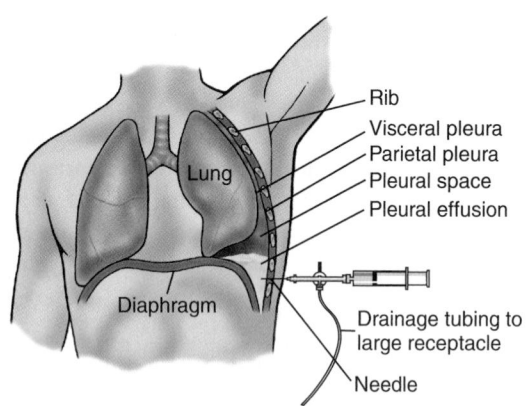

FIGURE 34-3 Thoracentesis. (Modified from Monahan FD, Neighbors M: *Foundations for clinical practice,* ed 2, Philadelphia, 1998, Saunders.)

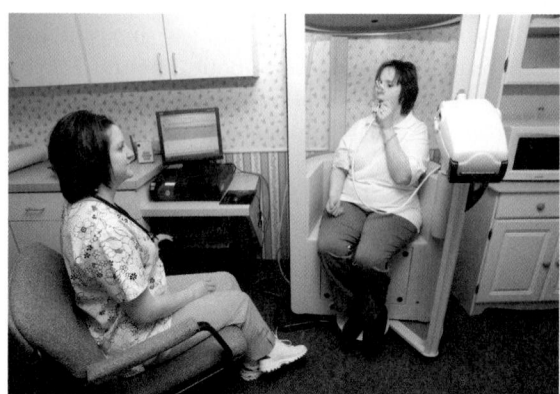

FIGURE 34-4 Pulmonary function testing.

◆ Pulse Oximetry

Pulse oximetry measures *(metry)* the oxygen *(oxi)* concentration in arterial blood. **Oxygen concentration** is the amount (percent) of hemoglobin containing oxygen. Measurements are used to prevent and treat hypoxia. The normal range is 95% to 100%. For example, if 97% of all the hemoglobin (100%) carries O_2, tissues get enough oxygen. If only 90% contains O_2, tissues do not get enough oxygen. However, an SpO_2 as low as 85% may be normal for persons with some chronic diseases.

A sensor attaches to a finger, toe, earlobe, nose, or forehead (Fig. 34-5). Light beams on one side of the sensor pass through the tissues. A detector on the other side measures the amount of light passing through the tissues. With this information, the oximeter measures the O_2 concentration. The value and pulse rate are shown. Oximeter alarms are set for continuous monitoring. An alarm sounds if:

▶ O_2 concentration is low
▶ The pulse is too fast or slow
▶ Other problems occur

A good sensor site is needed. Swollen sites are avoided. So are sites with skin breaks. Aging and vascular disease often cause poor circulation. Sometimes blood flow to the fingers or toes is poor. Then the earlobe, nose, and forehead sites are used.

Bright light, nail polish, fake nails, and movements affect measurements. Place a towel over the sensor to block bright light. Remove nail polish, or use another site. Do not use a finger site if the person has fake nails. Movements from shivering, seizures, or tremors affect finger sensors. The earlobe is a better site when there are such problems. Blood pressure cuffs affect blood flow. If using a finger site, do not measure blood pressure on that side.

Report and record measurements accurately. Use SpO_2 when recording the oxygen concentration value.

See *Focus on Children and Older Persons: Pulse Oximetry.*
See *Focus on Long-Term Care and Home Care: Pulse Oximetry.*
See *Delegation Guidelines: Pulse Oximetry.*
See *Promoting Safety and Comfort: Pulse Oximetry.*

FOCUS ON CHILDREN AND OLDER PERSONS

Pulse Oximetry

CHILDREN
The sensor is attached to the sole of a foot, palm of a hand, toe, or earlobe (Fig. 34-5, *B*). If the child moves a lot, the earlobe is a better site.

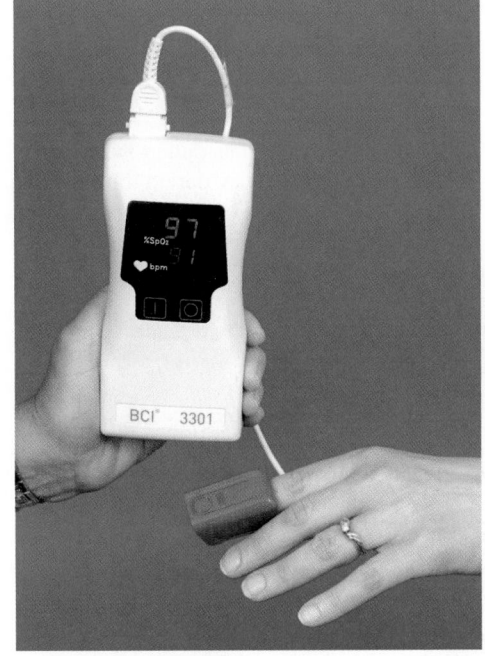
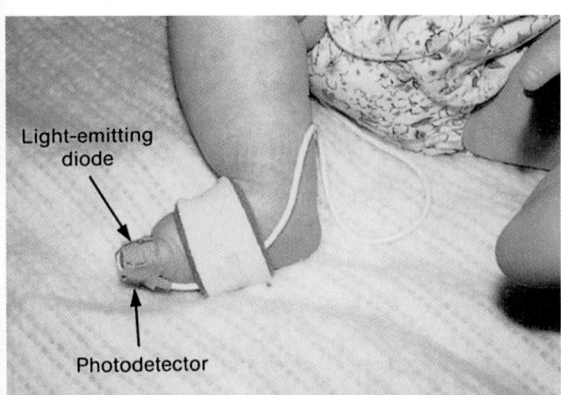

Light-emitting
diode

Photodetector

A

B

FIGURE 34-5 A, A pulse oximetry sensor is attached to a finger. **B,** The sensor is attached
to an infant's great toe. (**B** from Hockenberry MJ and Wilson D: *Wong's nursing care of
infants and children,* ed 8, St Louis, 2007, Mosby.)

FOCUS ON **LONG-TERM CARE** AND **HOME CARE**

Pulse Oximetry

HOME CARE

Oxygen concentration is often measured with vital signs. The
pulse oximeter is portable. It must be accurate. After applying
the sensor, check the person's pulse (apical or radial). Compare
it with the displayed pulse. The pulse rates should be the same.

PROMOTING SAFETY AND COMFORT: Pulse Oximetry

SAFETY

The person's condition can change rapidly. Pulse oximetry
does not lessen the need for good observations. Observe for
signs and symptoms of hypoxia (Box 34-2) and altered
respiratory system function (Box 34-3).

COMFORT

A clip-on sensor feels like a clothespin when applied to the
site. It should not hurt or cause discomfort. Ask the person to
tell you at once if it causes pain, discomfort, or too much
pressure on the site. The sensor site is changed every 4 hours
if continuous monitoring is ordered.

DELEGATION GUIDELINES: Pulse Oximetry

When assisting with pulse oximetry, you need this information
from the nurse and the care plan:
- What site to use
- How to use the equipment
- What sensor to use
- What type of tape to use
- The SpO$_2$ range that is normal for the person
- The alarm limits for SpO$_2$ and pulse rate for continuous
  monitoring:
  - Tell the nurse at once if the SpO$_2$ goes below the alarm limit
    (usually 95%)
  - Tell the nurse at once if the pulse rate goes above or below
    the alarm limit

- When to do the measurement
- What pulse site to use: apical or radial
- How often to check the sensor site (usually every 2 hours)
- What observations to report and record:
  - The date and time
  - The SpO$_2$ and display pulse rate
  - Apical or radial pulse rate
  - What the person was doing at the time
  - Oxygen flow rate (p. 595) and the device used (p. 594)
  - Reason for the measurement: routine or condition change
- When to report observations
- What specific patient or resident concerns to report at once

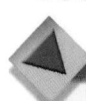

USING A PULSE OXIMETER

✔ Quality of Life *Remember to:*

- Knock before entering the person's room.
- Address the person by name.
- Introduce yourself by name and title.
- Explain the procedure to the person before beginning and during the procedure.

- Protect the person's rights during the procedure.
- Handle the person gently during the procedure.

PRE-PROCEDURE

1 Follow *Delegation Guidelines: Pulse Oximetry,* p. 587. See *Promoting Safety and Comfort: Pulse Oximetry,* p. 587.
2 Practice hand hygiene.
3 Collect the following before going to the person's room:
  - Oximeter and sensor
  - Nail polish remover
  - Cotton balls

- Tape
- Towel
4 Arrange your work area.
5 Decontaminate your hands.
6 Identify the person. Check the ID bracelet against your assignment sheet. Also call the person by name.
7 Provide for privacy.

PROCEDURE

8 Provide for comfort.
9 Remove nail polish from the fingernail or toenail. Use nail polish remover and a cotton ball.
10 Dry the site with a towel.
11 Clip or tape the sensor to the site.
12 Turn on the oximeter.
13 Set the high and low alarm limits for SpO_2 and pulse rate. Turn on audio and visual alarms. (This step is for continuous monitoring.)

14 Check the person's pulse (apical or radial) with the pulse on the display. The pulses should be equal. Tell the nurse if the pulses are not equal.
15 Read the SpO_2 on the display. Note the value on the flow sheet and your assignment sheet.
16 Leave the sensor in place for continuous monitoring. Otherwise, turn off the device and remove the sensor.

POST-PROCEDURE

17 Provide for comfort. (See the inside of the front book cover.)
18 Place the signal light within reach.
19 Unscreen the person.
20 Complete a safety check of the room. (See the inside of the front book cover.)

21 Return the device to its proper place (unless monitoring is continuous).
22 Decontaminate your hands.
23 Report and record the SpO_2, the pulse rate, and your other observations.

Sputum Specimens

Respiratory disorders cause the lungs, bronchi, and trachea to secrete mucus. Mucus from the respiratory system is called **sputum** when expectorated (*expelled*) through the mouth. Sputum specimens are studied for blood, microbes, and abnormal cells. See Chapter 30.

PROMOTING OXYGENATION

To get enough oxygen, air must move deep into the lungs. Air must reach the alveoli where O_2 and CO_2 are exchanged. Disease and injury can prevent air from reaching the alveoli. Pain and immobility interfere with deep breathing and coughing. So do narcotics. Therefore secretions collect in the airway and lungs. They interfere with air movement and lung function. Secretions also provide a place for microbes to grow and multiply. Infection is a threat.

Oxygen needs must be met. The following measures are common in care plans.

Positioning

Breathing is usually easier in semi-Fowler's and Fowler's positions. Persons with difficulty breathing often prefer sitting up and leaning over a table to breathe. This is called the **orthopneic position**. (*Ortho* means *sitting or standing. Pneic* means *breathing.*) Place a pillow on the table to increase the person's comfort (Fig. 34-6).

Frequent position changes are needed. Unless the doctor limits positioning, the person must not lie on one side for a long time. Secretions pool. The lungs cannot expand on that side. Position changes are needed at least every 2 hours. Follow the care plan.

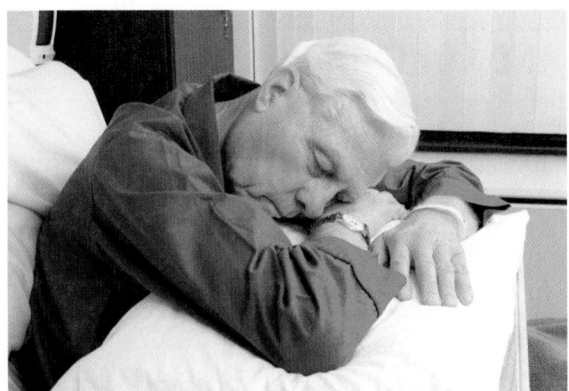

FIGURE 34-6 The person is in the orthopneic position. A pillow is on the overbed table for the person's comfort.

◢ Deep Breathing and Coughing

Deep breathing moves air into most parts of the lungs. Coughing removes mucus. Deep breathing and coughing exercises help persons with respiratory problems. They are done after surgery or injury and during bedrest. The exercises are painful after surgery or injury. Breaking an incision open while coughing is a fear.

Deep breathing and coughing help prevent pneumonia and atelectasis. *Atelectasis* is the collapse of a portion of the lung. It occurs when mucus collects in the airway. Air cannot get to a part of the lung. The lung collapses. Atelectasis is a risk after surgery. Bedrest, lung diseases, and paralysis are other risk factors.

Deep breathing and coughing are usually done every 2 hours while the person is awake. Sometimes they are done every hour while the person is awake.

See *Focus on Children and Older Persons: Deep Breathing and Coughing.*

See *Delegation Guidelines: Deep Breathing and Coughing.*

See *Promoting Safety and Comfort: Deep Breathing and Coughing.*

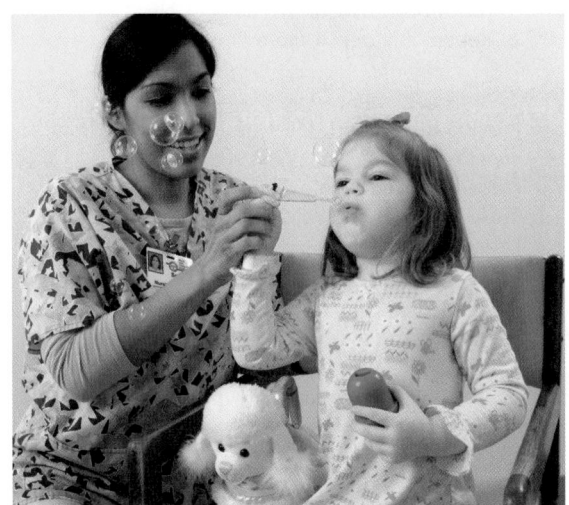

FIGURE 34-7 The child blows bubbles for a deep-breathing exercise.

ASSISTING WITH DEEP-BREATHING AND COUGHING EXERCISES

✔ **Quality of Life** *Remember to:*

- Knock before entering the person's room.
- Address the person by name.
- Introduce yourself by name and title.
- Explain the procedure to the person before beginning and during the procedure.

- Protect the person's rights during the procedure.
- Handle the person gently during the procedure.

PRE-PROCEDURE

1 Follow *Delegation Guidelines: Deep Breathing and Coughing,* p. 589. See *Promoting Safety and Comfort: Deep Breathing and Coughing,* p. 589.
2 Practice hand hygiene.

3 Identify the person. Check the ID bracelet against the assignment sheet. Also call the person by name.
4 Provide for privacy.

PROCEDURE

5 Lower the bed rail if up.
6 Help the person to a comfortable sitting position: dangling, semi-Fowler's, or Fowler's.
7 Have the person deep breathe:
  a Have the person place the hands over the rib cage (Fig. 34-8).
  b Have the person take a deep breath. It should be as deep as possible. Remind the person to inhale through the nose.
  c Ask the person to hold the breath for 2 to 3 seconds.
  d Ask the person to exhale slowly through pursed lips (Fig. 34-9). Ask the person to exhale until the ribs move as far down as possible.
  e Repeat this step 4 more times.

8 Ask the person to cough:
  a Have the person place both hands over the incision. One hand is on top of the other (Fig. 34-10, *A*). The person can hold a pillow or folded towel over the incision (Fig. 34-10, *B*).
  b Have the person take in a deep breath as in step 7.
  c Ask the person to cough strongly twice with the mouth open.

POST-PROCEDURE

9 Provide for comfort. (See the inside of the front book cover.)
10 Place the signal light within reach.
11 Raise or lower bed rails. Follow the care plan.
12 Unscreen the person.

13 Complete a safety check of the room. (See the inside of the front book cover.)
14 Decontaminate your hands.
15 Report and record your observations (Fig. 34-11).

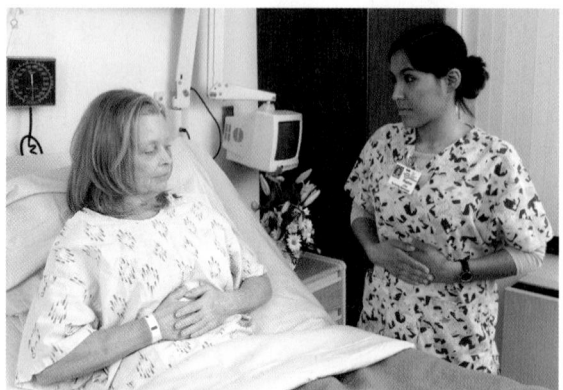

FIGURE 34-8 The hands are over the rib cage for deep breathing.

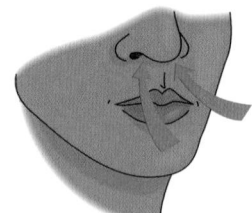 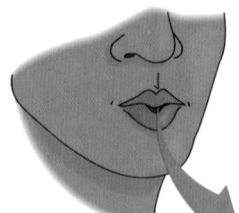

FIGURE 34-9 The person inhales through the nose and exhales through pursed lips during the deep-breathing exercise.

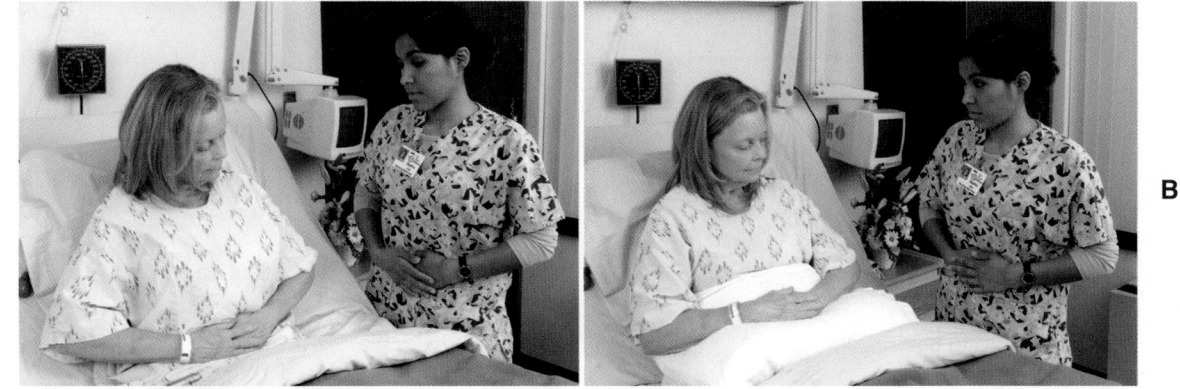

FIGURE 34-10 The person supports an incision for the coughing exercises. **A,** The hands are over the incision. **B,** A pillow is held over the incision.

	Date	Time	Nursing Margin	Other Depts Margin
3/15	0830		Assisted resident with deep-breathing and coughing exercises.	
			Resident performed exercises ×2. He states "It is getting easier every	
			day." Denied pain or discomfort. Requested to sit in his chair after	
			the exercises. Tray table with water pitcher and glass, tissues, and	
			a book within reach. Signal light within reach. Jean Hein, CNA	

FIGURE 34-11 Charting sample.

Incentive Spirometry

Incentive means to encourage. A *spirometer* is a machine that measures the amount *(volume)* of air inhaled. With incentive spirometry the person is encouraged to inhale until reaching a preset volume of air. Balls or bars in the machine let the person see air movement when inhaling (Fig. 34-12).

Incentive spirometry also is called *sustained maximal inspiration (SMI)*. Sustained means constant. *Maximal* means the most or the greatest. And *inspiration* relates to breathing in. SMI means inhaling as deeply as possible and holding the breath for a certain time. The breath is usually held for at least 3 seconds.

The goal is to improve lung function. Atelectasis is prevented or treated. Like yawning or sighing, breathing is long, slow, and deep. This moves air deep into the

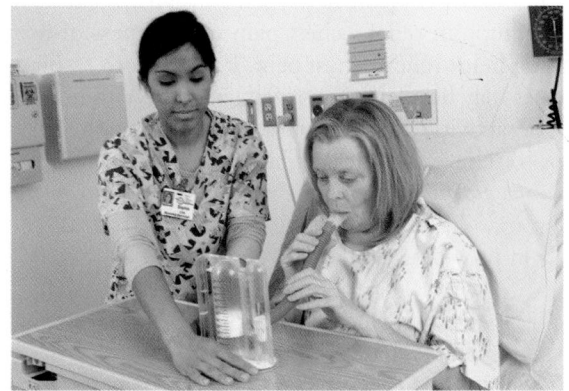

FIGURE 34-12 The person uses a spirometer.

DELEGATION GUIDELINES: Incentive Spirometry

Before assisting a person with incentive spirometry, you need this information from the nurse and the care plan:
- How often the person needs incentive spirometry
- How many breaths the person needs to take
- The desired height of the floating balls
- How to clean the mouthpiece
- When to replace the mouthpiece
- What observations to report and record:
  - How many breaths the person took
  - The height of the floating balls
  - If the person coughed after using the spirometer
  - How the person tolerated the incentive spirometry
- When to report observations
- What specific patient or resident concerns to report at once

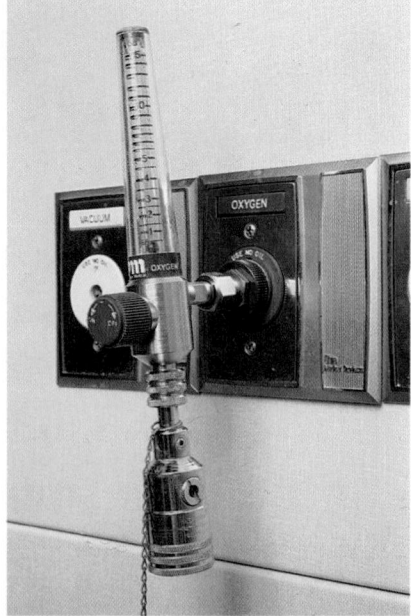

FIGURE 34-13 Wall oxygen outlet.

lungs. Secretions loosen. O_2 and CO_2 exchange occurs between the alveoli and the capillaries.

The device is used as follows:

1 The spirometer is placed upright.
2 The person exhales normally.
3 He or she seals the lips around a mouthpiece.
4 A slow, deep breath is taken until the balls rise to the desired height.
5 The breath is held for 3 to 6 seconds to keep the balls floating.
6 The person removes the mouthpiece and exhales slowly. The person may cough at this time.
7 After some normal breaths, the device is used again.
   See *Delegation Guidelines: Incentive Spirometry.*

ASSISTING WITH OXYGEN THERAPY

Disease, injury, and surgery often interfere with breathing. The amount of O_2 in the blood may be less than normal (hypoxemia). If so, the doctor orders oxygen therapy.

Oxygen is treated as a drug. The doctor orders the amount of oxygen to give, the device to use, and when to give it. Some people need oxygen constantly. Others need it for symptom relief—chest pain or shortness of breath. Oxygen helps relieve chest pain. Persons with respiratory diseases may have enough oxygen at rest. With mild exercise or activity, they become short of breath. Oxygen helps to relieve shortness of breath.

You do not give oxygen. The nurse and respiratory therapist start and maintain oxygen therapy. You assist the nurse in providing safe care.

Oxygen Sources

Oxygen is supplied as follows:
- *Wall outlet.* O_2 is piped into each person's unit (Fig. 34-13).
- *Oxygen tank.* The oxygen tank is placed at the bedside. Small tanks are used during emergencies and transfers. They also are used by persons who walk or use wheelchairs (Fig. 34-14). A gauge tells how much oxygen is left (Fig. 34-15). Tell the nurse if the tank is low.

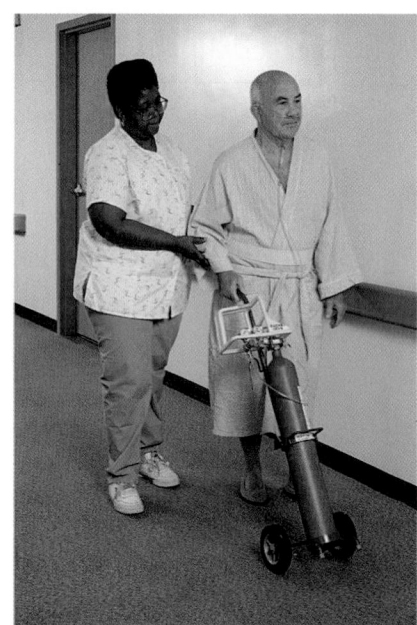

FIGURE 34-14 A portable oxygen tank is used when walking.

- *Oxygen concentrator.* The machine removes oxygen from the air (Fig. 34-16). A power source is needed. If the machine is not portable, the person stays near it. A portable oxygen tank is needed for power failures and mobility.
- *Liquid oxygen system.* A portable unit is filled from a stationary unit. The portable unit has enough oxygen for about 8 hours of use. A dial shows the amount of oxygen in the unit. Tell the nurse if the unit is low. The portable unit can be worn over the shoulder (Fig. 34-17). This allows the person to be mobile.

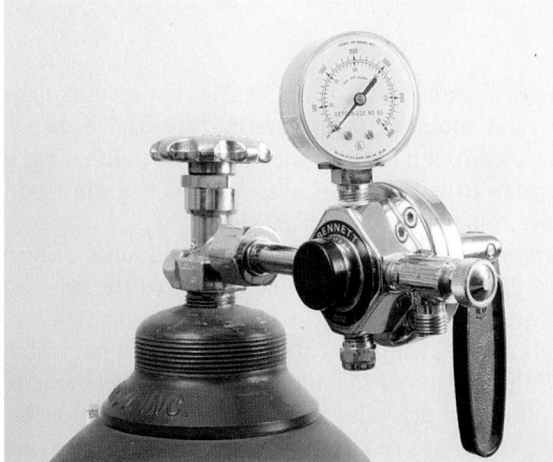

FIGURE 34-15 The gauge shows the amount of oxygen in the tank.

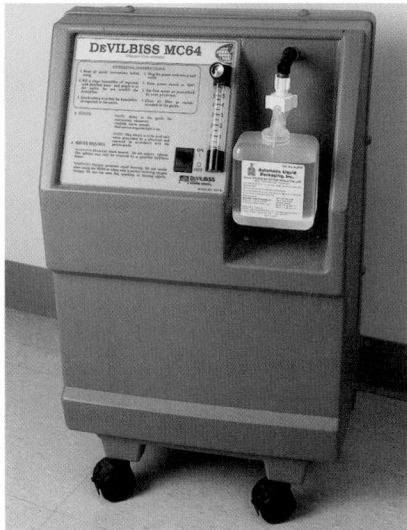

FIGURE 34-16 Oxygen concentrator.

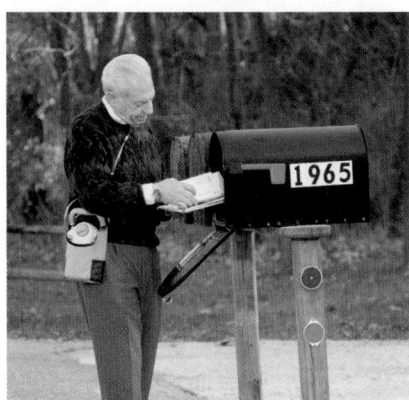

FIGURE 34-17 A portable liquid oxygen unit is worn over the shoulder. (Courtesy Covidien, formerly Tyco Healthcare, Mansfield, Mass.)

See *Focus on Long-Term Care and Home Care: Oxygen Sources*.

See *Promoting Safety and Comfort: Oxygen Sources*.

See *Teamwork and Time Management: Oxygen Sources*.

FOCUS ON **LONG-TERM CARE** AND **HOME CARE**

Oxygen Sources

HOME CARE

Oxygen tanks, oxygen concentrators, and liquid oxygen systems are used in home care. The type ordered depends on the person's needs. It is maintained by a medical supply company. Keep the company's name and phone number near the phone.

The patient and family must practice safety measures where oxygen is used and stored. This includes measures to prevent fires. See Box 34-4 and Chapter 11. Keep a fire extinguisher in the room.

BOX 34-4 **Safety Rules For Fire and Using Oxygen**

- Place "No Smoking" signs in the room and on the room door.
- Remove smoking materials from the room—cigarettes, cigars, pipes, matches, and lighters.
- Remove materials from the room that ignite easily—alcohol, nail polish remover, oils, greases.
- Keep oxygen sources and oxygen tubing away form heat sources and open flames. These include candles, stoves, heating ducts, radiators, heating pipes, space heaters, oil lamps, and kerosene heaters and lamps.
- Turn off electrical items before unplugging them.
- Use electrical items that are in good repair—shaver, radio, TV, music players, and others.
- Use only electrical items with three-prong plugs.
- Do not use materials that cause static electricity (wool and synthetic fabrics).
- Turn off the oxygen if a fire occurs. Get the person and family out of the home. Call the fire department.

PROMOTING SAFETY AND COMFORT: Oxygen Sources

SAFETY

Liquid oxygen is very cold. If touched, it can freeze the skin. Never tamper with the equipment. Doing so is unsafe and could damage the equipment. Follow agency procedures and the manufacturer's instructions when working with liquid oxygen.

TEAMWORK AND **TIME MANAGEMENT**

Oxygen Sources

Oxygen tanks and liquid oxygen systems only contain a certain amount of oxygen. When the oxygen level is low, another tank is needed or the liquid oxygen system is refilled. Always check the oxygen level when you are with or near persons using these oxygen sources. Report a low oxygen level to the nurse at once.

Oxygen Devices

The doctor orders the device to give oxygen. These devices are common:

▶ *Nasal cannula* (Fig. 34-18). The prongs are inserted into the nostrils. A band goes behind the ears and under the chin to keep the device in place. A cannula allows eating and drinking. Tight prongs can irritate the nose. Pressure on the ears and cheekbones is possible.

▶ *Simple face mask* (Fig. 34-19). It covers the nose and mouth. The mask has small holes in the sides. CO_2 escapes when exhaling.

▶ *Partial-rebreather mask* (Fig. 34-20). A bag is added to the simple face mask. The bag is for exhaled air. When breathing in, the person inhales oxygen and some exhaled air. Some room air also is inhaled. The bag should not totally deflate when inhaling.

▶ *Non-rebreather mask* (Fig. 34-21). It prevents exhaled air and room air from entering the bag. Exhaled air leaves through holes in the mask. When inhaling, only oxygen from the bag is inhaled. The bag must not totally collapse during inhalation.

▶ *Venturi mask* (Fig. 34-22). Precise amounts of oxygen are given. Color-coded adapters show the amount of oxygen given.

Talking and eating are hard to do with a mask. Listen carefully. Moisture can build up under the mask. Keep the face clean and dry. This helps prevent irritation from the mask. Masks are removed for eating. Usually oxygen is given by cannula during meals.

See *Focus on Children and Older Persons: Oxygen Devices.*

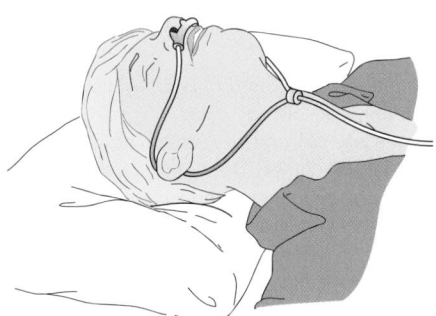
FIGURE 34-18 Nasal cannula.

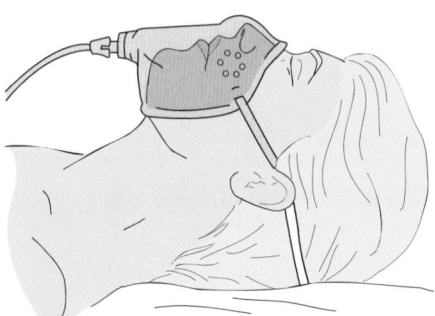
FIGURE 34-19 Simple face mask.

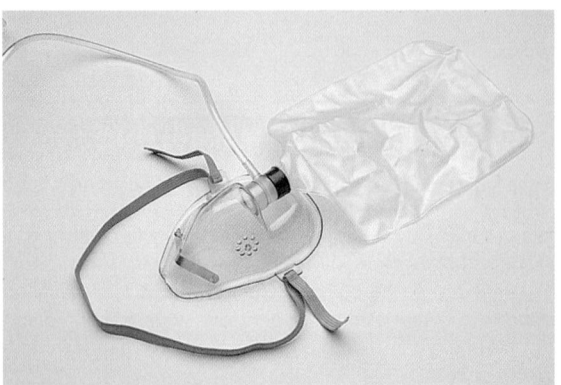
FIGURE 34-20 Partial-rebreather mask.

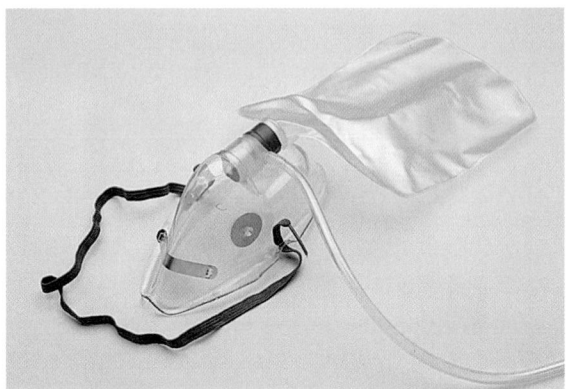
FIGURE 34-21 Non-rebreather mask.

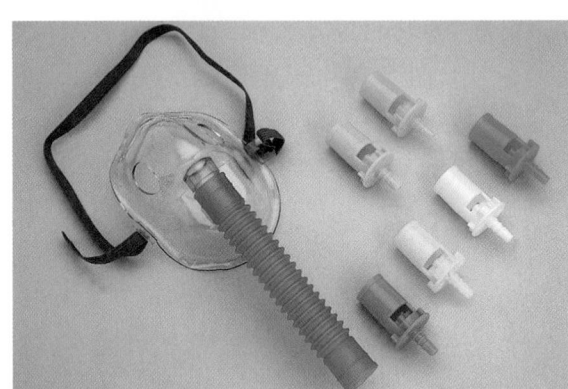
FIGURE 34-22 Venturi mask.

FOCUS ON CHILDREN AND OLDER PERSONS

Oxygen Devices

CHILDREN

Oxygen devices for children include cannulas, face masks, partial and non-rebreather masks, and Venturi masks. Oxygen hoods and mist tents also are used (Fig. 34-23).

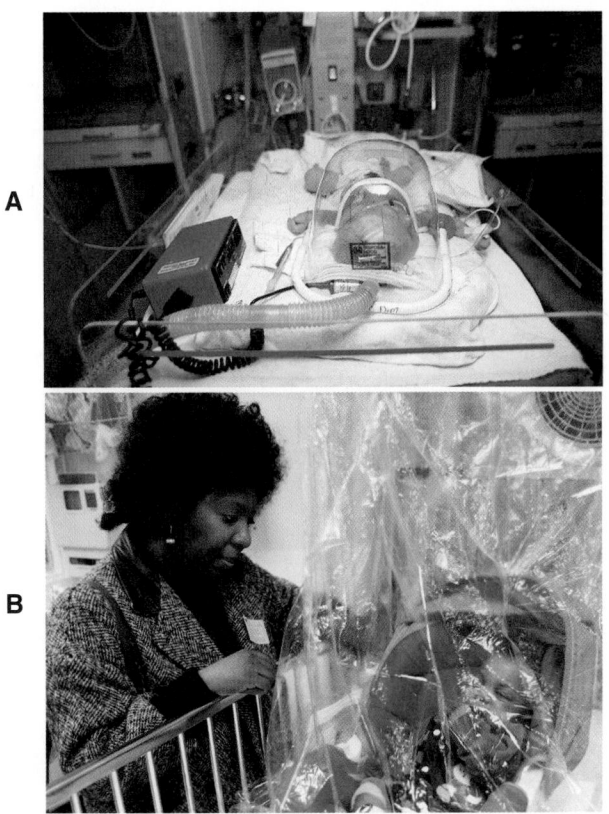

FIGURE 34-23 A, Oxygen hood. **B,** Mist tent. (From Hockenberry MJ and Wilson D: *Wong's nursing care of infants and children,* ed 8, St Louis, 2007, Mosby.)

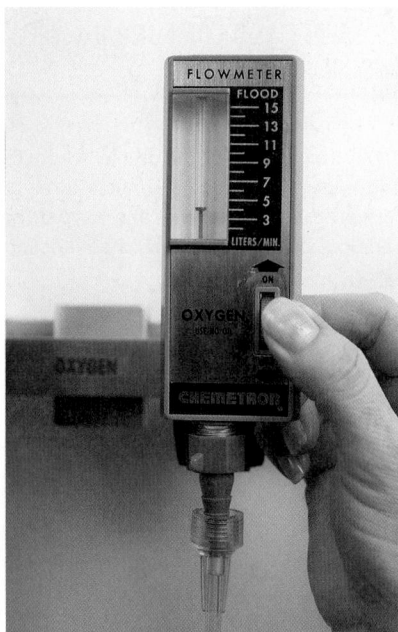

FIGURE 34-24 The flowmeter is used to set the oxygen flow rate.

Oxygen Flow Rates

The *flow rate* is the amount of oxygen given. It is measured in liters per minute (L/min). The doctor orders 2 to 15 liters of O_2 per minute. The nurse or respiratory therapist sets the flow rate (Fig. 34-24).

The nurse and care plan tell you the person's flow rate. When giving care and checking the person, always check the flow rate. Tell the nurse at once if it is too high or too low. A nurse or respiratory therapist will adjust the flow rate. Some states and agencies let nursing assistants adjust O_2 flow rates. Know your agency's policy.

◆ Oxygen Administration Set-Up

Oxygen is a dry gas. If not humidified (made moist), oxygen dries the airway's mucous membranes. Distilled water is added to the humidifier (Fig. 34-25). (Distilled water is pure. Dissolved salts were removed by a chemical process.)

When added to the humidifier, the distilled water creates water vapor. Oxygen picks up the water vapor as it flows into the system. Bubbling in the humidifier means that water vapor is being produced. Low flow rates (1 to 2 L/min) by cannula are not usually humidified.

See *Delegation Guidelines: Oxygen Administration Set-Up.*

See *Promoting Safety and Comfort: Oxygen Administration Set-Up,* p. 596.

See *Teamwork and Time Management: Oxygen Administration Set-Up,* p. 596.

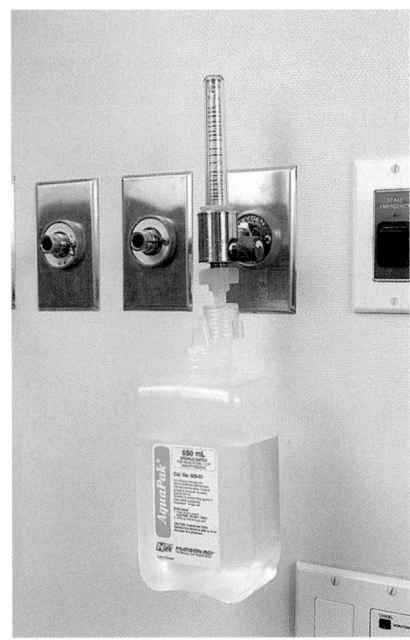

FIGURE 34-25 Oxygen administration system with humidifier.

DELEGATION GUIDELINES: Oxygen Administration Set-Up

If setting up oxygen is delegated to you, you need this information from the nurse:
- The person's name and room and bed number
- What oxygen device was ordered
- If humidification was ordered

PROMOTING SAFETY AND COMFORT: Oxygen
Administration Set-Up

SAFETY

You do not give oxygen. Tell the nurse when the oxygen administration system is set up. The nurse turns on the oxygen, sets the flow rate, and applies the oxygen device.

Practice medical asepsis. Make sure connecting tubing is not on the floor.

Oxygen Administration Set-Up

As you walk past the room of any person receiving oxygen, always check the humidifier. Make sure the humidifier is bubbling. Also make sure it has a enough water. Tell the nurse if there is no bubbling or if the water level is low.

SETTING UP FOR OXYGEN ADMINISTRATION

✔ Quality of Life *Remember to:*

- Knock before entering the person's room.
- Address the person by name.
- Introduce yourself by name and title.
- Explain the procedure to the person before beginning and during the procedure.
- Protect the person's rights during the procedure.
- Handle the person gently during the procedure.

PRE-PROCEDURE

1 Follow *Delegation Guidelines: Oxygen Administration Set-Up*, p. 595. See *Promoting Safety and Comfort: Oxygen Administration Set-Up.*
2 Practice hand hygiene.
3 Collect the following before going to the person's room:
   - Oxygen device with connecting tubing
   - Flowmeter
   - Humidifier (if ordered)
   - Distilled water (if using a humidifier)

4 Arrange your work area.
5 Decontaminate your hands.
6 Identify the person. Check the ID bracelet against the assignment sheet. Also call the person by name.

PROCEDURE

7 Make sure the flowmeter is in the *OFF* position.
8 Attach the flowmeter to the wall outlet or to the tank.
9 Fill the humidifier with distilled water.
10 Attach the humidifier to the bottom of the flowmeter.
11 Attach the oxygen device and connecting tubing to the humidifier. *Do not set the flowmeter. Do not apply the oxygen device on the person.*

12 Place the cap securely on the distilled water. Store the water according to agency policy.
13 Discard the packaging from the oxygen device and connecting tubing.

POST-PROCEDURE

14 Provide for comfort. (See the inside of the front book cover.)
15 Place the signal light within reach.
16 Decontaminate your hands.
17 Complete a safety check of the room. (See the inside of the front book cover.)

18 Tell the nurse when you are done. *The nurse will:*
   a *Turn on the oxygen and set the flow rate.*
   b *Apply the oxygen device on the person.*

Oxygen Safety

You assist the nurse with oxygen therapy. You do not give oxygen. You do not adjust the flow rate unless allowed by your state and agency. However, you must give safe care. Follow the rules in Box 34-5. Also follow the rules for fire and the use of oxygen (Chapter 11).

BOX 34-5 Safety Rules For Oxygen Therapy

- Never remove the oxygen device.
- Make sure the oxygen device is secure but not tight.
- Check for signs of irritation from the device. Check behind the ears, under the nose (cannula), and around the face (mask). Also check the cheekbones.
- Keep the face clean and dry when a mask is used.
- Never shut off the oxygen flow.
- Do not adjust the flow rate unless allowed by your state and agency.
- Tell the nurse at once if the flow rate is too high or too low.
- Tell the nurse at once if the humidifier is not bubbling.
- Secure tubing in place. Tape or pin it to the person's garment following agency policy.
- Make sure there are no kinks in the tubing.
- Make sure the person does not lie on any part of the tubing.
- Report signs and symptoms of hypoxia, respiratory distress, or abnormal breathing patterns to the nurse at once (see Boxes 34-2 and 34-3).
- Give oral hygiene as directed. Follow the care plan.
- Make sure the oxygen device is clean and free of mucus.
- Maintain an adequate water level in the humidifier.

REVIEW QUESTIONS

Circle the BEST answer.

1 Alcohol and narcotics affect oxygen needs because they
   a Depress the brain
   b Are pollutants
   c Cause allergies
   d Cause infection

2 Hypoxia is
   a Not enough oxygen in the blood
   b The amount of hemoglobin that affects oxygen
   c Not enough oxygen in the cells
   d The lack of carbon dioxide

3 An early sign of hypoxia is
   a Cyanosis
   b Increased pulse and respiratory rates
   c Restlessness
   d Dyspnea

4 A person can breathe deeply and comfortably only while sitting. This is called
   a Biot's respirations
   b Orthopnea
   c Bradypnea
   d Kussmaul respirations

5 The nurse tells you that a person has tachypnea. You know that the person's respirations are
   a Slow
   b Rapid
   c Absent
   d Difficult or painful

6 The person needs to rest after
   a A chest x-ray
   b A lung scan
   c Arterial blood gases
   d Pulmonary function tests

7 A person's SpO$_2$ is 98%. Which is *true?*
   a The pulse oximeter is wrong.
   b The pulse is 98 beats per minute.
   c The measurement is within normal range.
   d The person has respiratory depression.

8 Which is *not* a site for a pulse oximetry sensor?
   a Toe
   b Finger
   c Earlobe
   d Upper arm

9 You are assisting with deep breathing and coughing. Which is *false?*
   a The person inhales through pursed lips.
   b The person sits in a comfortable sitting position.
   c The person inhales deeply through the nose.
   d The person holds a pillow over an incision.

10 Deep-breathing and coughing exercises are ordered. The person has a productive cough. You need to remind the person to
   a Cover the nose and mouth when coughing
   b Use a face mask
   c Provide a sputum specimen
   d Inhale through the mouth

11 Which is useful for deep breathing?
   a Pulse oximeter
   b Incentive spirometry
   c Simple face mask
   d Partial-rebreather mask

12 When assisting with oxygen therapy, you can
   a Turn the oxygen on and off
   b Start the oxygen
   c Decide what device to use
   d Keep connecting tubing secure and free of kinks

Answers to these questions are on p. 781.

Respiratory Support and Therapies

OBJECTIVES

- Define the key terms and key abbreviations listed in this chapter
- Explain how to assist in the care of persons with artificial airways
- Describe the principles and safety measures for suctioning
- Explain how to assist in the care of persons on mechanical ventilation
- Explain how to assist in the care of persons with chest tubes

KEY TERMS

hemothorax Blood *(hemo)* in the pleural space *(thorax)*

intubation Inserting an artificial airway

mechanical ventilation Using a machine to move air into and out of the lungs

pleural effusion The escape and collection of fluid *(effusion)* in the pleural space

pneumothorax Air *(pneumo)* in the pleural space *(thorax)*

suction The process of withdrawing or sucking up fluid *(secretions)*

tracheostomy A surgically created opening *(stomy)* into the trachea *(tracheo)*

KEY ABBREVIATIONS

CO₂ Carbon dioxide

ET Endotracheal

O₂ Oxygen

SpO₂ Oxygen saturation

Some persons need artificial airways, suctioning, mechanical ventilation, and chest tubes. They need to recover from problems affecting the airway and lungs. The nurse may ask you to assist in their care.

ARTIFICIAL AIRWAYS

Artificial airways keep the airway patent (open). They are needed:

- When disease, injury, secretions, or aspiration obstructs the airway
- For mechanical ventilation (p. 601)
- By some persons who are semi-conscious or unconscious
- When the person is recovering from anesthesia

Intubation means inserting an artificial airway. Such airways are usually plastic and disposable. They come in adult, pediatric, and infant sizes. These airways are common:

- *Oropharyngeal airway*—inserted through the mouth and into the pharynx (Fig. 35-1, *A*, p. 600). A nurse or respiratory therapist inserts the airway.
- *Endotracheal (ET) tube*—inserted through the mouth or nose and into the trachea (Fig. 35-1, *B*, p. 600). A doctor inserts it using a lighted scope. Some RNs and respiratory therapists are trained to insert ET tubes. A cuff is inflated to keep the airway in place.
- *Tracheostomy tube*—inserted through a surgically created opening (stomy) into the trachea (tracheo) (Fig. 35-1, *C*, p. 600). Cuffed tubes are common. The cuff is inflated to keep the tube in place. Doctors perform tracheostomies.

Vital signs are checked often. Observe for hypoxia and other signs and symptoms. If an airway comes out or is dislodged, tell the nurse at once. Frequent oral hygiene is needed. Follow the care plan.

Gagging and choking feelings are common. Imagine something in your mouth, nose, or throat. Comfort and reassure the person. Remind the person that the airway helps breathing. Use touch to show you care.

Persons with ET tubes cannot speak. Some tracheostomy tubes allow speech. Paper and pencils, Magic Slates, and communication boards are ways to communicate. Hand signals, nodding the head, and hand squeezes are common for simple "yes" and "no" questions. Follow the care plan. *Always keep the signal light within reach.*

Tracheostomies

A **tracheostomy** is a surgically created opening *(stomy)* into the trachea *(tracheo)*. Tracheostomies are temporary or permanent for mechanical ventilation (p. 601). They are permanent when airway structures are surgically removed. Cancer, severe airway trauma, or brain damage may require a permanent tracheostomy.

A tracheostomy tube is made of plastic, silicone, or metal. It has three parts (Fig. 35-2, p. 600):

- The *obturator* has a round end. It is used to guide the insertion of the outer cannula (tube). Then it is removed. (The obturator is placed within easy reach in case the tracheostomy tube falls out and needs to be reinserted. It is taped to the wall or bedside stand.)
- The *inner cannula* is inserted and locked in place. It fits inside the outer cannula. It is removed for cleaning and mucus removal. This keeps the airway patent. (Some inner cannulas are disposable. Other tracheostomy tubes do not have inner cannulas.)
- The *outer cannula* is secured in place with ties around the neck or a Velcro collar. The outer cannula is not removed. It keeps the tracheostomy open.

The cuffed tracheostomy tube is used for mechanical ventilation. It provides a seal between the cannula and the trachea (see Fig. 35-1, *C*, p. 600). This prevents air from leaking around the tube. It also prevents aspiration. A nurse or respiratory therapist inflates and deflates the cuff.

The tube must not come out *(extubation)*. If not secure, it could come out with coughing or if pulled on. A loose tube moves up and down. It can damage the trachea.

The tube must remain patent (open). If able, the person coughs up secretions. Otherwise suctioning is needed. *Call for the nurse if you note signs and symptoms of hypoxia or respiratory distress. Also call the nurse if the outer cannula comes out.*

Nothing must enter the stoma. Otherwise the person can aspirate. These safety measures are needed:

- Dressings do not have loose gauze or lint.
- The stoma or tube is covered when outdoors. The person wears a stoma cover, scarf, or shirt or blouse that buttons at the neck. The cover prevents dust, insects, and other small particles from entering the stoma.
- The stoma is not covered with plastic, leather, or similar materials. They prevent air from entering the stoma. The person cannot breathe.
- Tub baths are taken. If showers are taken, a shower guard is worn. A hand-held nozzle is used to direct water away from the stoma.
- The person is assisted with shampooing. Water must not enter the stoma.
- The stoma is covered when shaving.
- Swimming is not allowed. Water will enter the tube or stoma.
- Medical-alert jewelry is worn. The person carries a medical alert ID card.

Follow Standard Precautions and the Bloodborne Pathogen Standard when assisting with tracheostomy care. The care is done daily or every 8 to 12 hours. It also

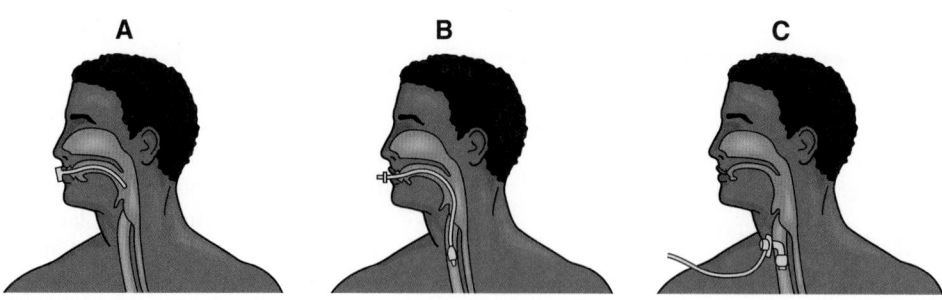

FIGURE 35-1 Artificial airways. **A,** Oropharyngeal airway. **B,** Endotracheal tube. **C,** Tracheostomy tube.

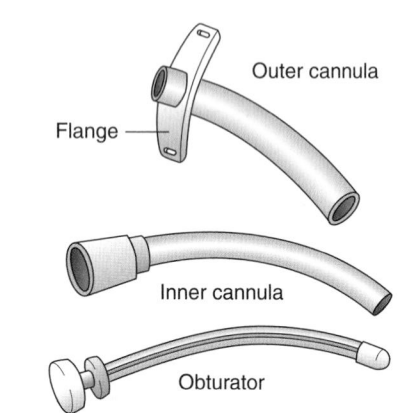

Outer cannula

Flange

Inner cannula

Obturator

FIGURE 35-2 Parts of a tracheostomy tube.

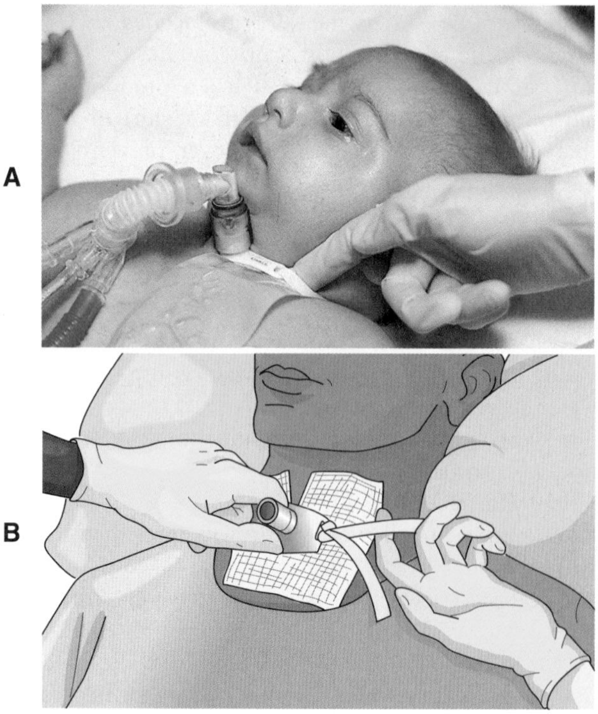

FOCUS ON CHILDREN AND OLDER PERSONS

Tracheostomies

CHILDREN

Some children have congenital defects. (*Congenitus* is a Latin word that means "to be born with.") Congenital defects are present at birth. Tracheostomies are needed for some congenital defects affecting the neck and airway.

Some infections cause swelling of the airway structures. This obstructs air flow. So does foreign body aspiration. These situations can require emergency tracheostomies.

Tracheostomy ties must be secure but not tight. Only a fingertip should slide under the ties (see Figure 35-3, *A*). Ties are too loose if you can slide your whole finger under them.

Assist the nurse by holding the child still. Position the child's head as the nurse directs.

PROMOTING SAFETY AND COMFORT: Tracheostomies

SAFETY

Mucus may contain microbes or blood. Follow Standard Precautions and the Bloodborne Pathogen Standard.

---

is done as needed for excess secretions, soiled ties or collar, or soiled or moist dressings. The care involves:

▶ Cleaning the inner cannula to remove mucus and keep the airway patent. (Some inner cannulas are disposable. They are discarded after one use. A new one is inserted.) Re-usable inner cannulas are cleaned with a small bottle brush or a pipe cleaner. The nurse tells you what cleaning agent to use—usually hydrogen peroxide or a mild soap.

▶ Cleaning the stoma to prevent infection and skin breakdown.

▶ Applying clean ties or a Velcro collar to prevent infection. Clean ties are applied before the dirty ones are removed. Hold the outer cannula in place when the nurse changes the ties or collar. Continue to do so until the nurse secures the new ties or collar. The ties or collar must be secure but not tight. For an adult, a finger should slide under the ties or collar (Fig. 35-3). See *Focus on Children and Older Persons: Tracheostomies.* See *Promoting Safety and Comfort: Tracheostomies.*

A

B

FIGURE 35-3 A, For children, only a fingertip is inserted under the ties. **B,** For an adult, a finger is inserted under the ties. (**A** from Hockenberry MJ and Wilson D: *Wong's nursing care of infants and children,* ed 8, St Louis, 2007, Mosby.)

SUCTIONING THE AIRWAY

Secretions can collect in the upper airway. Retained secretions:

▶ Obstruct air flow into and out of the airway
▶ Provide an environment for microbes
▶ Interfere with oxygen (O_2) and carbon dioxide (CO_2) exchange

Hypoxia can occur. Usually coughing removes secretions. Some persons cannot cough, or the cough is too weak to remove secretions. They need suctioning.

Suction is the process of withdrawing or sucking up fluid *(secretions)*. A suction source is needed—wall outlet or suction machine. A tube connects to a suction source at one end and to a suction catheter at the other end. The catheter is inserted into the airway. Secretions are withdrawn through the catheter.

The nose, mouth, and pharynx make up the upper airway. The trachea and bronchi are the lower parts of the airway. These routes are used to suction the airway:

▶ *Oropharyngeal*. The mouth *(oro)* and pharynx *(pharyngeal)* are suctioned. A suction catheter is passed through the mouth and into the pharynx. The Yankauer suction catheter is often used for thick secretions (Fig. 35-4).

▶ *Nasopharyngeal*. The nose *(naso)* and pharynx *(pharyngeal)* are suctioned. The suction catheter is passed through the nose into the pharynx.

▶ *Lower airway*. The suction catheter is passed through an ET or tracheostomy tube.

The person's lungs are hyperventilated before suctioning an ET or a tracheostomy tube. *Hyperventilate* means to be given extra *(hyper)* breaths *(ventilate)*. An Ambu bag is used (Fig. 35-5). The Ambu bag is attached to an oxygen source. Then the oxygen delivery device is removed from the ET or tracheostomy tube. The Ambu bag is attached to the ET or tracheostomy tube. To give a breath, the bag is squeezed with both hands. The nurse or respiratory therapist gives 3 to 5 breaths.

Oxygen is treated like a drug. You do not give drugs. Therefore you need to check if your state and agency allow you to use an Ambu bag attached to an oxygen source.

See *Focus on Children and Older Persons: Suctioning.*
See *Promoting Safety and Comfort: Suctioning.*

MECHANICAL VENTILATION

Weak muscle effort, airway obstruction, and damaged lung tissue cause hypoxia. Nervous system diseases and injuries can affect the respiratory center in the brain. Nerve damage interferes with messages between the lungs and the brain. Drug overdose depresses the brain. With severe problems, the person cannot breathe. Or normal

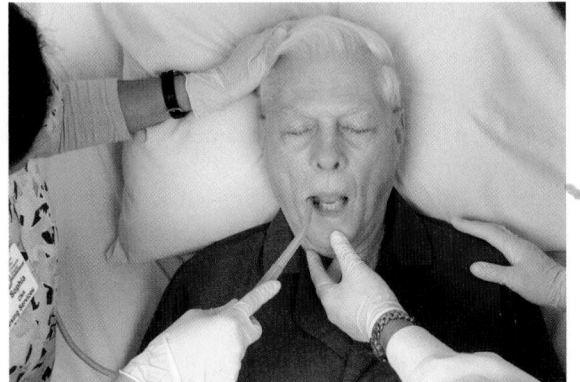

FIGURE 35-4 The Yankauer suction catheter is often used when there are large amounts of thick secretions.

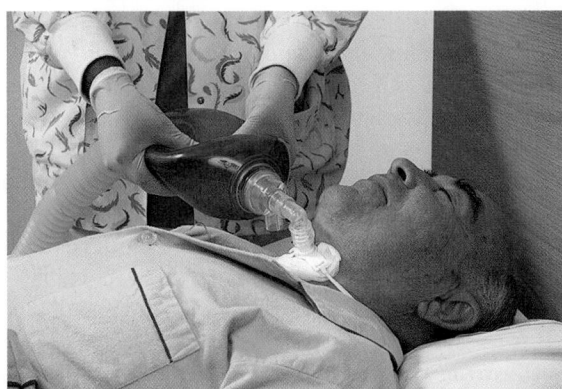

FIGURE 35-5 The Ambu bag is squeezed with two hands.

FOCUS ON **CHILDREN** AND **OLDER PERSONS**

Suctioning

CHILDREN
Suctioning may frighten children. They need clear, simple explanations about the procedure. As with other care, you many need to hold the child still. To do so, control the child's head and arm movements.

PROMOTING SAFETY AND COMFORT: Suctioning

SAFETY
If not done correctly, suctioning can cause serious harm. Suctioning removes oxygen from the airway. The person does not get oxygen during suctioning. Hypoxia and life-threatening problems can occur. They arise from the respiratory, cardiovascular, and nervous systems. Cardiac arrest can occur. Infection and airway injury are possible.

The nurse may ask you to assist with suctioning. However, you do not perform the suctioning procedure. Box 35-1, p. 602 lists the principles and safety measures for assisting with suctioning.

Always keep needed suction equipment and supplies at the bedside. When suctioning is needed, you do not have time to collect supplies from the supply area.

Mucus may contain microbes or blood. Follow Standard Precautions and the Bloodborne Pathogen Standard.

BOX 35-1 Principles and Safety Measures for Suctioning

- Review the procedure with the nurse. Know what the nurse expects you to do.
- Report coughing and the signs and symptoms of respiratory distress (Chapter 34) to the nurse. They signal the need for suctioning. Suctioning is done as needed, not on a schedule.
- Standard Precautions and Bloodborne Pathogen Standard are followed. Secretions can contain blood and are potentially infectious.
- Sterile technique is used (Chapter 14). This helps prevent microbes from entering the airway.
- The nurse tells you the catheter type and size needed. If too large, it can injure the airway.
- Needed suction supplies and equipment are kept at the bedside. They are ready when the person needs suctioning.
- Suction is not applied while inserting the catheter. When suction is applied, air is sucked out of the airway.
- The catheter is inserted smoothly. This helps prevent injury to mucous membranes.
- A suction cycle for an adult takes no more than 10 to 15 seconds. (Hold your breath during the suction cycle. This helps you experience what the person feels during suctioning.) For infants and children, the suction cycle is limited to 5 seconds. A suction cycle involves:
  - Inserting the catheter
  - Suctioning
  - Removing the catheter

- The catheter is cleared with sterile water or saline between suction cycles.
- The nurse waits 20 to 30 seconds between each suction cycle. Some agencies require waiting 60 seconds.
- The suction catheter is passed (inserted) no more than 3 times. Injury and hypoxia are risks each time the suction catheter is passed.
- Check the person's pulse, respirations, and pulse oximeter measurements before, during, and after the procedure. Also observe the person's level of consciousness. Tell the nurse at once if any of these occur:
  - A drop in pulse rate or a pulse rate less than 60 beats per minute.
  - Irregular cardiac rhythms.
  - A drop or rise in blood pressure.
  - Respiratory distress.
  - A drop in oxygen saturation (SpO_2). Normal range is 95% to 100% (Chapter 34).

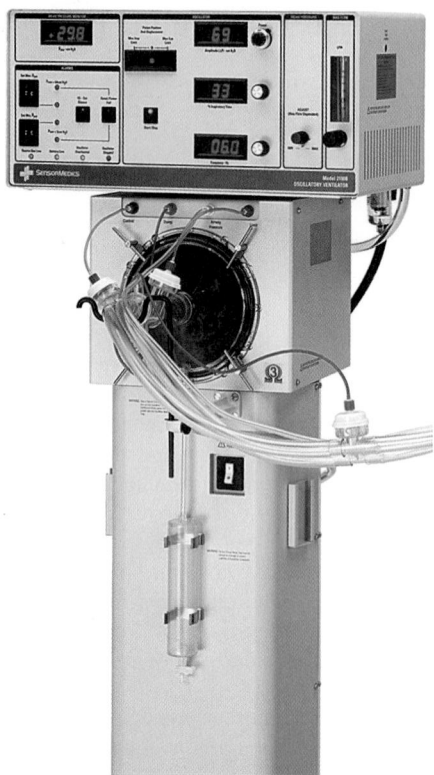

FIGURE 35-6 A mechanical ventilator. (Courtesy VIASYS Respiratory Care, Yorba Linda, Calif.)

blood oxygen levels are not maintained. Often mechanical ventilation is needed.

Mechanical ventilation is using a machine to move air into and out of the lungs (Fig. 35-6). Oxygen enters the lungs. Carbon dioxide leaves them. An ET or tracheostomy tube is needed for mechanical ventilation.

Alarms sound when something is wrong. One alarm means the person is disconnected from the ventilator. The nurse shows you how to reconnect the ET or tracheostomy tube. *When any alarm sounds, first check to see if the person's tube is attached to the ventilator. If not, attach it to the ventilator. The person can die if not attached to the ventilator.* Then tell the nurse at once about the alarm. Do not reset alarms.

Persons needing mechanical ventilation are very ill. Other problems and injuries are common. Some persons are confused, disoriented, or cannot think clearly. The machine and fear of dying frighten many. Some are relieved to get enough oxygen. Many fear needing the machine for life. Mechanical ventilation can be painful for those with chest injuries or chest surgery. Tubes and hoses restrict movement. This causes more discomfort.

The nurse may ask you to assist with the person's care. See Box 35-2.

See *Focus on Long-Term Care and Home Care: Mechanical Ventilation.*

See *Focus on Ethics and Laws: Mechanical Ventilation.*

BOX 35-2 **Care of Persons on Mechanical Ventilation**

- Keep the signal light within reach.
- Make sure hoses and connecting tubing have slack. They must not pull on the artificial airway.
- Answer signal lights promptly. The person depends on others for basic needs.
- Explain who you are and what you are going to do. Do this whenever you enter the room.
- Give the day, date, and time every time you give care.
- Report signs of respiratory distress or discomfort at once.
- Do not change settings on the machine or reset alarms.
- Follow the care plan for communication. The person cannot talk. Use agreed-upon hand or eye signals for "yes" and "no." Everyone must use the same signals. Otherwise, communication does not occur. Some persons can use paper and pencils, Magic Slates, communication boards, and hand signals.

- Ask questions that have simple answers. It may be hard to write long responses.
- Watch what you say and do. This includes when you are near and away from the person and family. They pay close attention to your verbal and non-verbal communication. Do not say or do anything that could upset the person.
- Use touch to comfort and reassure the person. Also tell the person about the weather, pleasant news events, and gifts and cards.
- Meet basic needs. Follow the care plan.
- Tell the person when you are leaving the room and when you will return.
- Complete a safety check before leaving the room. (See the inside of the front book cover.)

FOCUS ON LONG-TERM CARE AND HOME CARE

Mechanical Ventilation

LONG-TERM CARE

Mechanical ventilation is started in the hospital. Some people need it for a few hours or days. Others need it longer. They may require long-term care or subacute care. Often the person needs weaning from the ventilator. That is, the person needs to breathe without the machine. The respiratory therapist and RN plan the weaning process. Weaning can take many weeks.

HOME CARE

Home care is an option for some ventilator-dependent persons. The nurse teaches you how to care for the person. Family members learn how to assist with the person's care. Make sure you can reach the nurse by phone when in the person's home. Make sure delegated tasks are allowed by your state and agency.

FOCUS ON ETHICS AND LAWS

Mechanical Ventilation

A 54-year-old patient was in a hospital intensive care unit. He was on a ventilator with an endotracheal (ET) tube. A blocked ET tube led to a cardiac arrest. He was resuscitated, but was left with permanent brain damage. He will need 24-hour care for the rest of his life.

In a lawsuit, he and his wife claimed that nurses and a respiratory therapist:
- Did not properly assess him
- Did not determine that the ET tube was blocked
- Did not immediately call a doctor or an emergency code
    The jury found in favor of the patient. The final judgment was for over $5,000,000.

(*Sidney v Columbia St. David's*, October 2003.) With permission from *Medical Malpractice Verdicts, Settlements & Experts*, vol 19, no 9, September 2003, p. 18.

CHEST TUBES

Air, blood, or fluid can collect in the pleural space (sac or cavity). This occurs when the chest is entered because of injury or surgery.

- ▶ **Pneumothorax** is air (*pneumo*) in the pleural space (*thorax*).
- ▶ **Hemothorax** is blood (*hemo*) in the pleural space (*thorax*).
- ▶ **Pleural effusion** is the escape and collection of fluid (*effusion*) in the pleural space.

Pressure occurs when air, blood, or fluid collects in the pleural space. The pressure collapses the lung. Air cannot reach affected alveoli. O_2 and CO_2 are not exchanged. Respiratory distress and hypoxia result. Pressure on the heart threatens life. It affects the heart's ability to pump blood.

Hospital care is required. The doctor inserts chest tubes to remove the air, blood, or fluid (Fig. 35-7). The sterile procedure is done in surgery, in the emergency room, or at the bedside. A nurse assists.

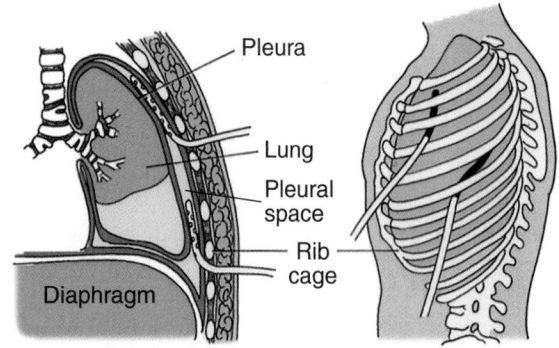

FIGURE 35-7 Chest tubes inserted into the pleural space. (Modified from Elkin MK, Perry AG, Potter PA: *Nursing interventions and clinical skills*, ed 4, St Louis, 2007, Mosby.)

Chest tubes attach to a drainage system (Fig. 35-8). The system must be airtight. Air must not enter the pleural space. Water-seal drainage keeps the system airtight. The bottles in Figure 35-9 show how the system works:

▶ A chest tube attaches to connecting tubing.
▶ Connecting tubing attaches to a tube in the drainage container.

▶ The tube in the drainage container extends under water. The water prevents air from entering the chest tube and then the pleural space.

See Box 35-3 for care of the person with chest tubes.

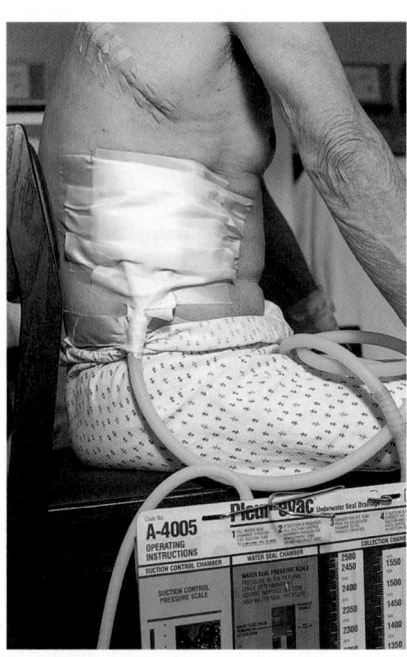

FIGURE 35-8 Chest tubes attached to a disposable water-seal drainage system. Chest tubes are inserted into the pleural space. (From Elkin MK, Perry AG, Potter PA: *Nursing interventions and clinical skills*, ed 4, St Louis, 2007, Mosby.)

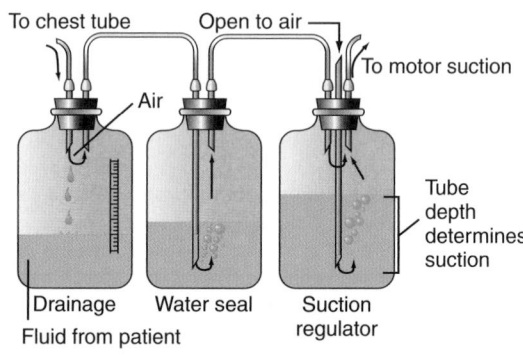

FIGURE 35-9 Water-seal drainage system. (From Lewis SM and others: *Medical-surgical nursing: assessment and management of clinical problems*, ed 6, St Louis, 2004, Mosby.)

BOX 35-3 Care of the Person With Chest Tubes

- Keep the drainage system below the chest.
- Measure vital signs as directed. Report vital sign changes at once.
- Report signs and symptoms of hypoxia and respiratory distress at once. Also report complaints of pain or difficulty breathing.
- Keep connecting tubing coiled on the bed. Allow enough slack so the chest tubes are not dislodged when the person moves. If tubing hangs in loops, drainage collects in the loops.
- Prevent tubing kinks. Kinks obstruct the chest tube. Air, blood, or fluid collects in the pleural space.
- Observe chest drainage. Report any change in chest drainage at once. This includes increases in drainage or the appearance of bright red drainage.
- Record chest drainage according to agency policy.

- Turn and position the person as directed. Be careful and gentle to prevent the chest tubes from dislodging.
- Assist with deep-breathing and coughing exercises as directed.
- Assist with incentive spirometry as directed.
- Note bubbling in the drainage system. Tell the nurse at once if bubbling increases, decreases, or stops.
- Tell the nurse at once if any part of the system is loose or disconnected.
- Keep sterile petrolatum gauze at the bedside. It is needed if a chest tube comes out.
- Call for help at once if a chest tube comes out. Cover the insertion site with sterile petrolatum gauze. Stay with the person. Follow the nurse's directions.
- Complete a safety check before leaving the room. (See the inside of the front book cover.)

Circle the BEST answer.

1. A person has a tracheostomy. Which is *false?*
   a The obturator is taped to the wall or bedside stand.
   b The nurse removes the inner cannula for cleaning.
   c The outer cannula must be secured in place.
   d The person must not cough.

2. A person with a tracheostomy can do the following *except*
   a Shampoo
   b Shave
   c Shower with a hand-held nozzle
   d Swim

3. A person has a tracheostomy. The nurse is changing the ties. You must
   a Remove the inner cannula
   b Clean the stoma
   c Remove the dressing
   d Hold the outer cannula in place

4. A person has a tracheostomy. You cannot slide a finger under the ties. This means that the ties
   a Are secure
   b Are too tight
   c Need to be replaced
   d Need to be removed

5. Which signals the need for suctioning?
   a A pulse rate of 90 beats per minute
   b Signs and symptoms of respiratory distress
   c The orthopneic position
   d Being unable to speak

6. Suctioning requires
   a Mechanical ventilation
   b Sterile technique
   c An artificial airway
   d Chest tubes

7. You are assisting the nurse with suctioning. You must
   a Insert the catheter no more than 3 times
   b Suction for no more than 10 to 15 minutes
   c Clear the suction catheter with water
   d Keep needed suction supplies at the bedside

8. You note the following while assisting with suctioning. Which should you report at once?
   a A pulse rate of 82 beats per minute
   b A regular heart rhythm
   c An SpO_2 of 92%
   d Thick secretions

9. A person requires mechanical ventilation. Which is *false?*
   a The person has an ET or tracheostomy tube.
   b The signal light must always be within reach.
   c Touch provides comfort and reassurance.
   d You can reset alarms on the ventilator.

10. An alarm sounds on a person's ventilator. What should you do *first?*
    a Reset the alarm.
    b Check to see if the airway is attached to the machine.
    c Call the nurse at once.
    d Ask the person what is wrong.

11. A person has a pneumothorax. This is
    a Fluid in the pleural space
    b Blood in the pleural space
    c Air in the pleural space
    d Secretions in the pleural space

12. Chest tubes are attached to water-seal drainage. You should do the following *except*
    a Tell the nurse if bubbling increases, decreases, or stops
    b Make sure tubing is not kinked
    c Keep the drainage system below the chest
    d Hang tubing in loops

Answers to these questions are on p. 781.

36 Rehabilitation and Restorative Nursing Care

OBJECTIVES

- Define the key terms and key abbreviations listed in this chapter
- Describe how rehabilitation and restorative care involve the whole person
- Identify the complications to prevent
- Identify the common reactions to rehabilitation
- Describe how rehabilitation can help the person with employment
- List the common rehabilitation programs and services
- Explain your role in rehabilitation and restorative care
- Explain how to promote quality of life

KEY TERMS

activities of daily living (ADL) The activities usually done during a normal day in a person's life

disability Any lost, absent, or impaired physical or mental function

prosthesis An artificial replacement for a missing body part

rehabilitation The process of restoring the person to his or her highest possible level of physical, psychological, social, and economic function

restorative aide A nursing assistant with special training in restorative nursing and rehabilitation skills

restorative nursing care Care that helps persons regain health, strength, and independence

KEY ABBREVIATIONS

ADL Activities of daily living

OBRA Omnibus Budget Reconciliation Act of 1987

Disease, injury, and surgery can affect body function. So can birth injuries and birth defects (Chapter 45). Often more than one function is lost. Losses are temporary or permanent. Eating, bathing, dressing, and walking are hard or seem impossible. Some persons cannot work. Others cannot care for children or family.

A **disability** is any lost, absent, or impaired physical or mental function. Causes are acute or chronic (Box 36-1).

▶ An *acute problem* has a short course. Recovery is complete. A fracture is an acute problem.

▶ A *chronic problem* has a long course. The problem is controlled—not cured—with treatment. Diabetes and arthritis are chronic health problems.

Disabilities are short-term or long-term. A leg fracture is short-term. The person has a cast. Crutches are used until the bone heals. A spinal cord injury is long-term if paralysis results.

The person may depend totally or in part on others for basic needs. The degree of disability affects how much function is possible.

A goal of health care is to prevent and reduce the degree of disability. Helping the person adjust is another goal. **Rehabilitation** is the process of restoring the person to his or her highest possible level of physical, psychological, social, and economic function. The focus is on improving abilities. This promotes function at the highest level of independence. For some persons the goal is to return to a job. For others, self-care is the goal. Sometimes improved function is not possible. Then the goal is to prevent further loss of function. This helps the person maintain the best possible quality of life.

Some persons return home after rehabilitation. The process may continue in home or community settings.

See *Focus on Long-Term Care and Home Care: Rehabilitation and Restorative Care.*

RESTORATIVE NURSING

Some persons are weak. Many cannot perform daily functions. They need restorative nursing care. **Restorative nursing care** is care that helps persons regain health, strength, and independence. Some illnesses are progressive. The person becomes more and more disabled. Restorative nursing programs:

▶ Help maintain the highest level of function
▶ Prevent unnecessary decline in function

Restorative nursing may involve measures that promote:

▶ Self-care
▶ Elimination
▶ Positioning
▶ Mobility
▶ Communication
▶ Cognitive function

Many persons need restorative nursing and rehabilitation. Often it is hard to separate them. In many agencies, they mean the same thing. Both focus on the whole person.

BOX 36-1 Common Health Problems Requiring Rehabilitation

- Amputation
- Birth defects
- Brain tumor
- Burns
- Cerebral palsy
- Chronic obstructive pulmonary disease
- Head injury
- Myocardial infarction (heart attack)
- Spinal cord injury
- Spinal cord tumor
- Stroke
- Substance abuse—drug, alcohol

FOCUS ON LONG-TERM CARE AND HOME CARE

Rehabilitation and Restorative Care

LONG-TERM CARE

Some nursing center residents have physical disabilities. Causes include strokes, fractures, amputations, and injuries. They need to regain function or adjust to a long-term disability. Often these residents return home.

Other residents have progressive illnesses. They become more and more disabled. The goals are to help them:

- Maintain their highest level of function
- Prevent unnecessary decline in function

Restorative Aides

Some agencies have restorative aides. A **restorative aide** is a nursing assistant with special training in restorative nursing and rehabilitation skills. These aides assist the nursing and health teams as needed.

Usually nursing assistants are promoted to restorative aide positions. Those chosen have excellent work ethics, job performance, and skills. Required training varies among states. If there are no state requirements, the agency provides needed training.

REHABILITATION AND THE WHOLE PERSON

A health problem has physical, psychological, and social effects. So does a disability. Suppose an illness left you paralyzed from the waist down. Answer these questions:

▶ Would you be angry, afraid, or depressed?
▶ How would you move about?
▶ How would you care for yourself?
▶ How would you care for your family?
▶ How would you worship, shop, or visit friends?
▶ What job could you do?
▶ How would you support yourself?

The person needs to adjust physically, psychologically, socially, and economically. Abilities—what the person can do—are stressed. Complications are prevented. They can cause further disability.

See *Focus on Children and Older Persons: Rehabilitation and the Whole Person,* p. 608.

Physical Aspects

Rehabilitation starts when the person first seeks health care. Complications are prevented. They can occur from bedrest, a long illness, or recovery from surgery or injury. Bowel and bladder problems are prevented. So are contractures and pressure ulcers. Good alignment, turning and repositioning, range-of-motion exercises, and supportive devices are needed (Chapters 15, 16, and 26). Good skin care also prevents pressure ulcers (Chapters 19 and 32).

Elimination

Some persons need bladder training (Chapter 21). The method depends on the person's problems, abilities, and needs. Some need bowel training (Chapter 22). Control of bowel movements and regular elimination are goals. Fecal impaction, constipation, and fecal incontinence are prevented. Follow the care plan and the nurse's instructions.

Self-Care

Self-care is a major goal. **Activities of daily living (ADL)** are the activities usually done during a normal day in a person's life. ADL include bathing, oral hygiene, dressing, eating, elimination, and moving about. The health team evaluates the person's ability to perform ADL. The need for self-help devices is considered.

Sometimes the hands, wrists, and arms are affected. Self-help devices are often needed. Equipment is changed, made, or bought to meet the person's needs.

▶ Eating devices include glass holders, plate guards, and silverware with curved handles or cuffs (Chapter 23). Some devices attach to splints (Fig. 36-1).

▶ Electric toothbrushes are helpful. They have back-and-forth brushing motions for oral hygiene.

▶ Longer handles attach to combs, brushes, and sponges. Or the devices have long handles (Fig. 36-3).

Self-help devices are useful for cooking, dressing, writing, phone calls, and other tasks. Some are shown in Figure 36-3.

Mobility

The person may need crutches or a walker, cane, or brace. Physical and occupational therapies are common for musculoskeletal and nervous system problems (Fig. 36-2). Some people need wheelchairs. If possible, they learn wheelchair transfers. Such transfers include to and from the bed, toilet, bathtub, sofa, and chair and in out of vehicles (Figs. 36-4 and 36-5, p. 610).

A **prosthesis** is an artificial replacement for a missing body part. The person learns how to use the artificial arm or leg (Chapter 39). The goal is for the device to be like the missing body part in function and appearance.

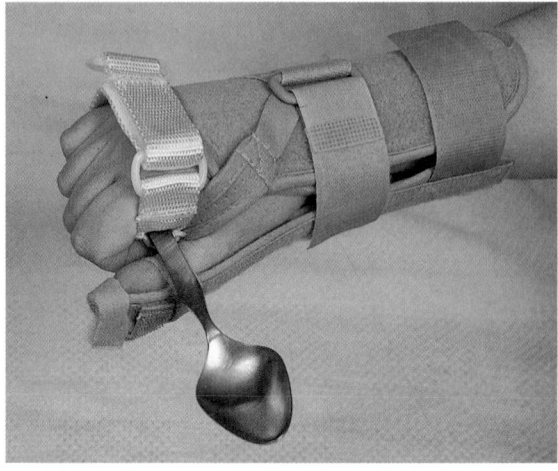

FIGURE 36-1 Eating device attached to a splint.

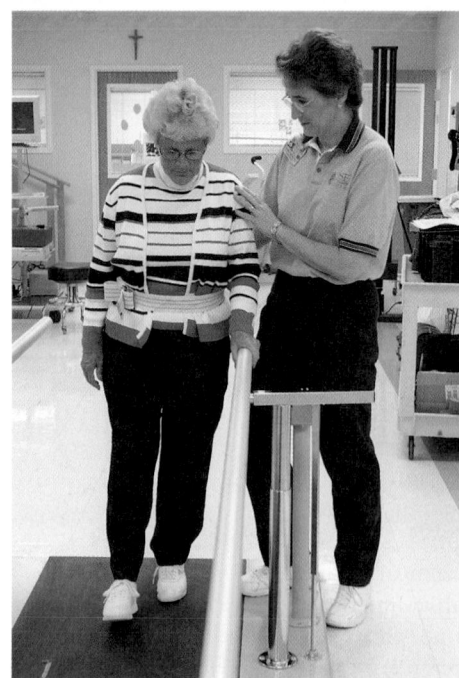

FIGURE 36-2 The person is assisted with walking in physical therapy.

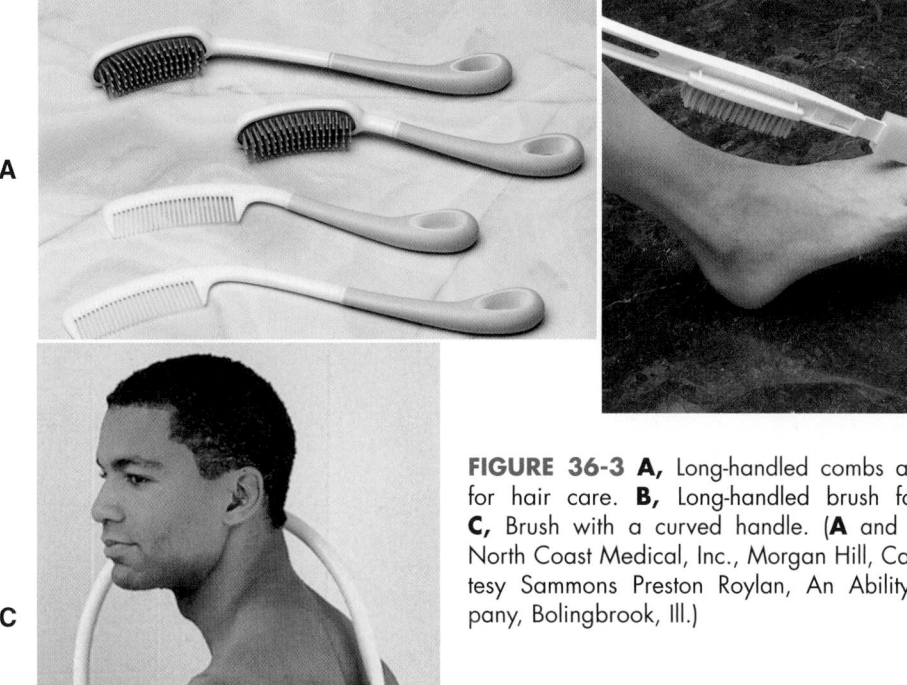

FIGURE 36-3 A, Long-handled combs and brushes for hair care. **B,** Long-handled brush for bathing. **C,** Brush with a curved handle. (**A** and **B** courtesy North Coast Medical, Inc., Morgan Hill, Calif.; **C** courtesy Sammons Preston Roylan, An AbilityOne Company, Bolingbrook, Ill.)

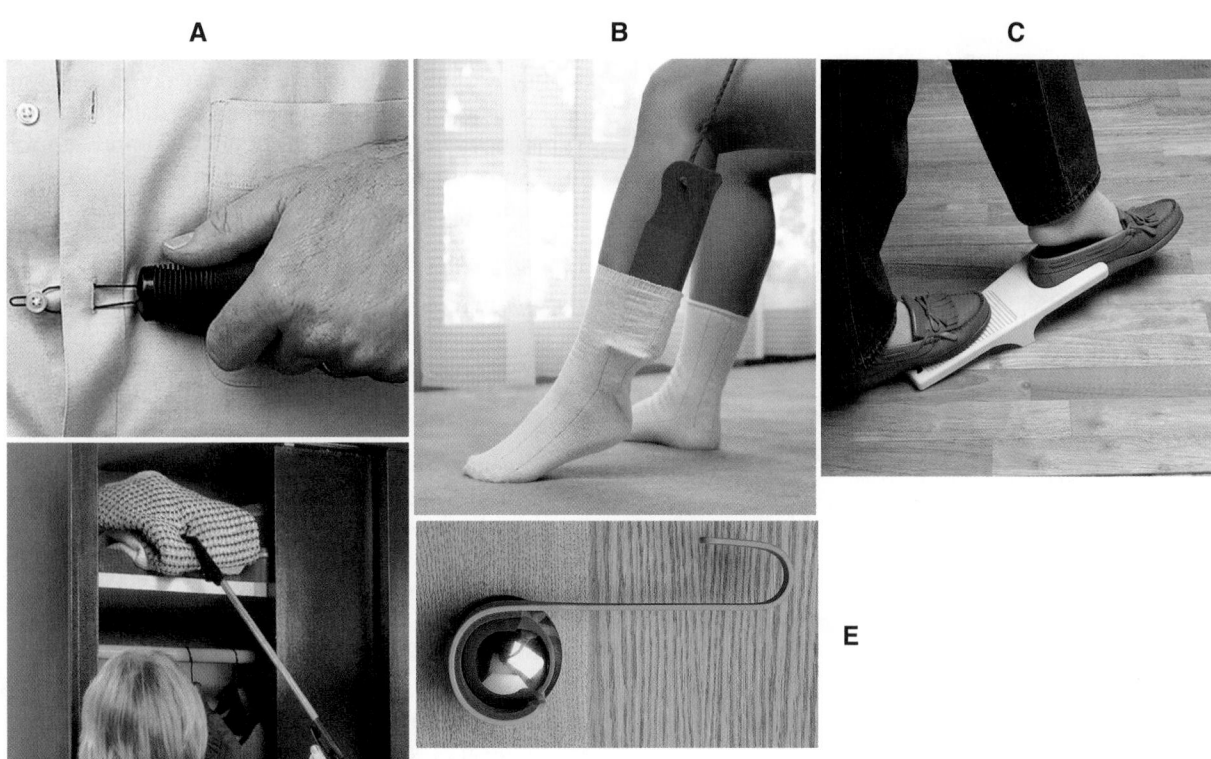

FIGURE 36-4 A, A button hook is used to button and zip clothing. **B,** A sock assist is used to pull on socks and stockings. **C,** A shoe remover is used to take off shoes. **D,** A reacher is helpful to remove items from high shelves. **E,** A doorknob turner increases leverage to help turn the knob. (**A, B, C,** and **E** courtesy North Coast Medical, Inc., Morgan Hill, Calif.; **D** courtesy Sammons Preston Roylan, An AbilityOne Company, Bolingbrook, Ill.)

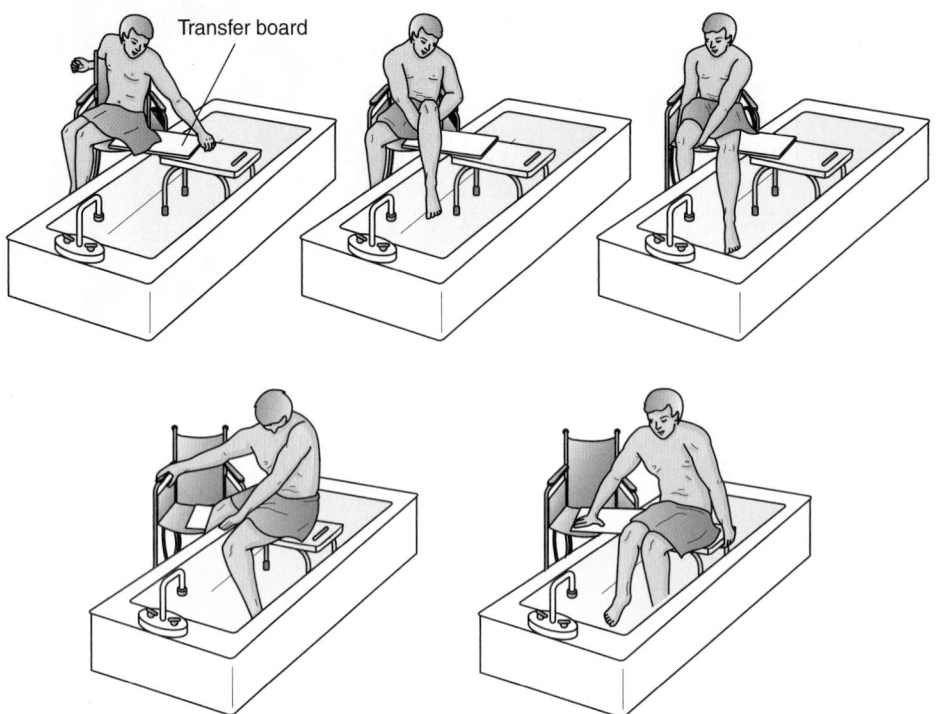

FIGURE 36-5 The person transfers from the wheelchair to the bathtub. A transfer board is used.

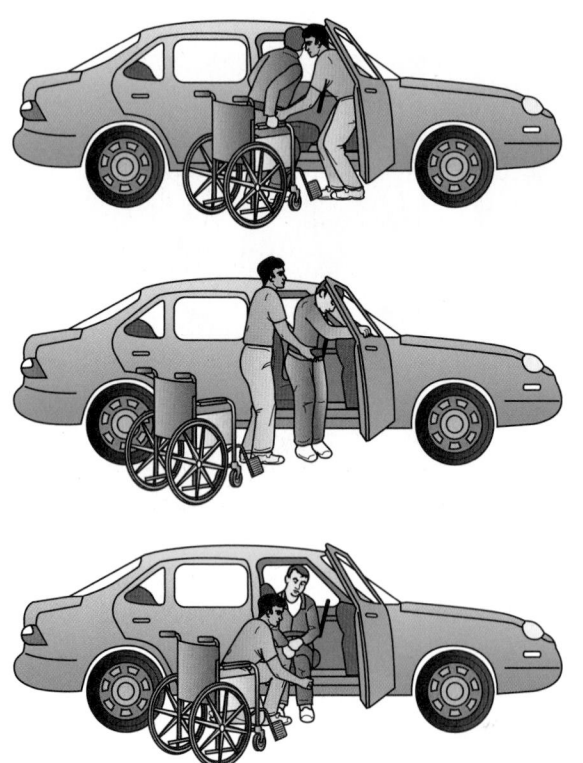

FIGURE 36-6 The person transfers from the wheelchair to the car.

Nutrition

Difficulty swallowing *(dysphagia)* may occur after a stroke. The person may need a dysphagia diet (Chapter 23). When possible, exercises are taught to improve swallowing. Some persons cannot swallow. They need enteral nutrition (Chapter 24).

Communication

Aphasia may occur from a stroke (Chapter 37). Aphasia means the inability to have normal speech. Speech therapy and communication devices are helpful (Chapter 7).

Mechanical Ventilation

Some persons need mechanical ventilation (Chapter 35). Some are weaned from the ventilator. That is, the person needs to breathe without the machine. The process may take many weeks. Other persons must learn to live with life-long mechanical ventilation.

Psychological and Social Aspects

A disability can affect function and appearance. Self-esteem and relationships may suffer. The person may feel unwhole, useless, unattractive, unclean, or undesirable. The person may deny the disability. The person may expect therapy to correct the problem. He or she may be depressed, angry, and hostile.

Successful rehabilitation depends on the person's attitude. The person must accept his or her limits and be motivated. The focus is on abilities and strengths. Despair and frustration are common. Progress may be slow. Learning a new task is a reminder of the disability. Old fears and emotions may recur.

Remind persons of their *progress*. They need help accepting disabilities and limits. Give support, reassurance, and encouragement. Psychological and social needs are part of the care plan. Spiritual support helps some persons.

Economic Aspects

Some persons cannot return to their jobs. The person is assessed for work skills, work history, interests, and talents. A job skill may be restored or a new one learned. The goal is for the person to become gainfully employed. Help is given finding a job.

THE REHABILITATION TEAM

Rehabilitation is a team effort. The person is the key team member. The family, doctor, nursing team, and other health team members help the person set goals and plan care. All help the person regain function and independence.

The team meets often to discuss the person's progress. Changes in the rehabilitation plan are made as needed. The person and family attend the meetings when possible. Families are important. They provide support and encouragement. Often they help with care when the person returns home.

Your Role

Every part of your job focuses on promoting the person's independence. Preventing decline in function also is a goal. The many procedures, care measures, and rules in this book apply. Safety, communication, legal, and ethical aspects apply. So do the measures in Box 36-2.

See *Focus on Communication: Your Role.*
See *Teamwork and Time Management: Your Role.*
See *Focus on Ethics and Laws: Your Role.*

FOCUS ON COMMUNICATION

Your Role

You may need to guide and direct the person during care measures. First listen to how the nurse or therapist guides and directs the person. Use those words. Hearing the same thing helps the person learn and remember what to do.

TEAMWORK AND TIME MANAGEMENT

Your Role

Rehabilitation can frustrate the person, you, and other nursing team members. Teamwork is not just about helping with care. It is also about giving emotional support to each other. It often helps to talk about your feelings. The nursing team can help you control or express your feelings. You may need to assist with other patients or residents for a while.

FOCUS ON ETHICS AND LAWS

Your Role

The person may not want to practice rehabilitation procedures or methods. He or she may want you to provide care instead. Personal choice is important. However, the person needs to follow the rehabilitation plan. Otherwise, he or she will not make progress. Do not let the person control you. Letting the person control you is the wrong thing to do. Report any problems at once.

BOX 36-2 Assisting With Rehabilitation and Restorative Care

- Follow the nurse's instructions carefully.
- Follow the person's care plan.
- Follow the person's daily routine.
- Provide for safety.
- Protect the person's rights. Privacy and personal choice are very important.
- Report early signs and symptoms of complications. They include pressure ulcers, contractures, and bowel and bladder problems.
- Keep the person in good alignment at all times.
- Turn and reposition the person as directed.
- Use safe transfer methods.
- Practice measures to prevent pressure ulcers.
- Perform range-of-motion exercises as instructed.
- Apply assistive devices as ordered.
- Do not pity the person or give sympathy.
- Encourage the person to perform ADL to the extent possible.
- Allow the person time to complete tasks. Do not rush the person.
- Give praise when even a little progress is made.
- Provide emotional support and reassurance.
- Try to understand and appreciate the person's situation, feelings, and concerns.
- Provide for spiritual needs.
- Practice the methods developed by the rehabilitation team. This helps you better assist the person.
- Practice the task that the person must do. This helps you guide and direct the person.
- Know how to apply the person's self-help devices.
- Know how to use and operate equipment used by the person.
- Stress what the person can do. Focus on abilities and strengths. Do not focus on disabilities and weaknesses.
- Remember that muscles will atrophy if not used. And contractures can develop.
- Have a hopeful outlook.

REHABILITATION PROGRAMS AND SERVICES

Rehabilitation begins when the person first needs health care. Often this in the hospital. Common rehabilitation programs include:

▶ *Cardiac rehabilitation*—for heart disorders (Chapter 40)
▶ *Brain injury rehabilitation*—for nervous system disorders including traumatic brain injury (Chapter 39)
▶ *Spinal cord rehabilitation*—for spinal cord injuries (Chapter 39)
▶ *Stroke rehabilitation*—after a stroke (Chapter 39)
▶ *Respiratory rehabilitation*—for respiratory system disorders such as chronic obstructive pulmonary disease, after lung surgery, for respiratory complications from other health problems (Chapter 40), and for mechanical ventilation (Chapter 35)
▶ *Musculoskeletal rehabilitation*—for fractures, joint replacement surgery, and so on (Chapter 39)
▶ *Rehabilitation for complex medical and surgical conditions*—for wound care (Chapter 32), diabetes (Chapter 41), burns (Chapter 49), and so on

Depending on the person's needs and problems, the process may continue after the person leaves the hospital. The person may need nursing center care. Some persons transfer to rehabilitation agencies. There are agencies for persons who are blind or deaf, have intellectual disabilities (mental retardation), are physically disabled, or have speech problems. Some agencies are for persons who are mentally ill. Many substance abuse programs are available.

Home care agencies also provide rehabilitation services. So do some assisted living residences (Chapter 48) and adult day care centers.

See *Focus on Children and Older Persons: Rehabilitation Services.*

See *Focus on Long-Term Care and Home Care: Rehabilitation Services.*

FOCUS ON **CHILDREN** AND **OLDER PERSONS**

Rehabilitation Services

CHILDREN
Federal laws require that schools provide needed therapies. In-school therapy is required to meet the child's learning needs.

FOCUS ON **LONG-TERM CARE** AND **HOME CARE**

Rehabilitation Services

LONG-TERM CARE
The Omnibus Budget Reconciliation Act of 1987 (OBRA) requires that nursing centers provide rehabilitation services. If not provided by center staff, the service is obtained from another source. For example, a center does not have a speech therapist. Instead, the service is obtained from a hospital or other agency.

The center must provide services required by a person's comprehensive care plan. If a person requires physical therapy, it must be provided. If a person requires occupational therapy, it must be provided. If a person requires speech therapy, it must be provided. Such services require a doctor's order.

HOME CARE
The rehabilitation team assesses the person's home setting (Box 36-3). Changes in the home are made as needed. Some persons require personal attendants 24 hours a day.

BOX 36-3 Home Assessment

OUTDOORS
- Where is parking located? How far is the parking area to the door?
- Where is the motor vehicle parked?
- Where is the mailbox?
- How wide are the doors?
- Can the person turn a key?
- Can the person open and close doors?
- Are ramps needed?
- Are hand rails needed?
- Are entrances lighted?
- Does the person have access to private or public transportation?
- Can the person drive a motor vehicle?
- How wide and high are ramps and sidewalks?

INDOORS
- Are there floor obstructions?
- Are there steps in the home? Where are they? How many are there?
- How is furniture arranged?
- Can the person use the furniture?
- Where are phones located?
- Can the person open and close windows?
- How are floors covered (wall-to-wall carpeting, tile, hardwood floors, throw rugs)?
- Can the person use a wheelchair throughout the home?
- Where is the fuse or circuit-breaker box located?
- Can the person control the heat?
- Are walkways, doors, and hallways wide enough for wheelchair use?
- Does the building have an elevator?

KITCHEN
- Can the person access the stove, sink, cupboards, storage areas, work space, refrigerator, and other appliances?
- How high is the sink and countertop?
- Is there an opening under the sink for wheelchair access?
- Can the person turn faucets on and off?
- Can the person use the microwave?
- Can the person reach stove knobs?
- Can the person reach appliances?

BATHROOM
- How high are the sink, toilet, shower, and tub?
- Can the person reach the faucets?
- Can the person turn the faucets on and off?

- Is there space for a wheelchair and other assistive devices?
- Can the person get into and out of the tub or shower?
- Are there safety bars by the toilet, shower, and tub?

BEDROOM
- How high is the person's bed?
- Can the person access the closet? Can the person reach rods and shelves?
- Can the person transfer in and out of bed safely? Is there space around the bed for the person to move?
- How is furniture arranged? Does it allow for a wheelchair or assistive devices?

SAFETY
- Is the house number clearly visible and readable during an emergency?
- Are deadbolts and locks secure? Can the person use them?
- Can the person see and talk to a visitor at the door without being seen?
- Are steps, porch, and entrances lighted?
- Are the steps, porch, and entrances protected from rain, sleet, and snow?
- Is there a non-slip doormat?
- Can the person use the phone?
- Are emergency phone numbers clearly posted?
- Can the person control water temperature?
- Do electrical outlets have childproof covers?
- Where are the smoke detectors? Are they working?
- Are rooms and hallways well-lighted?
- Can the person turn indoor and outdoor lighting on and off?
- Can the person exit the home in an emergency?
- Is oxygen used? Are safety measures for oxygen use in place?
- Can the person access the phone, TV, radio, and lights while in bed?
- Are space heaters used? Are safety measures in place?
- Does the person have good judgment for cooking and stove use?
- Is there a safe play area for children?
- Can the person safely dispose of blood, body fluids, secretions, and excretions?
- Is there a pest-free method of trash storage?

Modified from Hoeman SP: *Rehabilitation nursing: process, application, and outcomes*, ed 4, St Louis, 2007, Mosby.

QUALITY OF LIFE

Successful rehabilitation and restorative care improves the person's quality of life. A hopeful and winning outlook is needed. Promoting quality of life helps the person's attitude. The more the person can do alone, the better his or her quality of life. To promote quality of life:

▶ *Protect the right to privacy.* The person relearns old or practices new skills in private. No one needs to watch. They do not need to see mistakes, falls, spills, or clumsiness. Nor do they need to see anger or tears. Privacy protects dignity and promotes self-respect.

▶ *Encourage personal choice.* This gives the person control. Not being able to control body movements or functions is very frustrating. Allow and encourage persons to control their lives to the extent possible. Persons who are sad and depressed may not want to make choices. Encourage them to do so. It can help them feel in control of those things that affect them. Personal choice is important in planning care.

▶ *Protect the right to be free from abuse and mistreatment.* Sometimes improvement is not seen for weeks. Learning to use a self-help device takes time. Learning to speak again can take a long time. So can learning how to dress when there is paralysis. What seems simple is often very hard to do. Repeated explanations and demonstrations may have no or little results. You may become upset and short-tempered. Other staff or the family may have such behaviors. Protect the person from abuse and mistreatment. No one can shout, scream, or yell at the person. Nor can they call the person names. They cannot hit or strike the person. Unkind remarks are not allowed. Report signs of abuse or mistreatment to the nurse.

▶ *Learn to deal with your anger and frustration.* The person does not choose loss of function. If the process upsets you, think how the person must feel. Discuss your feelings with the nurse. The nurse can suggest ways to help you control or express your feelings. Perhaps you can assist other persons for a while.

▶ *Encourage activities.* Often a person worries about how others view the disability. Provide support and reassurance. Remind the person that others have disabilities. They can give support and understanding. Allow personal choice. Let the person do what interests him or her. The person usually chooses activities that he or she can do.

▶ *Provide a safe setting.* It must meet the person's needs. Needed changes are made. The overbed table, bedside stand, and signal light are moved to the person's strong side. If unable to use the signal light, another way is needed to communicate with the staff. The person may need a special chair. The rehabilitation team suggests these and other changes. They explain the need and purpose to the person and family.

▶ *Show patience, understanding, and sensitivity.* Progress may be slow and hard to see. The person may be upset and discouraged. Give support, encouragement, and praise when needed. Stress the person's abilities and strengths. Do not give pity or sympathy.

REVIEW QUESTIONS

Circle the BEST answer.

1 Rehabilitation and restorative nursing care focus on
  a What the person cannot do   c The whole person
  b What the person can do   d The person's rights

2 A person's rehabilitation begins with preventing
  a Angry feelings   c Illness and injury
  b Contractures and   d Loss of self-esteem
    pressure ulcers

3 A person has weakness on the right side. ADL are
  a Done by the person to the extent possible
  b Done by you
  c Postponed until the right side can be used
  d Supervised by a therapist

4 Persons with disabilities are likely to feel the following *except*
  a Undesirable   c Depressed
  b Angry and hostile   d Relief

5 Which statement is *false?*
  a Sympathy and pity help the person adjust.
  b You should know how to apply self-help devices.
  c You should know how to use equipment used in the person's care.
  d You need to convey hopefulness to the person.

6 During a therapy, a person asks to have music played. You should
  a Explain that music is not allowed
  b Choose some music
  c Ask the person to choose some music
  d Ask a therapist to choose some music

7 A person's right side is weak. You move the signal light to the left side. You have promoted quality of life by
  a Protecting the person from abuse and mistreatment
  b Allowing personal choice
  c Providing for safety
  d Taking part in activities

Circle T if the statement is true and F if it is false.

8 T F You should give praise even when slight progress is made.

9 T F A person's speech therapy should be done in private.

10 T F You tell a person that dessert is not allowed until exercises are done. This is abuse and mistreatment.

11 T F A person refuses to attend a concert at the nursing center. The person must attend. It is part of the rehabilitation plan.

12 T F Rehabilitation programs for older persons are usually slower paced than those for younger persons.

13 T F Nursing assistants and restorative aides are involved in the person's rehabilitation program.

14 T F You need to stress the person's abilities and strengths.

Answers to these questions are on p. 781.

Hearing, Speech, and Vision Problems

OBJECTIVES

- Define the key terms and key abbreviations listed in this chapter
- Describe the common ear disorders
- Describe how to communicate with persons who have hearing loss
- Explain the purpose of a hearing aid
- Describe how to care for hearing aids
- Describe the common speech disorders
- Explain how to communicate with speech-impaired persons
- Describe the common eye disorders
- Explain how to assist persons who are visually impaired or blind
- Explain how to protect an artificial eye from loss or damage
- Perform the procedure described in this chapter

PROCEDURE

- Caring For Eyeglasses

KEY TERMS

aphasia The total or partial loss *(a)* of the ability to use or understand language *(phasia)*; a language disorder resulting from damage to parts of the brain responsible for language

blind The absence of sight

braille A touch reading and writing system that uses raised dots for each letter of the alphabet; the first 10 letters also represent the numbers 0 through 9

Broca's aphasia Expressive aphasia; motor aphasia

cerumen Earwax

deafness Hearing loss in which it is impossible for the person to understand speech through hearing alone

expressive aphasia Difficulty expressing or sending out thoughts; motor aphasia, Broca's aphasia

expressive-receptive aphasia Difficulty expressing or sending out thoughts and difficulty understanding language; global aphasia, mixed aphasia

global aphasia Expressive-receptive aphasia; mixed aphasia

hearing loss Not being able to hear the normal range of sounds associated with normal hearing

low vision Eyesight that cannot be corrected with eyeglasses, contact lenses, drugs, or surgery

mixed aphasia Expressive-receptive aphasia; global aphasia

motor aphasia Expressive aphasia; Broca's aphasia

receptive aphasia Difficulty understanding language; Wernicke's aphasia

tinnitus A ringing, roaring, hissing, or buzzing sound in the ears or head

vertigo Dizziness

Wernicke's aphasia Receptive aphasia

KEY ABBREVIATIONS

AFB American Foundation for the Blind

AMD Age-related macular degeneration

ASL American Sign Language

NAD National Association of the Deaf

NIDCD National Institute on Deafness and Other Communication Disorders

Hearing, speech, and vision allow communication, learning, and moving about. They are important for self-care, work, and most activities. They also are important for safety and security needs. For example, you see dark clouds and hear tornado warning sirens. You know to seek shelter. With speech, you can alert others.

Many people have some degree of hearing or vision loss. Common causes are birth defects, accidents, infections, diseases, and aging.

EAR DISORDERS

The ear functions in hearing and balance. To review the structures and functions of the ear, see Box 37-1.

Otitis Media

Otitis media is infection *(itis)* of the middle *(media)* ear *(ot)*. It often begins with infections that cause sore throats or colds or with other respiratory infections that spread to the middle ear. Viruses and bacteria are causes.

Otitis media is acute or chronic. Chronic otitis media can damage the tympanic membrane (eardrum) or the ossicles (see Fig. 37-1). These structures are needed for hearing. Permanent hearing loss can occur.

Fluid builds up in the ear. Pain (earache) and hearing loss occur. So do fever and tinnitus. **Tinnitus** is a ringing, roaring, hissing, or buzzing sound in the ears or head. An untreated infection can travel to the brain and other structures in the head. The doctor orders antibiotics, drugs for pain relief, or drugs to relieve congestion.

See *Focus on Children and Older Persons: Otitis Media.*

Menière's Disease

Menière's disease involves the inner ear. It is a common cause of hearing loss. Usually one ear is affected. Symptoms include:

▶ **Vertigo** (dizziness)
▶ Tinnitus
▶ Hearing loss
▶ Pain or pressure in the affected ear

With Menière's disease, there is increased fluid in the inner ear. The increased fluid causes swelling and pressure in the inner ear. Symptoms occur suddenly. They can occur daily or just once a year. An attack can last several hours.

An attack usually involves vertigo, tinnitus, and hearing loss. Vertigo causes whirling and spinning sensations. The dizziness causes severe nausea and vomiting.

BOX 37-1 The Ear: Structures and Function

The *ear* is a sense organ (Fig. 37-1). It functions in hearing and balance. It has three parts: the *external ear, middle ear,* and *inner ear.*

The external ear (outer part) is called the *pinna* or *auricle.* Sound waves are guided through the external ear into the *auditory canal.* Glands in the auditory canal secrete a waxy substance called *cerumen.* The auditory canal extends about 1 inch to the *eardrum.* The eardrum *(tympanic membrane)* separates the external and middle ear.

The middle ear is a small space. It contains the *eustachian tube* and three small bones called *ossicles.* The eustachian tube connects the middle ear and the throat. Air enters the eustachian tube so that there is equal pressure on both sides of the eardrum. The ossicles amplify sound received from the eardrum and transmit the sound to the inner ear. The three ossicles are:
- The *malleus.* It looks like a hammer.
- The *incus.* It looks like an anvil.
- The *stapes.* It is shaped like a stirrup.

The inner ear consists of *semicircular canals* and the *cochlea.* The cochlea looks like a snail shell. It contains fluid. The fluid carries sound waves from the middle ear to the *auditory nerve.* The auditory nerve then carries the message to the brain.

The three semicircular canals are involved with balance. They sense the head's position and changes in position. They send messages to the brain.

FOCUS ON **CHILDREN** AND **OLDER PERSONS**

Otitis Media

CHILDREN

Otitis media is common in infants and children. It is most common between 4 months and 4 years of age. Infants cannot tell you about pain. For earaches, the child may:
- Tug or pull at the ears
- Roll the head back
- Cry a lot
- Be irritable
- Have fluid draining out of the ear
- Sleep poorly
- Have problems with balance
- Have trouble hearing
- Not respond to quiet sounds

Report signs and symptoms of an ear infection to the nurse.

OLDER PERSONS

Some persons with dementia cannot tell you they have pain or when something is wrong. Be alert for behavior changes. Report the following signs to the nurse. They may signal otitis media:
- Unusual irritability
- Problems sleeping
- Tugging or pulling at one or both ears
- Fever
- Fluid draining from the ear
- Balance problems
- Signs of hearing problems (p. 618)

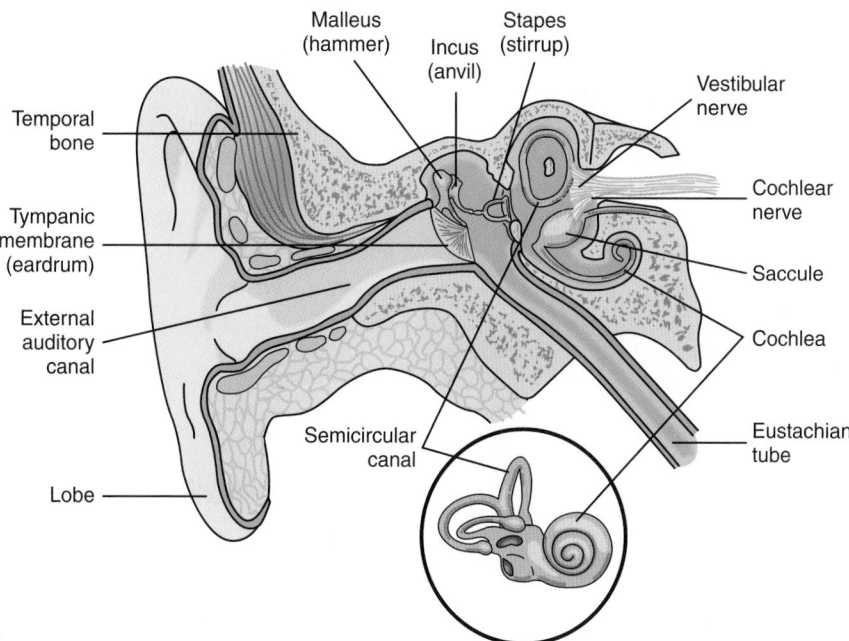

FIGURE 37-1 The ear.

Drugs, fluid restriction, a low-salt diet, and no alcohol or caffeine decrease fluid in the inner ear. Safety is needed during vertigo. The person must lie down. Falls are prevented. Bed rails are used according to the care plan. The person's head is kept still. The person avoids turning the head. To talk to the person, stand directly in front of him or her. When movement is necessary, move the person slowly. Sudden movements are avoided. So are bright or glaring lights. Assist with walking. The person should not walk alone in case vertigo occurs.

Hearing Loss

Hearing loss is not being able to hear the normal range of sounds associated with normal hearing. Losses are mild to severe. Deafness is the most severe form. **Deafness** is hearing loss in which it is impossible for the person to understand speech through hearing alone.

Hearing loss occurs in all age-groups. According to the National Institute on Aging, about one third (33%) of Americans between ages 65 and 74 have hearing problems. About half (50%) of persons age 85 years and older having hearing loss.

Common causes of hearing loss are:

▶ Damage to the outer, middle, or inner ear
▶ Damage to the auditory nerve

Risk factors that can damage the ear structures include:

▶ Aging
▶ Exposure to very loud sounds and noises—job-related noises, loud music, loud engines from vehicles, shooting firearms
▶ Drugs—antibiotics, too much aspirin
▶ Infections
▶ Reduced blood flow to the ear caused by high blood pressure, heart and vascular diseases, and diabetes
▶ Stroke
▶ Head injuries
▶ Tumors
▶ Heredity
▶ Birth defects

Temporary hearing loss can occur from earwax (cerumen). Hearing improves after the earwax is removed.

Clear speech, responding to others, safety, and awareness of surroundings require hearing. Many people deny hearing problems. They relate hearing loss to aging.

See *Focus on Communication: Hearing Loss.*
See *Promoting Safety and Comfort: Hearing Loss.*

FOCUS ON COMMUNICATION

Hearing Loss

The National Association of the Deaf (NAD) uses the terms *deaf* and *hard of hearing* to describe persons with hearing loss. Do not use the terms "deaf and dumb," "deaf-mute," or "hearing-impaired." Such terms offend persons who are deaf or hard of hearing.

PROMOTING SAFETY AND COMFORT: Hearing Loss

SAFETY

Do not try to remove earwax. This is done by a doctor or a nurse. Do not insert anything, including cotton swabs, into the ear.

Effects on the Person

A person may not notice gradual hearing loss. Others may see changes in the person's behavior or attitude. They may not relate the changes to hearing loss. Obvious signs and symptoms of hearing loss in children and adults include:

▶ Speaking too loudly
▶ Leaning forward to hear
▶ Turning and cupping the better ear toward the speaker
▶ Answering questions or responding inappropriately
▶ Asking for words to be repeated
▶ Asking others to speak louder or to speak more slowly and clearly
▶ Having trouble hearing over the phone
▶ Finding it hard to follow conversations when two or more people are talking
▶ Turning up the TV, radio, or music volume so loud that others complain
▶ Thinking that others are mumbling or slurring words
▶ Having problems understanding women and children

Psychological and social changes are less obvious. People may give wrong answers or responses. Therefore they tend to shun social events to avoid embarrassment. Often they feel lonely, bored, and left out. Only parts of conversations are heard. They may become suspicious. They think others are talking about them or are talking softly on purpose. Some control conversations to avoid responding or being labeled "senile" because of poor answers. Straining and working hard to hear can cause fatigue, frustration, and irritability.

Hearing is needed for speech. How you pronounce words and voice volume depend on how you hear yourself. Hearing loss may result in slurred speech. Words may be pronounced wrong. Some have monotone speech or drop word endings. It may be hard to understand what the person says. Do not assume or pretend that you understand what the person says. Otherwise serious problems can result. See "Speech Disorders" on p. 621.

See *Focus on Children and Older Persons: Effects on the Person.*

FOCUS ON CHILDREN AND OLDER PERSONS

Effects on the Person

CHILDREN

Some babies are born with hearing problems. Others develop hearing problems as they grow older. Hearing is needed for language development. Children learn to talk by imitating sounds and voices. Medical attention is needed if a child does not hear well or speak clearly. The National Institute on Deafness and Other Communication Disorders (NIDCD) has a hearing checklist for children (Box 37-2). The items checked "No" may signal hearing loss. Report concerns about a child's hearing to the nurse.

BOX 37-2 Hearing Checklist for Children

Items marked "No" may signal hearing loss.

Yes	No	Birth to 3 Months
___	___	Reacts to loud sounds.
___	___	Is soothed by a parent's voice.
___	___	Turns his or head to you when you speak.
___	___	Is awakened by loud voices or sounds.
___	___	Smiles when spoken to.
___	___	Seems to know the parent's voice and quiets down if crying.

Yes	No	3 to 6 Months
___	___	Looks upward or turns toward a new sound.
___	___	Responds to "no" and changes in tone of voice.
___	___	Imitates his or her own voice.
___	___	Enjoys rattles and other toys that make sounds.
___	___	Begins to repeat sounds. "Ooh," "aah," and "ba-ba" are examples.
___	___	Becomes scared by a loud voice.

Yes	No	6 to 10 Months
___	___	Responds to his or her own name, phones ringing, someone's voice. Responds even when such sounds are not loud.
___	___	Knows words for common things and sayings. Cup, shoe, and bye-bye are examples.
___	___	Makes babbling sounds, even when alone.
___	___	Starts to respond to requests. "Come here" is an example.
___	___	Looks at things or pictures when someone talks to them.

Yes	No	10 to 15 Months
___	___	Plays with his or her own voice. Enjoys the sound and feel of one's own voice.
___	___	Points or looks at familiar objects or people when asked to do so.
___	___	Imitates simple words and sounds. May use a few words with meaning.
___	___	Enjoys games like peek-a-boo and pat-a-cake.

Yes	No	15 to 18 Months
___	___	Follows simple directions. "Give me the ball" is an example.
___	___	Uses words he or she has learned. Uses them often.
___	___	Uses 2 to 3 words sentences to talk about and ask for things.
___	___	Knows 10 to 20 words.

Yes	No	18 to 24 Months
___	___	Understands simple "yes" and "no" questions. "Are you hungry?" is an example.
___	___	Understands simple phrases. "In the cup" and "on the table" are examples.
___	___	Enjoys being read to.
___	___	Points to pictures when asked.

Yes	No	24 to 36 Months
___	___	Understands "not now" and "no more."
___	___	Chooses things by size (big, little).
___	___	Follows simple directions. "Get your shoes" and "drink your milk" are examples.
___	___	Understands many action words. "Run" and "jump" are examples.

Yes	No	Other
___	___	Others in the family have a hearing problem. This includes brothers and sisters.
___	___	The mother had medical problems during pregnancy and delivery.
___	___	The baby's birth was premature.
___	___	The baby had physical problems at birth.
___	___	The child often rubs or pulls on the ear or ears.
___	___	The child had scarlet fever.
___	___	The child had meningitis.
___	___	The child had ear infections in the past year.
___	___	The child had colds, allergies, and ear infections.

Modified from National Institute on Deafness and Other Communication Disorders: *Your child's hearing development checklist: silence isn't always golden*, NIH Publication No. 95-4040, updated April 26, 2006, Bethesda, Md.

Communication

Persons with hearing loss may wear hearing aids or lip-read (speech-read). They watch facial expressions, gestures, and body language. Some people learn American Sign Language (ASL) (Figs. 37-2 and 37-3, p. 620). ASL uses signs made with the hands and other movements such as facial expressions, gestures, and postures. To promote communication, practice the measures in Box 37-3, p. 621. (Different sign languages are used in different countries and regions. For example, British Sign Language is different from ASL.)

Some people have *hearing assistance dogs* (hearing dogs). The dog alerts the person to sounds. Examples include phones, doorbells, smoke detectors, alarm clocks, sirens and on-coming cars.

Hearing Aids

Hearing aids are electronic devices that fit inside or behind the ear (Fig. 37-4, p. 621). They make sounds louder. They do not correct, restore, or cure hearing problems. Hearing ability does not improve. The person hears better because the device makes sounds louder. Background noise and speech are louder. The measures in Box 37-3 apply.

Hearing aids are battery-operated. Sometimes they do not seem to work properly. Try these simple measures:

▶ Check if the hearing aid is *on*. It has an *on* and *off* switch.
▶ Check the battery position.
▶ Insert a new battery if needed.
▶ Clean the hearing aid. *Follow the nurse's directions and the manufacturer's instructions.*

Hearing aids are turned off when not in use. And the battery is removed. These measures help prolong battery life. The person should not use hair spray or other hair care products while wearing a hearing aid. They can damage the device.

Hearing aids are costly. Handle and care for them properly. When not in the person's ear, store a hearing aid in its case. Place the case in the top drawer of the bedside stand. Report lost or damaged hearings aids to the nurse at once.

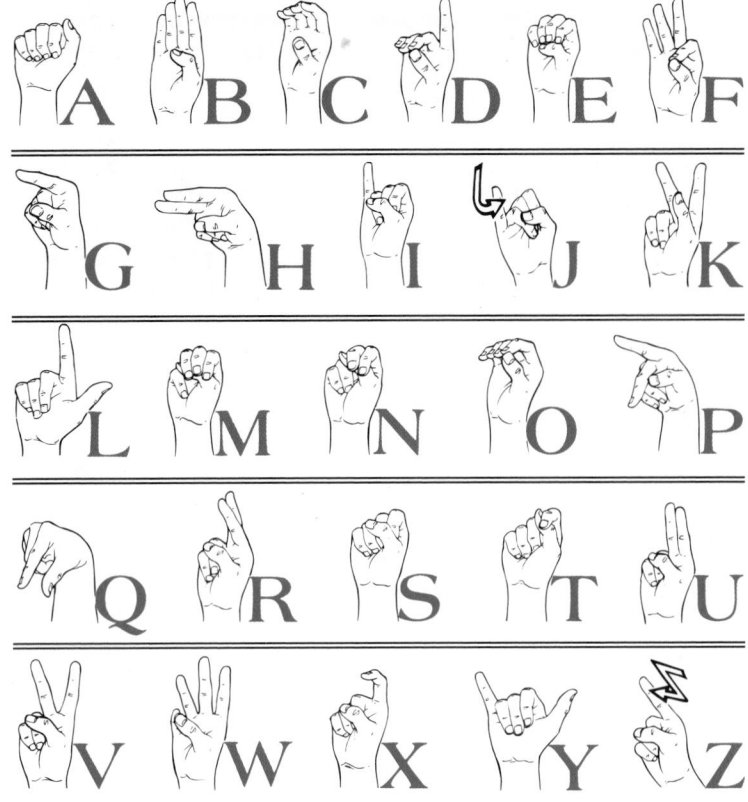

FIGURE 37-2 Manual alphabet. (Courtesy National Association of the Deaf, Silver Spring, Md.)

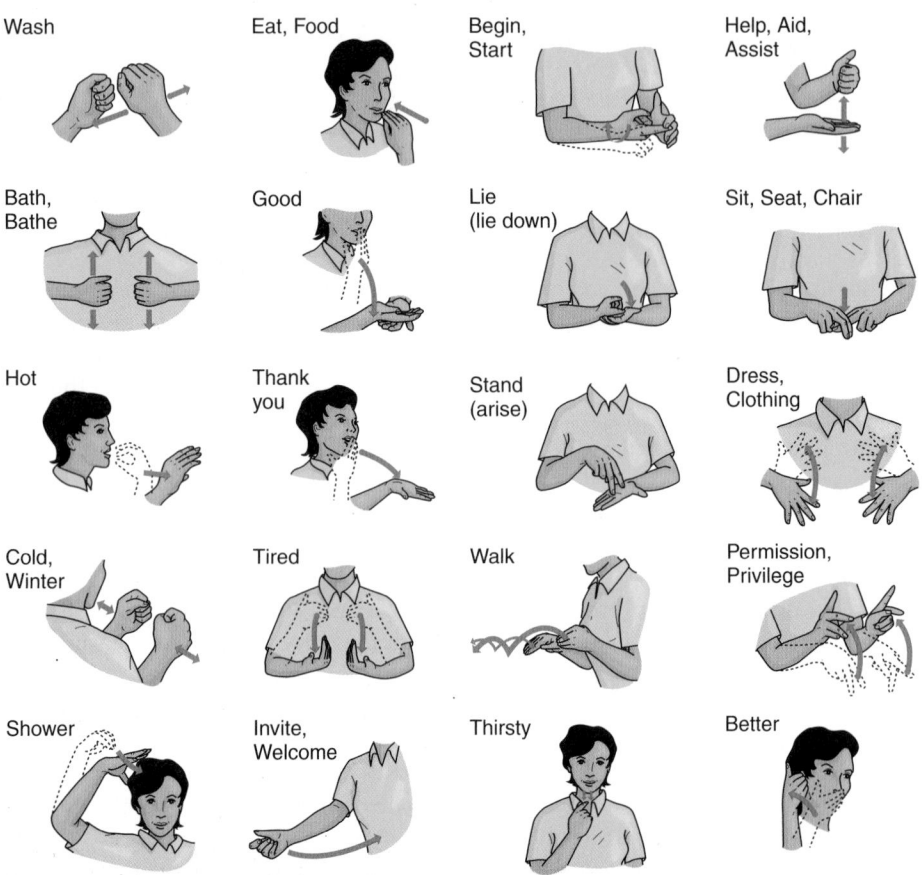

FIGURE 37-3 American Sign Language examples.

BOX 37-3 **Measures to Promote Hearing**

THE ENVIRONMENT

- Reduce or eliminate background noises. For example, turn off radios, stereos, music players, TVs, air conditioners, fans, and so on.
- Provide a quiet place to talk.
- Have the person sit in small groups or where he or she can hear best.

THE PERSON

- Have the person wear his or her hearing aid. It must be turned on and working.
- Have the person wear needed eyeglasses or contact lenses. The person needs to see your face for lip-reading (speech-reading).

YOU

- Gain attention. Alert the person to your presence. Raise an arm or hand, or lightly touch the person's arm. Do not startle or approach the person from behind.
- Position yourself at the person's level. If the person is sitting, you sit. If the person is standing, you stand.
- Face the person when speaking. Do not turn or walk away while you are talking. Do not talk to the person from the doorway or another room.
- Stand or sit in good light. Shadows and glares affect the person's ability to see your face clearly.
- Speak clearly, distinctly, and slowly.
- Speak in a normal tone of voice. Do not shout.
- Adjust the pitch of your voice as needed. Ask the person if he or she can hear you better:
  - If the person does not wear a hearing aid, lower the pitch if you are a female. Women's voices are higher-pitched and harder to hear than lower-pitched male voices.
  - If the person wears a hearing aid, raise the pitch slightly.
- Do not cover your mouth, smoke, eat, or chew gum while talking. Mouth movements are affected.
- Keep your hands away from your face. The person must be able to clearly see your face.
- Stand or sit on the side of the better ear.
- State the topic of conversation first.
- Tell the person when you are changing the subject. State the new subject of conversation.
- Use short sentences and simple words.
- Use gestures and facial expressions to give useful clues.
- Write out important names and words.
- Say things in another way if the person does not seem to understand.
- Keep conversations and discussions short. This avoids tiring the person.
- Repeat and rephrase statements as needed.
- Be alert to messages sent by your facial expressions, gestures, and body language.

Other Hearing Devices

Other devices can help the person with hearing loss. They include:

- *Telephone amplifying devices.* Special telephone receivers make sounds louder. Some phones work with hearing aids.
- *TV and radio listening systems.* These can be used with or without hearing aids. The person does not have to turn the TV or radio volume up high.

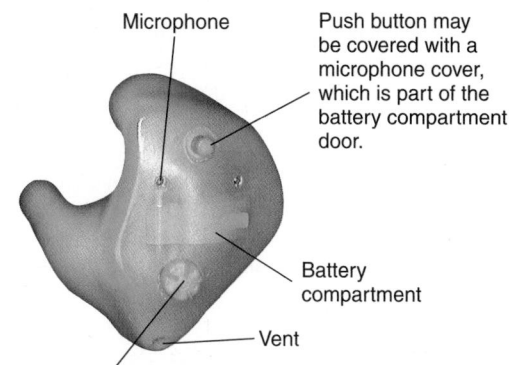

Microphone

Push button may be covered with a microphone cover, which is part of the battery compartment door.

Battery compartment

Vent

On/Off switch/Volume control

FIGURE 37-4 A hearing aid. (Courtesy Siemens Hearing Instruments, Inc., Piscataway, NJ.)

SPEECH DISORDERS

Speech is used to communicate with others. A speech disorder results in impaired or ineffective oral communication. Hearing loss, developmental disabilities (Chapter 45), and brain injury are common causes.

Aphasia, apraxia of speech, and dysarthria are common problems.

- *Aphasia.* See "Aphasia."
- *Apraxia* means not (*a*) to act, do, or perform (*praxia*). The person with *apraxia of speech* cannot use the speech muscles to produce understandable speech. The person understands speech and knows what to say. However, the brain cannot coordinate the speech muscles to make the words. Apraxia is caused by damage to the motor speech area in the brain.
- *Dysarthria* means difficult or poor (*dys*) speech (*arthria*). It is caused by damage to the nervous system. Mouth and face muscles are affected. Slurred speech, speaking slowly or softly, hoarseness, and drooling are among the problems that can occur.

To communicate with the speech-impaired person, practice the measures in Box 37-4, p. 622.

Some persons need speech rehabilitation. The goal is to improve the person's ability to communicate. The amount of improvement possible depends on many factors. They include the cause, amount, and area of brain damage and the person's age and health. The person's willingness and ability to learn are other factors. A speech-language pathologist and other health team members help the person:

- Improve affected language skills
- Use remaining abilities
- Restore language abilities to the extent possible
- Learn other methods of communicating
- Strengthen the muscles of speech

Aphasia

Aphasia is the total or partial loss (*a*) of the ability to use or understand language (*phasia*). Aphasia is a language disorder. It results from damage to parts of the brain responsible for language. Stroke, head injury, brain infec-

---

BOX 37-4 Measures to Communicate With the Speech-Impaired Person

THE PERSON
- Ask the person to repeat or rephrase statements if necessary.
- Repeat what the person has said. Ask if your understanding is correct.
- Ask the person to write down key words or the message.
- Ask the person to point, gesture, or draw to communicate key words.

YOU
- Follow the care plan. A consistent approach is needed.
- Provide a calm, quiet setting. Turn off the TV, radio, music, and other distractions.
- Include the person in conversations.
- Listen, and give the person your full attention.
- Use short, simple sentences.
- Repeat what you are saying as needed.
- Write down key words as needed.
- Speak to the person in a normal, adult tone. Do not treat or talk to the adult in a babyish or child-like way.
- Ask the person questions to which you know the answers. This helps you learn how the person speaks.
- Allow the person plenty of time to talk.
- Determine the subject being discussed. This helps you understand main points. Watch the person's lip movements.
- Watch facial expressions, gestures, and body language. They give clues about what is being said.
- Do not correct the person's speech.

BOX 37-5 The Eye: Structures and Functions

Receptors for vision are in the *eyes* (Fig. 37-5). The eye is easily injured. Bones of the skull, eyelids and eyelashes, and tears protect the eyes from injury. The eye has three layers:
- The *sclera*, the white of the eye, is the outer layer. It is made of tough connective tissue.
- The *choroid* is the second layer. Blood vessels, the *ciliary muscle*, and the *iris* make up the choroid. The iris gives the eye its color. The opening in the middle of the iris is the *pupil*. Pupil size varies with the amount of light entering the eye. The pupil constricts (narrows) in bright light. It dilates (widens) in dim or dark places.
- The *retina* is the inner layer. It has receptors for vision and the nerve fibers of the *optic nerve*.

Light enters the eye through the *cornea*. It is the transparent part of the outer layer that lies over the eye. Light rays pass to the *lens*, which lies behind the pupil. The light is then reflected to the retina. Light is carried to the brain by the optic nerve.

The *aqueous chamber* separates the cornea from the lens. The chamber is filled with a fluid called *aqueous humor*. The fluid helps the cornea keep its shape and position. The *vitreous body* is behind the lens. It is a gelatin-like substance that supports the retina and maintains the eye's shape.

---

tions, and cancer are common causes. Most people who have aphasia are middle-aged adults and older.

Expressive aphasia (motor aphasia, Broca's aphasia) relates to difficulty expressing or sending out thoughts. Thinking is clear. The person knows what to say but has difficulty or cannot speak the words. There are problems speaking, spelling, counting, gesturing, or writing. The person may:

▶ Omit small words such as "is," "and," "of," and "the."

▶ Speak in single words or short sentences. For example, the person may say "Walk dog." It can mean "I will take the dog for a walk" or "You take the dog for a walk."

▶ Put words in the wrong order. For example, instead of "bathroom," the person's says "room bath."

▶ Think one thing but say another. For example, the person wants food but asks for a book.

▶ Call people by the wrong names.

▶ Make up words.

▶ Produce sounds and no words.

▶ Cry or swear for no reason.

Receptive aphasia (Wernicke's aphasia) relates to difficulty understanding language. The person has trouble understanding what is said or read. The person may speak in long sentences that have no meaning. Because of difficulty understanding speech, the person may not be aware of his or her mistakes. People and common objects are not recognized. The person may not know how to use a fork, toilet, cup, TV, phone, or other items.

With *expressive aphasia*, the person has difficulty expressing or sending out thoughts. With *receptive aphasia*, the person has difficulty understanding language. Some people have both types. This is called **expressive-receptive aphasia (global aphasia, mixed aphasia)**. The person has problems speaking and understanding language.

The person with aphasia has many emotional needs. Frustration, depression, and anger are common. Communication is needed to function and relate to others. The person wants to communicate but cannot. You need to be patient and kind.

EYE DISORDERS

Vision loss occurs at all ages. Problems range from mild vision loss to complete blindness. **Blind** is the absence of sight. Vision loss is sudden or gradual in onset. One or both eyes are affected. See Box 37-5 for a review of the structures and functions of the eye.

Glaucoma

Glaucoma results in damage to the optic nerve. The eye produces a fluid that nourishes certain structures in the eye. The fluid normally drains from the eye. When the fluid cannot drain properly, fluid builds up in the eye and causes pressure on the optic nerve. The optic nerve is damaged. Vision loss with eventual blindness occurs.

Glaucoma can develop in one or both eyes. Onset is sudden or gradual. Peripheral vision (side vision) is lost. The person sees through a tunnel (Fig. 37-6). Other signs and symptoms vary. They include blurred vision and halos around lights. With sudden onset, the person has severe eye pain, nausea, and vomiting.

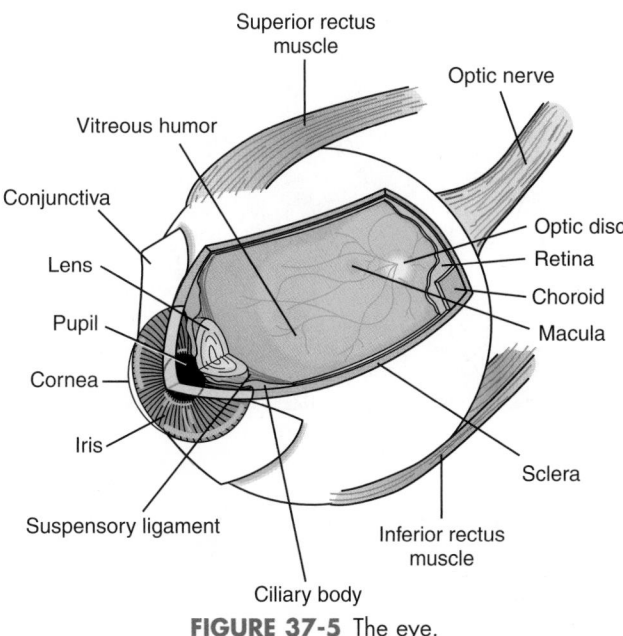

FIGURE 37-5 The eye.

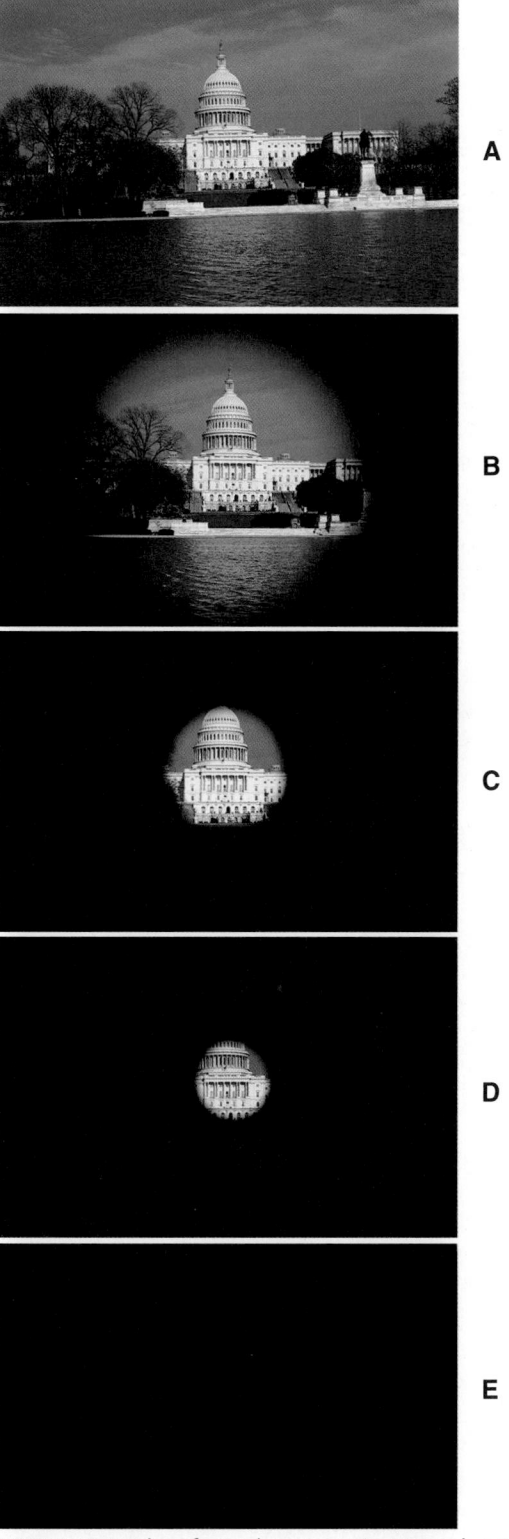

FIGURE 37-6 Vision loss from glaucoma. **A,** Normal vision. **B,** Loss of peripheral vision begins. **C, D,** and **E,** Vision loss continues, with eventual blindness.

Risk Factors

Glaucoma is a leading cause of vision loss in the United States. Persons at risk include:

▶ African Americans over 40 years of age
▶ Everyone over 60 years of age
▶ Those with a family history of the disease
▶ Those who have diabetes, high blood pressure, or heart disease
▶ Those who have eye diseases or eye injuries
▶ Those who have had eye surgery

Treatment

Glaucoma has no cure. Prior damage cannot be reversed. Drugs and surgery can control glaucoma and prevent further damage to the optic nerve.

Cataracts

A cataract is a clouding of the lens in the eye (Fig. 37-7, p. 624). Normally the lens is clear. Cataract comes from the Greek word that means *waterfall*. Trying to see is like looking through a waterfall. A cataract can occur in one or both eyes. Signs and symptoms include:

▶ Cloudy, blurry, or dimmed vision (Fig. 37-8, p. 624).
▶ Colors seem faded. Blues and purples are hard to see.
▶ Sensitivity to light and glares.
▶ Poor vision at night.
▶ Halos around lights.
▶ Double vision in one eye.

Risk Factors

Most cataracts are caused by aging. By age 80, more than 50% of all Americans have a cataract or have had cataract surgery. Diabetes, smoking, alcohol use, and prolong exposure to sunlight are risk factors. So is a family history of cataracts.

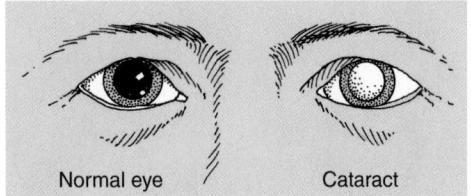

FIGURE 37-7 One eye is normal. The other has a cataract. (From Phipps WJ and others: *Medical-surgical nursing: concepts and clinical practice,* ed 5, St Louis, 1995, Mosby.)

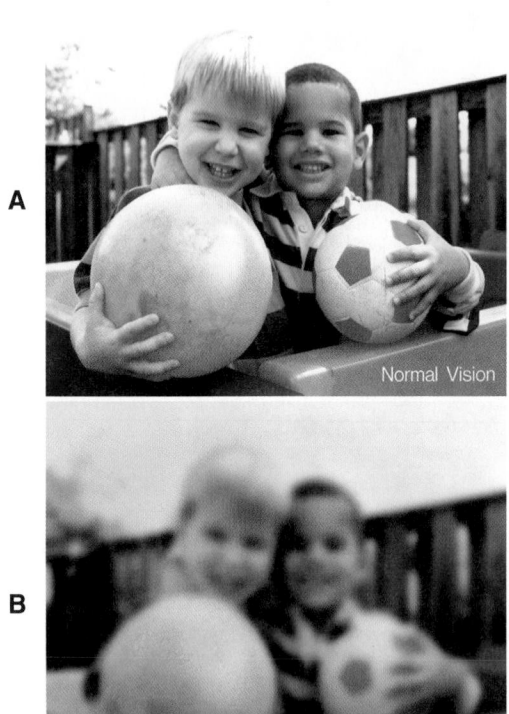

FIGURE 37-8 Vision loss from a cataract. **A,** Normal vision. **B,** Scene viewed with a cataract. (From National Eye Institute: *Cataract: what you should know,* Bethesda, Md, National Institutes of Health.)

Treatment

Surgery is the only treatment. Surgery is done when the cataract starts to interfere with daily activities. Driving, reading, and watching TV are examples.

Surgery involves removing the lens. Then a plastic lens is implanted. Vision improves after surgery. Post-operative care includes the following:

▶ Keep the eye shield or patch in place as directed. Some doctors allow the shield or patch off during the day if eyeglasses are worn. The shield or patch is worn for sleep, including naps.

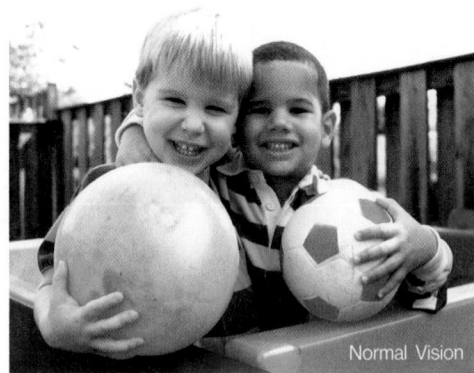

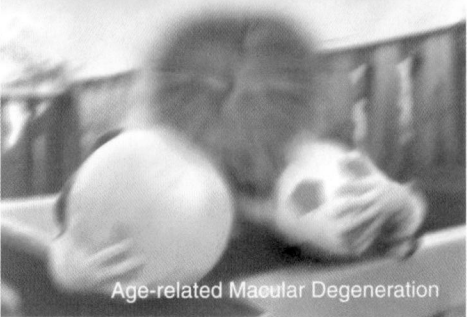

FIGURE 37-9 Vision loss from macular degeneration. **A,** Normal vision. **B,** Central vision is blurred. (From National Eye Institute: *Age-related macular degeneration: what you should know,* Bethesda, Md, National Institutes of Health.)

▶ Follow measures for persons who are visually impaired or blind when an eye shield or patch is worn (p. 626). The person may have vision loss in the other eye.
▶ Remind the person not to rub or press the affected eye.
▶ Do not let the person bend at the waist, pick up objects from the floor, or lift heavy objects. Assist the person with putting on socks or hose and footwear.
▶ Do not bump the eye.
▶ Do not shower or shampoo the person without a doctor's order.
▶ Place the overbed table and the bedside stand on the un-operative side.
▶ Place the signal light within reach.
▶ Report eye drainage or complaints of pain at once.

Age-Related Macular Degeneration

Age-related macular degeneration (AMD) is a disease that blurs central vision. *Central vision* is what you see "straight-ahead." It causes a blind spot in the center of vision (Fig. 37-9). Central vision is needed for reading, sewing, driving, and seeing faces and fine detail.

The disease damages the macula located in the center of the retina. The retina receives light and sends messages to the brain by way of the optic nerve. Normal signals are no longer sent to the brain. The disease is usually gradual in onset. Painless, it is the leading cause of blindness in persons 60 years of age and older.

The two types of AMD are:

▶ *Wet AMD*—Blood vessels behind the retina start to grow under the macula. These blood vessels leak blood and fluid. Loss of central vision occurs quickly. An early symptom is that straight lines appear wavy. Wet AMD is considered advanced. It is more severe than the dry form.

▶ *Dry AMD*—Light-sensitive cells in the macula slowly break down. Central vision in the affected eye gradually blurs. As dry AMD gets worse, a blurred spot is seen in the center of the eye. Central vision is gradually lost. Usually both eyes are affected.

Dry AMD is more common than wet AMD. People who have wet AMD had dry AMD first. Dry AMD can suddenly turn into wet AMD.

Risk Factors

AMD can occur during middle age. However, the risk increases with aging. Besides age, other risk factors include:

▶ Smoking.
▶ Obesity.
▶ Race. Whites are at greater risk than any other group.
▶ Family history. People with a family history of AMD are at higher risk than persons who do not have a family history.
▶ Gender. Women are at greater risk than men.
▶ Light-colored eyes.
▶ Exposure to sunlight.
▶ Cardiovascular disease. This includes high blood pressure, coronary artery disease, and stroke.

Treatment

When dry AMD is advanced, no treatment can prevent vision loss. For wet AMD, some treatments may stop or slow the progress of the disease. They may preserve what is left of the person's central vision. Laser surgery is an example.

The following measures can reduce the risk of AMD:

▶ Eating a healthy diet high in green leafy vegetables and fish
▶ Not smoking
▶ Maintaining a normal blood pressure
▶ Managing cardiovascular diseases
▶ Maintaining a normal weight
▶ Exercising
▶ Wearing sunglasses
▶ Regular eye exams

Diabetic Retinopathy

In diabetic retinopathy, the tiny blood vessels in the retina are damaged. A complication of diabetes, it is a leading cause of blindness. Usually both eyes are affected.

Vision blurs (Fig. 37-10). The person may see spots "floating" in vision. Often there are no early warning signs.

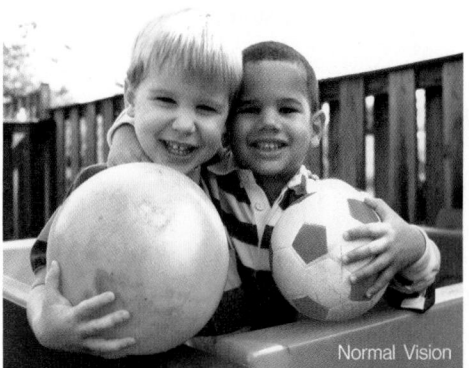
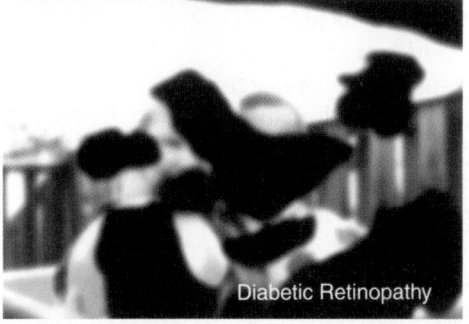

FIGURE 37-10 Vision loss from diabetic retinopathy. **A,** Normal vision. **B,** Vision with diabetic retinopathy. (From National Eye Institute: *Diabetic retinopathy: what you should know,* Bethesda, Md, National Institutes of Health.)

Risk Factors

Everyone with diabetes (Chapter 41) is at risk for diabetic retinopathy.

Treatment

The person needs to control his or her diabetes, blood pressure, and blood cholesterol. Advanced retinopathy is treated with laser surgery. Another surgery involves removing blood from the center of the eye.

The person with diabetic retinopathy may need low vision services.

Low Vision

Low vision is eyesight that cannot be corrected with eyeglasses, contact lenses, drugs, or surgery. Every day tasks are hard to do. Reading, shopping, cooking, watching TV, and writing are examples.

While wearing eyeglasses or contact lenses, the person with low vision has problems:

▶ Recognizing the faces of family and friends
▶ Doing tasks that require close vision—reading, cooking, sewing, and so on
▶ Picking out and matching the color of clothing
▶ Reading signs
▶ Doing things because lighting seems dimmer

Risk Factors

Persons at risk for low vision have:

► Eye diseases
► Glaucoma
► Cataracts
► Age-related macular degeneration
► Diabetes
► Eye injuries
► Birth defects

Treatment

The person learns how to use one or more visual and adaptive devices. The devices used depend on the person's needs. Examples include:

► Prescription reading glasses
► Large-print reading materials
► Magnifying aids for close vision
► Telescopic aids for far vision
► A black-felt tip marker for writing
► Paper with bold lines for writing
► Audio tapes
► Electronic reading machines
► Computer systems using large print
► Computer systems that talk
► Closed-circuit TV
► Phones, clocks, and watches with large numbers
► Phones designed for people who have low vision, are visually impaired, or blind
► Lighting that can be adjusted
► Dark-colored light switches and electrical outlets against light-colored walls
► Motion lights that turn on when the person enters a room

Impaired Vision and Blindness

Birth defects, accidents, and eye diseases are among the many causes of impaired vision and blindness. They also are complications of some diseases. Some people are totally blind. Others sense some light but have no usable vision. Still others have some usable vision but cannot read newsprint. The legally blind persons sees at 20 feet what a person with normal vision sees at 200 feet.

According to the American Foundation for the Blind (AFB), about 1.3 million Americans are legally blind. According to AFB reports, about 5.5 million older persons are blind or visually impaired.

Loss of sight is serious. Adjustments can be hard and long. Special education and training are needed. Moving about, performing daily activities, reading and writing, communicating with others, and using a dog guide are among the tasks the person needs to learn. All are needed for quality of life. So are the practices listed in Box 37-6. The person may need some of the devices used for low vision.

Rehabilitation programs help the person adjust to the vision loss and to learn to be independent. The goal is for the person to be as active as possible and to have quality of life. The person learns how to use visual and adaptive devices, braille, long canes, and dog guides.

See *Focus on Long-Term Care and Home Care: Impaired Vision and Blindness.*

FOCUS ON LONG-TERM CARE AND HOME CARE

Impaired Vision and Blindness

HOME CARE

The practices in Box 37-6 apply in the home setting. A safe setting is needed. Outdoor walks and stairs must be free of toys, ice, and snow. Furniture, closets, drawers, shelves, and other items are arranged to meet the person's needs. Always replace items where you found them; do not rearrange the person's belongings.

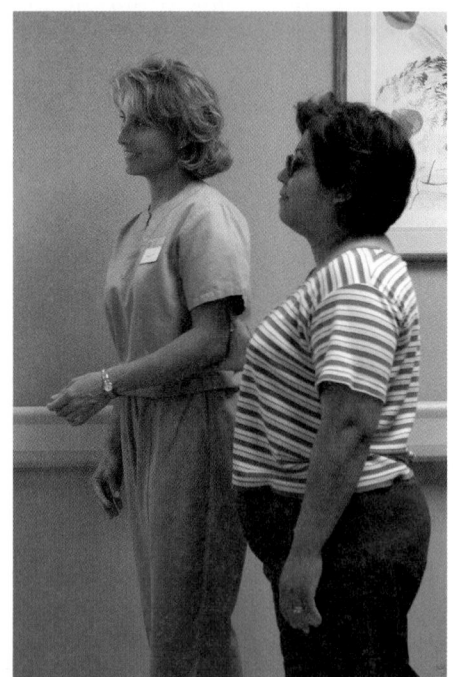

FIGURE 37-11 The blind person walks slightly behind the nursing assistant. She touches the assistant's arm lightly.

BOX 37-6 Caring for Blind and Visually Impaired Persons

THE ENVIRONMENT
- Report worn carpeting and other flooring.
- Keep furniture, equipment, and electrical cords out of areas where the person will walk.
- Keep table and desk chairs pushed in under the table or desk.
- Keep doors fully open or fully closed. This includes room, closet, cabinet, and other doors.
- Keep drawers fully closed.
- Report burnt out bulbs in rooms, lounges, dining areas, hallways, stairways, and other areas.
- Provide lighting as the person prefers. Tell the person when the lights are on or off.
- Adjust window coverings to prevent glares. Sunny days and bright, snowy days cause glares.
- Provide a consistent mealtime setting:
  - Avoid plates, napkins, placemats, and tablecloths with patterns and designs. These items should be solid colors and provide contrast. For example, place a white plate on a dark placemat or tablecloth.
  - Have the person sit in good light above the table where he or she will eat.
  - Place settings are always the same. The knife and spoon are to the right of the plate. The fork and napkin are to the left of the plate. The glass or cup is to the right of the plate if the person is right-handed. It is to the left of the plate if the person is left-handed.
  - Arrange main dishes, side dishes, seasonings, and condiments in a straight line or in a semi-circle just beyond the person's place setting. Arrange things in the same way for each meal.
  - Explain the location of food and beverages. Use the face of a clock (Chapter 23). Or guide the person's hand to each item on the tray or place setting.
  - Cut meat, open containers, butter bread, and perform other tasks as needed.
- Keep the signal light and TV, light, and other controls within the person's reach.
- Turn on night-lights in the person's room and bathroom. Make sure night-lights are on in hallways.
- Practice safety measures to prevent falls (Chapter 12).
- Orient the person to the room. Describe the layout. Also describe the location and purpose of furniture and equipment.
- Let the person move about. Let him or her touch and find furniture and equipment.
- Do not leave the person in the middle of a room. Make sure the person can reach a wall or furniture.
- Do not rearrange furniture and equipment.
- Tell the person when you are coming to a curb or steps. State if the steps are up or down.
- Inform the person of doors, turns, furniture, and other obstructions when assisting with ambulation.
- Complete a safety check before leaving the room. (See the inside of the front book cover.)

THE PERSON
- Have the person use railings when climbing stairs.
- Make sure the person wears comfortable shoes that fit correctly.

- Assist with walking as needed. Have the person lightly hold onto your arm just above the elbow (Fig. 37-11). Tell the person which arm is offered. Have the person walk about a half step behind you. Never push, pull, or guide the person in front of you. Walk at a normal pace.
- Let the person do as much for himself or herself as possible.
- Provide visual and adaptive devices. Follow the care plan.

YOU
- Face the person when speaking. Speak slowly and clearly.
- Use a normal tone of voice. Do not shout or speak loudly. Vision loss does not mean the person has hearing loss.
- Identify yourself when you enter the room. Give your name, title, and reason for being there. Do not touch the person until you have indicated your presence.
- Ask the person how much he or she can see. Do not assume the person is totally blind or that the person has some vision.
- Identify others. Explain where each person is located and what the person is doing.
- Address the person by name. This tells the person that you are directing a comment or question to him or her.
- Speak directly to the person. Do not just talk to family and friends who are present.
- Encourage the person to do as much for himself or herself as possible.
- Feel free to use words such as "see," "look," "read," or "watch TV."
- Feel free to refer to colors, sizes, shapes, patterns, designs, and so on.
- Describe people, places, and things thoroughly. Do not leave out a detail because you do not think it is important.
- Offer to help. Simply say "May I help you?" Respect the person's answer.
- Warn the person of dangers. Provide a calm and clear warning.
- Leave the person's belongings in the same place that you found them. Do not move or rearrange things.
- Greet the person by name when he or she enters a room. Tell the person who you are. Also identify others in the room.
- Listen to the person. Give the person verbal cues that you are listening. Say "yes," "ok," I see," "tell me more," "I don't understand," and so on.
- Answer the person's questions. Provide specific and descriptive responses.
- Give step-by-step explanations of procedures as you perform them. Say when the procedure is over.
- Give specific directions. Say "right behind you," "on your left," or "in front of you." Avoid phrases like "over here" or "over there."
- Tell the person when you are leaving the room or the area. If appropriate, tell the person where you are going. For example, "I'm going to go into your bathroom now."
- Tell the person when you are ending a conversation. For example, "I enjoyed hearing about your children. Thank you for sharing stories with me."
- Guide the person to a seat by placing your guiding arm on the seat. The person will move his or her hand down your arm to the seat.

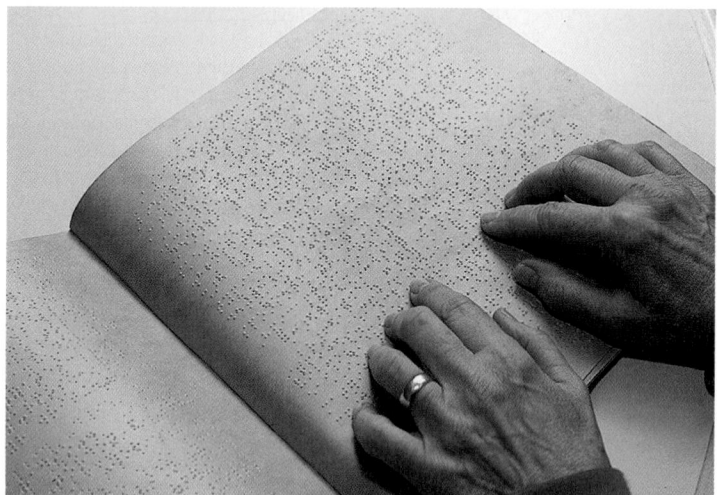

FIGURE 37-12 Braille.

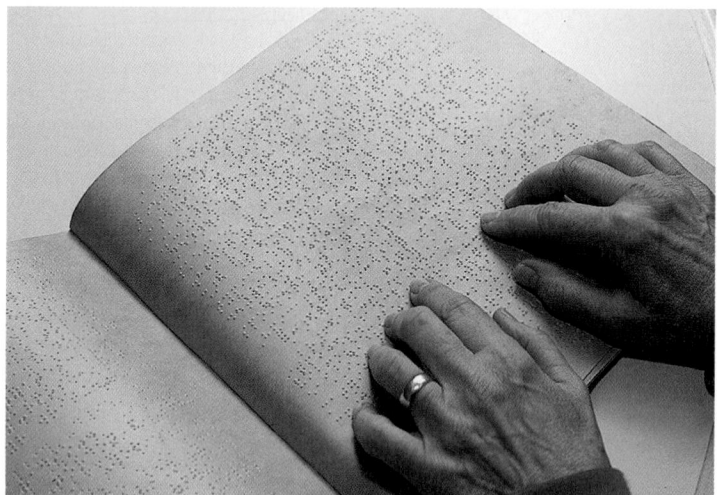

FIGURE 37-13 Braille is read by moving the fingers left to right across the braille lines.

Braille

Braille is a touch reading and writing system that uses raised dots for each letter of the alphabet (Fig. 37-12). The first 10 letters also represent the numbers 0 through 9. The person reads braille by moving the hands from left to right along each line of braille (Fig. 37-13).

Special devices allow computer access. A "braille display" sits on the person's desk. Using braille, the person can read information on the computer display. Braille printers allow the person to print computer information in braille. Braille keyboards also are available.

Mobility

Blind and visually impaired persons learn to move about using a long cane with a red tip or using a dog guide. Both are used worldwide by persons who are blind. The AFB describes them and measures to help as follows:

▶ Long canes are white or silver-grey. Some are a single piece of metal. Others can fold or collapse for storage. To assist a person using a long cane, announce your presence first. Ask if you can assist before trying to help. Do not interfere with the arm used to hold the cane. The person stores his or her cane. If you have to store the cane, tell the person where to find the cane.

▶ The dog guide sees for the person. The dog moves in response to commands from the master. Commands are disobeyed to avoid danger. For example, the master may want to cross the street. The dog guide disobeys the command if a vehicle is approaching. Do not pet, feed, or distract a dog guide. Such actions can place the person in danger.

Corrective Lenses

Eyeglasses and contact lenses can correct many vision problems. Some people wear eyeglasses for reading or seeing at a distance. Others wear them for all activities. Contact lenses are usually worn while awake. Some contacts can be worn day and night for up to 30 days.

◆ *Eyeglasses*

Lenses are hardened glass or plastic. Clean them daily and as needed. Wash glass lenses with warm water. Dry them with a lens cloth or cotton cloth. Plastic lenses scratch easily. Use special cleaning solutions and cloths.

See *Delegation Guidelines: Eyeglasses.*
See *Promoting Safety and Comfort: Eyeglasses.*

DELEGATION GUIDELINES: Eyeglasses

Cleaning eyeglasses is a routine care measure. Do not wait until the nurse tells you to clean them. Clean them daily and as needed.

When you need to clean eyeglasses, find out if a special cleaning solution is needed. Then follow the manufacturer's instructions.

PROMOTING SAFETY AND COMFORT: Eyeglasses

SAFETY
Eyeglasses are costly. Protect them from loss or damage. When not worn, put them in their case. Place the case in the top drawer of the bedside stand or in the drawer of the overbed table.

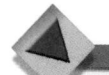

CARING FOR EYEGLASSES

✔ Quality of Life *Remember to:*

- Knock before entering the person's room.
- Address the person by name.
- Introduce yourself by name and title.
- Explain the procedure to the person before beginning and during the procedure.

- Protect the person's rights during the procedure.
- Handle the person gently during the procedure.

PRE-PROCEDURE

1 Follow *Delegation Guidelines: Eyeglasses.* See *Promoting Safety and Comfort: Eyeglasses.*
2 Practice hand hygiene.

3 Collect the following:
- Eyeglass case
- Cleaning solution or warm water
- Disposable lens cloth or cotton cloth

PROCEDURE

4 Remove the eyeglasses.
  a Hold the frames in front of the ear on both sides (Fig. 34-14, *A*, p. 630).
  b Lift the frames from the ears. Bring the eyeglasses down away from the face (Fig. 37-14, *B*, p. 630).
5 Clean the lenses with cleaning solution or warm water. Clean in a circular motion. Dry the lenses with the cloth.
6 If the person will not wear the eyeglasses:
  a Open the eyeglass case.
  b Fold the eyeglasses. Put them in the case. Do not touch the clean lenses.

  c Place the eyeglass case in the top drawer of the bedside stand. Or put it in the drawer of the overbed table.
7 If the person will wear the eyeglasses:
  a Unfold the eyeglasses.
  b Hold the frames at each side. Place them over the ears.
  c Adjust the eyeglasses so the nosepiece rests on the nose.
  d Return the eyeglass case to the top drawer in the bedside stand. Or put it in the drawer of the overbed table.

POST-PROCEDURE

8 Provide for comfort. (See the inside of the front book cover.)
9 Place the signal light within reach.
10 Return the cleaning solution to its proper place.
11 Discard the disposable cloth.

12 Complete a safety check of the room. (See the inside of the front book cover.)
13 Decontaminate your hands.
14 Report and record your observations.

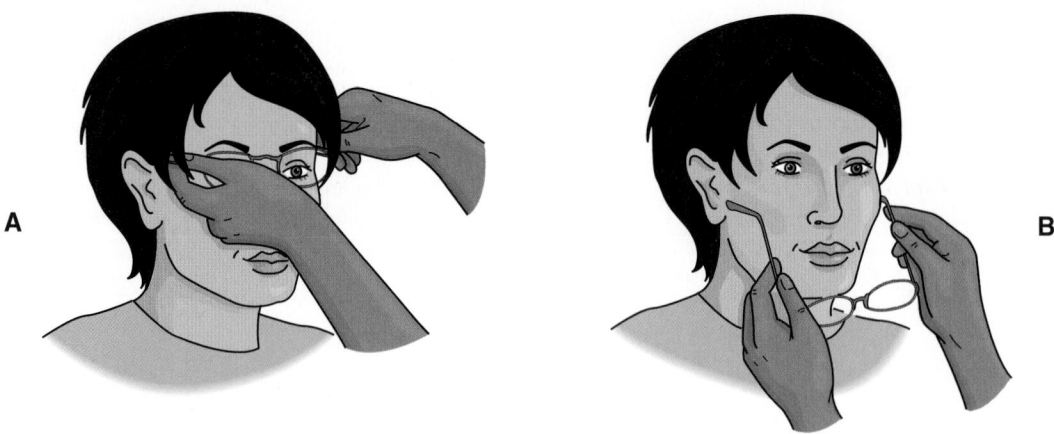

FIGURE 37-14 Removing eyeglasses. **A,** Hold the frames in the front of the ear on both sides. **B,** Lift the frames from the ears. Bring the eyeglasses down away from the face.

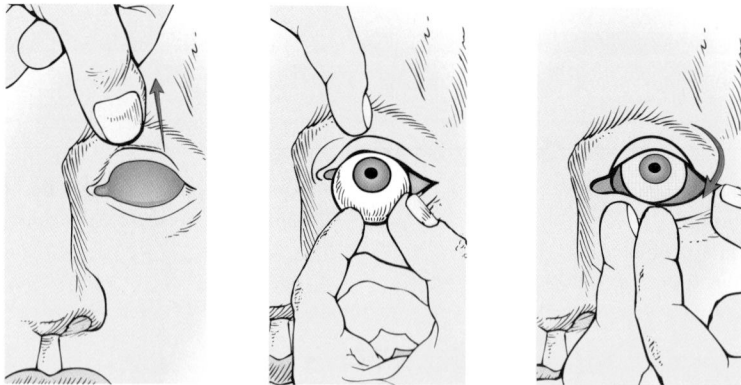

FIGURE 37-15 An ocular prosthesis is inserted. (From Lewis SM, Heitkemper MM, Dirksen SR: *Medical-surgical nursing: assessment and management of clinical problems,* ed 5, St Louis, 2000, Mosby.)

PROMOTING SAFETY AND COMFORT: Contact Lenses

SAFETY

Some agencies let nursing assistants remove and insert contact lenses. Others do not. Know your agency's policies. If allowed to insert and remove contacts, follow the agency's procedures.

Contact Lenses

Contact lenses fit on the eye. There are hard and soft contacts. Disposable lenses are discarded daily, weekly, or monthly. Contacts are cleaned, removed, and stored according to the manufacturer's instructions.

Report and record the following observations:
▶ Eye redness or irritation
▶ Eye drainage
▶ Complaints of eye pain, blurred or fuzzy vision, uncomfortable lenses
See *Promoting Safety and Comfort: Contact Lenses.*

Artificial Eyes

Removal of an eyeball is sometimes done because of injury or disease. The person is fitted with an ocular (eye) prosthesis (Fig. 37-15). It matches the other eye in color and shape. The person cannot see out of the artificial eye. The other eye may have normal, some, or no vision.

Some prostheses are permanent implants. Others are removable. If removable, the person may be taught to remove, clean, and insert it. This depends on the type of prosthesis and the person's needs.

PROMOTING SAFETY AND COMFORT: Artificial Eyes

SAFETY

When an artificial eye is removed, you must prevent chips and scratches. It must not fall on the floor or other hard surface. Always hold the eye over a towel or other soft surface.

The prosthesis is the person's property. Protect it from loss or damage.

See *Promoting Safety and Comfort: Artificial Eyes.*

Follow these measures if the eye is not inserted after removal:

▸ Wash the prosthesis with mild soap and warm water. Rinse well.
▸ Line a container with a soft cloth or 4 × 4 gauze. This prevents scratches and damage to the prosthesis.
▸ Fill the container with sterile water or saline (salt) solution.
▸ Place the prosthesis in the container. Close the container.
▸ Label the container with the person's name and room and bed number.
▸ Place the labeled container in the top drawer of the bedside stand.
▸ Wash the eye socket with warm water or saline. Use a washcloth or gauze square. Remove excess moisture with a gauze square.
▸ Wash the eyelid and eyelashes with warm water. Clean from the inner to the outer aspect of the eye (Chapter 19). Dry the eyelid.
▸ Rinse the eye with sterile water before the person inserts the eye.

REVIEW QUESTIONS

Circle the BEST answer.

1 A person with Menière's disease has
   a A middle ear infection
   b Vertigo
   c A hearing aid to correct the problem
   d A speech problem

2 Care of the person with Menière's disease includes preventing
   a Infection
   b Falls
   c Pain
   d Deafness

3 Which is *not* an obvious sign of hearing loss?
   a Loneliness and boredom
   b Speaking too loudly
   c Asking to repeat things
   d Answering questions poorly

4 You are talking to a person with hearing loss. You should do the following *except*
   a Speak clearly, distinctly, and slowly
   b Sit or stand in good light
   c Shout
   d Stand or sit on the side of the better ear

5 You are talking to a person with hearing loss. You can do the following *except*
   a State the topic
   b Change the subject if the person does not seem to understand
   c Use short sentences and simple words
   d Write out key words and names

6 A person wears a hearing aid. The hearing aid
   a Corrects the hearing problem
   b Makes sounds louder
   c Makes speech clearer
   d Lowers background noise

7 A person's hearing aid does not seem to be working. Your *first* action is to
   a See if it is turned on
   b Wash it with soap and water
   c Have it repaired
   d Remove the batteries

8 A person has aphasia. You know that
   a The person cannot use the muscles of speech
   b Mouth and face muscles are affected
   c The person has a language disorder
   d The person cannot speak

9 A person with receptive aphasia has trouble
   a Talking
   b Writing
   c Understanding messages
   d Using gestures

10 A person has a speech disorder. You should do the following *except*
   a Correct the person's speech
   b Have the person write key words
   c Ask the person to repeat or rephrase when necessary
   d Watch lip movements

Continued

11 A person has a cataract. Which is *false?*
  a Vision is cloudy, blurry, or dimmed.
  b Colors seem faded.
  c Central vision is lost.
  d The person is sensitive to light and glares.

12 A person had cataract surgery. You should do the following *except*
  a Follow measures for blind or visually impaired persons if an eye shield or patch is worn
  b Let the person bend to put on socks and shoes
  c Place the overbed table on the un-operative side
  d Have the person wear an eye shield or patch during naps

13 A person has age-related macular degeneration. Which is *true?*
  a There is a blind spot in the center of the eye.
  b Lost vision can be restored with surgery.
  c Peripheral (side) vision is lost.
  d Vision is blurry with spots.

14 These statements are about low vision. Which is *false?*
  a The person has usable vision.
  b Eyesight can be corrected.
  c The person needs visual or adaptive devices.
  d The person has problems doing things that require close vision.

15 You are caring for the following persons. Who is at risk for low vision?
  a The person with diabetic retinopathy
  b The person with global aphasia
  c The person with Menière's disease
  d The person who is blind

16 A person is not wearing eyeglasses. They should be
  a Soaked in a cleansing solution
  b Kept within the person's reach
  c Put in the eyeglass case
  d Placed on the overbed table

17 Braille involves
  a A long cane for walking
  b Raised dots arranged for letters of the alphabet
  c A dog guide
  d Special computers and printers

18 Which presents dangers to persons who are blind or visually impaired?
  a Drawers that are fully closed
  b Doors that are fully open
  c Burnt out bulbs
  d Night-lights

19 A person is blind. The person's mealtime setting should
  a Be the same for every meal
  b Provide variety for mental stimulation
  c Include plates, napkins, and placemats with designs
  d Be arranged like the face of a clock

20 A person is blind. You should do the following *except*
  a Identify yourself
  b Move equipment and furniture to provide variety
  c Explain procedures step by step
  d Have the person walk behind you

21 You are talking to a person who is blind or visually impaired. You should
  a Face the person when talking to him or her
  b Avoid words such as "see" and "look"
  c Avoid using colors when describing things
  d Assume that the person has no sight

22 You are giving directions to a blind person. You can say
  a "Over there."
  b "Right here."
  c "Across the room."
  d "On your left."

Answers to these questions are on p. 781.

Cancer, Immune System, and Skin Disorders

OBJECTIVES

- Define the key terms and key abbreviations listed in this chapter
- Explain the difference between benign tumors and cancer
- Identify cancer risk factors
- Identify the signs and symptoms of cancer
- Explain the common cancer treatments
- Describe the needs of a person with cancer
- Explain how immune system disorders occur
- Describe the common immune system disorders
- Explain how the human immunodeficiency virus is spread
- Identify the signs and symptoms of acquired immunodeficiency syndrome
- Explain how to assist in the care of persons with acquired immunodeficiency syndrome
- Describe the causes, signs and symptoms, and treatment of shingles

KEY TERMS

benign tumor A tumor that does not spread to other body parts; it can grow to a large size

cancer Malignant tumor

malignant tumor A tumor that invades and destroys nearby tissue and can spread to other body parts; cancer

metastasis The spread of cancer to other body parts

stomatitis Inflammation (itis) of the mouth (stomat)

tumor A new growth of abnormal cells; tumors are benign or malignant

KEY ABBREVIATIONS

AIDS Acquired immunodeficiency syndrome

HIV Human immunodeficiency virus

Understanding cancer and immune system and skin disorders gives meaning to the required care. Refer to Chapter 8 while you study this chapter.

CANCER

Cells reproduce for tissue growth and repair. Cells divide in an orderly way. Sometimes cell division and growth are out of control. A mass or clump of cells develops. This new growth of abnormal cells is called a **tumor.** Tumors are benign or malignant (Fig. 38-1):

▸ **Malignant tumors (cancer)** invade and destroy nearby tissue (Fig. 38-2). They can spread to other body parts. They may be life-threatening. Sometimes they grow back after removal.

▸ **Benign tumors** do not spread to other body parts. They can grow to a large size, but rarely threaten life. They usually do not grow back when removed.

Metastasis is the spread of cancer to other body parts (Fig. 38-3). Cancer cells break off the tumor and travel to other body parts. New tumors grow in other body parts. This occurs if cancer is not treated and controlled.

Cancer can occur almost anywhere. Common sites are the skin, lung and bronchus, colon and rectum, breast, prostate, uterus, ovary, urinary bladder, kidney, mouth and pharynx, pancreas, and thyroid gland. Cancer is the second leading cause of death in the United States.

See *Focus on Children and Older Persons: Cancer.*

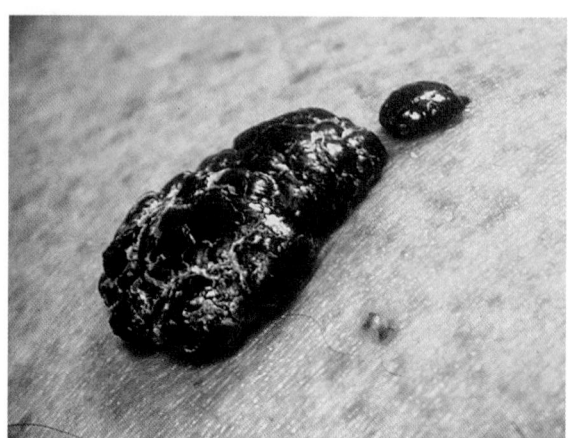

FIGURE 38-2 Malignant tumor on the skin. (From Belcher AE: *Cancer nursing,* St Louis, 1992, Mosby.)

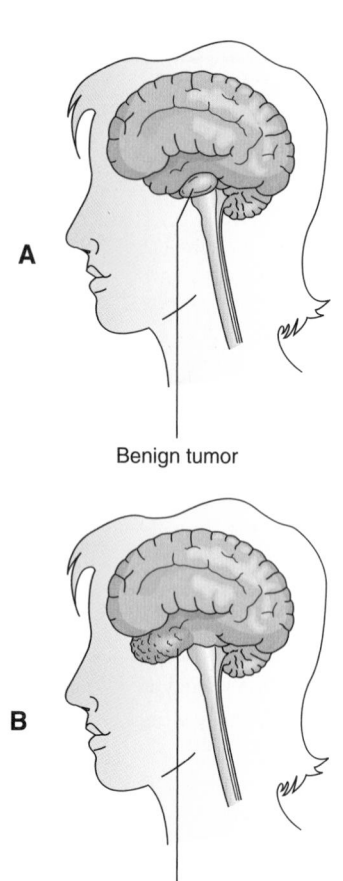

FIGURE 38-1 Tumors. **A,** A benign tumor grows within a local area. **B,** A malignant tumor invades other tissues.

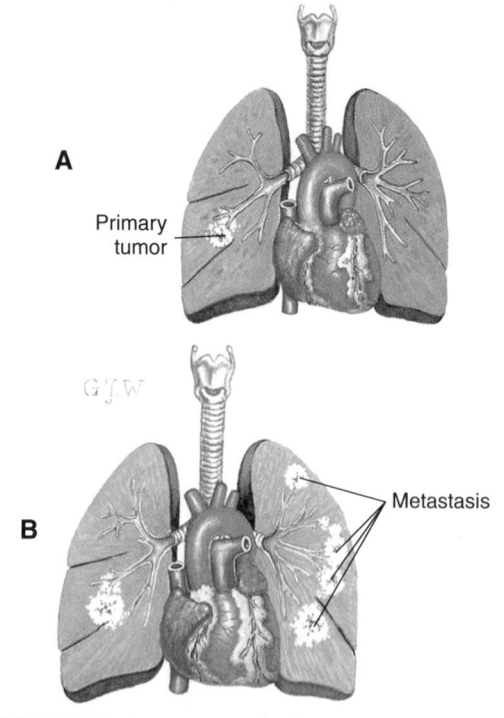

FIGURE 38-3 A, Tumor in the lung. **B,** Tumor has metastasized to the other lung. (Modified from Belcher AE: *Cancer nursing,* St Louis, 1992, Mosby.)

FOCUS ON CHILDREN AND OLDER PERSONS

Cancer

CHILDREN

Sites of cancer in children are the same as for adults. However, some cancers are more common in children. They include:

- Leukemia—a cancer of the blood. It develops in the bone marrow. The bone marrow is a spongy substance found inside bones. Blood cells are made in the bone marrow. Leukemia is the most common form of childhood cancer.
- Brain tumors.
- Lymphomas—tumors of the lymph tissue.
- Bone cancers.
- Liver cancers.
- Kidney cancers.
- Cancer of nerve cells.

Childhood cancers often occur suddenly. Often there are no symptoms. Childhood cancers have a high cure rate.

Risk Factors

Certain factors increase the risk of cancer. The National Cancer Institute describes these risk factors:

- *Growing older.* Cancer occurs in all age-groups. However, most cancers occur in persons over 65 years of age.
- *Tobacco.* This includes using tobacco (smoking, snuff, and chewing tobacco) and being around tobacco (second-hand smoke). This risk can be avoided.
- *Sunlight.* Sun, sunlamps, and tanning booths cause early aging of the skin and skin damage. These can lead to skin cancer. Time in the sun should be limited. Sunlamps and tanning booths should be avoided.
- *Ionizing radiation.* This can cause cell damage that leads to cancer. X-rays are one source. So is radon gas that forms in the soil and some rocks. People who work in mines are at risk for radon exposure. Radon is found in homes in some parts of the country. Radioactive fallout is another source. It can come from nuclear power plant accidents. It also can come from the production, testing, or use of atomic weapons.
- *Certain chemicals and other substances.* Painters, construction workers, and those in the chemical industry are at risk. Household substances also carry risks—paint, pesticides, used engine oil, and other chemicals.
- *Some viruses and bacteria.* Being infected with certain viruses increases the risk of the following cancers—cervical, liver, lymphoma, leukemia, Kaposi's sarcoma (a cancer associated with AIDS, p. 637), stomach.
- *Certain hormones.* Hormone replacement therapy for menopause may increase the risk of breast cancer. Diethylstilbestrol (DES), a form of estrogen, was given to some pregnant women between the early 1940s and 1971. Women who took the drug are at risk for breast cancer. Their daughters are at risk for a certain type of cervical cancer.
- *Family history of cancer.* Certain cancers tend to occur in families. They include melanoma and cancers of the breast, ovary, prostate, and colon.
- *Alcohol.* The risk of certain cancers increases with more than two drinks a day. Such cancers are of the mouth, throat, esophagus, larynx, liver, and breast. Women should have no more than one drink a day. Men should have no more than two drinks a day.
- *Poor diet, lack of physical activity, and being overweight.* A high fat diet increases the risk of cancers of the colon, uterus, and prostate. Lack of physical activity and being overweight increase the risk for cancers of the breast, colon, esophagus, kidney, and uterus.

Treatment

If detected early, cancer can be treated and controlled (Box 38-1). Treatment depends on the type of tumor, its site and size, and if it has spread. The goal of cancer treatment may be one of the following:

- Cure the cancer
- Control the disease
- Reduce symptoms for as long as possible

Some cancers respond to one type of treatment. Others respond best to two or more types. Cancer treatments also damage healthy cells and tissues. Side effects depend on the type and extent of the treatment.

Surgery

Surgery removes tumors. It is done to cure or control cancer. It also relieves pain from advanced cancer.

The person has some pain after surgery. The pain is controlled with pain-relief drugs. The person may feel weak or tired for a while. Some surgeries are very disfiguring. Self-esteem and body image are affected.

Radiation Therapy

Radiation therapy also is called *radiotherapy.* It kills cells. X-ray beams are aimed at the tumor. Sometimes radioactive material is implanted in or near the tumor.

Cancer cells and normal cells receive radiation. Both are destroyed. Radiation therapy:

- Destroys certain tumors.
- Shrinks a tumor before surgery.
- Destroys cancer cells that remain in an area after surgery.
- Controls tumor growth to prevent or relieve pain.

BOX 38-1 Some Signs and Symptoms of Cancer

- Thickening or lump in the breast or any other part of the body
- New mole or an obvious change in an existing mole
- A sore that does not heal
- Hoarseness or cough that does not go away
- Changes in bowel or bladder habits
- Discomfort after eating
- A hard time swallowing
- Weight gain or loss with no known reason
- Unusual bleeding or discharge
- Feeling weak or very tired

From National Cancer Institute: *What you need to know about cancer: an overview,* NIH Publication No. 05-1566, Bethesda Md, revised February, 2005, reprinted July, 2006.

Side effects depend on the body part being treated. Burns, skin breakdown, and hair loss can occur at the treatment site. The doctor may order special skin care measures. Fatigue is common. Extra rest is needed. Discomfort, nausea and vomiting, diarrhea, and loss of appetite (*anorexia*) are other side effects.

Chemotherapy

Chemotherapy involves drugs that kill cells. It is used to:
▶ Shrink a tumor before surgery.
▶ Kill cells that break off the tumor. The goal is to prevent metastasis.
▶ Relieve symptoms caused by the cancer.

Cancer cells and normal cells are affected. Side effects depend on the drug used:
▶ Hair loss (*alopecia*).
▶ Gastrointestinal irritation. Poor appetite, nausea, vomiting, and diarrhea can occur. **Stomatitis**, an inflammation (*itis*) of the mouth (*stomat*), may occur.
▶ Decreased production of blood cells. Bleeding and infection are risks. The person may feel weak and tired.

Hormone Therapy

Hormone therapy prevents cancer cells from getting or using hormones needed for their growth. Drugs are given that prevent the production of certain hormones. Organs or glands that produce a certain hormone are removed. For example, a breast cancer might need estrogen for growth. Then the ovaries are removed. A prostate cancer may need testosterone for growth. Then the testicles may be removed.

Side effects include fatigue, fluid retention, weight gain, hot flashes, nausea and vomiting, appetite changes, and blood clots. Fertility is affected in men and women. Men also may experience impotence (Chapter 46) and loss of sexual desire.

Biological Therapy

Biological therapy (*immunotherapy*) helps the immune system fight the cancer. It also protects the body from the side effects of cancer treatments.

Side effects include flu-like symptoms—chills, fever, muscle aches, weakness, loss of appetite, nausea, vomiting, and diarrhea. Bleeding, bruising, and swelling may occur. So can skin rashes.

The Person's Needs

Persons with cancer have many needs. They include:
▶ Pain relief or control
▶ Rest and exercise
▶ Fluids and nutrition
▶ Preventing skin breakdown
▶ Preventing bowel problems (Constipation occurs from pain-relief drugs. Diarrhea occurs from some cancer treatments.)
▶ Dealing with treatment side effects
▶ Psychological and social needs
▶ Spiritual needs
▶ Sexual needs

Psychological and social needs are great. Anger, fear, and depression are common. Some surgeries are disfiguring. The person may feel unwhole, unattractive, or unclean. The person and family need support.

Talk to the person. Do not avoid the person because you are uncomfortable. Cancer is not contagious. Use touch and listening to show that you care. Often the person needs to talk and have someone listen. Being there when needed is important. You may not have to say anything. Just listen.

Spiritual needs are important. A spiritual leader may provide comfort. To many people, spiritual needs are just as important as physical needs.

Persons dying of cancer often receive hospice care (Chapters 1 and 50). Support is given to the person and family.

IMMUNE SYSTEM DISORDERS

The immune system protects the body from microbes, cancer cells, and other harmful substances. The immune system defends against threats inside and outside the body.

Immune system disorders occur when there is a problem with the immune response. The response may be inappropriate, too strong, or lacking. *Autoimmune disorders* can occur. The immune system can cause disease by attacking the body's own (*auto*) normal cells, tissues, or organs. One of the following may occur:
▶ One or more types of body tissues are destroyed.
▶ An organ grows abnormally.
▶ There is a change in how an organ functions.

The organs and tissues commonly affected are:
▶ Red blood cells
▶ Blood vessels
▶ Connective tissue
▶ The endocrine glands (thyroid gland, pancreas)
▶ Muscles
▶ Joints
▶ Skin

Common autoimmune disorders include:
▶ *Graves' disease*—the most common form of hyperthyroidism. The immune system attacks the thyroid gland. The thyroid gland produces excess (*hyper*) amounts of the hormone thyroxine. Signs and symptoms include anxiety, problems sleeping, rapid heart rate, weight loss, and bulging of the eyeballs (Fig. 38-4).
▶ *Lupus*—an inflammatory disease affecting the blood cells, joints, skin, kidneys, lungs, heart, or brain. Lupus comes from the Latin word that means *wolf*. It was thought that the rash of lupus looked like a wolf bite (Fig. 38-5).
▶ *Multiple sclerosis* (Chapter 39)
▶ *Rheumatoid arthritis* (Chapter 39)
▶ *Type 1 diabetes* (Chapter 41)

Signs and symptoms depend on the type of disease. Fatigue, dizziness, not feeling well, and fever are common.

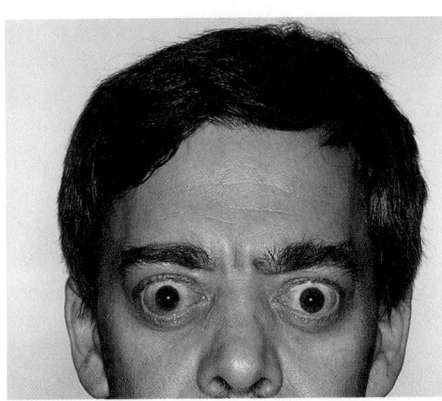

FIGURE 38-4 Bulging of the eyes occurs in Graves' disease. (From Belchetz PE, Hammond P: *Diabetes and endocrinology,* London, 2003, Mosby.)

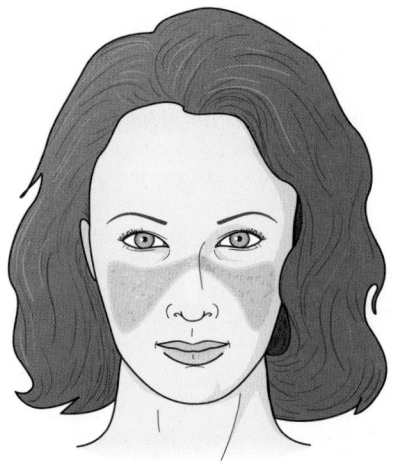

FIGURE 38-5 The rash from lupus is across the nose and cheeks. (Redrawn from National Institute of Arthritis and Musculoskeletal and Skin Diseases: *Do I have lupus?* Bethesda Md, National Institutes of Health.)

Most autoimmune disorders are chronic. Treatment depends on the type of disorder and the tissues and organs affected. Treatment is aimed at:

▶ Reducing symptoms
▶ Controlling the autoimmune response
▶ Maintaining the body's ability to fight disease

Acquired Immunodeficiency Syndrome

Acquired immunodeficiency syndrome (AIDS) is caused by a virus. The virus is called the *human immunodeficiency virus (HIV)*. It attacks the immune system. Therefore it destroys the body's ability to fight infections and certain cancers. Some infections are life-threatening.

The virus is spread through body fluids—blood, semen, vaginal secretions, and breast milk. HIV is not spread by saliva, tears, sweat, sneezing, coughing, insects, or causal contact. The virus is transmitted mainly by:

▶ Unprotected anal, vaginal, or oral sex with an infected person ("Unprotected" is without a new latex or polyurethane condom.)
▶ Needle and syringe sharing among IV drug users
▶ HIV-infected mothers before or during childbirth
▶ HIV-infected mothers through breast-feeding

The virus enters the bloodstream through the rectum, vagina, penis, mouth, or skin breaks. Small breaks in the vagina or rectum may occur when the penis, finger, or other objects are inserted. Gum disease can cause breaks in the gums. The virus can enter the bloodstream through these mucous membrane breaks (mouth, vagina, rectum). Breaks in the skin pose a risk. The virus can enter the bloodstream when infected body fluids come in contact with open skin areas. Babies can become infected during pregnancy, shortly after birth, or from breast-feeding.

The virus is carried in contaminated blood left in needles or syringes. When the devices are shared, contaminated blood enters the bloodstream. Needle-sticks pose a threat to the health team.

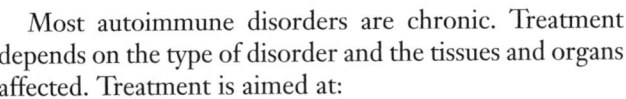

BOX 38-2 Signs and Symptoms of AIDS

- Appetite: loss of
- Cough
- Depression
- Diarrhea lasting more than a week
- Energy: lack of
- Fever
- Headache
- Memory loss, confusion, and forgetfulness
- Mouth or tongue:
  - Brown, red, pink, or purple spots or blotches
  - Sores or white patches
- Night sweats
- Pneumonia
- Shortness of breath
- Skin:
  - Rashes or flaky skin
  - Brown, red, pink, or purple spots or blotches on the skin, eyelids, or nose
- Swallowing: painful or difficult
- Swollen glands: neck, underarms, and groin
- Tiredness: may be extreme
- Vision loss
- Weight loss

The virus is very fragile. It cannot live outside the body. HIV is not spread by casual, everyday contact. Such contact includes using public telephones, restrooms, swimming pools, hot tubs, or water fountains. Other forms of casual contact include talking to, hugging, or dancing with an infected person. HIV is not transmitted by food prepared by the infected person.

Box 38-2 lists the signs and symptoms of AIDS. Some persons infected with HIV have symptoms within a few months. Others are symptom-free for more than 10 years. However, they carry the virus. They can spread it to others.

BOX 38-3 Caring for the Person With AIDS

- Practice Standard Precautions.
- Follow the Bloodborne Pathogen Standard.
- Provide daily hygiene. Avoid irritating soaps.
- Provide oral hygiene according to the care plan. A toothbrush with soft bristles is best.
- Provide oral fluids as ordered.
- Measure and record intake and output.
- Measure weight daily.
- Encourage deep-breathing and coughing exercises as ordered.
- Prevent pressure ulcers.
- Assist with range-of-motion exercises and ambulation as ordered.
- Encourage self-care as able. The person may need assistive devices (walker, commode, eating devices).
- Encourage the person to be as active as possible.
- Change linens and garments as often as needed when fever or night sweats are present.
- Be a good listener. Provide emotional support.

FOCUS ON CHILDREN AND OLDER PERSONS

Acquired Immunodeficiency Syndrome

OLDER PERSONS

Persons age 45 years and older are at risk. The Centers for Disease Control and Prevention (CDC) estimated that through 2005, there were over 221,000 cases of AIDS in persons age 45 years and older.

- *Ages 45 to 54—over 159,600 cases*
- *Ages 55 to 64—over 46,900 cases*
- *Ages 65 and older—14,500 cases*

Older persons get and spread HIV through sexual contact and IV drug use. However, many do not consider themselves to be at risk. Older persons tend to be less informed about the disease. And they tend not to practice safe sex. A blood transfusion between 1978 and 1985 increases the risk of HIV.

Aging and some diseases can mask the signs and symptoms of AIDS. Older persons are less likely to be tested for HIV/AIDS. Often the person dies without the disease being diagnosed. You must follow Standard Precautions and the Bloodborne Pathogen Standard.

The person with AIDS can develop other health problems. The immune system is damaged. Pneumonia, tuberculosis, Kaposi's sarcoma (a cancer), and nervous system damage are risks. Memory loss, loss of coordination, paralysis, mental health disorders, and dementia signal nervous system damage.

Many new drugs help slow the spread of HIV in the body. They also reduce complications and prolong life. AIDS has no vaccine and no cure at present. It is a life-threatening disease.

You may care for persons with AIDS or those who are HIV carriers (Box 38-3). You may have contact with the person's blood or body fluids. Protect yourself and others from the virus. Follow Standard Precautions and the Bloodborne Pathogen Standard. A person may have the HIV virus but no symptoms. In some persons, HIV or AIDS is not yet diagnosed.

See *Focus on Children and Older Persons: Acquired Immunodeficiency Syndrome*.

SKIN DISORDERS

There are many types of skin disorders. Alopecia, hirsutism, dandruff, lice, and scabies are discussed in Chapter 20. Skin tears and pressure ulcers are discussed in Chapter 32. Burns are discussed in Chapter 49. Shingles is discussed here.

Shingles

Shingles (*herpes zoster*) is caused by the same virus that causes chickenpox. The virus lies dormant in nerve tissue. (*Dormant* means to be *inactive*.) The virus can become active years later.

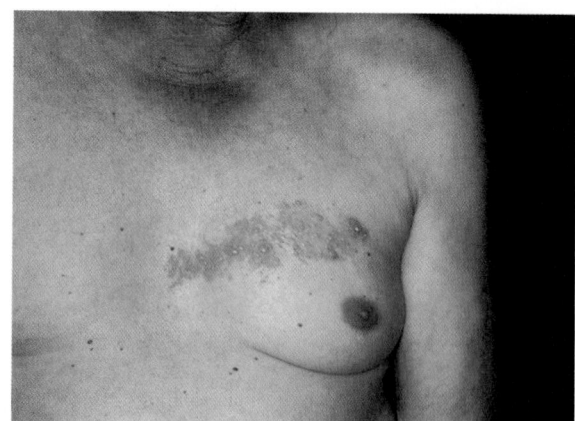

FIGURE 38-6 Shingles. (Courtesy of the Department of Dermatology, School of Medicine, University of Utah.)

The person has a rash or blisters on the skin. At first the person has a burning or tingling pain, numbness, or itching. This occurs in an area on one side of the body or one side of the face. After a few days or a week, a rash with fluid-filled blisters appears (Fig. 38-6). The person has mild to intense pain. Itching is a common complaint.

Shingles is most common in persons over 50 years of age. Persons who have had chickenpox are at risk. So are persons with weakened immune systems from HIV infection, cancer treatments, transplant surgeries, and stress.

The doctor orders anti-viral drugs and drugs for pain relief. For many healthy people, the blisters heal and pain is gone in 3 to 5 weeks. A vaccine is now available to prevent shingles.

REVIEW QUESTIONS

Circle the BEST answer.

1. A person has cancer. You know that
   a. The tumor will not threaten life
   b. The tumor can spread to other body parts
   c. The tumor is benign
   d. The person's mouth is inflamed

2. Which person has the greatest risk for cancer?
   a. The person who smokes
   b. The person who is physically active
   c. The person who limits time in the sun
   d. The person who is 40 years old

3. Which is *not* a warning sign of cancer?
   a. Painful, swollen joints
   b. A sore that does not heal
   c. Unusual bleeding or discharge
   d. Discomfort after eating

4. A person had surgery for cancer. The person's care will likely include
   a. Pain-relief measures
   b. Mouth care for stomatitis
   c. Skin care for burns at the treatment site
   d. Measures to prevent hair loss

5. A person receiving chemotherapy will likely experience
   a. Diarrhea
   b. Burns
   c. Skin breakdown
   d. Weight gain

6. Mrs. Jones has cancer. She is telling you about her treatments and how she feels. What should you do?
   a. Listen
   b. Change the subject
   c. Call for the nurse
   d. Ask about her feelings

7. HIV is spread through
   a. Body fluids
   b. Coughing and sneezing
   c. Using public telephones and restrooms
   d. Hugging or dancing with an infected person

8. HIV can enter the bloodstream in the following ways *except*
   a. Through gum disease
   b. Through the rectum, vagina, penis, mouth, or skin breaks
   c. Through needle-sharing
   d. Through swimming pools and hot tubs used by infected persons

9. Which of the following is used to prevent the spread of HIV and AIDS?
   a. Isolation Precautions
   b. Radiation therapy
   c. Chemotherapy
   d. Standard Precautions

10. A person has shingles. You will likely assist the nurse with measures to
    a. Prevent diarrhea
    b. Relieve pain
    c. Prevent skin breakdown
    d. Prevent weight loss

Circle T if the statement is true and F if the statement is false.

11. T F Cancer can occur suddenly in children without symptoms.

12. T F Cancer treatments damage healthy cells and tissues.

13. T F A person has an autoimmune disorder. The person's body has attacked its own cells, tissues, or organs.

14. T F Autoimmune disorders commonly affect the heart.

15. T F Autoimmune disorders are usually chronic.

16. T F A person infected with HIV does not have signs and symptoms. The person can spread the virus to others.

Answers to these questions are on p. 781.

Nervous System and Musculoskeletal System Disorders

OBJECTIVES

- Define the key terms and key abbreviations listed in this chapter
- Describe stroke and the care required
- Describe Parkinson's disease and the care required
- Describe multiple sclerosis and the care required
- Describe amyotrophic lateral sclerosis and the care required
- Describe head injury and spinal cord injury and the care required
- Describe autonomic dysreflexia and the care required
- Describe arthritis and the care required
- Explain how to assist in the care of persons after total joint replacement surgery
- Describe the care required for osteoporosis
- Explain how to assist in the care of persons in casts, in traction, and with hip pinnings
- Describe the effects of amputation

KEY TERMS

amputation The removal of all or part of an extremity

arthritis Joint *(arthr)* inflammation *(itis)*

arthroplasty The surgical replacement *(plasty)* of a joint *(arthr)*

closed fracture The bone is broken but the skin is intact; simple fracture

compound fracture An open fracture

fracture A broken bone

hemiplegia Paralysis on one side of the body

open fracture The broken bone has come through the skin; compound fracture

paraplegia Paralysis in the legs and lower trunk

quadriplegia Paralysis in the arms, legs, and trunk; tetraplegia

simple fracture Closed fracture

tetraplegia Quadriplegia

KEY ABBREVIATIONS

ADL Activities of daily living
ALS Amyotrophic lateral sclerosis
CVA Cerebrovascular accident
JRA Juvenile rheumatoid arthritis
MS Multiple sclerosis

PVS Persistent vegetative state
RA Rheumatoid arthritis
TBI Traumatic brain injury
TIA Transient ischemic attack

Understanding disorders of the nervous and muscu-loskeletal systems gives meaning to the required care. Refer to Chapter 8 while you study this chapter.

NERVOUS SYSTEM DISORDERS

Nervous system disorders can affect mental and physical function. They can affect the ability to speak, understand, feel, see, hear, touch, think, control bowels and bladder, and move.

Stroke

Stroke is a disease that affects the arteries that supply blood to the brain. It also is called a *brain attack* or *cerebro-vascular accident (CVA)*. It occurs when one of the following happens:

▶ A blood vessel in the brain bursts. Bleeding occurs in the brain (cerebral hemorrhage).
▶ A blood clot blocks blood flow to the brain.

Brain cells in the affected area do not get enough oxy-gen and nutrients. Brain cells die. Brain damage occurs. Functions controlled by that part of the brain are lost (Fig. 39-1).

BOX 39-1 Warning Signs of Stroke

- Sudden numbness or weakness of the face, arm, or leg, especially on one side of the body
- Sudden confusion, trouble speaking, or understanding speech
- Sudden trouble seeing in one or both eyes
- Sudden trouble walking, dizziness, loss of balance or coordination
- Sudden severe headache with no known cause

From National Institute for Neurological Disorders and Stroke: *What you need to know about stroke,* National Institutes of Health, NIH Publication No. 04-5517, Bethesda Md, updated June 19, 2007.

Stroke is the third leading cause of death in the United States. It is a leading cause of disability in adults. See Box 39-1 for warning signs. The person needs emergency care. Blood flow to the brain must be restored as soon as possible.

Sometimes warning signs last a few minutes. This is called a *transient ischemic attack (TIA)*. (*Transient* means temporary or short term. *Ischemic* means to hold back

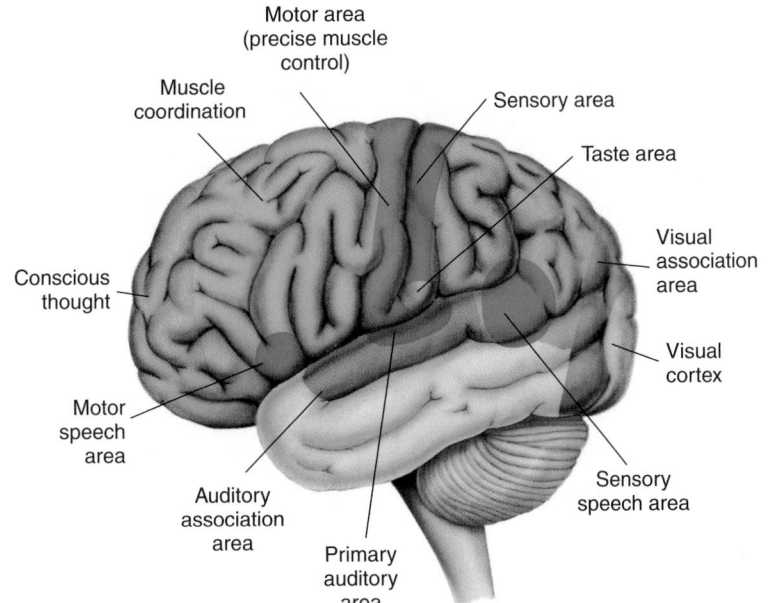

FIGURE 39-1 Functions lost from a stroke depend on the area of brain damage. (From Thibodeau GA, Patton KT: *The human body in health & disease,* ed 4, St Louis, 2005, Mosby.)

[ischein] blood *[hemic].*) Blood supply to the brain is interrupted for a short time. Sometimes a TIA occurs before a stroke. All stroke-like symptoms signal the need for emergency care.

Risk Factors

There are several risk factors for stroke. Some can be controlled, others cannot.

▶ *Age.* Older persons are at greater risk than younger persons.
▶ *Family history.* The risk increases if a parent, sister, or brother had a stroke.
▶ *Gender.* Both men and women are affected.
▶ *Race.* Blacks are at greater risk than other groups. This is because they have high rates of hypertension and diabetes.
▶ *Hypertension (high blood pressure).* This damages and weakens blood vessels. Clots can form. Or arteries can burst.
▶ *Heart disease.* Several heart diseases increase the risk of stroke. They include heart failure, heart attack, valve diseases, abnormal heart rhythms, and atherosclerosis (Chapter 40).
▶ *Smoking.* Blood vessels are damaged. The nicotine in cigarettes makes the heart work harder, increases the heart rate, and raises blood pressure. The amount of oxygen in the blood decreases.
▶ *Diabetes.* Blood vessels are damaged. The person is at risk for high blood pressure and blood clots.
▶ *High blood cholesterol.* Fatty materials build up on the walls of the artery and block blood flow.
▶ *Obesity.* The overweight person is at risk for high blood pressure, heart disease, diabetes, and high blood cholesterol.
▶ *Previous stroke or TIA.* Persons who had a stroke or a TIA are at great risk.

Signs and Symptoms

Stroke can occur suddenly. The person may have warning signs (see Box 39-1). The person also may have nausea, vomiting, and memory loss. Unconsciousness, noisy breathing, high blood pressure, slow pulse, redness of the face, and seizures may occur. So can **hemiplegia**—paralysis *(plegia)* on one side *(hemi)* of the body. The person may lose bowel and bladder control and the ability to speak. (See "Aphasia" in Chapter 37.)

Effects on the Person

If the person survives, some brain damage is likely. Functions lost depend on the area of brain damage (see Fig. 39-1). The effects of stroke include:

▶ Loss of face, hand, arm, leg, or body control
▶ Hemiplegia
▶ Changing emotions (crying easily or mood swings, sometimes for no reason)
▶ Difficulty swallowing (dysphagia)
▶ Aphasia or slowed or slurred speech (Chapter 37)

▶ Changes in sight, touch, movement, and thought
▶ Impaired memory
▶ Urinary frequency, urgency, or incontinence
▶ Loss of bowel control or constipation
▶ Depression and frustration

Behavior changes occur. The person may forget about or ignore the weaker side. This is called *neglect.* It is from the loss of vision or movement and feeling on that side. Sometimes thinking is affected. The person may not recognize or know how to use common items. Activities of daily living (ADL) and other tasks are hard to do. The person may forget what to do and how to do it. If the person does know, the body may not respond.

Rehabilitation starts at once. The person may depend in part or totally on others for care. The health team helps the person regain the highest possible level of function (Box 39-2).

See *Focus on Long-Term Care and Home Care: Stroke.*

BOX 39-2 Care of the Person With a Stroke

- The lateral (side-lying) position prevents aspiration.
- The bed is kept in semi-Fowler's position.
- The person is approached from the strong (unaffected) side. Objects are placed on the strong (unaffected) side. The person may have loss of vision on the affected side.
- Turning and repositioning are done at least every 2 hours.
- Assist devices are used for moving, turning, repositioning, and transfers.
- Incentive spirometry and deep breathing and coughing are encouraged.
- Contractures are prevented.
- Food and fluid needs are met. The person may need a dysphagia diet (Chapter 23).
- Elastic stockings prevent thrombi (blood clots) in the legs.
- Range-of-motion exercises prevent contractures. They also strengthen affected extremities.
- Elimination needs are met:
  - A catheter is inserted, or a bladder training program is started if needed.
  - A bowel training program is started if needed.
- Safety precautions are practiced:
  - The signal light is kept within reach. It is on the person's strong (unaffected) side.
  - The person is checked often if he or she cannot use the signal light. Follow the care plan.
  - Bed rails are used according to the care plan.
  - Falls are prevented.
- The person does as much self-care as possible. This includes turning, positioning, and transfers.
- Communication methods are established (Chapter 37).
- Speech, physical, and occupational therapies are ordered.
- Assistive and self-help devices are used as needed (Chapter 36).
- Ambulation aids are used as needed (Chapter 26).
- Support, encourage, and praise are given.
- A safety check is completed before leaving the room. (See the inside of the front book cover.)

Parkinson's Disease

Parkinson's disease is a slow, progressive disorder with no cure. The area of the brain that controls muscle movement is affected. Persons over the age of 50 are at risk. Signs and symptoms become worse over time (Fig. 39-2). They include:

▶ *Tremors*—often start in one finger and spread to the whole arm. Pill-rolling movements—rubbing the thumb and index finger—may occur. The person may have trembling in the hands, arms, legs, jaw, and face.

▶ *Rigid, stiff muscles*—in the arms, legs, neck, and trunk.

▶ *Slow movements*—the person has a slow, shuffling gait.

▶ *Stooped posture and impaired balance*—it is hard to walk. Falls are a risk.

▶ *Mask-like expression*—the person cannot blink and smile. A fixed stare is common.

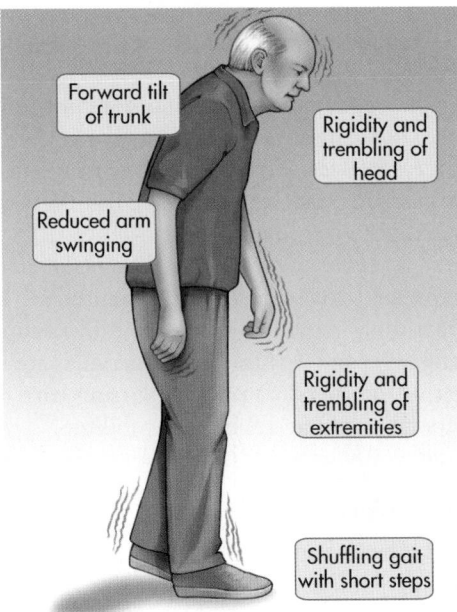

Forward tilt of trunk

Rigidity and trembling of head

Reduced arm swinging

Rigidity and trembling of extremities

Shuffling gait with short steps

FIGURE 39-2 Signs of Parkinson's disease. (From Thibodeau GA, Patton KT: *The human body in health & disease*, ed 4, St Louis, 2006, Mosby.)

Other signs and symptoms develop over time. They include swallowing and chewing problems, constipation, and bladder problems. Sleep problems, depression, and emotional changes (fear, insecurity) can occur. So can memory loss and slow thinking. The person may have slurred, monotone, and soft speech. Some people talk too fast or repeat what they say.

The doctor orders drugs to treat and control the disease. Exercise and physical therapy are ordered to improve strength, posture, balance, and mobility. Therapy is needed for speech and swallowing problems. The person may need help with eating and self-care. Normal elimination is a goal. Safety measures are needed to prevent falls and injury.

Multiple Sclerosis

Multiple sclerosis (MS) is a chronic disease. *Multiple* means many. *Sclerosis* means hardening or scarring. The myelin (which covers nerve fibers) in the brain and spinal cord is destroyed. Nerve impulses are not sent to and from the brain in a normal manner. Functions are impaired or lost. There is no cure.

Symptoms usually start between the ages of 20 and 40. More women are affected than men. Whites are at greater risk than other groups. A person's risk increases if a family member has MS.

Signs and symptoms depend on the damaged area. They may include:

▶ Vision problems—blurred or double vision, blindness in one eye

▶ Muscle weakness in the arms and legs

▶ Balance problems that affect standing and walking

▶ Tingling, prickling, or numb sensations

▶ Partial or complete paralysis

▶ Pain

▶ Speech problems

▶ Tremors

▶ Dizziness

▶ Problems with concentration, attention, memory, and judgment

▶ Depression

▶ Bowel and bladder problems

▶ Problems with sexual function

▶ Hearing loss

▶ Fatigue

▶ Coordination problems and clumsiness

MS can present as follows:

▶ *Relapsing-remitting*. The person has symptoms that last for a few weeks or a few months. The symptoms gradually disappear with partial or complete recovery. In other words, symptoms *remit* or the person is in *remission*. At some point, symptoms flare-up again (*relapse*).

▶ *Primary progressive*. The person's condition gradually declines with more and more symptoms. There are no remissions.

▶ *Secondary progressive.* Most people with relapsing-remitting MS enter this stage. Symptoms become worse. More symptoms occur with each flare-up. The person's condition declines.
▶ *Progressive-relapsing.* This occurs in persons with primary progressive MS. The person's condition gradually declines. Flare-ups occur. They leave new symptoms and more damage.

Persons with MS are kept active as long as possible and as independent as possible. The care plan reflects the person's changing needs. Skin care, hygiene, and range-of-motion exercises are important. So are turning, positioning, and deep breathing and coughing. Bowel and bladder elimination is promoted. Injuries and complications from bedrest are prevented.

See *Focus on Long-Term Care and Home Care: Multiple Sclerosis.*

Amyotrophic Lateral Sclerosis

Amyotrophic lateral sclerosis (ALS) attacks the nerve cells that control voluntary muscles. Commonly called *Lou Gehrig's disease,* it is rapidly progressive and fatal. (Lou Gehrig was a New York Yankees baseball player. He died of the disease in 1941.)

ALS affects more men than women. It usually strikes between 40 and 60 years of age. The person usually dies within 3 to 5 years after onset. Some survive for 10 or more years.

Motor nerve cells in the brain, brainstem, and spinal cord are affected. The cells degenerate or die. They stop sending messages to the muscles. The muscles weaken, waste away (atrophy), and twitch. Over time, the brain cannot start voluntary movements or control them. The person cannot move the arms, legs, and body. Muscles for speaking, chewing and swallowing, and breathing also are affected. Eventually muscles in the chest wall fail. The person needs a ventilator for breathing (Chapter 35).

The disease usually does not affect the mind, intelligence, or memory. Sight, smell, taste, hearing, and touch are not affected. Usually bowel and bladder functions remain intact.

ALS has no cure. Some drugs can slow disease progression. However, damage cannot be reversed. Persons with ALS are kept active as long as possible and as independent as possible. The care plan reflects the person's changing needs. The care plan may include:

▶ Physical, occupational, and speech/language therapies
▶ Range-of-motion exercises
▶ Braces, a walker, or a wheelchair for mobility
▶ Measures to relieve pain and promote comfort
▶ Communication methods
▶ Dysphagia diet or feeding tube
▶ Suctioning to remove excess fluids and saliva
▶ Mechanical ventilation
▶ Safety measures to prevent falls and injuries
▶ Psychological and social support
▶ Hospice care

Head Injury

Head injuries result from trauma to the scalp, skull, or brain. Some injuries are minor and do not need health care. Or the person is released from the hospital after emergency care.

Traumatic brain injury (TBI) occurs when a sudden trauma damages the brain. Brain tissue is bruised or torn. Bleeding can be in the brain or in nearby tissues. Spinal cord injuries are likely. Motor vehicle crashes, falls, and firearms are common causes. So are assaults and sports and recreation injuries.

Death can occur at the time of injury or afterwards. If the person survives TBI, some permanent damage is likely. Disabilities depend on the severity and location of the injury. They include:
▶ *Cognitive problems*—thinking, memory, and reasoning
▶ *Sensory problems*—sight, hearing, touch, taste, and smell
▶ *Communication problems*—expressing or understanding language
▶ *Behavior or mental health problems*—depression, anxiety, personality changes, aggressive behavior, socially inappropriate behavior
▶ *Stupor*—an unresponsive state; the person can be briefly aroused
▶ *Coma*—the person is unconscious, does not respond, is unaware, and cannot be aroused
▶ *Vegetative state*—the person is unconscious and unaware of surroundings; he or she has sleep-wake cycles and periods of being alert
▶ *Persistent vegetative state (PVS)*—the person is in a vegetative state for more than one month

Rehabilitation is required. Physical, occupational, speech/language, and mental health therapies are ordered depending on the person's needs. Nursing care depends on the person's needs and remaining abilities.

See *Focus on Children and Older Persons: Head Injury.*

Spinal Cord Injury

Spinal cord injuries can permanently damage the nervous system. Young adult men have the highest risk. Common causes are stab or gunshot wounds, motor vehicle crashes, falls, and sports injuries.

Problems depend on the amount of damage to the

FOCUS ON **CHILDREN** AND **OLDER PERSONS**

Head Injury

CHILDREN

Birth injuries are a major cause of head trauma in newborns. As children grow older, motor vehicle crashes, wheel-related sports (bikes, scooters, skates, skate boards), and falls are major causes of TBI.

Falls are a great danger for infants and toddlers. Falling down stairs and from windows are common accidents. See Chapters 11 and 12 for safety practices to prevent falls.

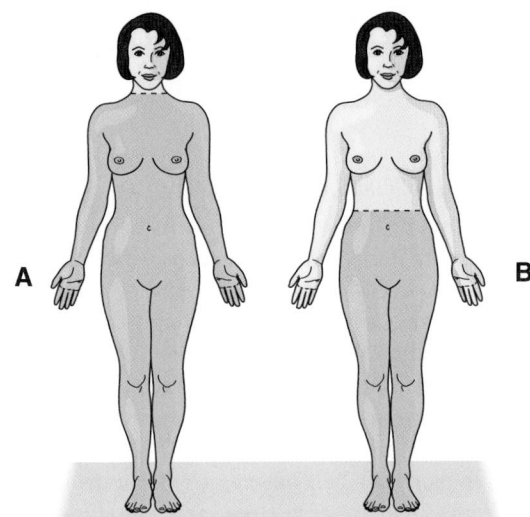

FIGURE 39-3 The *shaded areas* show the area of paralysis. **A,** Quadriplegia (tetraplegia). **B,** Paraplegia.

spinal cord and the level of injury. Damage to the spinal cord may be incomplete or complete:

▶ *Incomplete*—the spinal cord can still send messages to and from the brain. The person has some sensory (feeling) and motor (movement) function below the level of the injury.
▶ *Complete*—the spinal cord cannot send messages to and from the brain. The person has no sensory or motor function below the level of the injury.

The higher the level of injury, the more functions lost (Fig. 39-3):

▶ *Lumbar injuries*—sensory and muscle function in the legs is lost. The person has paraplegia. **Paraplegia** is paralysis in the legs and lower trunk. (*Para* means beside or beyond; *plegia* means paralysis.)
▶ *Thoracic injuries*—sensory and muscle function below the chest is lost. The person has paraplegia.
▶ *Cervical injuries*—sensory and muscle function of the arms, legs, and trunk are lost. Paralysis in the arms, legs, and trunk is called **quadriplegia** or **tetraplegia**. (*Quad* and *tetra* mean four.)

Cervical traction may be needed (p. 653). The person in cervical traction has a special bed. It keeps the spine

BOX 39-3 **Care of Persons With Paralysis**

- Prevent falls. Follow the care plan for safety measures and bed rail use.
- Keep the bed in the low position.
- Keep the signal light within reach. If unable to use the signal light, check the person often.
- Prevent burns. Check bath water, heat applications, and food for proper temperature.
- Turn and reposition the person at least every 2 hours. Follow the care plan.
- Prevent pressure ulcers. Follow the care plan.
- Maintain good alignment at all times. Use supportive devices according to the care plan.
- Follow bowel and bladder training programs.
- Keep intake and output records.
- Maintain muscle function and prevent contractures. Assist with range-of-motion exercises as directed.
- Assist with food and fluids as needed. Provide self-help devices as ordered.
- Give emotional and psychological support.
- Follow the person's rehabilitation plan.
- Complete a safety check of the room. (See the inside of the front book cover.)

straight at all times. Care measures are listed in Box 39-3. Emotional needs require attention. Reactions to paralysis and loss of function are often severe.

If the person survives, rehabilitation is necessary. Some rehabilitation centers focus on spinal cord injuries. The person learns to function at the highest possible level. He or she learns to use self-help, assistive, and other devices. Some persons return home and live independently. Others need long-term care, home care, or assisted-living settings.

Autonomic Dysreflexia

This syndrome affects persons with spinal cord injuries above the mid-thoracic level. There is uncontrolled stimulation of the sympathetic nervous system (Chapter 8). If untreated, stroke, heart attack, and death are risks. Report any of these signs and symptoms to the nurse at once:

▶ High blood pressure
▶ Throbbing or pounding headache
▶ Bradycardia—heart rate less than 60 beats per minute
▶ Blurred vision
▶ Sweating above the level of injury
▶ Flushing, reddening of the skin above the level of injury
▶ Cold, clammy skin below the level of injury
▶ "Goose bumps" *(piloerection)* below the level of injury
▶ Nasal congestion or stuffiness
▶ Nausea
▶ Anxiety

Autonomic dysreflexia is treated by raising the head of the bed 45 degrees or having the person sit upright if allowed. Once the cause is determined, it is removed. The

BOX 39-4 Preventing Autonomic Dysreflexia

- Monitor urinary output.
- If the person has a catheter:
  - Make sure the catheter is draining.
  - Make sure catheter tubing and drainage tubing are not kinked.
  - Empty the urinary drainage bag before it becomes too full. The bag should not overfill.
- Prevent urinary tract infections.
- Promote normal bowel elimination. Prevent constipation and fecal impaction.
- Prevent pressure ulcers.
- Prevent skin injuries—skin tears, cuts, bruises, blisters, and so on.
- Check the person's feet for ingrown toenails, blisters, pressure ulcers, and so on. Report any problems to the nurse.
- Prevent burns. This includes burns from hot water.
- Have the person wear clothing that is loose and comfortable. Avoid tight clothing.
- Make sure the person is not sitting or lying on wrinkled clothing or linens.
- Reposition the person at least every 2 hours. Avoid prolonged pressure from the bed or chair.
- Report menstrual cramps to the nurse.

PROMOTING SAFETY AND COMFORT: Autonomic Dysreflexia

SAFETY
Constipation and fecal impaction can cause autonomic dysreflexia. So can checking for an impaction and enemas. Do not perform these procedures if the person is at risk for autonomic dysreflexia. Such procedures are best done by a nurse.

most common causes are a full bladder, constipation or fecal impaction, and skin disorders. Measures to prevent autonomic dysreflexia are part of the person's care plan (Box 39-4).

See *Promoting Safety and Comfort: Autonomic Dysreflexia.*

MUSCULOSKELETAL DISORDERS

Musculoskeletal disorders affect movement. Activities of daily living, social activities, and quality of life are affected. Injury and age-related changes are common causes of musculoskeletal disorders.

Arthritis

Arthritis means joint *(arthr)* inflammation *(itis)*. It is the most common joint disease. Pain, swelling, and stiffness occur in the affected joints. The joints are hard to move. There are two basic types of arthritis.

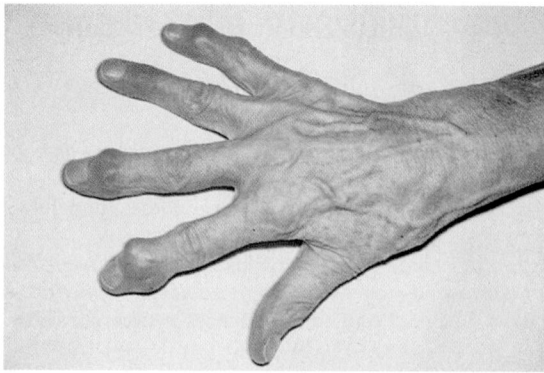

FIGURE 39-4 Bony growths called *Heberden nodes* occur in the finger joints. (From Kamal A, Brocklehurst JC: *A color atlas of geriatric medicine*, ed 2, St Louis, 1991, Mosby.)

Osteoarthritis (Degenerative Joint Disease)

This is the most common type of arthritis. Aging, being overweight, and joint injury are causes. Stress, muscle weakness, and heredity are other causes. The fingers, spine (neck and lower back), and weight-bearing joints (hips, knees, and feet) are often affected (Fig. 39-4).

Signs and symptoms include joint stiffness, pain, swelling, and tenderness. Joint stiffness occurs with rest and lack of motion. Pain occurs with weight-bearing and joint motion. Or pain can be constant or occur from lack of motion. Pain can affect rest, sleep, and mobility. Swelling is common after using the joint. Cold weather and dampness seem to increase symptoms.

There is no cure. Treatment involves:
- *Pain relief.* Drugs decrease swelling and inflammation and relieve pain.
- *Heat applications.* Heat relieves pain, increases blood flow to the part, and reduces swelling. Heat applications and warm baths or showers are helpful. So is water therapy in a heated pool. Sometimes cold applications are used after joint use.
- *Exercise.* Exercise decreases pain, increases flexibility, and improves blood flow. It helps with weight control and promotes fitness. Mental well-being improves. The person is taught what exercises to do.
- *Rest and joint care.* Good body mechanics, posture, and regular rest protect the joints. Relaxation methods are helpful. Canes and walkers provide support. Splints support weak joints and keep them in alignment. Adaptive and self-help devices for hands and wrists are useful for ADL. See Chapters 23 and 36.
- *Weight control.* Weight loss is stressed for person who are overweight. It reduces stress on weight-bearing joints. It also helps prevent further joint injury.
- *Healthy life-style.* Arthritis support programs can help the person develop a healthy outlook. Abilities and strengths are stressed. The focus is on fitness, exercise, rest, managing stress, and good nutrition.

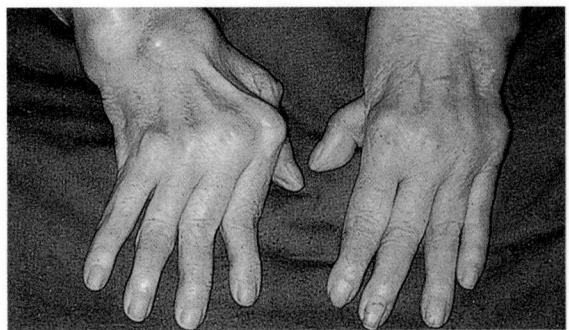

FIGURE 39-5 Deformities caused by rheumatoid arthritis. (From Stevens A, Lowe J: *Pathology: illustrated review in color,* ed 2, London, 2000, Mosby).

Falls are prevented. Help is given with ADL as needed. Toilet seat risers are helpful when hips and knees are affected. So are chairs with higher seats and armrests. Some people need joint replacement surgery.

Rheumatoid Arthritis

Rheumatoid arthritis (RA) is a chronic inflammatory disease. It causes joint pain, swelling, stiffness, and loss of function. More common in women than in men, it generally develops between the ages of 20 and 50.

RA occurs on both sides of the body. For example, if the right wrist is involved, so is the left wrist. The wrist and finger joints closest to the hand are often affected (Fig. 39-5). Other joints affected are the neck, shoulders, elbows, hips, knees, ankles, and feet. Joints are tender, warm, and swollen. Fatigue and fever are common. The person does not feel well. Symptoms may last for several years.

Other body parts may be affected. Decreased production of red blood cells and dry eyes and mouth are common. Inflammation of the linings of the heart, blood vessels, and lungs can occur but is rare.

RA varies from person to person. Some people have flare-ups and then feel better. In others, the disease is active most of the time.

Treatment goals are to:
- Relieve pain
- Reduce inflammation
- Slow down or stop joint damage
- Improve the person's sense of well-being and ability to function

The person's care plan may include:
- *Rest balanced with exercise.* More rest is needed when RA is active. More exercise is needed when it is not.
- *Proper positioning.* Contractures and deformities are prevented. Bed boards, a bed cradle, trochanter rolls, and pillows are used.
- *Joint care.* Good body mechanics and body alignment, wrist and hand splints, and self-help devices for ADL reduce stress on the joints. Walking aids may be needed.
- *Rest.* Short rest periods during the day are better than long times in bed.
- *Regular exercise.* The doctor and physical therapist prescribe an exercise program. Range-of-motion exercises are included. Exercise helps maintain healthy and strong muscles, joint mobility, and flexibility. Exercise also promotes sleep, reduces pain, and helps weight control.
- *Weight control.* Excess weight places stress on the weight-bearing joints. Exercise and a healthy diet help control weight.
- *Measures to reduce stress.* Relaxation, distraction, and regular rest help reduce stress. So does exercise.
- *Measure to prevent falls.* See Chapter 12.

Drugs are ordered for pain relief and to reduce inflammation. Heat and cold applications may be ordered. Some persons need joint replacement surgery.

Emotional support is needed. A good outlook is important. Persons with RA need to stay as active as possible. The more they can do for themselves, the better off they are. Give encouragement and praise. Listen when the person needs to talk.

See *Focus on Children and Older Persons: Rheumatoid Arthritis.*

Total Joint Replacement Surgery

Arthroplasty is the surgical replacement (*plasty*) of a joint (*arthro*). The damaged joint is removed and replaced with an artificial joint. The artificial joint is called a *prosthesis* (Fig. 39-6, p. 648).

Hip and knee replacements are the most common. Ankle, foot, shoulder, elbow, and finger joints also can be replaced. The surgery is done to relieve pain, restore or preserve joint function, or correct a deformed joint. See Box 39-5, p. 648 for care of the person after hip and knee replacement surgeries.

See *Focus on Ethics and Laws: Total Joint Replacement Surgery,* p. 648.

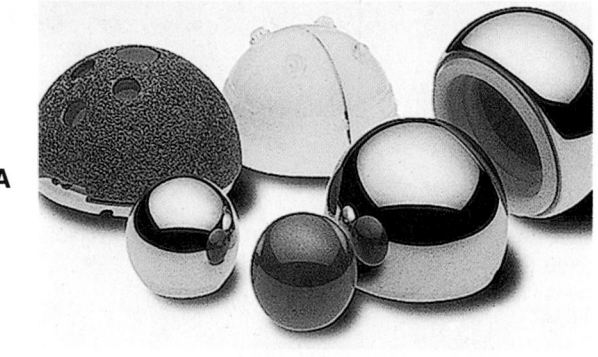

A

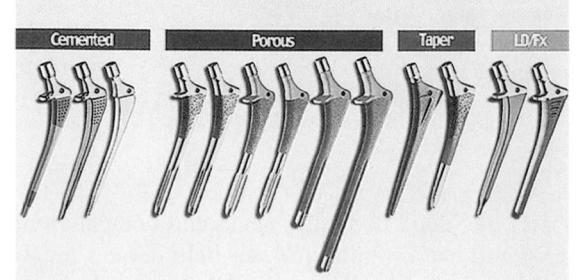

B

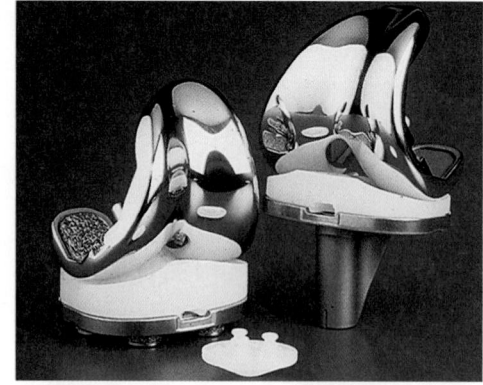

C

FIGURE 39-6 **A,** Hip replacement prosthesis. **B,** Hip replacement prosthesis stems. **C,** Knee replacement prosthesis. (Courtesy Zimmer, Inc., a Bristol-Meyers Squibb Company, Warsaw, Ind.)

BOX 39-5 Care of the Person After Total Joint Replacement Surgery—Hip and Knee

- Incentive spirometry and deep-breathing and coughing exercises to prevent respiratory complications.
- Elastic stockings to prevent thrombi (blood clots) in the legs.
- Exercises to strengthen the hip or knee. These are taught by a physical therapist.
- Measures to protect the hip (Fig. 39-7):
  - No turning of the feet or knees inward or outward.
  - No sitting in low chairs. A high, firm chair is used.
  - No crossing of the legs.
  - No bending at the hips more than 90 degrees.
  - Using long-handled devices for reaching and ADL.
  - Using a raised toilet seat.

- A positioning device placed between the legs—hip abduction wedge (abductor splint) or pillows. It is kept in place when turning in bed.
- Food and fluids for tissue healing and to restore strength.
- Safety measures to prevent falls.
- Measures to prevent infection. Wound, urinary tract, and skin infections must be prevented.
- Measures to prevent pressure ulcers.
- Assist devices for moving, turning, repositioning, and transfers.
- Assistance with walking and a walking aid. The person may need a cane, walker, or crutches.

FOCUS ON **ETHICS** AND **LAWS**

Total Joint Replacement Surgery

A patient and her husband filed suit in a Louisiana court against a hospital and two nursing aides. The patient had a total hip replacement in March 1994. The patient claimed that the following occurred while she was recovering from surgery.

- Two ladies came into her room to turn her. The ladies "raised her up high and then one of the ladies let go of the pad they were using to turn her and they dropped her."
- She was in severe pain when she was dropped and continued to have pain.
- She could not do any physical therapy or walk while in the hospital.
- She did not want to be discharged because of the severe pain after being dropped.

During a May 1994 office visit, the doctor noted that the patient had an abnormal gait. An x-ray showed that the hip prosthesis was dislocated. Two days later she had another surgery. The patient claimed that the dislocated hip was the result of negligence by the two nursing aides.

The nursing aides would testify that:

- They were in the process of transferring the patient from an orthopedic chair to bed.
- The hand of one nursing aide slipped. She let go of the sheet while they were pulling the patient onto the bed.
- The patient was already on the bed when the hand slipped.

- The patient was "not up in the air or dropped."
- The patient did not voice any complaints that she was hurting from the transfer.

The doctor testified that:

- The patient did not tell him about being dropped until she was in the hospital for the second surgery.
- When she told him of the incident, she said that:
  - "Within 24 hours of the first hip surgery, the bed dropped about two feet."
  - She had "sudden onset of pain in her hip."
- She was complaining of pain before and after the bed dropped.
- The dislocated hip may have resulted from the hip prosthesis design.

After the first surgery, physical therapy records showed that the patient was able to:

- Walk with a walker
- Do several exercises

The trial judge ruled in favor of the hospital and the nursing aides. The lawsuit was dismissed. The judge ruled that the patient did not prove that the dislocation was caused by nursing aides. The decision was appealed to a higher court. The Appellate Court reached the same decision.

(F. Guillot wife of/and R. Guillot v East Jefferson Hospital, Jane and Mary Doe, 2003.)

Do   **Do Not**

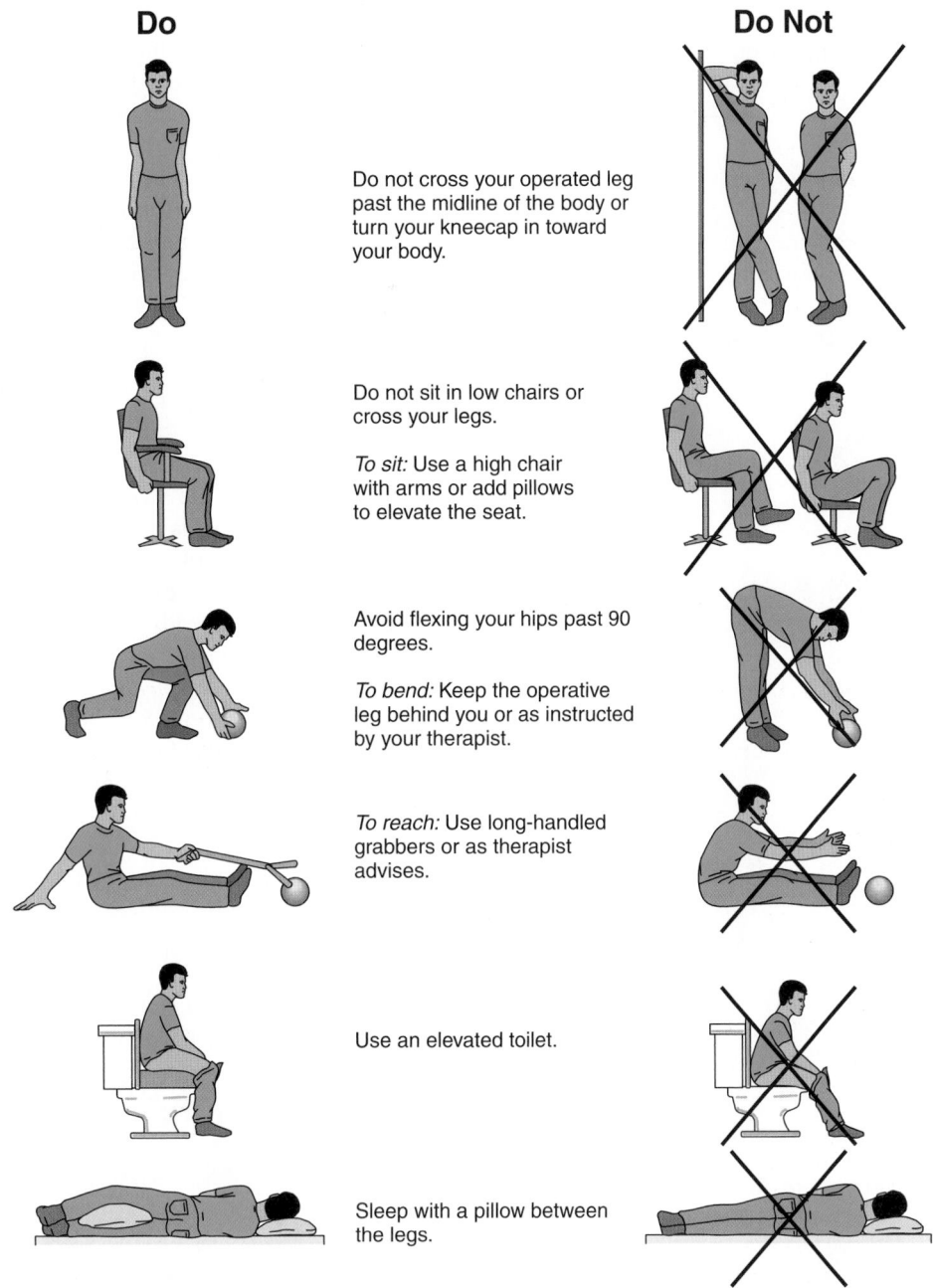

Do not cross your operated leg past the midline of the body or turn your kneecap in toward your body.

Do not sit in low chairs or cross your legs.

To sit: Use a high chair with arms or add pillows to elevate the seat.

Avoid flexing your hips past 90 degrees.

To bend: Keep the operative leg behind you or as instructed by your therapist.

To reach: Use long-handled grabbers or as therapist advises.

Use an elevated toilet.

Sleep with a pillow between the legs.

FIGURE 39-7 Measures to protect the hip after total hip replacement surgery. (Modified from Monahan FD and others: *Phipps' Medical-surgical nursing: health and illness perspectives*, ed 8, St Louis, 2007, Mosby.)

Osteoporosis

With osteoporosis, the bone *(osteo)* becomes porous and brittle *(porosis)*. Bones are fragile and break easily. Spine, hip, wrist, and rib fractures are common.

Older men and women are at risk. The risk for women increases after menopause. The ovaries do not produce estrogen after menopause. The lack of estrogen causes bone changes. So do low levels of dietary calcium.

All ethnic groups are at risk. Other risk factors include a family history of the disease, being thin or having a small frame, eating disorders (Chapter 43), tobacco use, alcoholism, lack of exercise, bedrest, and immobility. Exercise and activity are needed for bone strength. For bone to form properly, it must bear weight. If not, calcium is lost from the bone. The bone becomes porous and brittle.

Back pain, gradual loss of height, and stooped posture occur. Fractures are a major threat. With brittle bones, even slight activity can cause a fracture. Fractures can occur from turning in bed, getting up from a chair, or coughing. Fractures are great risks from falls and accidents.

Prevention is important. Doctors often order calcium and vitamin supplements. Estrogen is ordered for some women. Other preventive measures include:

▶ Exercising weight-bearing joints—walking, jogging, stair climbing
▶ Strength-training (lifting weights)
▶ No smoking
▶ Limiting alcohol and caffeine
▶ Back supports or corsets if needed for good posture
▶ Walking aids if needed
▶ Safety measures to prevent falls and accidents
▶ Good body mechanics
▶ Safe handling, moving, transfer, and turning and positioning procedures

Fractures

A **fracture** is a broken bone. Tissues around the fracture—muscles, blood vessels, nerves, and tendons—are injured. Fractures are open or closed (Fig. 39-8):

▶ **Closed fracture (simple fracture).** The bone is broken but the skin is intact.
▶ **Open fracture (compound fracture).** The broken bone has come through the skin.

Falls and accidents are causes. Bone tumors, metastatic cancer, and osteoporosis are other causes. Signs and symptoms of a fracture are:

▶ Pain
▶ Swelling
▶ Loss of function
▶ Limited or no movement of the part
▶ Movement where motion should not occur
▶ Deformity (the part is in an abnormal position)
▶ Bruising and skin color changes at the fracture site
▶ Bleeding (internal or external)

For healing, bone ends are brought into and held in normal position. This is called *reduction* or *fixation:*

▶ *Closed reduction or external fixation.* The doctor moves the bones back into place. The bone is not exposed.
▶ *Open reduction or internal fixation.* This requires surgery. The bone is exposed and moved into alignment. Nails, rods, pins, screws, plates, or wires keep the bone in place (Fig. 39-9).

After reduction, movement of the bone ends is prevented. This is done with a cast or traction. Other devices—splints, walking boots, external fixators—also are used (Fig. 39-10).

See *Focus on Children and Older Persons: Fractures.*

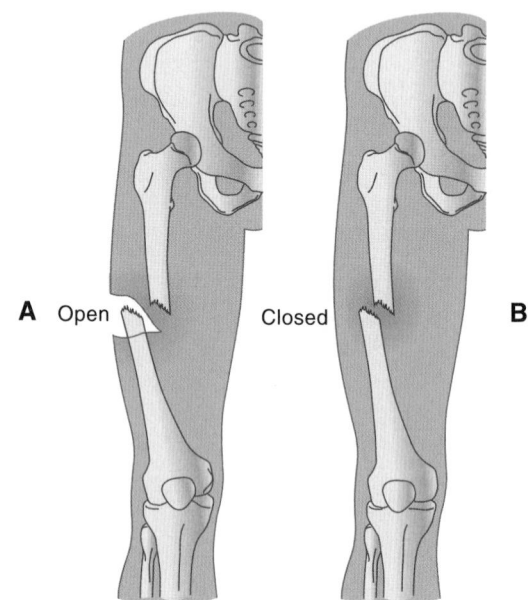

FIGURE 39-8 A, Open fracture. **B,** Closed fracture. (From Thibodeau GA, Patton KT: *The human body in health & disease,* ed 4, St Louis, 2005, Mosby.)

FOCUS ON **CHILDREN** AND **OLDER PERSONS**

Fractures

CHILDREN
Falls and accidents involving motor vehicles, bikes, skate boards, and roller blades are common causes of fractures in children. Fractures in infants may signal child abuse.

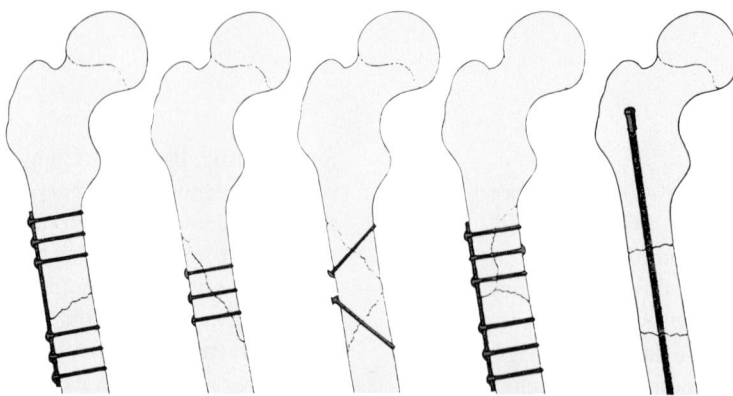

FIGURE 39-9 Devices used for open reduction of a fracture. (From Beare PG, Meyers JL: *Adult health nursing,* ed 3, St Louis, 1998, Mosby.)

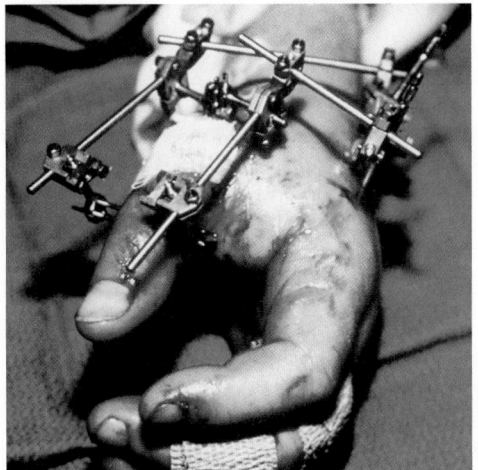

FIGURE 39-10 External fixator. (From Lewis SM, Heitkemper MM, Dirksen SR: *Medical-surgical nursing: assessment and management of clinical problems*, ed 7, St Louis, 2007, Mosby.)

Casts

Casts are made of plaster of paris, plastic, or fiberglass (Fig. 39-11). Before casting, the part is covered with stockinette or cotton padding. This protects the skin. Moistened cast rolls are wrapped around the part. Plastic and fiberglass casts dry quickly. A plaster of paris cast dries in 24 to 48 hours. It is odorless, white, and shiny when dry. When wet, it is gray and cool and has a musty smell. The nurse may ask you to assist with care (Box 39-6, p. 652).

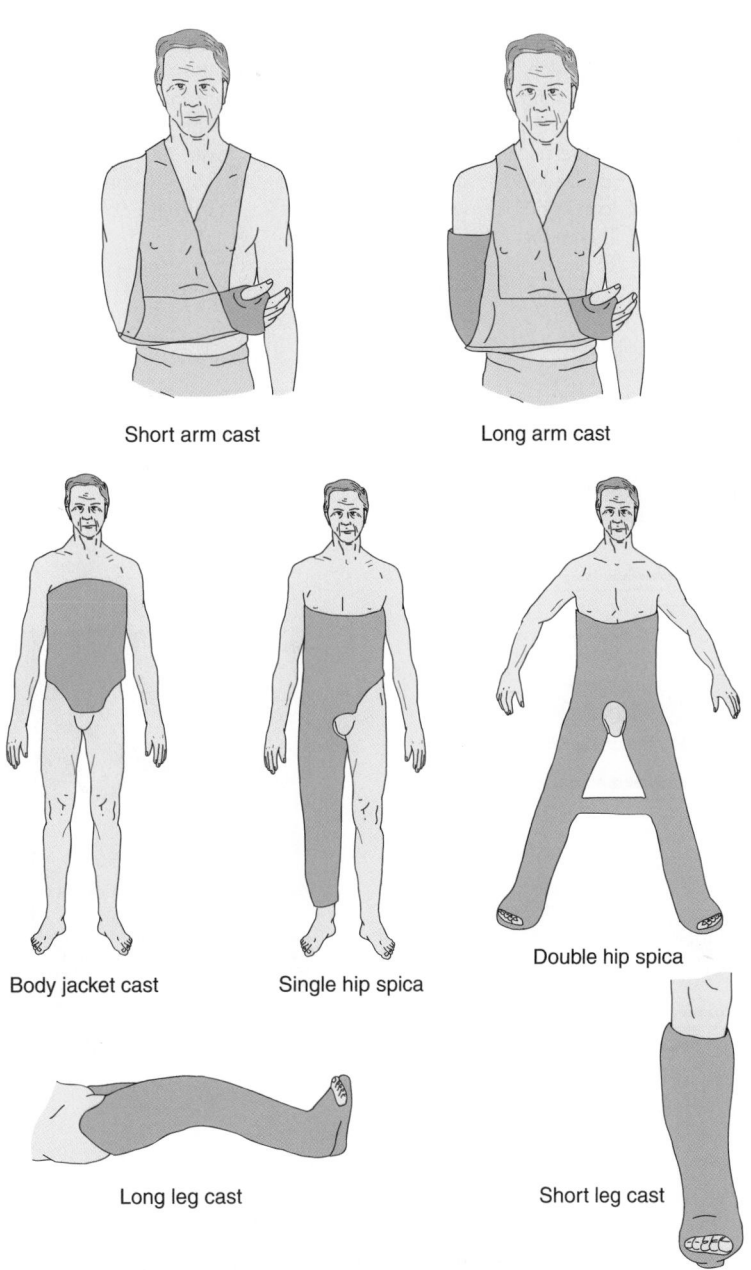

Short arm cast

Long arm cast

Body jacket cast

Single hip spica

Double hip spica

Long leg cast

Short leg cast

FIGURE 39-11 Common casts.

BOX 39-6 Rules for Cast Care

- Do not cover the cast with blankets, plastic, or other material. A cast gives off heat as it dries. Covers prevent the escape of heat. Burns can occur if heat cannot escape.
- Turn the person every 2 hours or as often as directed by the nurse and the care plan. All cast surfaces are exposed to the air at one time or another. Turning promotes even drying.
- Do not place a wet cast on a hard surface. It flattens the cast. The cast must keep its shape. Use pillows to support the entire length of the cast (Fig. 39-12).
- Support the wet cast with your palms when turning and positioning the person (Fig. 39-13). Fingertips can dent the cast. The dents can cause pressure areas that lead to skin breakdown.
- Report rough cast edges. The nurse will need to cover the cast edges with tape.
- Keep the cast dry. A wet cast loses its shape. Some casts are near the perineal area. The nurse may apply a waterproof material around the perineal area after the cast dries.
- Do not let the person insert anything into the cast. Itching under the cast causes an intense desire to scratch. Items used for scratching (pencils, coat hangers, knitting needles, back scratchers, and so on) can open the skin. An infection can develop. Scratching items can wrinkle the stockinette or cotton padding. Or scratching items can be lost into the cast. Both can cause pressure and lead to skin breakdown.
- Elevate a casted arm or leg on pillows. This reduces swelling.

- Have enough help when turning and repositioning the person. Plaster casts are heavy and awkward. Balance is lost easily.
- Position the person as directed.
- Provide a fracture pan if the person has a long leg or spica cast.
- Report these signs and symptoms at once:
  - Pain: means a pressure ulcer, poor circulation, or nerve damage
  - Swelling and a tight cast: mean reduced blood flow to the part
  - Pale skin: means reduced blood flow to the part
  - Cyanosis (bluish skin color): means reduced blood flow to the part
  - Odor: means infection
  - Inability to move the fingers or toes: means pressure on a nerve
  - Numbness: means pressure on a nerve or reduced blood flow to the part
  - Temperature changes: cool skin means poor circulation; hot skin means inflammation
  - Drainage on or under the cast: means infection or bleeding
  - Chills, fever, nausea, and vomiting: mean infection
- Complete a safety check before leaving the room. (See the inside of the front book cover.)

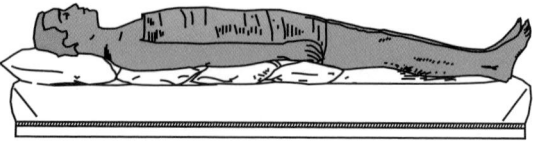
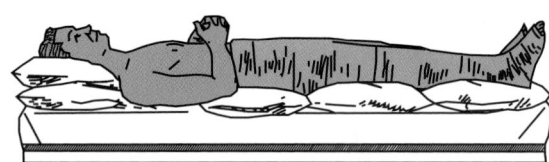
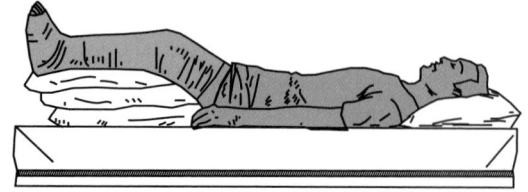

FIGURE 39-12 Pillows support the entire length of the wet cast. (From Harkness GA, Dincher JR: *Medical-surgical nursing: total patient care,* ed 10, St Louis, 1999, Mosby.)

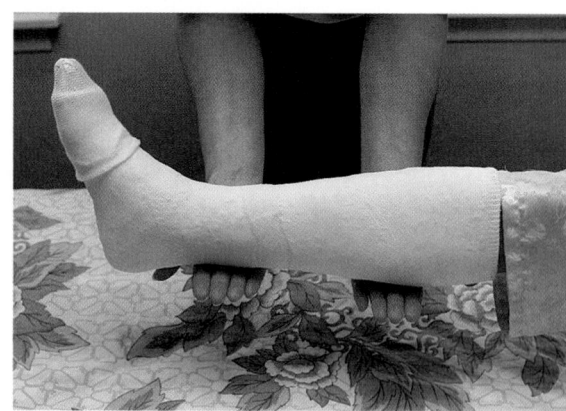

FIGURE 39-13 The cast is supported with the palms.

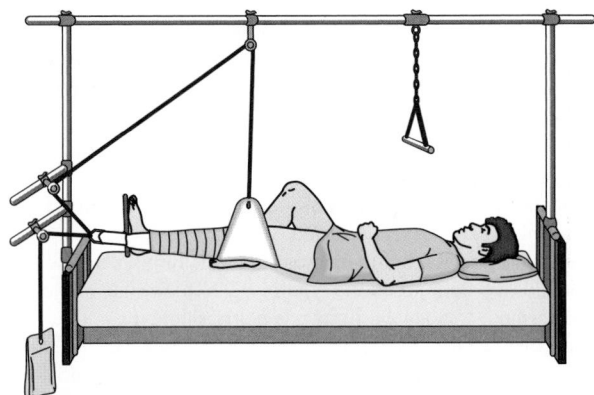

FIGURE 39-14 Traction set-up. Note the weights, pulleys, and ropes. (From Monahan FD and others: *Phipps' Medical-surgical nursing: health and illness perspectives,* ed 8, St Louis, 2007, Mosby.)

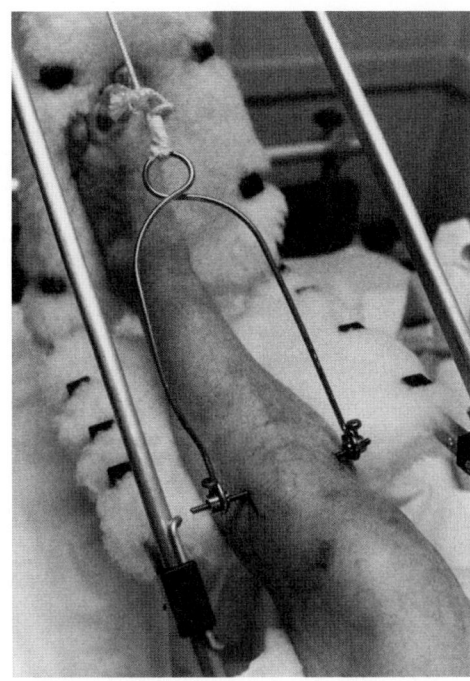

FIGURE 39-15 Skeletal traction is attached to the bone. (From Christensen BL, Kockrow EO: *Adult health nursing,* ed 4, St Louis, 2003, Mosby.)

BOX 39-7 Caring for Persons in Traction

- Keep the person in good alignment.
- Do not remove the traction.
- Keep the weights off the floor. Weights must hang freely from the traction set-up (see Fig. 39-14).
- Do not add or remove weights from the traction set-up.
- Check for frayed ropes. Report fraying to the nurse at once.
- Perform range-of-motion exercises for the uninvolved joints as directed.
- Position the person as directed. Usually only the back-lying position is allowed. Sometimes slight turning is allowed.
- Provide the fracture pan for elimination.
- Give skin care as directed.
- Put bottom linens on the bed from the top down. The person uses a trapeze to raise the body off the bed.
- Check pin, nail, wire, or tong sites for redness, drainage, and odors. Report any observations to the nurse at once.
- Observe for the signs and symptoms listed under cast care (see Box 39-6). Report them to the nurse at once.

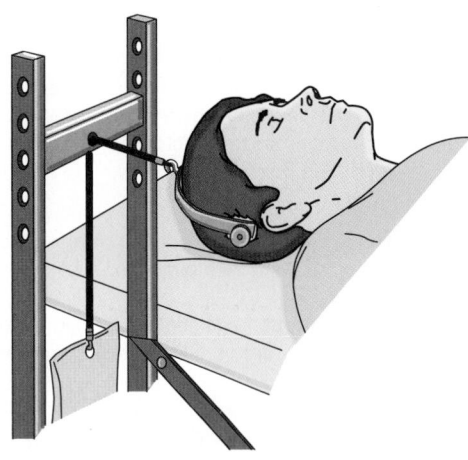

FIGURE 39-16 Tongs are inserted into the skull for cervical spine traction. (From Monahan FD and others: *Phipps' Medical-surgical nursing: health and illness perspectives,* ed 8, St Louis, 2007, Mosby.)

Traction

Traction reduces and immobilizes fractures. A steady pull from two directions keeps the bone in place. Traction also is used for muscle spasms and to correct deformities or contractures. Weights, ropes, and pulleys are used (Fig. 39-14). Traction is applied to the neck, arms, legs, or pelvis.

Skin traction is applied to the skin. Boots, wraps, tape, or splints are used. Weights are attached to the device (see Fig. 39-14). *Skeletal traction* is applied directly to the bone. Wires or pins are inserted through the bone (Fig. 39-15). For cervical traction, tongs are applied to the skull (Fig. 39-16). Weights are attached to the device.

The nurse may ask you to assist with the person's care (Box 39-7).

Hip Fractures

Fractured hips are common in older persons (Fig. 39-17, p. 654). Older women are at risk. Healing is slower in older people. Slow healing and other health problems affect the person's condition and care.

Post-operative problems present life-threatening risks. They include pneumonia, atelectasis (collapse of a part of a lung), urinary tract infections, and thrombi (blood clots) in the leg veins. Pressure ulcers, constipation, and confusion are other risks.

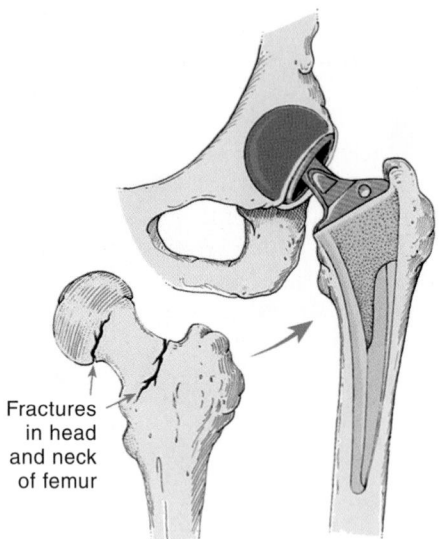

FIGURE 39-17 Hip fracture repaired with a prosthesis. (Modified from Christensen BL, Kockrow EO: *Adult health nursing,* ed 5, St Louis, 2006, Mosby.)

FOCUS ON LONG-TERM CARE AND HOME CARE

Hip Fractures

LONG-TERM CARE

Older persons often require rehabilitation after a hip fracture. If home care is not possible, the person requires subacute or long-term care. The person usually returns home after successful rehabilitation. Adduction, internal rotation, and severe hip flexion are avoided. See Box 39-8.

HOME CARE

The prosthesis can dislocate (move out of place) with adduction, internal rotation, and severe hip flexion. Such movements are avoided. See Box 39-8.

An occupational therapist helps the person learn self-care activities. Assistive devices are used for dressing and bathing (Chapter 36).

A physical therapist helps the person learn muscle-strengthening exercises. A walker is usually needed for ambulation.

BOX 39-8 Care of the Person With a Hip Fracture

- Give good skin care. Skin breakdown can occur rapidly.
- Follow the care plan to prevent pressure ulcers.
- Follow the care plan to prevent wound, skin, and urinary tract infections.
- Encourage incentive spirometry and deep-breathing and coughing exercises as directed.
- Turn and position the person as directed. Turning and positioning depend on the type of fracture and the surgery performed. Usually the person is not positioned on the operative side.
- Use trochanter rolls, pillows, and sandbags as directed. These prevent external rotation when the person is in bed.
- Keep the operated leg abducted at all times. The leg is abducted when the person is supine, being turned, or in a side-lying position. Use pillows (Fig. 39-18) or a hip abduction wedge (abductor splint) as directed. Do not exercise the affected leg.
- Provide a straight-back chair with armrests. The person needs a high, firm seat. A low, soft chair is not used.
- Place the chair on the unaffected side.
- Assist the nurse in transferring the person.
- Use assist devices for moving, turning, repositioning, and transfers.
- Do not let the person stand on the operated leg unless allowed by the doctor.
- Follow the care plan for when to elevate the leg. If the person has an internal fixation device, the leg is not elevated when the person sits in a chair. Elevating the leg puts strain on the device.
- Apply elastic stockings to prevent thrombi (blood clots) in the legs.
- Remind the person not to cross his or her legs.
- Assist with ambulation according to the care plan. The person uses a walker or crutches.
- Follow measures to protect the hip. See Box 35-5.
  - No turning of the feet or knees inward or outward.
  - No sitting in low chairs. A high, firm chair is used.
  - No crossing of the legs.
  - No bending at the hips more than 90 degrees.
  - Long-handled devices for reaching and ADL.
  - A raised toilet seat.
  - A positioning device between the legs—hip abduction wedge (abductor splint) or pillows. It is kept in place when turning in bed.
- Practice safety measures to prevent falls.

The fracture requires internal fixation (p. 650). Some hip fractures require partial or total hip replacement. Adduction, internal rotation, external rotation, and severe hip flexion are avoided after surgery. Rehabilitation is usually needed after a hip fracture. If home care is not possible, the person needs subacute or long-term care. Recovery can take 6 months. Some persons return home after successful rehabilitation. Others stay in long-term care centers. See Box 39-8 for the care required after surgery for a hip fracture.

See *Focus on Long-Term Care and Home Care: Hip Fractures.*

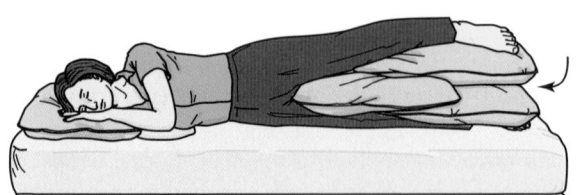

FIGURE 39-18 Pillows are used to keep the hip in abduction. (From Monahan FD and others: *Phipps' Medical-surgical nursing: health and illness perspectives,* ed 8, St Louis, 2007, Mosby.)

Loss of Limb

An **amputation** is the removal of all or part of an extremity. Most amputations involve a lower extremity. Severe injuries, tumors, severe infection, gangrene, and vascular disorders are common causes. Diabetes is a common cause of vascular changes that can lead to amputation.

Gangrene is a condition in which there is death of tissue. Causes include infection, injuries, and vascular disorders. Blood flow is affected. Tissues do not get enough oxygen and nutrients. Poisonous substances and wastes build up in the tissues. Tissue death results. Tissues become black, cold, and shriveled (Fig. 39-19). Surgery is needed to remove dead tissue. If untreated, gangrene spreads throughout the body. For example, in diabetes the toes are usually affected first. Unless the affected toes are removed, the gangrene spreads up the foot and to the knee. Gangrene can cause death.

Much support is needed. The amputation affects the person's life. Body image, appearance, daily activities, moving about, and work are some areas affected. Fear, shock, anger, denial, and depression are common emotions.

The person is fitted with a prosthesis—an artificial replacement for a missing body part (Fig. 39-20). First the stump is conditioned so the prosthesis fits. This involves shrinking and shaping the stump into a cone shape with bandages (Fig. 39-21). The person learns exercises to strengthen other limbs. Occupational and physical therapists help the person use the prosthesis.

The person may feel that the limb is still there. Aching, tingling, and itching are common sensations. Or the person may complain of pain in the amputated part. This is called *phantom limb pain*. This is a normal reaction. It may occur for a short time after surgery or for many years.

Lower limb amputations are common in older persons. Because of other health problems, many older persons cannot use a prosthesis. They need to use wheelchairs. After amputation, most older persons need long-term care on a temporary or permanent basis.

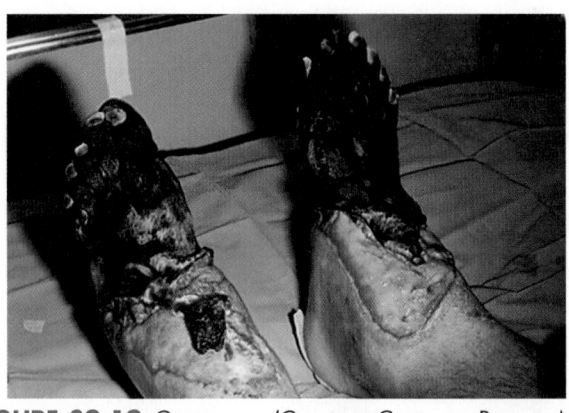

FIGURE 39-19 Gangrene. (Courtesy Cameron Bangs, MD. From Auerbach PS: *Wilderness medicine, management of wilderness and environmental emergencies*, ed 3, St Louis, 1995, Mosby.)

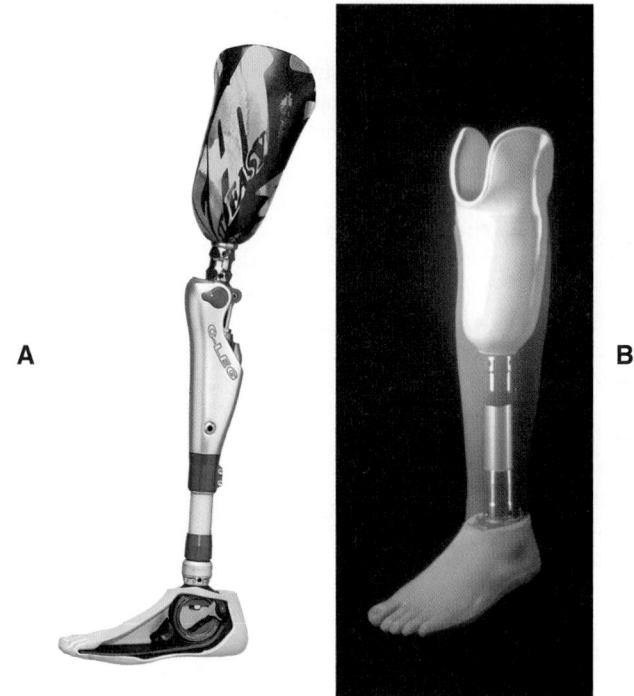

FIGURE 39-20 Leg prostheses. **A,** Above-the-knee prosthesis. **B,** Below-the-knee prostheses. (Courtesy Otto Bock Health Care, Minneapolis, Minn.)

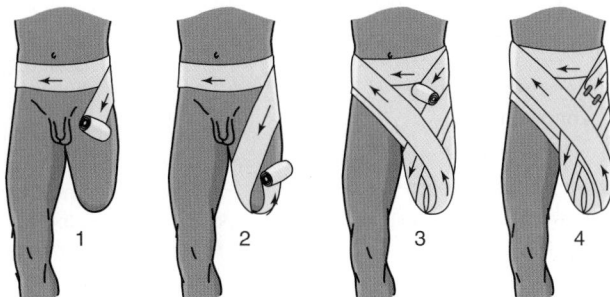

FIGURE 39-21 A mid-thigh amputation is bandaged to shrink and shape the stump. (From Monahan FD and others: *Phipps' Medical-surgical nursing: health and illness perspectives*, ed 8, St Louis, 2007, Mosby.)

REVIEW QUESTIONS

Circle the BEST answer.

1 A stroke also is called
   a A cerebrovascular accident
   b Aphasia
   c Hemiplegia
   d A transient ischemic attack

2 Warning signs of stroke occur
   a With exertion   c At rest
   b Suddenly   d Between the ages of
                              20 and 40

3 A person had a stroke. Which measure should you
   question?
   a Semi-Fowler's position
   b Range-of-motion exercises every 2 hours
   c Turn, reposition, and skin care every 2 hours
   d Bed in the highest horizontal position

4 A person has Parkinson's disease. Which is *false*?
   a The part of the brain controlling muscle movements
      is affected.
   b Mental function is affected first.
   c Tremors, slow movements, and a shuffling gait occur.
   d The person is protected from injury.

5 Parkinson's disease
   a Can be cured with drugs
   b Can be cured with surgery
   c Is a slow, progressive disorder
   d Progresses rapidly

6 A person has multiple sclerosis. Which is *false*?
   a There is no cure.
   b Only voluntary muscles are affected.
   c Symptoms begin in young adulthood.
   d Over time, the person depends on others for care.

7 A person has multiple sclerosis. Signs, symptoms, and
   the care required depend on the area of damage.
   a True
   b False

8 Amyotrophic lateral sclerosis affects nerve cells that
   control
   a Involuntary muscles   c The brain
   b Voluntary muscles   d The lungs

9 A person has amyotrophic lateral sclerosis. The care
   plan includes the following. Which should you
   question?
   a Range-of-motion exercises
   b Dysphagia diet
   c Walker for mobility
   d Measures to prevent confusion

10 Persons with head or spinal cord injuries require
   a Rehabilitation   c Long-term care
   b Speech therapy   d Chemotherapy

11 A person has tetraplegia following a spinal cord
   injury. Which care measure should you question?
   a Keep the bed in the low position.
   b Assist with active range-of-motion exercises.
   c Follow the bowel training program.
   d Turn and reposition every hour.

12 Autonomic dysreflexia occurs
   a After spinal cord injures
   b In Parkinson's disease
   c With Lou Gehrig's disease
   d Following stroke

13 Autonomic dysreflexia is usually triggered by
   a High blood sugar   c A full bladder
   b High blood pressure   d A virus

14 Arthritis affects
   a The joints   c The muscles
   b The bones   d The hips and knees

15 A person has arthritis. Care includes the following
   except
   a Preventing contractures   c A cast or traction
   b Range-of-motion   d Assisting with ADL
      exercises

16 A person had hip replacement surgery. Which measure
   should you question?
   a Provide a chair with a low seat.
   b Do not cross the legs.
   c Keep a hip abduction wedge between the legs.
   d Provide a long-handled brush for bathing.

17 A person with osteoporosis is at risk for
   a Fractures   c Phantom limb pain
   b An amputation   d Paralysis

18 A cast needs to dry. Which is *false*?
   a The cast is covered with blankets and plastic.
   b The person is turned so the cast dries evenly.
   c The entire cast is supported with pillows.
   d The cast is supported by the palms when lifted.

19 A person has an arm cast. The following are reported
   at once *except*
   a Pain, numbness, or inability to move the fingers
   b Chills, fever, nausea, or vomiting
   c Odor, cyanosis, or temperature changes of the skin
   d Pulse rate of 75 and urine output of 900 mL during
      your shift

20 A person is in traction. You should do the following
   except
   a Perform range-of-motion exercises as directed
   b Keep the weights off the floor
   c Remove the weights if the person is uncomfortable
   d Give skin care at frequent intervals

21 After a hip pinning, the operated leg is
   a Abducted at all times
   b Adducted at all times
   c Externally rotated at all times
   d Flexed at all times

22 After an amputation, the person
   a Is fitted with a prosthesis
   b Needs a wheelchair
   c Has quadriplegia
   d Needs arthroplasty

Answers to these questions are on p. 781.

Cardiovascular and Respiratory System Disorders

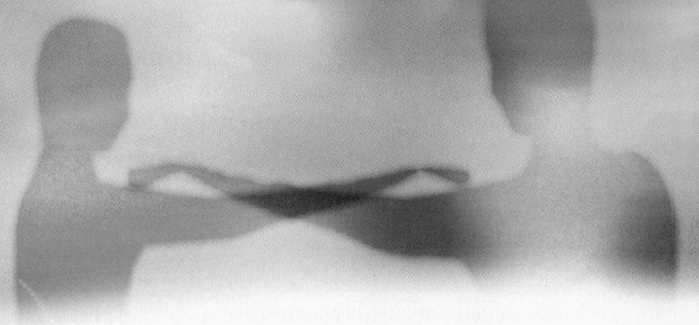

OBJECTIVES

- Define the key terms and key abbreviations listed in this chapter
- Describe congenital heart defects
- Identify the risk factors for hypertension
- Describe hypertension, its signs and symptoms, complications, and treatment
- Describe coronary artery disease and its risk factors
- Identify the complications of coronary artery disease
- Describe cardiac rehabilitation
- Describe angina, its signs and symptoms, and treatment

- Describe myocardial infarction, its signs and symptoms, and treatment
- Describe heart failure, its signs and symptoms, and treatment
- Describe chronic obstructive pulmonary disease, its signs and symptoms, and treatment
- Explain the difference between a cold and influenza
- Explain how influenza is treated
- Describe pneumonia, its signs and symptoms, and treatment
- Describe tuberculosis, its signs and symptoms, and treatment

KEY TERMS

congenital To be born with *(congenitus)*

hypertension The systolic pressure is 140 mm Hg or higher *(hyper)*, or the diastolic pressure is 90 mm Hg or higher; high blood pressure

pre-hypertension When the systolic pressure is between 120 and 139 mm Hg or the diastolic pressure is between 80 and 89 mm Hg

KEY ABBREVIATIONS

AMI Acute myocardial infarction

ASC Acute coronary syndrome

CAD Coronary artery disease

CDC Centers for Disease Control and Prevention

CHF Congestive heart failure

CO_2 Carbon dioxide

COPD Chronic obstructive pulmonary disease

MI Myocardial infarction

mm Hg Millimeters of mercury

O_2 Oxygen

TB Tuberculosis

C ardiovascular and respiratory system disorders are leading causes of death in the United States. Many people have these disorders. Refer to Chapter 8 while you study this chapter.

CARDIOVASCULAR DISORDERS

Problems occur in the heart or blood vessels. Circulatory ulcers were discussed in Chapter 32.

See *Focus on Children and Older Persons: Cardiovascular Disorders.*

FOCUS ON **CHILDREN** AND **OLDER PERSONS**

Cardiovascular Disorders

CHILDREN

Some babies are born with congenital heart defects. (**Congenital** comes from the Latin word *congenitus*. It means to *be born with*.) Defects occur during pregnancy as the baby's heart develops. One or more defects can occur in:

- A part of the heart
- The heart valves
- The blood vessels near the heart
  Depending on the defect, blood flow:
- Slows down
- Goes in the wrong direction
- Goes to the wrong place
- Is blocked completely
  In most cases, the cause is unknown. Risk factors include:
- Heredity. A parent with a congenital heart defect is at risk of having a child with one.
- The mother had a viral infection during pregnancy. German measles (rubella) is a common cause.
- The mother has diabetes.
- The mother took some types of drugs during pregnancy.
- The mother had repeated exposure to some chemicals or x-rays during pregnancy.
- The mother used alcohol or street drugs during pregnancy. The common signs of congenital heart defects are:
- Heart sounds other than "lub-dub" when you take an apical pulse.
- A bluish tint to the skin, lips, and fingernails. "Blue baby" is a term that refers to a child with this sign.
- Fast breathing.
- Shortness of breath.
- Poor feeding. The infant tires easily while nursing.
- Poor weight gain.
- Tiring easily during exercise or activity. Be alert for this sign in older children.
  Some heart defects are found during pregnancy. Others are found when the child is very young. Some defects are not diagnosed until the child is older. Treatment may involve:
- Drugs.
- Correcting the defect by using a catheter. A catheter is inserted into a blood vessel and then into the heart.
- Surgery.
- A heart transplant.
  With successful treatment, many children with heart defects grow into healthy adults. Some need life-long treatment.

Hypertension

With **hypertension** *(high blood pressure)*, the resting blood pressure is too high. The systolic pressure is 140 mm Hg (millimeters of mercury) or higher *(hyper)*. Or the diastolic pressure is 90 mm Hg or higher. Such measurements must occur several times. **Pre-hypertension** is when the systolic pressure is between 120 and 139 mm Hg or the diastolic pressure is between 80 and 89 mm Hg. The person with pre-hypertension will likely develop hypertension in the future. Most people have high blood pressure some time during their lives. See Box 40-1 for risk factors.

Narrowed blood vessels are a common cause. The heart pumps with more force to move blood through narrowed vessels. Kidney disorders, head injuries, some pregnancy problems, and adrenal gland tumors are causes.

A person can have high blood pressure for many years without knowing it. That is why hypertension is called "the silent killer." Usually hypertension is found when blood pressure is measured. Signs and symptoms develop over time. Headache, blurred vision, dizziness, and nose bleeds occur. Hypertension can lead to stroke, hardening of the arteries, heart attack, heart failure, kidney failure, and blindness.

Life-style changes can lower blood pressure. A diet low in fat and salt, a healthy weight, and regular exercise are needed. No smoking is allowed. Alcohol and caffeine are limited. Managing stress and sleeping well also lower blood pressure. Certain drugs can lower blood pressure.

BOX 40-1   Risk Factors for Hypertension

FACTORS YOU *CANNOT* CHANGE

- *Age*—45 years or older for men; 55 years or older for women
- *Gender*—younger men are at greater risk than younger women; the risk increases for women after menopause
- *Race*—African-Americans are at greater risk than whites
- *Family history*—tends to run in families

FACTORS YOU *CAN* CHANGE

- *Being overweight*—related to diet, lack of exercise, and atherosclerosis
- *Stress*—increased sympathetic nervous system activity
- *Tobacco use*—nicotine narrows blood vessels
- *High-salt diet*—sodium causes fluid retention; increased fluid raises blood volume
- *Excessive alcohol*—increases chemical substances in the body that increase blood pressure
- *Lack of exercise*—increases the risk of being overweight
- *Atherosclerosis*—arteries narrow because of fatty build-up in the vessels
- *Pre-hypertension*—blood pressure can be controlled with life-style changes and drugs

Coronary Artery Disease

The coronary arteries are in the heart. They supply the heart with blood. In coronary artery disease (CAD), the coronary arteries become hardened and narrow. One or all are affected. Therefore the heart muscle gets less blood and oxygen. CAD also is called *coronary heart disease* and *heart disease.*

The most common cause is atherosclerosis (Fig. 40-1). Plaque—made up of fat, cholesterol, and other substances—collects on the arterial walls. The narrowed arteries block blood flow. Blockage may be total or partial. Blood clots also can form along the plaque and block blood flow.

The major complications of CAD are angina, myocardial infarction (heart attack), irregular heartbeats, and sudden death. The more risk factors, the greater the chance of CAD and its complications. These risk factors *cannot* be controlled:

▶ Gender—men are at greater risk than women
▶ Age—in men, the risk increases after age 45; in women, the risk increases after age 55
▶ Family history
▶ Race—African-Americans are at greater risk than other groups

These factors *can* be controlled:

▶ Being overweight
▶ Lack of exercise
▶ High blood cholesterol
▶ Hypertension
▶ Smoking
▶ Diabetes
▶ Stress (anger, worry, arguing)

CAD can be treated. The goals of treatment are to:

▶ Relieve symptoms (see "Angina")
▶ Slow or stop atherosclerosis
▶ Lower the risk of blood clots forming
▶ Widen or bypass clogged arteries
▶ Reduce cardiac events (see "Angina" and "Myocardial Infarction")

Persons with CAD need to make life-style changes. The person must quit smoking, exercise, and reduce stress. The person must eat a healthy diet to reduce high

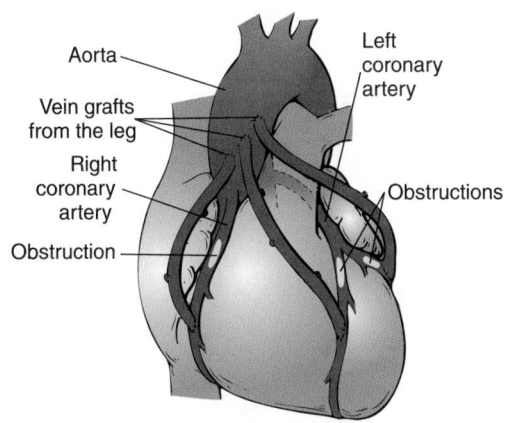

Triple bypass

FIGURE 40-2 Coronary artery bypass surgery. (Modified from Thibodeau GA, Patton KT: *The human body in health & disease,* ed 4, St Louis, 2005, Mosby.)

blood pressure, lower blood cholesterol, and maintain a healthy weight. If overweight, the person must lose weight.

Some persons need drugs to decrease the heart's workload and relieve symptoms. Other drugs are given to prevent a heart attack or sudden death. Drugs also can delay the need for medical and surgical procedures that open or bypass diseased arteries (Fig. 40-2).

Cardiac Rehabilitation

Persons with complications from CAD may need cardiac rehabilitation (cardiac rehab). The cardiac rehab team includes doctors (the person's doctor, a heart specialist, a heart surgeon), nurses, exercise specialists, physical and occupational therapists, dietitians, and psychologists or psychiatrists.

Cardiac rehab has two parts:

▶ Exercise training. The person learns how to exercise safely. Exercises are done to strengthen muscles and improve stamina (staying power, endurance). The exercise plan is based on the person's abilities, needs, and interests.
▶ Education, counseling, and training. The person learns about his or her heart condition and how to reduce the risk of future problems. The person learns how to adjust to a new life-style and how to deal with fears about the future.

Angina

Angina *(pain)* is chest pain. It is from reduced blood flow to part of the heart muscle (myocardium). It occurs when the heart needs more oxygen. Normally blood flow to the heart increases when the need for oxygen increases. Exertion, a heavy meal, stress, and excitement increase the heart's need for oxygen. So does smoking and exposure to very hot or cold temperatures. In CAD, narrowed vessels prevent increased blood flow.

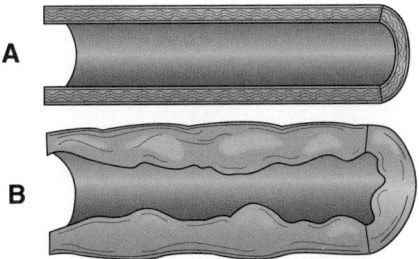

FIGURE 40-1 A, Normal artery. **B,** Plaque on the artery wall in atherosclerosis.

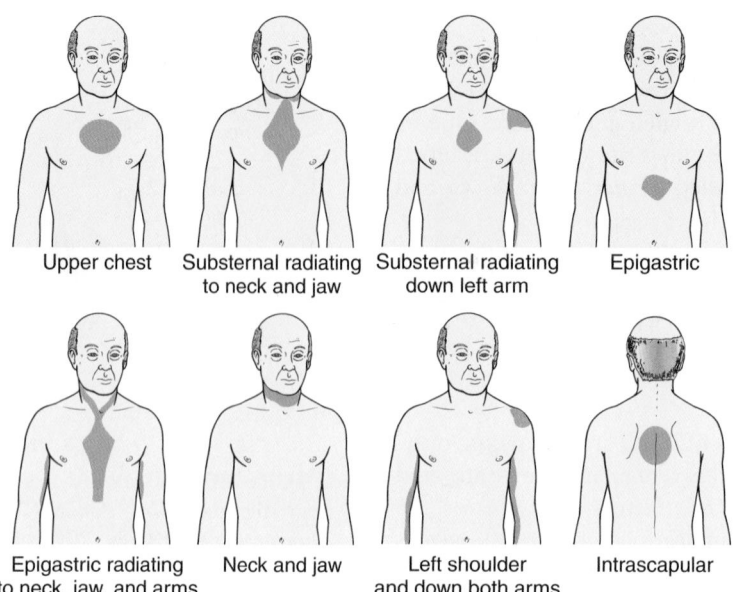

Upper chest | Substernal radiating to neck and jaw | Substernal radiating down left arm | Epigastric

Epigastric radiating to neck, jaw, and arms | Neck and jaw | Left shoulder and down both arms | Intrascapular

FIGURE 40-3 *Shaded areas* show where the pain of angina is located. (From Lewis SM, Heitkemper MM, Dirksen SR: *Medical-surgical nursing: assessment and management of clinical problems,* ed 7, St Louis, 2007, Mosby.)

Chest pain is described as a tightness, pressure, squeezing, or burning in the chest (Fig. 40-3). Pain can occur in the shoulders, arms, neck, jaw, or back. Pain in the jaw, neck, and down one or both arms is common. The person may be pale, feel faint, and perspire. Dyspnea is common. Nausea, fatigue, and weakness may occur. Some persons complain of "gas" or indigestion. Rest often relieves symptoms in 3 to 15 minutes. Rest reduces the heart's need for oxygen. Therefore normal blood flow is achieved. Heart damage is prevented.

Besides rest, a nitroglycerin tablet is taken when angina occurs. It is placed under the tongue. There it dissolves and is rapidly absorbed into the bloodstream. Tablets are kept within the person's reach at all times. The person takes a tablet and then tells the nurse. Some persons have nitroglycerin patches. These are applied and removed by the nurse.

Things that cause angina are avoided. These include over-exertion, heavy meals and over-eating, and emotional stress. The person needs to stay indoors during cold weather or during hot, humid weather. Exercise programs are helpful. They are supervised by the doctor.

See "Coronary Artery Disease" for the treatment of angina. The goal is to increase blood flow to the heart. Doing so may prevent or lower the risk of heart attack and death. Chest pain lasting longer than a few minutes and that is not relieved by rest and nitroglycerin may signal heart attack. The person needs emergency care.

Myocardial Infarction

Myocardial refers to the heart muscle. *Infarction* means tissue death. With myocardial infarction (MI), part of the heart muscle dies. Sudden cardiac death *(sudden cardiac arrest)* can occur (Chapter 49).

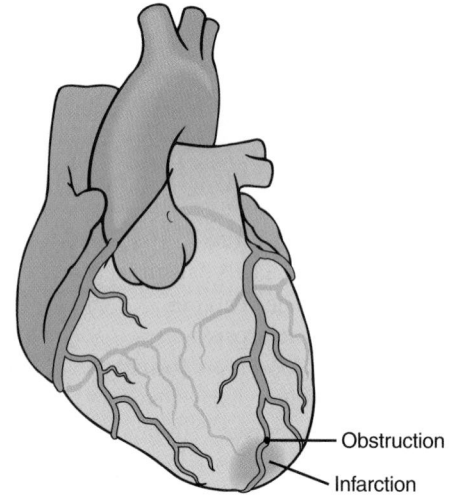

Obstruction

Infarction

FIGURE 40-4 Myocardial infarction. (Modified from Lewis SM, Heitkemper MM, Dirksen SR: *Medical-surgical nursing: assessment and management of clinical problems,* ed 7, St Louis, 2007, Mosby.)

MI also is called:
► Heart attack
► Acute myocardial infarction (AMI)
► Acute coronary syndrome (ACS)
► Coronary
► Coronary thrombosis
► Coronary occlusion

In MI, blood flow to the heart muscle is suddenly blocked. A thrombus (blood clot) blocks blood flow in an artery with atherosclerosis. The area of damage may be small or large (Fig. 40-4).

BOX 40-2 Signs and Symptoms of Myocardial Infarction

- Chest pain
  - Sudden, severe; usually on the left side
  - Described as crushing, stabbing, or squeezing; some describe it as someone sitting on the chest
  - More severe and lasts longer than angina
  - Not relieved by rest and nitroglycerin
- Pain or numbness in one or both arms, the back, neck, jaw, or stomach
- Indigestion or "heartburn"
- Dyspnea
- Nausea
- Dizziness
- Perspiration and cold, clammy skin
- Pallor or cyanosis
- Blood pressure: low
- Pulse: weak and irregular
- Fear, apprehension, and a feeling of doom

CAD, angina, and previous MI are risk factors. Signs and symptoms are listed in Box 40-2. MI is an emergency. Efforts are made to:

▶ Relieve pain
▶ Restore blood flow to the heart
▶ Stabilize vital signs
▶ Give oxygen
▶ Calm the person
▶ Prevent life-threatening problems

If the person survives, he or she may need medical or surgical procedures to open or bypass the diseased artery. Cardiac rehabilitation is needed. The goals are to:

▶ Recover and resume normal activities
▶ Prevent another MI
▶ Prevent complications such as heart failure or sudden cardiac arrest

See *Focus on Long-Term Care and Home Care: Myocardial Infarction.*

Heart Failure

Heart failure or congestive heart failure (CHF) occurs when the heart is weakened and cannot pump normally. Blood backs up. Tissue congestion occurs.

When the left side of the heart cannot pump blood normally. Blood backs up into the lungs. Respiratory congestion occurs. The person has dyspnea, increased sputum, cough, and gurgling sounds in the lungs. Also, the rest of the body does not get enough blood. Signs and symptoms occur from the effects on other organs. Poor blood flow to the brain causes confusion, dizziness, and fainting. The kidneys produce less urine. The skin is pale. Blood pressure falls.

When the right side of the heart cannot pump blood normally. Blood backs up into the venous system. Feet and ankles swell. Neck veins bulge. Liver congestion affects liver function. The abdomen becomes congested with fluid. The right side of the heart pumps less blood to the lungs. Normal blood flow does not occur from the lungs to the left side of the heart. The left side has less

---

FOCUS ON LONG-TERM CARE AND HOME CARE

Myocardial Infarction

HOME CARE
Cardiac rehabilitation continues. The person may go to a gym, health club, or hospital fitness center. Some persons go to indoor malls for walking. Normal activities are increased slowly. The person returns to work with the doctor's approval.

---

blood to pump to the body. As with left-sided heart failure, organs receive less blood. The signs and symptoms described for left-sided failure occur.

A very severe form of heart failure is *pulmonary edema* (fluid in the lungs). It is an emergency. The person can die.

A damaged or weakened heart usually causes heart failure. CAD, MI, hypertension, age, diabetes, and irregular heart rhythms are common causes. So are damaged heart valves and kidney disease.

Drugs strengthen the heart. They also reduce the amount of fluid in the body. A sodium-controlled diet is ordered. Oxygen is given. Semi-Fowler's position is preferred for breathing. The person must reduce the risk factors for CAD. If acutely ill, the person needs hospital care.

You assist with these aspects of the person's care:

▶ Promoting rest and activity as ordered
▶ Measuring intake and output
▶ Measuring weight daily
▶ Assisting with pulse oximetry
▶ Restricting fluids as ordered
▶ Promoting a diet that is low in sodium, fat, and cholesterol
▶ Preventing skin breakdown and pressure ulcers
▶ Performing range-of-motion exercises
▶ Assisting with other exercises as ordered
▶ Assisting with transfers and ambulation
▶ Assisting with self-care activities
▶ Maintaining good alignment
▶ Applying elastic stockings

Many older persons have heart failure. They are at risk for skin breakdown. Tissue swelling, poor circulation, and fragile skin combine to increase the risk of pressure ulcers. Good skin care and regular position changes are needed.

See *Focus on Children and Older Persons: Heart Failure.*

FOCUS ON CHILDREN AND OLDER PERSONS

Heart Failure

CHILDREN
Congenital heart defects can cause heart failure in children.

OLDER PERSONS
Many older persons suffer from heart failure. Some need home care or long-term care.

Older persons are at risk for skin breakdown. Tissue swelling, poor circulation, and fragile skin combine to increase the risk of pressure ulcers. Good skin care and regular position changes are needed.

RESPIRATORY DISORDERS

The respiratory system brings oxygen (O_2) into the lungs and removes carbon dioxide (CO_2) from the body. Respiratory disorders interfere with this function and threaten life.

Chronic Obstructive Pulmonary Disease

Three disorders are grouped under chronic obstructive pulmonary disease (COPD). They are chronic bronchitis, emphysema, and asthma. These disorders interfere with O_2 and CO_2 exchange in the lungs. They obstruct airflow. Lung function is gradually lost.

Cigarette smoking is the most important risk factor for COPD. Pipe, cigar, and other smoking tobaccos are also risk factors. So is exposure to second-hand smoke. Not smoking is the best way to prevent COPD. COPD has no cure.

COPD affects the airways and alveoli (Chapter 8). Less air gets into the lungs; less air goes out of the lungs. The following changes occur:

▶ The airways and alveoli (air sacs) become less elastic. They are like old rubber bands.
▶ The walls between many of the alveoli are destroyed.
▶ Walls of the airway become thick, inflamed, and swollen.
▶ The airways secrete more mucus than usual. The excess mucus clogs the airways.

Chronic Bronchitis

Chronic bronchitis occurs after repeated episodes of bronchitis. Bronchitis means inflammation (*itis*) of the bronchi (*bronch*). Smoking is the major cause. Infection, air pollution, and industrial dusts are risk factors.

Smoker's cough in the morning is often the first symptom. At first the cough is dry. Over time, the person coughs up mucus. Mucus may contain pus. The cough becomes more frequent. The person has difficulty breathing and tires easily. Mucus and inflamed breathing passages obstruct airflow into the lungs. The body cannot get normal amounts of oxygen.

The person must stop smoking. Oxygen therapy and breathing exercises are often ordered. Respiratory tract infections are prevented. If one occurs, the person needs prompt treatment.

Emphysema

In emphysema, the alveoli enlarge. They become less elastic. They do not expand and shrink normally with breathing in and out. As a result, some air is trapped in the alveoli when exhaling. Trapped air is not exhaled. Over time, more alveoli are involved. O_2 and CO_2 exchange cannot occur in affected alveoli. As more air is trapped in the lungs, the person develops a *barrel chest* (Fig. 40-5).

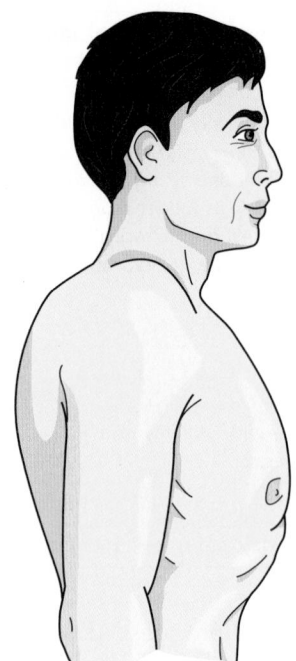

FIGURE 40-5 Barrel chest from emphysema.

Smoking is the most common cause. Air pollution and industrial dusts are risk factors.

The person has shortness of breath and a cough. At first, shortness of breath occurs with exertion. Over time, it occurs at rest. Sputum may contain pus. Fatigue is common. The person works hard to breathe in and out. And the body does not get enough oxygen. Breathing is easier when the person sits upright and slightly forward (Chapter 34).

The person must stop smoking. Respiratory therapy, breathing exercises, oxygen, and drug therapy are ordered.

Asthma

The airway becomes inflamed and narrow. Extra mucus is produced. Dyspnea results. Wheezing and coughing are common. So are pain and tightening in the chest. Symptoms are mild to severe.

Asthma usually is triggered by allergies. Other triggers include air pollutants and irritants, smoking and second-hand smoke, respiratory infections, exertion, and cold air.

Sudden attacks (*asthma attacks*) can occur. There is shortness of breath, wheezing, coughing, rapid pulse, sweating, and cyanosis. The person gasps for air and is very frightened. Fear makes the attack worse.

Asthma is treated with drugs. Severe attacks may require emergency care. The person and family learn how to prevent asthma attacks. Repeated attacks can damage the respiratory system.

TABLE 40-1 Cold vs the Flu

SYMPTOMS	COLD	FLU
Fever	Rare	Usually high (100° to 102° F); lasts 3 to 4 days
Headache	Rare	Common
General aches & pains	Slight	Usual; often severe
Fatigue; weakness	Sometimes	Usual; can last 2 to 3 weeks
Extreme exhaustion	Never	Usual; at the beginning of the illness
Stuffy nose	Common	Sometimes
Sneezing	Usual	Sometimes
Sore throat	Common	Sometimes
Chest discomfort; cough	Mild to moderate; hacking cough	Common; can be severe
Complications	Sinus congestion; middle ear infection (otitis media); asthma	Bronchitis; pneumonia; can be life-threatening

Modified from National Institute of Allergy and Infectious Disease: *Is it a cold or the flu?* Bethesda, Md, September 2005, National Institutes of Health.

Influenza

Influenza *(flu)* is a respiratory infection. See Table 40-1 for the differences between a *cold* and the *flu*. Caused by viruses, flu season is usually from November through March. According to the Centers for Disease Control and Prevention (CDC), about 36,000 people die every year from the flu and its complications. Most deaths occur in older persons. Older persons with lung or heart diseases are at great risk.

Treatment involves fluids, rest, and relief of symptoms. The doctor orders drugs for symptom relief and to shorten the flu episode. Most people are better in about one week.

Coughing and sneezing spread flu viruses. Standard Precautions are followed. The flu vaccine is the best way to prevent the disease. The CDC recommends the flu vaccine for persons who:

▶ Are 50 years of age and older
▶ Have chronic heart, lung, or kidney diseases
▶ Have diabetes
▶ Have immune system problems
▶ Have a severe form of anemia (a decrease in hemoglobin in the blood)
▶ Will be more than 3 months pregnant during the flu season
▶ Are nursing center or assisted-living residents
▶ Are in close contact with children 0 to 23 months of age
 Pneumonia is a common complication.
 See *Focus on Children and Older Persons: Influenza.*

Pneumonia

Pneumonia is an inflammation and infection of lung tissue. (*Pneumo* means lungs.) Affected tissues fill with fluid. O_2 and CO_2 exchange is affected.

Bacteria, viruses, and other microbes are causes. Microbes reach the lungs by being inhaled, aspirated, or carried in the blood to the lungs from an infection elsewhere in the body. Children under 2 years of age and adults over 65 years of age are at risk. Older adults are at

---

FOCUS ON CHILDREN AND OLDER PERSONS

Influenza

OLDER PERSONS

Older persons may not have the signs and symptoms listed in Table 40-1. The following may signal flu in older persons:
- Changes in mental status
- Worsening of other health problems
- A body temperature below the normal range
- Fatigue
- Decreased appetite and fluid intake

---

great risk of dying from the disease. Smoking, aging, stroke, bedrest, immobility, chronic diseases, and tube feedings are among the factors that increase the risk of pneumonia.

Onset may be sudden. The person is very ill. High fever, chills, painful cough, chest pain on breathing, and rapid pulse occur. Shortness of breath and rapid breathing also occur. Cyanosis may be present. Sputum is thick and white, green, yellow, or rust colored. The color depends on the cause. Other signs and symptoms are nausea, vomiting, headache, tiredness, and muscle aches.

Drugs are ordered for infection and pain. Fluid intake is increased because of fever and to thin secretions. Thin secretions are easier to cough up. Intravenous therapy and oxygen may be needed. Semi-Fowler's position eases breathing. Rest is important. Standard Precautions are followed. Isolation Precautions are used depending on the cause. Mouth care is important. Frequent linen changes are needed because of fever.

See *Focus on Children and Older Persons: Pneumonia,* p. 664.

Tuberculosis

Tuberculosis (TB) is a bacterial infection in the lungs. It also can occur in the kidneys, bones, joints, nervous system (including the spine), muscles, and other parts of the body. If TB is not treated, the person can die.

TB is spread by airborne droplets with coughing,

FOCUS ON **CHILDREN** AND **OLDER PERSONS**

Pneumonia

CHILDREN
Pneumonia occurs in children of all ages. It is more common in infants and toddlers.

OLDER PERSONS
Changes from aging, diseases, and decreased mobility increase the risk of pneumonia in older persons. Decreased mobility after surgery also is a risk factor.

Aspiration pneumonia is common in older persons. Dysphagia, decreased cough and gag reflexes, and nervous system disorders are risk factors. So are substances that depress the brain—narcotics, sedatives, alcohol, and drugs for anesthesia.

Older persons may not have the typical signs and symptoms. Drugs and other diseases can mask signs and symptoms. Older persons may show signs of confusion, dehydration, and rapid respirations.

FOCUS ON **LONG-TERM CARE** AND **HOME CARE**

Tuberculosis

LONG-TERM CARE
Increased numbers of nursing center residents have active TB. Infected long ago, the TB becomes active because general health declines with aging. Other older people become newly infected from lengthy, extended contact with those already infected.

sneezing, speaking, singing, or laughing (Chapter 14). Nearby persons can inhale the bacteria. Those who have close, frequent contact with an infected person are at risk. TB is more likely to occur in close, crowded areas. Age, poor nutrition, and HIV (human immunodeficiency virus) infection are other risk factors.

TB can be present in the body but not cause signs and symptoms. An active infection may not occur for many years. Only persons with an active infection can spread the disease to others.

Chest x-rays and TB testing can detect the disease. Signs and symptoms are tiredness, loss of appetite, weight loss, fever, and night sweats. Cough and sputum production increase over time. Sputum may contain blood. Chest pain occurs.

Drugs for TB are given. Standard Precautions and Isolation Precautions are needed (Chapter 14). The person must cover the mouth and nose with tissues when sneezing, coughing, or producing sputum. Tissues are flushed down the toilet, placed in a biohazard bag, or placed in a paper bag and burned. Hand washing after contact with sputum is essential.

See *Focus on Long-Term Care and Home Care: Tuberculosis.*

REVIEW QUESTIONS

Circle the BEST answer.

1 A person has a congenital heart defect. This means that the person
   a Needs heart surgery
   b Has damaged heart values
   c Has blocked coronary arteries
   d Was born with the defect

2 A person has hypertension. You know that the person's systolic blood pressure is
   a Over 140 mm Hg
   b Over 120 mm Hg
   c Over 90 mm Hg
   d Over 80 mm Hg

3 Which is *not* a complication of hypertension?
   a Stroke
   b Heart attack
   c Renal failure
   d Diabetes

4 A person has hypertension. Treatment will likely include the following *except*
   a No smoking and regular exercise
   b A high-sodium diet
   c A low-calorie diet if the person is obese
   d Drugs to lower blood pressure

5 A person has angina. Which is *true?*
   a There is heart muscle damage.
   b Pain is described as crushing, stabbing, or squeezing.
   c Pain is relieved with rest and nitroglycerin.
   d Pain is always on the left side of the chest.

6 Cardiac rehabilitation involves
   a Exercise
   b Surgery
   c Catheter procedures
   d Receiving a vaccine

7 A person is having a myocardial infarction. Which is *false?*
   a The person is having a heart attack.
   b This is an emergency.
   c The person may have a cardiac arrest.
   d The person does not have enough blood to provide needed oxygen.

8 The pain of myocardial infection is usually
   a On the left side of the chest
   b On the right side of the chest
   c In the upper abdomen
   d In the mid-back region

9 A person has heart failure. Which measure should you question?
   a Encourage fluids.
   b Measure intake and output.
   c Measure weight daily.
   d Perform range-of-motion exercises.

10 The most common cause of COPD is
   a Smoking
   b Allergies
   c Being overweight
   d A high-sodium diet

11 A person has emphysema. Which is *false?*
   a The person has dyspnea.
   b The person has an infection.
   c Breathing is usually easier sitting upright and slightly forward.
   d Sputum may contain pus.

12 The flu virus is spread by
   a Coughing and sneezing
   b The fecal-oral route
   c Blood
   d Needle sharing

13 A person has pneumonia. You know that this is
   a An inflammation of the airway
   b Narrowing of the airway
   c An inflammation and infection of lung tissue
   d A bacterial infection in the lungs

14 Which position is usually best for the person with pneumonia?
   a Supine
   b Prone
   c Semi-Fowler's
   d Trendelenburg's

15 Tuberculosis is spread by
   a Coughing and sneezing
   b Contaminated drinking water
   c Contact with wound drainage
   d The fecal-oral route

16 A person has TB. You had contact with the person's sputum. What should you do?
   a Wash your hands.
   b Put on gloves.
   c Use an alcohol-based hand rub.
   d Tell the nurse.

Answers to these questions are on p. 782.

CHAPTER
41 Digestive and Endocrine System Disorders

OBJECTIVES

- Define the key terms and key abbreviations listed in this chapter
- Describe gastroesophageal reflux disease and the care required
- Describe the care required for vomiting
- Describe diverticular disease and the care required
- Describe gallstones and the care required
- Describe hepatitis and the care required
- Describe diabetes and the care required

KEY TERMS

emesis Vomitus

hyperglycemia High *(hyper)* sugar *(glyc)* in the blood *(emia)*

hypoglycemia Low *(hypo)* sugar *(glyc)* in the blood *(emia)*

jaundice Yellowish color of the skin or whites of the eyes

vomitus Food and fluids expelled from the stomach through the mouth; emesis

KEY ABBREVIATIONS

GERD Gastroesophageal reflux disease
HBV Hepatitis B virus
I&O Intake and output
IV Intravenous

BOX 41-2 **Signs and Symptoms of Hepatitis**

- Jaundice (yellowish color of the skin or whites of the eyes)
- Fatigue, weakness
- Pain and discomfort: abdominal, joint, muscles
- Appetite: loss of
- Nausea and vomiting
- Diarrhea
- Bowel movements: light, clay-colored
- Urine: dark
- Fever and chills
- Headache
- Itching
- Weight loss
- Skin rash

FOCUS ON **CHILDREN** AND **OLDER PERSONS**

Hepatitis A

CHILDREN

Hepatitis A is more common in pre-school and school-age children. Children in day care are at risk. Poor hygiene after bowel movements leads to contaminated eating and drinking vessels. Also, young children often put their hands into their mouths.

Hepatitis A

This type is spread by the fecal-oral route. The hepatitis A virus is ingested when eating or drinking contaminated food or water. It is also ingested when eating or drinking from a contaminated vessel. Causes include poor sanitation, crowded living conditions, poor nutrition, poor hygiene, and anal sex.

Treatment involves rest, a healthy diet, fluids, and no alcohol. Recovery takes about 8 weeks.

Persons with fecal incontinence, confusion, and dementia can cause contamination. Carefully look for contaminated items and areas.

Handle bedpans, feces, and rectal thermometers carefully. Good hand washing is needed by everyone, including the person. Assist with hand washing after bowel movements. The hepatitis A vaccine provides protection against the disease.

See *Focus on Children and Older Persons: Hepatitis A.*

Hepatitis B

Hepatitis B is caused by the hepatitis B virus (HBV). It is present in the blood and body fluids (saliva, semen, vaginal secretions) of infected persons. It is spread by:

- IV drug use and sharing needles
- Accidental needle sticks
- Sex without a condom, especially anal sex
- Contaminated tools used for tattoos or body piercings
- Sharing a toothbrush, razor, or nail clippers with an infected person

For the HBV vaccine, see Chapter 14. The doctor orders drugs to treat chronic hepatitis B.

Hepatitis C

This type is spread by blood contaminated with the hepatitis C virus. A person may have the virus but no symptoms. Serious liver disease and damage may show up years later. Even without symptoms, the person can transmit the disease. Hepatitis C is treated with drugs. The virus is spread by:

- Blood contaminated with the virus
- IV drug use and sharing needles
- Inhaling cocaine through contaminated straws
- Contaminated tools used for tattoos or body piercings
- High-risk sexual activity—sex with an infected person, multiple sex partners
- Sharing a toothbrush, razor, or nail clippers with an infected person

Hepatitis D and Hepatitis E

Hepatitis D occurs only in people infected with hepatitis B. It is spread the same way as HBV.

Hepatitis E is spread through food or water contaminated by feces from an infected person. It is spread by the fecal-oral route. This disease is not common in the United States.

THE ENDOCRINE SYSTEM

The endocrine system is made up of glands. The endocrine glands secrete hormones that affect other organs and glands. Diabetes is the most common endocrine disorder.

Diabetes

In this disorder the body cannot produce or use insulin properly. Insulin is needed for glucose to move from the blood into the cells. The cells need glucose for energy. The pancreas secretes insulin. Without enough insulin, sugar builds up in the blood. Blood glucose (sugar) is high. Cells do not have enough sugar for energy and cannot function.

Risk factors include a family history of the disease. For type 1, whites are at greater risk than non-whites. Type 2 is more common in older and overweight persons. These ethnic groups are at risk for type 2:

- African-Americans
- Native Americans
- Hispanics

Signs and Symptoms

Signs and symptoms of diabetes are:

- Being very thirsty
- Urinating often
- Feeling very hungry or tired
- Losing weight without trying
- Having sores that heal slowly
- Having dry, itchy skin
- Losing feeling or tingling in the feet
- Blurred vision

Types of Diabetes

There are three types of diabetes:

▶ *Type 1*—occurs most often in children, teenagers, and young adults. The pancreas produces little or no insulin. Onset is rapid.

▶ *Type 2*—can occur at any age, even during childhood. Persons over 45 years of age are at risk. Being overweight, lack of exercise, and hypertension are risk factors. The pancreas secretes insulin. However, the body cannot use it well. Onset is slow. Infections are frequent. Wounds heal slowly. Gum disease (Chapter 19) is common.

▶ *Gestational diabetes*—develops during pregnancy. (Gestation comes from *gestare*. It means to *bear*.) It usually goes away after the baby is born. However, the mother is at risk for type 2 diabetes later in life.

Complications

Diabetes must be controlled to prevent complications. They include blindness, renal failure, nerve damage, and damage to the gums and teeth. Heart and blood vessel diseases are very serious problems. They can lead to stroke, heart attack, and slow healing. Foot and leg wounds and ulcers are very serious (Chapter 32). Infection and gangrene can occur. Sometimes amputation is necessary.

Treatment

Type 1 is treated with daily insulin therapy, healthy eating (Chapter 23), and exercise. Type 2 is treated with healthy eating and exercise. Many persons with type 2 take oral drugs. Some need insulin. Overweight persons need to lose weight. Types 1 and 2 involve controlling blood pressure, cholesterol, and the risk factors for coronary artery disease.

Good foot care is needed. Corns, blisters, calluses, and other foot problems can lead to an infection and amputation (Chapter 32).

The person's blood sugar level can fall too low or go too high. Blood glucose is monitored daily or 3 or 4 times a day for:

▶ **Hypoglycemia** means low (*hypo*) sugar (*glyc*) in the blood (*emia*).

▶ **Hyperglycemia** means high (*hyper*) sugar (*glyc*) in the blood (*emia*).

See Table 41-1 for the causes, signs, and symptoms of hypoglycemia and hyperglycemia. Both can lead to death if not corrected. You must call for the nurse at once.

See *Focus on Children and Older Persons: Treatment*.

FOCUS ON **CHILDREN** AND **OLDER PERSONS**

Treatment

CHILDREN

You may prepare meals for a child with diabetes. Follow the child's diet carefully. Also prepare snacks for the child to take to school. The snack is needed in case the child's blood sugar level drops.

TABLE 41-1 Hypoglycemia and Hyperglycemia

	CAUSES	SIGNS AND SYMPTOMS
Hypoglycemia (low blood sugar)	Too much insulin or diabetic drugs Omitting or missing a meal Delayed meal Eating too little food Increased exercise Vomiting Drinking alcohol	Hunger Fatigue; weakness Trembling; shakiness Sweating Headache Dizziness Faintness Pulse: rapid Blood pressure: low Respirations: rapid and shallow Motions: clumsy and jerky Tingling around the mouth Confusion Vision: changes in Skin: cold and clammy Convulsions Unconsciousness

TABLE 41-1 Hypoglycemia and Hyperglycemia—cont'd

	CAUSES	SIGNS AND SYMPTOMS
Hyperglycemia (high blood sugar)	Undiagnosed diabetes Not enough insulin or diabetic drugs Eating too much food Too little exercise Emotional stress Infection or sickness	Weakness Drowsiness Thirst Dry mouth (very) Hunger Urination: frequent Leg cramps Face: flushed Breath odor: sweet Respirations: slow, deep, and labored Pulse: rapid, weak Blood pressure: low Skin: dry Vision: blurred Headache Nausea and vomiting Convulsions Coma

REVIEW QUESTIONS

Circle the BEST answer.

1 A person has gastroesophageal reflux disease. Which nursing measure should you question?
   a Person to wear loose clothing
   b Supine position after meals
   c Person to have small meals
   d No smoking or alcohol

2 A person with gastroesophageal reflux disease has the following food choices. Which is best for the person?
   a Baked chicken
   b Pasta with tomato sauce
   c Pizza
   d Salad with orange slices

3 A person is vomiting. How should you position the person?
   a Supine
   b Prone
   c Semi-Fowler's
   d With the head turned to the side

4 Vomiting is dangerous because of
   a Aspiration
   b Diverticular disease
   c Fluid loss
   d Jaundice

5 Vomitus looks like coffee grounds. You need to report this at once because it signals
   a Bleeding
   b Gastroesophageal reflux disease
   c Gallstones
   d A ruptured pouch

6 A person has diverticular disease. You will likely assist the nurse with
   a Preventing diarrhea
   b Giving antibiotics
   c Giving enemas
   d Preventing constipation

7 Gallbladder attacks usually occur
   a On awakening
   b During a fast
   c After a fatty meal
   d When the person is lying down

8 Which is *not* a sign of gallstones?
   a Jaundice
   b Pain under the right shoulder
   c Clay-colored stools
   d Hoarseness and choking sensation

9 Hepatitis is an inflammation of the
   a Liver
   b Gallbladder
   c Pancreas
   d Stomach

10 Hepatitis A is spread by
   a Needle sharing
   b IV drug use
   c Contaminated blood
   d The fecal-oral route

11 Hepatitis requires
   a Sterile gloves
   b Double bagging
   c Standard Precautions
   d Masks, gowns, and goggles

12 Which is *not* a sign of diabetes?
   a Increased urine production
   b Weight gain
   c Hunger
   d Increased thirst

13 A person with diabetes needs the following *except*
   a Exercise
   b Good foot care
   c A sodium-controlled diet
   d Healthy eating

14 A person with diabetes is vomiting after a meal. The person is at risk for
   a Hypoglycemia
   b Hyperglycemia
   c Jaundice
   d Bleeding

Answers to these questions are on p. 782.

42 Urinary and Reproductive System Disorders

OBJECTIVES

- Define the key terms and key abbreviations listed in this chapter
- Describe urinary tract infections and the care required
- Describe prostate enlargement and the care required
- Describe urinary diversions and the care required
- Describe renal calculi and the care required
- Explain the difference between acute renal failure and chronic renal failure and the care required
- Describe sexually transmitted diseases and the care required

KEY TERMS

diuresis The process *(esis)* of passing *(di)* urine *(ur)*; large amounts of urine are produced—1000 to 5000 mL a day

dysuria Difficult or painful *(dys)* urination *(uria)*

hematuria Blood *(hemat)* in the urine *(uria)*

oliguria Scant *(olig)* urine *(uria)*

pyuria Pus *(py)* in the urine *(uria)*

urinary diversion A new pathway for urine to exit the body

urostomy A surgically created opening *(stomy)* between the ureter *(uro)* and the abdomen

KEY ABBREVIATIONS

AIDS Acquired immunodeficiency syndrome

BPH Benign prostatic hyperplasia

HIV Human immunodeficiency virus

mL Milliliter

STD Sexually transmitted disease

TURP Transurethral resection of the prostate

UTI Urinary tract infection

URINARY SYSTEM DISORDERS

Understanding urinary and reproductive disorders gives meaning to the required care. Refer to Chapter 8 while you study this chapter.

URINARY SYSTEM DISORDERS

The kidneys, ureters, bladder, and urethra are the major urinary system structures. Disorders can occur in these structures. Men can develop prostate problems.

Urinary Tract Infections

Urinary tract infections (UTIs) are common. Infection in one area can involve the entire system. Microbes can enter the system through the urethra. Catheterization, urological exams, intercourse, poor perineal hygiene, immobility, and poor fluid intake are common causes. UTI is a common healthcare-associated infection (Chapter 14).

Women are at high risk. Microbes can easily enter the short female urethra. Prostate gland secretions help protect men from UTIs. However, an enlarged prostate increases the risk of UTI in older men.

Older persons are at high risk for UTIs. Incomplete bladder emptying, perineal soiling from fecal incontinence, poor fluid intake, and poor nutrition increase the risk of UTI in older men and women.

Cystitis

Cystitis is a bladder *(cyst)* infection *(itis)*. It is caused by bacteria. The following signs and symptoms are common:

► Urinary frequency
► **Oliguria**—scant *(olig)* urine *(uria)*
► Urgency
► **Dysuria**—difficult or painful *(dys)* urination *(uria)*
► Pain or burning on urination
► Foul-smelling urine
► **Hematuria**—blood *(hemat)* in the urine *(uria)*
► **Pyuria**—pus *(py)* in the urine *(uria)*
► Fever

Antibiotics are ordered. Fluids are encouraged—usually 2000 mL (milliliters) per day. If untreated, cystitis can lead to pyelonephritis.

Pyelonephritis

Pyelonephritis is inflammation *(itis)* of the kidney *(nephr)* pelvis *(pyelo)*. Infection is the most common cause. Cloudy urine may contain pus, mucus, and blood. Chills, fever, back pain, and nausea and vomiting occur. So do the signs and symptoms of cystitis. Treatment involves antibiotics and fluids.

Prostate Enlargement

The prostate is a gland in men. It lies in front of the rectum and just below the bladder (Chapter 8). The prostate also surrounds the urethra. In young men, the prostate is about the size of a walnut. The prostate grows larger (enlarges) as the man grows older. This is called benign prostatic hyperplasia (BPH). (*Benign* means non-malignant. *Hyper*

means excessive. *Plasia* means formation or development.) Benign prostatic hypertrophy is another name for enlarged prostate. (*Trophy* means growth.)

Usually BPH does not cause problems until after age 50. Most men in their 60s, 70s, and 80s have some symptoms of BPH.

BPH causes urinary problems. The enlarged prostate presses against the urethra. This obstructs urine flow through the urethra. Bladder function is gradually lost. These problems are common:

► A weak urine stream
► Frequent voidings of small amounts of urine
► Urgency and leaking or dribbling of urine
► Frequent urination at night
► Urinary retention (The man cannot void. Urine remains in the bladder.)

Treatment depends on the extent of the problem. For mild BPH, the doctor may order drugs. Drugs can shrink the prostate or stop its growth. Some microwave and laser treatments destroy the excess prostate tissue.

Transurethral resection of the prostate (TURP) is a common surgical procedure. A lighted scope is inserted through the penis. The scope has a wire loop. The doctor uses the loop to cut tissue and seal blood vessels. The removed tissue is flushed out of the bladder at the end of the surgery. A special catheter is inserted and left in place for a few days. Flushing fluid enters the bladder through the catheter. Urine and the flushing fluid flow out of the bladder through the same catheter. Some bleeding and blood clots are normal. After surgery, the person's care plan may include the following:

► No straining or sudden movements
► Drinking at least 8 cups of water daily to flush the bladder
► No straining to have a bowel movement
► A balanced diet to prevent constipation
► No heavy lifting

Urinary Diversions

Sometimes the urinary bladder is surgically removed. Cancer and bladder injuries are common reasons. When the bladder is removed, urine must still leave the body. A new pathway—**urinary diversion**—is needed for urine to exit the body.

Often an ostomy is involved. A **urostomy** is a surgically created opening *(stomy)* between the ureter *(uro)* and the abdomen (Fig. 42-1, p. 674). The nurse provides care after surgery. You may care for persons with long-standing urostomies. The persons assists with care as able.

A pouch is applied over the stoma (Fig. 42-2, p. 674). Urine drains through the stoma into the pouch. Pouches are changed every 5 to 7 days. A pouch is replaced anytime it leaks. Skin irritation, breakdown, and infection can occur if urine leaks onto the skin. See "The Person With an Ostomy" in Chapter 22.

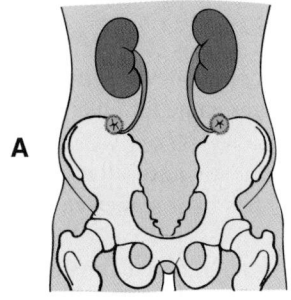 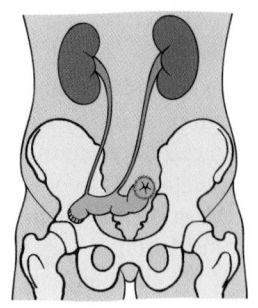

FIGURE 42-1 Urostomies. **A,** Both ureters are brought through the skin onto the abdomen. The person has two stomas. **B,** The ileal conduit. A small section of the small intestine is removed. One end is sutured closed. The other end is brought through the skin onto the abdomen to form a stoma. The ureters are attached to this part of the small intestine. (From Beare PA, Myers JL: *Principles and practices of adult health nursing*, ed 3, St Louis, 1998, Mosby.)

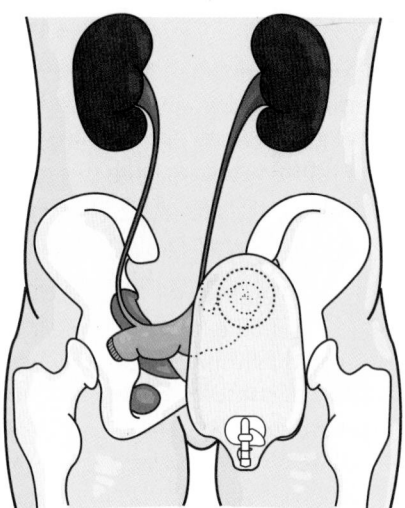

FIGURE 42-2 Urostomy pouch.

Renal Calculi

Renal calculi are kidney (renal) stones (calculi). White men between the ages of 20 and 40 years are at risk. Bedrest, immobility, and poor fluid intake are risk factors. Stones vary in size (Fig. 42-3). Some are as small as grains of sand or as large as pearls. Some are as big as golf balls. Signs and symptoms include:

▶ Severe, cramping pain in the back and side just below the ribs (Fig. 42-4)
▶ Pain in the abdomen, thigh, and urethra
▶ Nausea and vomiting
▶ Fever and chills
▶ Dysuria—difficult or painful *(dys)* urination *(uria)*
▶ Urinary frequency
▶ Urinary urgency
▶ Burning on urination
▶ Oliguria—scant *(olig)* urine *(uria)*
▶ Hematuria—blood *(hemat)* in the urine *(uria)*
▶ Cloudy urine
▶ Foul-smelling urine

Drugs are given for pain relief. The person needs to drink 2000 to 3000 mL of fluid a day. Increased fluids help stones pass from the body through the urine. All urine is strained (Chapter 30). Surgical removal of the stone may be necessary. Some dietary changes can prevent stones.

Renal Failure

In renal failure (kidney failure), the kidneys do not function or are severely impaired. Waste products are not removed from the blood. The body retains fluid. Heart failure and hypertension easily result. Renal failure may be acute or chronic. The person is very ill.

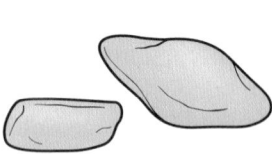

Smooth

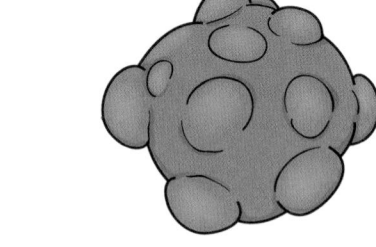

Golf-ball-sized and brown

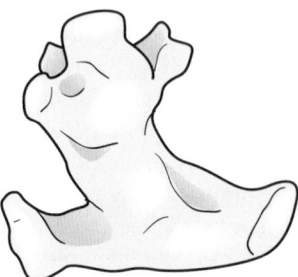

Staghorn

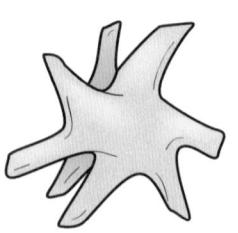

Jagged and yellow

FIGURE 42-3 Kidney stones.

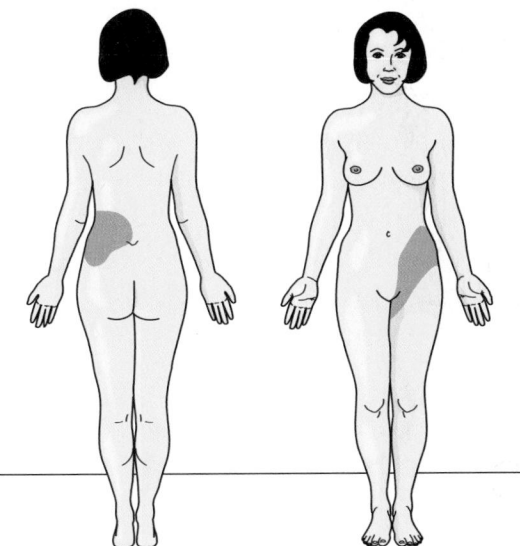

FIGURE 42-4 *Shaded areas* show where the pain from kidney stones is located.

BOX 42-1 Signs and Symptoms of Chronic Renal Failure

- Skin:
  - Color: yellow, tan, or dusky
  - Dry, itchy
  - Thin, brittle
- Bruises
- Breath: bad breath (*halitosis*)
- Mouth: inflammation of (*stomatitis*)
- Nausea
- Vomiting
- Appetite: loss of
- Weight loss
- Diarrhea or constipation
- Urine output: decreased
- Bleeding tendencies
- Infection: susceptible to
- Hypertension
- Heart failure
- Gastric ulcers
- Gastrointestinal bleeding
- Pulse: irregular
- Breathing: abnormal patterns
- Legs and feet: burning sensation in
- Muscles: twitching and cramps
- Fatigue
- Sleep disorders
- Headache
- Convulsions
- Confusion
- Coma

Acute Renal Failure

Acute renal failure is sudden. There is severe decreased blood flow to the kidneys. Causes include severe injury or bleeding, myocardial infarction (heart attack), heart failure, burns, infection, and severe allergic reactions. Hospital care is needed.

At first, *oliguria* (scant amount of urine) occurs. Urine output is less than 400 mL in 24 hours. This phase lasts a few days to 2 weeks. Then **diuresis** occurs. *Diuresis* means the process (*esis*) of passing (*di*) urine (*ur*). Large amounts of urine are produced—1000 to 5000 mL a day. Kidney function improves and returns to normal during the recovery phase. This can take from 1 month to 1 year. Some persons develop chronic renal failure.

Every system is affected by the build-up of waste products in the blood. Death can occur.

Treatment involves drugs, restricted fluids, and diet therapy. The diet is high in carbohydrates. It is low in protein and potassium. The care plan will likely include:

▶ Measuring and recording urine output every hour. Report an output of less than 30 mL per hour to the nurse at once.
▶ Measuring and recording intake and output.
▶ Restricting fluid intake.
▶ Measuring weight daily.
▶ Turning and repositioning at least every 2 hours.
▶ Measures to prevent pressure ulcers.
▶ Frequent oral hygiene.
▶ Measures to prevent infection.
▶ Deep-breathing and coughing exercises.
▶ Measures to meet emotional needs.

Chronic Renal Failure

The kidneys cannot meet the body's needs. Nephrons in the kidney are destroyed over many years. Hypertension

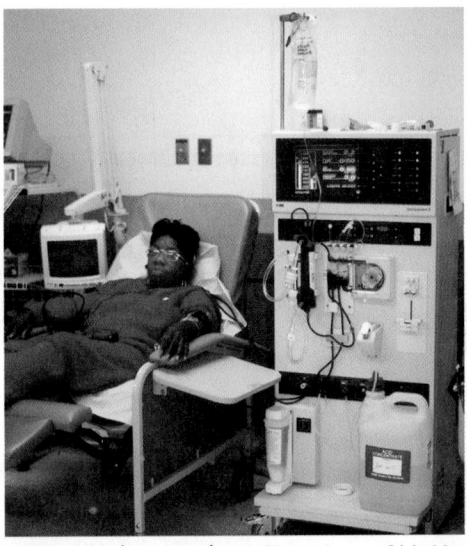

FIGURE 42-5 Dialysis machine. (From Lewis SM, Heitkemper MM, Dirksen SR: *Medical-surgical nursing: assessment and management of clinical problems,* ed 6, St Louis, 2004, Mosby.)

and diabetes are common causes. Infections, urinary tract obstructions, and tumors are other causes.

Signs and symptoms appear when 75% of kidney function is lost (Box 42-1). Every body system is affected as waste products build up in the blood.

Treatment includes fluid restriction, diet therapy, drugs, and dialysis. *Dialysis* is the process of removing waste products from the blood.

▶ *Hemodialysis* removes waste and fluid by filtering the blood (*hemo*) through an artificial kidney (Fig. 42-5).
▶ *Peritoneal dialysis* uses the lining of the abdominal cavity (*peritoneal membrane*) to remove waste and fluid from the blood (Fig. 42-6, p. 676).

You will assist the nurse in the care of persons with chronic renal failure. See Box 42-2, p. 676.

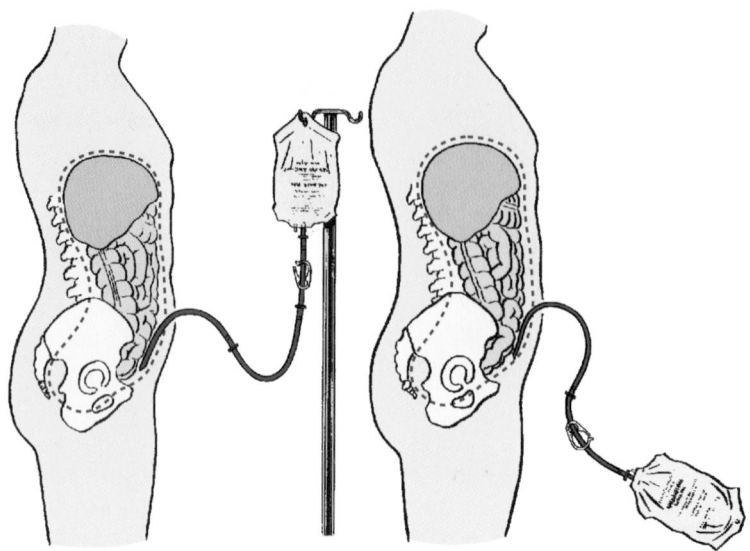

FIGURE 42-6 Peritoneal dialysis system. (From Tucker S and others: *Patient care standards: collaborative practice planning guides,* ed 6, St Louis, 1996, Mosby.)

BOX 42-2 Care of the Person in Chronic Renal Failure

- A diet low in protein, potassium, and sodium
- Fluid restriction
- Measuring blood pressure in the supine, sitting, and standing positions
- Measuring daily weight
- Measuring and recording intake and output
- Turning and repositioning
- Measures to prevent pressure ulcers
- Range-of-motion exercises
- Measures to prevent itching (bath oils, lotions, creams)
- Measures to prevent injury and bleeding
- Frequent oral hygiene
- Measures to prevent infection
- Measures to prevent diarrhea or constipation
- Measures to meet emotional needs
- Measures to promote rest

REPRODUCTIVE DISORDERS

Sexual activities involve the structures and functions of the reproductive system. The male reproductive system:

▶ Produces and transports sperm
▶ Deposits sperm in the female reproductive tract
▶ Secretes hormones
The female reproductive system:
▶ Produces eggs (ova)
▶ Secretes hormones
▶ Protects and nourishes the fetus during pregnancy

Aging affects the structures and functions of the reproductive system (Chapter 46). Many injuries, diseases, and surgeries can affect reproductive structures and functions.

Sexually Transmitted Diseases

A sexually transmitted disease (STD) is spread by oral, vaginal, or anal sex (Table 42-1). Some people do not have signs and symptoms or are not aware of an infection. Others know but do not seek treatment because of embarrassment.

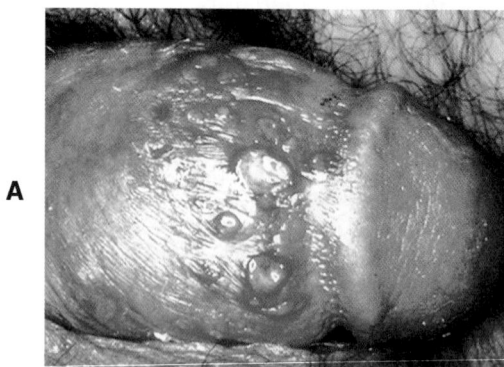
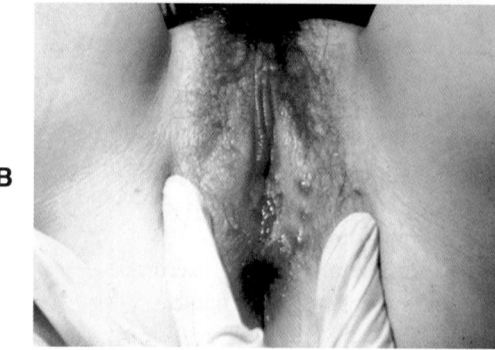

FIGURE 42-7 Herpes. **A,** Sores on the penis. **B,** Sores on the female perineum. (Courtesy United States Public Health Service, Washington, DC.)

TABLE 42-1 Sexually Transmitted Diseases

DISEASE	SIGNS AND SYMPTOMS	TREATMENT
Herpes	Painful, blister-like sores on or near the genitals, mouth, or anus (Fig. 42-7) The sores may have a watery discharge Pain, itching, burning, and tingling in the affected area Vaginal discharge Pain during urination or intercourse Fever Swollen glands	No known cure Anti-viral drugs
Genital warts	*Male*—Warts in or on the penis, anus, genitalia, mouth, or throat *Female*—Warts in or on the vagina, cervix, labia, anus, mouth, or throat	Application of special ointment that causes the warts to dry up and fall off Surgical removal may be necessary if the ointment is not effective
HIV/AIDS	See Chapter 38.	See Chapter 38.
Gonorrhea	Burning and pain on urination Urinary frequency and urgency Genital discharge (vagina, urethra, rectum)	Antibiotic drugs
Chlamydia	May not show symptoms Discharge from the penis or vagina Burning or pain on urination Testicular pain or swelling Vaginal bleeding Rectal inflammation and/or discharge Pain during intercourse Diarrhea Nausea Abdominal pain Fever	Antibiotic drugs
Pubic lice	Intense itching	Over-the-counter or prescription lice treatment Washing or dry-cleaning all exposed clothing, bedding, and towels
Trichomoniasis (occurs in women; men are carriers)	No symptoms in men Frothy, thick, foul-smelling, yellow vaginal discharge Genital itching and irritation Burning and pain on urination Genital swelling	Metronidazole
Syphilis	*Stage 1*—10 to 90 days after exposure • Painless sores (chancres) on the penis, in the vagina, or on the genitalia; the chancre may also be on the lips or inside of the mouth, or anywhere on the body *Stage 2*—About 3 to 6 weeks after the sores • General fatigue, loss of appetite, nausea, fever, headache, rash, swollen glands, sore throat, bone and joint pain, hair loss, lesions on the lips and genitalia • Symptoms may come and go for many years *Stage 3*—3 to 15 years after infection • Central nervous system damage (including paralysis), heart damage, blindness, liver damage, mental health problems, death	Penicillin and other antibiotic drugs

STDs often occur in the genital and rectal areas. They also occur in the ears, mouth, nipples, throat, tongue, eyes, and nose. Using condoms helps prevent the spread of STDs, especially the human immunodeficiency virus (HIV) and acquired immunodeficiency syndrome (AIDS). (HIV and AIDS are discussed in Chapter 38.) Some STDs are also spread through skin breaks, by contact with infected body fluids (blood, semen, saliva), or by contaminated blood or needles.

Standard Precautions and the Bloodborne Pathogen Standard are followed.

Circle the BEST answer.

1 A person has cystitis. This is a
   a Kidney infection
   b Kidney stone
   c Urinary diversion
   d Bladder infection

2 The person with cystitis needs to drink about
   a 500 mL daily
   b 1000 mL daily
   c 1500 mL daily
   d 2000 mL daily

3 Benign prostatic hyperplasia causes urinary problems because
   a The person has a weak urine stream
   b The person voids frequently at night
   c The enlarged prostate presses against the urethra
   d Voidings are in small amounts

4 Mr. Jones had a transurethral resection of the prostate. His care plan includes the following. Which should you question?
   a No sudden movements
   b No heavy lifting
   c No straining to have a bowel movement
   d No oral fluids

5 A person has a urostomy. This means that the person
   a Has a new pathway for urine to exit the body
   b Needs dialysis
   c Had surgery for an enlarged prostate
   d Has pyuria

6 A person has renal calculi. When the person voids, you need to
   a Strain all urine
   b Empty the pouch
   c Collect a urine specimen
   d Change the urinary drainage bag

7 A person has renal failure. Which statement is *false*?
   a Waste products are removed from the blood.
   b The body retains fluid.
   c Every body system is affected.
   d Diuresis follows oliguria.

8 A person has chronic renal failure. The care includes the following *except*
   a A diet low in protein, potassium, and sodium
   b Measuring urine output every hour
   c Measures to prevent pressure ulcers
   d Measuring weight daily

9 These statements are about STDs. Which is *false*?
   a They are usually spread by sexual contact.
   b They can affect the genital area and other body parts.
   c Signs and symptoms are obvious.
   d Some result in death.

10 STDs require
    a Masks and protective eyewear
    b Gowns
    c Double bagging
    d Standard Precautions

Answers to these questions are on p. 782.

Mental Health Problems

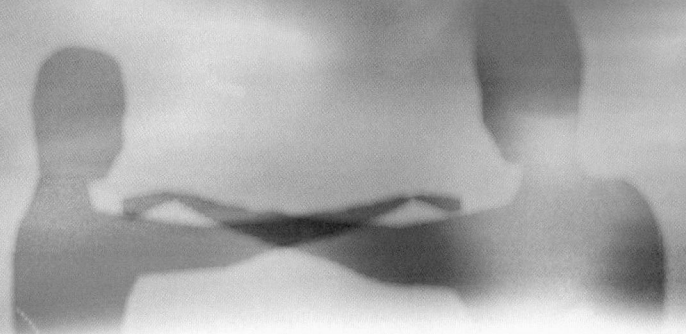

OBJECTIVES

- Define the key terms and key abbreviations listed in this chapter
- Explain the difference between mental health and mental illness
- List the causes of mental illness
- Explain how personality develops
- Describe four anxiety disorders
- Explain the defense mechanisms used to relieve anxiety

- Describe common phobias
- Explain schizophrenia
- Describe bipolar disorder and depression
- Describe personality disorders
- Describe substance abuse
- Describe eating disorders
- Describe suicide and the persons at risk
- Describe the care required by persons with mental health disorders

KEY TERMS

affect Feelings and emotions

anxiety A vague, uneasy feeling in response to stress

compulsion Repeating an act over and over again

conscious Awareness of the environment and experiences; the person knows what is happening and can control thoughts and behaviors

defense mechanism An unconscious reaction that blocks unpleasant or threatening feelings

delusion A false belief

delusion of grandeur An exaggerated belief about one's importance, wealth, power, or talents

delusion of persecution A false belief that one is being mistreated, abused, or harassed

ego The part of the personality dealing with reality; deals with thoughts, feelings, reasoning, good sense, and problem solving

emotional illness Mental disorder, mental illness, psychiatric disorder

flashback Reliving the trauma in thoughts during the day and in nightmares during sleep

hallucination Seeing, hearing, smelling, or feeling something that is not real

id The part of the personality at the unconscious level; concerned with pleasure

mental Relating to the mind; something that exists in the mind or is done by the mind

Continued

KEY TERMS — cont'd

mental disorder Emotional illness, mental illness, psychiatric disorder

mental health The person copes with and adjusts to everyday stresses in ways accepted by society

mental illness A disturbance in the ability to cope with or adjust to stress; behavior and function are impaired; emotional illness, mental disorder, psychiatric disorder

obsession A recurrent, unwanted thought, idea, or image

panic An intense and sudden feeling of fear, anxiety, terror, or dread

paranoia A disorder (*para*) of the mind (*noia*); false beliefs (delusions) and suspicion about a person or situation

personality The set of attitudes, values, behaviors, and traits of a person

phobia An intense fear

psychiatric disorder Emotional illness, mental disorder, mental illness

psychosis A state of severe mental impairment

stress The response or change in the body caused by any emotional, physical, social, or economic factor

stressor The event or factor that causes stress

subconscious Memory, past experiences, and thoughts of which the person is not aware; they are easily recalled

suicide To kill oneself

suicide contagion Exposure to suicide or suicidal behaviors within one's family, one's peer group, or media reports of suicide

superego The part of the personality concerned with right and wrong

unconscious Experiences and feelings that cannot be recalled

withdrawal syndrome The person's physical and mental response after stopping or severely reducing the use of a substance that was used regularly

KEY ABBREVIATIONS

AIDS Acquired immunodeficiency syndrome
BPD Borderline personality disorder
CNA Certified nursing assistant
HIV Human immunodeficiency virus
NIAAA National Institute on Alcohol Abuse and Alcoholism

NIMH National Institute of Mental Health
OCD Obsessive-compulsive disorder
PTSD Post-traumatic stress disorder
STD Sexually transmitted disease

The whole person has physical, social, psychological, and spiritual parts. Each part affects the other.

- A physical problem has social, mental, and spiritual effects.
- A mental health problem can affect the person physically, socially, and spiritually.
- A social problem can have physical, mental health, and spiritual effects.

BASIC CONCEPTS

Physical illnesses range from mild to severe. The common cold is at one extreme. A life-threatening illness is at the other extreme. Mental health problems have the same extremes.

Mental Health

Mental relates to the mind. It is something that exists in the mind or is done by the mind. Therefore mental health involves the mind. Mental health and mental illness involve stress:

- **Stress**—is the response or change in the body caused by any emotional, physical, social, or economic factor.
- **Mental health**—means that the person copes with and adjusts to everyday stresses in ways accepted by society.

- **Mental illness**—is a disturbance in the ability to cope with or adjust to stress. Behavior and function are impaired. **Mental disorder, emotional illness,** and **psychiatric disorder** also mean mental illness.

Causes of mental health disorders include:

- Not being able to cope or adjust to stress
- Chemical imbalances
- Genetics
- Drug or substance abuse
- Social and cultural factors

Personality

Personality is the set of attitudes, values, behaviors, and traits of a person. Personality starts to develop at birth. It is affected by many factors. They include genes, culture, environment, parenting, and social experiences.

Maslow's theory of basic needs (Chapter 7) affects personality development. Lower-level needs must be met before higher-level needs. Physical needs are met before safety and security, love and belonging, self-esteem, and self-actualization needs. A child who grows up hungry, neglected, cold, or abused will not feel safe and secure. Higher-level needs cannot be met. Unmet needs at any age affect personality development.

Growth and development also affect personality development (Chapter 9). They occur in a sequence, order, and pattern. Certain tasks must be accomplished at each stage. Each stage lays the foundation for the next stage.

Freud's Theory of Personality Development

Freud's theory of personality development involves three levels of awareness:

▶ **Conscious**—awareness of the environment and experiences. The person knows what is happening. He or she can control thoughts and behavior.

▶ **Subconscious**—memory, past experiences, and thoughts of which the person is not aware. They are easily recalled.

▶ **Unconscious**—experiences and feelings that cannot be recalled.

His theory also involves the id, ego, and superego. The **id** part of the personality is at the unconscious level. The id is concerned with pleasure. The need for pleasure must be satisfied almost right away. The id deals with hunger, comfort, sex, and warmth. People are not aware that they believe and act in ways to satisfy the id.

The **ego** deals with reality, with what is happening in the person's world. Thoughts, feelings, reasoning, good sense, and problem solving occur in the ego. The ego decides what to do and when.

The **superego** is concerned with right and wrong. Morals and values are in the superego. The superego judges what the ego thinks and does. It is like a parent helping a child look at behaviors.

ANXIETY DISORDERS

Anxiety is a vague, uneasy feeling in response to stress. The person may not know why or the cause. The person senses danger or harm—real or imagined. The person acts to relieve the unpleasant feeling. Often anxiety occurs when needs are not met.

Some anxiety is normal. Persons with mental health problems have higher levels of anxiety. Signs and symptoms depend on the degree of anxiety (Box 43-1).

Anxiety level depends on the stressor. A **stressor** is the event or factor that causes stress. It can be physical, emotional, social, or economic. Past experiences affect how a person reacts. So does the number of stressors. A stressor may produce mild anxiety. Anxiety can be higher at another time.

Coping and defense mechanisms are used to relieve anxiety. Some are healthy. Others are not—eating, drinking, smoking, and fighting are examples. Healthy ways to cope include discussing the problem, exercising, playing music, taking a hot bath, and wanting to be alone.

Defense mechanisms are unconscious reactions that block unpleasant or threatening feelings (Box 43-2). Used by everyone, defense mechanisms protect the ego. Some use of defense mechanisms is normal. With mental health problems, they are used poorly.

BOX 43-1 Signs and Symptoms of Anxiety

- A "lump" in the throat
- "Butterflies" in the stomach
- Pulse: rapid
- Respirations: rapid
- Blood pressure: increased
- Speech: rapid
- Voice changes
- Mouth: dry
- Sweating

- Nausea
- Diarrhea
- Urinary frequency and urgency
- Attention span: poor
- Directions: difficulty following
- Sleep: difficulty
- Appetite: loss of

BOX 43-2 Defense Mechanisms

Compensation. *Compensate* means to make up for, replace, or substitute. The person makes up for or substitutes a strength for a weakness.
EXAMPLE: Not good in sports, a child develops another talent.

Conversion. *Convert* means to change. An emotion is shown as a physical symptom or changed into a physical symptom.
EXAMPLE: Not wanting to read out loud in school, a child complains of a headache.

Denial. *Deny* means refusing to accept or believe something that is true. The person refuses to face or accept unpleasant or threatening things.
EXAMPLE: After a heart attack, a person continues to smoke.

Displacement. *Displace* means to move or take the place of. An individual moves behaviors or emotions from one person, place, or thing to a safe person, place, or thing.
EXAMPLE: Angry at your boss, you yell at a friend.

Identification. *Identify* means to relate or recognize. A person assumes the ideas, behaviors, and traits of another person.
EXAMPLE: A neighbor is a high school cheerleader. A little girl practices cheerleading in her backyard.

Projection. *Project* means to blame another. An individual blames another person or object for unacceptable behaviors, emotions, ideas, or wishes.
EXAMPLE: Sleeping too long, a worker blames the traffic when late for work.

Rationalization. *Rational* means sensible, reasonable, or logical. An acceptable reason or excuse is given for behaviors or actions. The real reason is not given.
EXAMPLE: Often late for work, an employee does not get a raise. The employee thinks "My boss doesn't like me."

Reaction formation. A person acts in a way opposite to what he or she truly feels.
EXAMPLE: A worker does not like his boss. He buys the boss an expensive gift.

Regression. *Regress* means to move back or to retreat. The person retreats or moves back to an earlier time or condition.
EXAMPLE: A 3-year-old wants a baby bottle when a new baby comes into the family.

Repression. *Repress* means to hold down or keep back. The person keeps unpleasant or painful thoughts or experiences from the conscious mind. They cannot be recalled or remembered.
EXAMPLE: A child was sexually abused. Now 33 years old, there is no memory of the event.

Panic Disorder

Panic is the highest level of anxiety. **Panic** is an intense and sudden feeling of fear, anxiety, terror, or dread. Onset is sudden with no obvious reason. The person cannot function. Signs and symptoms of anxiety are severe (see Box 43-1). The person may also have:

▶ Chest pain
▶ Shortness of breath
▶ Rapid heart rate ("heart pounding")
▶ Numbness and tingling in the hands
▶ Dizziness
▶ A smothering sensation
▶ Feeling of impending doom or loss of control

The person may feel that he or she is having a heart attack, losing his or her mind, or on the verge of death. Attacks can occur at any time, even during sleep.

Panic attacks can last for 10 minutes or longer. They can occur often. Panic disorder can last for a few months or for many years.

Many people avoid places where panic attacks occurred. For example, a person had a panic attack in a shopping mall. Malls are avoided.

Phobias

Phobia means an intense fear. The person has an intense fear of an object, situation, or activity that has little or no actual danger. Common phobias are fear of:

▶ Being in an open, crowded, or public place (agoraphobia—*agora* means marketplace)
▶ Being in pain or seeing others in pain (algophobia—*algo* means pain)
▶ Water (aquaphobia—*aqua* means water)
▶ Being in or being trapped in an enclosed or narrow space (claustrophobia—*claustro* means closing)
▶ The slightest uncleanliness (mysophobia—*myso* means anything that is disgusting)
▶ Night or darkness (nyctophobia—*nycto* means night or darkness)
▶ Fire (pyrophobia—*pyro* means fire)
▶ Strangers (xenophobia—*xeno* means strange)

The person avoids what is feared. When faced with the fear, the person has high anxiety. He or she cannot function.

Obsessive-Compulsive Disorder

An **obsession** is a recurrent, unwanted thought, idea, or image. **Compulsion** is repeating an act over and over again (a ritual). The act may not make sense. However, the person has much anxiety if the act is not done.

Common rituals are hand washing, constant checking to make sure the stove is off, cleaning, and counting things to a certain number. Such activities can take over [h]our every day. They are very distressing and affect [   ] life. Some persons with obsessive-compulsive disor- [   ]CD) also have depression, eating disorders, sub- [   ] abuse, and other anxiety disorders.

BOX 43-3 Signs and Symptoms of Post-Traumatic Stress Disorder

- Startles easily
- Emotionally numb—especially to those with whom the person used to be close
- Difficulty trusting people
- Difficulty feeling close to people
- Loss of interest in things he or she used to enjoy
- Problems being affectionate
- Feelings of intense guilt
- Irritability
- Avoiding situations that are reminders of the harmful event
- Difficulty around the anniversary of the harmful event
- Gets mad easily
- Outbursts of anger
- Problems sleeping
- Increasingly aggressive
- Becoming more violent
- Physical symptoms:
  - Headache
  - Gastrointestinal distress
  - Immune system problems
  - Dizziness
  - Chest pain
  - Discomfort in other body parts

Post-Traumatic Stress Disorder

Post-traumatic stress disorder (PTSD) occurs after a terrifying ordeal. The ordeal involved physical harm or the threat of physical harm. Signs and symptoms of PTSD are listed in Box 43-3. PTSD can develop:

▶ After being harmed
▶ After a loved one was harmed
▶ After seeing a harmful event happen to loved ones or strangers

PTSD can result from many traumatic events. They include:

▶ War
▶ A terrorist attack
▶ Mugging
▶ Rape
▶ Torture
▶ Kidnaping
▶ Being held captive
▶ Child abuse
▶ A crash—vehicle, train, plane
▶ Bombing
▶ A natural disaster—flood, tornado, hurricane

Most people with PTSD have flashbacks. A **flashback** is reliving the trauma in thoughts during the day and in nightmares during sleep. A flashback may involve images, sounds, smells, or feelings. They are often triggered by everyday things. A door slamming is an example. During a flashback, the person may lose touch with reality. He or she may believe that the trauma is happening all over again.

Signs and symptoms usually develop about 3 months after the harmful event. However, they may not emerge until years later. Some people recover within 6 months. PTSD lasts longer in other people. The condition may become chronic.

PTSD can develop at any age including during childhood. The person may also suffer from depression, substance abuse, and other anxiety disorders.

SCHIZOPHRENIA

Schizophrenia means split *(schizo)* mind *(phrenia)*. It is a severe, chronic, disabling brain disorder. It involves:

▶ **Psychosis**—a state of severe mental impairment. The person does not view the real or unreal correctly.

▶ **Delusion**—a false belief. For example, the person believes that a radio station is broadcasting the person's thoughts.

▶ **Hallucination**—seeing, hearing, smelling, or feeling something that is not real. A person may see animals, insects, or people that are not real. "Voices" are the most common type of hallucination in schizophrenia. "Voices" may comment on behavior, order the person to do things, warn of danger, or talk to other voices.

▶ **Paranoia**—a disorder *(para)* of the mind *(noia)*. The person has false beliefs (delusions). He or she is suspicious about a person or situation. For example, a person may believe that others are cheating, harassing, poisoning, spying upon, or plotting against him or her.

▶ **Delusion of grandeur**—an exaggerated belief about one's importance, wealth, power, or talents. For example, a man believes he is Superman. Or a woman believes she is the Queen of England.

▶ **Delusion of persecution**—the false belief that one is being mistreated, abused, or harassed. A person may believe that someone is "out to get" him or her.

The person with schizophrenia has severe mental impairment *(psychosis)*. Thinking and behavior are disturbed. The person has false beliefs *(delusions)*. He or she also has *hallucinations*—the person sees, hears, smells, or feels things that are not real. The person has problems relating to others. He or she may be *paranoid*—the person is suspicious about a person or situation. The person may have difficulty organizing thoughts. Responses are inappropriate. Communication is disturbed. The person may ramble or repeat what another says. Sometimes speech cannot be understood. He or she may make up words. The person may withdraw—the person lacks interest in others. He or she is not involved with people or society.

Disorders of movement occur. These include:

▶ Being clumsy and uncoordinated

▶ Involuntary movements

▶ Grimacing

▶ Unusual mannerisms

▶ Sitting for hours without moving, speaking, or responding

Some persons regress. To *regress* means to retreat or move back to an earlier time or condition. For example, a 5-year-old wets the bed when there is a new baby. This is normal. Healthy adults do not act like infants or children.

In men, the symptoms usually begin in the late teens or early 20s. In women, symptoms usually begin in the mid-20s and early 30s. People with schizophrenia do not tend to be violent. However, if a person with paranoid schizophrenia becomes violent, it is often directed at family members. The violence usually occurs at home. Some persons with schizophrenia attempt suicide (p. 687).

MOOD DISORDERS

Mood or **affect** relates to feelings and emotions. Mood (or affective) disorders involve feelings, emotions, and moods.

Bipolar Disorder

Bipolar means two *(bi)* poles or ends *(polar)*. The person with bipolar disorder has severe extremes in mood, energy, and ability to function (Box 43-4). There are emotional lows *(depression)* and emotional highs *(mania)*. The disorder also is called manic-depressive illness. The person may:

▶ Be more depressed than manic

▶ Be more manic than depressed

▶ Alternate between depression and mania

BOX 43-4 **Signs and Symptoms of Bipolar Disorder**

MANIA (MANIC EPISODE)	DEPRESSION (DEPRESSIVE EPISODE)
Increased energy, activity, and restlessness	Lasting sad, anxious, or empty mood
Excessively "high," overly good mood	Feelings of hopelessness
Extreme irritability	Feelings of guilt, worthlessness, or helplessness
Racing thoughts and talking very fast	Loss of interest or pleasure in activities once enjoyed
Jumping from one idea to another	Loss of interest in sex
Easily distracted; problems concentrating	Decreased energy; a feeling of fatigue or being "slowed down"
Little sleep needed	Problems concentrating, remembering, or making decisions
Unrealistic beliefs in one's abilities and powers	Restlessness or irritability
Poor judgment	Sleeping too much, or unable to sleep
Spending sprees	Change in appetite
A lasting period of behavior that is different from usual	Unintended weight loss or gain
Increased sexual drive	Chronic pain or other symptoms not caused by physical illness or injury
Drug abuse (particularly cocaine, alcohol, and sleeping pills)	Thoughts of death or suicide
Aggressive behavior	Suicide attempts
Denial that anything is wrong	

BOX 43-5 Signs and Symptoms of Depression in Older Persons

- Fatigue and lack of interest
- Inability to experience pleasure
- Feelings of uselessness, hopelessness, and helplessness
- Decreased sexual interest
- Increased dependency
- Anxiety
- Slow or unreliable memory
- Paranoia
- Agitation
- Focus on the past
- Thoughts of death and suicide
- Difficulty completing activities of daily living
- Changes in sleep patterns
- Poor grooming
- Withdrawal from people and interests
- Muscle aches, abdominal pain, and headaches
- Nausea and vomiting
- Dry mouth

From Meiner SB and Lueckenotte AG: *Gerontologic nursing*, ed 3, St Louis, 2006, Mosby.

The disorder tends to run in families. It usually develops in the late teens or in early adulthood. The disorder requires life-long management.

See Box 43-4 for the signs and symptoms of mania and depression. They can range from mild to severe. Mood changes are called "episodes." Bipolar disorder can damage relationships and affect school or work performance. Some people are suicidal.

Major Depression

Depression involves the body, mood, and thoughts. Symptoms affect work, study, sleep, eating, and other activities. The person is very sad. He or she loses interest in daily activities.

Depression may occur because of a stressful event such as death of a partner, parent, or child. Divorce and loss of job are other stressful events. Some physical disorders can cause depression. Stroke, myocardial infarction (heart attack), cancer, and Parkinson's disease are examples. Hormonal factors may cause depression in women—menstrual cycle changes, pregnancy, miscarriage, after birth (post-partum depression), and before and during menopause.

See *Focus on Children and Older Persons: Major Depression.*

PERSONALITY DISORDERS

Personality disorders involve rigid and maladaptive behaviors. To *adapt* means to change or adjust. *Mal* means bad, wrong, or ill. *Maladaptive* means to change or adjust in the wrong way. Because of their behaviors, those with personality disorders cannot function well in society. Personality disorders include:

▸ *Antisocial personality disorder.* The person is at least 18 years old and has poor judgment. The person lacks responsibility and is hostile. The person is not loyal to any person or group. Morals and ethics are lacking. The person lies or cons others for personal gain or pleasure. Others are blamed for actions and behaviors. The rights of others do not matter. The person has no guilt. He or she does not learn from experiences or punishment. The person is often in trouble with the police.

▸ *Borderline personality disorder (BPD).* The person has problems with moods, interpersonal relationships, self-image, and behavior. The person has intense bouts of anger, depression, and anxiety that last hours or most of the day. Aggression, self-injury, and drug or alcohol abuse may occur. The person may greatly admire and love family and friends and then suddenly shift to intense anger and dislike. The person may have other mental health disorders.

SUBSTANCE ABUSE AND ADDICTION

Substance abuse or addiction occurs when a person overuses or depends on alcohol or drugs. The person's physical and mental health are affected. The welfare of others is affected too.

Substances involved in abuse and addiction affect the nervous system. Some depress the nervous system. Others stimulate it. All affect the mind and thinking.

See *Focus on Ethics and Laws: Substance Abuse and Addiction.*

Alcoholism and Alcohol Abuse

Alcohol slows down brain activity. It affects alertness, judgment, coordination, and reaction time. Over time, heavy drinking damages the brain, central nervous system, liver, heart, kidneys, and stomach. It causes changes in the heart and blood vessels. It also can cause forgetfulness and confusion.

According to the National Institute on Alcohol Abuse and Alcoholism (NIAAA), *alcoholism* (alcohol dependence) includes these symptoms:

▸ *Craving.* The person has a strong need or urge to drink.
▸ *Loss of control.* The person cannot stop drinking once drinking has begun.
▸ *Physical dependence.* The person has withdrawal symptoms when he or she stops drinking. They include nausea, sweating, shakiness, and anxiety.
▸ *Tolerance.* The person needs to drink greater amounts of alcohol to get "high."

FOCUS ON **ETHICS** AND **LAWS**

Substance Abuse and Addiction

A certified nursing assistant (CNA) worked at a nursing home in Arizona. The following occurred during a 6-week period:

- The police were called to an altercation between the CNA and her ex-husband in the facility's parking lot. The CNA left the facility without notifying a supervisor.
- The CNA left her assigned unit and could not be found. The police were called. The CNA was found in her car in the facility parking lot with a boyfriend. They were in possession of drug paraphernalia. The CNA was arrested. She also lost her job.
- The CNA was arrested during a routine traffic stop. She had drugs and drug paraphernalia in the vehicle.
- The CNA was charged in a court of law with the following:
  - Possession and use of marijuana—a felony
  - Used or possessed drug paraphernalia with intent to use—a felony
  - Driving with a suspended license—a misdemeanor

When the CNA did not appear for her pre-trial hearing, a warrant went out for her arrest. And the CNA did not respond to communications sent to her from the Arizona State Board of Nursing.

The Arizona State Board of Nursing found that the CNA's actions violated the state's Nurse Practice Act. The Board revoked her nursing assistant certificate. She could apply for reinstatement after a 5 year period.

(Arizona State Board of Nursing, January 25, 2006. NOTE: Names withheld by request of the Arizona State Board of Nursing.)

Alcoholism is a chronic disease. It lasts throughout life. Life-style and genetics are risk factors. Some people turn to alcohol for relief from life stresses—retirement, lowered income, loss of job, failing health, loneliness, or the deaths of loved ones or friends. The craving for alcohol can be as strong as the need for food or water. An alcoholic will continue to drink despite serious family, health, or legal problems.

Alcoholism can be treated. Counseling and drugs are used to help the person stop drinking. The person must avoid all alcohol to avoid a relapse.

Alcohol abuse is just as harmful as alcoholism. A person who abuses alcohol drinks too much but is not dependent on alcohol.

Problems linked to alcoholism and alcohol abuse include:

- Not being able to meet work, school, or family responsibilities
- Motor vehicle crashes
- Drunk-driving arrests
- Drinking-related medical conditions

Drinking occasionally or regularly does not mean a drinking problem. According to the NIAAA, a person needs help if he or she:

- Drinks to calm nerves, forget worries, or reduce depression
- Has lost interest in food
- Gulps drinks down fast
- Lies or tries to hide drinking habits

FOCUS ON **CHILDREN** AND **OLDER PERSONS**

Alcoholism and Alcohol Abuse

CHILDREN

According to a 2003 NIAAA report, nearly half (50 out of 100) of the adolescents in the United States have had a least one drink by the eighth grade. Over 20 percent (20 out of 100) of those same children report having been "drunk." Among 12th graders, 30 percent (30 out of 100) report drinking on 3 or more occasions each month. About 30 percent of the 12th graders reported "binge" drinking—having 5 or more drinks on one occasion within the past 2 weeks.

Underage drinking is illegal. It also poses a high risk to the child and society.

- *Traffic crashes.* There are more alcohol-related traffic crashes among drivers between the ages of 16 and 20 than among those 21 and older.
- *Fatal crashes.* Motor vehicle crashes are the leading cause of death among persons aged 15 to 20. For alcohol-involved drivers, the rate of fatal crashes for those between 16 and 20 is more than twice the rate for those 21 and over.
- *Suicide.* Alcohol use interacts with depression and stress to increase the risk of suicide. Suicide is the third leading cause of death among persons aged 14 to 25.
- *Sexual assault and rape.* These crimes occur most often in late adolescence and early adulthood. They usually occur during a date. The likelihood of sexual assault by the male increases with alcohol use by:
  - The offender
  - The victim
  - Both the offender and the victim
- *High-risk sex.* This includes multiple sex partners and not using condoms. Unwanted pregnancy and sexually transmitted diseases (STDs) are risks. STDs include HIV (human immunodeficiency virus) and AIDS (acquired immunodeficiency syndrome).
- *Brain damage.* Adolescents are at risk for alcohol-induced brain damage. Alcohol may affect brain development. Learning, memory, and job performance may be affected.
- *Alcohol abuse and dependence.* Youthful drinking increases the risk of alcohol abuse or dependence later in life.

OLDER PERSONS

Alcohol effects vary with age. Even small amounts can make older persons feel "high." Older persons are at risk for falls, vehicle crashes, and other injuries from drinking. They have:

- Slower reaction times
- Hearing and vision problems
- A lower tolerance for alcohol

Older people tend to take more drugs than younger persons. Mixing alcohol with some drugs can be harmful, even fatal. Alcohol also makes some health problems worse. High blood pressure is an example.

- Drinks alone more often
- Has hurt oneself or someone else while drinking
- Was drunk more than 3 or 4 times in one year
- Needs more alcohol to get "high"
- Feels irritable, resentful, or unreasonable when not drinking
- Has medical, social, or money problems caused by drinking

See *Focus on Children and Older Persons: Alcoholism and Alcohol Abuse.*

Drug Abuse and Addiction

Drugs interfere with normal brain function. While they create powerful feelings of pleasure, they have long-term effects on the brain. At some point, changes in the brain can turn drug abuse into addiction.

▶ *Drug abuse*—is the overuse of a drug for non-medical or non-therapy effects.

▶ *Drug addition*—is a chronic, relapsing brain disease. The person has an overwhelming desire to take a drug. The person repeatedly takes the drug because of its effect. Usually the effect is altered mental awareness. The person has to have the drug. Often higher doses are needed. The person cannot stop taking the drug without treatment.

A diagnosis of drug abuse or addiction is based on three or more of the following. They must have occurred any time during a 12-month period.

▶ The substance is often taken in larger amounts. Or it is taken over a longer period than intended.

▶ The person has a constant desire for the substance. Or the person cannot cut down or control substance use.

▶ A great deal of time is spent using the substance or recovering from its effects. Or a great deal of time is spent trying to obtain the substance. For example, the person visits many doctors to obtain the substance. Or he or she drives long distances to get the substance.

▶ The person gave up or reduced important social, occupational, or recreational activities because of substance abuse.

▶ The person continues to use the substance. The person does so despite knowing that a constant or recurring problem is caused by or made worse by using the substance. The problem may be physical or psychological.

▶ The person has tolerance to the substance:
  ▶ Increased amounts are needed to achieve intoxication or the desired effect.
  ▶ Continued use of the same amount has a greatly reduced effect on the person.

▶ Withdrawal from the substance (*withdraw* means to stop, remove, or take away):
  ▶ The withdrawal syndrome is that expected for the drug. (**Withdrawal syndrome** is the person's physical and mental response after stopping or severely reducing the use of a substance that was used regularly. The body responds with anxiety, restlessness, insomnia, irritability, impaired attention, and physical illness.)
  ▶ The same (or similar) substance is taken to relieve or avoid withdrawal symptoms.

Drug abuse and addiction affect social and mental function. Drug abuse and addiction are linked to crimes, violence, and motor vehicle crashes.

There also are physical effects. The following can occur from one use, high doses, or prolonged use:

▶ HIV and AIDS
▶ Cardiovascular disease
▶ Stroke
▶ Sudden death
▶ Hepatitis
▶ Lung disease
▶ Cancer

Legal and illegal drugs are abused (Box 43-6). Legal drugs are approved for use in the United States. Doctors prescribe them. Illegal drugs are not approved for use. They are obtained through illegal means. Often legal drugs also are obtained through illegal means.

BOX 43-6 Commonly Abused Drugs

Anabolic steroids (Anadrol, Oxandrin, Durabolin, Depo-Testosterone, Equipoise)—roids, juice

Amphetamine (Biphetamine, Dexedrine)—bennies, black beauties, crosses, hearts, LA turnaround, speed, truck drivers, uppers

Barbiturates (Amytal, Nembutal, Seconal, Phenobarbital)—barbs, reds, red birds, phennies, tooies, yellows, yellow jackets

Benzodiazepines (Ativan, Halcion, Librium, Valium, Xanax)—candy, downers, sleeping pills, tranks

Cocaine—coke, snow, flake, blow, C, candy, Charlie, crack, rock, toot

Codeine (Emperin with Codeine, Fiorinal with Codeine, Robitussin A-C, Tylenol with Codeine)—Captain Cody, schoolboy, doors & fours, loads, pancakes and syrup

Fentanyl (Actiq, Duragesic, Sublimaze)—Apache, China girl, China white, dance fever, friend, goodfella, jackpot, murder 8, TNT, Tango and Cash

Flunitrazepam (Rohypnol)—forget-me pill, Mexican Valium, R2, Roche, roofies, roofinol, rope, rophies

GHB (gamma-hydroxybutyrate)—G, Georgia home boy, grievous bodily harm, liquid ecstasy

Hashish—boom, chronic, gangster, hash, hash oil, hemp

Heroin—smack, H, skag, junk, brown sugar, horse, skunk, white horse, dope

Inhalants—whippets, poppers, snappers

Ketamine (Ketalar SV)—cat Valiums, K, Special K, vitamin K

LSD (lysergic acid diethylamide)—acid, blotter, boomer, cubes, microdot, yellow sunshines

Marijuana—pot, dope, ganja, weed, grass, blunt, herb, joints, Mary Jane, reefer, sinsemilla, skunk

MDMA (methylenedioxy-methamphetamine)—Adam, clarity, ecstasy, Eve, lover's speed, peace, STP, X, XTC

Mescaline—buttons, cactus, mesc, peyote

Methamphetamine—speed, meth, chalk, ice, crystal, glass, crank, fire, go fast

Methaqualone (Quaalude, Sopor, Parest)—ludes, mandrex, quad, quay

Ritalin—JIF, MPH, R-ball, Skippy, the smart drug, vitamin R

Morphine (Roxanol, Duramorph)—M, Miss Emma, monkey, white stuff

PCP (Phencyclidine)—angel dust, boat, hog, love boat, peace pill

Psilocybin—magic mushroom, purple passion, shrooms

Opium (laudanum, paregoric)—big O, black stuff, block, gum, hop

Oxycontin—oxy, O.C., killer

Vicodin—vike, Watson-387

Modified from National Institute on Drug Abuse, *Commonly abused drugs,* National Institutes of Health, Bethesda, Md, May 17, 2007.

Treatment depends on the drug and the person. A drug treatment program combines various therapies and services to meet the person's needs. The person's age, race, culture, sexual orientation, and gender are considered. So are issues such as pregnancy, parenting, housing, employment, and physical and sexual abuse.

Drug abuse and addiction are chronic problems. Relapses can occur. A short-term, one-time treatment is often not enough. Treatment is a long-term process.

EATING DISORDERS

Eating disorders involve disturbances in eating behaviors. The two common eating disorders are anorexia nervosa and bulimia nervosa.

Anorexia Nervosa

Anorexia means no (*a*) appetite (*orexis*). *Nervosa* relates to nerves or emotions. Anorexia nervosa occurs when a person has an intense fear of weight gain or obesity. It occurs mainly in teenage girls and young women.

The person believes she is fat despite being dangerously thin (Fig. 43-1). Poor eating habits include:

▶ Avoiding food and meals
▶ Choosing a few foods and eating them in small amounts
▶ Weighing and measuring food

Intense exercise and vomiting are common. Some people abuse laxatives and enemas to rid the body of food. Laxatives are drugs that rid the intestines of feces through defecation.

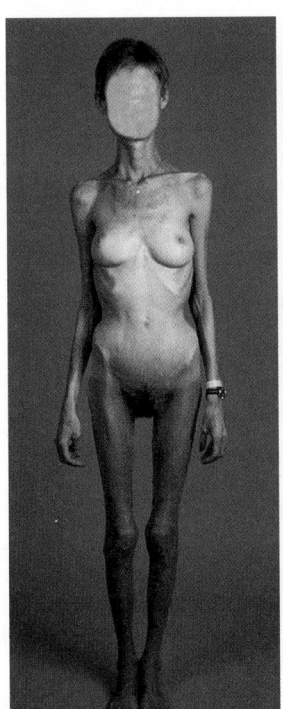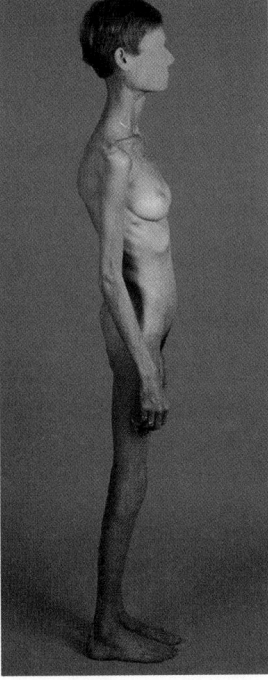

FIGURE 43-1 A person with anorexia nervosa. (Courtesy George D. Comerci, MD, Tuscon, Arizona. In Jarvis C: *Physical examination and health assessment,* ed 4, Philadelphia, 2004, Saunders.)

Diuretic abuse also may occur. These drugs cause the kidneys to produce large amounts of urine. Extra fluid in the body is lost. Weight loss results.

The person has a poor self-image and may avoid people. Sleep problems and depression may occur. The person may not have monthly menstrual periods. Serious health problems can result. Death is a risk from cardiac arrest or suicide.

Bulimia Nervosa

Bulimia comes from the Greek words for ox (*bous*) and hunger (*limos*). It occurs mainly in teenage girls and young women.

Binge eating occurs. That is, the person eats large amounts of food. Then the body is purged (rid) of the food eaten to prevent weight gain. Vomiting, laxatives, enemas, diuretics, fasting, and intense exercise are some methods used.

SUICIDE

Suicide means to kill oneself. According to a 2004 National Institute of Mental Health (NIMH) report:

▶ Suicide was the 11th leading cause of death in the United States.
▶ There were more suicides than homicides.
▶ There were more deaths due to suicide than from HIV and AIDS.
▶ Suicide by firearms was the most common method for men and women. More than half of all suicides involved firearms. Most firearm suicides were by men.
▶ Hanging is the second most common suicide method for men. For women, the second most common method is self-poisoning. This includes drug overdose.
▶ More men than women die by suicide. Of all the suicide deaths, most were white males.
▶ The highest rate of suicide was among white men aged 85 years and older.
▶ Suicide was the third leading cause of death among persons aged 15 to 20.
▶ There are about 8 to 25 attempted suicides for each suicide death.
▶ Women attempt suicide more often than men. However, more men die from suicide. Their methods (firearms, hanging) are more lethal.
▶ Some disorders that run in families increase the risk of suicide behaviors. The disorders are bipolar disorder, major depression, schizophrenia, alcoholism, substance abuse, and certain personality disorders.
▶ Over half the people who commit suicide have a mood disorder. Major depression and bipolar disorder are examples.
▶ Younger persons who commit suicide often have both a substance abuse disorder and depression.
▶ Among American Indians and Alaskan natives, depression and alcohol use and abuse are the most common risk factors for completed suicide.

BOX 43-7 Risk Factors for Suicide

- Depression and other mental health disorders
- Substance abuse disorder
- Stressful life events (in combination with other risk factors)
- Prior suicide attempt
- Family history of a mental health disorder or substance abuse
- Family history of suicide
- Family violence (including physical or sexual abuse)
- Firearms in the home
- Incarceration
- Exposure to suicidal behavior of others (family, peers, media figures)

From National Institute of Mental Health: *Suicide in the U.S.: statistics and prevention,* National Institutes of Health, NIH publication No. 03-4594, revised December 2007, updated April 20, 2007.

▶ Alcohol and substance abuse problems contribute to suicidal behavior. Persons who abuse substances:
  ▶ Often have a number of risk factors for suicide.
  ▶ Are likely to have depression.
  ▶ Are likely to have social and financial problems.
  ▶ Are likely to be impulsive.
  ▶ Tend to engage in high-risk behaviors that result in self-harm.

People think about suicide when they are feel hopeless or when they cannot see solutions to their problems. Suicide is most often linked to:
▶ Depression
▶ Alcohol or substance abuse
▶ Stressful events (Major losses and jail are examples.)

Risk factors for suicide are listed in Box 43-7. *If a person mentions or talks about suicide, take the person seriously. Call for the nurse at once. Do not leave the person alone.*

Agencies that treat persons with mental health problems must identify persons at risk for suicide. They must:
▶ Identify specific factors or features that increase or decrease the risk for suicide.
▶ Meet the person's immediate safety needs.
▶ Provide the most appropriate setting for treating the person.
▶ Provide crisis information to the person and family. A crisis "hotline" phone number is an example.

See *Focus on Children and Older Persons: Suicide.*
See *Focus on Long-Term Care and Home Care: Suicide.*

FOCUS ON LONG-TERM CARE AND HOME CARE
Suicide
HOME CARE
A firearm in the home is a risk factor for suicide. So are other lethal weapons. If a patient talks about suicide, find out if there are firearms and other weapons in the home. Find out what kind, how many, and where they are located. Report all information to the nurse at once.

If the person is in danger, call 911.

FOCUS ON CHILDREN AND OLDER PERSONS
Suicide
OLDER PERSONS
According to NIMH, older persons have higher suicide rates than younger persons. Older white males have the highest rates. Among white males 65 and older, the risk goes up with age. White men 85 and older have the highest suicide rates. Some older persons are less likely to recover from a suicide attempt.

Many older persons suffer from depression (p. 684). Depression often occurs with other serious illnesses. Heart disease, stroke, diabetes, cancer, and Parkinson's disease are examples. The person also may have social and financial problems.

Most older victims did not report depression to their doctors. Or depression was not detected by the doctors.

Suicide Contagion
The NIMH defines **suicide contagion** as exposure to suicide or suicidal behaviors within the family, peer group, or media reports of suicide. The exposure has lead to an increase in suicide and suicidal behaviors in persons at risk for suicide. Adolescents and young adults are at risk for suicide contagion.

Following suicide exposure, those close to the victim should be evaluated by a mental health professional. They include family, friends, peers, and co-workers. Persons at risk for suicide need mental health services.

CARE AND TREATMENT
Treatment of mental health problems involves having the person explore his or her thoughts and feelings. This is done through psychotherapy and behavior, group, occupational, art, and family therapies. Often drugs are ordered.

The care plan reflects the person's needs. The needs of the total person must be met. This includes physical, safety and security, and emotional needs.

Communication is important. Be alert to nonverbal communication. This includes the person's nonverbal communication and your own.

See *Focus on Ethics and Laws: Care and Treatment,* p. 689.

FOCUS ON **ETHICS** AND **LAWS**

Care and Treatment

A patient sued a hospital after she set her bed and herself on fire. The patient was in the hospital for alcohol abuse and mental illness. She had a history of mental illness, suicide threats, and alcohol abuse.

While in the hospital, the following occurred:

- Many packs of cigarettes were taken from her.
- Arm, leg, and waist restraints were applied when she became agitated. She was also given a sedative.
- After she calmed down, some restraints were removed at her request. They were removed from her right wrist, left ankle, and waist.
- She asked to go outside to smoke. A nurse left after asking her to wait a few minutes.

- While the nurse was out of the room, the patient set her bed on fire with a cigarette and lighter.
- The patient suffered severe burns to her left arm and chest. (The burns required skin grafting. Scars were left at the burn and skin graft sites.)

The patient's lawsuit claimed negligence because:

- The nurse left her.
- Restraints were removed.
- The cigarettes and lighter were not found.

The jury found in favor of the patient. She was awarded $350,000 for past and future pain, suffering, and disfigurement.

(Wilson v Boscobel Area Health Care Center.) With permission from Medical Malpractice Verdicts, Settlements & Experts; Lewis Laska, editor. 901 Church St. Nashville TN, 37203-3411. 1-800-298-6288.

REVIEW QUESTIONS

Circle the BEST answer.

1 Stress is
 a The way a person copes with and adjusts to everyday living
 b A response or change in the body caused by some factor
 c A mental illness
 d A thought or idea

2 Personality is
 a The id and the ego
 b A person's attitudes, values, behaviors, and traits
 c How a person copes with stress
 d A false thought or idea

3 Defense mechanisms are used to
 a Blame others
 b Make excuses for behavior
 c Return to an earlier time
 d Block unpleasant feelings

4 These statements are about defense mechanisms. Which is *false?*
 a Mentally healthy persons use them.
 b They relieve anxiety.
 c They prevent mental illness.
 d Persons with mental illness use them.

5 A phobia is
 a The event that causes stress
 b A false belief
 c An intense fear of something
 d Feelings and emotions

6 A person cleans and cleans. This behavior is
 a A delusion
 b A hallucination
 c A compulsion
 d An obsession

7 A person has nightmares about a trauma. The person is having
 a Phobias
 b Panic attacks
 c Flashbacks
 d Anxiety

8 A woman believes she is married to a rock singer. This is called a
 a Fantasy
 b Delusion of grandeur
 c Delusion of persecution
 d Hallucination

9 A man believes that someone is trying to kill him. This belief is called a
 a Fantasy
 b Delusion of grandeur
 c Delusion of persecution
 d Hallucination

10 These statements are about schizophrenia. Which is *false?*
 a It is a brain disorder.
 b It can be cured with drugs and therapy.
 c Thinking and behavior are disturbed.
 d Suicide is a risk.

Continued

11 Bipolar disorder means that the person
   a Is very suspicious
   b Has anxiety
   c Is very unhappy and feels unwanted
   d Has severe mood swings

12 In bipolar disorder, an "emotional high" is called
   a Depression
   b Psychosis
   c An obsession
   d Mania

13 These statements are about antisocial personality disorder. Which is *false?*
   a The person is at least 18 years old.
   b The person blames others.
   c The person lies or cons others for pleasure.
   d The person is loyal to others.

14 Substances involved in abuse and addiction affect the
   a Circulatory system
   b Respiratory system
   c Nervous system
   d Immune system

15 These statements are about alcoholism. Which is *false?*
   a The person has a strong craving for alcohol.
   b The disease lasts throughout life.
   c After treatment, the person can have a social drink.
   d The person physically depends on alcohol.

16 These statements are about drug addiction. Which is *false?*
   a It is a chronic brain disease.
   b Higher doses of the drug may be needed.
   c The person has to have the drug.
   d The person can stop taking the drug without treatment.

17 A person has withdrawal syndrome. This means that
   a The person has a physical and mental response when the drug is not taken
   b The person needs higher doses of the drug
   c The effect is reduced with the same amount of drug
   d The person has a relapse after treatment

18 Which is not common in eating disorders?
   a Weight gain
   b Vomiting after eating
   c Intense exercise
   d Taking drugs to rid the body of water and feces

19 Which group has the highest suicide rate?
   a White men over 85 years of age
   b Teenagers and young adults between the ages of 15 and 20
   c Men
   d Women

20 The most common method of suicide involves
   a Firearms
   b Hanging
   c Self-poisoning
   d Drug overdose

21 Most persons who commit suicide have
   a A mood disorder
   b Schizophrenia
   c An eating disorder
   d Suicide contagion

22 A hospital patient talks about suicide. What should you do?
   a Call for the nurse.
   b Identify factors that increase the risk of suicide.
   c Ask what method the person intends to use.
   d Restrain the person.

Circle T if the statement is true and F if it is false.

23 T F Some anxiety is normal.

24 T F Anxiety is an intense and sudden feeling of fear or dread.

25 T F Anxiety is a false belief.

26 T F Panic is the highest level of anxiety.

27 T F Memories in the subconscious can be recalled.

28 T F Depression is common in older persons.

29 T F HIV, AIDS, and sudden death can occur from one use of a substance.

30 T F A person is talking about suicide. You can leave the person alone to get the nurse.

Answers to these questions are on p. 782.

Confusion and Dementia

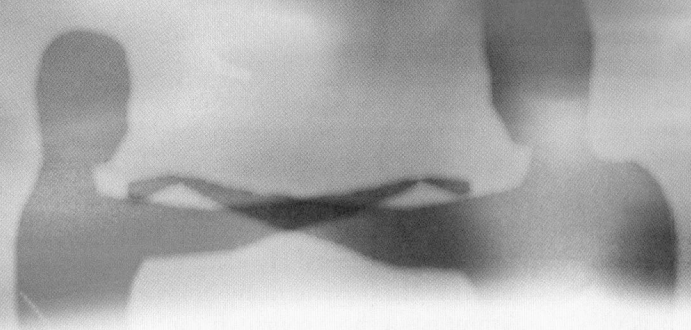

OBJECTIVES

- ▣ Define the key terms and key abbreviations listed in this chapter
- ▣ Describe confusion and its causes
- ▣ List the measures that help confused persons
- ▣ Explain the differences between delirium, depression, and dementia
- ▣ Describe Alzheimer's disease (AD)
- ▣ Describe the signs, symptoms, and behaviors of AD
- ▣ Explain the care required by persons with AD and other dementias
- ▣ Describe the effects of AD on the family
- ▣ Explain validation therapy

KEY TERMS

cognitive function Involves memory, thinking, reasoning, ability to understand, judgment, and behavior
delirium A state of temporary but acute mental confusion
delusion A false belief
dementia The loss of cognitive function that interferes with routine personal, social, and occupational activities
hallucination Seeing, hearing, smelling, or feeling something that is not real
pseudodementia False (*pseudo*) dementia
sundowning Signs, symptoms, and behaviors of AD increase during hours of darkness

KEY ABBREVIATIONS

AD Alzheimer's disease
ADL Activities of daily living
LNA Licensed nursing assistant
MCI Mild cognitive impairment
MID Multi-infarct dementia
OBRA Omnibus Budget Reconciliation Act of 1987

Changes in the brain and nervous system occur with aging (Box 44-1). Certain diseases affect the brain. Changes in the brain can affect cognitive function. (*Cognitive* relates to knowledge.) Quality of life is affected. **Cognitive function** involves:

▶ Memory
▶ Thinking
▶ Reasoning
▶ Ability to understand
▶ Judgment
▶ Behavior

CONFUSION

Confusion has many causes. Diseases, infections, hearing and vision loss, and drug side effects are some causes. So is brain injury. With aging, there is reduced blood supply to the brain. Personality and mental changes can result. Memory and the ability to make good judgments are lost. A person may not know people, the time, or the place. Some people gradually lose the ability to perform daily activities. Behavior changes are common. The person may be angry, restless, depressed, and irritable.

Acute confusion (delirium) occurs suddenly. It is usually temporary. Causes include infection, illness, injury, drugs, and surgery. Treatment is aimed at the cause.

Confusion caused by physical changes cannot be cured. Some measures help to improve function (Box 44-2). You must meet the person's basic needs.

DEMENTIA

Dementia is the loss of cognitive function that interferes with routine personal, social, and occupational activities. (*De* means from. *Mentia* means mind.) The person may have changes in personality, mood, or behavior. Dementia is a group of symptoms that may occur with certain diseases or conditions.

Dementia is not a normal part of aging. Most older people do not have dementia. Some early warning signs include:

▶ Recent memory loss that affects job skills
▶ Problems with common tasks (for example, dressing, cooking, driving)
▶ Problems with language; forgetting simple words
▶ Getting lost in familiar places
▶ Misplacing things and putting things in odd places (for example, putting a watch in the oven)
▶ Personality changes
▶ Poor or decreased judgment (for example, going outdoors in the snow without shoes)
▶ Loss of interest in life

If changes in the brain have not occurred, some dementias can be reversed. When the cause is removed, so are the signs and symptoms. Treatable causes include:

▶ Drugs and alcohol
▶ Delirium and depression
▶ Tumors

▶ Heart, lung, and blood vessel problems
▶ Head injuries
▶ Infection
▶ Vision and hearing problems

Permanent dementias result from changes in the brain. They have no cure. Function declines over time. Causes of permanent dementia are listed in Box 44-3. Alzheimer's disease is the most common type of permanent dementia.

Pseudodementia means false (*pseudo*) dementia. The person has signs and symptoms of dementia. However, there are no changes in the brain. This can occur with delirium and depression.

Delirium and Depression

Delirium and depression can be mistaken for dementia. **Delirium** is a state of temporary but acute mental confusion. Onset is sudden. It is common in older persons with acute or chronic illnesses. Infections, heart and lung diseases, and poor nutrition are common causes. So are hormone disorders. Hypoglycemia is also a cause (Chapter 41). Alcohol and many drugs can cause delirium. Delirium has a short course. It can last for a few hours to as long as 1 month.

Delirium signals physical illness in older persons and in persons with dementia. It is an emergency. The cause must be found and treated. Signs and symptoms include:

▶ Anxiety
▶ Disorientation
▶ Tremors
▶ Hallucinations (p. 695)
▶ Delusions (p. 695)
▶ Attention problems
▶ Decline in level of consciousness
▶ Memory problems

Depression is the most common mental health problem in older persons. It is often overlooked. Depression, aging, and some drug side effects have similar signs and symptoms. See Chapter 43 for signs and symptoms of depression in older persons.

BOX 44-1 Changes in the Nervous System From Aging

- Nerve cells are lost.
- Nerve conduction slows.
- Responses and reaction times are slower.
- Reflexes are slower.
- Vision and hearing decrease.
- Taste and smell decrease.

- Touch and sensitivity to pain decrease.
- Blood flow to the brain is reduced.
- Sleep patterns change.
- Memory is shorter.
- Forgetfulness occurs.
- Dizziness can occur.

BOX 44-2 Caring for the Confused Person

- Follow the person's care plan.
- Provide for safety.
- Face the person. Speak clearly.
- Call the person by name every time you are in contact with him or her.
- State your name. Show your name tag.
- Give the date and time each morning. Repeat as needed during the day or evening.
- Explain what you are going to do and why.
- Give clear, simple directions and answers to questions.
- Ask clear and simple questions. Give the person time to respond.
- Keep calendars and clocks with large numbers in the person's room and in nursing areas (Fig. 44-1). Remind the person of holidays, birthdays, and special events.
- Have the person wear eyeglasses and hearing aids as needed.
- Use touch to communicate (Chapter 7).
- Place familiar objects and pictures within the person's view.

- Provide newspapers, magazines, TV, and radio. Read to the person if appropriate.
- Discuss current events with the person.
- Maintain the day-night cycle.
  - Open window coverings during the day. Close them at night.
  - Use night-lights at night. Use them in rooms, bathrooms, hallways, and other areas.
  - Have the person wear regular clothes during the day—not sleepwear.
- Provide a calm, relaxed, and peaceful setting. Prevent loud noises, rushing, and congested hallways and dining rooms.
- Follow the person's routine. Meals, bathing, exercise, TV, bedtime, and other activities have a schedule. This promotes a sense of order and what to expect.
- Break tasks into small steps when helping the person.
- Do not rearrange furniture or the person's belongings.
- Encourage the person to take part in self-care.
- Be consistent.

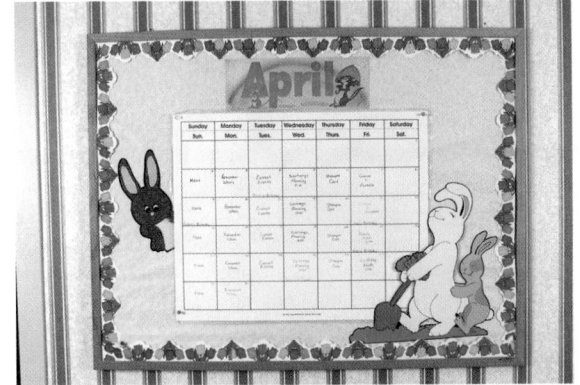

FIGURE 44-1 A large calendar can help confused persons.

BOX 44-3 Causes of Permanent Dementia

- Alcohol-related dementia and Korsakoff's syndrome
- Alzheimer's disease
- AIDS-related dementia
- Brain tumors
- Cerebrovascular disease
- Huntington's disease (a nervous system disease)
- Multi-infarct dementia (MID) (many (multi) strokes leave areas of damage (infarct))
- Multiple sclerosis
- Parkinson's disease
- Stroke
- Syphilis
- Trauma and head injury

Mild Cognitive Impairment

Mild cognitive impairment (MCI) is a type of memory change. People with MCI have on-going memory problems but do not have other losses like confusion, attention problems, and difficulty with language. The person may develop Alzheimer's disease.

ALZHEIMER'S DISEASE

Alzheimer's disease (AD) is a brain disease. Nerve cells that control intellectual and social function are damaged. These functions are affected:

▶ Memory
▶ Thinking
▶ Reasoning
▶ Judgment
▶ Language
▶ Behavior
▶ Mood
▶ Personality

The person has problems with work and everyday functions. Problems with family and social relationships occur. There is a steady decline in memory and mental function.

AD is gradual in onset. It gets worse and worse over time. Persons with AD usually live 8 to 10 years after diagnosis. Some persons live as few as 3 years. Others as long as 20 years. Some people in their 40s and 50s have AD. However, it usually occurs after the age of 60. The risk increases with age. It is often diagnosed around the age of 80. Nearly half of persons age 85 and older have AD.

The cause is unknown. A family history of AD increases a person's risk of developing the disease. More women than men have AD. Women live longer than men.

BOX 44-4 Signs of AD

WARNING SIGNS
- Asking the same question over and over again.
- Repeating the same story—word for word, again and again.
- Forgetting how to cook, how to make repairs, or how to play cards. The person forgets activities that were once done regularly and with ease.
- Losing the ability to pay bills or balance a checkbook.
- Getting lost in familiar places. Or misplacing household objects.
- Neglecting to bathe. Or wearing the same clothes over and over again. Meanwhile, the person insists that a bath was taken or that clothes are clean.
- Relying on someone else to make decisions or answer questions that he or she would have handled.

OTHER SIGNS
- Forgets recent events, conversations, and appointments.
- Forgets simple directions.
- Forgets names (including family members).
- Forgets the names of everyday things (clock, radio, TV, and so on).
- Forgets words, loses train of thought.
- Substitutes unusual words and names for what is forgotten.
- Speaks in a native language.
- Curses or swears.

- Misplaces things; puts things in odd places.
- Has problems writing checks.
- Gives away large amounts of money.
- Does not recognize or understand numbers.
- Has problems following conversations.
- Has problems reading and writing.
- Becomes lost in familiar settings.
- Forgets where he or she is.
- Does not know how to get back home.
- Wanders from home.
- Cannot tell or understand time or dates.
- Cannot solve everyday problems (iron is left on, stove burners left on, food burning on the stove, and so on).
- Cannot perform everyday tasks (dressing, bathing, brushing teeth, and so on).
- Distrusts others.
- Is stubborn.
- Withdraws socially.
- Is restless.
- Becomes suspicious.
- Becomes fearful.
- Does not want to do things.
- Sleeps more than usual.

Warning signs written by Eric Pfeiffer, MD, the director of the University of South Florida Suncoast Alzheimer's and Gerontology Center. Reprinted with permission.

BOX 44-5 Stages of Alzheimer's Disease

STAGE 1: MILD AD
- Memory loss—forgetfulness; forgets recent events
- Problems finding words, finishing thoughts, following directions, and remembering names
- Poor judgment; bad decisions (including when driving)
- Disoriented to time and place
- Lack of spontaneity—less outgoing or interested in things
- Blames others for mistakes, forgetfulness, and other problems
- Moodiness
- Problems performing everyday tasks

STAGE 2: MODERATE AD
- Restlessness—increases during the evening hours
- Sleep problems
- Memory loss increases—may not know family and friends
- Dulled senses—cannot tell the difference between hot and cold; cannot recognize dangers
- Fecal and urinary incontinence
- Needs help with activities of daily living (ADL)—bathing, feeding, and dressing self; afraid of bathing; will not change clothes
- Loses impulse control—foul language, poor table manners, sexual aggression, rudeness

- Movement and gait problems—walks slowly, has a shuffling gait
- Communication problems—cannot follow directions; problems with reading, writing, and math; speaks in short sentences or single words; statements may not make sense
- Repeats motions and statements—moves things back and forth constantly; says the same thing over and over again
- Agitation—behavior may be violent

STAGE 3: SEVERE AD
- Seizures (Chapter 49)
- Cannot speak—may groan, grunt, or scream
- Does not recognize self or family members
- Depends totally on others for all ADL
- Disoriented to person, time, and place
- Totally incontinent of urine and feces
- Cannot swallow—choking and aspiration are risks
- Sleep problems increase
- Becomes bed bound—cannot sit or walk
- Coma
- Death

Signs of AD

The classic sign of AD is *gradual loss of short-term memory*. At first, the only symptom may be forgetfulness. Box 44-4 lists the warning signs and other signs of AD.

Stages of AD

Signs and symptoms become more severe as the disease progresses. The disease ends in death. AD is often described in terms of 3 stages (Box 44-5). The Alzheimer's Association describes seven stages:

- *No impairment.* The person does not show signs of memory problems.
- *Very mild cognitive decline.* The person thinks that he or she has memory lapses. Familiar words or names are forgotten. The person does not know where to find keys, eyeglasses, or other objects. These problems are not apparent to family, friends, or the health team.
- *Mild cognitive decline.* Family, friends, and others notice problems. The person has problems with memory or concentration and with words or names. The person loses or misplaces something valuable. Functioning in social or work settings declines.
- *Moderate cognitive decline.* Memory of recent or current events declines. There are problems with shopping, paying bills, and managing money. The person may withdraw or be quiet in social situations.
- *Moderately severe decline.* The person has major memory problems. There may be confusion about the date or day of the week. He or she may need help choosing the correct clothing to wear. The person knows his or her own name, a partner's name, and children's names. Usually help is not needed with eating or elimination.
- *Severe cognitive decline.* Memory problems are worse. Personality and behavior changes develop—delusions, hallucinations, repetitive behavior. The person needs much help with daily activities, including dressing and elimination. Names may be forgotten, but faces may be recognized. Sleep problems, incontinence (urinary and fecal), and wandering are common.
- *Very severe decline.* The person cannot respond to his or her environment, speak, or control movement. The person cannot walk without help. Over time, he or she cannot sit up without support or hold the head up. Muscles become rigid. Swallowing is impaired.

Behaviors

The following behaviors are common with AD.

Wandering

Persons with AD are not oriented to person, time, and place. They may wander away and not find their way back. Wandering may be by foot, car, bike, or other means. They may be with you one moment and gone the next.

Judgment is poor. They cannot tell what is safe or dangerous. Life-threatening accidents are great risks. They can walk into traffic or into a nearby river, lake, ocean, or forest. If not properly dressed, heat or cold exposure is a risk.

Wandering may have no cause. Or the person may be looking for something or someone—the bathroom, the bedroom, a child, or a partner. Pain, drug side effects, stress, restlessness, and anxiety are possible causes. Sometimes finding the cause prevents wandering.

Safe Return Program. For persons living at home, the Alzheimer's Association has a *Safe Return Program.* The program is nationwide. It serves to identify and safely return persons who wander or become lost. A small fee is charged. A family member completes a form and provides a photo. These are entered into a national database. The person receives an ID (wallet card, bracelet or necklace, clothing labels).

Anyone finding a person can call the Safe Return number on the ID. Safe Return then calls the family member or caregiver. Some persons are reported missing. Safe Return can provide the person's information and photo to the police.

Sundowning

With **sundowning**, signs, symptoms, and behaviors of AD increase during hours of darkness. It occurs in the late afternoon and evening hours. As daylight ends and darkness starts, confusion and restlessness increase. So do anxiety, agitation, and other symptoms. Behavior is worse after the sun goes down. It may continue throughout the night.

Sundowning may relate to being tired or hungry. Poor light and shadows may cause the person to see things that are not there. Persons with AD may be afraid of the dark.

Hallucinations

A **hallucination** is seeing, hearing, smelling, or feeling something that is not real. Senses are dulled. Affected persons see animals, insects, or people that are not present. Some hear voices. They may feel bugs crawling or feel that they are being touched.

Sometimes the problem is caused by impaired vision or hearing. The person needs to wear eyeglasses and hearing aids as prescribed.

Delusions

Delusions are false beliefs. People with AD may think they are some other person. Some believe they are in jail, are being killed, or are being attacked. A person may believe that the caregiver is someone else. Many other false beliefs can occur.

Catastrophic Reactions

These are extreme responses. The person reacts as if there is a disaster or tragedy. The person may scream, cry, or be agitated or combative. These reactions are common from too many stimuli. Eating, music or TV playing, and being asked questions all at once can overwhelm the person.

Agitation and Restlessness

The person may pace, hit, or yell. Common causes are pain or discomfort, anxiety, lack of sleep, and too many or too few stimuli. Hunger and the need to eliminate also are causes. A calm, quiet setting helps calm the person. So does meeting basic needs.

Caregivers can cause these behaviors. A caregiver may rush the person or be impatient. Or mixed verbal and nonverbal messages are sent. For example, a caregiver may talk too fast or too loud. Caregivers always need to look at how their behaviors affect other persons.

Aggression and Combativeness

These behaviors include hitting, pinching, grabbing, biting, or swearing. They may result from agitation and restlessness. They frighten others.

Sometimes these behaviors are personality traits. Or pain, fatigue, too much stimulation, caregiver stress, and feeling lost or abandoned are causes. The behaviors can occur during care measures (bathing, dressing) that upset or frighten the person. See Chapter 7 for dealing with the angry person. See Chapter 11 for workplace violence. Also follow the person's care plan.

Screaming

Persons with AD have communication problems. At first, it is hard to find the right words. As AD progresses, the person speaks in short sentences or in words. Often speech is not understandable.

The person screams to communicate. This is common in persons who are very confused and have poor communication skills. The person may scream a word or a name. Or the person just makes screaming sounds.

Possible causes include hearing and vision problems, pain or discomfort, fear, and fatigue. Too much or not enough stimulation is another cause. The person may react to a caregiver or family member by screaming.

Sometimes these measures are helpful:

▶ Providing a calm, quiet setting
▶ Playing soft music
▶ Having the person wear hearing aids and eyeglasses
▶ Having a family member or favorite caregiver comfort and calm the person
▶ Using touch to calm the person

Abnormal Sexual Behaviors

Sexual behaviors are labeled abnormal because of how and when they occur. Persons with AD are not oriented to person, time, and place. Sexual behaviors may involve the wrong person, the wrong place, and the wrong time. Also, persons with AD cannot control behavior.

Healthy persons do not undress or expose themselves in front of others. They do not masturbate or engage in sexual pleasures in public. They know their sexual partners. Persons with AD often mistake someone else for a sexual partner. The person kisses and hugs the other person.

Some behaviors are not sexual. Touching, scratching, and rubbing the genitals can signal infection, pain, or discomfort in the urinary or reproductive systems. Poor hygiene is another cause. So is being wet or soiled from urine or feces.

The nurse encourages the person's sexual partner to show affection. Their normal practices are encouraged. Examples include hand holding, hugging, kissing, and touching. When a person masturbates in public, lead the person to his or her room. Provide for privacy and safety. Good hygiene prevents itching. Clean the person quickly and thoroughly after elimination. Do not let the person stay wet or soiled.

The nurse assesses the person for urinary or reproductive system problems. The doctor is contacted as necessary.

Repetitive Behaviors

Repetitive means to repeat over and over again. Persons with AD repeat the same motions over and over again. For example, the person folds the same napkin over and over. Or the person says the same words over and over. Or the same question is asked. Such behaviors do not harm the person. However, they can annoy caregivers and the family.

Harmless acts are allowed. Music, picture books, exercise, and movies are distracting. Taking the person for a walk can help. Such measures help when words or questions are repeated.

CARE OF PERSONS WITH AD AND OTHER DEMENTIAS

Usually the person is cared for at home until symptoms are severe. Adult day care may help. Often assisted living or nursing center care is required. Sometimes hospital care is needed for other illnesses. You may care for persons with AD or other dementias in such settings. The person and family need your support and understanding.

People with AD do not choose to be forgetful, incontinent, agitated, or rude. Nor do they choose to have other behaviors, signs, and symptoms of the disease. They cannot control what is happening to them. The disease causes the behaviors. *The disease is responsible, not the person.*

Currently AD has no cure. Symptoms worsen over many years. The rate varies from person to person. Over time, persons with AD depend on others for care. Safety, hygiene, nutrition and fluids, elimination, and activity needs must be met. So must comfort and sleep needs. The person's care plan will include many of the measures listed in Box 44-6.

Comfort and safety are important. Good skin care and alignment prevent skin breakdown and contractures. You must treat these persons with dignity and respect. They have the same rights as persons who are alert and active. Talk to them in a calm voice. Always explain what you are going to do. Massage, soothing touch, music, and aromatherapy are comforting and relaxing. Range-of-motion exercises are also important. The person may need hospice care as death nears (Chapter 50).

The person can have other health problems and injuries. However, the person may not be aware of pain, fever, constipation, incontinence, or other signs and symptoms. Carefully observe the person. Report any change in the person's usual behavior to the nurse.

Infection is a risk. The person cannot fully tend to self-care. Infection can occur from poor hygiene. This includes poor skin care, oral hygiene, and perineal care after bowel and bladder elimination. Inactivity and immobility can cause pneumonia and pressure ulcers.

The person needs to feel useful, worthwhile, and active. This promotes self-esteem. Therapists work with

BOX 44-6 Care of Persons With AD and Other Dementias

ENVIRONMENT
- Follow established routines.
- Avoid changing rooms or roommates.
- Place picture signs by room doors, bathrooms, dining rooms, and other areas (Fig. 44-2, p. 698).
- Keep personal items where the person can see them.
- Stay within the person's sight to the extent possible.
- Place memory aids (large clocks and calendars) where the person can see them.
- Keep noise levels low.
- Play music and show movies from the person's past.
- Select tasks and activities that fit the person's cognitive abilities and interests.

COMMUNICATION
- Approach the person in a calm, quiet manner.
- Approach the person from the front. Do not approach the person from the side or the back. This can startle the person.
- Call the person by name. Have the person's attention before you start speaking.
- Identify other people by their names. Avoid pronouns (he, she, them, and so on).
- Follow the rules of communication (Chapters 5 and 7).
- Practice measures to promote communication (Chapter 7).
- Use gestures or cues. Point to objects.
- Speak in a calm, gentle voice.
- Speak slowly. Use simple words and short sentences.
- Let the person speak. Do not interrupt or rush the person.
- Give the person time to respond.
- Do not criticize, correct, or interrupt the person.
- Present one idea, question, or instruction at a time.
- Ask simple questions having simple answers. Do not ask complex questions.
- Do not present the person with many questions.
- Provide simple explanations of all procedures and activities.
- Give consistent responses.
- Practice measures to promote hearing (Chapter 37).
- Practice measures to communicate with speech-impaired persons (Chapter 37).
- Practice measures for blind and visually impaired persons (Chapter 37).

SAFETY
- Remove harmful, sharp, and breakable objects from the area. This includes knives, scissors, glass, dishes, razors, and tools.
- Provide plastic eating and drinking utensils. This helps prevent breakage and cuts.
- Place safety plugs in electric outlets.
- Keep cords and electric equipment out of reach.
- Remove electric appliances from the bathroom. Examples include hair dryers, curling irons, make-up mirrors, and electric shavers.
- Store personal care items (shampoo, deodorant, lotion, and so on) in a safe place.
- Keep childproof caps on medicine containers and household cleaners.
- Store household cleaners and drugs in locked storage areas.
- Store dangerous equipment and tools in a safe place.
- Remove knobs from stoves or place childproof covers on the knobs.
- Remove dangerous appliances and power tools from the home.
- Remove firearms from the home.
- Store car keys in a safe place.
- Supervise the person who smokes.
- Store cigarettes, cigars, pipes, matches, and other smoking materials in a safe place.
- Practice safety measures to prevent falls (Chapter 12).
- Practice safety measures to prevent fires (Chapter 11).
- Practice safety measures to prevent burns (Chapter 11).
- Practice safety measures to prevent poisoning (Chapter 11).
- Lock all doors to kitchens, utility rooms, and housekeeping closets. Keep them locked.

WANDERING
- Follow agency policy for locking doors and windows. Locks are often placed at the top and bottom of doors (Fig. 44-3, p. 698). The person is not likely to look for a lock in such places.
- Keep door alarms and electronic doors turned on. The alarm goes off when the door is opened. Respond to door alarms at once.
- Follow agency policy for fire exits. Everyone must be able to leave the building if there is a fire.
- Make sure the person wears an ID bracelet or Safe Return ID at all times.
- Exercise the person as ordered. Adequate exercise often reduces wandering.
- Involve the person in activities—folding napkins, dusting a table, sorting socks, rolling yarn, sweeping, sanding blocks of wood, or watering plants.
- Do not use restraints. Restraints require a doctor's order. They also tend to increase confusion and disorientation.
- Do not argue with the person who wants to leave. The person does not understand what you are saying.
- Go with the person who insists on going outside. Make sure he or she is properly dressed. Guide the person inside after a few minutes (Fig. 44-4, p. 698).
- Let the person wander in enclosed areas. The agency may have enclosed areas where the person can walk about (Fig. 44-5, p. 699). They provide a safe place for the person to wander.

SUNDOWNING
- Complete treatments and activities early in the day.
- Provide a calm, quiet setting late in the day.
- Do not restrain the person.
- Encourage exercise and activity early in the day.
- Meet nutrition needs. Hunger can increase restlessness.
- Promote elimination. The need to eliminate can increase restlessness.
- Do not try to reason with the person. He or she cannot understand what you are saying.
- Do not ask the person to tell you what is bothering him or her. Communication is impaired. The person does not understand what you are asking. He or she cannot think or speak clearly.

HALLUCINATIONS AND DELUSIONS
- Make sure the person wears eyeglasses and hearing aids as needed. Follow the care plan.
- Do not argue with the person. He or she does not understand what you are saying.
- Reassure the person. Tell him or her that you will provide protection from harm.
- Distract the person with some item or activity. Taking the person for a walk may be helpful.
- Turn off TV or movies when violent and disturbing programs are on. The person may believe that the story is real.
- Use touch to calm and reassure the person (Fig. 44-6, p. 699).

Continued

BOX 44-6 Care of Persons With AD and Other Dementias—cont'd

HALLUCINATIONS AND DELUSIONS—cont'd

- Eliminate noises that the person could misinterpret. TV, radio, stereos, furnaces, air conditioners, and other things could affect the person.
- Check lighting. Make sure there are no glares, shadows, or reflections.
- Cover or remove mirrors. The person could misinterpret his or her reflection.

SLEEP

- Develop a regular bedtime. Keep the bedtime at the same time each evening.
- Follow bedtime rituals.
- Use night-lights so the person can see. Use them in rooms, hallways, bathrooms, and other areas. They help prevent accidents and disorientation.
- Limit caffeine during the day.
- Discourage naps during the day.
- Reduce noises.

BASIC NEEDS

- Meet food and fluid needs (Chapters 23). Provide finger foods. Cut food and pour liquids as needed.
- Provide good skin care (Chapters 19 and 32). Keep the person's skin free of urine and feces.
- Promote urinary and bowel elimination (Chapters 21 and 22).
- Provide incontinence care as needed (Chapters 21 and 22).
- Promote exercise and activity during the day (Chapter 26). This helps reduce wandering and sundowning behaviors. The person may also sleep better.
- Reduce intake of coffee, tea, and cola drinks. These contain caffeine. Caffeine is a stimulant. It can increase restlessness, confusion, and agitation.

- Provide a quiet, restful setting. Soft music is better than loud TV programs.
- Play music during care activities such as bathing and during meals.
- Promote personal hygiene (Chapter 19). Do not force the person into a shower or tub. People with AD are often afraid of bathing. Try bathing the person when he or she is calm. Use the person's preferred bathing method (tub bath, shower). Provide privacy and keep the person warm. Do not rush the person.
- Provide oral hygiene (Chapter 19).
- Choose clothing that is comfortable and simple to put on. Front opening garments are easy to put on. Pullover tops are harder to put on. And the person may become frightened when his or her head is inside the pullover top.
- Select clothing that closes with Velcro. Such items are easy to put on and take off. Buttons, zippers, snaps, and other closures can frustrate the person.
- Offer simple clothing choices (Fig. 44-7). Let the person choose between two shirts or two blouses, two pants or two slacks, and so on.
- Lay clothing out in the order it will be put on. Hand the person one clothing item at a time. Tell or show the person what to do. Do not rush him or her.
- Have equipment ready for any procedure. This reduces the amount of time the person is involved in care measures.
- Observe for signs and symptoms of health problems (Chapter 6).
- Prevent infection (Chapter 14).

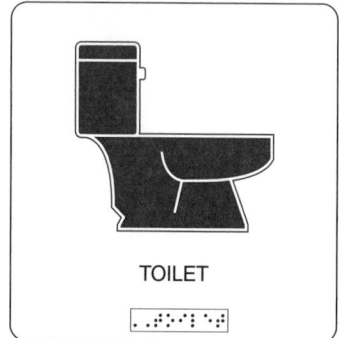 

FIGURE 44-2 Signs give cues to persons with dementia.

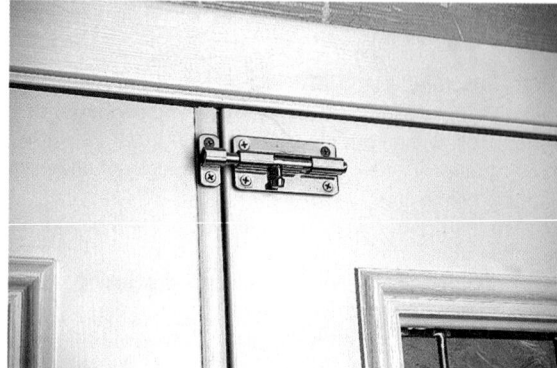

FIGURE 44-3 A slide lock is at the top of the door.

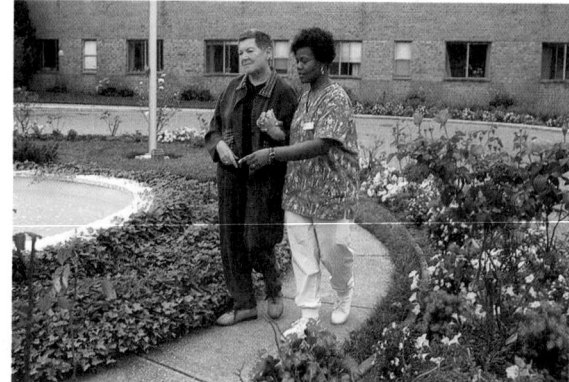

FIGURE 44-4 Walk outside with the person who wanders. Then guide the person back inside after a few minutes.

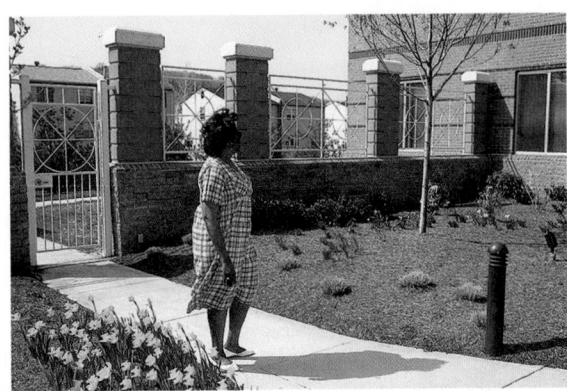

FIGURE 44-5 An enclosed garden allows persons with AD to wander in a safe setting.

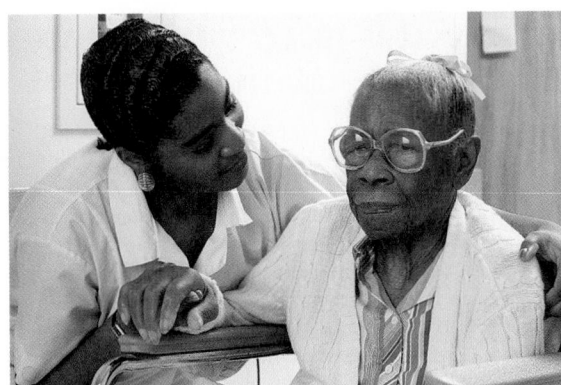

FIGURE 44-6 Use touch to calm the person.

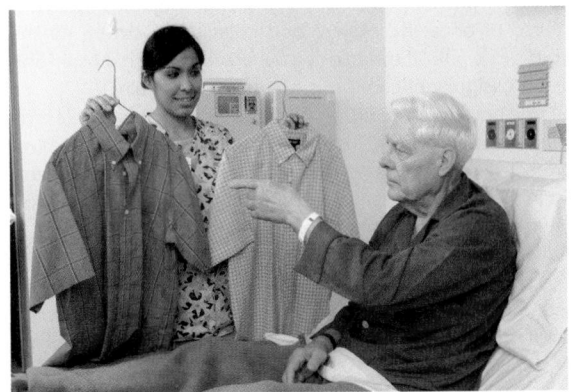

FIGURE 44-7 The person with AD is offered simple clothing choices.

one person, a small group, or a large group. Therapies and activities focus on the person's strengths and past successes. For example:

- A woman used to cook. She helps clean fruit.
- A man was a good dancer. Activities are planned so he can dance.
- A man likes to clean. He helps with dusting.

Supervised activities meet the person's needs and cognitive abilities. The person's interests are considered. Activities are based on what the person enjoys and can do. Some people like crafts, exercise, gardening, and listening and moving to music. Others like sing-alongs, reminiscing, and board games. Some like to string beads, fold towels, or roll dough.

See *Focus on Communication: Care of Persons With AD and Other Dementias.*

See *Teamwork and Time Management: Care of Persons With AD and Other Dementias.*

See *Focus on Long-Term Care and Home Care: Care of Persons With AD and Other Dementias.*

See *Focus on Ethics and Laws: Care of Persons With AD and Other Dementias.*

FOCUS ON LONG-TERM CARE AND HOME CARE
Care of Persons With AD and Other Dementias

LONG-TERM CARE

Many nursing centers have special units for persons with AD and other dementias. Some units are secured. This means that entrances and exits are locked. Persons in these units have a safe setting to move about in. They cannot wander away. Some persons have aggressive behaviors that disrupt or threaten others. They may need a secured unit.

According to the Omnibus Budget Reconciliation Act of 1987 (OBRA), secured units are physical restraints. The center must follow OBRA rules. They must use the least restrictive approach. A dementia diagnosis and a doctor's order are needed to place a person on a secured unit. At least every 90 days, the health team reviews the person's need for a secured unit. The person's rights are always protected.

At some point, the secured unit is no longer needed for safe care. For example, the person's condition progresses from stage 2 to stage 3. The person cannot sit or walk. Wandering is not a concern. The person is transferred to another unit.

Licensing and accrediting agencies have standards of care for special care units. Staff must have special training in the care of persons with dementia. The unit must have programs that promote dignity, personal freedom, and safety.

Quality of life is important for all persons with confusion and dementia. Nursing center residents have rights under OBRA. They may not know or be able to exercise their rights. However, the family knows the person's rights. They want those rights protected. They want respect and dignity for the loved one.

The person has the right to privacy and confidentiality. Protect the person from exposure. Only those involved in the person's care are present for care and procedures. The person is allowed to visit in private. Protect confidentiality. Do not share information about the person's care and condition with others.

Personal choice is important. If able, simple choices are encouraged. For example, a person chooses to wear a shirt or sweater. Watching or not watching TV may be a simple choice. The family makes choices if the person cannot. They choose bath times, menus, clothing, activities, and other care.

The person has the right to keep and use personal items. Some items provide comfort. A pillow, blanket, afghan, or sweater may have meaning to the person. The person may not know why or even recognize the item. Still, it is important. Keep personal items safe. Protect the person's property from loss or damage.

These persons must be kept free from abuse, mistreatment, and neglect. Caring for persons with confusion and dementia is often very frustrating. Some behaviors are hard to deal with. Family and staff can become short-tempered and angry. Protect the person from abuse. Report any signs and symptoms of abuse to the nurse at once. Be patient and calm when caring for these persons. Talk with the nurse if you are becoming upset. Sometimes an assignment change is needed for a while.

All persons have the right to be free from restraints. Restraints require a doctor's order. They are used only if it is the best way to protect the person. They are not used for staff convenience. Restraints can make confusion and demented behaviors worse. The nurse tells you when to use restraints.

Activity and a safe setting promote quality of life (see Box 44-6). Safe, calm, and quiet activities are needed. The recreational therapist and other health team members will find activities that are best for each person. These are part of the person's care plan.

FOCUS ON ETHICS AND LAWS
Care of Persons With AD and Other Dementias

While a licensed nursing assistant (LNA) was feeding a nursing home resident with Alzheimer's disease, the resident threw the tray on the floor. The LNA called the resident a degrading name and swore at her.

The Board of Nursing concluded that the LNA abused and improperly cared for the resident. The unprofessional conduct violated the Administrative Rules of the Board of Nursing because of:
* Abuse or neglect of a patient
* Performing unsafe or unacceptable patient care
* Failing to conform to acceptable standards of practice
* Engaging in conduct likely to harm the public
  The nursing assistant's license was reprimanded.
  (Author note: A reprimand means that the Board considered her conduct to be improper. However, the Board did not limit her right to work as an LNA.)

(State of Vermont Board of Nursing in regard to K. Blaufox, 2000.)

The Family

The person may live at home or with a partner, children, or other family members. The family gives care. Or someone stays with the person. Health care is sought when the family cannot deal with the situation or meet the person's needs. Home health care may help for a while. Adult day care is an option. Long-term care is needed when:
▶ Family members cannot meet the person's needs
▶ The person no longer knows the caregiver
▶ Family members have health problems
▶ Money problems occur
▶ The person's behavior presents dangers to self and others

Diagnostic tests, doctor's visits, drugs, and home care are costly. So is long-term care. The person's medical care can drain family finances.

The family has special needs. Caring for the person at home or in a nursing center is stressful. There are physical, emotional, social, and financial stresses. Adult children are in the *sandwich generation.* They are caught between their own children who need attention and an ill parent who needs care. Caring for two families is stressful. Often adult children have jobs too.

Caregivers can suffer from anger, anxiety, depression, and sleeplessness. Some cannot concentrate or are irritable. They can develop health problems. They need to take care of their own health. A healthy diet, exercise, and plenty of rest are needed. Asking for help is important. The caregiver needs to feel free to ask family and friends for help.

Caregivers need much support and encouragement. Many join AD support groups. The groups are sponsored by hospitals, nursing centers, and the Alzheimer's Association. The Alzheimer's Association has chapters in cities and towns across the country. Support groups offer encouragement and advice. People in similar situations share their feelings, anger, frustration, guilt, and other emotions. They also share coping and caregiving ideas.

The family often feels hopeless. No matter what is done, the person only gets worse. Much time, money, energy, and emotion are needed to care for the person. Anger and resentment may result. Guilt feelings are common. The family also knows that the person did not choose the disease. They know that the person does not choose to have its signs, symptoms, and behaviors. Sometimes behaviors are embarrassing. The family may be upset and angry that the loved one cannot show love or affection.

The family is an important part of the health team. They help plan the person's care whenever possible. They need to learn how to bathe, feed, dress, and give oral hygiene to the person. They also need to learn how to provide a safe setting. The nurse and support group help the family learn how to give necessary care.

Some family members take part in unit activities. For many persons, family members provide comfort. They also need support and understanding from the health team.

See *Focus on Long-Term Care and Home Care: The Family.*

FOCUS ON LONG-TERM CARE AND HOME CARE

The Family

HOME CARE

Home care is an option for many families. They may need someone to prepare the person's meals. Help is often needed with bathing and elimination. Someone needs to supervise the person while family members work, do errands, and have time to themselves. The amount and kind of care depend on the person's needs and the family's ability to provide care.

Validation Therapy

Validation therapy may be part of the person's care plan. The therapy is based on these principles:

▶ All behavior has meaning.
▶ Development occurs in a sequence, order, and pattern (Chapter 9). Certain tasks must be completed during a stage of development. A stage cannot be skipped. Each stage is the basis of the next stage.
▶ If a person does not successfully complete a stage of development, unresolved issues and emotions may surface later in life.
▶ A person may return to the past to resolve such issues and emotions.
▶ Caregivers need to listen and provide empathy.
▶ Attempts are not made to correct the person's thoughts or bring the person back to reality. For example:
  ▶ While going from room to room, Mrs. Bell calls for her daughter. In reality, her daughter died 20 years ago. The caregiver does not tell Mrs. Bell that her daughter died. Instead, the caregiver says: "Tell me about your daughter."
  ▶ Mrs. Brown sits all day on a bench by the window. She says that she is at the train station waiting to meet her husband. In reality, her husband was killed during World War II. Buried in England, he never returned home. The caregiver does not remind Mrs. Brown of what happened. Instead, the caregiver encourages Mrs. Brown to talk about her husband.
  ▶ Mr. Garcia was 3 years old when his father died. He holds a ball constantly. He is very upset when anyone tries to remove it from his hand. He calls for his father and repeats "play ball, play ball." The caregiver does not remind Mr. Garcia that he is 80 years old and that his father died many years ago. Instead, the caregiver says, "Tell me about playing ball."

The health team decides if validation therapy might help a person. If so, it will be part of the person's care plan. Proper use of validation therapy requires special training. If the therapy is used in your agency, you will receive the training needed to use it correctly.

REVIEW QUESTIONS

Circle the BEST answer.

1 Cognitive function relates to the following *except*
   a Memory loss and personality
   b Thinking and reasoning
   c Ability to understand
   d Judgment and behavior

2 A person is confused after surgery. The confusion is likely to be
   a Permanent
   b Temporary
   c Caused by an infection
   d Caused by a brain injury

3 A person is confused. The care plan includes the following. Which should you question?
   a Restrain in bed at night.
   b Give clear, simple directions.
   c Use touch to communicate.
   d Open drapes during the day.

4 A person has delusions. A delusion is
   a A false belief
   b An illness caused by changes in the brain
   c Seeing, hearing, or feeling something that is not real
   d Alzheimer's disease

5 A person has AD. Which is *true?*
   a AD occurs only in older persons.
   b Diet and drugs can cure the disease.
   c AD and delirium are the same.
   d AD ends in death.

6 The following are common in persons with AD *except*
   a Memory loss, poor judgment, and sleep disturbances
   b Loss of impulse control and loss of the ability to communicate
   c Wandering, delusions, and hallucinations
   d Paralysis, dyspnea, and pain

7 Sundowning means that
   a The person becomes sleepy when the sun sets
   b Behaviors become worse in the late afternoon and evening hours
   c Behavior improves at night
   d The person goes to bed when the sun sets

8 A person with AD is screaming. You know that this is
   a An agitated reaction
   b A way to communicate
   c Caused by a delusion
   d A repetitive behavior

9 AD support groups do the following *except*
   a Provide care
   b Offer encouragement and care ideas
   c Provide support for the family
   d Promote the sharing of feelings and frustrations

10 A person with AD tends to wander. You should do the following *except*
   a Make sure door alarms are turned on
   b Make sure an ID bracelet is worn
   c Assist with exercise as ordered
   d Tell the person where to wander safely

11 Safety is important for the person with AD. Which is *false?*
   a Safety plugs are placed in electrical outlets.
   b Cleaners and drugs are kept locked up.
   c The person can keep smoking materials.
   d Sharp and breakable objects are removed from the person's setting.

12 You are caring for a person with AD. Which is *false?*
   a You can reason with the person.
   b Touch can calm and reassure the person.
   c A calm, quiet setting is important.
   d Help is needed with ADL.

Answers to these questions are on p. 782.

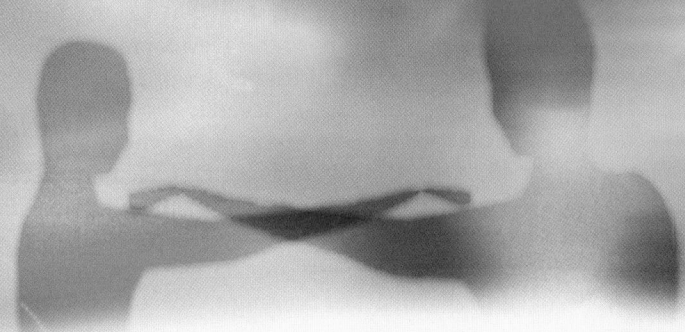

CHAPTER

45

Developmental Disabilities

OBJECTIVES

- Define the key terms and key abbreviations listed in this chapter
- Identify the areas of function limited by a developmental disability
- Explain how a developmental disability affects the child and family across the life span
- Explain when developmental disabilities occur
- Describe the causes of developmental disabilities
- Explain how various developmental disabilities affect a person's function

KEY TERMS

developmental disability (DD) A disability occurring before 22 years of age

diplegia Similar body parts are affected on both sides of the body

spastic Uncontrolled contractions of skeletal muscles

KEY ABBREVIATIONS

AAMR American Association on Mental Retardation

ADA Americans With Disabilities Act of 1990

CP Cerebral palsy

DD Developmental disability

DS Down syndrome

IQ Intelligence Quotient

OBRA Omnibus Budget Reconciliation Act of 1987

703

Many diseases, illnesses, and injuries cause disabilities in adulthood. A disability occurring before 22 years of age is a **developmental disability (DD)**. Causes of DD occur before, during, or after birth. Childhood illness and injuries can result in disabilities.

Some infants have birth defects. A birth defect can involve a body structure or function. Or it can affect metabolism. The defects result in disabilities or death. Causes of birth defects include:

► Genetic problems
► Problems with the number of chromosomes
► Problems with the structure of chromosomes
► Problems during pregnancy:
  ► Rubella (German measles)
  ► Untreated or uncontrolled diabetes
  ► Contact with dangerous chemicals
  ► Using drugs
  ► Using alcohol
  ► Smoking

A DD can be a physical or mental impairment or both. It is severe and permanent. Function is limited in three or more life skills:

► Self-care
► Understanding and expressing language
► Learning
► Mobility
► Self-direction
► Capacity for independent living
► Economic self-sufficiency (supporting oneself financially)

Developmentally disabled children become adults. They are not children forever. They need life-long assistance, support, and special services in these areas:

► Housing
► Employment
► Education
► Civil and human rights protection
► Health care

Independence to the extent possible is the goal for these persons. This includes having a job and living in the community. There are many resources to assist the person and family. Such support includes:

► Assistive and self-help devices
► Education
► Job training
► Personal assistive services
► Home and vehicle changes
► Financial assistance
► Physical therapy
► Occupational therapy
► Speech and language therapy
► Respiratory therapy
► Recreation therapy
► Assistance with hearing and vision

The disability affects the child and family throughout life. The person does not remain an infant or child. He or she becomes a teenager, young adult, middle-age adult, and older adult. Both the child and parents grow older. Often it is harder to care for an older child or adult. It may be hard to handle or move the person. A parent may become ill, injured, or disabled or die. Yet the disabled person still needs care.

Changes from aging occur (Chapter 10). However, the onset of aging may occur earlier when developmental disabilities are severe.

Persons with developmental disabilities have the same rights as every citizen in the United States. They have the right to live, learn, work, and enjoy life. The Americans With Disabilities Act of 1990 (ADA) further protects their rights. So does the Developmental Disabilities Assistance and Bill of Rights Act of 2000.

Some children are severely disabled. They need long-term care in centers for those who are developmentally disabled. Some adults with DD need nursing center care. They are further protected by the Omnibus Budget Reconciliation Act of 1987 (OBRA). OBRA requires that centers provide age-appropriate activities for them. Staff must have special training to meet their care needs.

INTELLECTUAL DISABILITIES (MENTAL RETARDATION)

Intellectual disabilities involve low intellectual function. Adaptive behavior is impaired. (*Intellectual* function relates to learning, thinking, and reasoning. *Adapt* means to change or adjust.)

See *Focus on Communication: Intellectual Disabilities (Mental Retardation)*.

The American Association on Mental Retardation (AAMR) describes mental retardation (intellectual disabilities) as:

► An IQ score of about 70 or below. (IQ means Intelligence Quotient.) The person learns at a slower rate than normal. The ability to learn is less than normal.
► A significant limit in at least one adaptive behavior. Adaptive behaviors are skills needed to function in everyday life—to live, work, and play. They involve communication, reading and writing, and money concepts. Social skills involve interpersonal skills, responsibility, not being tricked by others, following rules, and obeying laws. Personal activities of daily living include eating, dressing, mobility, and elimination. Other needed skills include preparing meals, taking drugs, using the phone, managing money, using transportation, housekeeping, job skills, and maintaining a safe setting.
► The condition being present before 18 years of age.

Brain development is impaired. It can occur before birth, during birth, or before the age of 18 years. Causes are listed in Box 45-1.

Intellectual disabilities range from mild to severe. Some persons are mildly affected. They are slow to learn in school. As adults, they can function in society with some support. For example, help is needed finding a job.

■ ■ ■
■   ■

Intellectual Disabilities (Mental Retardation)

Mental retardation is a common term that means intellectual disabilities. However, the term is offensive to others and is outdated. While still widely used, "intellectual disabilities" is the newer term preferred by the Arc of the United States. The Arc is a national organization focused on people with mental retardation and related developmental disabilities.

In June of 2003, the President's Committee on Mental Retardation was changed to the President's Committee for People with Intellectual Disabilities. The name was changed to:
- Update and improve the image of people with mental retardation
- Help reduce discrimination against such persons
- Reduce confusion between the terms "mental illness" and "mental retardation"

Avoid using "mental retardation" and "mentally retarded." Instead use the terms "intellectual disabilities" or "intellectually disabled."

Support is not needed every day. Some people need much support every day at home and at work. Still others need constant support in all areas.

The Arc of the United States believes that persons with intellectual disabilities must be able to enjoy and maintain a good quality of life. A good quality of life involves friendships, health and safety, and the right to make choices and take risks.

The Arc believes that children should live in a family. They should learn and play with children without disabilities. As adults, they should control their lives to the greatest extent possible. They should speak, make choices, and act for themselves. They should live in a home and have friends. They should do meaningful work and enjoy adult activities.

The Arc recognizes the sexuality of persons with intellectual disabilities and related developmental disabilities. They have physical, emotional, and social needs and desires. Reproductive organs develop. Some have life partners. Others marry and have children. Some persons can control their sexual urges. Others cannot. The type and location of sexual responses may be inappropriate. Also, sometimes persons with intellectual disabilities are sexually abused. The following are among the Arc's beliefs:
▶ The right to dignity and respect
▶ The right to privacy and confidentiality
▶ The right to chose friendships and emotional relationships
▶ The right to sexual expression
▶ The right to learn about sex, sexual abuse, safe sex, and sexually transmitted diseases
▶ The right to protection from sexual harassment, sexual and other abuses, and sexual relationships with staff members
▶ The right to sexual relationships, including marriage
▶ The right to choose birth control or to have and raise children

---

BOX 45-1 Causes of Intellectual Disabilities (Mental Retardation)

GENETIC CONDITIONS
- Abnormal genes from parents
- Errors when genes combine
- Gene disorders caused during pregnancy by infections, over-exposure to x-rays, and other factors
- Down syndrome
- Fragile X syndrome

PROBLEMS DURING PREGNANCY
- Alcohol use (fetal alcohol syndrome)
- Drug use
- Smoking
- Malnutrition (*mal* means bad)
- Rubella (German measles)
- Diabetes
- Lack of oxygen to the brain
- Sexually transmitted diseases (syphilis, genital herpes, chlamydia, AIDS)
- Rh blood disease

PROBLEMS AT BIRTH
- Prematurity
- Low birth weight
- Head injury
- Lack of oxygen to the brain

PROBLEMS AFTER BIRTH
- Childhood diseases (whooping cough, chicken pox, measles, Hib disease, meningitis, encephalitis)
- Head injuries
- Near drowning
- Lead poisoning
- Poisoning (alcohol, ammonia, bleaches, detergent, household cleaners and polishes, gasoline, kerosene, lighter fluid, drugs, lye, paint thinners and removers, pesticides, turpentine, weed killers, mercury and so on)
- Shaken baby syndrome
- Malnutrition
- Dehydration
- Reye's syndrome (a disease caused by drugs that contain aspirin)
- Poor health care

Modified from *Causes and prevention of mental retardation,* The Arc of the United States, May 2005, Silver Spring, Md, and *Preventing mental retardation: a guide to the causes of mental retardation,* The Arc of the United States, 2001, Silver Spring, Md.)

DOWN SYNDROME

Down syndrome (DS) is named for the doctor who identified the syndrome. DS is the most common genetic cause of mild to moderate intellectual disabilities (mental retardation). It is caused by an error in cell division. At fertilization, a male sex cell (sperm) unites with a female sex cell (ovum). Each cell has 23 chromosomes. When they unite, the cell has 46 chromosomes. In DS, an extra 21st chromosome is present. The fertilized cell has 47 chromosomes. Thus DS occurs at fertilization.

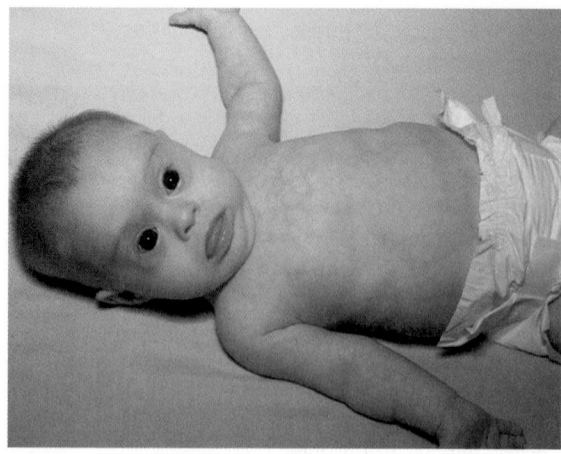

FIGURE 45-1 An infant with Down syndrome. (From Hockenberry MJ, Wilson D: *Wong's nursing care of infants and children*, ed 8, St Louis, 2007, Mosby.)

The DS child has certain features caused by the extra chromosome (Fig. 45-1):

- Small head
- Oval-shaped eyes that slant upward
- Flat face
- Short, wide neck
- Large tongue
- Wide, flat nose
- Small ears
- Short stature
- Short, wide hands with stubby fingers
- Low muscle tone

Many children with DS have heart defects and thyroid gland problems. They tend to have hearing and vision problems. They are at risk for ear and respiratory infections. Leukemia is a risk. (Leukemia is a malignant disease in which there is an abnormal increase in the number of white blood cells.) Dementia may appear in adults with DS.

Persons with DS need speech, language, physical, and occupational therapies. Most learn self-care skills. They also need health and sex education. Weight gain and constipation are problems. They need a healthy diet and regular exercise.

CEREBRAL PALSY

Cerebral palsy (CP) is a term applied to a group of disorders involving muscle weakness or poor muscle control (*palsy*). The defect is in the motor region of the brain (*cerebral*). Abnormal movements, posture, and coordination result. The defects result from brain damage. It occurs before, during, or within a few years after birth. Lack of oxygen to the brain is the usual cause. Brain defects (from faulty brain development) are other causes. There is no cure.

Infants at risk include those who:

- Are premature
- Have low birth weight

- Do not cry within the first 5 minutes after birth
- Need mechanical ventilation
- Have bleeding in the brain
- Have heart, kidney, or spinal cord defects
- Have blood problems
- Have seizures
- Have fetal alcohol syndrome

Brain damage in infancy and early childhood also can result in CP. Lack of oxygen to the brain can occur from:

- Choking
- Poisoning
- Near drowning
- Head injuries from accidents, falls, or child abuse (including shaken baby syndrome)
- Encephalitis and meningitis
- Rubella (German measles)

Body movements and body parts are affected. These types are the most common:

- *Spastic cerebral palsy.* Spastic comes from *spastikos*. It means to draw in. **Spastic** means uncontrolled contractions of skeletal muscles. Muscles contract or shorten. They are stiff and cannot relax. One or both sides of the body may be involved. Posture, balance, and movement are affected. The arms may be affected. If so, there are problems with eating, writing, dressing, and other activities of daily living.
- *Athetoid cerebral palsy.* The person cannot control movements. *Athetoid* comes from *athetos.* It means not fixed. The person has constant, slow, weaving, or writhing motions. These occur in the trunk, arms, hands, legs, and feet. Sometimes the tongue, face, and neck muscles are involved. Drooling and grimacing result.

Certain terms describe the body parts involved:

- *Hemiplegia.* The arm and leg on one side are paralyzed.
- *Diplegia. Di* means twice. **Diplegia** means that similar body parts are affected on both sides of the body. Both arms or both legs are paralyzed. The legs are commonly involved.
- *Quadriplegia.* Both arms and both legs are paralyzed. So are the trunk and neck muscles.

The person with CP can have many other impairments. They include:

- Intellectual disabilities (mental retardation)
- Learning disabilities
- Hearing impairments
- Speech impairments
- Vision impairments
- Drooling
- Bladder and bowel control problems
- Seizures
- Difficulty swallowing
- Attention deficit hyperactivity disorder (short attention span, poor concentration, increased activity)
- Breathing problems from poor posture
- Pressure ulcers from immobility

Care needs depend on the degree of brain damage. Disabilities and impairments range from mild to severe.

Some persons are very intelligent. Others have severe intellectual disabilities. The goal is for the person to be as independent as possible. Physical, occupational, and speech therapies can help. Some persons need braces and use crutches. Others need wheelchairs. Some need eyeglasses and hearing aids. Drugs can control seizures. Surgery and drugs can help some muscle problems.

AUTISM

Autism begins in early childhood. It can be diagnosed by 3 years of age. (*Autos* means self.) It is a brain disorder with no cure. The child has:

▶ Problems with social skills
▶ Verbal and nonverbal communication problems
▶ Repetitive behaviors and routines and narrow interests (*Repetitive* means to repeat or repeated.)

Autism is more common in boys than in girls. The cause is unknown. Genetics and environmental factors may be involved.

The disorder can range from mild to severe. Signs of autism are listed in Box 45-2. With therapy, the person can learn to change or control behaviors. Many therapies are used. They include:

▶ Behavior modification
▶ Speech and language therapy
▶ Music therapy
▶ Auditory therapy
▶ Sensory therapies
▶ Physical therapy
▶ Occupational therapy
▶ Drug therapy
▶ Diet therapy
▶ Communication therapy
▶ Recreation therapy

The person needs to develop social and work skills. Children with autism become adults. Some adults work and live independently. Others need support from family and community services. Some live in group homes or residential facilities.

Persons with autism may have other disorders. Intellectual disabilities and seizures are common.

SPINA BIFIDA

Spina bifida is a defect of the spinal column. (*Spina* means backbone. *Bifid* means split in two parts.) The defect occurs during the first month of pregnancy. Hydrocephalus often occurs with spina bifida (p. 708).

Bones of the spinal column are called *vertebrae*. They protect the spinal cord. In spina bifida, vertebrae do not form properly. This leaves a split in the vertebrae. The split leaves the spinal cord unprotected. Only a membrane covers the spinal cord. The spinal cord contains nerves. The nerves send messages to and from the brain. If the spinal cord is unprotected, nerve damage occurs. Affected body parts do not function properly. Paralysis may occur. Bowel and bladder problems are common. Infection is a threat.

Spina bifida can occur anywhere in the spine. The

BOX 45-2 Signs of Autism

- Shows no interest in other people
- Makes little or no eye contact
- Wants to be alone
- Has trouble understanding the feelings of others
- Has trouble talking about his or her own feelings
- Does not like to be held or cuddled; screams to be put down
- Over-reacts to touch
- Shows little reaction to pain
- Has frequent tantrums for no apparent reason
- Does not notice when others try to talk to him or her
- May not know how to talk, play, or relate to others
- May not talk
- Has slow language development
- Talks later than other children
- Repeats what others say at the moment or later
- Repeats words or phrases
- May not understand gestures (such as waving good-bye)
- Has a voice that sounds flat
- Cannot control voice volume (loudness or softness)
- Does not start or maintain conversations
- Stands too close to people when talking to them
- Stays with one topic of conversation for too long
- Has difficulty listening to what others say
- May act deaf
- Does not respond to his or her name
- Repeats actions over and over again
- Has routines where things stay the same
- Does not like change
- Repeats body movements (hand flapping, hand twisting, rocking)
- Has strong attachment to one item, idea, activity, or person
- Is very active or very quiet

---

lower back is the most common site. Types of spinal bifida include:

▶ *Spina bifida occulta. Occult* means hidden. The vertebrae are closed. A defect occurs in the vertebrae closure. In other words, the defect is hidden. The spinal cord and nerves are normal. The person has a dimple or tuft of hair on the back (Fig. 45-2, p. 708). Often there are no symptoms. Foot weakness and bowel and bladder problems can occur.

▶ *Spina bifida cystica. Cystica* means pouch or sac. Part of the spinal column is in the pouch or sac. A membrane or a thin layer of skin covers the sac. It looks like a large blister. The pouch is easily injured. Infection is a threat. There are two types of spina bifida cystica (Fig. 45-3, p. 708):

▶ *Meningocele. Meningo* comes from *meninx.* It means membrane. *Cele* means hernia or swelling. Meninges are the connective tissue that covers and protects the brain and spinal cord. Cerebrospinal fluid also protects the brain and spinal cord. The sac contains meninges and cerebrospinal fluid (see Fig. 45-3, *A,* and Fig. 45-4, p. 708). The sac does not contain nerve tissue. The spinal cord and nerves are usually normal. Nerve damage usually does not occur. Surgery corrects the defect.

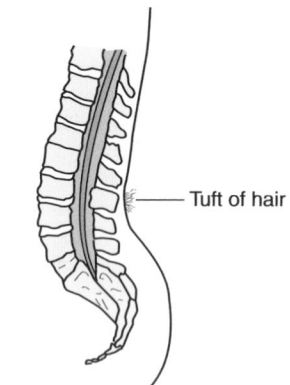

FIGURE 45-2 Spina bifida occulta.

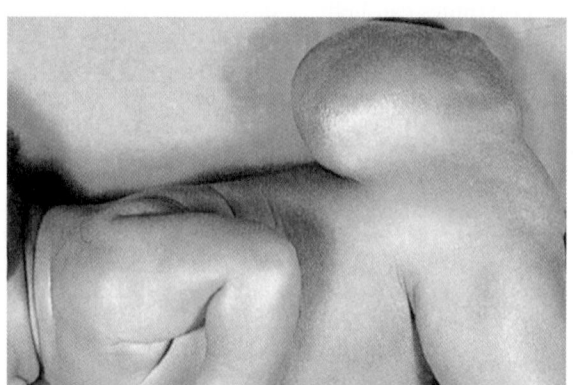

FIGURE 45-4 Meningocele. (From Zitelli BJ, Davis HW: *Atlas of pediatric physical diagnosis*, St Louis, 1987, Gower Medical Publishing.)

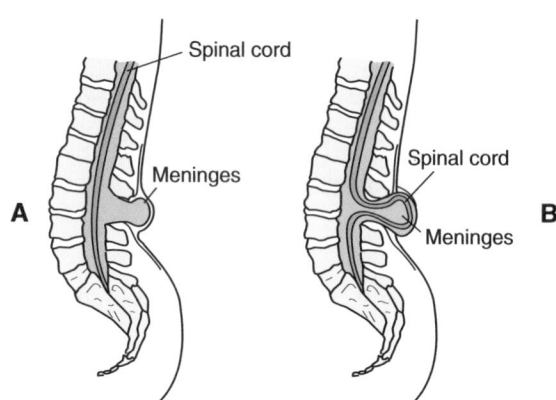

FIGURE 45-3 A, Meningocele. **B,** Meningomyelocele.

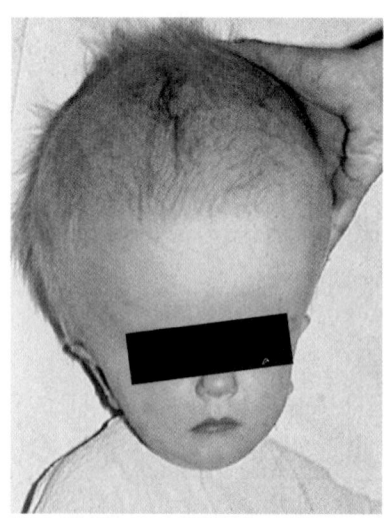

FIGURE 45-5 Hydrocephalus. (From Hart CA, Broadhead RL: *Color atlas of pediatric infectious diseases*, London, 1992, Mosby-Wolfe.)

▶ *Myelomeningocele* (or *meningomyelocele*). *Myelo* means spinal cord. The pouch contains nerves, spinal cord, meninges, and cerebrospinal fluid (see Fig. 45-3, *B*). Nerve damage occurs. Loss of function occurs below the level of damage. Leg paralysis and lack of sensation are common problems. So is the lack of bowel and bladder control. The defect is closed with surgery. Some children walk with braces or crutches. Others use wheelchairs.

Some children have learning problems. They may have problems with attention, language, reading, and math. They are at high risk for gastrointestinal disorders and mobility problems. Skin breakdown, depression, and social and sexual issues are other risks.

HYDROCEPHALUS

With hydrocephalus, cerebrospinal fluid collects in and around the brain. (*Hydro* means water. *Cephalo* means head.) The head enlarges (Fig. 45-5). Pressure inside the head increases. Intellectual disabilities (mental retardation) and neurological damage occur without treatment.

A shunt is placed in the brain. It allows cerebrospinal fluid to drain from the brain. The shunt is a long flexible tube. It goes from the brain into a body cavity (Fig. 45-6). Usually it drains into the abdomen or a heart chamber. The shunt must remain open (*patent*). If blocked, the cerebrospinal fluid cannot drain from the brain.

The person can have many problems. Vision problems, seizures, and learning disabilities can occur.

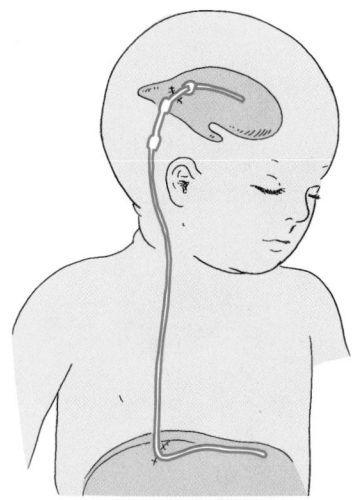

FIGURE 45-6 A shunt drains fluid from the brain. (From Hockenberry MJ, Wilson D: *Wong's nursing care of infants and children*, ed 8, St Louis, 2007, Mosby.)

REVIEW QUESTIONS

Circle the BEST answer.

1 All developmental disabilities occur
   a At birth   c During pregnancy
   b From trauma   d Before 22 years of age

2 These statements are about developmental disabilities. Which is *true*?
   a Self-care, learning, and mobility are always affected.
   b The disability is severe and permanent.
   c Physical and intellectual impairment occur together.
   d The person cannot hold a job.

3 The person with intellectual disabilities
   a Has delayed development of sexual organs
   b Does not have the skills to live, work, and play
   c Needs care in a special setting
   d Learns at a slower rate than normal

4 Intellectual disabilities
   a Are always severe
   b Can occur before, during, or after birth
   c Are caused by an extra chromosome
   d Affect the motor region of the brain

5 Down syndrome occurs
   a At fertilization
   b During the first month of pregnancy
   c Any time before, during, or after birth
   d From trauma

6 The person with Down syndrome always has some degree of
   a Cerebral palsy   c Impaired mobility
   b Autism   d Intellectual disability

7 Cerebral palsy is usually caused by
   a An extra chromosome
   b High fever
   c Lack of oxygen to the brain
   d Infection during pregnancy

8 The person with spastic type of cerebral palsy has problems with
   a Learning
   b Drooling
   c Posture, balance, and movement
   d Weaving motions of the trunk, arms, and legs

9 Autism begins
   a At fertilization   c At birth
   b During pregnancy   d In early childhood

10 The person with autism has
   a Impaired movement
   b Social and communication problems
   c Diplegia and brain damage
   d Intellectual disabilities

11 Spina bifida involves
   a Nerve damage
   b A defect in the spinal column
   c Seizures
   d Intellectual disabilities

12 Which is common in spina bifida?
   a Short attention span
   b Hearing and vision problems
   c Seizures
   d Bowel and bladder problems

13 Hydrocephalus often occurs with
   a Down syndrome   c Spina bifida
   b Cerebral palsy   d Autism

14 Hydrocephalus is treated with
   a Braces and crutches   c Drugs
   b A shunt   d Social services

Answers to these questions are on p. 782.

CHAPTER
46 Sexuality

OBJECTIVES

- Define the key terms and key abbreviations listed in this chapter
- Describe sex, sexuality, and sexual relationships
- Explain why sexuality is important throughout life
- Explain how injury and illness can affect sexuality
- Explain how aging can affect sexuality in older persons
- Explain how the nursing team can promote sexuality
- Explain why some persons become sexually aggressive
- Describe how to deal with sexually aggressive persons

KEY TERMS

bisexual A person who is attracted to both sexes

erectile dysfunction (ED) Impotence

heterosexual A person who is attracted to members of the other sex

homosexual A person who is attracted to members of the same sex

impotence The inability of the male to have an erection; erectile dysfunction

sex Physical activities involving the reproductive organs; done for pleasure or to have children

sexuality The physical, emotional, social, cultural, and spiritual factors that affect a person's feelings and attitudes about his or her sex

transgender A broad term used to describe people who express their sexuality or gender in other than the expected way; persons who are undergoing hormone therapy or surgery for sexual reassignment (female to male; male to female)

transsexual A person who believes that he or she is a member of the other sex

transvestite A person who dresses and behaves like the other sex for emotional and sexual relief; cross-dresser

KEY ABBREVIATIONS

CNA Certified nursing assistant
ED Erectile dysfunction

OBRA Omnibus Budget Reconciliation Act of 1987

Patients and residents are viewed as whole persons. They have physical and safety needs. They also have love and belonging, self-esteem, and self-actualization needs. Their physical, emotional, social, and spiritual needs are considered.

Sexuality involves the whole person. Illness, injury, and aging can affect sexuality.

SEX AND SEXUALITY

Sex is the physical activities involving the reproductive organs (Box 46-1, p. 712). It is done for pleasure or to have children. **Sexuality** is the physical, emotional, social, cultural, and spiritual factors that affect a person's feelings and attitudes about his or her sex. Sexuality involves the personality and the body. It affects how a person behaves, thinks, dresses, and responds to others.

Sexuality develops when a baby's sex is known. It is shown in names, colors, and toys. Blue is for boys and pink for girls. Dolls are for girls. Trains are for boys. By the age of 2, children know their own sex. Three-year-olds know the sex of other children. They learn male and female roles from adults (Fig. 46-4, p. 713). Children learn that boys and girls each behave in certain ways.

As children grow older, interest increases about the body and how it works. Teens are more aware of sex and the body. Their bodies respond to stimulation. They engage in sexual behaviors. They kiss, embrace, pet, or have intercourse. Pregnancy and sexually transmitted diseases (Chapter 42) are great risks.

Sex has more meaning as young adults mature. Attitudes and feelings are important. Partners are selected. They decide about sex before marriage and birth control.

Sexuality is important throughout life. Attitudes and sex needs change with aging. They are affected by life events. These include divorce, death of a partner, injury, illness, and surgery.

SEXUAL RELATIONSHIPS

A **heterosexual** is attracted to members of the other sex. Men are attracted to women. Women are attracted to men. Sexual behavior is male-female.

A **homosexual** is attracted to members of the same sex. Men are attracted to men. Women are attracted to women. *Gay* refers to homosexuality. Homosexual men are called *gay men. Lesbian* refers to a female homosexual. Before the 1960s and 1970s, many gay persons were secret about their sexual orientation. Now many gay persons openly express their sexual preferences and relationships.

Bisexuals are attracted to both sexes. Some have same-gender and male-female behaviors. They often marry and have children. They may seek a same-gender relationship or experience outside of marriage.

Transvestites dress and behave like the other sex for emotional and sexual relief. Commonly called *cross-dressers*, most are men. Often they marry and are heterosexual. They dress as men most of the time. They usually dress as women in private. Some dress completely as women. Others focus on bras and panties. The sex partner may not know about the practice. Some partners take part in cross-dressing activities. Some transvestites have same-gender friends with similar interests.

Transsexuals believe that they are members of the other sex. A male believes that he is a female in a man's body. A female believes that she is a male in a woman's body. They often feel "trapped" in the wrong body. Most have always had these feelings. As children they usually behave like the other sex. Many seek mental health treatment. Some have sex-change operations.

Transgender is a broad term used to describe people who express their sexuality or gender in other than the expected way. The term also is used to describe persons who are undergoing hormone therapy or surgery for sexual reassignment (female to male; male to female).

INJURY, ILLNESS, AND SURGERY

Injury, illness, and surgery can affect sexual function. Sometimes the nervous, circulatory, and reproductive systems are involved. One or more systems may be affected. Sexual ability may change. Most chronic illnesses affect sexual function. Heart disease, stroke, and chronic obstructive pulmonary disease are examples.

Reproductive system surgeries have physical and mental effects. Removal of the uterus, ovaries, or a breast affects women. Prostate or testes removal affects erections.

Impotence (erectile dysfunction; ED) is the inability of the male to have an erection. Diabetes, spinal cord injuries, and multiple sclerosis are causes. So are prostate problems and alcoholism. Heart and circulatory disorders, drugs, drug abuse, and psychological factors are other causes. Some drugs for high blood pressure cause impotence. So do other drugs. Some drugs treat impotence.

Emotional changes are common. The person may feel unclean, unwhole, unattractive, or mutilated. Attitudes may change. The person may feel unfit for closeness and love. Therefore some problems are emotional. Time and understanding are helpful. So is a caring partner. Some need counseling.

Changes in sexual function greatly impact the person. Fear, anger, worry, and depression are common. They are seen in the person's behavior and comments. The person's feelings are normal and expected. Follow the care plan. It has measures to help the person deal with his or her feelings.

BOX 46-1 **The Reproductive System: Body Structure and Function**

THE MALE REPRODUCTIVE SYSTEM

The male reproductive system is shown in Figure 46-1. The *testes (testicles)* are the male sex glands. Sex glands also are called *gonads*. The two testes are oval or almond-shaped glands. The testes are suspended between the thighs in a sac called the *scrotum*. Male sex cells are produced in the testes. Male sex cells are called *sperm* cells.

Testosterone, the male hormone, is produced in the testes. This hormone is needed for reproductive organ function. It also is needed for the development of the male secondary sex characteristics (Chapter 9).

Sperm travel from the testis to the *epididymis*. The epididymis is a coiled tube on top and to the side of the testis. From the epididymis, sperm travel through a tube called the *vas deferens*. Each vas deferens joins a seminal vesicle. The two seminal vesicles store sperm and produce *semen*. Semen is a fluid that carries sperm from the male reproductive tract. The ducts of the seminal vesicles unite to form the *ejaculatory duct*. It passes through the prostate gland.

The *prostate gland* lies just below the bladder. It is shaped like a donut. The gland secretes fluid into the semen. As the ejaculatory ducts leave the prostate, they join the *urethra*. The urethra runs through the prostate gland. The urethra is the outlet for urine and semen. The urethra is contained within the penis.

The *penis* is outside of the body and has *erectile* tissue. When a man is sexually excited, blood fills the erectile tissue. The penis enlarges and becomes hard and erect. The erect penis can enter a female's vagina. The semen, which contains sperm, is released into the vagina.

THE FEMALE REPRODUCTIVE SYSTEM

Figure 46-2 shows the female reproductive system. The female gonads are two almond-shaped glands called *ovaries*. An ovary is on each side of the uterus in the abdominal cavity.

The ovaries contain *ova* or eggs. Ova are the female sex cells. One *ovum* (egg) is released monthly during the woman's reproductive years. Release of an ovum is called *ovulation*.

The ovaries secrete the female hormones *estrogen* and *progesterone*. These hormones are needed for reproductive system function. They also are needed for the development of secondary sex characteristics in the female (Chapter 9).

When an ovum is released from an ovary, it travels through a *fallopian tube*. There are two fallopian tubes, one on each side. The tubes are attached at one end to the uterus. The ovum travels through the fallopian tube to the *uterus*.

The *uterus* is a hollow, muscular organ shaped like a pear. It is in the center of the pelvic cavity behind the bladder and in front of the rectum. The main part of the uterus is the *fundus*. The neck

or narrow section of the uterus is the *cervix*. Tissue lining the uterus is called the *endometrium*. The endometrium has many blood vessels. If sex cells from the male and female unite into one cell, that cell implants into the endometrium. There the cell grows into a baby. The uterus serves as a place for the *fetus* (unborn baby) to grow and receive nourishment.

The *cervix* of the uterus projects into a muscular canal called the *vagina*. The vagina opens to the outside of the body. It is just behind the urethra. The vagina receives the penis during intercourse. It also is part of the birth canal. Glands in the vaginal wall keep it moistened with secretions.

The external female genitalia are called the *vulva* (Fig. 46-3):
* The *mons pubis* is covered with hair in the adult female.
* The *labia majora* and *labia minora* are two folds of tissue on each side of the vaginal opening.
* The *clitoris* is a small organ composed of erectile tissue. It becomes hard when sexually stimulated.

Menstruation

The endometrium is rich in blood to nourish the cell that grows into a *fetus*. If pregnancy does not occur, the endometrium breaks up. It is discharged from the body through the vagina. This process is called *menstruation*. Menstruation occurs about every 28 days. Therefore it is called the *menstrual cycle*.

The first day of the menstrual cycle begins with menstruation. Blood flows from the uterus through the vaginal opening. Menstrual flow usually lasts 3 to 7 days. Ovulation occurs during the next phase. An ovum matures in an ovary and is released. Ovulation usually occurs on or about day 14 of the cycle.

Meanwhile, estrogen and progesterone (the female hormones) are secreted by the ovaries. These hormones cause the endometrium to thicken for pregnancy. If pregnancy does not occur, the hormones decrease in amount. This causes the blood supply to the endometrium to decrease. The endometrium breaks up. It is discharged through the vagina. Another menstrual cycle begins.

Fertilization

To reproduce, a male sex cell (sperm) must unite with a female sex cell (ovum). The uniting of the sperm and ovum into one cell is called *fertilization*. A sperm has 23 chromosomes. An ovum has 23 chromosomes. When the two cells unite, the fertilized cell has 46 chromosomes.

During intercourse, millions of sperm are deposited into the vagina. Sperm travel up the cervix, through the uterus, and into the fallopian tubes. If a sperm and an ovum unite in a fallopian tube, fertilization results. Pregnancy occurs. The fertilized cell travels down the fallopian tube to the uterus. After a short time, the fertilized cell implants in the thick endometrium and grows during pregnancy.

FIGURE 46-1 Male reproductive system.

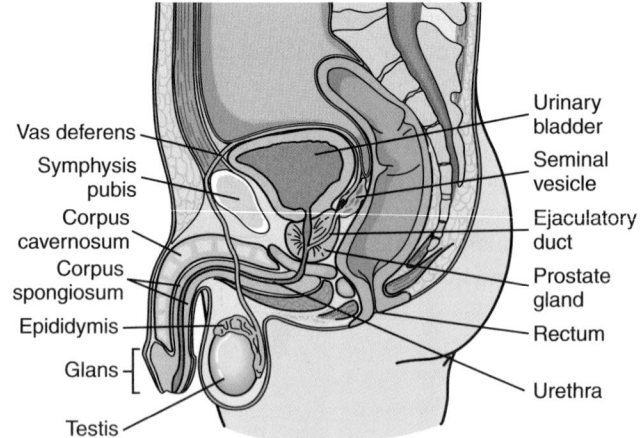

Vas deferens

Symphysis pubis

Corpus cavernosum

Corpus spongiosum

Epididymis

Glans

Testis

Urinary bladder

Seminal vesicle

Ejaculatory duct

Prostate gland

Rectum

Urethra

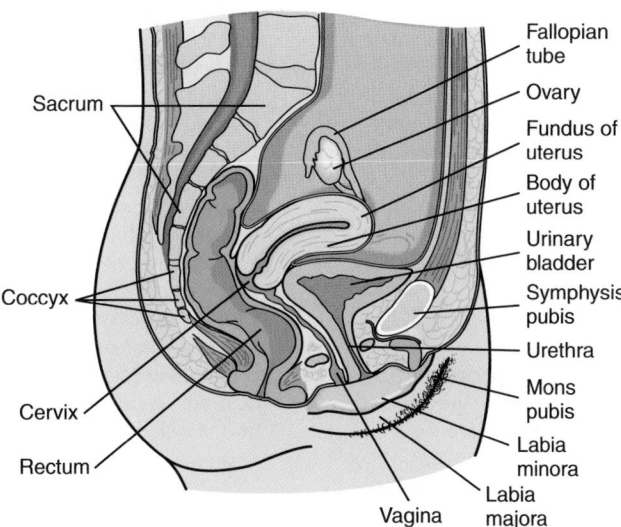

FIGURE 46-2 Female reproductive system.

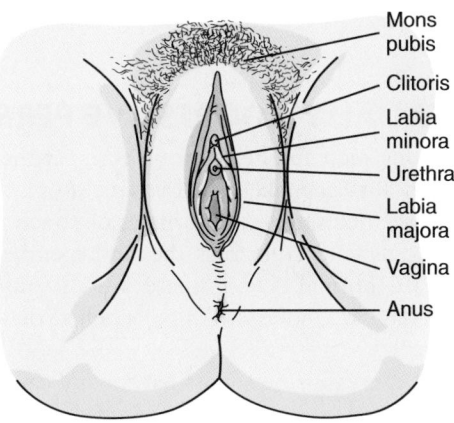

FIGURE 46-3 External female genitalia.

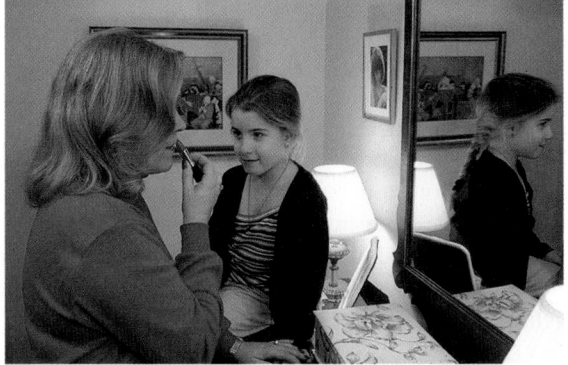

FIGURE 46-4 This little girl is learning female roles from her mother.

SEXUALITY AND OLDER PERSONS

Reproductive organs change with aging (Chapter 10). Frequency of sex decreases for many older persons. Reasons relate to weakness, fatigue, and pain. Reduced mobility, aging, and chronic illness are factors.

Some older people do not have intercourse. This does not mean loss of sexual needs or desires. Often needs are expressed in other ways. They hold hands, touch, caress, and embrace. These bring closeness and intimacy.

Sexual partners are lost through death, divorce, and relationship break-ups. Or a partner needs hospital or nursing center care. These situations occur in adults of all ages.

See *Focus on Children and Older Persons: Sexuality and Older Persons.*

MEETING SEXUAL NEEDS

The nursing team promotes the meeting of sexual needs. The measures in Box 46-2 (p. 714) may be part of the person's care plan.

See *Focus on Long-Term Care and Home Care: Meeting Sexual Needs,* p. 714.

FOCUS ON **CHILDREN AND OLDER PERSONS**
Sexuality and Older Persons

OLDER PERSONS
Love, affection, and intimacy are needed throughout life. Older persons love, fall in love, hold hands, and embrace. Many have intercourse.

Older persons have many losses. Children leave home. Family and friends die. People retire. Health problems occur. Strength decreases. Appearance changes. It helps to feel close to another person.

BOX 46-2 Promoting Sexuality

- Let the person practice grooming routines. Assist as needed. For women, this includes applying makeup, nail polish, and cologne. Many women shave their legs and underarms and pluck eyebrows. Men may use after-shave lotion and cologne. Hair care is important to men and women.
- Let the person choose clothing. Hospital gowns (patient gowns) embarrass both men and women. Street clothes are worn if the person's condition permits.
- Protect the right to privacy. Do not expose the person. Drape and screen the person.
- Accept the person's sexual relationships. The person may not share your sexual attitudes, values, or practices. The person may have a homosexual, premarital, or extramarital relationship. Do not judge or gossip about relationships.
- Allow privacy. You can usually tell when people want to be alone. If the person has a private room, close the door for privacy. Some agencies have *Do Not Disturb* signs for doors. Let the person and partner know how much time they have alone. For example, remind them about meal times, drugs, and treatments. Tell other staff members that the person wants time alone.

- Knock before you enter any room. This is a simple courtesy that shows respect for privacy.
- Consider the person's roommate. Privacy curtains provide little privacy. They do not block sound. Arrange for privacy when the roommate is out of the room. Sometimes roommates offer to leave for a while. If the roommate cannot leave, the nurse finds a private area.
- Allow privacy for masturbation. It is a normal form of sexual expression. Close the privacy curtain and the door. Knock before you enter any room. This saves you and the person embarrassment. Sometimes confused persons masturbate in public areas. Lead the person to a private area. Or distract him or her with an activity.

FOCUS ON LONG-TERM CARE AND HOME CARE

Meeting Sexual Needs

LONG-TERM CARE

Married couples in nursing centers can share the same room. This is a requirement of the Omnibus Budget Reconciliation Act of 1987 (OBRA). The couple has lived together a long time. Long-term care is no reason to keep them apart. They can share the same bed if their conditions permit. A double, queen-size, or king-size bed is provided by the couple or the center.

Single persons may develop relationships. They are allowed time together, not kept apart (Fig. 46-5).

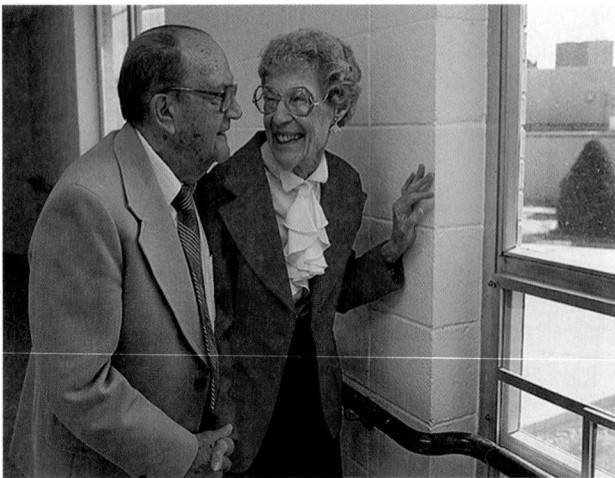

Figure 46-5 Relationships develop in nursing centers.

THE SEXUALLY AGGRESSIVE PERSON

Some persons want the health team to meet their sexual needs. They flirt or make sexual advances or comments. Some expose themselves, masturbate, or touch the staff. This can anger and embarrass the staff member. These reactions are normal. Often there are reasons for the person's behavior. Understanding this helps you deal with the matter.

Sexually aggressive behaviors have many causes. They include:
- Nervous system disorders
- Confusion, disorientation, and dementia
- Drug side effects
- Fever
- Poor vision

The person may confuse someone with his or her partner. Or the person cannot control behavior. The cause is changes in mental function. The healthy person controls sexual urges. Changes in the brain make control difficult. Sexual behavior in these cases is usually innocent.

Sometimes touch serves to gain attention. For example, Mr. Green cannot speak. He cannot move his right side. Your buttocks are near him. To get your attention, he touches your buttocks. His behavior is not sexual.

Sometimes masturbation is a sexually aggressive behavior. Some persons touch and fondle the genitals for sexual pleasure. However, urinary or reproductive system disorders can cause genital soreness or itching. So can poor hygiene and being wet or soiled from urine or feces. Touching genitals could signal a health problem.

The Sexually Aggressive Person

Confronting the sexually aggressive person is difficult. This is true for young and older staff and for new and experienced staff. Ask yourself these questions:
- Does the person have a health problem that affects impulse control? If yes, the behavior may not have a sexual purpose.
- Is the person's behavior on purpose? Is the intent sexual? If yes, you must confront the behavior. Be direct and matter-of-fact. For example, you can say:
  - "You brushed your hand across my breast (or other body part) two times this morning. Please don't do that again."
  - "No, I cannot kiss you. It would be unprofessional for me to do so."
  - "You exposed yourself to me again today. Please do not do that again."

The sexually aggressive person needs the nurse's attention. Discuss the matter with the nurse. Report what happened and when. Also report what you said and did. The nurse must deal with the problem. If other staff are reporting such behaviors, the nurse views the problem in a broader and different way.

Protecting the Person

A certified nursing assistant (CNA) had his certificate revoked by the Arizona State Board of Nursing. The Board found that he violated the state's Nurse Practice Act because of the following actions:
- He was convicted of Driving Under the Influence in April 2002.
- In September 2002, he agreed to a $150 penalty on his CNA certificate for several incidents of resident abuse. He also admitted to removing an impaction from a female resident, which he knew was not within the scope of CNA duties.
- While employed at a nursing home, the following incidents occurred from November 14 through November 23, 2005:
  - A female resident reported that he was "rough with her and hurt her groin." The resident demanded a transfer to another facility.
  - An alert and oriented resident reported that the CNA "raped her by placing his hand inside of her private parts." The resident also stated that she "could smell alcohol on his breath."
  - His employment was terminated for policy violation and "causing a resident undo stress and fear when he assisted her to expel an impaction."
- While employed in a group home, it was reported that he violated agency policy regarding alcohol use. He was employed by the group home during August–December 2005.

He can apply for re-instatement of his certificate after a 5 year period.

(Arizona State Board of Nursing, May, 18, 2006. NOTE: Names withheld by request of the Arizona State Board of Nursing.)

Sometimes the purpose of touch is sexual. For example, a man wants to prove that he is attractive and can perform sexually. You must be professional about the matter.

▶ Ask the person not to touch you. State the places where you were touched.
▶ Tell the person that you will not do what he or she wants.
▶ Tell the person what behaviors make you uncomfortable. Politely ask the person not to act that way.
▶ Allow privacy if the person is becoming aroused. Provide for safety. Complete a safety check of the room (see the inside of the front book cover). Tell the person when you will return.
▶ Discuss the matter with the nurse. The nurse can help you understand the behavior.
▶ Follow the care plan. It has measures to deal with sexually aggressive behaviors. They are based on the cause of the behavior. Many agencies have classes to help staff deal with such behavior.

See *Focus on Communication: The Sexually Aggressive Person*.

Protecting the Person

The person must be protected from unwanted sexual comments and advances. This is sexual abuse (Chapter 3). Tell the nurse right away. No one should be allowed to sexually abuse another person. This includes staff members, patients, residents, family members or other visitors, and volunteers.

See *Focus on Ethics and Laws: Protecting the Person*.

SEXUALLY TRANSMITTED DISEASES

Some diseases are spread by sexual contact. They are discussed in Chapter 42.

Circle the BEST answer.

1 Sex involves
 a The organs of reproduction
 b Attitudes and feelings
 c Cultural and spiritual factors
 d Masturbation

2 Sexuality is important to
 a Small children
 b Teenagers and young adults
 c Middle-age adults
 d Persons of all ages

3 Impotence is
 a When menstruation stops
 b A reaction to illness
 c Not being able to achieve an erection
 d No sexual activity

4 Reproductive organs change with aging.
 a True
 b False

5 Mr. and Mrs. Green live in a nursing center. Which will *not* promote their sexuality?
 a Allowing their normal grooming routines
 b Having them wear patient gowns
 c Allowing them privacy
 d Accepting their relationship

6 Two residents are holding hands. Nursing staff should keep them apart.
 a True
 b False

7 Mr. and Mrs. Green want some time alone. The nursing team can do the following *except*
 a Close the room door
 b Put a *Do Not Disturb* sign on the door
 c Tell other staff that they want some time alone
 d Close the privacy curtain so no one can hear them

8 Mr. and Mrs. Green should each have a room. This is an OBRA requirement.
 a True
 b False

9 A person is masturbating in the dining room. You should do the following *except*
 a Cover the person and quietly take the person to his or her room
 b Scold the person
 c Provide privacy
 d Tell the nurse

10 A person touches you sexually and asks for a kiss. You should do the following *except*
 a Discuss the matter with the nurse
 b Do what the person asks
 c Explain that the behaviors make you uncomfortable
 d Ask the person not to touch you

Answers to these questions are on p. 782.

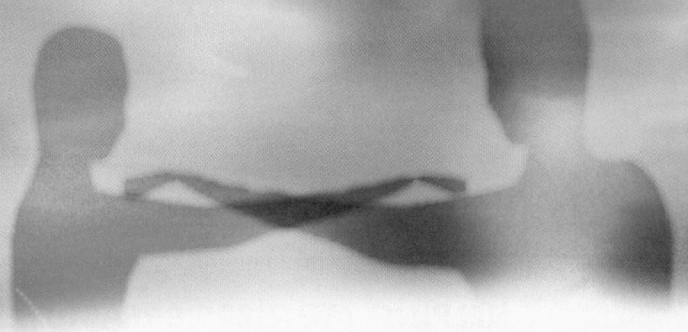

Caring For Mothers and Newborns

OBJECTIVES

- Define the key terms and key abbreviations listed in this chapter
- Describe how to meet an infant's safety and security needs
- Identify the signs and symptoms of illness in infants
- Explain how to help mothers with breast-feeding
- Describe three forms of baby formulas
- Explain how to bottle-feed babies
- Explain how to burp a baby
- Describe how to give cord care
- Describe the purposes of circumcision, needed observations, and the required care
- Explain how to bathe infants
- Explain why infants are weighed
- Describe the care needed by mothers after childbirth
- Perform the procedures described in this chapter

PROCEDURES

- Cleaning Baby Bottles
- Diapering the Baby
- Giving the Baby a Sponge Bath
- Giving the Baby a Tub Bath
- Weighing the Infant

KEY TERMS

breast-feeding Feeding a baby milk from the mother's breasts; nursing

circumcision The surgical removal of foreskin from the penis

episiotomy Incision *(otomy)* into the perineum

lochia The vaginal discharge that occurs after childbirth

meconium A dark green to black, tarry bowel movement

nursing Breast-feeding

postpartum After *(post)* childbirth *(partum)*

umbilical cord The structure that connects the mother and fetus; it carries blood, oxygen, and nutrients from the mother to the fetus

KEY ABBREVIATIONS

C Centigrade

C-section Cesarean section

F Fahrenheit

HIV Human immunodeficiency virus

mm Millimeter

Mothers and newborns usually have short hospital stays. Some need home care after discharge. Common reasons for home care include that the mother:

► Has complications before or after childbirth
► Has health problems
► Needs help with other young children in the home
► Had a multiple birth (twins, triplets, and so on)
► Needs help with meals and housekeeping

Babies are helpless. They depend on others for their basic needs. Babies have physical, safety and security, and love and belonging needs. A review of growth and development will help you care for babies (Chapter 9).

INFANT SAFETY AND SECURITY

Babies cannot protect themselves. They need to feel safe and secure. They feel secure when warm and when wrapped and held snugly. Babies cry to communicate. They cry when wet, hungry, hot or cold, tired, uncomfortable, or in pain. To promote safety and security, respond to their cries—feed them when hungry, change diapers as needed, comfort them, talk to them, and so on. See Chapter 11 for infant safety measures. Also follow the measures in Box 47-1.

Nursery equipment must be safe and in good repair. Use the guidelines in Box 47-2 (p. 720) to check nursery equipment in an agency or home setting.

Signs and Symptoms of Illness

Babies can become ill quickly. Signs and symptoms may be sudden. You must be very alert. Report any of the signs and symptoms in Box 47-3, p. 721 to the nurse at once. Be alert to any change in the baby's behavior—sleep pattern, cry, appetite, activity.

Tell the nurse when a sign or symptom began. You may need to measure the child's temperature, pulse, and respirations (Chapter 25). The nurse tells you what temperature site to use—tympanic, rectal, temporal artery, or axillary. Apical pulses are taken on infants and young children.

HELPING MOTHERS BREAST-FEED

Breast-feeding (nursing) is feeding a baby milk from the mother's breasts.

► The baby can feed at the mother's breast.
► The mother can pump milk from her breasts. The baby is fed breast-milk from a bottle.

Babies usually breast-feed 1½ to 2½ hours during the first month (8 to 12 times a day). They are fed on demand. That is, they are fed when hungry, not on a schedule. Breast milk is digested faster than formula. Therefore breast-feeding is needed more often.

Babies nurse for a short time the first few days (5 to 10 minutes at each breast). Eventually, nursing time takes 10 to 20 minutes at each breast. The rate varies for each baby. The following signal that the first breast is empty:

► The baby's sucking slows.
► The baby pulls off the breast.
► The baby is no longer interested in feeding.

Nurses help new mothers learn to breast-feed. They also teach breast care. Mothers and babies learn how to nurse in a very short time. Tell the nurse if the mother or baby is having problems breast-feeding.

Mothers may need help getting ready to breast-feed. They may need help with hand washing and positioning. Assist as needed. Make sure the signal light is within reach before you leave the room. Also provide for privacy. Follow the care plan and the measures in Box 47-4, p. 721 to help with breast-feeding.

See *Focus on Long-Term Care and Home Care: Helping Mothers Breast-Feed.*

Text continued on p. 723

BOX 47-1 Infant Safety

GENERAL SAFETY
- Follow the safety measures listed in Chapter 11.
- Keep the baby warm. Check windows for drafts. Close windows securely.
- Keep your fingernails short. Do not wear fake nails. Long nails can scratch the baby.
- Do not wear rings or bracelets. Jewelry can scratch the baby.
- Respond to the baby's crying. Babies cry when hungry, uncomfortable, wet, frightened, tired, or when they want attention. They communicate by crying. Responding to their cries helps them feel safe and secure.
- Keep one hand on the baby at all times. Do not use safety straps on changing tables. The baby can roll off the table and strangle on the straps. See Chapter 11.
- Keep pins and small objects out of the baby's reach.
- Do not shake powders directly over the baby. The powder can get into the baby's eyes and lungs. Shake some on your hand away from the baby.
- Use infant seats safely:
  - Restrain the baby in the seat.
  - Do not leave the baby unattended when the seat is on a raised surface.
- Do not tie a pacifier around the baby's neck.

HOLDING A BABY
- Use both hands to lift a newborn. Use one hand to support the head and upper back. Use your other hand to support the legs. Do not lift a newborn by the arms.
- Hold the baby securely. Use the cradle hold, football hold, or shoulder hold (Fig. 47-1).
- Support the baby's head and neck when lifting or holding the baby. Neck support is necessary for the first 3 months after birth.
- Handle the baby with gentle, smooth movements. Avoid sudden or jerking movements. Do not startle the baby.
- Hold and cuddle infants. It is comforting and helps them learn to feel love and security.

CRIB AND FURNITURE SAFETY
- Tighten all nuts, bolts, and screws on cribs, high chairs, and other infant furniture. Do this often.
- Check mattress hooks to make sure none are bent, broken, or open.
- Make sure the mattress is not covered with plastic.
- Make sure the crib is within hearing distance of the caregivers.
- Place the crib away from heat sources (radiators, registers).
- Place the crib away from other furniture.
- Do not put a pillow, quilts, or soft toys in the crib. They can cause suffocation.
- Do not lay an infant on soft bedding products. This includes fluffy, plush products such as sheepskin, quilts, comforters, pillows, and toys. These soft products can cover the baby's nose and mouth and cause suffocation.
- Do not place infants on an adult or child's bed, water bed, bunk bed, or beanbag chair or pillow. The following are risks:
  - Death from entrapment. The baby can get trapped between the bed and the wall; between the bed and another object; or between the bed frame, head board, or foot board.
  - Death from suffocation in soft bedding. This includes pillows, quilts, and comforters.
  - Death from suffocation after falling onto piles of clothing, plastic bags, pillows, cushions, or other soft materials.
- Do not place the child in a high chair until he or she can sit well with support.

SLEEP
- Remove bibs and necklaces before naps and bedtime.
- Lay babies on their backs for sleep. *Do not lay babies on their stomachs for sleep. This can interfere with chest expansion and breathing. The baby can suffocate.* Infants can lay on their sides and stomachs when awake.
- Make sure there is no soft bedding under the baby.

A   **B**   **C**

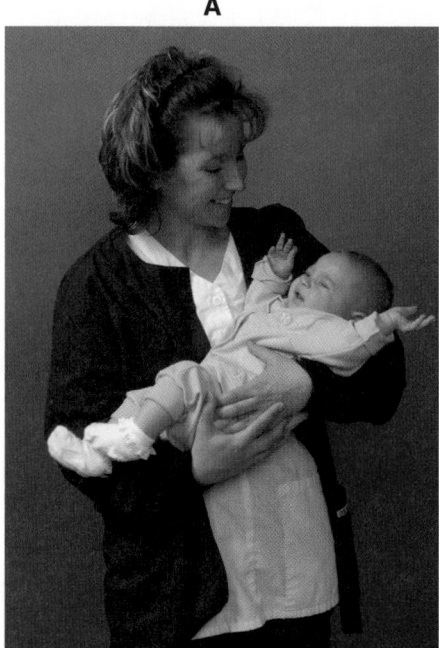 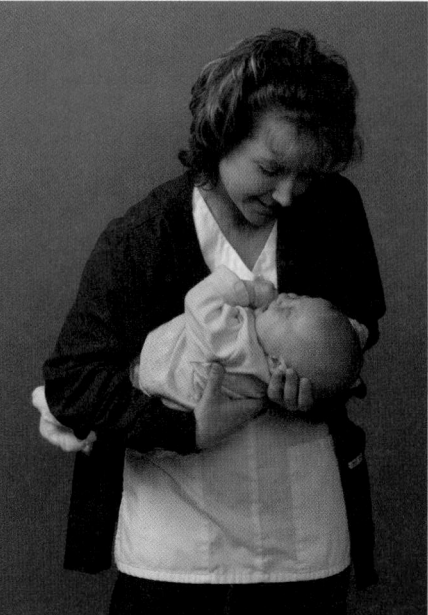 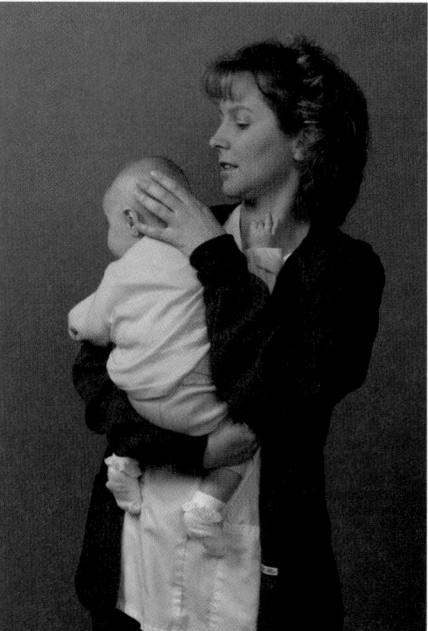

FIGURE 47-1 Holding a baby. **A,** The cradle hold. **B,** The football hold. **C,** The shoulder hold.

BOX 47-2 Safety Guide for New or Used Nursery Equipment

CRIBS

- Slats are spaced no more than 2⅜ inches (60 millimeters [mm]) apart.
- No slats are missing, loose, or cracked.
- The mattress fits snugly—less than a 2-finger width between the edge of mattress and crib side.
- The mattress support is securely attached to the head and foot boards.
- Corner posts are no higher than ¹/₁₆ inch (1.5 mm). This prevents entanglement of clothing or other objects worn by the child.
- There are no cutouts in the headboard and footboard. Cut-outs allow head entrapment.
- Drop-side latches cannot be easily released by the baby.
- Drop-side latches securely hold the side rails in the raised position.
- All screws, bolts, and other hardware are present and tight.

CRIB TOYS

- Strings or cords do not dangle into the crib.
- A crib gym or mobile has a label warning to remove the device from the crib when one of the following occurs:
  - The child can push on the hands and knees
  - The child reaches 5 months of age
- Toy parts are too large to be a choking hazard.

GATES AND ENCLOSURES

- Gate openings are too small to entrap a child's head or neck.
- The gate has a pressure bar or other fastener that will resist forces exerted by a child.

HIGH CHAIRS

- The high chair has a "crotch" strap that must be used when restraining a child in a high chair.
- The high chair has restraining straps that are independent of the tray.
- The tray locks securely.
- Buckles on straps are easy to fasten and unfasten.
- The high chair has a wide, stable base.
- Caps or plugs on tubing are firmly attached and cannot be pulled off and choke a child.
- A folding high chair has an effective locking device. The locking device keeps the chair from collapsing.

PLAYPENS

- Playpens or travel cribs have top rails that automatically lock when lifted into the normal use position.
- The playpen does not have a rotating hinge in the center of the top rails.
- A drop-side mesh playpen or mesh crib has a label about never leaving a side in the down position.
- Playpen mesh has small weave (less than ¼ inch openings).
- The mesh has no tears, holes, or loose threads.
- The mesh is securely attached to the top rail and floor-plate.
- A wooden playpen has slats spaced no more than 2⅜ inches (60 mm) apart.

RATTLES, SQUEEZE TOYS, AND TEETHERS

- Rattles, squeeze toys, and teethers have handles too large to lodge in the baby's throat.
- Squeeze toys do not contain a squeaker that could detach and choke a baby.
- Rattles do not have ball-shaped ends.

TOY CHESTS

- The toy chest has no latch to entrap the child within the chest.
- The toy chest has a spring-loaded lid support that will not require periodic adjustment. It supports the lid in any position to prevent lid slam.
- The chest has ventilation holes or spaces in the front and sides or under the lid. The ventilation holes are in case the child gets caught inside.

WALKERS

- The walker has safety features to help prevent a fall down stairs.

BACK CARRIERS

- Leg openings are small enough to prevent the child from slipping out.
- Leg openings are large enough to prevent chafing.
- The folding mechanism has frame joints.
- There is a padded covering over the metal frame near the baby's face.

BASSINETS AND CRADLES

- The item has a sturdy bottom and a wide base for stability.
- The item has smooth surfaces—no protruding staples or other hardware that could injure the baby.
- Legs have strong, effective locks to prevent folding while in use.
- The mattress is firm and fits snugly.
- Wood or metal cradles have slats spaced no more than 2⅜ inches (60 mm) apart.

CARRIER SEATS

- The item has a wide, sturdy base for stability.
- The item has non-skid feet to prevent slipping.
- Supporting devices lock securely.
- The seat has a crotch and waist strap.
- The buckle or strap is easy to use.

CHANGING TABLES

- The table has safety straps to prevent falls.
- The table has drawers or shelves that are easy to reach without leaving the baby unattended.

HOOK-ON CHAIRS

- The chair has a restraining strap.
- The chair has a clamp that locks onto the table for added security.
- Caps or plugs on tubing are firmly attached and cannot be pulled off and choke a child.
- The hook-on chair has a warning never to place the chair where the child can push off with the feet.

PACIFIERS

- The item has no ribbons, strings, cords, or yarn attached.
- The shield is large and firm enough so it cannot fit into the child's mouth.
- The guard or shield has ventilation holes. The holes allow the baby to breath if the shield does get into the mouth.
- The pacifier nipple has no holes or tears that might cause it to break off in the baby's mouth.

STROLLERS AND CARRIAGES

- There is a wide base to prevent tipping.
- The seat belt and crotch strap securely attach to the frame.
- The seat buckle is easy to use.
- Brakes securely lock the wheels.
- The shopping basket is low on the back. It is located directly over or in front of the rear wheels.
- When used in the carriage position, the leg openings can be closed.

Modified from the U.S. Consumer Product Safety Commission: *The safe nursery*, CPSC 202, Washington DC.

BOX 47-3 Signs and Symptoms of Illness in Babies

- The baby has jaundice—a yellowish color to the skin and whites of the eyes.
- The baby looks sick.
- The baby has redness or drainage around the cord stump (p. 729) or circumcision (p. 730).
- The baby has a fever (Chapter 25).
- The baby is limp and slow to respond.
- The baby is hard to wake up.
- The baby is less active than usual.
- The baby cries all the time or does not stop crying.
- The baby is flushed, pale, or perspiring.
- The baby has noisy, rapid, difficult, or slow respirations.
- The baby is coughing or sneezing.
- The baby has reddened or irritated eyes.
- The baby turns his or her head to one side or puts a hand to one ear (signs of an earache).
- The baby screams for a long time.
- The baby is feeding poorly or has skipped feedings.
- The baby has vomited most of the feeding or vomits between feedings.
- The baby has watery stools or hard, formed stools.
- Stools are light-colored, green, or foul-smelling.
- The baby has fewer wet diapers.
- The baby has a rash.

FOCUS ON LONG-TERM CARE AND HOME CARE

Helping Mothers Breast-Feed

HOME CARE

When the mother is nursing, stay within hearing distance in case she needs help.

The nursing mother needs good nutrition. When planning meals or grocery shopping, remember that:

- Calorie intake may increase. The nurse tells you what the mother's calorie intake needs to be.
- She should have 3 servings a day from the milk, yogurt, and cheese group. She can drink whole, 2 percent, or skim milk. The nurse tells you if more servings are needed.
- She needs foods high in calcium.
- She can eat the foods she likes. The baby may become fussy or gassy or have cramping or diarrhea after she eats a certain food. She should avoid that food for a while. Onions, garlic, spices, cabbage, brussel sprouts, asparagus, and beans are examples.
- Chocolate, cola beverages, coffee, and tea contain caffeine. They are used in moderation. Caffeine can cause the baby to be fussy or gassy. The baby may become agitated or have sleep problems.
- She should not drink alcohol.

BOX 47-4 Helping with Breast-Feeding

- Practice hand hygiene and Standard Precautions. Remember, HIV (human immunodeficiency virus) can be transmitted through breast milk (Chapter 38).
- Place milk, juice, or water near the mother. Most mothers become thirsty while breast-feeding.
- Help the mother wash her hands. She needs clean hands before handling her breasts.
- Help the mother to a comfortable position. The cradle position, side-lying position, and football hold are the basic positions for breast-feeding (Fig. 47-2, p. 722).
- Change the baby's diaper if necessary. Bring the baby to the mother.
- Make sure the mother holds the baby close to her breast.
- Have the mother use her nipple to stroke the baby's cheek or lower lip. This stimulates the *rooting reflex*. The baby turns his or her head toward the breast and starts to suck.
- Make sure the baby's nose is not blocked by the mother's breast. One nostril must be clear for breathing. If the nose seems blocked, have the mother do one of the following:
  - Reposition the baby. She can raise the baby's hips. Or she can move the baby's head back slightly.
  - Use her thumb to keep breast tissue away from the baby's nose (Fig. 47-3, p. 722).
- Give her a baby blanket to cover the baby and her breast. This promotes privacy.
- Encourage nursing from both breasts at each feeding. If the last feeding ended at the right breast, the next feeding is started at the right breast. The mother can use a ribbon or diaper pin on her bra strap to remind her which breast to start with.
- Remind her how to remove the baby from the breast. To break the suction between the baby and the breast, she can insert a finger into a corner of the baby's mouth (Fig. 47-4, p. 722).

- Help the mother burp the baby (p. 725). The baby is burped after nursing at one breast. Then the baby is burped after nursing at the other breast.
- Remind the mother to air dry her nipples after a feeding.
- Change the baby's diaper after the feeding.
- Lay the baby in the crib if he or she has fallen asleep. *Lay the baby on his or her back. Do not lay the baby on his or her stomach.*
- Help the mother prevent dry and cracked nipples. Follow the nurse's directions and the care plan.
  - Milk is left on the nipple after a feeding. The milk is allowed to air dry.
  - The mother applies prescribed cream after each feeding if the nipples are cracked. Remind her to wash her breasts with water before a feeding to remove the cream.
  - Soap is not used to clean the breasts and nipples.
  - Breasts and nipples are washed and dried gently.
- Help the mother straighten clothing after the feeding if necessary.
- Remind the mother to wash her breasts with a clean wash cloth and warm water. Soap is not used. It can cause the nipples to dry and crack. Nipples are air dried after washing to prevent cracking and soreness.
- Encourage the mother to wear a nursing bra day and night. The bra supports the breasts and promotes comfort.
- Encourage the mother to place nursing pads in the bra. The pads absorb leaking milk.

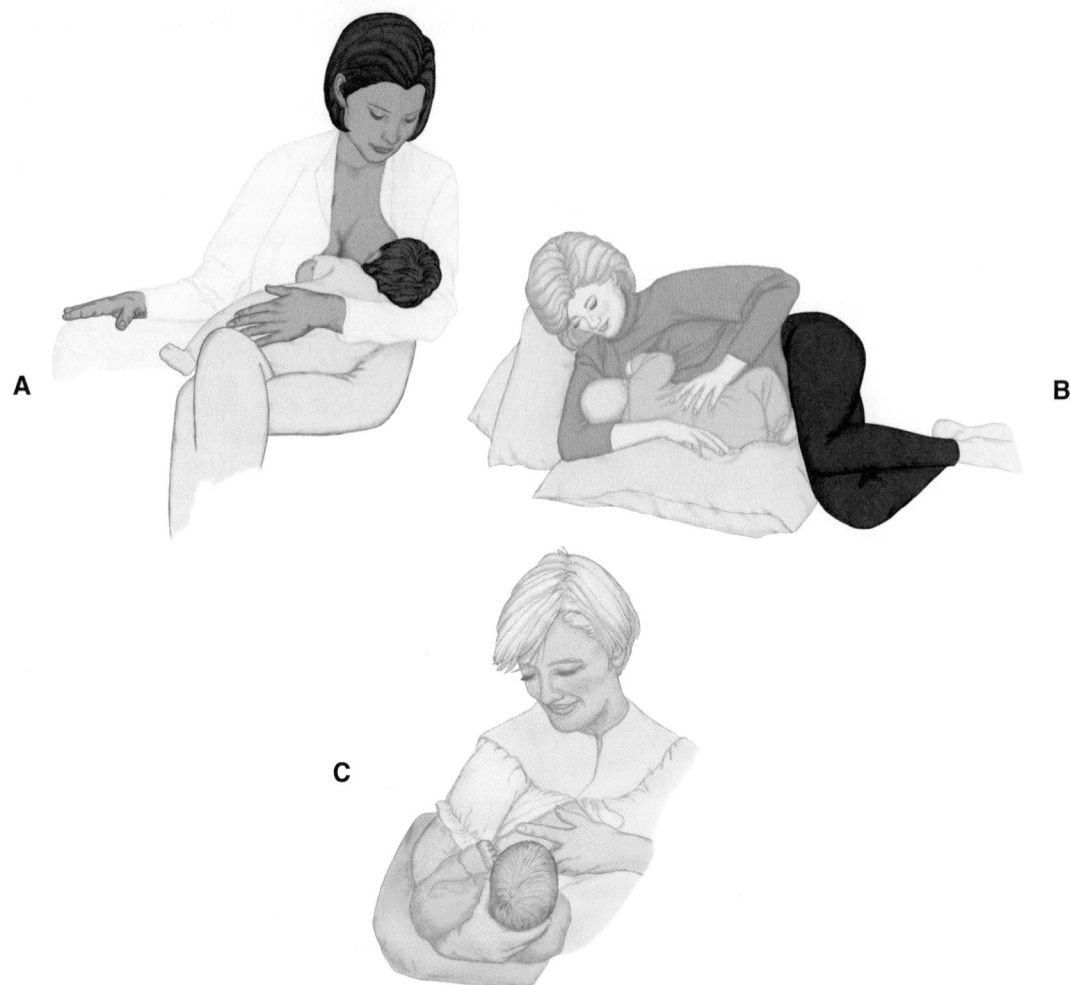

FIGURE 47-2 Basic breast-feeding positions. **A,** Cradle position. **B,** Side-lying position. **C,** Football hold. (From James SR, Ashwill JW, Droske SC: *Nursing care of children: principles and practice,* ed 2, Philadelphia, 2002, Saunders.)

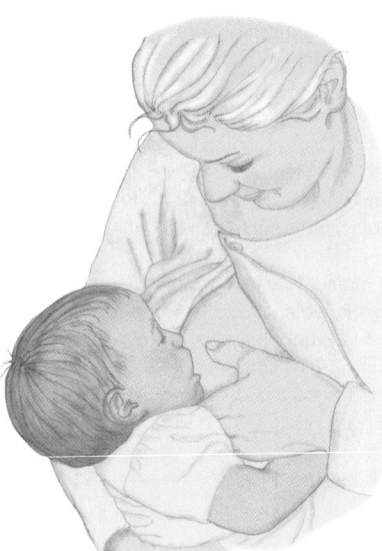

FIGURE 47-3 The mother supports her breast with one hand. The thumb is on top of the breast to keep breast tissue away from the baby's nose. (From James SR, Ashwill JW, Droske SC: *Nursing care of children: principles and practice,* ed 2, Philadelphia, 2002, Saunders.)

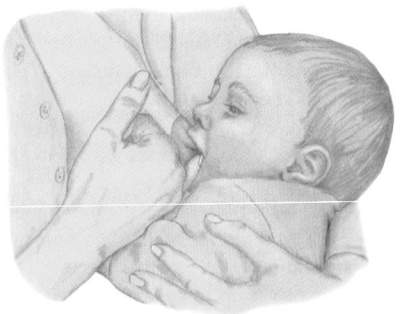

FIGURE 47-4 The mother inserts a finger into the corner of the baby's mouth to remove the baby from the breast. (From James SR, Ashwill JW, Droske SC: *Nursing care of children: principles and practice,* ed 2, Philadelphia, 2002, Saunders.)

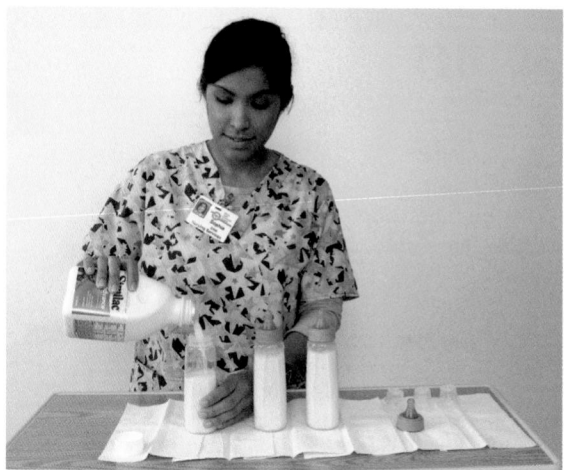

FIGURE 47-5 Ready-to-feed formula is poured from the can into the bottle. A funnel is used to prevent spilling.

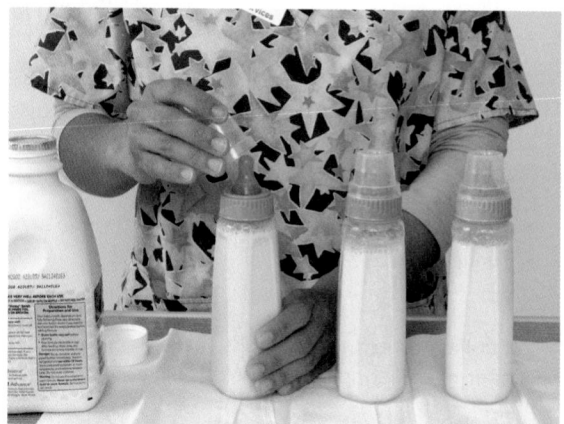

FIGURE 47-6 Bottles are capped for storage in the refrigerator.

◆ BOTTLE-FEEDING BABIES

Formula is given to babies who are not breast-fed. The doctor prescribes the formula. It provides the nutrients the infant needs.

Formula comes in three forms.

▶ *Ready-to-feed.* It is ready to use. It is poured from the can into the baby bottle (Fig. 47-5). The can may have more than 1 feeding. Refrigerate the can after opening it. Use the contents within 24 hours.

▶ *Powdered.* Container directions tell how much powder and water to use.

▶ *Liquid concentrate.* Container directions tell you how much liquid and water to use.

Bottles are prepared one at a time, or in batches for the whole day.

▶ Boil water for 1 minute or as directed by the nurse.

▶ Follow the container directions carefully. Measure exact amounts.

▶ Cap extra bottles (Fig. 47-6). Store them in the refrigerator. Use stored bottles within 24 hours.

Protect the baby from infection. Wash formula containers before opening them. Also, baby bottles, caps, nipples, and other items must be as clean as possible. Disposable equipment is used in hospitals. Reusable equipment is common in homes. It is carefully washed in hot, soapy water or in a dishwasher. Complete rinsing is needed to remove all soap. Some bottles have plastic liners that are discarded after one use.

See *Focus on Long-Term Care and Home Care: Cleaning Baby Bottles.*

See *Promoting Safety and Comfort: Cleaning Baby Bottles.*

FOCUS ON LONG-TERM CARE AND HOME CARE

Cleaning Baby Bottles

HOME CARE

Some homes have well water. The nurse may have you do one of the following:

- Place baby bottles, caps, and nipples in boiling water for 5 to 10 minutes.
- Use "terminal heating:"
  - Fill the bottles with prepared formula.
  - Cap the bottles loosely.
  - Place the filled bottles in a pan of water. The water should reach half-way up the bottles.
  - Bring the water to a gentle boil for about 25 minutes.

PROMOTING SAFETY AND COMFORT: Cleaning Baby Bottles

SAFETY

Baby bottles, caps, nipples, and other items must be thoroughly rinsed to remove all soap. Otherwise, the baby takes in soap with the feeding. This can cause serious stomach and intestinal irritation.

CLEANING BABY BOTTLES

PRE-PROCEDURE

1 See *Promoting Safety and Comfort: Cleaning Baby Bottles*, p. 723.
2 Practice hand hygiene.
3 Collect the following:
   • Bottles, nipples, and caps
   • Funnel

   • Can opener
   • Bottle brush
   • Dishwashing soap
   • Other items used to prepare formula
   • Towel

PROCEDURE

4 Wash the bottles, nipples, caps, funnel, and can opener in hot, soapy water. Wash other items used to prepare formula.
5 Clean inside baby bottles with the bottle brush (Fig. 47-7).
6 Squeeze hot, soapy water through the nipples (Fig. 47-8). This removes formula.

7 Rinse all items thoroughly in hot water. Squeeze hot water through the nipples to remove soap.
8 Lay a clean towel on the counter.
9 Stand bottles upside down to drain. Place nipples, caps, and other items on the towel. Let the items dry.

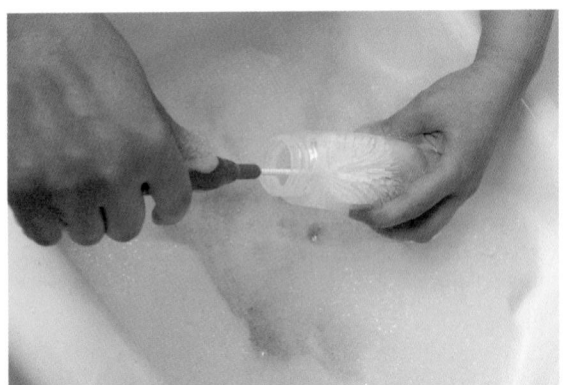

FIGURE 47-7 A bottle brush is used to clean inside a baby bottle.

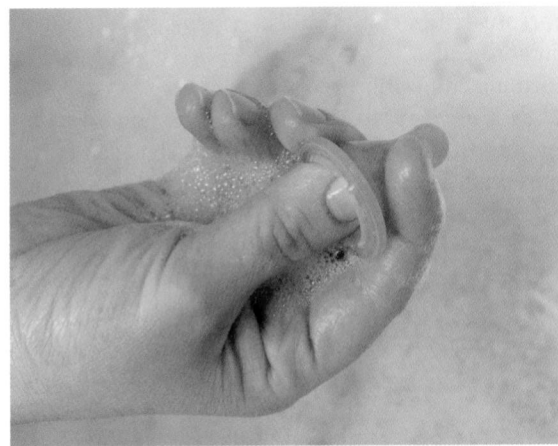

FIGURE 47-8 Water is squeezed through the nipple during washing and rinsing.

Feeding the Baby

Bottle-fed babies usually want to be fed every 2 to 4 hours. They are fed on demand. The amount of formula taken increases as they grow older. The nurse or the mother tells you how much formula a baby needs at each feeding. Babies usually take as much formula as they need. The baby stops sucking and turns away from the bottle when satisfied.

Most babies do not like cold formula out of the refrigerator. Warm a bottle before the feeding. Do one of the following:
▶ Warm it in a pan of water on the stove. Use low heat. Turn the bottle often.
▶ Hold the bottle under warm running tap water.

The formula should feel warm. To test the temperature, sprinkle a few drops on the inside of your wrist (Fig. 47-9). The guidelines in Box 47-5 will help you bottle-feed babies.

See *Promoting Safety and Comfort: Feeding the Baby.*

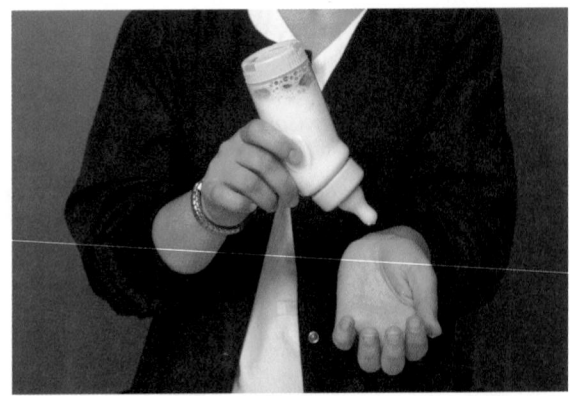

FIGURE 47-9 Formula should feel warm on the inside of your wrist.

BOX 47-5 Bottle-Feeding Babies

- Warm a refrigerated bottle. The formula should feel warm to the inside of your wrist.
- Assume a comfortable position for the feeding.
- Hold the baby close to you. Relax and snuggle the baby.
- Stroke the baby's cheek or lip with the nipple. The baby's head will turn to the nipple.
- Tilt the bottle so that the neck of the bottle and the nipple are always full (Fig. 47-10). Otherwise some air is in the neck or nipple. The baby sucks air into the stomach. The air causes cramping and discomfort.
- Do not prop the bottle and lay the baby down for the feeding (Fig. 47-11).
- Burp the baby after every 2 to 3 ounces of formula. Also burp the baby at the end of the feeding.
- Do not leave the baby alone with a bottle.
- Do not force the baby to finish the bottle.
- Discard remaining formula. Do not save or reheat it for another feeding.
- Wash the bottle, cap, and nipple after the feeding (see procedure: *Cleaning Baby Bottles*.

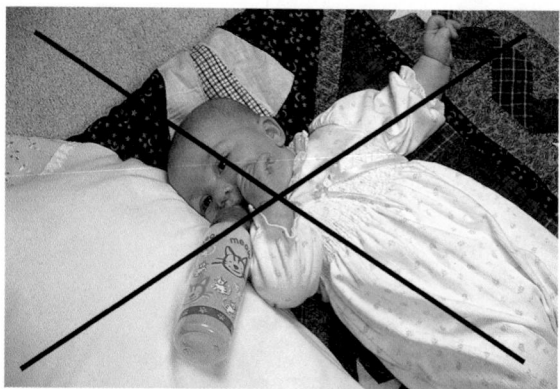

FIGURE 47-11 Do **NOT** prop the bottle to feed the baby.

PROMOTING SAFETY AND COMFORT: Feeding the Baby

SAFETY

Do not set the bottle out to warm at room temperature. This takes too long and allows the growth of microbes. Do not heat formula in microwave ovens. The formula can heat unevenly and burn the baby's mouth.

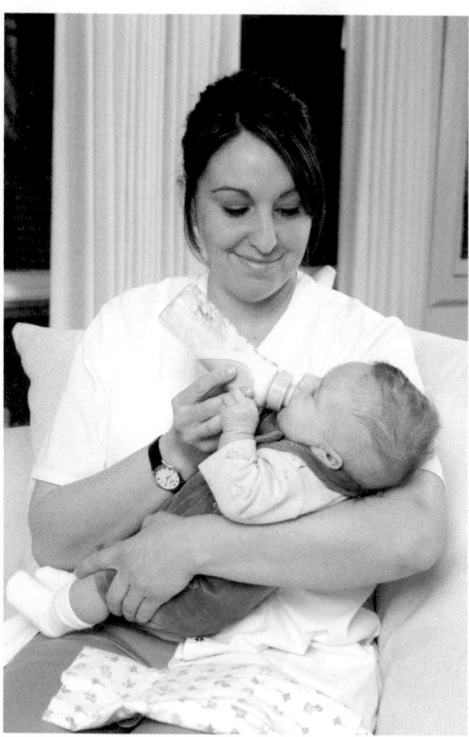

FIGURE 47-10 The bottle is tilted so that formula fills the bottle neck and nipple.

BURPING THE BABY

Babies take in air during feedings. Air in the stomach and intestines causes cramping and discomfort. This can lead to vomiting. Burping helps to get rid of the air. Most babies burp mid-way and after a feeding.

Burping a baby also is called *bubbling*. You pat or rub the baby's back with circular motions. Do this for 2 or 3 minutes. Figure 47-12 (p. 726) shows how to position the baby for burping.

▶ *Over the shoulder.* First place a clean diaper or towel over your shoulder. This protects your clothing if the baby "spits up." Then hold the infant over your shoulder.

▶ *On your lap.* Support the baby in a sitting position on your lap. Hold the towel or diaper in front of the baby. *Remember to support the infant's head and neck for the first 3 months after birth.*

▶ *On the baby's stomach.* First place a clean diaper or towel on your lap where the baby's head will be. Position the baby on your lap with his or her stomach down.

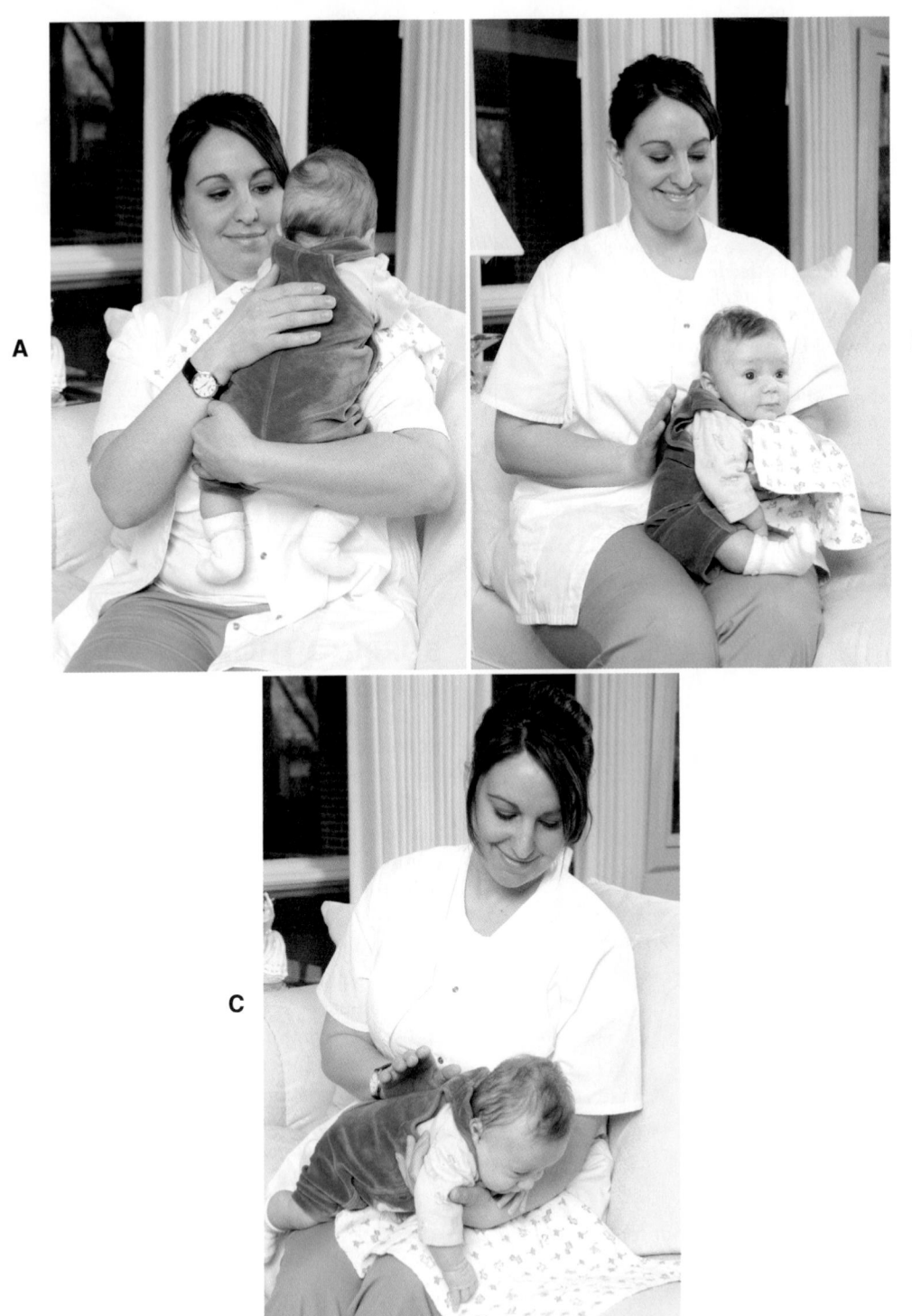

FIGURE 47-12 Burping a baby. **A,** The baby is held over the shoulder. **B,** The baby is supported in the sitting position. **C,** The baby is laid on the stomach.

◆ DIAPERING

In the first 1 or 2 days after birth, newborns have meconium stools. **Meconium** is a dark green to black, tarry bowel movement. By day 3, stools are greenish brown to yellowish brown in color and less sticky. By day 4, the baby has milk stools:

▶ *Breast-fed babies.* Stools are yellow and seedy-looking. They are soft or runny. Breast-fed babies usually have a bowel movement with every feeding.

▶ *Bottle-fed babies.* Stools are yellow to brown. Bottle-fed babies have fewer stools than breast-fed babies, and their stools are firmer. They may have 1 or 2 stools a day.

Over time, an elimination pattern develops. Some babies have 1, 2, or 3 stools a day. Stools are usually soft and unformed. Hard, formed stools signal constipation. Watery stools mean diarrhea. Diarrhea is very serious in infants. Their fluid balance is upset quickly (Chapter 23). Tell the nurse at once if you suspect constipation or diarrhea.

Babies wet at least 6 to 8 times a day. Diapers are changed when wet or when stools are present.

Cloth diapers are re-used. With Velcro fasteners, no diaper pins are needed. The danger of sticking the baby or yourself with a diaper pin is avoided. To care for cloth diapers:

▶ Rinse a soiled cloth diaper in the toilet.
▶ Store soiled diapers in a diaper pail.
▶ Wash them daily or every 2 days.
▶ Do not wash them with other laundry items.
▶ Wash them in hot water. Use a baby laundry detergent.
▶ Put them through the wash cycle a second time without detergent. This helps remove all soap.
▶ Hang them outside to dry if possible. This gives them a fresh, clean smell. Otherwise, dry them in the dryer.

Disposable diapers are secured with Velcro or tape strips. Fold soiled diapers so the soiled area is on the inside. Then discard the diaper in the trash container. Do not flush it down the toilet. Using disposable diapers costs more than using cloth ones.

Changing diapers often helps prevent diaper rash. Moisture, stools, and urine irritate the baby's skin. When changing diapers, make sure the baby is clean and dry before applying a clean diaper. If a diaper rash develops, tell the nurse at once. The nurse tells you what to do.

See *Delegation Guidelines: Diapering a Baby.*
See *Promoting Safety and Comfort: Diapering a Baby.*

DELEGATION GUIDELINES: Diapering a Baby

Before changing a baby's diaper, you need this information from the nurse and the care plan:

- The size and type of diaper to use (cloth or disposable)
- If you need to give cord care (p. 729) or circumcision care (p. 730)
- What lotion or cream to use
- What observations to report and record:
  - Color, amount, consistency, and odor of stools
  - Condition of the baby's skin and genital area
  - Redness or irritation of the skin or genital area
  - Blood or discharge on the diaper
- When to report observations
- What specific concerns about the baby to report at once

PROMOTING SAFETY AND COMFORT: Diapering a Baby

SAFETY

Disposable diapers present safety hazards to babies. Babies can choke on the tab papers that cover the tape strips. Keep the tab papers away from the baby. Discard them as soon as possible.

Older babies can tear and pull disposable diapers apart. They can choke or suffocate on the plastic if they put the plastic in their noses or mouths. Observe babies closely. Change any torn or damaged diaper at once.

You must keep the baby safe during diapering. The baby may squirm, wiggle, or kick and cry. To prevent falls:

- Gather all needed supplies before you begin.
- Place the baby on a firm surface. If the baby is on a table, make sure it is sturdy.
- Always keep one hand on a baby who is on a table or other raised surface.
- Never look away from the baby.

If using diaper pins for cloth diapers, the pins must point away from the abdomen. If a pin opens, a pin pointing toward the abdomen can pierce the skin and damage organs.

DIAPERING THE BABY

✔ Quality of Life *Remember to:*

- Knock before entering the baby's room.
- Address the baby and parents by name.
- Introduce yourself by name and title.
- Explain the procedure to the parents before beginning and during the procedure.
- Protect the baby's rights during the procedure.
- Handle the baby gently during the procedure.

Continued

DIAPERING THE BABY—cont'd

PRE-PROCEDURE

1 Follow *Delegation Guidelines: Diapering a Baby*, p. 727. See *Promoting Safety and Comfort: Diapering a Baby*, p. 727.
2 Practice hand hygiene.
3 Collect the following:
   • Gloves
   • Clean diaper

   • Waterproof changing pad
   • Washcloth
   • Disposable wipes or cotton balls
   • Basin of warm water
   • Baby soap
   • Baby lotion or cream

PROCEDURE

4 Put on the gloves.
5 Place the changing pad under the baby.
6 Unfasten the dirty diaper. Place diaper pins out of the baby's reach.
7 Wipe the genital area with the front of the diaper (Fig. 47-13). Wipe from the front to the back.
8 Fold the diaper so urine and feces are inside. Set the diaper aside.
9 Clean the genital area from front to back. Use a wet washcloth, disposable wipes, or cotton balls. Wash with mild soap and water for a large amount of feces or if the baby has a rash. Rinse thoroughly and pat the area dry.
10 Clean the circumcision (p. 730). Give cord care.
11 Apply cream or lotion to the genital area and buttocks. Do not use too much. Caking can occur.
12 Raise the baby's legs. Slide a clean diaper under the buttocks.

13 Fold a cloth diaper as follows:
   a For a boy: the extra thickness is in the front (Fig. 47-14, A).
   b For a girl: the extra thickness is at the back (Fig. 47-14, B).
   c Bring the diaper between the baby's legs.
14 Make sure the diaper is snug around the hips and abdomen.
   a It is loose near the penis if the circumcision has not healed.
   b It is below the umbilicus if the cord stump has not healed.
15 Secure the diaper in place. Use the tape strips or Velcro on disposable diapers (Fig. 47-15, A). Make sure the tabs stick in place. Use baby pins or Velcro for cloth diapers. Pins point away from the abdomen (Fig. 47-15, B).
16 Apply a diaper cover or plastic pants if cloth diapers are worn.
17 Put the baby in the crib, infant seat, or other safe location.

POST-PROCEDURE

18 Rinse feces from the cloth diaper in the toilet.
19 Store used cloth diapers in a covered pail. Put a disposable diaper and paper tabs in the trash.
20 Remove the gloves. Practice hand hygiene.

21 Put on clean gloves.
22 Clean and return other items to their proper location.
23 Remove the gloves. Practice hand hygiene.
24 Report and record your observations.

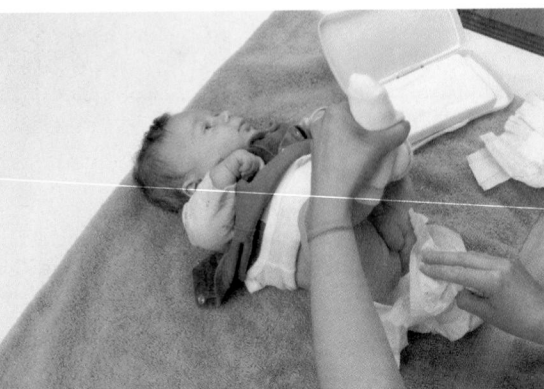 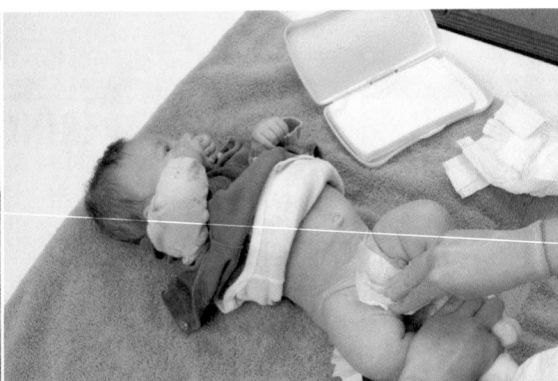

FIGURE 47-13 The front of the diaper is used to clean the genital area.

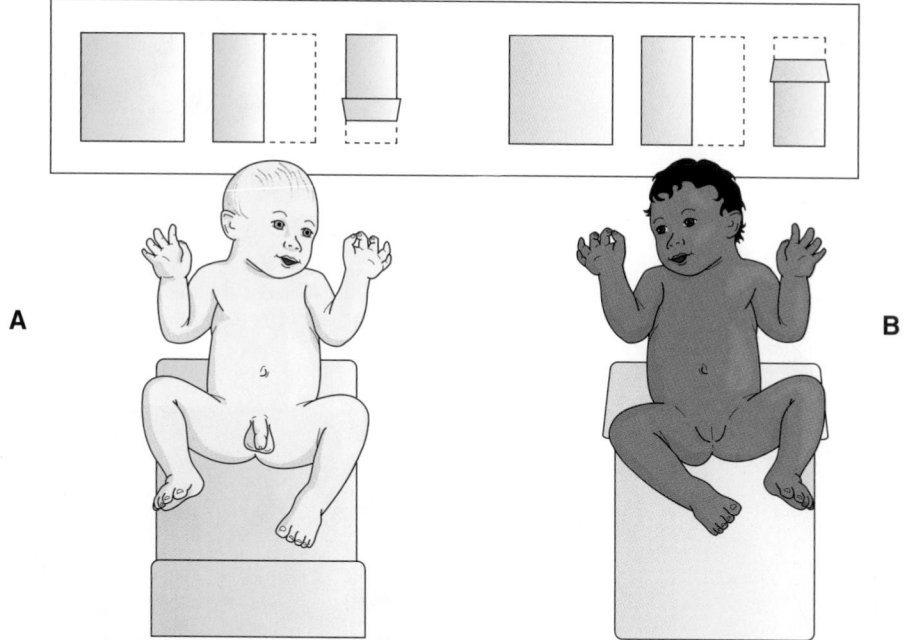

FIGURE 47-14 A, A cloth diaper is folded in front for boys. **B,** The diaper has a fold in the back for girls.

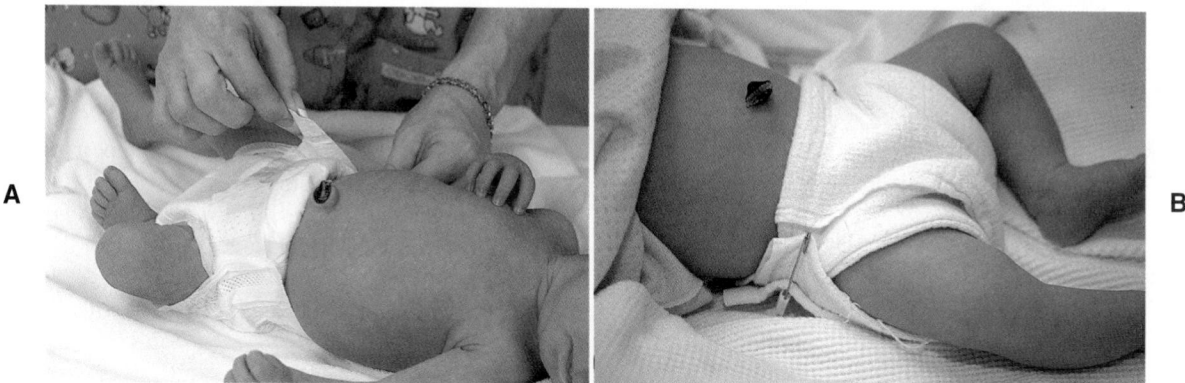

FIGURE 47-15 Securing a diaper. **A,** A disposable diaper is secured in place with tape strips. **B,** Diaper pins secure a cloth diaper. Pins point away from the abdomen. *NOTE:* The diapers in **A** and **B** are below the cord.

CARE OF THE UMBILICAL CORD

The **umbilical cord** connects the mother and the fetus (unborn baby). It carries blood, oxygen, and nutrients from the mother to the fetus (Fig. 47-16, p. 730). The cord is not needed after birth. Shortly after delivery, the doctor clamps and cuts the cord. A cord stump is left on the baby (see Fig. 47-15). The stump dries up and falls off about 2 weeks after birth. Slight bleeding can occur when the cord comes off.

The cord provides a place for microbes to grow. You need to keep it clean and dry. Cord care is done at each diaper change. Cord care is continued for 1 or 2 days after the cord comes off. It involves the following:

▶ Keep the stump clean and dry. Do not get the stump wet.

▶ Keep the diaper below the cord as in Figure 47-15. This prevents the diaper from irritating the stump. It also keeps the cord from becoming wet from urine.

▶ Give sponge baths until the cord falls off. Then the baby can have a tub bath.

▶ Do not pull the cord off—even if looks ready to fall off.

▶ Report the following to the nurse:
   ▶ Swelling, redness, odor, or drainage from the stump
   ▶ Bleeding from the cord or navel area
   ▶ Fever

See *Promoting Safety and Comfort: Care of the Umbilical Cord* (p. 730).

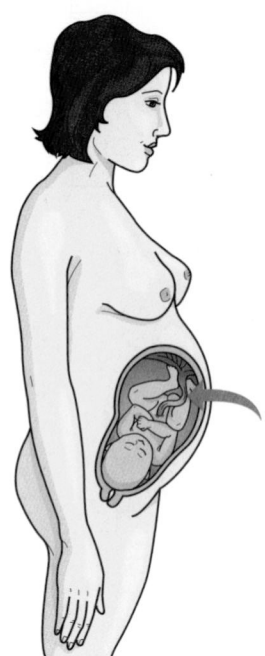

FIGURE 47-16 The umbilical cord connects the mother and fetus.

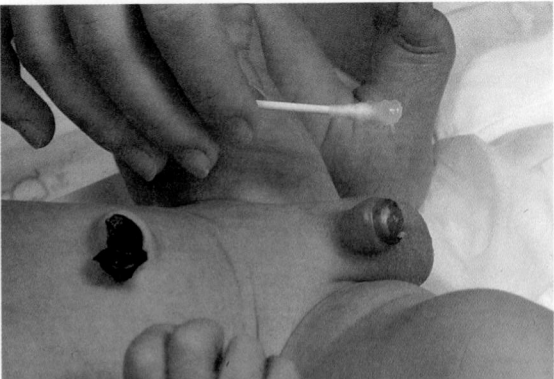

FIGURE 47-17 Petrolatum jelly is applied to the circumcised penis.

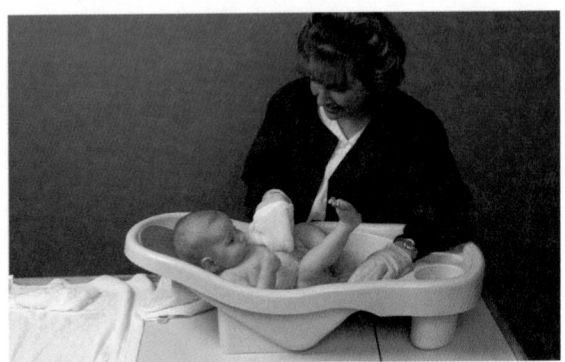

FIGURE 47-18 The baby is given a tub bath in a baby bath tub.

PROMOTING SAFETY AND COMFORT: Care of the Umbilical Cord

SAFETY

A common cord care practice involved wiping the base of the stump with alcohol at every diaper change. The alcohol promoted drying. It is now thought that the stump heals faster if left to air dry. When giving cord care, follow the nurse's directions. The nurse may have you wash the stump with soap and water if it is dirty or sticky. If so, dry it thoroughly after washing.

CARE OF THE CIRCUMCISION

Boys are born with foreskin on the penis. The surgical removal of foreskin from the penis is called a **circumcision** (Chapter 21). The procedure allows good hygiene. It is thought to:

▶ Prevent urinary tract infections in infants
▶ Lower the risk of cancer of the penis
▶ Decrease the risk of sexually transmitted diseases

The procedure is usually done before the baby leaves the hospital. Circumcision is a religious ceremony in the Jewish faith.

The penis will look red, swollen, and sore. However, the circumcision should not interfere with voiding. Carefully observe for signs of bleeding and infection. There should be no swelling, odor, or drainage. Also check the diaper for bleeding. Report any concerns to the nurse at once. The area should heal in 7 to 10 days.

Circumcision care involves the following:

▶ Clean the penis at each diaper change. This is very important after a bowel movement.

▶ Use mild soap and water, plain water, or commercial wipes as the nurse directs.
▶ Apply a petrolatum gauze dressing or petrolatum jelly to the penis as the nurse directs. This protects the penis from urine and feces. It also prevents the penis from sticking to the diaper. Use a cotton swab to apply the petrolatum jelly (Fig. 47-17).
▶ Apply the diaper loosely. This prevents the diaper from irritating the penis.

◆ BATHING AN INFANT

A bath is important for hygiene. Though babies do not get very dirty, they need good skin care. Baths comfort and relax babies. They also provide a wonderful time to hold, touch, and talk to babies. Stimulation is important for development. Being touched and held helps babies learn safety, security, and love and belonging.

Planning for the bath is important. You cannot leave the baby alone if you forget something. Gather needed equipment, supplies, and the baby's clothes before you start the bath. Everything you need must be within your reach.

There are two bath procedures for babies. Sponge baths are given until the cord stump falls off and the umbilicus and circumcision heal. *Keep the stump dry.* The tub bath is given after the cord site and circumcision heal (Fig. 47-18). A baby bath tub is used.

See *Focus on Long-Term Care and Home Care: Bathing an Infant.*

See *Delegation Guidelines: Bathing an Infant.*

See *Promoting Safety and Comfort: Bathing an Infant.*

Bathing an Infant

HOME CARE

Bath time is part of the baby's daily routine. Some mothers bathe their babies in the morning. Others do so in the evening. Evening baths have important advantages.

- The bath is comforting and relaxing. This helps some babies sleep longer at night.
- Working fathers are usually home in the evening. The evening bath lets them be involved.

Sometimes fathers bathe babies so mothers can rest or tend to other children. Follow the family's routine when working in the home.

DELEGATION GUIDELINES: Bathing an Infant

Before bathing an infant, you need this information from the nurse and the care plan:

- How often to bathe the baby. Babies do not need baths everyday.
- What type of bath to give—sponge bath or tub bath.
- What water temperature to use—usually 100° to 105° F (Fahrenheit) (37.7° to 40.5° C [centigrade]).
- When to bathe the infant.
- If you should use baby soap or plain water. Usually soap is not used unless the baby is dirty or smells.
- If you should apply lotion after the bath.
- What observations to report and record:
  - Bruising
  - Rashes
  - Skin irritation
  - Redness
  - Swelling
  - Open skin areas
  - See "Care of the Umbilical Cord," p. 729
  - See "Care of the Circumcision," p. 730
- When to report observations.
- What specific concerns about the baby to report at once.

PROMOTING SAFETY AND COMFORT: Bathing an Infant

SAFETY

To protect an infant during a bath, follow these safety measures.

- Turn up the thermostat and close windows and doors about 20 minutes before the bath. Room temperature should be 75° to 80° F for the bath. The room may be too warm for you. Remove a sweater or lab coat or roll up your sleeves before starting the bath.
- Measure bath water temperature with a bath thermometer. The nurse tells you what temperature to use (usually 100° to 105° F [37.7° to 40.5° C]). Or test water temperature with the inside of your wrist (Fig. 47-19). The water should feel warm and comfortable to your wrist. Babies have delicate skin and are easily burned.
- Never leave the baby alone on a table or in the bath tub.
- Always keep one hand on the baby if you must look away for a moment.
- Hold the baby securely during the bath. Babies are very slippery when they are wet. A wet, squirming baby is hard to hold.

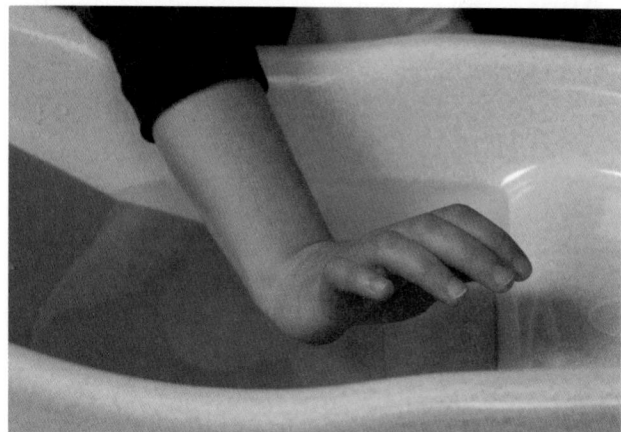

FIGURE 47-19 The inside of the wrist is used to test bath water temperature.

GIVING THE BABY A SPONGE BATH

✔ **Quality of Life** *Remember to:*

- Knock before entering the baby's room.
- Address the baby and parents by name.
- Introduce yourself by name and title.
- Explain the procedure to the parents before beginning and during the procedure.

- Protect the baby's rights during the procedure.
- Handle the baby gently during the procedure.

PRE-PROCEDURE

1 Follow *Delegation Guidelines: Bathing an Infant.* See *Promoting Safety and Comfort: Bathing an Infant.*
2 Practice hand hygiene.
3 Place the following items in your work area:
   - Bath basin
   - Bath thermometer
   - Bath towel
   - Two hand towels
   - Receiving blanket

- Washcloth
- Clean diaper
- Clean clothing for the baby
- Cotton balls
- Baby soap (if needed)
- Baby shampoo
- Baby lotion
- Gloves

Continued

GIVING THE BABY A SPONGE BATH—cont'd

PROCEDURE

4 Fill the bath basin with warm water. Water temperature should be 100° to 105° F (37.7° to 40.5° C). Measure water temperature with the bath thermometer or use the inside of your wrist. The water should feel warm and comfortable on your wrist.

5 Provide for privacy.

6 Identify the baby following agency policy.

7 Put on gloves.

8 Undress the baby. Leave the diaper on.

9 Wash the baby's eye lids (Fig. 47-20):
   a Dip a cotton ball into the water.
   b Squeeze out excess water.
   c Wash one eye lid from the inner part to the outer part.
   d Repeat this step for the other eye with a new cotton ball.

10 Moisten the washcloth and make a mitt (Chapter 19). Clean the outside of the ear and then behind the ear. Repeat this step for the other ear. Be gentle.

11 Rinse and squeeze out the washcloth. Make a mitt with the washcloth.

12 Wash the baby's face (Fig. 47-21). Clean inside the nostrils with the washcloth. *Do not use cotton swabs to clean inside the nose.* Pat the face dry.

13 Pick up the baby. Hold the baby over the bath basin using the football hold. Support the baby's head and neck with your wrist and hand.

14 Wash the baby's head (Fig. 47-22):
   a Squeeze a small amount of water from the washcloth onto the baby's head.
   b Apply a small amount of baby shampoo to the head.
   c Wash the head with circular motions.
   d Rinse the head by squeezing water from a washcloth over the baby's head. Rinse thoroughly. Do not get soap in the baby's eyes.
   e Use a small hand towel to dry the head.

15 Lay the baby on the table.

16 Remove the diaper.

17 Wash the front of the body. Also wash the arms, hands, and fingers, and the legs, feet, and toes. Use a washcloth. Or wash the baby with your hands. Do not get the cord wet. Rinse thoroughly. Pat dry. Be sure to wash and dry all creases and folds.

18 Turn the baby to the prone position. Wash the back and buttocks. Use a washcloth or your hands.

19 Give cord care. Clean the circumcision.

20 Apply baby lotion as directed by the nurse.

21 Remove the gloves. Decontaminate your hands.

22 Put a clean diaper and clean clothes on the baby.

23 Wrap the baby in the receiving blanket. Put the baby in the crib or other safe area.

POST-PROCEDURE

24 Decontaminate your hands. Put on gloves.

25 Clean and return equipment and supplies to the proper place. Do this step when the baby is settled.

26 Remove the gloves. Practice hand hygiene.

27 Complete a safety check of the room. (See the inside of the front book cover.)

28 Report and record your observations.

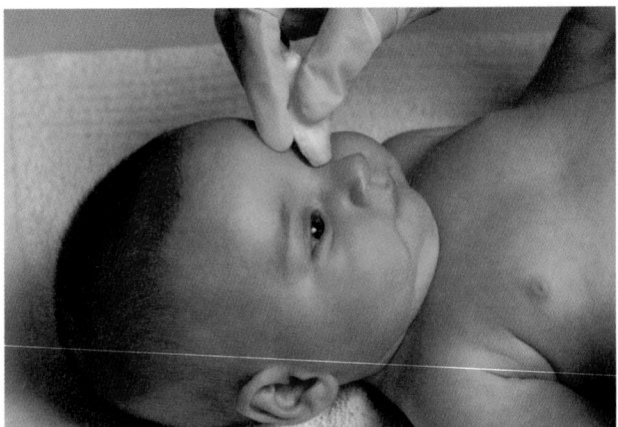

FIGURE 47-20 Wash the baby's eyes with cotton balls. The eye lids are cleaned from the inner to the outer part.

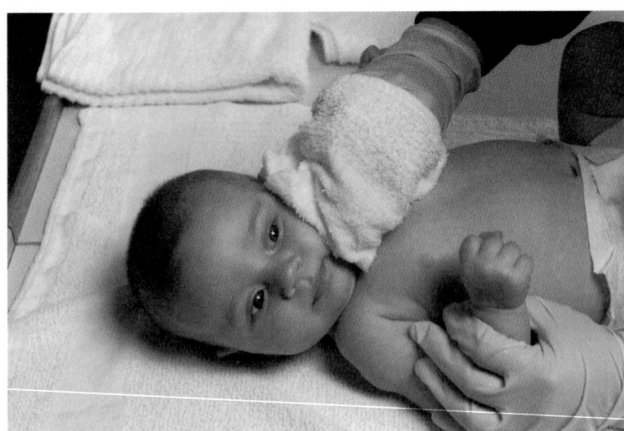

FIGURE 47-21 The baby's face is washed with a mitted washcloth.

GIVING THE BABY A TUB BATH

✔**Quality of Life** *Remember to:*

- Knock before entering the baby's room.
- Address the baby and parents by name.
- Introduce yourself by name and title.
- Explain the procedure to the parents before beginning and during the procedure.

- Protect the baby's rights during the procedure.
- Handle the baby gently during the procedure.

PROCEDURE

1 Follow steps 1 through 16 in procedure: *Giving the Baby a Sponge Bath* (p. 731). Use a baby bath tub.
2 Hold the baby as in Figure 47-23:
   a Place one hand under the baby's shoulders. Your thumb should be over the baby's shoulder. Your fingers should be under the arm.
   b Support the buttocks with your other hand. Slide your hand under the thighs. Hold the far thigh with your other hand.
3 Lower the baby into the water feet first.
4 Wash the front of the baby's body. Also wash the arms, hands, and fingers, and the legs, feet, and toes. Wash all folds and creases.

5 Wash the genital area. Rinse thoroughly.
6 Reverse your hold. Use your other hand to hold the baby.
7 Wash the baby's back and buttocks. Rinse thoroughly.
8 Reverse your hold again. Hold the baby with your other hand.
9 Lift the baby out of the water and onto a towel.
10 Wrap the baby in the towel. Also cover the baby's head.
11 Pat the baby dry. Dry all folds and creases.
12 Follow steps 20-28 in procedure: *Giving the Baby a Sponge Bath* (p. 732).

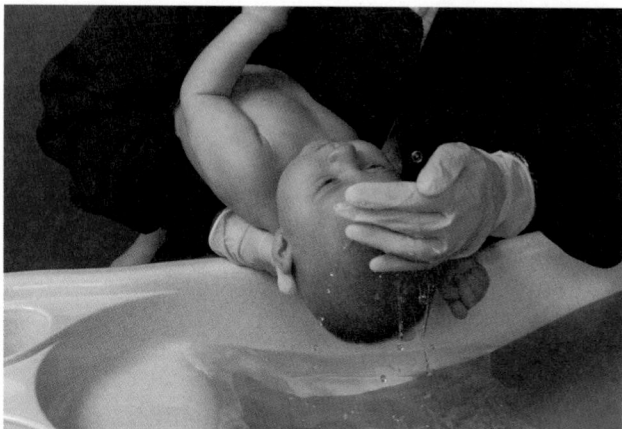
FIGURE 47-22 The baby's head is washed over the bath basin.

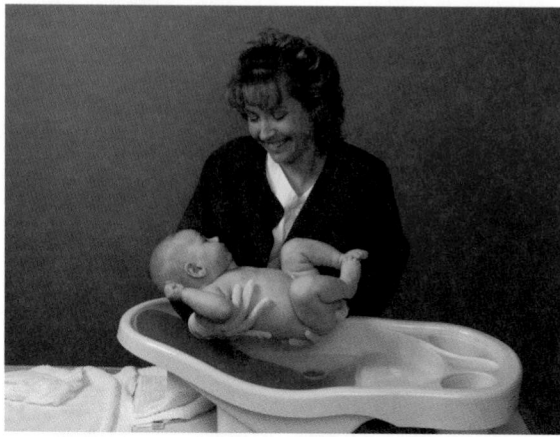
FIGURE 47-23 The baby is held for the tub bath.

NAIL CARE

The baby's fingernails and toenails are kept short. Otherwise, the baby can scratch himself or herself and others. Nails are best cut when the baby is sleeping. The baby is quiet and will not squirm or fuss. Use infant nail clippers and a soft emery board.

▶ Hold the finger or toe with one hand.
▶ Press the skin under the nail. This moves the skin out of the way to avoid pinching or cutting the skin.
▶ Trim the nails with an infant nail clipper:
   ▶ Fingernails: clip following the natural shape of the nail.
   ▶ Toenails: clip straight across as for an adult (Chapter 20).
▶ Smooth rough or sharp edges with a soft emery board.

◆ WEIGHING INFANTS

The infant's birth weight is the baseline for measuring growth. The nurse uses weight measurements in the assessment step of the nursing process. They also are used to measure the amount of breast milk taken during breast-feeding. The baby is weighed before and after breast-feeding. The difference in the weights is the amount of milk taken in during breast-feeding. It tells the nurse if the baby is getting enough milk.

See *Delegation Guidelines: Weighing Infants.*
See *Promoting Safety and Comfort: Weighing Infants.*

Before weighing an infant, you need this information from the nurse and the care plan:
- When to weigh the baby
- If the baby is breast-fed or bottle-fed—breast-fed babies wear the same diaper, clothes, and blanket for each weight measurement (before and after the feeding)
- When to report the weight measurement
- What specific concerns about the baby to report at once

SAFETY

You must meet the baby's safety needs. Protect the baby from chills. Keep the room warm and free of drafts. Also protect the baby from falling. Always keep a hand over the baby when taking the weight measurement. Remember to keep one hand on the baby if you need to look away.

WEIGHING THE INFANT

✔ Quality of Life *Remember to:*

- Knock before entering the baby's room.
- Address the baby and parents by name.
- Introduce yourself by name and title.
- Explain the procedure to the parents before beginning and during the procedure.

- Protect the baby's rights during the procedure.
- Handle the baby gently during the procedure.

PRE-PROCEDURE

1 Follow *Delegation Guidelines: Weighing Infants.* See *Promoting Safety and Comfort: Weighing Infants.*
2 Practice hand hygiene.

3 Collect the following:
- Baby scale (Fig. 47-24)
- Paper for the scale
- Items for diaper changing (see procedure: *Diapering the Baby*, p. 727)
- Gloves

PROCEDURE

4 Identify the baby following agency policy.
5 Place the paper on the scale. Adjust the scale to zero (0).
6 Put on the gloves.
7 Undress the baby and remove the diaper. Clean the genital area.
8 Lay the baby on the scale. Keep one hand over the baby to prevent falling.

9 Read the digital display or move the pointer until the scale is balanced.
10 Note the measurement.
11 Remove the gloves, and decontaminate your hands. Put on clean gloves.
12 Diaper and dress the baby. Lay the baby in the crib.
13 Discard the soiled diaper.
14 Remove and discard the gloves. Practice hand hygiene.

POST-PROCEDURE

15 Return the scale to its proper place.
16 Decontaminate your hands.
17 Report and record your observations.

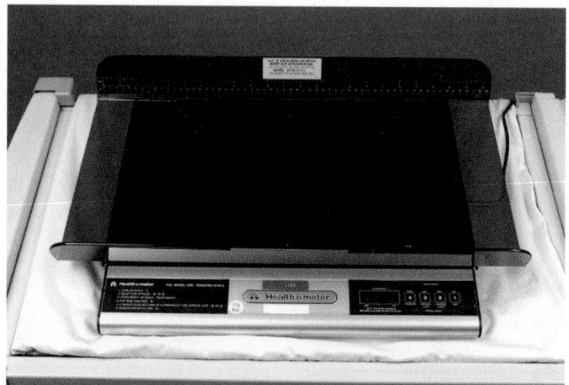

FIGURE 47-24 Digital infant scale.

CARE OF THE MOTHER

Postpartum means after (*post*) childbirth (*partum*). The postpartum period starts with birth of the baby. It ends 6 weeks later. The mother's body returns to its normal state during this time. The mother adjusts physically and emotionally to childbirth.

The uterus returns almost to its pre-pregnant size. This is called *involution of the uterus*. If the mother does not breast-feed, she can expect a menstrual period within 3 to 8 weeks. Breast-feeding is not an effective method of birth control. Without birth control measures, the mother can get pregnant again.

A vaginal discharge occurs after childbirth. It is called **lochia**. (Lochia comes from the Greek word *lochos*. It means *childbirth*.) Lochia consists of blood and other matter left in the uterus from childbirth. The lochia changes color and decreases in amount during the postpartum period.

▶ *Lochia rubra*—is dark or bright red (*rubra*) discharge. Mainly blood, it is seen during the first 3 to 4 days.

▶ *Lochia serosa*—is pinkish brown (*serosa*) drainage. It lasts until about 10 days after birth.

▶ *Lochia alba*—is whitish (*alba*) drainage. It continues for 2 to 6 weeks after birth.

Lochia increases with breast-feeding and activity. When she stands after lying or sitting, the mother may feel a gush of lochia. She wears a sanitary napkin to absorb the lochia. Normally, lochia smells like menstrual flow. Foul-smelling lochia signals an infection.

Good perineal care is important. Sanitary pads are changed often. When wiping after elimination, the mother wipes from front to back. Sanitary napkins are applied and removed from front to back. Good hand washing is essential after perineal care, changing sanitary napkins, and elimination. Standard Precautions and the Bloodborne Pathogen Standard are followed.

Some mothers have episiotomies. An **episiotomy** is an incision (*otomy*) into the perineum. (*Episeion* means *pubic region*.) The doctor performs this procedure during childbirth. It increases the size of the vaginal opening for the baby. The incision is sutured after delivery. The doctor may order sitz baths for comfort and hygiene (Chapter 33). Like other incisions, complications can develop. These include infection and wound separation (*dehiscence*). Tell the nurse at once if the mother complains of pain, discomfort, or a discharge.

Some mothers deliver by *cesarean section (C-section)*. The doctor makes an incision into the abdominal wall. The baby is delivered through the incision. This is done when:

▶ The baby must be delivered to save the baby's or mother's life.

▶ The baby is too large to pass through the birth canal.

▶ The mother has a vaginal infection that could be transmitted to the baby.

▶ A normal vaginal delivery will be difficult for the baby or mother.

The C-section incision needs to heal. See Chapter 32 for wound healing and wound care.

The mother has emotional reactions after childbirth. Hormone changes, lifestyle changes, and lack of sleep can cause mood swings. So can frequent visits and telephone calls from family and friends. Some interfere or offer advice and opinions about parenting. The mother can help herself by resting when the baby sleeps. She needs time for herself and her partner. She may feel better after pampering herself with a shower, washing and styling her hair, and getting dressed. These can be done while the baby sleeps.

Complications can occur during pregnancy, labor, and delivery. They also can occur in the postpartum period. Report any sign or symptom listed in Box 47-6 to the nurse at once.

BOX 47-6 Signs and Symptoms of Postpartum Complications

- Temperature of 100.4° F or greater
- Pain: abdominal or perineal
- Discharge:
  - Foul smelling from the vagina
  - From an episiotomy
  - From a C-section incision
- Bleeding: from an episiotomy or C-section incision
- Redness, swelling: episiotomy or C-section incision
- Saturating a sanitary napkin within 1 hour of application
- Lochia:
  - Red lochia after lochia has changed color to pinkish-brown or white
  - Lochia with large clots
- Urination: burning
- Leg pain, tenderness, or swelling
- Sadness or feelings of depression
- Breast pain, tenderness, or swelling

Circle the best answer.

1 A baby's head and neck are supported for the first
   a 7 to 10 days
   b Month
   c 3 months
   d 6 months

2 When holding a newborn you should do the following *except*
   a Hold the infant securely
   b Cuddle the infant
   c Sing and talk to the infant
   d Hold the infant on his or her stomach

3 You observe the following. Which is considered normal?
   a The baby looks flushed and is perspiring.
   b The baby has watery stools.
   c The baby's eyes are red and irritated.
   d The baby spits up a small amount when burped.

4 A baby is breast-fed. The mother should do the following *except*
   a Wash her hands
   b Hold the baby close to her breast
   c Stimulate the rooting reflex
   d Clean her breasts with soap and water

5 A breast-fed baby is burped
   a Every 5 minutes
   b After nursing from one breast
   c After nursing from both breasts
   d After half the formula is taken

6 A baby is bottle-fed. You do the shopping. Which formula should you buy?
   a The one that is on sale
   b The ready-to-feed type
   c The one ordered by the doctor
   d The powdered form

7 You are to warm a baby bottle. Which is *true?*
   a The bottle is warmed in the microwave.
   b The formula is left out to warm at room temperature.
   c The formula should feel warm on the inside of your wrist.
   d The formula is warmed in a pan for 5 minutes.

8 When bottle-feeding a baby, you should
   a Burp the baby every 5 minutes
   b Save remaining formula for the next feeding
   c Tilt the bottle so that formula fills the neck of the bottle and the nipple
   d Leave the baby alone with the bottle

9 A newborn's cord has not yet healed. The diaper should be
   a Loose over the cord
   b Snug over the cord
   c Below the cord
   d Disposable

10 A circumcision is cleaned
   a Once a day
   b When the baby has a bowel movement
   c Three times a day
   d At every diaper change

11 Bath water for a newborn should be
   a 85° to 90° F
   b 90° to 95° F
   c 95° to 100° F
   d 100° to 105° F

12 Which should you use to wash a baby's nose?
   a A mitted washcloth
   b Alcohol wipes
   c A cotton swab
   d Cotton balls

13 A mother has a red vaginal discharge the first few days after childbirth. This
   a Is a menstrual period
   b Signals a postpartum complication
   c Is lochia rubra
   d Is from her episiotomy

14 A cesarean delivery involves
   a A vaginal incision
   b A perineal incision
   c An abdominal incision
   d A normal delivery through the birth canal

Circle T if the statement is true and F if it is false.

15 **T F** A baby's crib should be within hearing distance of caregivers.

16 **T F** A baby needs a pillow for sleep.

17 **T F** A baby is placed on his or her back for sleep.

18 **T F** Crib rails are up at all times when the baby is in the crib.

19 **T F** A baby's diapers are changed whenever they are wet.

20 **T F** A baby's cord and circumcision have not healed. The baby should have a sponge bath.

21 **T F** Cotton swabs are used to clean a baby's ears.

22 **T F** A baby is being breast-fed. The baby is weighed with the diaper on.

Answers to these questions are on p. 782.

Assisted Living

OBJECTIVES

- Define the key terms and key abbreviations listed in this chapter
- Identify the purpose of assisted living
- Identify the person's rights
- Identify the types of assisted living residences and the living areas offered
- Describe the physical and environmental requirements for assisted living
- Describe the requirements for assisted living staff
- Describe the requirements for persons who want to live in an assisted living residence

- Explain the purpose of a service plan
- Explain how to assist with housekeeping and laundry
- Identify food safety measures
- Explain how to assist with drugs
- Identify the reasons for transferring, discharging, or evicting a person
- Explain how to promote quality of life

KEY TERMS

assisted living residence Provides housing, personal care, support services, health care, and social activities in a home-like setting

medication reminder Reminding the person to take drugs, observing them being taken as prescribed, and charting that they were taken

service plan A written plan listing the services needed by the person and who provides them

KEY ABBREVIATIONS

AARP American Association of Retired Persons
AD Alzheimer's disease
ADL Activities of daily living
ALF Assisted living facility
ALR Assisted living residence

M

any older people do not need nursing center care. However, they cannot or do not want to live alone. Some need help with self-care. Some have physical or cognitive problems and disabilities. Still others need help taking drugs.

Assisted living offers quality of life with independence and companionship. An **assisted living residence (ALR)** provides housing, personal care, support services, health care, and social activities in a home-like setting. Some needs are scheduled, such as taking drugs at certain times. Others are unscheduled—elimination, transfers, getting a snack, or taking a walk.

ALRs also are called *assisted living facilities (ALFs)* or *assisted living homes*. Many other names are used.

Like nursing centers, ALRs must follow state laws. State laws vary. Common requirements are described in this chapter.

See *Promoting Safety and Comfort: Assisted Living*.

PURPOSE

People are living longer, and there are more older people than before. Men and women lose life partners through death. Divorce rates are high. Some remarry; others do not. Some persons have never married. Today's older persons had some birth control options. Many had small families. And the United States is a mobile society. Children grow-up and move away from their families. For these reasons, many older persons live alone and without family in the area. Often there is no one nearby to help them.

According to the American Association of Retired Persons (AARP), most assisted living residents need help with two or more activities of daily living (ADL). They commonly need help with taking drugs, bathing, dressing, elimination, transferring, and eating. At least half of them are cognitively impaired.

Some ALRs are part of nursing centers or retirement communities. Others are separate facilities. State laws for ALRs must be followed. Resident's rights are part of such laws (Box 48-1, p. 740). So are licensing requirements.

Living Areas

Living areas vary. A small apartment has a bedroom, bathroom, living area, kitchen, and laundry area (Figs. 48-1 and 48-2, p. 740). Some people just want a bedroom and bathroom. Others share a bedroom and a bathroom with a roommate. Box 48-2 (p. 741) lists the requirements and features of assisted living units. Box 48-3 (p. 741) lists environmental requirements.

Alzheimer's Care Units

Some residents have Alzheimer's disease (AD) or other dementias (Chapter 44). State requirements must be met. They relate to care, the setting, staffing, activities, safety, and the family's role in meeting the person's needs.

Persons with AD have poor judgment. They cannot

follow directions. And they tend to wander. A safe setting is needed. They need supervision and help leaving the building in an emergency.

The person needs a comfortable routine and schedule. Activities provide stimulation and promote the person's highest level of function. The activities must be things the person once enjoyed doing and can still do to a limited and safe extent.

Staff must have training about AD and other dementias. Many states require on-going or annual training.

STAFF REQUIREMENTS

Staff requirements vary from state to state. Some require that the staff complete a nursing assistant training and competency evaluation program. Others require training in the following areas:

▶ The needs and goals of ALR residents
▶ Promoting dignity, independence, and resident rights
▶ Using service plans
▶ Ethics, privacy, and confidentiality of records and information
▶ Hygiene and infection control
▶ Nutrition and menu planning
▶ Food preparation, service, and storage
▶ Housekeeping and sanitation
▶ Preventing and reporting abuse and neglect
▶ Incident reports
▶ Fire, emergency, and disaster plans
▶ Assisting with drugs
▶ Early signs of illness and the need for health care
▶ Safety measures
▶ Communication skills
▶ Special needs of persons with AD and other dementias
▶ Cardiopulmonary resuscitation and first aid (Chapter 49)

Criminal background and fingerprint checks are common staff requirements. The ALR cannot employ a person with a criminal record.

RESIDENT REQUIREMENTS

Assisted living is for persons needing some help with ADL. They do not need 24-hour nursing care. And they are not bedridden. Some persons are paralyzed or chronically ill.

BOX 48-1 Assisted Living Resident's Rights

Persons who live in an assisted living facility keep the rights they have had all their lives. They also gain special rights under state laws and regulations.

The basic rights for residents are outlined below. If a person cannot exercise these rights, family members, legal representatives, or consumer advocates (ombudsmen) can act on the resident's behalf to protect and promote these basic rights.

FAIRNESS AND DIGNITY
- Visit the facility before signing a contract.
- Review a copy of the admission agreement.
- Receive written information about all services and their costs, and the policies and procedures governing the facility.
- Be free from discrimination because of age, race, religion, physical or mental disability, gender, sexual orientation, financial status, nationality, or family status.
- Be treated with courtesy, respect, and dignity.
- Be informed and given a copy of the resident's personal rights in a language that is understandable.
- Be given information on how residents and others can file complaints.

Safety
- Live in a safe and clean setting.
- Keep and use personal belongings without loss or theft.
- Be free from punishment, humiliation, intimidation, isolation, or retaliation.
- Have personal belongings stored safely.

FREEDOM
- Be free from physical, emotional, and verbal abuse and neglect.
- Be free from restraining devices.
- Take part in religious, social, community, and other activities.
- Leave the facility and return without unreasonable restriction.
- Be free from unjustified room transfers or discharge (eviction) from the facility.

SELF-DETERMINATION
- Choose one's doctor, pharmacist, and other health care providers.
- Be given all information about one's condition, care, and needs.
- Make one's wishes known about personal care and medical treatment. Have advance directives, such as powers of attorney for health care.
- Take part in the development of one's own plan for care and services.
- Refuse treatment or services.
- Express preferences with respect to room, roommates, food, and activities.
- Use personal belongings and furnishings as space permits.
- Manage and control personal finances, or be given a written record of all transactions.
- Voice grievances to the facility staff, family, licensing agency, the ombudsman program, or any other person without fear of reprisal or retaliation.
- File complaints and have them properly addressed and resolved.
- Organize and take part in a resident council and recommend changes and improvements in the facility's policies and services.
- Receive help in exercising the right to vote.
- Move from the facility.

PRIVACY
- Have personal privacy, including visits, phone calls, and unopened mail.
- Have reasonable access to phones in making or receiving confidential calls.
- Communicate privately and freely with any person.
- Have the guarantee of privacy during bathing, medical treatment, and personal care.
- Have the ALR maintain confidential records.

The most pertinent laws are found in the California Health and Safety Code. The most relevant regulations are in the California Code of Regulations.

Modified from the California Advocates for Nursing Home Reform, RCFS/Assisted living fact sheets: resident's rights CANRH 2001.0203, San Francisco.

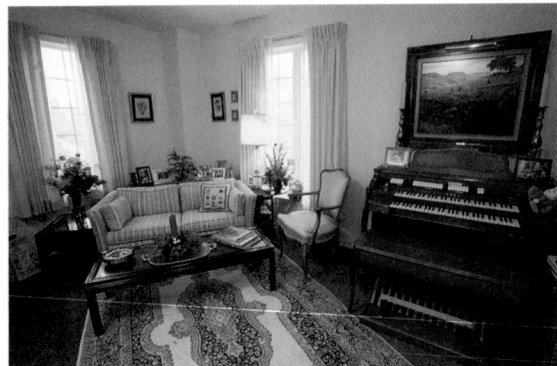

FIGURE 48-1 A living area in an assisted living apartment.

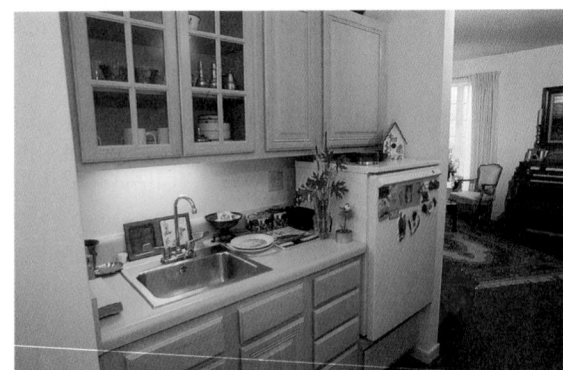

FIGURE 48-2 A kitchen in an assisted living apartment.

BOX 48-2 Requirements and Features of Assisted Living Units

- A door that locks; the person keeps a key
- A telephone jack
- A 24-hour emergency communication system in the person's room
- A window or door that provides natural light
- Wheelchair access
- Lighted common areas
- A window or door that allows safe exit in an emergency
- A mailbox for each person
- A bathroom that provides privacy:
  - A sink in the bathroom or in the next room (sink is not used for food preparation)
  - A bathtub or shower that has a shower curtain and non-slip surfaces
  - Ventilation or a window that opens
  - Grab bars for the toilet and bathtub or shower
  - Other assistive devices needed for safety and identified in the service plan
- Smoke detectors
- A bed (frame and mattress) that is clean and in good repair
- Adequate general and task lighting
- An easy chair
- A table and chair for meals
- Adjustable window covers that provide privacy
- A dresser or storage space for clothing and personal items
- Appliances for food—sink, stove, refrigerator with freezer, and storage for food and cooking items

BOX 48-3 Environmental Requirements

- The ALR is clean, safe, orderly, odor-free, and in good repair.
- The ALR is free of insects and rodents.
- Garbage is stored in covered containers lined with plastic bags. Bags are removed from the ALR at least once a week.
- Hot water temperatures are between 95° F and 120° F in areas used by residents.
- The hot and cold water supply meets hygiene needs.
- Common bathrooms have toilet paper, soap, and cloth towels, paper towels, or a dryer.
- Clean linens are handled, transported, and stored to prevent contamination.
- Soiled linen and clothing are stored in closed containers away from food, kitchen, and dining areas.
- Oxygen containers are stored according to the manufacturer's instructions.
- Cleaning solutions, insecticides, and other hazardous substances are stored in their original containers. They are in locked cabinets in rooms separate from food, dining areas, and drugs.
- Pets or animals are controlled to protect residents and maintain sanitation.
- Employees have access to a first aid kit.

However, they do not need help with complex medical problems. If nursing services are needed, home health care is arranged.

Mobility is often a requirement. The person walks or is mobile with a wheelchair or motor scooter. The person must be able to leave the building in an emergency. Stable health is another requirement. Only limited health care or treatment is needed.

Assisted living is not for people who have greater care needs or require skilled nursing services.

Service Plan

A **service plan** is a written plan listing the services needed by the person and who provides them. It also addresses how much help is needed. The plan relates to ADL, activities and social services, dietary needs, taking drugs, and special needs. Health services are included.

For example, a person needs help getting dressed. The service plan states that you will assist the person. The service plan also states that a nurse will replace the person's catheter. The person needs physical therapy after a hip fracture. The service plan states a physical therapist will visit. And the person needs help taking drugs. A family member will assist the person.

The plan is reviewed every 6 months and when the person's condition, wants, or service needs change. Services are added or reduced as the person's needs change.

SERVICES

ALRs usually offer these services:

- 3 meals a day
- Help with ADL—bathing, dressing, grooming, toileting, eating, walking
- Housekeeping
- Linen and personal laundry
- A 24-hour emergency communication system to use for an emergency or to call for help
- 24-hour security
- 24-hour supervision
- Transportation
- Social, educational, recreational, and religious services
- Help with shopping, banking, and money management
- Some health services
- Exercise and wellness programs
- Medication (drug) management or help taking drugs

Meals

Three meals a day and snacks are provided. The time between the evening meal and breakfast usually is no more than 14 hours. It can be longer if there is a nutritious evening snack. Special dietary needs are met. Menus are posted for residents to review.

Residents are encouraged to eat in the dining room with other persons. They can eat in their rooms if they want to. Special eating utensils are provided as needed. So is help with eating, opening cartons, buttering bread, cutting meat, and so on (Chapter 23).

Housekeeping

The following housekeeping measures help prevent infection. They also keep living units neat and clean.

▶ Dust furniture at least weekly.
▶ Vacuum floors at least weekly and as needed.
▶ Wipe up spills right away.
▶ Use a dust mop or broom to sweep. Use a dustpan to collect dust and crumbs.
▶ Sweep daily or more often as needed.
▶ Make sure toilets are flushed after each use.
▶ Rinse the sink after washing, shaving, or oral hygiene.
▶ Clean the tub or shower after each use.
▶ Remove and dispose of hair from the sink, tub, or shower.
▶ Hang towels to dry. Or place them in a hamper.
▶ Clean bathroom surfaces every day. Use a disinfectant or water and detergent to clean all surfaces. They include:
  ▶ The toilet bowl, seat, and outside areas of the toilet
  ▶ The floor
  ▶ The sides, walls, and curtain or door of the tub or shower
  ▶ Towel racks and toilet tissue, toothbrush, and soap holders
  ▶ The sink and mirror
  ▶ Windowsills
▶ Mop or vacuum the bathroom floor every day.
▶ Empty bathroom wastebaskets every day.
▶ Put out clean towels and washcloths every day.
▶ Wash bath mats, the wastebasket, and laundry hamper every week.
▶ Replace toilet and facial tissue as needed.
▶ Open bathroom windows for a short time. Also use air fresheners.

Food Safety

Certain measures are needed when handling, preparing, and storing food. They protect against infection. See Chapter 23. Also practice these measures:

▶ Handle meat and poultry safely. Follow the safe handling instructions on food labels (Fig. 48-3).
▶ Protect left-over foods. Place left-over food in small containers. Cover containers with lids, foil, or plastic wrap. Date and refrigerate containers as soon as possible.
▶ Use left-over food within 2 or 3 days.
▶ Wash eating and cooking items. Use liquid detergent and hot water. Wash glasses and cups first. Follow with silverware, plates, bowls, and then pots and pans. Rinse items well with hot water.
▶ Place washed eating and cooking items in a drainer to dry. Air-drying is more aseptic than towel drying.
▶ Rinse dishes before loading them into a dishwasher. Use dishwasher soap.

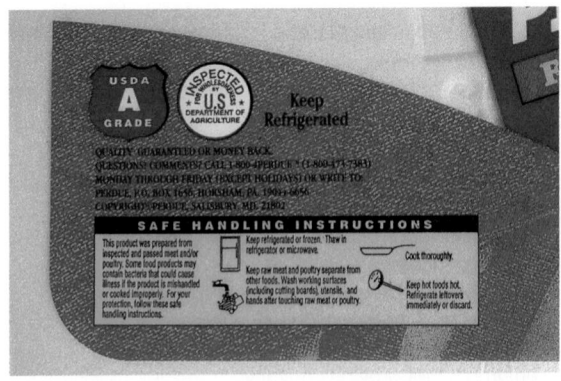

FIGURE 48-3 Safe handling instructions for meat and poultry. They are required by the U.S. Department of Agriculture.

▶ Do not wash pots and pans and cast iron, wood, and some plastic items in a dishwasher.
▶ Clean kitchen appliances, counters, tables, and other surfaces after each meal. Use hot, soapy water and paper towels or clean cloths.
▶ Remove grease spills and splashes. Use a liquid surface cleaner.
▶ Clean sinks with a sink cleaner.
▶ Dispose of garbage, left-overs, and other soiled supplies after each meal. A garbage disposal is best for food and liquid garbage. Do not put bones in the garbage disposal.
▶ Recycle paper, boxes, cans, and plastic containers according to the ALR policy.
▶ Empty garbage at least once a day.

Laundry

Laundry services include providing clean linens. Residents can use a washing machine, dryer, iron, and ironing board for personal laundry. When assisting with laundry, follow these guidelines:

▶ Wear gloves when handling soiled laundry (see *Promoting Safety and Comfort: Assisted Living*, p. 739).
▶ Follow the person's preferences.
▶ Follow care label directions.
▶ Sort items by color and fabric. Separate white, colored, and dark items. Separate sturdy and delicate fabrics.
▶ Empty pockets.
▶ Fasten buttons, zippers, snaps, hooks, and other closures.
▶ Wash heavily soiled items separately.
▶ Follow detergent directions.
▶ Select the correct wash cycle and water temperature. Follow care label directions and the person's preferences.
▶ Select the correct drying temperature and cycle. Follow care label directions and the person's preferences.
▶ Fold, hang, or iron clothes as the person prefers. See *Teamwork and Time Management: Laundry*.

TEAMWORK AND TIME MANAGEMENT

Laundry

Residents may share washers and dryers. If assisting with laundry, remove clothes from washers and dryers promptly. Other residents and staff may want to use them. You may find another person's laundry left in a washer or dryer when you are ready to use the machine. First, try to find the person who left the laundry. Politely tell the person that the washer or dryer is done and that you are ready to use the machine. Offer to remove laundry from the machine if the staff member or resident is busy. If you cannot find the staff member or resident, do the following:

- *Laundry left in a washer*—place the wet laundry on a clean surface. Do not put the laundry in the dryer. Some items may need to dry flat or hang to dry. Some fabrics may need certain dryer settings. Or the resident may have drying preferences.
- *Laundry left in a dryer*—fold the laundry. Place the folded laundry on a clean surface.

While laundry is in the washer or dryer, use the time for other tasks. You can assist with ADL, do housekeeping tasks, prepare meals, and so on.

Nursing Services

Some ALRs provide limited nursing services. The nurse assesses each person and monitors health. The nurse supervises tasks delegated to caregivers. If a person cannot manage his or her own drugs, the nurse gives them.

Medication Assistance

Drugs must be taken as prescribed. The six rights of drug administration are:

▶ The right drug
▶ The right dose (amount)
▶ The right route (by mouth, injection, applied to the skin, inhalation, vaginally, or rectally)
▶ The right time
▶ The right person
▶ The right documentation

Your role in assisting with drugs depends on your state's laws, ALR policy, and your training and education. It may involve one or more of the following. *Remember, you do not give drugs (Chapter 2). Also remember that the person has the right to refuse to take prescribed drugs.*

▶ Reminding the person it is time to take a drug
▶ Reading the drug label to the person
▶ Opening containers for persons who cannot do so
▶ Checking the dosage against the drug label
▶ Providing water, juice, milk, crackers, applesauce, or other food and fluids as needed
▶ Making sure the person takes the right drug, the right amount, at the right time, and in the right way
▶ Charting that the person took or refused to take the drug (right documentation)
▶ Storing drugs

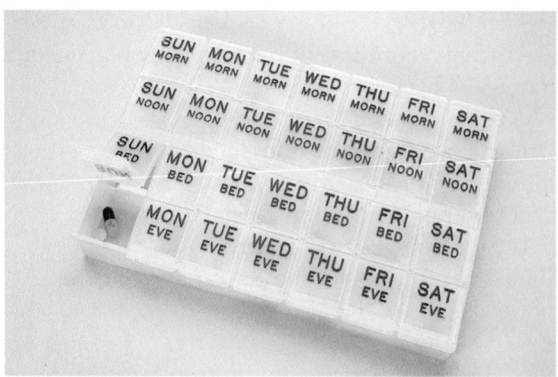

FIGURE 48-4 Pill organizer.

FOCUS ON COMMUNICATION

Medication Assistance

You may be allowed to assist the person with drugs. To remind a person to take his or her drugs, you can say:

- "Ms. Epstein, it's time to take your 8 o'clock pills."
- "Mr. Ladd, you'll need to take your pills in about 10 minutes."
- "Mrs. Young, are you ready to take your pills?"
To read a drug label to a person, read the following:
- The name of the person on the drug label
- The name of the drug
- How to take the drug (by mouth, with food, with a full glass of water, apply to the skin, rectally, and so on)
- The dosage
- When to take the drug (before meals, with meals, after meals, and so on)
- How often to take the drug
- Warnings and other information on the drug label

Residents manage and take their own drugs if able. This is called *self-directed medication management*. The person knows drugs by name, color, or shape. The person knows what drugs to take, the correct doses, and when and how to take them. The person is able to question changes in the usual drug routine. For example, the person comments that a pill is not broken in half. Or the person says that a pill looks different. Report comments or questions to the nurse.

Pill organizers are often used (Fig. 48-4). They have sections for days and times. Some are for a week. Others are for a month. The person, a family member or legal representative, or a nurse prepares the pill organizer. The person then takes the drugs on the right day and at the right time.

Some people need medication reminders. A **medication reminder** means reminding the person to take drugs, observing them being taken as prescribed, and charting that they were taken.

See *Focus on Communication: Medication Assistance.*

Medication Record

A medication record is kept for each person needing help with drugs. The record includes:

▶ The person's name
▶ Drug name, dose, directions, and route of administration
▶ Date and time to take the drug
▶ Date and time help was given
▶ Signature or initials of the person assisting

Drug Errors

Report any drug error to the nurse. Also complete an incident report. An error means one or more of the following:

▶ Taking another person's drugs
▶ Taking the wrong drug
▶ Taking the wrong dose
▶ Taking a drug at the wrong time
▶ Taking a drug by the wrong route
▶ Not taking a drug when ordered

Storing Drugs

Drugs are kept in a secure place. This prevents others from taking them. If the ALR stores the drugs, they are kept in a locked container, cabinet, or area.

Some persons manage and store their own drugs. This is on the service plan. If the room is shared, each person's ability to safely have drugs is assessed. If safety is a factor, drugs are kept in a locked container.

Drugs must have the original pharmacy label. They are stored as directed on the label. For example, some drugs are refrigerated. Others are kept away from light. The label also has an expiration date. Expired or discontinued drugs are disposed of following ALR procedures.

Activities and Recreation

Residents are urged to take part in activity and recreational programs. Social, physical, and community activities promote well-being and independence. An activities director plans, organizes, and conducts the ALR's activity program. These activities are put on a weekly or monthly calendar. The calendar also tells about community events and activities.

Special Services and Safety Needs

Sometimes emergencies occur. Some people need help getting out of bed or transferring to a wheelchair. Then they can leave the building with little or no help.

Other people cannot walk or use a wheelchair or motor scooter. They need attendants. If an attendant is needed, the ALR and the person agree on how and who will meet the person's needs. An attendant is needed 24 hours a day.

TRANSFER, DISCHARGE, AND EVICTION

Residents can be transferred, discharged, or evicted. State laws require that the ALR tell the person about the action. Reasons for such action are:

▶ The ALR can no longer meet the person's health needs. The person is a threat to the health and safety of self or others. Or the ALR cannot provide needed care.
▶ The person fails to pay for services as agreed upon.
▶ The person fails to comply with ALR policies or rules.
▶ The person wants to transfer.
▶ The ALR closes.

Circle the BEST answer.

1 ALRs provide the following *except*
  a Nursing care
  b Housing
  c Help with activities of daily living
  d Support services

2 These statements are about ALRs. Which is *false*?
  a Each person has a private apartment.
  b Some have Alzheimer's disease care units.
  c 24-hour security is provided.
  d Three meals a day are provided.

3 Which statement is *false*?
  a Residents can refuse care.
  b Residents must plan and organize their own activities.
  c Residents are able to lock their doors.
  d An emergency communication system is provided.

4 Which of these violates an assisted living resident's rights?
  a Covering the person during personal care
  b Giving the person mail that was not opened
  c Keeping information confidential
  d Choosing activities for the person

5 A person wants to attend a concert. Which statement is *true*?
  a The concert must be approved by the ALR.
  b The person must return by 10 PM.
  c An attendant must go with the person.
  d The ALR must respect the person's choice.

6 Assisted living staff must
  a Complete a nursing assistant training and competency evaluation program
  b Meet state requirements
  c Assist with drugs
  d Provide transportation

7 ALRs often require the following *except*
  a That persons be mobile
  b That persons have stable health
  c That persons require only limited care
  d That persons speak English

8 A service plan
  a Describes nursing care needs
  b Describes the services needed and who provides them
  c Lists the drugs the person needs to take
  d Lists service fees and charges

9 Assisted living residents are encouraged to eat
  a In their rooms
  b In the dining room
  c At home
  d At community events

10 You assist with housekeeping. Which is *false*?
  a Dusting and vacuuming are done at least weekly.
  b Spills are wiped up right away.
  c Bathroom surfaces are cleaned daily.
  d Spills and splashes are wiped up after meals.

11 You assist with food. Which is *false*?
  a Safe handling instructions are followed.
  b Left-over food is used in 3 to 5 days.
  c Garbage is emptied at least once a day.
  d Pots and pans are washed by hand.

12 You assist with laundry. Which is *true*?
  a Care label directions are followed.
  b Clothes are washed in hot water.
  c Clothes are ironed.
  d All white fabrics are washed together.

13 Usually assisted living staff are allowed to
  a Give drugs
  b Give medication reminders
  c Refill drugs
  d Prepare pill organizers

14 Drugs are kept
  a In the person's closet
  b In the person's drawer
  c In a locked container, cabinet, or area
  d By the family

15 The ALR cannot provide a person with all needed services. Which is *true*?
  a The ALR must hire more staff.
  b The family must provide the needed care.
  c The ALR can ask the person to transfer.
  d The person's service plan needs to change.

Answers to these questions are on p. 782.

OBJECTIVES

- Define the key terms and key abbreviations listed in this chapter
- Describe the rules of emergency care
- Identify the signs of sudden cardiac arrest and the emergency care required
- Describe the signs, symptoms, and emergency care for hemorrhage
- Identify the signs, symptoms, and emergency care for shock
- Describe the causes and types of seizures and how to care for a person during a seizure
- Describe the causes, types, and emergency care for burns
- Identify the common causes and emergency care for fainting
- Describe the signs, symptoms, and emergency care for stroke
- Explain how to promote quality of life during emergencies
- Perform the procedures described in this chapter

PROCEDURES

- Adult CPR—One Rescuer
- Adult CPR—Two Rescuers
- Adult CPR With AED—Two Rescuers
- Child CPR—One Rescuer
- Child CPR With AED—Two Rescuers
- Infant CPR—One Rescuer
- Infant CPR—Two Rescuers

KEY TERMS

anaphylaxis A life-threatening sensitivity to an antigen

cardiac arrest See "sudden cardiac arrest"

convulsion See "seizure"

fainting The sudden loss of consciousness from an inadequate blood supply to the brain

first aid Emergency care given to an ill or injured person before medical help arrives

hemorrhage The excessive loss of blood in a short time

respiratory arrest Breathing stops but heart action continues for several minutes

seizure Violent and sudden contractions or tremors of muscle groups; convulsion

shock Results when organs and tissues do not get enough blood

sudden cardiac arrest (SCA) The heart and breathing stop suddenly and without warning; cardiac arrest

KEY ABBREVIATIONS

ABC Airway, breathing, circulation

ABCD Airway, breathing, circulation, defibrillation

AED Automated external defibrillator

AHA American Heart Association

BLS Basic life support

CPR Cardiopulmonary resuscitation

EMS Emergency Medical Services

RRT Rapid response team

SCA Sudden cardiac arrest

SIDS Sudden infant death syndrome

VF Ventricular fibrillation

V-fib Ventricular fibrillation

Emergencies can occur anywhere. Sometimes you can save a life if you know what to do. You are encouraged to take a first aid course and a basic life support (BLS) course. These courses prepare you to give emergency care.

The basic life support procedures in this chapter are given as basic information. They do not replace certification training. You need a basic life support course for health care providers.

EMERGENCY CARE

First aid is the emergency care given to an ill or injured person before medical help arrives. Its goals are to:

▶ Prevent death

▶ Prevent injuries from becoming worse

For emergencies in out-of-hospital settings, the Emergency Medical Services (EMS) system is activated. Emergency personnel (paramedics, emergency medical technicians) rush to the scene. They treat, stabilize, and transport persons with life-threatening problems. Their ambulances have emergency drugs, equipment, and supplies. They communicate with doctors in hospital emergency departments. The doctors tell them what to do. To activate the EMS system, do one of the following:

▶ Dial 911

▶ Call the local fire or police department

▶ Call the phone operator

Each emergency is different. The rules in Box 49-1 (p. 748) apply to any emergency. Hospitals and other agencies have procedures for emergencies. Rapid response teams (RRTs) are called to the bedside when a person shows warning signs of a life-threatening condition. An RRT may include a doctor, an RN, and a respiratory therapist. The RRT's goal is to prevent death.

See *Focus on Long-Term Care and Home Care: Emergency Care*, p. 748.

See *Teamwork and Time Management: Emergency Care*, p. 748.

See *Promoting Safety and Comfort: Emergency Care*, p. 748.

BASIC LIFE SUPPORT FOR ADULTS

When the heart and breathing stop, the person is clinically dead. Blood is not circulated through the body. Heart, brain, and other organ damage occurs within minutes. The American Heart Association's (AHA) BLS procedures support breathing and circulation.

Chain of Survival for Adults

The AHA's basic life support courses teach the adult *Chain of Survival*. These actions are taken for heart attack (Chapter 40), sudden cardiac arrest, p. 748, respiratory arrest, stroke (Chapter 39 and p. 766), and choking (Chapter 11). They also apply to other life-threatening problems. They are done as soon as possible. Any delay reduces the person's chance of surviving.

Chain of Survival actions for the adult are:

▶ *Early access to emergency cardiovascular care.* This means activating the EMS system or RRT. Hospitals and nursing centers call special codes for life-threatening emergencies.

▶ *Early CPR.*

▶ *Early defibrillation.* See p. 752.

▶ *Early advanced care.* This is given by EMS staff or the RRT, doctors, and nurses. They give drugs and perform life-saving measures.

BOX 49-1 **Rules of Emergency Care**

- Know your limits. Do not do more than you are able. Do not perform an unfamiliar procedure. Do what you can under the circumstances.
- Stay calm. This helps the person feel more secure.
- Know where to find emergency supplies.
- Follow Standard Precautions and the Bloodborne Pathogen Standard to the extent possible.
- Check for life-threatening problems. Check for breathing, a pulse, and bleeding.
- Keep the person lying down or as you found him or her. Moving the person could make an injury worse.
- Move the person only if the setting is unsafe (for example: a burning building or car, a building that might collapse, stormy conditions with lightning, in water, near electrical wires, and on so).
- Perform necessary emergency measures.
- Call for help. Or have someone activate the EMS system. *Do not hang up until the operator has hung up.* Give the operator the following information:
  - Your location: street address and city, cross streets or roads, and landmarks
- Phone number you are calling from
- What seems to have happened (for example: heart attack, crash, fire)—police, fire equipment, and ambulances may be needed
- How many people need help
- Conditions of victims, obvious injuries, and life-threatening situations
- What aid is being given
- Do not remove clothes unless you have to. If you must remove clothing, tear or cut garments along the seams.
- Keep the person warm. Cover the person with a blanket, coats, or sweaters.
- Reassure the person. Explain what is happening and that help was called.
- Do not give the person food or fluids.
- Keep onlookers away. They invade privacy, and tend to stare, give advice, and comment about the person's condition. The person may think the situation is worse than it really is.

FOCUS ON LONG-TERM CARE AND HOME CARE

EMERGENCY CARE

In nursing centers, a nurse decides when to activate the EMS system or RRT. The nurse tells you how to help. If a person has stopped breathing or is in sudden cardiac arrest, the nurse may start cardiopulmonary resuscitation (CPR) (p. 749). Some centers allow nursing assistants to start CPR. Others do not. Know your center's policy about CPR.

Death is expected in persons with terminal illnesses. Usually these persons are not resuscitated (Chapter 50). This information is in the care plan.

TEAMWORK AND TIME MANAGEMENT

Emergency Care

Onlookers can threaten privacy and confidentiality. During an emergency, your main concern is the person's illness or injuries. You cannot give care and manage onlookers at the same time. Ask someone else to deal with the onlookers. If someone else is giving care, keep onlookers away from the person.

Sudden Cardiac Arrest

Sudden cardiac arrest (SCA) or cardiac arrest is when the heart and breathing stop suddenly and without warning. Permanent brain and other organ damage occurs unless circulation and breathing are restored. There are three major signs of SCA:

▶ No response.
▶ No breathing. The person may have *agonal gasps* or *agonal respirations* early during SCA. (*Agonal* means to

PROMOTING SAFETY AND COMFORT: Emergency Care

SAFETY

During emergencies, contact with blood, body fluids, secretions, and excretions is likely. Follow Standard Precautions and the Bloodborne Pathogen Standard to the extent possible.

COMFORT

Mental comfort is important during emergencies. Help the person feel safe and secure. Provide reassurance and explanations about care. Use a calm approach.

struggle. Agonal is used in relation to death and dying.) Agonal gasps do not bring enough oxygen into the lungs. Consider agonal gasps to mean "no breathing."
▶ No pulse.

The person's skin is cool, pale, and gray. The person is not coughing or moving.

SCA can occur anywhere and at any time—while driving, shoveling snow, playing golf or tennis, watching TV, eating, or sleeping. Common causes include heart disease, drowning, electric shock, severe injury, choking, and drug overdose. These causes lead to an abnormal heart rhythm called ventricular fibrillation (p. 752). The heart cannot pump blood. A normal rhythm must be restored or the person will die.

Respiratory Arrest

Respiratory arrest is when breathing stops but heart action continues for several minutes. If breathing is not restored, cardiac arrest occurs. Causes of respiratory arrest include:

▶ Drowning
▶ Stroke
▶ Choking
▶ Drug overdose
▶ Electric shock (including lightning strikes)
▶ Smoke inhalation
▶ Suffocation
▶ Heart attack
▶ Coma
▶ Other injuries

Cardiopulmonary Resuscitation for Adults

When the heart and breathing stop, the person is clinically dead. Blood is not circulated through the body. Brain and other organ damage occurs within minutes.

Cardiopulmonary resuscitation (CPR) must be started at once when a person has SCA. CPR supports breathing and circulation. It provides blood and oxygen to the heart, brain, and other organs until advanced emergency care is given. CPR involves four parts—the ABCDs of CPR:

▶ **A**irway
▶ **B**reathing
▶ **C**irculation
▶ **D**efibrillation

CPR procedures require speed, skill, and efficiency. Airway, breathing, and circulation procedures are done until a defibrillator is available.

See *Promoting Safety and Comfort: Cardiopulmonary Resuscitation for Adults.*

PROMOTING SAFETY AND COMFORT: Cardiopulmonary Resuscitation for Adults

SAFETY

The discussion and procedures that follow assume that the person does not have injuries from trauma. If injuries are present, special measures are needed to position the person and open the airway. Such measures are learned during a BLS certification course.

Airway

The respiratory passages (airway) must be open to restore breathing. The airway is often obstructed (blocked) during SCA. The person's tongue falls toward the back of the throat and blocks the airway. The head tilt-chin lift method opens the airway (Fig. 49-1):

▶ Position the person supine on a hard, flat surface.
▶ Kneel or stand at the person's side.
▶ Place the palm of one hand on the forehead.
▶ Tilt the head back by pushing down on the forehead with your palm.
▶ Place the fingers of your other hand under the lower jaw. Use your index and middle fingers. Do not use your thumb.
▶ Lift the jaw. This brings the chin forward.
▶ Do not close the person's mouth. The mouth should be slightly open unless you need to do mouth-to-nose breathing (p. 750).

Breathing

Air is not inhaled when breathing stops. The person must get oxygen. If not, permanent heart, brain, and other organ damage occurs. The person is given *breaths*. That is, a rescuer inflates the person's lungs.

Before giving breaths, check for *adequate breathing* (Fig. 49-2). Agonal gasping is not adequate breathing. After opening the airway, take 5 to 10 seconds (but no more than 10 seconds) to check for adequate breathing.

▶ Open the airway with the head tilt-chin lift method.
▶ Place your ear over the person's mouth and nose.
▶ Observe the person's chest.
▶ *Look* to see if the chest rises and falls.
▶ *Listen* for the escape of air.
▶ *Feel* for the flow of air on your cheek.

When you start CPR, give 2 breaths first. Each breath should take 1 second. *You should see the chest rise with each breath.* Then two breaths are given after every 30 chest compressions (p. 751).

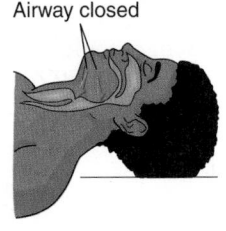
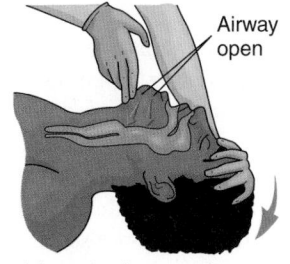

Airway closed

Airway open

FIGURE 49-1 The head tilt-chin lift method opens the airway. One hand is on the person's forehead. Pressure is applied to tilt the head back. The chin is lifted with the fingers of the other hand.

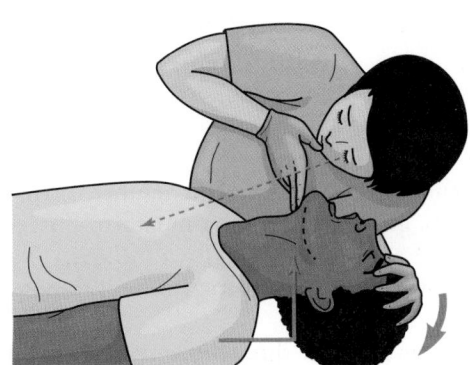

FIGURE 49-2 Checking for adequate breathing. *Look* to see if the chest rises and falls. *Listen* for the escape of air. *Feel* for the flow of air on your cheek.

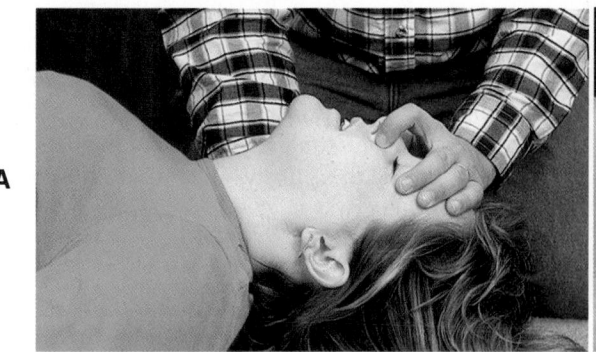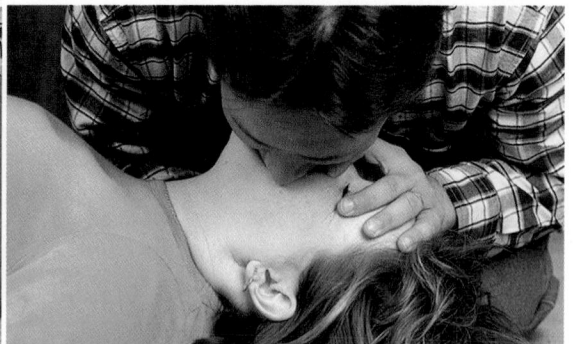

FIGURE 49-3 Mouth-to-mouth breathing. **A,** The person's airway is opened. The nostrils are pinched shut. **B,** The person's mouth is sealed by the rescuer's mouth.

Mouth-to-Mouth Breathing. One way to give breaths is mouth-to-mouth breathing (Fig. 49-3). You place your mouth over the person's mouth. Contact with the person's blood, body fluids, secretions, or excretions is likely. To give mouth-to-mouth breathing:

▶ Keep the airway open with the head tilt-chin lift method.
▶ Pinch the person's nostrils shut. Use your thumb and index finger. Use the hand on the forehead. Shutting the nostrils prevents air from escaping through the nose.
▶ Take a breath. A regular breath is needed, not a deep breath.
▶ Place your mouth tightly over the person's mouth. Seal the person's mouth with your lips.
▶ Blow air into the person's mouth. You should see the chest rise as the lungs fill with air. You should also hear air escape when the person exhales.
▶ Repeat the head tilt-chin lift method if the person's chest did not rise.
▶ Remove your mouth from the person's mouth. Then take in a quick breath.
▶ Give another breath. You should see the chest rise.

Mouth-to-Barrier Device Breathing. Mouth-to-barrier device breathing is used whenever possible. A barrier device is placed over the person's mouth and nose (Fig. 49-4). It prevents contact with the person's mouth and blood, body fluids, secretions, or excretions. The seal must be tight.

A face shield is replaced with a face mask as soon as possible. If using a face mask, seal the face mask against the person's face. Then open the airway with the head tilt-chin lift method.

The Ambu bag (Chapter 35) is another barrier device. It is used to give oxygen during mouth-to-barrier device breathing.

Mouth-to-Nose Breathing. Mouth-to-nose breathing is used when:

▶ You cannot ventilate through the person's mouth.
▶ You cannot open the mouth.
▶ Your mouth is too small to make a tight seal for mouth-to-mouth breathing.
▶ The mouth or jaw is severely injured.

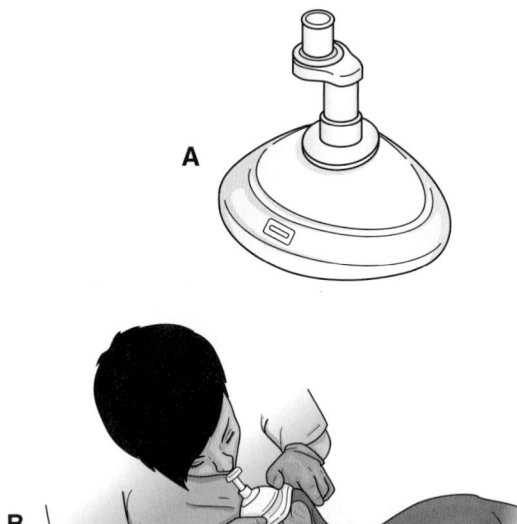

FIGURE 49-4 **A,** Barrier device. **B,** The barrier device is in place.

▶ The person is bleeding from the mouth.
▶ You are rescuing a drowning victim.

The mouth is closed for mouth-to-nose breathing. The head tilt-chin lift method opens the airway. Pressure is placed on the chin to close the mouth. To give a breath, place your mouth over the person's nose and blow air into the nose (Fig. 49-5). After giving a breath, remove your mouth from the person's nose.

Mouth-to-Stoma Breathing. Some people breathe through *stomas* (openings) in their necks (Fig. 49-6). To give *mouth-to-stoma breathing*:

▶ Keep the person's mouth closed.
▶ Do not tilt the person's head back.
▶ Seal your mouth around the stoma.
▶ Blow air into the stoma (Fig. 49-7).

Before giving mouth-to-mouth or mouth-to-nose breathing, always check to see if the person has a stoma. Other breathing methods are not effective if the person has a stoma.

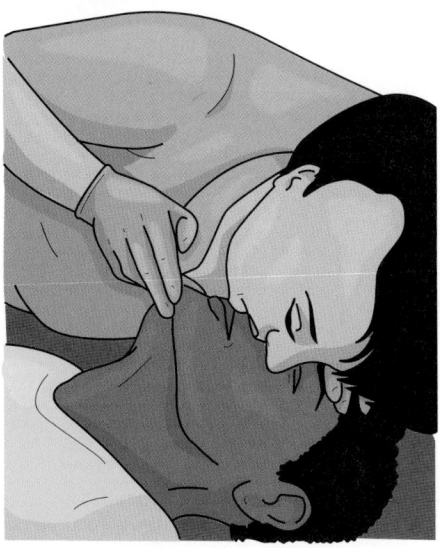

FIGURE 49-5 Mouth-to-nose breathing.

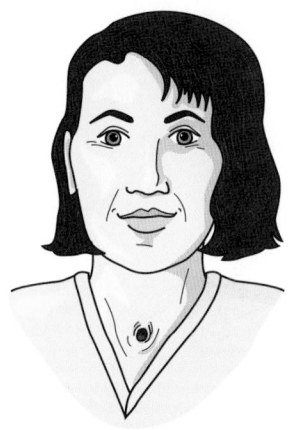

FIGURE 49-6 A stoma in the neck. The person breathes in and out of the stoma.

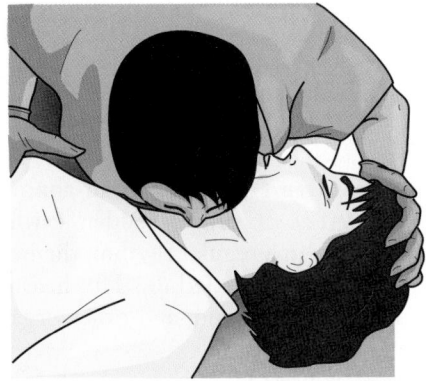

FIGURE 49-7 Mouth-to-stoma breathing.

Circulation

The heart, brain, and other organs must receive blood. Otherwise, permanent damage results. In cardiac arrest, the heart has stopped beating. Blood must be pumped through the body in some other way. Chest compressions force blood through the circulatory system.

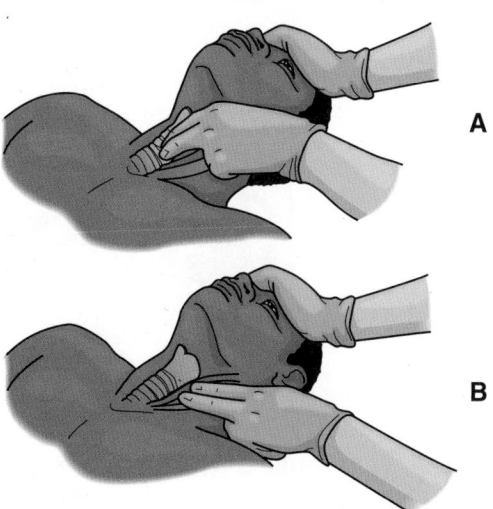

FIGURE 49-8 Locating the carotid pulse. **A,** Two fingertips are placed on the trachea. **B,** The fingertips are moved down into the groove of the neck to the carotid artery.

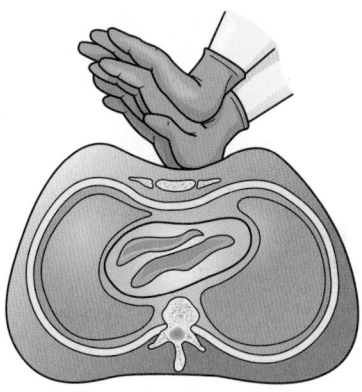

FIGURE 49-9 The heart lies between the sternum and the spinal column. The heart is compressed when pressure is applied to the sternum.

Before starting chest compressions, check for a pulse. Use the carotid artery on the side near you. To find the carotid pulse, place 2 or 3 fingertips on the trachea (windpipe). Then slide your fingertips down off the trachea to the groove of the neck (Fig. 49-8). While checking for a pulse, also look for signs of circulation. See if the person has started breathing or is coughing or moving.

The heart lies beneath the sternum (breastbone) and the spinal column. When pressure is applied to the sternum, the sternum is depressed. This compresses the heart between the sternum and spinal column (Fig. 49-9). For effective chest compressions, the person must be supine on a hard, flat surface—floor or backboard. You are positioned at the person's side.

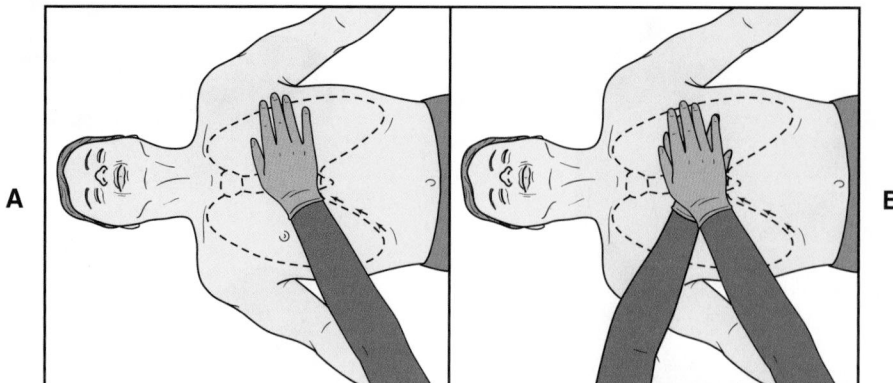

FIGURE 49-10 Proper hand position for CPR. **A,** The heel of the dominant hand is placed in the center of the chest between the nipples. **B,** The heel of the non-dominant hand is placed on top of the dominant hand.

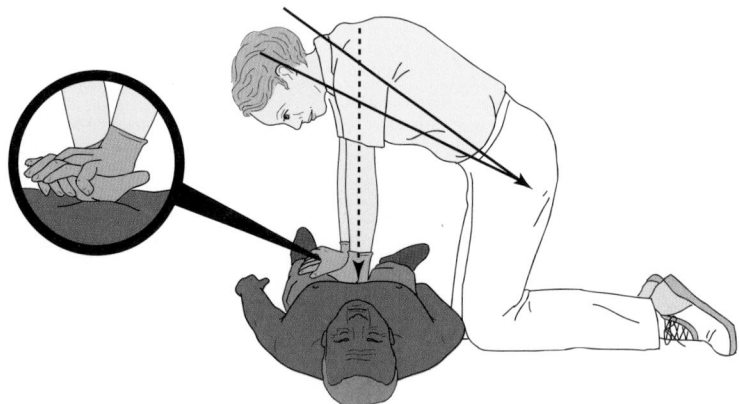

FIGURE 49-11 Giving chest compressions. The arms are straight. The shoulders are over the hands.

Hand position also is important for effective chest compressions (Fig. 49-10). You use the heels of your hands—one on top of the other—for chest compressions. For proper placement:

▶ Expose the person's chest. Remove clothing or move it out of the way. You need to be able to see the person's bare skin for proper hand position.
▶ Place the heel of one hand (usually your dominant hand) in the center of the bare chest. The heel of this hand is placed on the sternum between the nipples.
▶ Place the heel of your other hand on top of the heel of the first hand.

To give chest compressions, your arms are straight. Your shoulders are directly over your hands (Fig. 49-11). Exert firm downward pressure to depress the adult sternum about 1½ to 2 inches. Then release pressure without removing your hands from the chest. Releasing pressure allows the chest to recoil—to return to its normal position. Recoil lets the heart fill with blood.

The AHA recommends that you:

▶ Give compressions at a rate of 100 per minute.
▶ Push hard, and push fast.
▶ Push deeply into the chest.

▶ Interrupt chest compressions only when necessary. Interruptions should be less than 10 seconds. When there are no chest compressions, blood does not flow to the heart, brain, and other organs.

Defibrillation

Ventricular fibrillation (VF, V-fib) is an abnormal heart rhythm (Fig. 49-12). It causes sudden cardiac arrest. Rather than beating in a regular rhythm, the heart shakes and quivers like a bowl of Jell-O. The heart does not pump blood. The heart, brain, and other organs do not receive blood and oxygen.

A *defibrillator* is used to deliver a shock to the heart. The shock stops the VF. This allows the return of a regular heart rhythm. Defibrillation as soon as possible after the onset of VF increases the person's chance of survival.

The AHA recommends the following cycle for adults:

▶ Immediate defibrillation if the person's collapse is witnessed.
▶ One shock and then immediate CPR—5 cycles of 30 compressions and 2 breaths.
▶ Check for a heart rhythm.

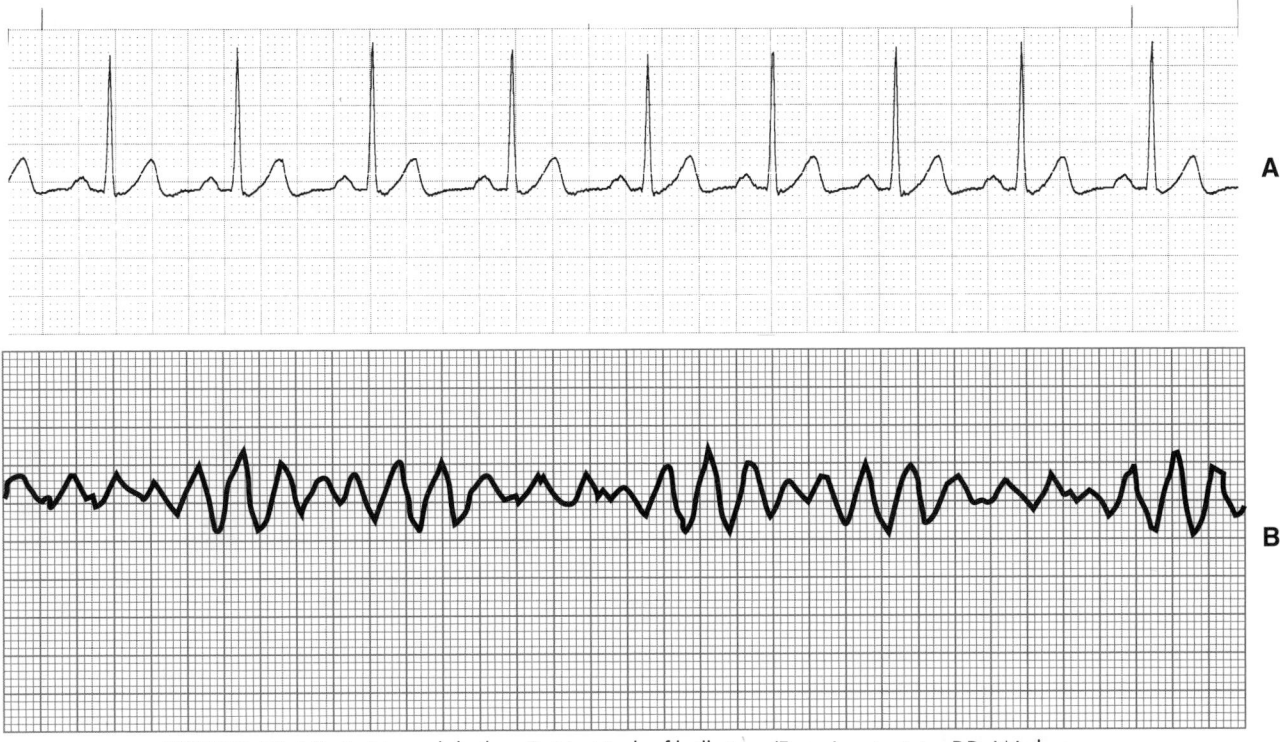

FIGURE 49-12 A, Normal rhythm. **B,** Ventricular fibrillation. (From Ignatavicius DD, Workman ML: *Medical-surgical nursing: critical thinking for collaborative care,* ed 5, St Louis, 2006, Saunders.)

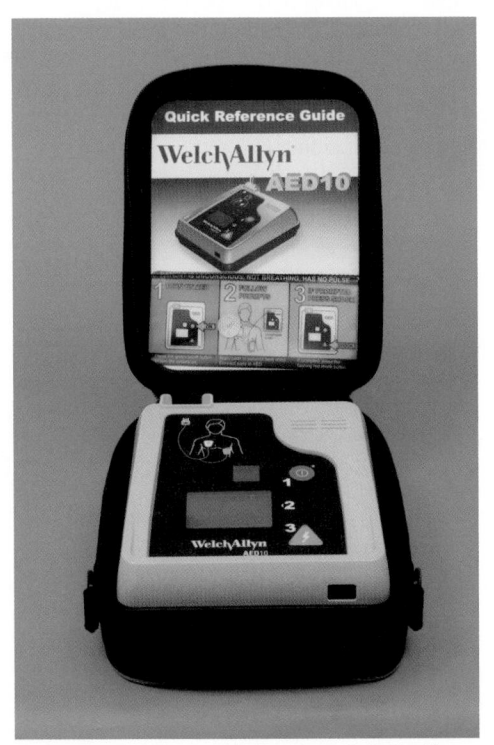

FIGURE 49-13 An automated external defibrillator (AED).

> ## FOCUS ON **CHILDREN** AND **OLDER PERSONS**
>
> ### Defibrillation
>
> #### CHILDREN
> The shock dosage for children 8 years and older is the same as the adult dosage. Lower shock dosages are used for children aged 1 to 8 years.
>
> Some AEDs are designed for adults and children. There may be a key or switch for child dosages. Always follow the manufacturer's instructions.

Automated external defibrillators (AEDs) are found in hospitals, nursing centers, dental offices, and other health care agencies (Fig. 49-13). They are on airplanes and in airports, health clubs, malls, and many other public places. Many people have them in their homes.

You will learn how to use an AED in the AHA's basic life support course for healthcare providers.

See *Focus on Children and Older Persons: Defibrillation.*

Performing Adult CPR

CPR is done only for cardiac arrest. You must determine if cardiac arrest or fainting has occurred. *CPR is done if the person does not respond, is not breathing, and has no pulse.*

CPR is done alone or with another person. When done alone, giving breaths and chest compressions are done by the one rescuer. With two rescuers, one person gives breaths and the other gives chest compressions. The second rescuer uses the AED if one is available.

See *Promoting Safety and Comfort: Performing Adult CPR.*

PROMOTING SAFETY AND COMFORT: Performing Adult CPR

SAFETY

Never practice CPR on another person. Serious damage can be done. Mannequins are used to learn and practice CPR.

Make sure you have a safe setting for CPR. Move the person only if the setting is unsafe (see Box 49-1).

The person must be on a hard, flat surface for CPR. If the person is in bed, place a board under the person. Or move the person to the floor.

ADULT CPR—ONE RESCUER

PROCEDURE

1 Check if the person is responding. Tap or gently shake the person, call the person by name, and shout "Are you OK?"

2 Call for help. Activate the EMS system or the agency's RRT.

3 Get or ask someone to bring an AED if available.

4 Position the person supine on a hard, flat surface. Logroll the person so there is no twisting of the spine. Place the arms alongside the body.

5 Open the airway. Use the head tilt-chin lift method.

6 Check for adequate breathing. *Look* to see if the chest rises and falls. *Listen* for the escape of air. *Feel* for the flow of air on your cheek. This should take 5 to 10 seconds.

7 Give 2 breaths if the person is not breathing adequately. Each breath should take only 1 second. Each breath must make the chest rise. (If the first breath does not make the chest rise, try opening the airway again. Use the head tilt-chin lift method.)

8 Check for a carotid pulse. This should take 5 to 10 seconds. Use your other hand to keep the airway open with the head tilt-chin lift method. Start chest compressions if there are no signs of circulation.

9 Expose the person's chest.

10 Give chest compressions at a rate of 100 per minute. Give 30 chest compressions followed by 2 breaths. Establish a regular rhythm, and count out loud—try "1 and, 2 and, 3 and, 4 and," so on to 30.

11 Check for a carotid pulse every few minutes. Also check for breathing, coughing, and moving.

12 Continue CPR if the person has no signs of circulation. Continue the cycle of 30 compressions and 2 breaths until the AED arrives.

13 Do the following if the person has signs of circulation:
  a Check for breathing.
  b Position the person in the recovery position (p. 756) if the person is breathing.
  c Monitor breathing and circulation.

14 Do the following if the person has signs of circulation but breathing is absent:
  a Give 1 breath every 5 to 6 seconds. This is at a rate of 10 to 12 breaths per minute.
  b Monitor circulation.

ADULT CPR—TWO RESCUERS

PROCEDURE

1 *Rescuer 1:* Check if the person is responding. Tap or gently shake the person, call the person by name, and shout "Are you OK?"
2 *Rescuer 2:*
  a Activate the EMS system or the agency's RRT.
  b Get a defibrillator (AED) if one is available. Ready the AED.
3 *Rescuer 1:* Position the person supine on a hard, flat surface. Logroll the person so there is no twisting of the spine. Place the arms alongside the body.
4 *Rescuer 2:*
  a Open the airway. Use the head tilt-chin lift method.
  b Check for adequate breathing. *Look* to see if the chest rises and falls. *Listen* for the escape of air. *Feel* for the flow of air on your cheek.
  c Check for a carotid pulse and for breathing, coughing, and moving. This should take 5 to 10 seconds. Use your other hand to keep the airway open with the head tilt-chin lift method.
5 Perform 2-person CPR if there are no signs of circulation (Fig. 49-14). (*NOTE:* For children, give 15 compressions followed by 2 breaths.)
  a *Rescuer 1:* Give chest compressions at a rate of 100 per minute—30 chest compressions. Establish a regular rhythm, and count out loud—try "1 and, 2 and, 3 and, 4 and," so on to 30.

  b *Rescuer 2:* Give 2 breaths after every 30 chest compressions.
  c Change positions every 2 minutes or after 5 cycles of 30 compressions and 2 breaths. The switch should take no more than 5 seconds.
6 Check for a carotid pulse and for breathing, coughing, and moving every few minutes.
7 Continue CPR if the person has no signs of circulation. Continue the cycle of 30 compressions and 2 breaths until the AED arrives. Check for circulation every few minutes.
8 Do the following if the person has signs of circulation:
  a Check for breathing.
  b Position the person in the recovery position (p. 756) if the person is breathing.
  c Monitor breathing and circulation.
9 Do the following if the person has signs of circulation but breathing is absent:
  a Give 1 breath every 5 to 6 seconds. This is at a rate of 10 to 12 breaths per minute.
  b Monitor circulation.

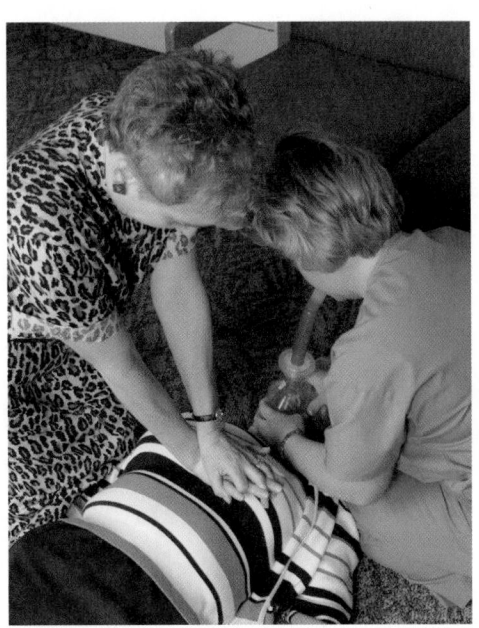

FIGURE 49-14 Two people perform CPR.

ADULT CPR WITH AED—TWO RESCUERS

PROCEDURE

1 *Rescuer 1:* Check if the person is responding. Tap or gently shake the person, call the person by name, and shout "Are you OK?"

2 *Rescuer 2:* Activate the EMS system or the agency's RRT. Get a defibrillator (AED), and get it ready.

3 *Rescuer 1:* Position the person supine on a hard, flat surface. Logroll the person so there is no twisting of the spine. Place the arms alongside the body.

4 *Rescuer 1:*
  a Open the airway. Use the head tilt-chin lift method.
  b Check for adequate breathing. *Look* to see if the chest rises and falls. *Listen* for the escape of air. *Feel* for the flow of air on your cheek.
  c Give 2 breaths if the person is not breathing adequately. Each breath should take only 1 second. Each breath must make the chest rise. (If a breath does not make the chest rise, try opening the airway again. Use the head tilt-chin lift method.)
  d Check for a carotid pulse. This should take 5 to 10 seconds. Use your other hand to keep the airway open with the head tilt-chin lift method.
  e Expose the person's chest.
  f Give chest compressions at a rate of 100 per minute. Give 30 chest compressions followed by 2 breaths. Establish a regular rhythm, and count out loud—try "1 and, 2 and, 3 and, 4 and," so on to 30.
  g Give 2 breaths.

5 *Rescuer 2:*
  a Open the case with the AED.
  b Turn on the AED.
  c Attach adult electrode pads to the person's chest. Follow the instructions and diagram provided with the AED.
  d Attach the connecting cables to the AED.
  e Clear away from the person. Make sure no one is touching the person.
  f Let the AED check the person's heart rhythm.
  g Make sure everyone is clear of the person if the AED advises a "shock."
  h Press the "SHOCK" button if the AED advises a "shock."

6 *Rescuers 1 and 2:*
  a Perform 2-person CPR:
    (1) One rescuer gives chest compressions at a rate of 100 per minute—30 chest compressions followed by 2 breaths. Establish a regular rhythm, and count out loud—try "1 and, 2 and, 3 and, 4 and," so on to 30.
    (2) The other rescuer gives 2 breaths after every 30 chest compressions.

7 Repeat steps 5 e, f, g, and h after 2 minutes of CPR (5 cycles of 30 compressions and 2 breaths). Then continue CPR.

Recovery Position

The recovery position is used when the person is breathing and has a pulse but is not responding (Fig. 49-15). The position helps keep the airway open and prevents aspiration.

Logroll the person into the recovery position. Keep the head, neck, and spine straight. A hand supports the head. *Do not use this position if the person might have neck injuries or other trauma.*

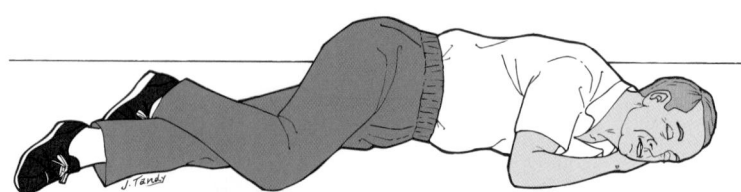

FIGURE 49-15 Recovery position.

BASIC LIFE SUPPORT FOR CHILDREN AND INFANTS

The AHA defines a child and an infant as follows:

▶ *Child*—from 1 year of age to puberty. Puberty is marked by secondary sex characteristics in males and females (Chapter 9).
▶ *Infant*—from birth (outside of the delivery room) until 1 year (12 months) of age.

Chain of Survival for Children and Infants

Sudden infant death syndrome (SIDS) is the sudden, unexplained death of an infant younger than 1 year old. It is the leading cause of death in children between 1 month and 1 year of age. Most SIDS deaths occur in babies between 2 months and 4 months of age. It occurs during sleep.

Cardiac arrest caused by heart disease is rare in children. More common causes involve respiratory diseases or injuries that lead to respiratory arrest or circulatory failure. Motor vehicle crashes, drowning, burns, smoke inhalation, and guns are major death-producing injuries.

The AHA's pediatric *Chain of Survival* involves these steps:

▶ Preventing cardiac arrest
▶ Early and effective CPR
▶ Rapid activation of the EMS system or the agency's RRT
▶ Early and effective advanced life support

◆ CPR for Children and Infants

The AHA's CPR guidelines for children and infants differ from adult guidelines (Box 49-2). The procedures also differ. Remember to use barrier devices for breathing whenever possible.

Text continued on p. 761

BOX 49-2 CPR Rules for Children and Infants

CHILDREN

• Give only enough air to make the child's chest rise. If the child is very small, use less air than for larger children and adults.
• Give 2 breaths that make the child's chest rise. If a breath does not make the chest rise:
  • Try again to open the airway.
  • Give a breath. The breath should make the chest rise.
• Hand position for chest compressions is the same as for adults (p. 751).
• Use 1 or 2 hands for chest compressions if the child is very small (Fig. 49-16, p. 758).
• Give chest compressions with enough pressure to press down ⅓ to ½ the depth of the chest.
• Count the pulse for at least 5 seconds but no more than 10 seconds. For the heart rate per minute:
  • 5 seconds: multiply the number by 12
  • 10 seconds: multiply the number by 6
• Start CPR if the child's heart rate is less than 60 beats per minute with signs of poor circulation. For example, the child's skin color is poor.
• Give compressions at the rate of 100 per minute:
  • 1 rescuer—30 compressions followed by 2 breaths
  • 2 rescuers—15 compressions followed by 2 breaths
• Activate the EMS system.
  • After 5 cycles of CPR if you are alone
  • At once if you witness a sudden collpase
• Use an AED as soon as possible for:
  • Any in-hospital cardiac arrest
  • A witnessed, sudden collapse of a child in an out-of-hospital setting
• Provide 5 cycles of CPR before using an AED if not in a hospital setting.
• Push hard, and push fast. Give compressions at a rate of 100 per minute.

INFANTS

• Use the head tilt-chin lift method to open the airway. Often the tongue obstructs the airway when it falls into the throat (Fig. 49-17, p. 759).
  • Place one hand on the infant's forehead.
  • Use your palm to push the head back.
  • Place the fingers of your other hand under the bony part of the lower jaw. This is near the chin. Do not press in deep.
  • Use your fingers (not your thumb) to lift the jaw to bring the chin forward. The head should be in a neutral ("sniffing") position.
  • Do not close the infant's mouth completely.
• Use the mouth-to-mouth-to-nose method to give breaths (Fig. 49-18, p. 759). This is the preferred method. Use the mouth-to-mouth method if you cannot cover the infant's nose and mouth with your mouth. To give mouth-to-mouth-to-nose breaths:
  • Keep the airway open with the head tilt-chin lift method.
  • Cover the infant's nose and mouth with your mouth. Make sure you have a tight seal.
  • Blow air into the infant's nose and mouth.
• Give 2 breaths that make the infant's chest rise. If a breath does not make the chest rise:
  • Try again to open the airway.
  • Give a breath. The breath should make the chest rise.
• Use the brachial artery to check for a pulse (Fig. 49-19, p. 759):
  • Place the index and middle fingers on the inside of the infant's upper arm. Finger placement is between the elbow and shoulder.
  • Press gently for 5 to 10 seconds.
• Count the pulse for at least 5 seconds but no more than 10 seconds. For the heart rate per minute:
  • 5 seconds: multiply the number by 12
  • 10 seconds: multiply the number by 6

Adapted from: *BLS for healthcare providers: student manual,* © Copyright 2005, American Heart Association.   *Continued*

BOX 49-2 **CPR Rules for Children and Infants—cont'd**

INFANTS—cont'd
- Start CPR if the child's heart rate is less than 60 beats per minute with signs of poor circulation. For example, the child's skin color is poor.
- Locate hand position for chest compressions (Fig. 49-20, p. 760):
  - Draw an imaginary line between the nipples. Find the sternum (breastbone).
  - Place 2 fingers on the sternum just below the imaginary line.
- Give chest compressions as follows:
  - Press on the lower half of the sternum.
  - Use enough pressure to press down ⅓ to ½ the depth of the chest.
- Give compressions at a rate of 100 per minute:
  - 1 rescuer—30 compressions followed by 2 breaths
  - 2 rescuers—15 compressions followed by 2 breaths

- Use the 2 thumb-encircling hands method for chest compressions when there are 2 rescuers (Fig. 49-21, p. 760):
  - Draw an imaginary line between the nipples. Find the sternum (breastbone).
  - Place both thumbs just below the imaginary line. The thumbs are side by side in the center of the chest. (Thumbs may overlap. The infant may be small. Or you may have large hands.)
  - Encircle the infant's chest with your hands.
  - Support the infant's back with your fingers. Use both hands.
  - Press down on the sternum with your thumbs (⅓ to ½ the depth of the chest). Squeeze the chest with your fingers.
- Activate the EMS system:
  - If you are alone: after 5 cycles of CPR. Then return to the infant and continue CPR.
  - If you are alone and witness an infant suddenly collapse: at once. Then return to the infant and start CPR.
  - If the infant is small and not injured: carry the infant to the phone. You can start or continue CPR faster after calling 911.

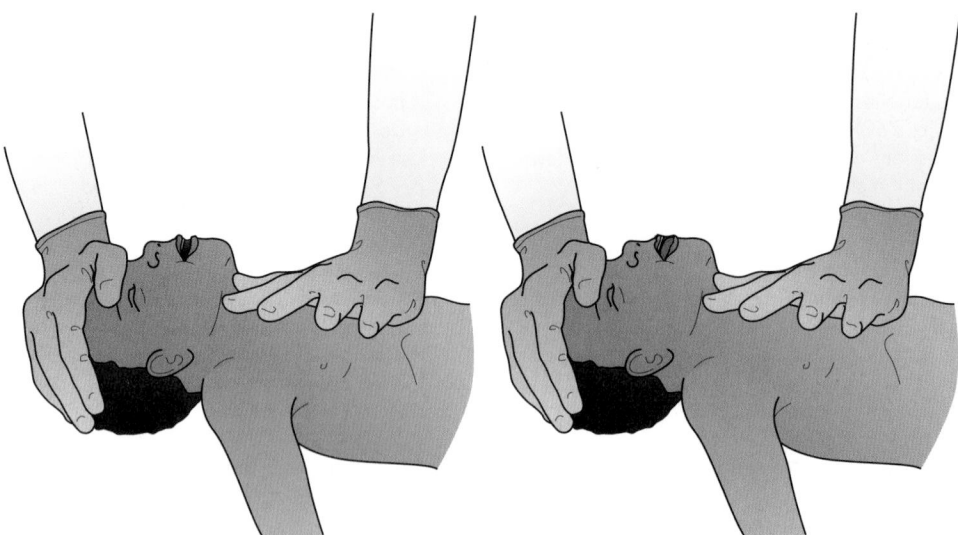

FIGURE 49-16 The heel of one hand can be used for CPR if the child is very small. The fingers are off the chest.

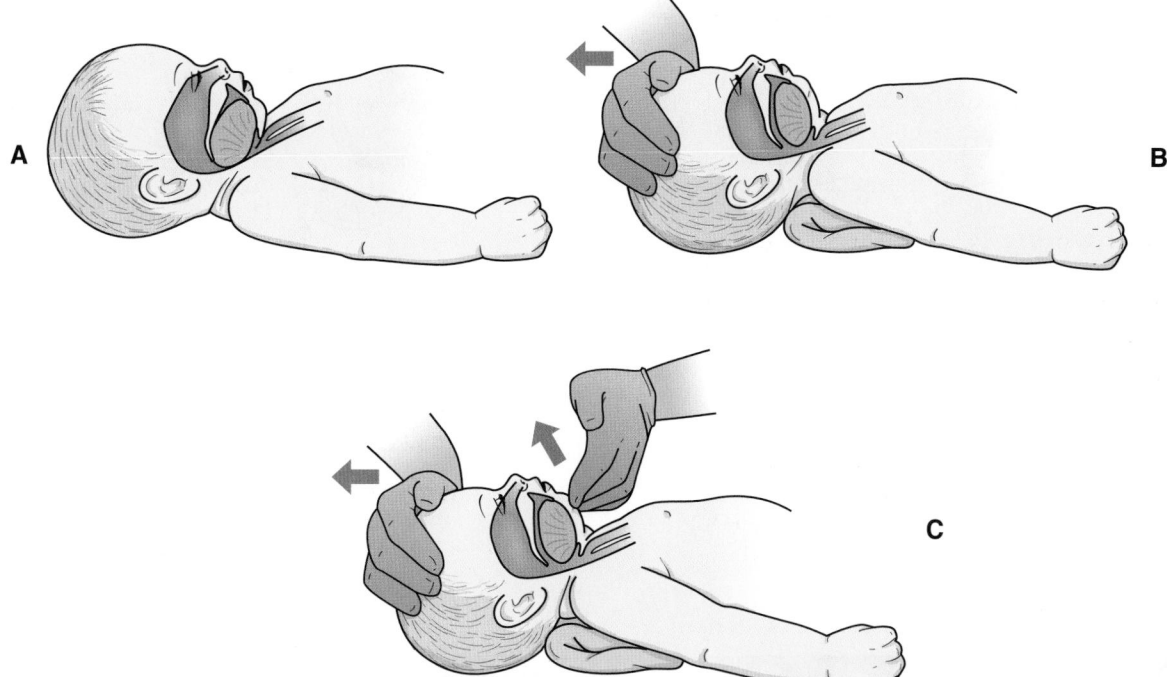

FIGURE 49-17 The head tilt-chin lift method for infants. **A,** The tongue is at the back of the throat, obstructing the airway. **B,** One hand is on the infant's forehead. The palm is used to push the head back. **C,** The fingers of the other hand are under the bony part of the lower jaw. This is near the chin. The fingers are used to lift the jaw to bring the chin forward. The head is in a neutral ("sniffing") position.

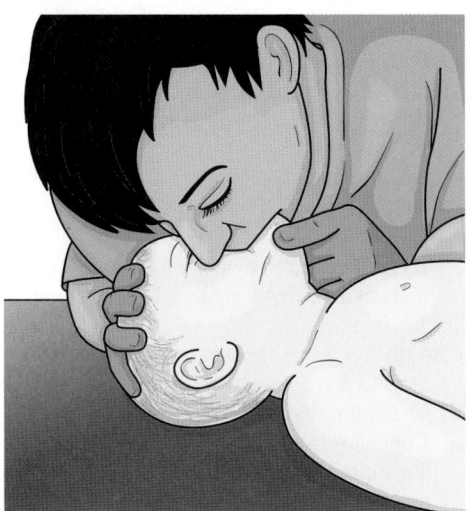

FIGURE 49-18 Mouth-to-mouth-to nose breathing. The infant's nose and mouth are covered to give breaths.

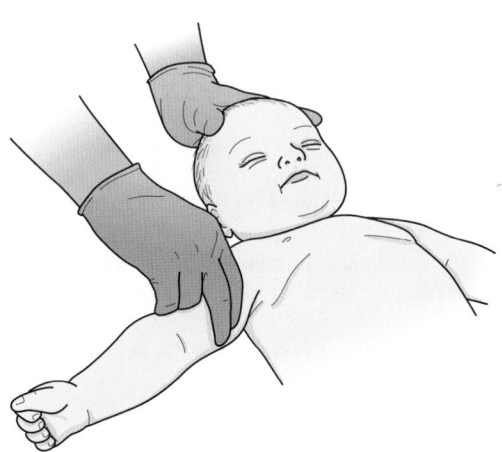

FIGURE 49-19 Locating the infant's brachial pulse.

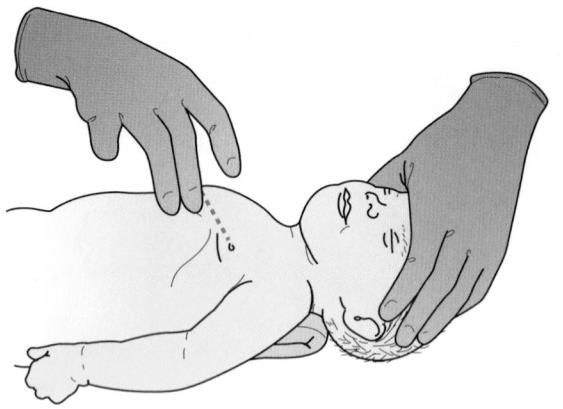

FIGURE 49-20 Locating hand position for infant chest compressions. Draw an imaginary line between the nipples. Find the sternum (breastbone). Place 2 fingers on the sternum just below the imaginary line.

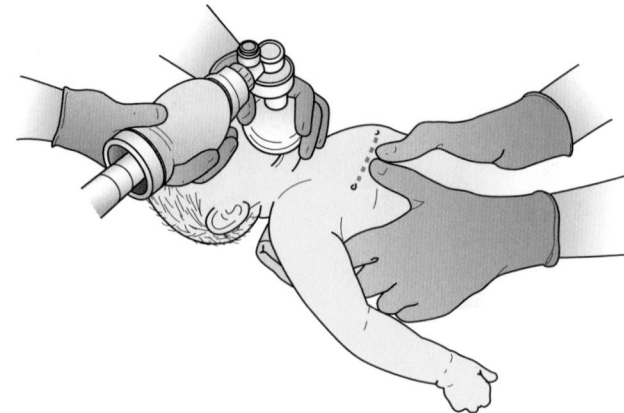

FIGURE 49-21 The 2 thumb-encircling hands method for chest compressions.

CHILD CPR—ONE RESCUER

PROCEDURE

1 Check if the child is responding. Tap or shake the child, call the child by name, and shout "Are you OK?"
2 Call for help. If someone responds, ask the person to:
  a Activate the EMS system or the agency's RRT.
  b Get an AED if one is available.
3 Position the child supine on a hard, flat surface. Logroll the child so there is no twisting of the spine. Place the arms alongside the body.
4 Open the airway. Use the head tilt-chin lift method.
5 Check for adequate breathing. This should take 5 to 10 seconds.
  a *Look* to see if the chest rises and falls.
  b *Listen* for the escape of air.
  c *Feel* for the flow of air on your cheek.
6 Give a total of 2 breaths if the child is not breathing. Each breath should take only 1 second. Each breath should make the chest rise. If a breath does not make the chest rise:
  a Re-open the airway with a the head tilt-chin lift method.
  b Give another breath.
7 Check the carotid pulse. This should take 5 to 10 seconds. Use your other hand to keep the airway open with the head tilt-chin lift method.

8 Expose the child's chest.
9 Start chest compressions if:
  a The child has no pulse.
  b The heart rate is less than 60 beats per minute and there are signs of poor circulation.
10 Give chest compressions at a rate of 100 per minute. Give 30 compressions followed by 2 breaths. Establish a regular rhythm, and count out loud—try "1 and, 2 and, 3 and, 4 and," so on to 30.
11 Do the following, if not already done, after 5 cycles of CPR:
  a Activate the EMS system.
  b Get an AED if one is available.
  c Use the AED.
12 Check for a shockable rhythm with the AED.
  a For a shockable rhythm: Give 1 shock. Then start CPR.
  b If the rhythm is not shockable:
    (1) Start CPR.
    (2) Check the rhythm after every 5 cycles of CPR.
    (3) Continue steps 12b (1) and (2) until advanced life support is available or the child starts to move.

Child CPR—Two Rescuers

When two rescuers give child CPR, 15 compressions are given followed by 2 breaths (15:2). The compression rate is 100 per minute. See procedure: *Adult CPR—Two Rescuers*, p. 755. Use the following procedure if an AED is available.

 CPR for Infants

The BLS sequence for infants does not involve defibrillation. The ABCs of CPR for children are:
▶ Airway
▶ Breathing
▶ Circulation

CHILD CPR WITH AED—TWO RESCUERS

PROCEDURE

1 *Rescuer 1:* Check if the child is responding. Tap or gently shake the child, call the child by name, and shout "Are you OK?"

2 *Rescuer 2:* Activate the EMS system or the agency's RRT. Get an (AED), and get it ready.

3 *Rescuer 1:* Position the child supine on a hard, flat surface. Logroll the child so there is no twisting of the spine. Place the arms alongside the body.

4 *Rescuer 1:*
  a Open the airway. Use the head tilt-chin lift method.
  b Check for adequate breathing. *Look* to see if the chest rises and falls. *Listen* for the escape of air. *Feel* for the flow of air on your cheek.
  c Give a total of 2 breaths if the child is not breathing. Each breath should take only 1 second. Each breath should make the chest rise. If a breath does not make the chest rise:
    (1) Re-open the airway with the head tilt-chin lift method.
    (2) Give another breath.
  d Check for a carotid pulse. This should take 5 to 10 seconds. Use your other hand to keep the airway open with the head tilt-chin lift method.
  e Expose the child's chest.
  f Start chest compressions if:
    (1) The child has no pulse.
    (2) The heart rate is less than 60 beats per minute and there are signs of poor circulation.
  g Give chest compressions at a rate of 100 per minute. Give 30 chest compressions followed by 2 breaths. Establish a regular rhythm, and count out loud—try "1 and, 2 and, 3 and, 4 and," so on to 15.
  h Give 2 breaths.

5 *Rescuer 2:*
  a Open the case with the AED.
  b Turn on the AED.
  c Attach child electrode pads if available. Follow the instructions and diagram provided with the AED.
  d Switch the AED to the child setting (if available).
  e Attach the connecting cables to the AED.
  f Clear away from the child. Make sure no one is touching the child.
  g Let the AED check the child's heart rhythm.
  h Make sure everyone is clear of the child if the AED advises a "shock."
  i Press the "SHOCK" button if the AED advises a "shock."

6 *Rescuers 1 and 2:*
  a Perform 2-person CPR:
    (1) One rescuer gives chest compressions at a rate of 100 per minute—15 chest compressions followed by 2 breaths. Establish a regular rhythm, and count out loud—try "1 and, 2 and, 3 and, 4 and," so on to 15.
    (2) The other rescuer gives 2 breaths after every 15 chest compressions.

7 Repeat steps 5 f, g, h, and i after 2 minutes of CPR (5 cycles of 15 compressions and 2 breaths). Then continue CPR.

INFANT CPR—ONE RESCUER

PROCEDURE

1 Check if the infant is responding. Tap the infant's foot, and shout "Are you OK?" (*NOTE:* Infants cannot answer you. However, shouting should startle the responsive infant.)
2 Call for help. If someone responds, ask the person to activate the EMS system or the agency's RRT.
3 Position the child supine on a hard, flat surface. Logroll the child so there is no twisting of the spine. Place the arms alongside the body.
4 Open the airway. Use the head tilt-chin lift method.
5 Check for adequate breathing. This should take 5 to 10 seconds.
  a *Look* to see if the chest rises and falls.
  b *Listen* for the escape of air.
  c *Feel* for the flow of air on your cheek.
6 Give a total of 2 breaths if the child is not breathing. Each breath should take only 1 second. Each breath should make the chest rise. If a breath does not make the chest rise:
  a Re-open the airway with a the head tilt-chin lift method.
  b Give another breath.

7 Check the brachial pulse. This should take 5 to 10 seconds. Use your other hand to keep the airway open with the head tilt-chin lift method.
8 Expose the child's chest.
9 Start chest compressions if:
  a The child has no pulse.
  b The heart rate is less than 60 beats per minute and there are signs of poor circulation.
10 Give chest compressions at a rate of 100 per minute. Give 30 compressions followed by 2 breaths. Establish a regular rhythm, and count out loud—try "1 and, 2 and, 3 and, 4 and," so on to 30.
11 Activate the EMS system after 5 cycles of CPR. Do this if not already done.
12 Continue CPR.

INFANT CPR—TWO RESCUERS

PROCEDURE

1 *Rescuer 1:* Check if the infant is responding. Tap the infant's foot, and shout "Are you OK?" (*NOTE:* Infants cannot answer you. However, shouting should startle the responsive infant.)
2 *Rescuer 2:* Activate the EMS system or the agency's RRT.
3 *Rescuer 1* (at the infant's side): Position the infant supine on a hard, flat surface. Logroll the infant so there is no twisting of the spine. Place the arms alongside the body.
4 *Rescuer 2* (at the infant's head):
  a Open the airway. Use the head tilt-chin lift method.
  b Check for adequate breathing. *Look* to see if the chest rises and falls. *Listen* for the escape of air. *Feel* for the flow of air on your cheek.

  c Check for a brachial pulse and for breathing, coughing, and moving. This should take 5 to 10 seconds. Use your other hand to keep the airway open with the head tilt-chin lift method.
5 Perform 2-person CPR if there are no signs of circulation:
  a *Rescuer 1:* Give chest compressions at a rate of 100 per minute—15 chest compressions followed by 2 breaths. Use the 2 thumb-encircling hands method. Establish a regular rhythm, and count out loud—try "1 and, 2 and, 3 and, 4 and," so on to 15.
  b *Rescuer 2:* Give 2 breaths after every 15 chest compressions.
  c Change positions every 2 minutes or after 5 cycles of 15 compressions and 2 breaths. The switch should take no more than 5 seconds.

◆ *Rescue Breathing*

Respiratory arrest can occur in infants and children (p. 749). Rescue breathing is done if breathing stops, but heart action continues. To provide rescue breathing:

▶ Open the airway. Use the head tilt-chin lift method.
▶ Give 1 breath every 3 to 5 seconds. Breaths are given at a rate of 12 to 20 per minute.
▶ Take 1 second to give a breath.
▶ Make sure the chest rises with each breath.
▶ Check the pulse every 2 minutes. Use the brachial pulse for infants. Use the carotid pulse for children.

HEMORRHAGE

Life and body functions require an adequate blood supply. If a blood vessel is cut or torn, bleeding occurs. The larger the blood vessel, the greater the bleeding and blood loss. **Hemorrhage** is the excessive loss of blood in a short time. If bleeding is not stopped, the person will die.

Hemorrhage is internal or external. You cannot see internal hemorrhage. The bleeding is inside body tissues and body cavities. Pain, shock, vomiting blood, coughing up blood, and loss of consciousness signal internal hemorrhage. There is little you can do for internal bleeding.

▶ Follow the rules in Box 49-1. This includes activating the EMS system.
▶ Keep the person warm, flat, and quiet until help arrives.
▶ Do not give fluids.

If not hidden by clothing, external bleeding is usually seen. Bleeding from an artery occurs in spurts. There is a steady flow of blood from a vein. To control external bleeding:

▶ Follow the rules in Box 49-1. This includes activating the EMS system.
▶ Do not remove any objects that have pierced or stabbed the person.
▶ Elevate the affected part—hand, arm, foot, or leg.
▶ Place a sterile dressing directly over the wound. Or use any clean material (handkerchief, towel, cloth, or sanitary napkin).
▶ Apply pressure with your hand directly over the bleeding site (Fig. 49-22). Do not release pressure until bleeding stops.
▶ If direct pressure does not control bleeding, apply pressure over the artery above the bleeding site (Fig. 49-23). For example, if bleeding is from the lower arm, apply pressure over the brachial artery.
▶ Bind the wound when bleeding stops. Tape or tie the dressing in place. You can tie the dressing with such things as clothing, a scarf, a necktie, or a belt.
See *Promoting Safety and Comfort: Hemorrhage.*

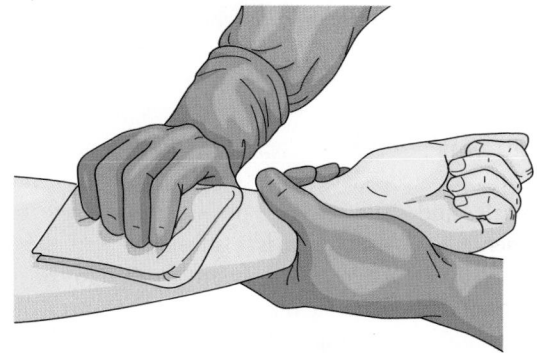

FIGURE 49-22 Direct pressure is applied to the wound to stop bleeding.

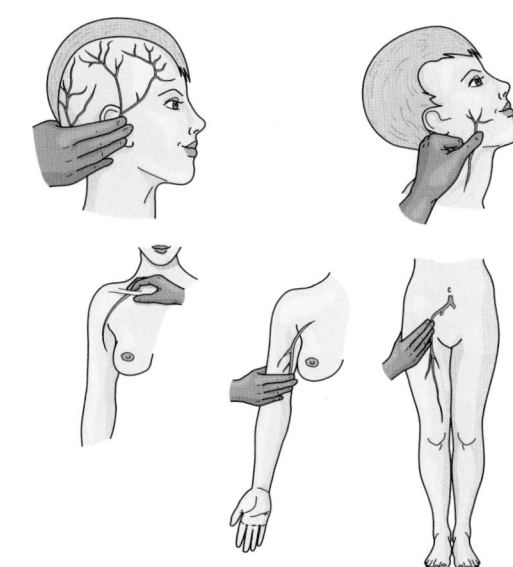

FIGURE 49-23 Pressure points to control bleeding.

PROMOTING SAFETY AND COMFORT: Hemorrhage

SAFETY

Contact with blood is likely with hemorrhage. Follow Standard Precautions and the Bloodborne Pathogen Standard to the extent possible. Wear gloves if possible. Practice hand hygiene as soon as you can.

SHOCK

Shock results when organs and tissues do not get enough blood. Blood loss, heart attack (myocardial infarction), burns, and severe infection are causes. Signs and symptoms include:

▶ Low or falling blood pressure
▶ Rapid and weak pulse
▶ Rapid respirations
▶ Cold, moist, and pale skin
▶ Thirst
▶ Restlessness
▶ Confusion and loss of consciousness as shock worsens

Shock is possible in any person who is acutely ill or severely injured. Follow the rules in Box 49-1. Maintain an open airway and control bleeding.

Anaphylactic Shock

Some people are allergic or sensitive to foods, insects, chemicals, and drugs. Many people are allergic to the drug penicillin. An *antigen* is a substance that the body reacts to. The body releases chemicals to fight or attack the antigen. The person may react with an area of redness, swelling, or itching. Or the reaction can involve the entire body.

Anaphylaxis is a life-threatening sensitivity to an antigen. (*Ana* means without. *Phylaxis* means protection.) It can occur within seconds. Signs and symptoms include:

▶ Sweating
▶ Shortness of breath
▶ Low blood pressure
▶ Irregular pulse
▶ Respiratory congestion
▶ Swelling of the larynx (laryngeal edema)
▶ Hoarseness
▶ Dyspnea

Anaphylactic shock is an emergency. The EMS system must be activated. The person needs special drugs to reverse the allergic reaction. Keep the person lying down and the airway open. Start CPR if cardiac arrest occurs.

SEIZURES

Seizures (convulsions) are violent and sudden contractions or tremors of muscle groups. Movements are uncontrolled. The person may lose consciousness. Seizures are caused by an abnormality in the brain. Causes include head injury during birth or from trauma, high fever, brain tumors, poisoning, and nervous system disorders. Lack of blood flow to the brain, seizure disorders, and epilepsy are other causes.

Epilepsy

Epilepsy is a brain disorder in which clusters of nerve cells sometimes signal abnormally. There are brief changes in the brain's electrical function. The person can have strange sensations, emotions, and behaviors. Sometimes there are seizures, muscle spasms, and loss of consciousness.

A single seizure does not mean epilepsy. In epilepsy, seizures recur. The person has a permanent brain injury or defect.

Children and young adults are commonly affected. However, epilepsy can develop at any time in a person's life. It can occur with any problem affecting the brain. Such causes include:

▶ Brain injury before, during, or after birth
▶ Problems with brain development before birth
▶ The mother having an injury or infection during pregnancy
▶ Head injury (accidents, gun shot wounds, sports injuries, falls, blows to the head)
▶ Poor nutrition

▶ Brain tumor
▶ Childhood fevers
▶ Poisoning—such as lead and alcohol
▶ Infection—such as meningitis and encephalitis
▶ Stroke

There is no cure at this time. Doctors order drugs to prevent seizures. The drugs control seizures in many people. For others, drug therapy does not work.

When controlled, epilepsy usually does not affect learning and activities of daily living. Activity and job limits occur in severe cases. For example, a person has seizures at any time. The person may not be allowed to drive. This may limit job choices. Also the person is at risk for accidents and injuries. Safety measures are needed. They are needed for the home, workplace, transportation, and recreation.

Types of Seizures

The major types of seizures are:

▶ *Partial seizure.* Only one part of the brain is involved. A body part may jerk. Or the person has a hearing or vision problem or stomach discomfort. The person does not lose consciousness.
▶ *Generalized tonic-clonic seizure (grand mal seizure).* This type has two phases. In the *tonic phase*, the person loses consciousness. If standing or sitting, the person falls to the floor. The body is rigid because all muscles contract at once. The *clonic phase* follows. Muscle groups contract and relax. This causes jerking and twitching movements. Urinary and fecal incontinence may occur. A deep sleep is common after the seizure. Confusion and headache may occur on awakening.
▶ *Generalized absence (petit mal) seizure.* This type usually lasts a few seconds. There is loss of consciousness, twitching of the eyelids, and staring. No first aid is necessary. However, you should guide the person away from dangers—stairs, streets, a hot stove, fireplaces, and so on.

Emergency Care

You cannot stop a seizure. However you can protect the person from injury:

▶ Follow the rules in Box 49-1. This includes activating the EMS system.
▶ Do not leave the person alone.
▶ Lower the person to the floor. This protects the person from falling.
▶ Note the time the seizure started.
▶ Place something soft under the person's head (Fig. 49-24). It prevents the person's head from striking the floor. You can use a pillow, a cushion, or a folded blanket, towel, or jacket. Or cradle the person's head in your lap.
▶ Loosen tight jewelry and clothing (ties, scarves, collars, necklaces) around the person's neck.
▶ Turn the person onto his or her side. Make sure the head is turned to the side.

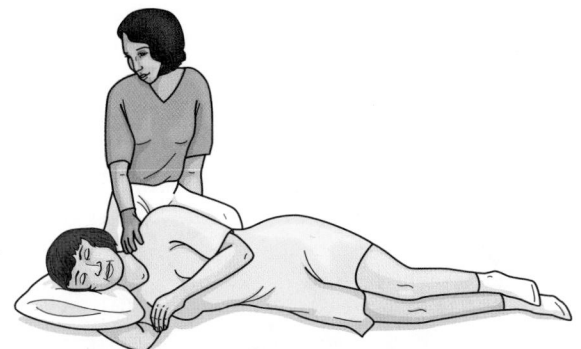

FIGURE 49-24 A pillow protects the person's head during a seizure.

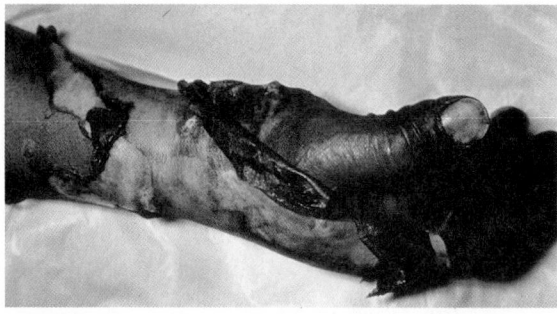

FIGURE 49-25 Full thickness burn. (From Ignatavicius DD, Workman ML: *Medical-surgical nursing: critical thinking for collaborative care,* ed 5, St Louis, 2006, Saunders.)

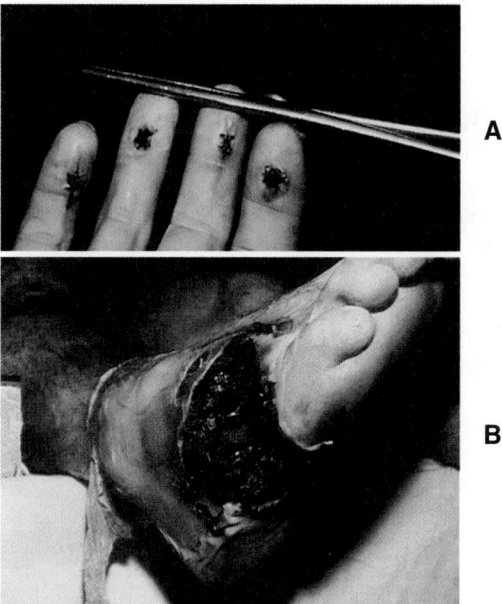

FIGURE 49-26 An electrical burn. **A,** The electrical current enters through the hand. **B,** The electrical current exits through the foot. (From Sanders M: *Mosby's paramedic textbook,* St Louis, 1994, Mosby.)

▶ Do not put any object or your fingers between the person's teeth. The person can bite down on your fingers during the seizure.

▶ Do not try to stop the seizure or control the person's movements.

▶ Move furniture, equipment, and sharp objects away from the person. He or she may strike these objects during the seizure.

▶ Note the time when the seizure ends.

▶ Make sure the mouth is clear of food, fluids, and saliva after the seizure.

▶ Provide BLS if the person is not breathing after the seizure.

BURNS

Burns can severely disable a person (Fig. 49-25). They can also cause death. Most burns occur in the home. Infants and children are at risk. So are older persons. Common causes of burns and fires are:

▶ Scalds from hot liquids

▶ Playing with matches and lighters

▶ Electrical injuries (Fig. 49-26)

▶ Cooking accidents (barbecues, microwaves, stoves, ovens)

▶ Falling asleep while smoking

▶ Fireplaces

▶ Space heaters

▶ No smoke detectors or non-functioning smoke detectors

▶ Sunburn

▶ Chemicals

The skin has two layers: the dermis and epidermis. Burns are described as partial thickness and full thickness:

▶ *Partial thickness burns*—involve the epidermis and part of the dermis. They are very painful. Nerve endings are exposed.

▶ *Full thickness burns*—involve the entire epidermis and dermis. Fat, muscle, and bone may be injured or destroyed. These burns are not painful. Nerve endings are destroyed.

Some burns are minor; others are severe. Severity depends on burn size and depth, the body part involved, and the person's age. Burns to the face, eyes, ears, hands, and feet are more serious than burns to an arm or leg. Infants, young children, and older persons are at high risk for death.

Emergency care of burns includes the following:

▶ Follow the rules in Box 49-1. This includes activating the EMS system.

▶ Do not touch the person if he or she is in contact with an electrical source. Have the power source turned off, or remove the electrical source. Use an object that does not conduct electricity (rope or wood) to remove the electrical source.

▶ Remove the person from the fire or burn source.

▶ Stop the burning process. Put out flames with water or roll the person in a blanket. Or smother flames with a coat, sheet, or towel.

List continued on p. 766.

- ▶ Do not remove burned clothing.
- ▶ Remove hot clothing that is not sticking to the skin. If you cannot remove hot clothing, cool the clothing with water.
- ▶ Remove jewelry and any tight clothing that is not sticking to the skin.
- ▶ Provide rescue breathing and CPR as needed.
- ▶ Cover burns with sterile, cool, moist coverings. Or use towels, sheets, or any other clean cloth. Keep the covering wet.
- ▶ Do not put oil, butter, salve, or ointments on the burns.
- ▶ Cover the person with a blanket or coat to prevent heat loss.
  See *Focus on Children and Older Persons: Burns.*

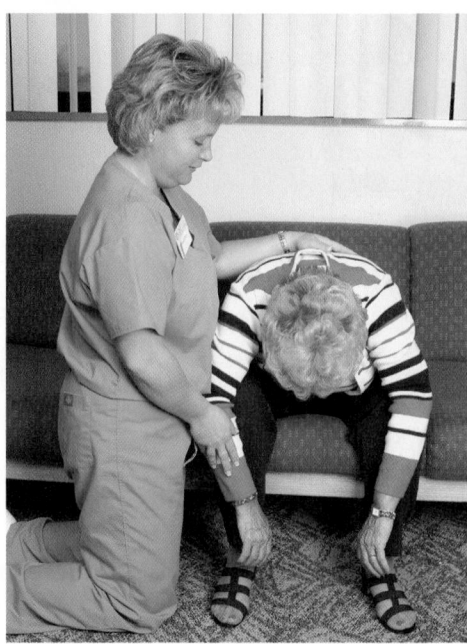

FIGURE 49-27 The person bends forward and lowers her head between her knees to prevent fainting.

FOCUS ON CHILDREN AND OLDER PERSONS

Burns

CHILDREN
Infants and children are at risk for burns. Severe burns can be fatal. Remember, infants and young children do not know the difference between safety and danger. They cannot protect themselves. They rely on adults for protection.

OLDER PERSONS
Older persons are at risk for burns. Severe burns can be fatal. Spilling hot liquids is a common cause of burns in older persons. Weakness and poor coordination put some older persons at risk. They need to be careful when handling hot liquids and when cooking.

FAINTING

Fainting is the sudden loss of consciousness from an inadequate blood supply to the brain. Hunger, fatigue, fear, and pain are common causes. Some people faint at the sight of blood or injury. Standing in one position for a long time and being in a warm, crowded room are other causes. Dizziness, perspiration, and blackness before the eyes are warning signals. The person looks pale. The pulse is weak. Respirations are shallow if consciousness is lost. Emergency care for fainting includes the following:

- ▶ Have the person sit or lie down before fainting occurs.
- ▶ If sitting, the person bends forward and places the head between the knees (Fig. 49-27).
- ▶ If the person is lying down, raise the legs.
- ▶ Loosen tight clothing (belts, ties, scarves, collars, and so on).
- ▶ Keep the person lying down if fainting has occurred. Raise the legs.
- ▶ Do not let the person get up until symptoms have subsided for about 5 minutes.
- ▶ Help the person to a sitting position after recovery from fainting. Observe for fainting.

STROKE

Stroke (cerebrovascular accident) occurs when the brain is suddenly deprived of its blood supply (Chapter 39). Usually only part of the brain is affected. A stroke may be caused by a thrombus, an embolus, or hemorrhage if a blood vessel in the brain ruptures.

Signs of stroke vary (Chapter 39). They depend on the size and location of brain injury. Loss of consciousness or semi-consciousness, rapid pulse, labored respirations, high blood pressure, and hemiplegia are signs of a stroke. The person may have slurred speech or aphasia (the inability to have normal speech). Loss of vision in one eye, unsteadiness, and falling also are signs. Seizures may occur.

Emergency care includes the following:

- ▶ Follow the rules in Box 49-1. This includes activating the EMS system.
- ▶ Position the person in the recovery position on the affected side (see Fig. 49-15). The affected side is limp, and the cheek appears puffy.
- ▶ Raise the head without flexing the neck.
- ▶ Loosen tight clothing (belts, ties, scarves, collars, and so on).
- ▶ Keep the person quiet and warm.
- ▶ Reassure the person.
- ▶ Provide CPR if necessary.
- ▶ Provide emergency care for seizures if necessary.

QUALITY OF LIFE

Protect quality of life during emergencies. Treat the person with dignity and respect.

Protect the right to privacy and confidentiality. Do not expose the person unnecessarily. You may be in a place where you cannot close doors or window coverings. The person may be in a lounge, dining area, or public place. Do what you can to provide privacy.

Protect the person from onlookers. (See *Teamwork and Time Management: Emergency Care* on p. 748.) People are curious. They want to know what happened, the extent of injuries or illness, and if the person will be okay. Only doctors diagnose. You can make observations about signs and symptoms. The doctor determines what is wrong with the person. Do not discuss the situation. Information about the person's care, treatment, and condition is confidential.

Protect the right to personal choice. Choices are few in emergencies. They are given when possible. Hospital care may be required. The person has the right to choose a hospital.

Protect personal items from loss and damage. Dentures, eyeglasses, and hearing aids are often lost or broken in emergencies. Watches and jewelry are easily lost. Clothing may be torn or cut. Be very careful to protect the person's property. In public places, personal items are given to the police or EMS personnel.

Physical and psychological safety is important. Protect the person from further injury. For example, protect the person from falls after a stroke. Protect the person's head during a seizure. The person needs to feel safe and secure. Reassurance, explanations about care, and a calm approach are helpful.

REVIEW QUESTIONS

Circle the BEST answer.

1 The goals of first aid are to
   a Call for help and keep the person warm
   b Prevent death and prevent injuries from becoming worse
   c Stay calm and give emergency care
   d Calm the person and keep bystanders away

2 When giving first aid, you should
   a Be aware of your own limits
   b Move the person
   c Give the person fluids
   d Remove clothing

3 Sudden cardiac arrest is
   a The same as stroke
   b The sudden stopping of heart action and breathing
   c The sudden loss of consciousness
   d When organs and tissues do not get enough blood

4 Which is *not* a sign of sudden cardiac arrest?
   a No pulse
   b No breathing
   c A sudden drop in blood pressure
   d Unconsciousness

5 Mouth-to-mouth breathing for an adult involves the following *except*
   a Pinching the nostrils shut
   b Placing your mouth tightly over the person's mouth
   c Blowing air into the mouth as you exhale
   d Covering the nose with your mouth

6 Chest compressions are performed on an adult. The chest is compressed
   a ½ to 1 inch with the index and middle fingers
   b 1 to 1½ inches with the heel of one hand
   c 1½ to 2 inches with two hands
   d With one hand in the middle of the sternum

7 Which does *not* determine adequate breathing?
   a Looking to see if the chest rises and falls
   b Counting respirations for 30 seconds
   c Listening for the escape of air
   d Feeling for the flow of air

8 Which pulse is used during adult CPR?
   a The apical pulse
   b The brachial pulse
   c The carotid pulse
   d The femoral pulse

9 How many breaths are given when CPR is started?
   a 1   c 3
   b 2   d 4

10 You are doing adult CPR alone. Which is *true*?
   a Give 2 breaths after every 15 compressions.
   b Give 2 breaths after every 30 compressions.
   c Give 1 breath after every 5 compressions.
   d Give 2 breaths when you are tired from giving compressions.

Continued

11 Two rescuers are giving adult CPR. Breaths are given
  a After every compression
  b After every 5 compressions
  c After every 15 compressions
  d After every 30 compressions

12 For infant and child CPR, chest compressions are given at a rate of
  a 60 per minute   c 80 per minute
  b 75 per minute   d 100 per minute

13 For 1 rescuer child or infant CPR
  a 5 compressions are given followed by 2 breaths
  b 10 compressions are given followed by 2 breaths
  c 15 compressions are given followed by 2 breaths
  d 30 compressions are given followed by 2 breaths

14 Arterial bleeding
  a Cannot be seen   c Is dark red
  b Occurs in spurts   d Oozes from the wound

15 A person is hemorrhaging from the left forearm. Your first action is to
  a Lower the arm
  b Apply pressure to the brachial artery
  c Apply direct pressure to the wound
  d Tape a dressing in place

16 Which is *not* a sign of shock?
  a High blood pressure
  b Rapid pulse
  c Rapid respirations
  d Cold, moist, and pale skin

17 A person in shock needs
  a BLS procedures
  b To be kept lying down
  c Clothes removed
  d The recovery position

18 These statements relate to tonic-clonic seizures. Which is *false*?
  a There is contraction of all muscles at once.
  b Incontinence may occur.
  c The seizure lasts 5 seconds.
  d There is loss of consciousness.

19 A person was burned. There are no complaints or signs of pain. You know that
  a The burn is minor
  b The burn is partial thickness
  c The burn is full thickness
  d It is an electrical burn

20 Burns are covered with
  a A clean, moist cloth or dressing
  b Butter, oil, or salve
  c Water
  d Nothing

21 A person is about to faint. Which is *false*?
  a Take the person outside for fresh air.
  b Have the person sit or lie down.
  c Loosen tight clothing.
  d Raise the legs if the person is lying down.

22 A person is having a stroke. Emergency care involves the following *except*
  a Positioning the person on the affected side
  b Giving the person sips of water
  c Loosening tight clothing
  d Keeping the person quiet and warm.

Answers to these questions are on p. 782.

The Dying Person

OBJECTIVES

- Define the key terms and key abbreviations listed in this chapter
- Describe terminal illness
- Describe the factors that affect attitudes about death
- Describe how different age-groups view death
- Describe the five stages of dying
- Explain how to meet the needs of the dying person and family
- Describe hospice care
- Explain the purpose of the Patient Self-Determination Act
- Explain what is meant by a "Do Not Resuscitate" order
- Identify the signs of approaching death and the signs of death
- Explain how to assist with postmortem care
- Perform the procedure described in this chapter

PROCEDURE

- Assisting With Postmortem Care

KEY TERMS

advance directive A document stating a person's wishes about health care when that person cannot make his or her own decisions

autopsy The examination of the body after death

postmortem care Care of the body after *(post)* death *(mortem)*

reincarnation The belief that the spirit or soul is reborn in another human body or in another form of life

rigor mortis The stiffness or rigidity *(rigor)* of skeletal muscles that occurs after death *(mortis)*

terminal illness An illness or injury for which there is no reasonable expectation of recovery

KEY ABBREVIATIONS

CPR Cardiopulmonary resuscitation

DNR Do Not Resuscitate

NG Nasogastric

OBRA Omnibus Budget Reconciliation Act of 1987

Sometimes death is sudden. Often it is expected. Health team members see death often. Many are unsure of their feelings about death. Dying persons and the subject of death cause them discomfort. Death and dying mean helplessness and failure to cure. They also remind us that our loved ones and we will die.

Your feelings about death affect the care you give. You will help meet the dying person's physical, psychological, social, and spiritual needs. Therefore you must understand the dying process. Then you can approach the dying person with caring, kindness, and respect.

See *Teamwork and Time Management: The Dying Person.*

TERMINAL ILLNESS

Many illnesses and diseases have no cure. Some injuries are so serious that the body cannot function. Recovery is not expected. The disease or injury ends in death. An illness or injury for which there is no reasonable expectation of recovery is a **terminal illness.**

Doctors cannot predict the exact time of death. A person may have days, months, weeks, or years to live. People expected to live for a short time have lived for years. Others expected to live longer have died sooner than expected.

Modern medicine has found cures or has prolonged life in many cases. Research will bring new cures. However, hope and the will to live strongly influence living and dying. Many people have died for no apparent reason when they have lost hope or the will to live.

ATTITUDES ABOUT DEATH

Experiences, culture, religion, and age influence attitudes about death. Many people fear death. Others do not believe they will die. Some look forward to and accept death. Attitudes about death often change as a person grows older and with changing circumstances.

Dying people often need hospital, nursing center, hospice, or home care. The family is often involved in the person's care. They usually gather at the bedside to comfort the person and each other. When death occurs, the funeral director is called. He or she takes the body to the funeral home to prepare it for funeral practices.

Many adults and children never have had contact with a dying person. Nor have they been present at the time of death. Some have not attended a visitation (wake) or funeral. They have not seen the process of dying and death. Therefore it is frightening, morbid, and a mystery.

Culture and Religion

Practices and attitudes about death differ among cultures. See *Caring About Culture: Death Rites.* In some cultures, dying people are cared for at home by the family. Some families prepare the body for burial.

Attitudes about death are closely related to religion. Some believe that life after death is free of suffering and hardship. They also believe in reunion with loved ones. Many believe sins and misdeeds are punished in the afterlife. Others do not believe in the afterlife. To them, death is the end of life.

There also are religious beliefs about the body's form after death. Some believe the body keeps its physical form. Others believe that only the spirit or soul is present in the afterlife. **Reincarnation** is the belief that the spirit or soul is reborn in another human body or in another form of life.

Many people strengthen their religious beliefs when dying. Religion provides comfort for the dying person and the family.

Many religions practice rites and rituals during the dying process and at the time of death. Prayers, blessings, and scripture readings are common in many religions.

TEAMWORK AND TIME MANAGEMENT

The Dying Person

The nurse may need to spend a lot of time with the dying person. Often it is a busy time before and after someone dies. Offer to take equipment and supplies to and from the room. Also offer to help with other patients and residents.

Death Rites

In *Vietnam,* quality of life is more important than length of life because of beliefs in reincarnation. Less suffering in the next life is expected. Therefore dying persons are helped to recall past good deeds and to achieve a fitting mental state. Death at home is preferred over death in the hospital. Upon death, the body is washed and wrapped in clean, white sheets. In some areas a coin or jewels (a wealthy family) and rice (a poor family) are put in the dead person's mouth. This is from the belief that they will help the soul go through encounters with gods and devils and the soul will be born rich in the next life. Relatives sew small pillows to place under the body's neck, feet, and wrists. The body is placed in a coffin for in-ground burial.

The *Chinese* have an aversion to death and anything concerning death. Autopsy and disposal of the body are not prescribed by religion. Donating body parts is encouraged. The eldest son makes all arrangements. The body is buried in a coffin. After 7 years, the body is exhumed and cremated. The urn, containing the ashes, is buried in the tomb. White or yellow and black clothing is worn for mourning.

In *India,* Hindu persons are often accepting of God's will. The person's desire to be clear-headed as death nears must be assessed in planning medical treatment. A time and place for prayer are essential for the family and the person. Prayer helps them deal with anxiety and conflict. The Hindu priest reads from Holy Sanskrit books. Some priests tie strings (meaning a blessing) around the neck or wrist. After death, the son pours water into the mouth of the deceased. Blood transfusions, organ transplants, and autopsies are allowed. Cremation is preferred. Reincarnation is a Hindu belief.

From D'Avanzo CE, Geissler EM: *Pocket guide to cultural health assessment,* ed 3, St Louis, 2003, Mosby.

Age

Adults fear pain and suffering, dying alone, and the invasion of privacy. They also fear loneliness and separation from loved ones. They worry about the care and support of those left behind. Adults often resent death because it affects plans, hopes, dreams, and ambitions.

See *Focus on Children and Older Persons: Attitudes About Death.*

THE STAGES OF DYING

Dr. Elisabeth Kübler-Ross described five stages of dying.

► *Stage 1: Denial.* The person refuses to believe that he or she is dying. "No, not me" is a common response. The person believes a mistake was made. Information about the illness or injury is not heard. The person cannot deal with any problem or decision about the matter. This stage can last for a few hours, days, or much longer. Some people are still in denial when they die.

► *Stage 2: Anger.* The person thinks "Why me?" There is anger and rage. Dying persons envy and resent those with life and health. Family, friends, and the health team are often targets of anger. The person blames others and finds fault with those who are loved and needed the most. It is hard to deal with the person during this stage. Anger is normal and healthy. Do not take the person's anger personally. Control any urge to attack back or avoid the person.

Attitudes About Death

CHILDREN

Infants and toddlers do not understand the nature or meaning of death. They are aware of or sense that something is different. They sense that a caregiver is absent or that there is a different caregiver. They also sense changes in when and how their needs are met. They may feel a sense of loss.

Between 2 and 6 years old, children think death is temporary. Death can be reversed. The dead person continues to live and function in some ways. The dead person can come back to life. These ideas come from fairy tales, cartoons, movies, video games, and TV. For example, a cartoon character is injured and dies. Later the character comes back to life, whole and intact. Children this age often blame themselves when someone or something dies. To them, death is punishment for being bad. They know when family members or pets die. They notice dead birds or bugs. Answers to questions about death often cause fear and confusion. Children who are told "He is sleeping" may be afraid to go to sleep.

Between 6 and 11 years, children learn that death is final. They do not think that they will die. Death happens to other people, especially adults. It can be avoided. Children relate death to punishment and body mutilation. It also involves witches, ghosts, goblins, and monsters.

By age 11, children more fully understand death. Death is still viewed as something that happens to other people. One's own death is viewed as an event in the distant future. Without correct information, they may have some wrong ideas. However, understanding increases as they grow older and have more experiences with death.

OLDER PERSONS

Older persons usually have fewer fears than younger adults. They know death will occur. They have had more experiences with dying and death. Many have lost family and friends. Some welcome death as freedom from pain, suffering, and disability. Death also means reunion with those who have died. Like younger adults, they often fear dying alone.

► *Stage 3: Bargaining.* Anger has passed. The person now says "Yes, me, but. . . ." Often the person bargains with God for more time. Promises are made in exchange for more time. The person may want to see a child marry, see a grandchild, have one more Christmas, or live for some other event. Usually more promises are made as the person makes "just one more" request. You may not see this stage. Bargaining is usually private and spiritual.

► *Stage 4: Depression.* The person thinks "Yes, me" and is very sad. The person mourns things that were lost and the future loss of life. The person may cry or say little. Sometimes the person talks about people and things that will be left behind.

► *Stage 5: Acceptance.* The person is calm and at peace. The person has said what needs to be said. Unfinished business is completed. The person accepts death. This stage may last for many months or years. Reaching the acceptance stage does not mean death is near.

Dying persons do not always pass through all five stages. A person may never get beyond a certain stage. Some move back and forth between stages. For example, Mr. Jones reached acceptance but moves back to bargaining. Then he moves forward to acceptance. Some people stay in one stage.

PSYCHOLOGICAL, SOCIAL, AND SPIRITUAL NEEDS

Dying people have psychological, social, and spiritual needs. They may want family and friends present. They may want to talk about their fears, worries, and anxieties. Some want to be alone. Often they need to talk during the night. Things are quiet. There are few distractions, and there is more time to think. You need to listen and use touch.

▶ *Listening.* The person needs to talk and share worries and concerns. Let the person express feelings and emotions in his or her own way. Do not worry about saying the wrong thing or finding comforting words. You do not need to say anything. Being there for the person is what counts.

▶ *Touch.* Touch shows caring and concern when words cannot. Sometimes the person does not want to talk but needs you nearby. Do not feel that you need to talk. Silence, along with touch, is a powerful and meaningful way to communicate.

Some people may want to see a spiritual leader. Or they want to take part in religious practices. Provide privacy during prayer and spiritual moments. Be courteous to the spiritual leader. The person has the right to have religious objects nearby—medals, pictures, statues, writings, and so on. Handle these valuables with care and respect.

See *Focus on Communication: Psychological and Spiritual Needs.*

PHYSICAL NEEDS

Dying may take a few minutes, hours, days, or weeks. Body processes slow. The person is weak. Changes occur in levels of consciousness. To the extent possible, independence is allowed. As the person weakens, basic needs are met. The person may depend on others for basic needs and activities of daily living. Every effort is made to promote physical and psychological comfort. The person is allowed to die in peace and with dignity.

FOCUS ON COMMUNICATION

Psychological and Spiritual Needs

You may not know what to say to the dying person. That is hard for many experienced health team members. Unless you have been near death yourself, do not say "I understand what you are going through." The statement is a communication barrier. Instead you can say:

• "Would you like to talk? I have time to listen."
• "You seem sad. How can I help?"
• "Is it okay if I quietly sit with you for a while?"

Vision, Hearing, and Speech

Vision blurs and gradually fails. The person naturally turns toward light. A darkened room may frighten the person. The eyes may be half-open. Secretions may collect in the eye corners.

Because of failing vision, explain what you are doing to the person or in the room. The room should be well lit. However, avoid bright lights and glares.

Good eye care is essential (Chapter 19). If the eyes stay open, a nurse may apply a protective ointment. Then the eyes are covered with moist pads to prevent injury.

Hearing is one of the last functions lost. Many people hear until the moment of death. Even unconscious persons may hear. Always assume that the person can hear. Speak in a normal voice. Provide reassurance and explanations about care. Offer words of comfort. Avoid topics that could upset the person.

Speech becomes harder. It may be hard to understand the person. Sometimes the person cannot speak. Anticipate the person's needs. Do not ask questions that need long answers. Ask "yes" or "no" questions. These should be few in number. Despite speech problems, you must talk to the person.

Mouth, Nose, and Skin

Oral hygiene promotes comfort. Give routine mouth care if the person can eat and drink. Frequent oral hygiene is given as death nears and when taking oral fluids is difficult. Oral hygiene is needed if mucus collects in the mouth and the person cannot swallow.

Crusting and irritation of the nostrils can occur. Nasal secretions, an oxygen cannula, and an NG (nasogastric) tube are common causes. Carefully clean the nose. Apply lubricant as directed by the nurse and the care plan.

Circulation fails and body temperature rises as death nears. The skin feels cool, pale, and mottled (blotchy). Perspiration increases. Skin care, bathing, and preventing pressure ulcers are necessary. Linens and gowns are changed whenever needed. Although the skin feels cool, only light bed coverings are needed. Blankets may make the person feel warm and cause restlessness.

Elimination

Urinary and fecal incontinence may occur. Use incontinence products or bed protectors as directed. Give perineal care as needed. Constipation and urinary retention are common. Enemas and catheters may be needed. Provide catheter care according to the care plan.

Comfort and Positioning

Skin care, personal and oral hygiene, back massages, and good alignment promote comfort. Some persons have severe pain. The nurse gives pain relief drugs ordered by the doctor. Frequent position changes and supportive devices promote comfort. Turn the person slowly and gently. Semi-Fowler's position is usually best for breathing problems.

The Person's Room

Provide a comfortable and pleasant room. It should be well lit and well ventilated. Remove unnecessary equipment. Some equipment is upsetting to look at (suction machines, drainage containers). If possible, keep these items out of the person's sight.

Mementos, pictures, cards, flowers, and religious items provide comfort. Arrange them within the person's view. The person and family arrange the room as they wish. This helps meet love, belonging, and self-esteem needs. The room should reflect the person's choices.

THE FAMILY

This is a hard time for the family. It may be very hard to find comforting words. Show you care by being available, courteous, and considerate. Use touch to show your concern.

The family usually is allowed to stay as long as they wish. Sometimes family members stay during the night. The health team makes them as comfortable as possible.

Respect the right to privacy. The person and family need time together. However, do not neglect care because the family is present. Most agencies let family members help give care. Or you can suggest that they take a break for a beverage or meal.

The family may be very tired, sad, and tearful. Watching a loved one die is very painful. So is dealing with the eventual loss of that person. The family goes through stages like the dying person. They need support, understanding, courtesy, and respect. A spiritual leader may provide comfort. Communicate this request to the nurse at once.

HOSPICE CARE

Hospice care focuses on the physical, emotional, social, and spiritual needs of dying persons and their families (Chapter 1). It is not concerned with cure or life-saving measures. Pain relief and comfort are stressed. The goal is to improve the dying person's quality of life.

A hospice may be part of a hospital, nursing center, or home care agency. It may be a separate agency. Many hospices offer home care. The sponsoring agency provides hospice training for the health team.

Follow-up care and support groups for survivors are hospice services. Hospice also provides support for the health team to deal with a person's death.

LEGAL ISSUES

Much attention is given to the right to die. Many people do not want machines or other measures keeping them alive. Consent is needed for any treatment. When able, the person makes care decisions. Some people make end-of-life wishes known.

The Patient Self-Determination Act

The Patient Self-Determination Act and the Omnibus Budget Reconciliation Act of 1987 (OBRA) give persons the right to accept or refuse medical treatment. They also give the right to make advance directives. An **advance directive** is a document stating a person's wishes about health care when that person cannot make his or her own decisions. Advance directives usually forbid certain care if there is no hope of recovery. Living wills and durable power of attorney for health care are common advance directives.

These laws protect quality of care. Quality of care cannot be less because of the person's advance directives.

Health care agencies must inform all persons of the right to advance directives on admission. This information is in writing. The medical record must document whether or not the person has made them.

Living Wills

A living will is a document about measures that support or maintain life when death is likely. Tube feedings, ventilators, and CPR (cardiopulmonary resuscitation) are examples. A living will may instruct doctors:

▶ Not to start measures that prolong dying
▶ To remove measures that prolong dying

Durable Power of Attorney for Health Care

This advance directive gives the power to make health care decisions to another person. Usually this is a family member, friend, or lawyer. When a person cannot make health care decisions, the person with durable power of attorney can do so.

"Do Not Resuscitate" Orders

When death is sudden and unexpected, efforts are made to save the person's life. Basic life support (Chapter 49) is given. The agency's RRT is activated. Doctors, nurses, and other staff rush to the person. They bring emergency and life-saving equipment. CPR and other life-support measures are continued until the person is resuscitated or until the doctor declares the person dead.

Doctors often write "Do Not Resuscitate" (DNR) or "No Code" orders for terminally ill persons. This means that the person will not be resuscitated. The person is allowed to die with peace and dignity. The orders are written after consulting with the person and family. The family and doctor make the decision if the person is not mentally able to do so. Some advance directives address resuscitation.

You may not agree with care and resuscitation decisions. However, you must follow the person's or family's wishes and the doctor's orders. These may be against your personal, religious, and cultural values. If so, discuss the matter with the nurse. An assignment change may be needed.

QUALITY OF LIFE

A person has the right to die in peace and with dignity. Box 50-1 contains the dying person's bill of rights.

See *Focus on Long-Term Care and Home Care: Quality of life.*

BOX 50-1 A Dying Patient's Bill of Last Rights

- *The Right to BE IN CONTROL.* Grant me the right to make as many decisions as possible regarding my care. Please do not take choices from me. Let me make my own decisions.
- *The Right to HAVE A SENSE OF PURPOSE.* I have lost my job. I can no longer fulfill my role in my family. Please help me find some sense of purpose in my last days.
- *The Right to REMINISCE.* There has been pleasure in my life, moments of pride, moments of love. Please give some time to recollect those moments. And please listen to my recollections.
- *The Right to TOUCH AND BE TOUCHED.* Sometimes I need distance. Yet sometimes I have a strong need to be close. When I want to reach out, please come to me and hold me as I hold you.
- *The Right to LAUGH.* People often—far too often—come to me wearing masks of seriousness. Although I am dying, I still need to laugh. Please laugh with me and help others to laugh as well.
- *The Right to BE ANGRY AND SAD.* It is difficult to leave behind all my attachments and all that I love. Please allow me the opportunity to be angry and sad.
- *The Right to HAVE A RESPECTED SPIRITUALITY.* Whether I am questioning or affirming, doubting or praising, I sometimes need your ear, a non-judging ear. Please let my spirit travel its own journey, without judging its direction.
- *The Right to HEAR THE TRUTH.* If you withhold the truth from me, you will treat me as if I am no longer living. I am still living, and I need to know the truth about my life. Please help me find that truth.
- *The Right to BE IN DENIAL.* If I hear the truth and choose not to accept it, that is my right.
  Honor these Rights. One day you too will want the same Rights.

Modified from *The Hospice RN: Patient's bill of rights: a dying patient's bill of last rights.*

Quality of Life

LONG-TERM CARE

The dying person also has these rights under OBRA:

- *The right to privacy before and after death.* Do not expose the person unnecessarily. The person has the right not to have his or her body seen by others. Proper draping and screening are important.
- *The right to visit others in private.* If the person is too weak to leave the room, the roommate may have to do so. The nurse and social worker develop a plan that satisfies everyone. Moving the dying person to a private room provides privacy. The family can also stay as long as they like.
- *The right to confidentiality before and after death.* Only those involved in care need to know the person's diagnosis and condition. The final moments and cause of death also are kept confidential. So are statements, conversations, and family reactions.
- *The right to be free from abuse, mistreatment, and neglect.* Some health team members avoid dying persons. They are uncomfortable with death and dying. Others have religious or cultural beliefs about being near dying people. Neglect is possible. So is abuse or mistreatment. Family, friends, or staff may be sources of such actions. The dying person may be too weak to report the abuse or mistreatment. Or the person may feel that the punishment is deserved for needing so much care. The person has the right to receive kind and respectful care before and after death. Always report signs of abuse, mistreatment, or neglect to the nurse at once.
- *Freedom from restraint.* Restraints are used only if ordered by the doctor. Dying persons are often too weak to pose dangers to themselves or others.
- *The right to have personal possessions.* You must protect the person's property. The person may want photos and religious items nearby. Protect the person's property from loss or damage before and after death. They may be family treasures or mementos.
- *The right to a safe and home-like setting.* Dying persons depend on others for safety. Everyone must keep the setting safe and home-like. The center is the person's home. Try to keep equipment and supplies out of view. The room also should be free from unpleasant odors and noises. Do your best to keep the room neat and clean.
- *The right to personal choice.* The person has the right to be involved in treatment and care. The dying person may refuse treatment. Advance directives are common. Some persons cannot make treatment decisions. The family or legal representative does so. The decision may be to allow the person to die with peace and dignity. The health team must respect choices to refuse treatment or not prolong life.

Signs of Death

HOME CARE

Death often occurs in the home setting. Before the body is taken to the funeral home, the person must be pronounced dead. This is a legal requirement. So is contacting the coroner or medical examiner. State laws and agency policies vary. If a person dies at home, call the nurse. The nurse decides what to do.

SIGNS OF DEATH

There are signs that death is near. These signs may occur rapidly or slowly:

- Movement, muscle tone, and sensation are lost. This usually starts in the feet and legs. When mouth muscles relax, the jaw drops. The mouth may stay open. The facial expression is often peaceful.
- Peristalsis and other gastrointestinal functions slow down. Abdominal distention, fecal incontinence, nausea, and vomiting are common.
- Body temperature rises. The person feels cool or cold, looks pale, and perspires heavily.
- Circulation fails. The pulse is fast, weak, and irregular. Blood pressure starts to fall.
- The respiratory system fails. Slow or rapid and shallow respirations are observed. Mucus collects in the airway. This causes the *death rattle* that is heard.
- Pain decreases as the person loses consciousness. However, some people are conscious until the moment of death.

The signs of death include no pulse, no respirations, and no blood pressure. The pupils are fixed and dilated. A doctor determines that death has occurred. He or she pronounces the person dead.

See *Focus on Long-Term Care and Home Care: Signs of Death.*

◄ CARE OF THE BODY AFTER DEATH

Care of the body after (*post*) death (*mortem*) is called **postmortem care.** A nurse gives postmortem care. You may be asked to assist. Postmortem care begins when the doctor pronounces the person dead.

Postmortem care is done to maintain a good appearance of the body. Discoloration and skin damage are prevented. Valuables and personal items are gathered for the family. The right to privacy and the right to be treated with dignity and respect apply after death.

Within 2 to 4 hours after death, rigor mortis develops. **Rigor mortis** is the stiffness or rigidity (*rigor*) of skeletal muscles that occurs after death (*mortis*). The body is positioned in normal alignment before rigor mortis sets in. The family may want to see the body. The body should appear in a comfortable and natural position for this viewing.

In some agencies, the body is prepared only for viewing by the family. The funeral director completes postmortem care.

Sometimes an autopsy is done. An **autopsy** is the examination of the body after death. (*Autos* means *self. Opsis* means *view.*) Its purpose is to determine the cause of death. The coroner or medical examiner can order an autopsy. Or the family can request one. Follow agency procedures when an autopsy is to be done. Postmortem care is not done. Doing so could remove or destroy evidence.

Postmortem care involves moving the body. For example, soiled areas are bathed and the body is placed in good alignment. Moving the body can cause remaining air in the lungs, stomach, and intestines to be expelled. When air is expelled, sounds are produced. Do not let these sounds alarm or frighten you. They are normal and expected.

See *Delegation Guidelines: Postmortem Care.*
See *Promoting Safety and Comfort: Postmortem Care.*

When assisting with postmortem care, you need this information from the nurse:
- If dentures will be inserted or placed in a denture cup
- If tubes and dressings will be removed or left in place
- If rings will be removed or left in place
- If the family wants to view the body
- Special agency policies and procedures

SAFETY
Standard Precautions and the Bloodborne Pathogen Standard are followed. You may have contact with blood, body fluids, secretions, or excretions.

ASSISTING WITH POSTMORTEM CARE

PRE-PROCEDURE

1 Follow *Delegation Guidelines: Postmortem Care*, p. 775. See *Promoting Safety and Comfort: Postmortem Care*, p. 775.
2 Practice hand hygiene.
3 Collect the following:
   - Postmortem kit (shroud or body bag, gown, ID tags, gauze squares, safety pins)
   - Bed protectors
   - Wash basin
   - Bath towel and washcloths
   - Denture cup
   - Tape
   - Dressings
   - Gloves
   - Cotton balls
   - Valuables envelope
4 Provide for privacy.
5 Raise the bed for good body mechanics.
6 Make sure the bed is flat.

PROCEDURE

7 Put on the gloves.
8 Position the body supine. Arms and legs are straight. A pillow is under the head and shoulders. Or raise the head of the bed 15 to 20 degrees if this is agency policy.
9 Close the eyes. Gently pull the eyelids over the eyes. Apply moist cotton balls gently over the eyelids if the eyes will not stay closed.
10 Insert dentures if it is agency policy to do so. If not, put them in a labeled denture cup.
11 Close the mouth. If necessary, place a rolled towel under the chin to keep the mouth closed.
12 Follow agency policy for jewelry. Remove all jewelry, except for wedding rings if this is agency policy. List the jewelry that you removed. Place the jewelry and the list in a valuables envelope.
13 Place a cotton ball over the rings. Tape them in place.
14 Remove drainage containers.
15 Remove tubes and catheters. Use the gauze squares as needed.
16 Bathe soiled areas with plain water. Dry thoroughly.
17 Place a bed protector under the buttocks.
18 Remove soiled dressings. Replace them with clean ones.
19 Put a clean gown on the body. Position the body as in step 8.
20 Brush and comb the hair if necessary.
21 Cover the body to the shoulders with a sheet if the family will view the body.
22 Gather the person's belongings. Put them in a bag labeled with the person's name. Make sure you include eyeglasses, hearing aids, and other valuables.
23 Remove supplies, equipment, and linens. Straighten the room. Provide soft lighting.
24 Remove the gloves. Decontaminate your hands.
25 Let the family view the body. Provide for privacy. Return to the room after they leave.
26 Decontaminate your hands. Put on gloves.
27 Fill out the ID tags. Tie one to the ankle or to the right big toe.
28 Place the body in the body bag or cover it with a sheet. Or apply the shroud (Fig. 50-1).
   a Position the shroud under the body.
   b Bring the top down over the head.
   c Fold the bottom up over the feet.
   d Fold the sides over the body.
   e Pin or tape the shroud in place.
29 Attach the second ID tag to the shroud, sheet, or body bag.
30 Leave the denture cup with the body.
31 Pull the privacy curtain around the bed. Or close the door.

POST-PROCEDURE

32 Remove the gloves. Decontaminate your hands.
33 Strip the unit after the body has been removed. Wear gloves for this step.
34 Remove the gloves. Decontaminate your hands.
35 Report the following:
   - The time the body was taken by the funeral director
   - What was done with jewelry, other valuables, and personal items
   - What was done with dentures

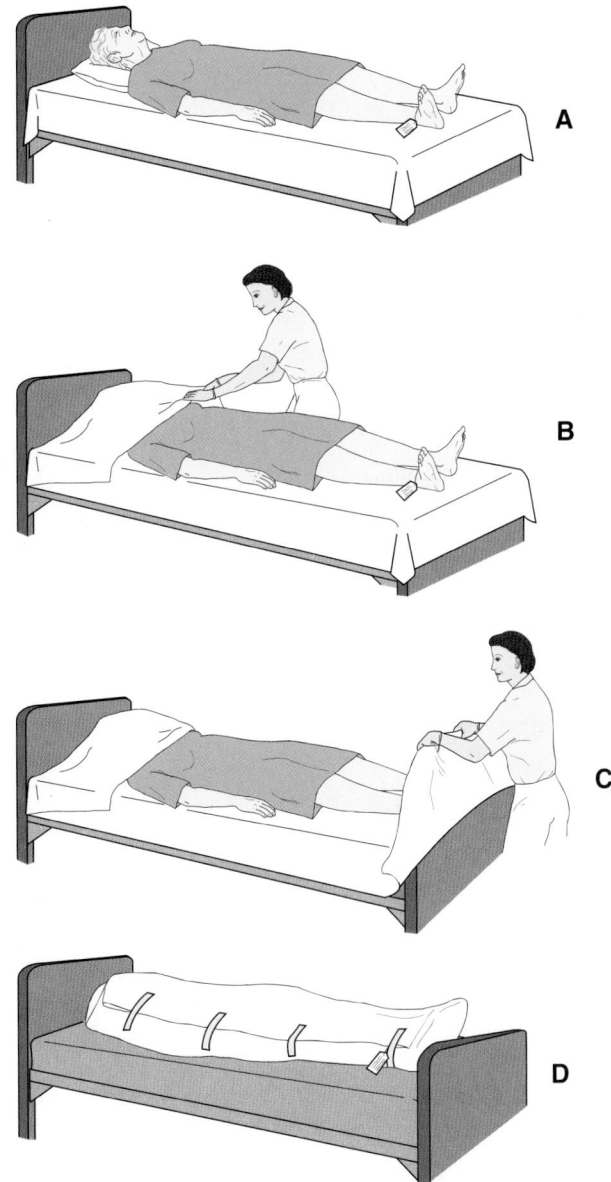

FIGURE 50-1 Applying a shroud. **A,** Position the shroud under the body. **B,** Bring the top of the shroud down over the head. **C,** Fold the bottom up over the feet. **D,** Fold the sides over the body. Tape or pin the sides together. Attach the ID tag.

Circle the BEST answer.

1 Which is *true?*
   a Death from terminal illness is sudden and unexpected.
   b Doctors know when death will occur.
   c An illness is terminal when there is no reasonable hope of recovery.
   d All severe injuries end in death.

2 These statements relate to attitudes about death. Which is *false?*
   a Dying people are often cared for in health care agencies.
   b Religion influences attitudes about death.
   c Infants and toddlers understand death.
   d Young children often blame themselves when someone dies.

3 Reincarnation is the belief that
   a There is no afterlife
   b The spirit or soul is reborn into another human body or another form of life
   c The body keeps its physical form in the afterlife
   d Only the spirit or soul is present in the afterlife

4 Children between the ages of 2 and 6 years view death as
   a Temporary
   b Final
   c Adults do
   d Going to sleep

5 Adults and older persons usually fear
   a Dying alone
   b Reincarnation
   c The five stages of dying
   d Advance directives

6 Persons in the stage of denial
   a Are angry
   b Make "deals" with God
   c Are sad and quiet
   d Refuse to believe they are dying

7 A dying person tries to gain more time during the stage of
   a Anger
   b Bargaining
   c Depression
   d Acceptance

8 When caring for the dying person, you should
   a Use touch and listen
   b Do most of the talking
   c Keep the room darkened
   d Speak in a loud voice

9 As death nears, the last sense lost is
   a Sight
   b Taste
   c Smell
   d Hearing

10 The dying person's care includes the following *except*
   a Eye care
   b Mouth care
   c Active range-of-motion exercises
   d Position changes

11 The dying person is positioned in
   a The supine position
   b The Fowler's position
   c Good body alignment
   d The dorsal recumbent position

12 A "DNR" order was written. This means that
   a CPR will not be done
   b The person has a living will
   c Life-prolonging measures will be carried out
   d The person is kept alive as long as possible

13 Which are *not* signs of approaching death?
   a Increased body temperature and rapid pulse
   b Loss of movement and muscle tone
   c Increased pain and blood pressure
   d Slow or rapid and shallow respirations and the death rattle

14 The signs of death are
   a Convulsions and incontinence
   b No pulse, respirations, or blood pressure
   c Loss of consciousness and convulsions
   d The eyes stay open, no muscle movements, and the body is rigid

15 Postmortem care is done
   a After rigor mortis sets in
   b After the doctor pronounces the person dead
   c When the funeral director arrives for the body
   d After the family has viewed the body

Answers to these questions are on p. 782.

Review Question Answers

Chapter 1:
Introduction to
Health Care
Agencies
1 d
2 b
3 a
4 b
5 b
6 a
7 a
8 a
9 b
10 a
11 a
12 a
13 c
14 d

Chapter 2:
The Nursing
Assistant
1 b
2 c
3 c
4 d
5 c
6 b
7 c
8 c
9 c
10 b
11 a
12 a
13 b
14 c
15 b

Chapter 3:
Ethics and Laws
1 b
2 c
3 d
4 a
5 c
6 c
7 c
8 d
9 a
10 d
11 c
12 b
13 a
14 d
15 b

16 d
17 a
18 a
19 b
20 a
21 c
22 b
23 c
24 c

Chapter 4:
Work Ethics
1 T
2 T
3 F
4 T
5 T
6 T
7 F
8 F
9 T
10 F
11 c
12 d
13 a
14 d
15 b
16 d
17 c
18 c
19 d
20 c
21 b
22 a
23 a
24 b
25 c
26 d
27 c
28 a
29 d
30 d

Chapter 5:
Communicating
With the Health
Team
1 a
2 c
3 d
4 b
5 c
6 c
7 d
8 d

9 b
10 c
11 a
12 d
13 b
14 b

Chapter 6:
Assisting with the
Nursing Process
1 a
2 d
3 b
4 c
5 d
6 b
7 a
8 c
9 c
10 b
11 c
12 d

Chapter 7:
Understanding
the Person
1 c
2 d
3 c
4 b
5 a
6 d
7 a
8 d
9 a
10 c
11 b
12 d
13 c
14 a
15 c
16 a
17 d
18 a
19 d
20 c
21 d
22 b
23 b
24 c

Chapter 8:
Body Structure
and Function
1 a
2 b
3 d

4 c
5 c
6 a
7 b
8 c
9 d
10 d
11 b
12 a
13 b
14 b
15 b
16 c
17 d
18 a
19 d
20 a
21 b

Chapter 9:
Growth and
Development
1 b
2 c
3 b
4 a
5 b
6 c
7 b
8 a
9 c
10 c
11 c
12 c
13 a
14 b
15 c
16 a
17 d
18 c

Chapter 10:
Care of the Older
Person
1 b
2 c
3 a
4 d
5 c
6 b
7 c
8 a
9 b
10 a
11 b

12 d
13 c
14 d
15 c
16 a
17 d
18 b
19 a
20 b
21 d
22 c
23 c
24 b
25 c
26 a
27 a
28 b
29 a
30 b

Chapter 11:
Safety
1 b
2 a
3 d
4 c
5 c
6 a
7 d
8 b
9 c
10 d
11 a
12 a
13 c
14 c
15 d
16 b
17 a
18 b
19 b
20 c
21 b
22 d
23 b
24 b
25 a
26 b
27 c
28 c
29 b
30 d

Chapter 12:
Preventing Falls
1 a
2 d
3 c
4 a
5 a
6 c
7 d
8 c
9 a
10 b
11 a
12 c
13 c
14 a

Chapter 13:
Promoting a
Restraint-Free
Environment
1 F
2 F
3 F
4 T
5 T
6 T
7 T
8 T
9 F
10 F
11 F
12 T
13 F
14 T
15 F
16 d
17 a
18 c
19 b
20 c
21 a
22 d
23 c
24 c
25 d

Chapter 14:
Preventing
Infection
1 F
2 T
3 T
4 F
5 F
6 F
7 F
8 T

9 T
10 b
11 d
12 d
13 b
14 a
15 b
16 a
17 d
18 c
19 a
20 d
21 c
22 a
23 d
24 b
25 d
26 c
27 b
28 a

Chapter 15:
Body Mechanics
1 d
2 b
3 a
4 a
5 a
6 c
7 c
8 b
9 a
10 b
11 c
12 a

Chapter 16:
Safely Handling,
Moving, and
Transferring the
Person
1 b
2 a
3 a
4 b
5 a
6 b
7 a
8 a
9 a
10 a
11 b
12 a
13 d
14 b
15 c
16 c

Chapter 17:
The Person's Unit
1 c
2 d
3 a
4 b
5 d
6 a
7 b
8 d
9 c
10 b
11 c
12 c
13 T
14 T
15 F
16 T
17 T
18 T
19 T
20 T
21 F
22 F

Chapter 18:
Bedmaking
1 F
2 T
3 F
4 T
5 T
6 F
7 T
8 b
9 d
10 b
11 a
12 b
13 a
14 d
15 c

Chapter 19:
Personal Hygiene
1 T
2 T
3 F
4 F
5 F
6 F
7 F
8 T
9 F
10 F
11 F
12 F
13 T
14 T

15 T
16 d
17 d
18 b
19 b
20 c
21 c
22 d

Chapter 20:
Grooming
1 d
2 b
3 c
4 a
5 d
6 d
7 b
8 d
9 b
10 F
11 T
12 T
13 F
14 F

Chapter 21:
Urinary
Elimination
1 b
2 d
3 a
4 b
5 a
6 a
7 d
8 a
9 a
10 a
11 a
12 b
13 a
14 d
15 c

Chapter 22:
Bowel Elimination
1 a
2 b
3 d
4 a
5 c
6 a
7 a
8 c
9 d
10 d

Chapter 23:
Nutrition and
Fluids
1 b
2 a
3 a
4 d
5 d
6 c
7 a
8 c
9 a
10 c
11 d
12 a
13 c
14 c
15 c
16 b
17 b
18 c
19 d
20 b
21 c
22 d
23 T
24 F
25 F
26 T
27 F
28 F
29 F
30 F
31 T
32 F
33 F
34 T
35 T

Chapter 24:
Nutritional
Support & IV
Therapy
1 c
2 a
3 a
4 b
5 d
6 a
7 a
8 a
9 a
10 c
11 a
12 b
13 a
14 d
15 b
16 b
17 b
18 a

**Chapter 25:
Measuring
Vital Signs**
1 c
2 b
3 a
4 c
5 b
6 a
7 a
8 b
9 b
10 c
11 b
12 d
13 a
14 b

**Chapter 26:
Exercise and
Activity**
1 b
2 b
3 c
4 b
5 c
6 b
7 c
8 a
9 a
10 c
11 b
12 F
13 F
14 F
15 T

**Chapter 27:
Comfort, Rest,
and Sleep**
1 a
2 c
3 d
4 c
5 a
6 b
7 c
8 d
9 b
10 c
11 d
12 a
13 b
14 T
15 F
16 T

**Chapter 28:
Admissions,
Transfers, and
Discharges**
1 F
2 F
3 F
4 T
5 T
6 F
7 F
8 F
9 T
10 F
11 F
12 T
13 T
14 T
15 F
16 T
17 T
18 T

**Chapter 29:
Assisting With
the Physical
Examination**
1 b
2 d
3 c
4 b
5 c

**Chapter 30:
Collecting and
Testing Specimens**
1 d
2 b
3 a
4 c
5 d
6 b
7 a
8 d
9 a
10 b
11 c
12 a
13 d
14 a

**Chapter 31:
The Person
Having Surgery**
1 c
2 b
3 b
4 a
5 a
6 c
7 c
8 a
9 b
10 c
11 d
12 a
13 b
14 a
15 d
16 a
17 F
18 T
19 F
20 F
21 T
22 T
23 T
24 F
25 T
26 T

**Chapter 32:
Wound Care**
1 a
2 c
3 a
4 c
5 b
6 b
7 b
8 d
9 c
10 a
11 a
12 b
13 a
14 a
15 d
16 b
17 d
18 c
19 b
20 a
21 d
22 c
23 b
24 d
25 a
26 c

**Chapter 33:
Heat and Cold
Applications**
1 d
2 b
3 b
4 b
5 c
6 d
7 d
8 a
9 d
10 c
11 a
12 b

**Chapter 34:
Oxygen Needs**
1 a
2 c
3 c
4 b
5 b
6 d
7 c
8 d
9 a
10 a
11 b
12 d

**Chapter 35:
Respiratory
Support and
Therapies**
1 d
2 d
3 d
4 b
5 b
6 b
7 d
8 c
9 a
10 b
11 c
12 d

**Chapter 36:
Rehabilitation
and Restorative
Nursing Care**
1 c
2 b
3 a
4 d
5 a

**Chapter 37:
Speech, Hearing,
and Vision
Disorders**
1 b
2 b
3 a
4 b
5 b
6 b
7 a
8 c
9 c
10 a
11 c
12 b
13 a
14 b
15 a
16 c
17 b
18 c
19 a
20 b
21 a
22 d

**Chapter 38:
Cancer, Immune
System, and Skin
Disorders**
1 b
2 a
3 a
4 a
5 a
6 a
7 a
8 d
9 d
10 b
11 T
12 T
13 T
14 F
15 T
16 T

Chapter 33 continued:
6 c
7 c
8 T
9 T
10 T
11 F
12 T
13 T
14 T

Chapter 39:
Nervous System and Musculoskeletal Disorders
1. a
2. b
3. d
4. b
5. c
6. b
7. a
8. b
9. d
10. a
11. b
12. a
13. c
14. a
15. c
16. a
17. a
18. a
19. d
20. c
21. a
22. a

Chapter 40:
Cardiovascular and Respiratory Disorders
1. d
2. a
3. d
4. b
5. c
6. a
7. d
8. a
9. a
10. a
11. b
12. a
13. c
14. c
15. a
16. a

Chapter 41:
Digestive and Endocrine Disorders
1. b
2. a
3. d
4. a
5. a
6. d
7. c
8. d
9. a
10. d
11. c
12. b
13. c
14. a

Chapter 42:
Urinary and Reproductive Disorders
1. d
2. d
3. c
4. d
5. a
6. a
7. a
8. b
9. c
10. d

Chapter 43:
Mental Health Problems
1. b
2. b
3. d
4. c
5. c
6. c
7. c
8. b
9. c
10. b
11. d
12. d
13. d
14. c
15. c
16. d
17. a
18. a
19. a
20. a
21. a

22. a
23. T
24. F
25. F
26. T
27. T
28. T
29. T
30. F

Chapter 44:
Confusion and Dementia
1. a
2. b
3. a
4. a
5. d
6. d
7. b
8. b
9. a
10. d
11. c
12. a

Chapter 45:
Developmental Disabilities
1. d
2. b
3. d
4. b
5. a
6. d
7. c
8. c
9. d
10. b
11. b
12. d
13. c
14. b

Chapter 46:
Sexuality
1. a
2. d
3. c
4. a
5. b
6. b
7. d
8. b
9. b
10. b

Chapter 47:
Caring for Mothers and Newborns
1. c
2. d
3. d
4. d
5. b
6. c
7. c
8. c
9. c
10. d
11. d
12. a
13. c
14. c
15. T
16. F
17. T
18. T
19. T
20. T
21. F
22. T

Chapter 48:
Assisted Living
1. a
2. a
3. b
4. d
5. d
6. b
7. d
8. b
9. b
10. d
11. b
12. a
13. b
14. c
15. c

Chapter 49:
Basic Emergency Care
1. b
2. a
3. b
4. c
5. d
6. c
7. b
8. c
9. b
10. b
11. d
12. d
13. d
14. b
15. c
16. a
17. b
18. c
19. c
20. a
21. a
22. b

Chapter 50:
The Dying Person
1. c
2. c
3. b
4. a
5. a
6. d
7. b
8. a
9. d
10. c
11. c
12. a
13. c
14. b
15. b

National Nurse Aide Assessment Program (NNAAP™) Written Examination Content Outline

The NNAAP Written Examination is comprised of seventy (70) multiple choice questions. Ten (10) of these questions are pre-test (non-scored) questions on which statistical information will be collected.

I. Physical Care Skills

A. Activities of Daily Living. . . . . .14% of exam
   1. Hygiene
   2. Dressing and Grooming
   3. Nutrition and Hydration
   4. Elimination
   5. Rest/Sleep/Comfort
B. Basic Nursing Skills. . . . . .35% of exam
   1. Infection Control
   2. Safety/Emergency
   3. Therapeutic/Technical Procedures
   4. Data Collection and Reporting
C. Restorative Skills . . . . .8% of exam
   1. Prevention
   2. Self Care/Independence

II. Psychosocial Care Skills

A. Emotional and Mental Health
   Needs . . . . .10% of exam
B. Spiritual and Cultural Needs. . . . .4% of exam

III. Role of the Nurse Aide

A. Communication . . . . .7% of exam
B. Client Rights . . . . .7% of exam
C. Legal and Ethical Behavior . . . . . .5% of exam
D. Member of the Health Care
   Team. . . . . .10% of exam

National Nurse Aide Assessment Program (NNAAP™) Skills Evaluation

List of Skills

1. Washes hands
2. Measures and records weight of ambulatory client
3. Provides mouth care
4. Dresses client with affected (weak) right arm
5. Transfers client from bed to wheelchair
6. Assists client to ambulate
7. Cleans and stores dentures
8. Performs passive range-of-motion (ROM) for one shoulder
9. Performs passive range-of-motion (ROM) for one knee and one ankle
10. Measures and records urinary output
11. Assists client with use of bedpan
12. Provides perineal care (peri-care) for incontinent client
13. Provides catheter care
14. Measures and records oral temperature with a non-mercury glass thermometer
15. Counts and records radial pulse
16. Counts and records respirations
17. Measures and records blood pressure (two-step procedure)
18. Puts one knee-high elastic stocking on client
19. Makes an occupied bed
20. Provides foot care on one foot
21. Provides fingernail care on one hand
22. Feeds client who cannot feed self
23. Positions client on side
24. Gives modified bed bath (face and one arm, hand and underarm)
25. Shampoos client's hair in bed

Numeric Identifier_____

MINIMUM DATA SET (MDS) — *VERSION 2.0*
FOR NURSING HOME RESIDENT ASSESSMENT AND CARE SCREENING

BASIC ASSESSMENT TRACKING FORM

SECTION AA. IDENTIFICATION INFORMATION

1.	RESIDENT NAME⊙				
		a. (First)	b. (Middle Initial)	c. (Last)	d. (Jr/Sr)
2.	GENDER⊙	1. Male		2. Female	
3.	BIRTHDATE⊙	☐☐ — ☐☐ — ☐☐☐☐			
		Month	Day	Year	
4.	RACE/ ETHNICITY⊙	1. American Indian/Alaskan Native	4. Hispanic		
		2. Asian/Pacific Islander	5. White, not of		
		3. Black, not of Hispanic origin	Hispanic origin		
5.	SOCIAL SECURITY⊙ AND MEDICARE NUMBERS⊙ [C in 1ˢᵗ box if non med. no.]	a. Social Security Number ☐☐☐ — ☐☐ — ☐☐☐☐			
		b. Medicare number (or comparable railroad insurance number) ☐☐☐☐☐☐☐☐☐☐			
6.	FACILITY PROVIDER NO.⊙	a. State No. ☐☐☐☐☐☐☐☐☐☐			
		b. Federal No. ☐☐☐☐☐☐☐☐☐☐			
7.	MEDICAID NO. ["+" if pending, "N" if not a Medicaid recipient]⊙	☐☐☐☐☐☐☐☐☐☐☐☐			

8. REASONS FOR ASSESSMENT

[Note—Other codes do not apply to this form]

a. Primary reason for assessment
1. Admission assessment (required by day 14)
2. Annual assessment
3. Significant change in status assessment
4. Significant correction of prior full assessment
5. Quarterly review assessment
10. Significant correction of prior quarterly assessment
0. *NONE OF ABOVE*

b. *Codes for assessments required for Medicare PPS or the State*
1. *Medicare 5 day assessment*
2. *Medicare 30 day assessment*
3. *Medicare 60 day assessment*
4. *Medicare 90 day assessment*
5. *Medicare readmission/return assessment*
6. *Other state required assessment*
7. *Medicare 14 day assessment*
8. *Other Medicare required assessment*

9. Signatures of Persons who Completed a Portion of the Accompanying Assessment or Tracking Form

I certify that the accompanying information accurately reflects resident assessment or tracking information for this resident and that I collected or coordinated collection of this information on the dates specified. To the best of my knowledge, this information was collected in accordance with applicable Medicare and Medicaid requirements. I understand that this information is used as a basis for ensuring that residents receive appropriate and quality care, and as a basis for payment from federal funds. I further understand that payment of such federal funds and continued participation in the government-funded health care programs is conditioned on the accuracy and truthfulness of this information, and that I may be personally subject to or may subject my organization to substantial criminal, civil, and/or administrative penalties for submitting false information. I also certify that I am authorized to submit this information by this facility on its behalf.

Signature and Title	Sections	Date
a.		
b.		
c.		
d.		
e.		
f.		
g.		
h.		
i.		
j.		
k.		
l.		

GENERAL INSTRUCTIONS

Complete this information for submission with all full and quarterly assessments (Admission, Annual, Significant Change, State or Medicare required assessments, or Quarterly Reviews, etc.)

⊙ = Key items for computerized resident tracking

☐ = When box blank, must enter number or letter   [a.] = When letter in box, check if condition applies

MDS 2.0 September, 2000

Resident _____   Numeric Identifier _____

MINIMUM DATA SET (MDS) — *VERSION 2.0*
FOR NURSING HOME RESIDENT ASSESSMENT AND CARE SCREENING

BACKGROUND (FACE SHEET) INFORMATION AT ADMISSION

SECTION AB. DEMOGRAPHIC INFORMATION

1.	DATE OF ENTRY	Date the stay began. Note — Does not include readmission if record was closed at time of temporary discharge to hospital, etc. In such cases, use prior admission date

☐ ☐ — ☐ ☐ — ☐ ☐ ☐ ☐
Month   Day   Year

2.	ADMITTED FROM (AT ENTRY)	1. Private home/apt. with no home health services 2. Private home/apt. with home health services 3. Board and care/assisted living/group home 4. Nursing home 5. Acute care hospital 6. Psychiatric hospital, MR/DD facility 7. Rehabilitation hospital 8. Other
3.	LIVED ALONE (PRIOR TO ENTRY)	0. No 1. Yes 2. In other facility
4.	ZIP CODE OF PRIOR PRIMARY RESIDENCE	☐ ☐ ☐ ☐ ☐
5.	RESIDENTIAL HISTORY 5 YEARS PRIOR TO ENTRY	(***Check all settings*** resident **lived in** during 5 years prior to date of entry given in item AB1 above) Prior stay at this nursing home — a. Stay in other nursing home — b. Other residential facility—board and care home, assisted living, group home — c. MH/psychiatric setting — d. MR/DD setting — e. *NONE OF ABOVE* — f.
6.	LIFETIME OCCUPATION(S) [Put "/" between two occupations]	☐ ☐ ☐ ☐ ☐ ☐ ☐ ☐ ☐ ☐ ☐ ☐ ☐ ☐ ☐ ☐ ☐
7.	EDUCATION (*Highest Level Completed*)	1. No schooling 5. Technical or trade school 2. 8th grade/less 6. Some college 3. 9-11 grades 7. Bachelor's degree 4. High school 8. Graduate degree
8.	LANGUAGE	(*Code for correct response*) **a.** Primary Language 0. English 1. Spanish 2. French 3. Other **b. If other, specify**
9.	MENTAL HEALTH HISTORY	Does resident's RECORD indicate any history of mental retardation, mental illness, or developmental disability problem? 0. No 1. Yes
10.	CONDITIONS RELATED TO MR/DD STATUS	(***Check all conditions*** that are related to MR/DD status that were manifested before age 22, and are likely to continue indefinitely) Not applicable—no MR/DD (Skip to AB11) — a. MR/DD with organic condition Down's syndrome — b. Autism — c. Epilepsy — d. Other organic condition related to MR/DD — e. MR/DD with no organic condition — f.
11.	DATE BACKGROUND INFORMATION COMPLETED	☐ ☐ — ☐ ☐ — ☐ ☐ ☐ ☐ Month Day Year

SECTION AC. CUSTOMARY ROUTINE

1.	CUSTOMARY ROUTINE (*In year prior to DATE OF ENTRY* to this nursing home, or year last in community if now being admitted from another nursing home)	(***Check all that apply.*** If all information UNKNOWN, check last box only.)

CYCLE OF DAILY EVENTS

Stays up late at night (e.g., after 9 pm)	a.
Naps regularly during day (at least 1 hour)	b.
Goes out 1+ days a week	c.
Stays busy with hobbies, reading, or fixed daily routine	d.
Spends most of time alone or watching TV	e.
Moves independently indoors (with appliances, if used)	f.
Use of tobacco products at least daily	g.
NONE OF ABOVE	h.

EATING PATTERNS

Distinct food preferences	i.
Eats between meals all or most days	j.
Use of alcoholic beverage(s) at least weekly	k.
NONE OF ABOVE	l.

ADL PATTERNS

In bedclothes much of day	m.
Wakens to toilet all or most nights	n.
Has irregular bowel movement pattern	o.
Showers for bathing	p.
Bathing in PM	q.
NONE OF ABOVE	r.

INVOLVEMENT PATTERNS

Daily contact with relatives/close friends	s.
Usually attends church, temple, synagogue (etc.)	t.
Finds strength in faith	u.
Daily animal companion/presence	v.
Involved in group activities	w.
NONE OF ABOVE	x.
UNKNOWN—Resident/family unable to provide information	y.

SECTION AD. FACE SHEET SIGNATURES

SIGNATURES OF PERSONS COMPLETING FACE SHEET:

a. Signature of RN Assessment Coordinator   Date

I certify that the accompanying information accurately reflects resident assessment or tracking information for this resident and that I collected or coordinated collection of this information on the dates specified. To the best of my knowledge, this information was collected in accordance with applicable Medicare and Medicaid requirements. I understand that this information is used as a basis for ensuring that residents receive appropriate and quality care, and as a basis for payment from federal funds. I further understand that payment of such federal funds and continued participation in the government-funded health care programs is conditioned on the accuracy and truthfulness of this information, and that I may be personally subject to or may subject my organization to substantial criminal, civil, and/or administrative penalties for submitting false information. I also certify that I am authorized to submit this information by this facility on its behalf.

Signature and Title	Sections	Date
b.		
c.		
d.		
e.		
f.		
g.		

☐ = When box blank, must enter number or letter   ☐a. = When letter in box, check if condition applies

Resident_____ Numeric Identifier_____

MINIMUM DATA SET (MDS) — *VERSION 2.0*
FOR NURSING HOME RESIDENT ASSESSMENT AND CARE SCREENING
FULL ASSESSMENT FORM
(Status in last 7 days, unless other time frame indicated)

SECTION A. IDENTIFICATION AND BACKGROUND INFORMATION

1.	RESIDENT NAME	
		a. (First)　　b. (Middle Initial)　　c. (Last)　　d. (Jr/Sr)

2.	ROOM NUMBER	☐☐☐☐☐

3.	ASSESS-MENT REFERENCE DATE	a. *Last day of MDS observation period*
		☐☐ — ☐☐ — ☐☐☐☐
		Month　　Day　　Year
		b. Original (0) or corrected copy of form (enter number of correction)

4a.	DATE OF REENTRY	Date of reentry from most recent temporary discharge to a hospital in last 90 days (or since last assessment or admission if less than 90 days)
		☐☐ — ☐☐ — ☐☐☐☐
		Month　　Day　　Year

5.	MARITAL STATUS	1. Never married　　3. Widowed　　5. Divorced 2. Married　　4. Separated

6.	MEDICAL RECORD NO.	☐☐☐☐☐☐☐☐☐☐

7.	CURRENT PAYMENT SOURCES FOR N.H. STAY	(*Billing Office to indicate; check all that apply in last 30 days*)
		Medicaid per diem　a.　　VA per diem　f.
		Medicare per diem　b.　　Self or family pays for full per diem　g.
		Medicare ancillary part A　c.　　Medicaid resident liability or Medicare co-payment　h.
		Medicare ancillary part B　d.　　Private insurance per diem (including co-payment)　i.
		CHAMPUS per diem　e.　　Other per diem　j.

8.	REASONS FOR ASSESS-MENT [*Note—If this is a discharge or reentry assessment, only a limited subset of MDS items need be completed*]	a. Primary reason for assessment 　1. Admission assessment (required by day 14) 　2. Annual assessment 　3. Significant change in status assessment 　4. Significant correction of prior full assessment 　5. Quarterly review assessment 　6. Discharged—return not anticipated 　7. Discharged—return anticipated 　8. Discharged prior to completing initial assessment 　9. Reentry 　10. Significant correction of prior quarterly assessment 　0. *NONE OF ABOVE* b. *Codes for assessments required for Medicare PPS or the State* 　1. *Medicare 5 day assessment* 　2. *Medicare 30 day assessment* 　3. *Medicare 60 day assessment* 　4. *Medicare 90 day assessment* 　5. *Medicare readmission/return assessment* 　6. *Other state required assessment* 　7. *Medicare 14 day assessment* 　8. *Other Medicare required assessment*

9.	RESPONSI-BILITY/ LEGAL GUARDIAN	(*Check all that apply*)
		Legal guardian　a.　　Durable power attorney/financial　d.
		Other legal oversight　b.　　Family member responsible　e.
		Durable power of attorney/health care　c.　　Patient responsible for self　f.
			NONE OF ABOVE　g.

10.	ADVANCED DIRECTIVES	(*For those items with supporting* documentation *in the medical record,* check all that apply)
		Living will　a.　　Feeding restrictions　f.
		Do not resuscitate　b.　　Medication restrictions　g.
		Do not hospitalize　c.　　Other treatment restrictions　h.
		Organ donation　d.
		Autopsy request　e.　　*NONE OF ABOVE*　i.

SECTION B. COGNITIVE PATTERNS

1.	COMATOSE	(*Persistent vegetative state/no discernible consciousness*) 0. No　　1. Yes　　(**If yes, skip to Section G**)
2.	MEMORY	(*Recall of what was learned or known*) a. Short-term memory OK—seems/appears to recall after 5 minutes 　0. Memory OK　　1. Memory problem b. Long-term memory OK—seems/appears to recall long past 　0. Memory OK　　1. Memory problem

3.	MEMORY/ RECALL ABILITY	(*Check all that resident was* **normally able to recall during** *last 7 days*)
		Current season　a.　　That he/she is in a nursing home　d.
		Location of own room　b.
		Staff names/faces　c.　　*NONE OF ABOVE* are recalled　e.

4.	COGNITIVE SKILLS FOR DAILY DECISION-MAKING	(*Made decisions regarding tasks of daily life*) 0. *INDEPENDENT*—decisions consistent/reasonable 1. *MODIFIED INDEPENDENCE*—some difficulty in new situations only 2. *MODERATELY IMPAIRED*—decisions poor; cues/supervision required 3. *SEVERELY IMPAIRED*—never/rarely made decisions

5.	INDICATORS OF DELIRIUM— PERIODIC DISOR-DERED THINKING/ AWARENESS	(*Code for behavior in the* **last 7 days**.) [*Note: Accurate assessment requires conversations with staff and family who have direct knowledge of resident's behavior over this time*]. 0. Behavior not present 1. Behavior present, not of recent onset 2. Behavior present, over last 7 days appears different from resident's usual functioning (e.g., new onset or worsening)
		a. EASILY DISTRACTED—(e.g., difficulty paying attention; gets sidetracked)
		b. PERIODS OF ALTERED PERCEPTION OR AWARENESS OF SURROUNDINGS—(e.g., moves lips or talks to someone not present; believes he/she is somewhere else; confuses night and day)
		c. EPISODES OF DISORGANIZED SPEECH—(e.g., speech is incoherent, nonsensical, irrelevant, or rambling from subject to subject; loses train of thought)
		d. PERIODS OF RESTLESSNESS—(e.g., fidgeting or picking at skin, clothing, napkins, etc; frequent position changes; repetitive physical movements or calling out)
		e. PERIODS OF LETHARGY—(e.g., sluggishness; staring into space; difficult to arouse; little body movement)
		f. MENTAL FUNCTION VARIES OVER THE COURSE OF THE DAY—(e.g., sometimes better, sometimes worse; behaviors sometimes present, sometimes not)

6.	CHANGE IN COGNITIVE STATUS	Resident's cognitive status, skills, or abilities have changed as compared to status of **90 days ago** (or since last assessment if less than 90 days) 0. No change　　1. Improved　　2. Deteriorated

SECTION C. COMMUNICATION/HEARING PATTERNS

1.	HEARING	(*With hearing appliance, if used*) 0. *HEARS ADEQUATELY*—normal talk, TV, phone 1. *MINIMAL DIFFICULTY* when not in quiet setting 2. *HEARS IN SPECIAL SITUATIONS ONLY*—speaker has to adjust tonal quality and speak distinctly 3. *HIGHLY IMPAIRED*/absence of useful hearing

2.	COMMUNI-CATION DEVICES/ TECH-NIQUES	(*Check all that apply* during last 7 days)
		Hearing aid, present and used　a.
		Hearing aid, present and not used regularly　b.
		Other receptive comm. techniques used (e.g., lip reading)　c.
		NONE OF ABOVE　d.

3.	MODES OF EXPRESSION	(*Check all used* by resident to make needs known)
		Speech　a.　　Signs/gestures/sounds　d.
		Writing messages to express or clarify needs　b.　　Communication board　e.
			Other　f.
		American sign language or Braille　c.　　*NONE OF ABOVE*　g.

4.	MAKING SELF UNDER-STOOD	(*Expressing information content—however able*) 0. *UNDERSTOOD* 1. *USUALLY UNDERSTOOD*—difficulty finding words or finishing thoughts 2. *SOMETIMES UNDERSTOOD*—ability is limited to making concrete requests 3. *RARELY/NEVER UNDERSTOOD*

5.	SPEECH CLARITY	(*Code for speech in the* **last 7 days**) 0. *CLEAR SPEECH*—distinct, intelligible words 1. *UNCLEAR SPEECH*—slurred, mumbled words 2. *NO SPEECH*—absence of spoken words

6.	ABILITY TO UNDER-STAND OTHERS	(*Understanding verbal information content—however able*) 0. *UNDERSTANDS* 1. *USUALLY UNDERSTANDS*—may miss some part/intent of message 2. *SOMETIMES UNDERSTANDS*—responds adequately to simple, direct communication 3. *RARELY/NEVER UNDERSTANDS*

7.	CHANGE IN COMMUNI-CATION/ HEARING	Resident's ability to express, understand, or hear information has changed as compared to status of **90 days ago** (or since last assessment if less than 90 days) 0. No change　　1. Improved　　2. Deteriorated

☐ = When box blank, must enter number or letter　　a. = When letter in box, check if condition applies

MDS 2.0 September, 2000

Resident _____ Numeric Identifier _____

SECTION D. VISION PATTERNS

1.	VISION	(Ability to see in adequate light and with glasses if used) 0. *ADEQUATE*—sees fine detail, including regular print in newspapers/books 1. *IMPAIRED*—sees large print, but not regular print in newspapers/books 2. *MODERATELY IMPAIRED*—limited vision; not able to see newspaper headlines, but can identify objects 3. *HIGHLY IMPAIRED*—object identification in question, but eyes appear to follow objects 4. *SEVERELY IMPAIRED*—no vision or sees only light, colors, or shapes; eyes do not appear to follow objects	
2.	VISUAL LIMITATIONS/ DIFFICULTIES	Side vision problems—decreased peripheral vision (e.g., leaves food on one side of tray, difficulty traveling, bumps into people and objects, misjudges placement of chair when seating self)	a.
		Experiences any of following: sees halos or rings around lights; sees flashes of light; sees "curtains" over eyes	b.
		NONE OF ABOVE	c.
3.	VISUAL APPLIANCES	Glasses; contact lenses; magnifying glass 0. No 1. Yes	

SECTION E. MOOD AND BEHAVIOR PATTERNS

1.	INDICATORS OF DEPRES- SION, ANXIETY, SAD MOOD	(Code for indicators observed in last 30 days, irrespective of the assumed cause) 0. Indicator not exhibited in last 30 days 1. Indicator of this type exhibited up to five days a week 2. Indicator of this type exhibited daily or almost daily (6, 7 days a week)

VERBAL EXPRESSIONS OF DISTRESS

a. Resident made negative statements—e.g., "*Nothing matters; Would rather be dead; What's the use; Regrets having lived so long; Let me die*"

b. Repetitive questions—e.g., "*Where do I go; What do I do?*"

c. Repetitive verbalizations— e.g., calling out for help, ("*God help me*")

d. Persistent anger with self or others—e.g., easily annoyed, anger at placement in nursing home; anger at care received

e. Self deprecation—e.g., "*I am nothing; I am of no use to anyone*"

f. Expressions of what appear to be unrealistic fears—e.g., fear of being abandoned, left alone, being with others

g. Recurrent statements that something terrible is about to happen—e.g., believes he or she is about to die, have a heart attack

h. Repetitive health complaints—e.g., persistently seeks medical attention, obsessive concern with body functions

i. Repetitive anxious complaints/concerns (non-health related) e.g., persistently seeks attention/ reassurance regarding schedules, meals, laundry, clothing, relationship issues

SLEEP-CYCLE ISSUES

j. Unpleasant mood in morning

k. Insomnia/change in usual sleep pattern

SAD, APATHETIC, ANXIOUS APPEARANCE

l. Sad, pained, worried facial expressions—e.g., furrowed brows

m. Crying, tearfulness

n. Repetitive physical movements—e.g., pacing, hand wringing, restlessness, fidgeting, picking

LOSS OF INTEREST

o. Withdrawal from activities of interest—e.g., no interest in long standing activities or being with family/friends

p. Reduced social interaction

2.	MOOD PERSIS- TENCE	One or more indicators of depressed, sad or anxious mood were not easily altered by attempts to "cheer up", console, or reassure the resident over last 7 days 0. No mood indicators 1. Indicators present, easily altered 2. Indicators present, not easily altered
3.	CHANGE IN MOOD	Resident's mood status has changed as compared to status of 90 days ago (or since last assessment if less than 90 days) 0. No change 1. Improved 2. Deteriorated

4.	BEHAVIORAL SYMPTOMS	(A) Behavioral symptom frequency in last 7 days 0. Behavior not exhibited in last 7 days 1. Behavior of this type occurred 1 to 3 days in last 7 days 2. Behavior of this type occurred 4 to 6 days, but less than daily 3. Behavior of this type occurred daily (B) Behavioral symptom alterability in last 7 days 0. Behavior not present OR behavior was easily altered 1. Behavior was not easily altered	(A)	(B)
		a. WANDERING (moved with no rational purpose, seemingly oblivious to needs or safety)		
		b. VERBALLY ABUSIVE BEHAVIORAL SYMPTOMS (others were threatened, screamed at, cursed at)		
		c. PHYSICALLY ABUSIVE BEHAVIORAL SYMPTOMS (others were hit, shoved, scratched, sexually abused)		
		d. SOCIALLY INAPPROPRIATE/DISRUPTIVE BEHAVIORAL SYMPTOMS (made disruptive sounds, noisiness, screaming, self-abusive acts, sexual behavior or disrobing in public, smeared/threw food/feces, hoarding, rummaged through others' belongings)		
		e. RESISTS CARE (resisted taking medications/ injections, ADL assistance, or eating)		

5.	CHANGE IN BEHAVIORAL SYMPTOMS	Resident's behavior status has changed as compared to status of 90 days ago (or since last assessment if less than 90 days) 0. No change 1. Improved 2. Deteriorated	

SECTION F. PSYCHOSOCIAL WELL-BEING

1.	SENSE OF INITIATIVE/ INVOLVE- MENT	At ease interacting with others	a.
		At ease doing planned or structured activities	b.
		At ease doing self-initiated activities	c.
		Establishes own goals	d.
		Pursues involvement in life of facility (e.g., makes/keeps friends; involved in group activities; responds positively to new activities; assists at religious services)	e.
		Accepts invitations into most group activities	f.
		NONE OF ABOVE	g.
2.	UNSETTLED RELATION- SHIPS	Covert/open conflict with or repeated criticism of staff	a.
		Unhappy with roommate	b.
		Unhappy with residents other than roommate	c.
		Openly expresses conflict/anger with family/friends	d.
		Absence of personal contact with family/friends	e.
		Recent loss of close family member/friend	f.
		Does not adjust easily to change in routines	g.
		NONE OF ABOVE	h.
3.	PAST ROLES	Strong identification with past roles and life status	a.
		Expresses sadness/anger/empty feeling over lost roles/status	b.
		Resident perceives that daily routine (customary routine, activities) is very different from prior pattern in the community	c.
		NONE OF ABOVE	d.

SECTION G. PHYSICAL FUNCTIONING AND STRUCTURAL PROBLEMS

1.	(A) ADL SELF-PERFORMANCE—(Code for resident's PERFORMANCE OVER ALL SHIFTS during last 7 days—Not including setup)

0. *INDEPENDENT*—No help or oversight —OR— Help/oversight provided only 1 or 2 times during last 7 days

1. *SUPERVISION*—Oversight, encouragement or cueing provided 3 or more times during last 7 days —OR— Supervision (3 or more times) plus physical assistance provided only 1 or 2 times during last 7 days

2. *LIMITED ASSISTANCE*—Resident highly involved in activity; received physical help in guided maneuvering of limbs or other nonweight bearing assistance 3 or more times — OR—More help provided only 1 or 2 times during last 7 days

3. *EXTENSIVE ASSISTANCE*—While resident performed part of activity, over last 7-day period, help of following type(s) provided 3 or more times: —Weight-bearing support — Full staff performance during part (but not all) of last 7 days

4. *TOTAL DEPENDENCE*—Full staff performance of activity during entire 7 days

8. *ACTIVITY DID NOT OCCUR* during entire 7 days

(B) ADL SUPPORT PROVIDED—(Code for MOST SUPPORT PROVIDED OVER ALL SHIFTS during last 7 days; code regardless of resident's self-performance classification)

0. No setup or physical help from staff
1. Setup help only
2. One person physical assist
3. Two+ persons physical assist
8. ADL activity itself did not occur during entire 7 days

			(A) SELF-PERF	(B) SUPPORT
a.	BED MOBILITY	How resident moves to and from lying position, turns side to side, and positions body while in bed		
b.	TRANSFER	How resident moves between surfaces—to/from: bed, chair, wheelchair, standing position (EXCLUDE to/from bath/toilet)		
c.	WALK IN ROOM	How resident walks between locations in his/her room		
d.	WALK IN CORRIDOR	How resident walks in corridor on unit		
e.	LOCOMO- TION ON UNIT	How resident moves between locations in his/her room and adjacent corridor on same floor. If in wheelchair, self-sufficiency once in chair		
f.	LOCOMO- TION OFF UNIT	How resident moves to and returns from off unit locations (e.g., areas set aside for dining, activities, or treatments). If facility has only one floor, how resident moves to and from distant areas on the floor. If in wheelchair, self-sufficiency once in chair		
g.	DRESSING	How resident puts on, fastens, and takes off all items of street clothing, including donning/removing prosthesis		
h.	EATING	How resident eats and drinks (regardless of skill). Includes intake of nourishment by other means (e.g., tube feeding, total parenteral nutrition)		
i.	TOILET USE	How resident uses the toilet room (or commode, bedpan, urinal); transfer on/off toilet, cleanses, changes pad, manages ostomy or catheter, adjusts clothes		
j.	PERSONAL HYGIENE	How resident maintains personal hygiene, including combing hair, brushing teeth, shaving, applying makeup, washing/drying face, hands, and perineum (EXCLUDE baths and showers)		

Resident _____   Numeric Identifier _____

2.	BATHING	How resident takes full-body bath/shower, sponge bath, and transfers in/out of tub/shower (EXCLUDE washing of back and hair.) **Code for most dependent** in self-performance and support. (A) BATHING SELF-PERFORMANCE codes appear below		(A)	(B)
		0. Independent—No help provided			
		1. Supervision—Oversight help only			
		2. Physical help limited to transfer only			
		3. Physical help in part of bathing activity			
		4. Total dependence			
		8. Activity itself did not occur during entire 7 days (*Bathing support codes are as defined in Item 1, code B above*)			

3.	TEST FOR BALANCE (see training manual)	(*Code for ability during test in the last 7 days*) 0. Maintained position as required in test 1. Unsteady, but able to rebalance self without physical support 2. Partial physical support during test; or stands (sits) but does not follow directions for test 3. Not able to attempt test without physical help		
		a. Balance while standing		
		b. Balance while sitting—position, trunk control		

4.	FUNCTIONAL LIMITATION IN RANGE OF MOTION (see training manual)	(*Code for limitations during last 7 days that interfered with daily functions or placed resident at risk of injury*) (A) RANGE OF MOTION 0. No limitation 1. Limitation on one side 2. Limitation on both sides	(B) VOLUNTARY MOVEMENT 0. No loss 1. Partial loss 2. Full loss	(A)	(B)
		a. Neck			
		b. Arm—Including shoulder or elbow			
		c. Hand—Including wrist or fingers			
		d. Leg—Including hip or knee			
		e. Foot—Including ankle or toes			
		f. Other limitation or loss			

5.	MODES OF LOCOMO-TION	(*Check all that apply* during last 7 days)			
		Cane/walker/crutch	a.	Wheelchair primary mode of locomotion	d.
		Wheeled self	b.		
		Other person wheeled	c.	NONE OF ABOVE	e.

6.	MODES OF TRANSFER	(*Check all that apply* during last 7 days)			
		Bedfast all or most of time	a.	Lifted mechanically	d.
		Bed rails used for bed mobility or transfer	b.	Transfer aid (e.g., slide board, trapeze, cane, walker, brace)	e.
		Lifted manually	c.	NONE OF ABOVE	f.

7.	TASK SEGMENTA-TION	Some or all of ADL activities were broken into subtasks during **last 7 days** so that resident could perform them 0. No 1. Yes	

8.	ADL FUNCTIONAL REHABILITA-TION POTENTIAL	Resident believes he/she is capable of increased independence in at least some ADLs	a.
		Direct care staff believe resident is capable of increased independence in at least some ADLs	b.
		Resident able to perform tasks/activity but is very slow	c.
		Difference in ADL Self-Performance or ADL Support, comparing mornings to evenings	d.
		NONE OF ABOVE	e.

9.	CHANGE IN ADL FUNCTION	Resident's ADL self-performance status has changed as compared to status of **90 days ago** (or since last assessment if less than 90 days) 0. No change 1. Improved 2. Deteriorated	

SECTION H. CONTINENCE IN LAST 14 DAYS

1.	CONTINENCE SELF-CONTROL CATEGORIES (*Code for resident's PERFORMANCE OVER ALL SHIFTS*) 0. CONTINENT—Complete control [includes use of indwelling urinary catheter or ostomy device that does not leak urine or stool] 1. *USUALLY CONTINENT*—BLADDER, incontinent episodes once a week or less; BOWEL, less than weekly 2. *OCCASIONALLY INCONTINENT*—BLADDER, 2 or more times a week but not daily; BOWEL, once a week 3. *FREQUENTLY INCONTINENT*—BLADDER, tended to be incontinent daily, but some control present (e.g., on day shift); BOWEL, 2-3 times a week 4. *INCONTINENT*—Had inadequate control BLADDER, multiple daily episodes; BOWEL, all (or almost all) of the time	
a.	BOWEL CONTI-NENCE	Control of bowel movement, with appliance or bowel continence programs, if employed	
b.	BLADDER CONTI-NENCE	Control of urinary bladder function (if dribbles, volume insufficient to soak through underpants), with appliances (e.g., foley) or continence programs, if employed	

2.	BOWEL ELIMINATION PATTERN	Bowel elimination pattern regular—at least one movement every three days	a.	Diarrhea	c.
				Fecal impaction	d.
		Constipation	b.	NONE OF ABOVE	e.

3.	APPLIANCES AND PROGRAMS	Any scheduled toileting plan	a.	Did not use toilet room/commode/urinal	f.
		Bladder retraining program	b.	Pads/briefs used	g.
		External (condom) catheter	c.	Enemas/irrigation	h.
		Indwelling catheter	d.	Ostomy present	i.
		Intermittent catheter	e.	NONE OF ABOVE	j.

4.	CHANGE IN URINARY CONTI-NENCE	Resident's urinary continence has changed as compared to status of **90 days ago** (or since last assessment if less than 90 days) 0. No change 1. Improved 2. Deteriorated	

SECTION I. DISEASE DIAGNOSES

Check only those diseases that have a relationship to current ADL status, cognitive status, mood and behavior status, medical treatments, nursing monitoring, or risk of death. (Do not list inactive diagnoses)

1.	DISEASES	(*If none apply, CHECK the NONE OF ABOVE box*)			
		ENDOCRINE/METABOLIC/NUTRITIONAL		Hemiplegia/Hemiparesis	v.
				Multiple sclerosis	w.
		Diabetes mellitus	a.	Paraplegia	x.
		Hyperthyroidism	b.	Parkinson's disease	y.
		Hypothyroidism	c.	Quadriplegia	z.
		HEART/CIRCULATION		Seizure disorder	aa.
		Arteriosclerotic heart disease (ASHD)	d.	Transient ischemic attack (TIA)	bb.
		Cardiac dysrhythmias	e.	Traumatic brain injury	cc.
		Congestive heart failure	f.	**PSYCHIATRIC/MOOD**	
		Deep vein thrombosis	g.	Anxiety disorder	dd.
		Hypertension	h.	Depression	ee.
		Hypotension	i.	Manic depression (bipolar disease)	ff.
		Peripheral vascular disease	j.	Schizophrenia	gg.
		Other cardiovascular disease	k.	**PULMONARY**	
		MUSCULOSKELETAL		Asthma	hh.
		Arthritis	l.	Emphysema/COPD	ii.
		Hip fracture	m.	**SENSORY**	
		Missing limb (e.g., amputation)	n.	Cataracts	jj.
		Osteoporosis	o.	Diabetic retinopathy	kk.
		Pathological bone fracture	p.	Glaucoma	ll.
		NEUROLOGICAL		Macular degeneration	mm.
		Alzheimer's disease	q.	**OTHER**	
		Aphasia	r.	Allergies	nn.
		Cerebral palsy	s.	Anemia	oo.
		Cerebrovascular accident (stroke)	t.	Cancer	pp.
		Dementia other than Alzheimer's disease	u.	Renal failure	qq.
				NONE OF ABOVE	rr.

2.	INFECTIONS	(*If none apply, CHECK the NONE OF ABOVE box*)			
		Antibiotic resistant infection (e.g., Methicillin resistant staph)	a.	Septicemia	g.
				Sexually transmitted diseases	h.
		Clostridium difficile (c. diff.)	b.	Tuberculosis	i.
		Conjunctivitis	c.	Urinary tract infection **in last 30 days**	j.
		HIV infection	d.	Viral hepatitis	k.
		Pneumonia	e.	Wound infection	l.
		Respiratory infection	f.	NONE OF ABOVE	m.

3.	OTHER CURRENT OR MORE DETAILED DIAGNOSES AND ICD-9 CODES	a. _____			•	
		b. _____			•	
		c. _____			•	
		d. _____			•	
		e. _____			•	

SECTION J. HEALTH CONDITIONS

1.	PROBLEM CONDITIONS	(*Check all problems present* in last 7 days unless other time frame is indicated)			
		INDICATORS OF FLUID STATUS		Dizziness/Vertigo	f.
				Edema	g.
		Weight gain or loss of 3 or more pounds within a 7 day period	a.	Fever	h.
				Hallucinations	i.
				Internal bleeding	j.
		Inability to lie flat due to shortness of breath	b.	Recurrent lung aspirations in **last 90 days**	k.
		Dehydrated; output exceeds input	c.	Shortness of breath	l.
				Syncope (fainting)	m.
		Insufficient fluid; did **NOT** consume all/almost all liquids provided during **last 3 days**	d.	Unsteady gait	n.
				Vomiting	o.
		OTHER		NONE OF ABOVE	p.
		Delusions	e.		

Resident _____   Numeric Identifier _____

2.	PAIN SYMPTOMS	(Code the **highest level of pain** present in the **last 7 days**)		
		a. FREQUENCY with which resident complains or shows evidence of pain 0. No pain (**skip to J4**) 1. Pain less than daily 2. Pain daily	**b. INTENSITY** of pain 1. Mild pain 2. Moderate pain 3. Times when pain is horrible or excruciating	

3.	PAIN SITE	(If pain present, **check all sites** that apply in **last 7 days**)				
		Back pain	a.	Incisional pain	f.	
		Bone pain	b.	Joint pain (other than hip)	g.	
		Chest pain while doing usual activities	c.	Soft tissue pain (e.g., lesion, muscle)	h.	
		Headache	d.	Stomach pain	i.	
		Hip pain	e.	Other	j.	

4.	ACCIDENTS	(**Check all that apply**)			
		Fell in **past 30 days**	a.	Hip fracture in **last 180 days**	c.
		Fell in **past 31-180 days**	b.	Other fracture in **last 180 days**	d.
				NONE OF ABOVE	e.

5.	STABILITY OF CONDITIONS	Conditions/diseases make resident's cognitive, ADL, mood or behavior patterns unstable—(fluctuating, precarious, or deteriorating)	a.
		Resident experiencing an acute episode or a flare-up of a recurrent or chronic problem	b.
		End-stage disease, 6 or fewer months to live	c.
		NONE OF ABOVE	d.

SECTION K. ORAL/NUTRITIONAL STATUS

1.	ORAL PROBLEMS	Chewing problem	a.
		Swallowing problem	b.
		Mouth pain	c.
		NONE OF ABOVE	d.

2.	HEIGHT AND WEIGHT	Record (**a.**) height in inches and (**b.**) weight in pounds. Base weight on most recent measure in **last 30 days**; measure weight consistently in accord with standard facility practice—e.g., in a.m. after voiding, before meal, with shoes off, and in nightclothes
		a. HT (in.) **b.** WT (lb.)

3.	WEIGHT CHANGE	**a. Weight loss**—5 % or more in **last 30 days**; or 10 % or more in **last 180 days** 0. No 1. Yes	
		b. Weight gain—5 % or more in **last 30 days**; or 10 % or more in **last 180 days** 0. No 1. Yes	

4.	NUTRITIONAL PROBLEMS	Complains about the taste of many foods	a.	Leaves 25% or more of food uneaten at most meals	c.
		Regular or repetitive complaints of hunger	b.	NONE OF ABOVE	d.

5.	NUTRITIONAL APPROACHES	(**Check all that apply in last 7 days**)			
		Parenteral/IV	a.	Dietary supplement between meals	f.
		Feeding tube	b.	Plate guard, stabilized built-up utensil, etc.	g.
		Mechanically altered diet	c.	On a planned weight change program	h.
		Syringe (oral feeding)	d.		
		Therapeutic diet	e.	NONE OF ABOVE	i.

6.	PARENTERAL OR ENTERAL INTAKE	(**Skip to Section L if neither 5a nor 5b is checked**)
		a. Code the proportion of **total calories** the resident received through parenteral or tube feedings in the **last 7 days** 0. None 3. 51% to 75% 1. 1% to 25% 4. 76% to 100% 2. 26% to 50%
		b. Code the average **fluid intake** per day by IV or tube in **last 7 days** 0. None 3. 1001 to 1500 cc/day 1. 1 to 500 cc/day 4. 1501 to 2000 cc/day 2. 501 to 1000 cc/day 5. 2001 or more cc/day

SECTION L. ORAL/DENTAL STATUS

1.	ORAL STATUS AND DISEASE PREVENTION	Debris (soft, easily movable substances) present in mouth prior to going to bed at night	a.
		Has dentures or removable bridge	b.
		Some/all natural teeth lost—does not have or does not use dentures (or partial plates)	c.
		Broken, loose, or carious teeth	d.
		Inflamed gums (gingiva); swollen or bleeding gums; oral abcesses; ulcers or rashes	e.
		Daily cleaning of teeth/dentures or daily mouth care—by resident or staff	f.
		NONE OF ABOVE	g.

SECTION M. SKIN CONDITION

			Number at Stage
1.	ULCERS (Due to any cause)	(Record the number of ulcers at each ulcer stage—regardless of cause. If none present at a stage, record "0" (zero). Code all that apply during **last 7 days**. Code 9 = 9 or more.) [**Requires full body exam.**]	
		a. Stage 1. A persistent area of skin redness (without a break in the skin) that does not disappear when pressure is relieved.	
		b. Stage 2. A partial thickness loss of skin layers that presents clinically as an abrasion, blister, or shallow crater.	
		c. Stage 3. A full thickness of skin is lost, exposing the subcutaneous tissues - presents as a deep crater with or without undermining adjacent tissue.	
		d. Stage 4. A full thickness of skin and subcutaneous tissue is lost, exposing muscle or bone.	

2.	TYPE OF ULCER	(For each type of ulcer, **code for the highest stage in the last 7 days** using scale in item M1—i.e., 0=none; stages 1, 2, 3, 4)	
		a. Pressure ulcer—any lesion caused by pressure resulting in damage of underlying tissue	
		b. Stasis ulcer—open lesion caused by poor circulation in the lower extremities	

3.	HISTORY OF RESOLVED ULCERS	Resident had an ulcer that was resolved or cured **in LAST 90 DAYS** 0. No 1. Yes	

4.	OTHER SKIN PROBLEMS OR LESIONS PRESENT	(**Check all that apply** during **last 7 days**)	
		Abrasions, bruises	a.
		Burns (second or third degree)	b.
		Open lesions other than ulcers, rashes, cuts (e.g., cancer lesions)	c.
		Rashes—e.g., intertrigo, eczema, drug rash, heat rash, herpes zoster	d.
		Skin desensitized to pain or pressure	e.
		Skin tears or cuts (other than surgery)	f.
		Surgical wounds	g.
		NONE OF ABOVE	h.

5.	SKIN TREATMENTS	(**Check all that apply** during **last 7 days**)	
		Pressure relieving device(s) for chair	a.
		Pressure relieving device(s) for bed	b.
		Turning/repositioning program	c.
		Nutrition or hydration intervention to manage skin problems	d.
		Ulcer care	e.
		Surgical wound care	f.
		Application of dressings (with or without topical medications) other than to feet	g.
		Application of ointments/medications (other than to feet)	h.
		Other preventative or protective skin care (other than to feet)	i.
		NONE OF ABOVE	j.

6.	FOOT PROBLEMS AND CARE	(**Check all that apply** during **last 7 days**)	
		Resident has one or more foot problems—e.g., corns, callouses, bunions, hammer toes, overlapping toes, pain, structural problems	a.
		Infection of the foot—e.g., cellulitis, purulent drainage	b.
		Open lesions on the foot	c.
		Nails/calluses trimmed during **last 90 days**	d.
		Received preventative or protective foot care (e.g., used special shoes, inserts, pads, toe separators)	e.
		Application of dressings (with or without topical medications)	f.
		NONE OF ABOVE	g.

SECTION N. ACTIVITY PURSUIT PATTERNS

1.	TIME AWAKE	(**Check appropriate time periods over last 7 days**) Resident awake all or most of time (i.e., naps no more than one hour per time period) in the:			
		Morning	a.	Evening	c.
		Afternoon	b.	NONE OF ABOVE	d.

(If resident is comatose, skip to Section O)

2.	AVERAGE TIME INVOLVED IN ACTIVITIES	(**When awake and not receiving treatments or ADL care**) 0. Most—more than 2/3 of time 2. Little—less than 1/3 of time 1. Some—from 1/3 to 2/3 of time 3. None	

3.	PREFERRED ACTIVITY SETTINGS	(**Check all settings** in which activities are **preferred**)			
		Own room	a.		
		Day/activity room	b.	Outside facility	d.
		Inside NH/off unit	c.	NONE OF ABOVE	e.

4.	GENERAL ACTIVITY PREFERENCES (adapted to resident's current abilities)	(**Check all PREFERENCES** whether or not activity is currently available to resident)			
		Cards/other games	a.	Trips/shopping	g.
		Crafts/arts	b.	Walking/wheeling outdoors	h.
		Exercise/sports	c.	Watching TV	i.
		Music	d.	Gardening or plants	j.
		Reading/writing	e.	Talking or conversing	k.
		Spiritual/religious activities	f.	Helping others	l.
				NONE OF ABOVE	m.

MDS 2.0 September, 2000

Resident_____ Numeric Identifier _____

5.	PREFERS CHANGE IN DAILY ROUTINE	Code for resident preferences in daily routines 0. No change 1. Slight change 2. Major change	
		a. Type of activities in which resident is currently involved	
		b. Extent of resident involvement in activities	

SECTION O. MEDICATIONS

1.	NUMBER OF MEDICA-TIONS	(*Record the number of different medications used in the last 7 days;* enter "0" if none used)	
2.	NEW MEDICA-TIONS	(*Resident currently receiving medications that were initiated during the last 90 days*) 0. No 1. Yes	
3.	INJECTIONS	(*Record the number of DAYS injections of any type received during the last 7 days; enter "0" if none used*)	
4.	DAYS RECEIVED THE FOLLOWING MEDICATION	(*Record the number of DAYS during last 7 days; enter "0" if not used. Note—enter "1" for long-acting meds used less than weekly*)	
		a. Antipsychotic	**d.** Hypnotic
		b. Antianxiety	**e.** Diuretic
		c. Antidepressant	

SECTION P. SPECIAL TREATMENTS AND PROCEDURES

1.	SPECIAL TREAT-MENTS, PROCE-DURES, AND PROGRAMS	**a. SPECIAL CARE—Check** treatments or programs received during the last 14 days	

TREATMENTS				
			Ventilator or respirator	l.
Chemotherapy	a.		**PROGRAMS**	
Dialysis	b.		Alcohol/drug treatment program	m.
IV medication	c.		Alzheimer's/dementia special care unit	n.
Intake/output	d.			
Monitoring acute medical condition	e.		Hospice care	o.
Ostomy care	f.		Pediatric unit	p.
Oxygen therapy	g.		Respite care	q.
Radiation	h.		Training in skills required to return to the community (e.g., taking medications, house work, shopping, transportation, ADLs)	r.
Suctioning	i.			
Tracheostomy care	j.			
Transfusions	k.		NONE OF ABOVE	s.

b. THERAPIES - Record the number of days and total minutes each of the following therapies was administered (for at least 15 minutes a day) in the last 7 calendar days (Enter 0 if none or less than 15 min. daily) [Note—count only post admission therapies]
(A) = # of days administered for **15 minutes or more**
(B) = total # of minutes provided in last 7 days

	DAYS (A)	MIN (B)
a. Speech - language pathology and audiology services		
b. Occupational therapy		
c. Physical therapy		
d. Respiratory therapy		
e. Psychological therapy (by any licensed mental health professional)		

2.	INTERVEN-TION PROGRAMS FOR MOOD, BEHAVIOR, COGNITIVE LOSS	(**Check all interventions or strategies used in last 7 days**—no matter where received)	
		Special behavior symptom evaluation program	a.
		Evaluation by a licensed mental health specialist in **last 90 days**	b.
		Group therapy	c.
		Resident-specific deliberate changes in the environment to address mood/behavior patterns—e.g., providing bureau in which to rummage	d.
		Reorientation—e.g., cueing	e.
		NONE OF ABOVE	f.

3.	NURSING REHABILITA-TION/ RESTOR-ATIVE CARE	Record the NUMBER OF DAYS each of the following rehabilitation or restorative techniques or practices was **provided to the resident for more than or equal to 15 minutes per day in the last 7 days** (Enter 0 if none or less than 15 min. daily.)	
		a. Range of motion (passive)	**f.** Walking
		b. Range of motion (active)	**g.** Dressing or grooming
		c. Splint or brace assistance	**h.** Eating or swallowing
		TRAINING AND SKILL PRACTICE IN:	**i.** Amputation/prosthesis care
		d. Bed mobility	**j.** Communication
		e. Transfer	**k.** Other

4.	DEVICES AND RESTRAINTS	(*Use the following codes for last 7 days:*) 0. Not used 1. Used less than daily 2. Used daily	
		Bed rails	
		a. — Full bed rails on all open sides of bed	
		b. — Other types of side rails used (e.g., half rail, one side)	
		c. Trunk restraint	
		d. Limb restraint	
		e. Chair prevents rising	
5.	HOSPITAL STAY(S)	Record number of times resident was admitted to hospital with an overnight stay **in last 90 days** (or since last assessment if less than 90 days). (*Enter 0 if no hospital admissions*)	
6.	EMERGENCY ROOM (ER) VISIT(S)	Record number of times resident visited ER without an overnight stay **in last 90 days** (or since last assessment if less than 90 days). (*Enter 0 if no ER visits*)	
7.	PHYSICIAN VISITS	In the **LAST 14 DAYS** (or since admission if less than 14 days in facility) how many days has the physician (or authorized assistant or practitioner) examined the resident? (*Enter 0 if none*)	
8.	PHYSICIAN ORDERS	In the **LAST 14 DAYS** (or since admission if less than 14 days in facility) how many days has the physician (or authorized assistant or practitioner) changed the resident's orders? Do not include order renewals without change. (Enter 0 if none)	
9.	ABNORMAL LAB VALUES	Has the resident had any abnormal lab values during the **last 90 days** (or since admission)? 0. No 1. Yes	

SECTION Q. DISCHARGE POTENTIAL AND OVERALL STATUS

1.	DISCHARGE POTENTIAL	**a.** Resident expresses/indicates preference to return to the community 0. No 1. Yes	
		b. Resident has a support person who is positive towards discharge 0. No 1. Yes	
		c. Stay projected to be of a short duration— discharge projected **within 90 days** (do not include expected discharge due to death) 0. No 2. Within 31-90 days 1. Within 30 days 3. Discharge status uncertain	

2.	OVERALL CHANGE IN CARE NEEDS	Resident's overall self sufficiency has changed significantly as compared to status of **90 days ago** (or since last assessment if less than 90 days)
		0. No change 1. Improved—receives fewer 2. Deteriorated—receives
		                     supports, needs less more support
		                     restrictive level of care	

SECTION R. ASSESSMENT INFORMATION

1.	PARTICIPA-TION IN ASSESS-MENT	a. Resident:	0. No	1. Yes	
		b. Family:	0. No	1. Yes	2. No family
		c. Significant other:	0. No	1. Yes	2. None

2. SIGNATURE OF PERSON COORDINATING THE ASSESSMENT:

a. Signature of RN Assessment Coordinator (sign on above line)

b. Date RN Assessment Coordinator signed as complete					
Month		Day		Year	

Resident _____   Numeric Identifier _____

SECTION T. THERAPY SUPPLEMENT FOR MEDICARE PPS

1.	SPECIAL TREAT-MENTS AND PROCE-DURES	**a. RECREATION THERAPY**—*Enter number of days and total minutes of recreation therapy administered (**for at least 15 minutes a day**) in the last 7 days* (*Enter 0 if none*)

		DAYS (A)	MIN (B)

(A) = # of days administered for 15 minutes or more
(B) = total # of minutes provided in last 7 days

Skip unless this is a Medicare 5 day or Medicare readmission/ return assessment.

b. ORDERED THERAPIES—*Has physician ordered any of following therapies to begin in FIRST 14 days of stay—physical therapy, occupational therapy, or speech pathology service?*
0. No   1. Yes

If not ordered, skip to item 2

c. Through day 15, provide an estimate of the number of days when at least 1 therapy service can be expected to have been delivered.

d. Through day 15, provide an estimate of the number of therapy minutes (across the therapies) that can be expected to be delivered?

2.	WALKING WHEN MOST SELF SUFFICIENT	*Complete item 2 if ADL self-performance score for TRANSFER (G.1.b.A) is 0,1,2, or 3 AND at least one of the following are present:*

• Resident received physical therapy involving gait training (P.1.b.c)
• Physical therapy was ordered for the resident involving gait training (T.1.b)
• Resident received nursing rehabilitation for walking (P.3.f)
• Physical therapy involving walking has been discontinued within the past 180 days

Skip to item 3 if resident did not walk in last 7 days

(FOR FOLLOWING FIVE ITEMS, BASE CODING ON THE EPISODE WHEN THE RESIDENT WALKED THE FARTHEST WITHOUT SITTING DOWN. INCLUDE WALKING DURING REHABILITATION SESSIONS.)

a. Furthest distance walked without sitting down during this episode.

0. 150+ feet   3. 10-25 feet
1. 51-149 feet   4. Less than 10 feet
2. 26-50 feet

b. Time walked without sitting down during this episode.

0. 1-2 minutes   3. 11-15 minutes
1. 3-4 minutes   4. 16-30 minutes
2. 5-10 minutes   5. 31+ minutes

c. Self-Performance in walking during this episode.

0. *INDEPENDENT*—No help or oversight
1. *SUPERVISION*—Oversight, encouragement or cueing provided
2. *LIMITED ASSISTANCE*—Resident highly involved in walking; received physical help in guided maneuvering of limbs or other nonweight bearing assistance
3. *EXTENSIVE ASSISTANCE*—Resident received weight bearing assistance while walking

d. Walking support provided associated with this episode (code regardless of resident's self-performance classification).

0. No setup or physical help from staff
1. Setup help only
2. One person physical assist
3. Two+ persons physical assist

e. Parallel bars used by resident in association with this episode.

0. No   1. Yes

3.	CASE MIX GROUP	Medicare					State					

SECTION V. RESIDENT ASSESSMENT PROTOCOL SUMMARY

Numeric Identifier _____

Resident's Name:	Medical Record No.:

1. Check if RAP is triggered.

2. For each triggered RAP, use the RAP guidelines to identify areas needing further assessment. Document relevant assessment information regarding the resident's status.

   • Describe:
   — Nature of the condition (may include presence or lack of objective data and subjective complaints).
   — Complications and risk factors that affect your decision to proceed to care planning.
   — Factors that must be considered in developing individualized care plan interventions.
   — Need for referrals/further evaluation by appropriate health professionals.

   • Documentation should support your decision-making regarding whether to proceed with a care plan for a triggered RAP and the type(s) of care plan interventions that are appropriate for a particular resident.

   • Documentation may appear anywhere in the clinical record (e.g., progress notes, consults, flowsheets, etc.).

3. Indicate under the <u>Location of RAP Assessment Documentation</u> column where information related to the RAP assessment can be found.

4. For each triggered RAP, indicate whether a new care plan, care plan revision, or continuation of current care plan is necessary to address the problem(s) identified in your assessment. The Care Planning Decision column must be completed within 7 days of completing the RAI (MDS and RAPs).

A. RAP PROBLEM AREA	(a) Check if triggered	Location and Date of RAP Assessment Documentation	(b) Care Planning Decision—check if addressed in care plan
1. DELIRIUM			
2. COGNITIVE LOSS			
3. VISUAL FUNCTION			
4. COMMUNICATION			
5. ADL FUNCTIONAL/ REHABILITATION POTENTIAL			
6. URINARY INCONTINENCE AND INDWELLING CATHETER			
7. PSYCHOSOCIAL WELL-BEING			
8. MOOD STATE			
9. BEHAVIORAL SYMPTOMS			
10. ACTIVITIES			
11. FALLS			
12. NUTRITIONAL STATUS			
13. FEEDING TUBES			
14. DEHYDRATION/FLUID MAINTENANCE			
15. DENTAL CARE			
16. PRESSURE ULCERS			
17. PSYCHOTROPIC DRUG USE			
18. PHYSICAL RESTRAINTS			

B. _____

1. Signature of RN Coordinator for RAP Assessment Process

2. ☐☐ — ☐☐ — ☐☐☐☐ Month Day Year

3. Signature of Person Completing Care Planning Decision

4. ☐☐ — ☐☐ — ☐☐☐☐ Month Day Year

MDS 2.0 September, 2000

RESIDENT ASSESSMENT PROTOCOL TRIGGER LEGEND FOR REVISED RAPS (FOR MDS VERSION 2.0)

Key:
- ● = One item required to trigger
- ❷ = Two items required to trigger
- ★ = One of these three items, plus at least one other item required to trigger
- @ = When both ADL triggers present, maintenance takes precedence

Proceed to RAP Review once triggered

MDS ITEM		CODE	Delirium	Cognitive Loss/Dementia	Visual Function	Communication	ADL-Rehabilitation Trigger A @	ADL-Maintenance Trigger B @	Urinary Incontinence and Indwelling Catheter	Psychosocial Well-Being	Mood State	Behavioral Symptoms	Activities Trigger A	Activities Trigger B	Falls	Nutritional Status	Feeding Tubes	Dehydration/Fluid Maintenance	Dental Care	Pressure Ulcers	Psychotropic Drug Use	Physical Restraints	
B2a	Short term memory	1		●																			B2a
B2b	Long term memory	1		●																			B2b
B4	Decision making	1,2,3		●																			B4
B4	Decision making	3				●																	B4
B5a to B5f	Indicators of delirium	2	●																		●		B5a to B5f
B6	Change in cognitive status	2	●																		●		B6
C1	Hearing	1,2,3				●																	C1
C4	Understood by others	1,2,3				●																	C4
C6	Understand others	1,2,3		●		●																	C6
C7	Change in communication	2																			●		C7
D1	Vision	1,2,3			●																		D1
D2a	Side vision problem	√			●																		D2a
E1a to E1p	Indicators of depression, anxiety, sad mood	1,2									●												E1a to E1p
E1n	Repetitive movement	1,2																			●		E1n
E1o	Withdrawal from activities	1,2								●													E1o
E2	Mood persistence	1,2									●												E2
E3	Change in mood	2	●																		●		E3
E4aA	Wandering	1,2,3											●										E4aA
E4aA - E4eA	Behavioral symptoms	1,2,3										●											E4aA - E4eA
E5	Change in behavioral symptoms	1										●											E5
E5	Change in behavioral symptoms	2	●																		●		E5
F1d	Establishes own goals	√								●													F1d
F2a to F2d	Unsettled relationships	√								●													F2a to F2d
F3a	Strong id, past roles	√								●													F3a
F3b	Lost roles	√								●													F3b
F3c	Daily routine different	√								●													F3c
G1aA - G1jA	ADL self-performance	1,2,3,4					●																G1aA - G1jA
G1aA	Bed mobility	2,3,4,8																		●			G1aA
G2A	Bathing	1,2,3,4					●																G2A
G3b	Balance while sitting	1,2,3																		●			G3b
G6a	Bedfast	√																		●			G6a
G8a,b	Resident, staff believe capable	√					●																G8a,b
H1a	Bowel incontinence	1,2,3,4																		●			H1a
H1b	Bladder incontinence	2,3,4							●														H1b
H2b	Constipation	√																			●		H2b
H2d	Fecal impaction	√																			●		H2d
H3c,d,e	Catheter use	√							●														H3c,d,e
H3g	Use of pads/briefs	√							●														H3g
I1i	Hypotension	√																			●		I1i
I1j	Peripheral vascular disease	√																		●			I1j
I1ee	Depression	√																			●		I1ee
I1jj	Cataracts	√			●																		I1jj
I1ll	Glaucoma	√			●																		I1ll
I2j	UTI	√																●					I2j
I3	Dehydration diagnosis	276.5																●					I3
J1a	Weight fluctuation	√																●					J1a
J1c	Dehydrated	√																●					J1c
J1d	Insufficient fluid	√																●					J1d
J1f	Dizziness	√													●						●		J1f
J1h	Fever	√																●					J1h
J1i	Hallucinations	√																			●		J1i
J1j	Internal bleeding	√																●					J1j
J1k	Lung aspirations	√																			●		J1k
J1m	Syncope	√																			●		J1m

RESIDENT ASSESSMENT PROTOCOL TRIGGER LEGEND FOR REVISED RAPS (FOR MDS VERSION 2.0)

Key:
- ● = One item required to trigger
- ❷ = Two items required to trigger
- ★ = One of these three items, plus at least one other item required to trigger
- @ = When both ADL triggers present, maintenance takes precedence

Proceed to RAP Review once triggered

MDS ITEM		CODE	Delirium	Cognitive Loss/Dementia	Visual Function	Communication	ADL-Rehabilitation Trigger A @	ADL-Maintenance Trigger B @	Urinary Incontinence and Indwelling Catheter	Psychosocial Well-Being	Mood State	Behavioral Symptoms	Activities Trigger A	Activities Trigger B	Falls	Nutritional Status	Feeding Tubes	Dehydration/Fluid Maintenance	Dental Care	Pressure Ulcers	Psychotropic Drug Use	Physical Restraints	Ref
J1n	Unsteady gait	√																			●		J1n
J4a,b	Fell	√													●						●		J4a,b
J4c	Hip fracture	√																			●		J4c
K1b	Swallowing problem	√																			●		K1b
K1c	Mouth pain	√																	●				K1c
K3a	Weight loss	1														●							K3a
K4a	Taste alteration	√														●							K4a
K4c	Leave 25% food	√														●							K4c
K5a	Parenteral/IV feeding	√														●		●					K5a
K5b	Feeding tube	√															●	●					K5b
K5c	Mechanically altered	√														●							K5c
K5d	Syringe feeding	√														●							K5d
K5e	Theraputic diet	√														●							K5e
L1a,c,d,e	Dental	√																	●				L1a,c,d,e
L1f	Daily cleaning teeth	Not √																	●				L1f
M2a	Pressure ulcer	2,3,4														●							M2a
M2a	Pressure ulcer	1,2,3,4																		●			M2a
M3	Previous pressure ulcer	1																		●			M3
M4e	Impaired tactile sense	√																		●			M4e
N1a	Awake morning	√											❷										N1a
N2	Involved in activities	0											❷										N2
N2	Involved in activities	2,3								●													N2
N5a,b	Prefers change in daily routine	1,2								●													N5a,b
O4a	Antipsychotics	1-7																			★		O4a
O4b	Antianxiety	1-7													●						★		O4b
O4c	Antidepressants	1-7													●						★		O4c
O4e	Diuretic	1-7																●					O4e
P4c	Trunk restraint	1,2													●							●	P4c
P4c	Trunk restraint	2																		●			P4c
P4d	Limb restraint	1,2																				●	P4d
P4e	Chair prevents rising	1,2																				●	P4e

Useful Spanish Vocabulary and Phrases*

CHAPTER 2: THE NURSING ASSISTANT

Miss	señorita (seh-nyoh-ree-tah)
Mrs.	señora (seh-nyoh-rah)
Mr.	señor (seh-nyohr)
Hello!	¡Hola! (Oh-lah)
I am going to cover you.	Lo voy acubrir. (Loh boy ah-koo-breer)

CHAPTER 3: WORK ETHICS

Excuse me.	Con permiso. (kohn pehr-mee-soh)
Good morning, sir.	Buenos días, señor. (Boo-eh-nohs dee-ahs, seh-nyohr)
Good afternoon!	¡Buenas tardes! (Boo-eh-nahs tahr-dehs)
How may I help you?	¿En qué puedo servirle? (Ehn keh poo-eh-doh sehr-beer-leh)
Thank you for talking to me!	¡Gracias por hablar conmigo! (Grah-see-ahs pohr ah-blahr kohn-mee-goh)
Good morning, Mrs. Ortiz!	!Buenos días, señora Ortiz! (Boo-eh-nohs dee-ahs, seh-nyo-rah ohr-tees)
Good morning, doctor!	!Buenos días, doctor! (Boo-eh-nohs dee-ahs, dohk-tohr)
You are welcome.	De nada. (Deh nah-dah)
Good afternoon!	!Buenas tardes! (Boo-eh-nahs tahr-dehs)
employ	emplear (ehm-pleh-ahr)
My name is . . .	Mi nobres es . . . /Me llamo . . . (Mee nohm-breh ehs/ Meh yah-moh)
Please!	¡Por favor! (Pohr fah-bohr)
Thank you!	¡Gracias! (Grah-see-ahs)
Thank you very much!	¡Muchas gracias! (Moo-chahs grah-see-ahs)
What can I help you with?	¿En qué puedo ayudarlo? (Ehn keh poo-eh-doh ah-yoo-dahr-loh)
Yes, sir.	Sí, señor. (See, seh-nyohr)

---

*This appendix is presented for your convenience. Please note: This listing does not include all chapters; only those for which vocabulary and phrases directly relate to the content in this textbook.
Translations taken from Joyce EV, Villanueva ME: *Say it in Spanish: A Guide for Health Care Professionals*, ed 3, St. Louis, 2003, Saunders.

CHAPTER 5: COMMUNICATING WITH THE HEALTH TEAM

Number	English	Spanish	Pronunciation	Number	English	Spanish	Pronunciation
1	one	uno	(oo-noh)	17	seventeen	diecisiete	(dee-ehs-ee-see-eh-teh)
2	two	dos	(dohs)	18	eighteen	dieciocho	(dee-ehs-ee-oh-choh)
3	three	tres	(trehs)	19	nineteen	diecinueve	(dee-ehs-ee-noo-eh-beh)
4	four	cuatro	(koo-ah-troh)	20	twenty	veinte	(beh-een-teh)
5	five	cinco	(seen-koh)	30	thirty	treinta	(treh-een-tah)
6	six	seis	(seh-ees)	40	forty	cuarenta	(koo-ah-rehn-tah)
7	seven	siete	(see-eh-teh)	50	fifty	cincuenta	(seen-koo-ehn-tah)
8	eight	ocho	(oh-choh)	60	sixty	sesenta	(seh-sehn-tah)
9	nine	nueve	(noo-eh-beh)	70	seventy	setenta	(seh-tehn-tah)
10	ten	diez	(dee-ehs)	80	eighty	ochenta	(oh-chehn-tah)
11	eleven	once	(ohn-seh)	90	ninety	noventa	(noh-behn-tah)
12	twelve	doce	(doh-seh)	100	one hundred	cien	(see-ehn)
13	thirteen	trece	(treh-seh)				
14	fourteen	catorce	(kah-tohr-seh)				
15	fifteen	quince	(keen-seh)				
16	sixteen	dieciséis	(dee-ehs-ee-seh-ees)				

Time	Standard	Military (hours P.M.)
one o'clock	la una (la oo-nah)	las trece horas (lahs treh-seh oh-rahs)
two o'clock	las dos (lahs dohs)	las catorce horas (lahs kah-tohr-seh oh-rahs)
three o'clock	las tres (lahs trehs)	las quince horas (lahs keen-seh oh-rahs)
four o'clock	las cuatro (lahs koo-ah-troh)	las dieciséis horas (lahs dee-ehs-ee-seh-ees oh-rahs)
five o'clock	las cinco (lahs seen-koh)	las diecisiete horas (lahs dee-ehs-ee-see-eh-teh oh-rahs)
six o'clock	las seis (lahs seh-ees)	las dieciocho horas (lahs dee-ehs-ee-oh-choh oh-rahs)
seven o'clock	las siete (lahs see-eh-teh)	las diecinueve horas (lahs dee-ehs-ee-noo-eh-beh oh-rahs)
eight o'clock	las ocho (lahs oh-choh)	las veinte horas (lahs beh-een-teh oh-rahs)
nine o'clock	las nueve (lahs noo-eh-beh)	las veintiuna horas (lahs beh-een-tee-oo-nah oh-rahs)
ten o'clock	las diez (lahs dee-ehs)	las veintidós horas (lahs beh-een-tee-dohs oh-rahs)
eleven o'clock	las once (lahs ohn-seh)	las veintitrés horas (lahs beh-een-tee-trehs oh-rahs)
twelve o'clock/ midnight	las doce/la media noche (lahs doh-seh/lah meh-dee-ah non-cheh)	las cero horas (lahs seh-roh-oh-rahs) las veinticuatro horas (lahs beh-een-tee-koo-ah-troh oh-rahs)

abdomen	abdomen (ahb-doh-mehn)	which?	¿cuál? (koo-ahl)
communication	comunicación (koh-moo-nee-kah-see-ohn)	who?	¿quién? (kee-ehn)
black	negro (neh-groh)	how many?	¿cuántos? (koo-ahn-tohs)
blue	azul (ah-sool)	how much?	¿cuánto? (koo-ahn-toh)
clear	claro (klah-roh)	no, not	no (noh)
green	verde (behr-deh)	no one, nobody	nadie (nah-dee-eh)
red	rojo (roh-hoh)	nothing	nada (nah-dah)
yellow	amarillo (ah-mah-ree-yoh)	never, not ever	nunca, jamás (noon-kah, hah-mahs)
white	blanco (blahn-koh)	neither	tampoco (tahm-poh-koh)
Monday	lunes (loo-nehs)	neither. . . . nor	ni. . . . ni (nee. . . . nee)
Tuesday	martes (mahr-tehs)	not one, not any	ninguno (neen-goo-noh)
Wednesday	miércoles (mee-ehr-koh-lehs)	without	sin (seen)
Thursday	jueves (hoo-eh-behs)	Every two hours.	Cada dos horas. (Kah-dah dohs oh-rahs)
Friday	viernes (bee-ehr-nehs)	Hello, I'm John Goodguy.	Hola, soy John Goodguy. (Oh-lah, soh-ee John Goodguy)
Saturday	sábado (sah-bah-doh)	Hello, Mrs. Mora.	Hola, se–ora Mora. (Oh-lah, seh-nyoh-rah Moh-rah)
Sunday	domingo (doh-meen-goh)	How are you?	¿Cómo está? (Koh-moh ehs-tah)
what?	¿qué?/¿qué tal? (keh/keh tahl)	How do you feel?	¿Cómo te sientes? (Koh-moh teh see-ehn-tehs)
when?	¿cuándo? (koo-ahn-doh)	How do you feel now?	¿Cómo se siente ahora? (Koh-moh seh see-ehn-teh ah-oh-rah)
where?	¿dónde? (dohn-deh)		
why?	¿por qué? (pohr keh)		
for whom?	¿para quién? (pah-rah kee-ehn)		
for what?	¿para qué? (pah-rah keh)		

CHAPTER 6: ASSISTING WITH THE NURSING PROCESS

Do you know where we are?	¿Sabe dónde está? (Sah-beh dohn-deh ehs-tah)
Do you know the day?	¿Qué día es hoy? (Keh dee-ah ehs oh-ee)
Where does it hurt?	¿Dónde le duele? (Don-deh leh doo-eh-leh)
Point.	Apunte./Señale. (Ah-poon-teh/Seh-nyah-leh)
Did you fall?	¿Se cay—? (Seh kah-yoh)
Do you have any symptoms: nausea, dizziness, other unusual feelings?	¿Tiene algún síntoma como náuseas, vértigo, otra sensación rara? (Tee-eh-neh ahl-goon seen-toh-mah koh-moh nah-oo-seh-ahs, behr-tee-goh, oh-trah sehn-sah-see-ohn rah-rah)
Does the pain move from one place to another?	¿El dolor se mueve de un lugar a otro? (Ehl doh-lohr seh moo-eh-beh deh oon loo-gahr ah oh-trah)
Does the pain get better if you stop and rest?	¿Se mejora el dolor si se detiene y descansa? (Seh meh-hoh-rah ehl doh-lohr see seh deh-tee-eh-neh ee dehs-kahn-sah)
Has the pain gotten worse or gotten better?	¿Se ha puesto el dolor peor o mejor? (Seh ah poo-ehs-toh ehl doh-lohr peh-ohr oh meh-hohr)
How often do you have the pain?	¿Qué tan seguido tiene el dolor? (Keh tahn seh-gee-doh tee-eh-neh ehl doh-lohr)
How severe is the pain?	¿Qué tan severo es el dolor? (Keh tahn seh-beh-roh ehs ehl doh-lohr)
On a scale from 1 [insignificant] to 10 [unbearable]	En una escala del 1 [insignificante] al 10 [intolerable]: (Ehn oo-nah ehs-kah-lah dehl oo-noh [een-seeg-nee-fee-kahn-teh] ahl deeehs [een-toh-leh-rah-bleh])
Is the pain there all the time, or does it come and go?	¿Está el dolor allí todo el tiempo, o va y viene? (Ehs-tah ehl doh-lohr ah-yee toh-doh ehl tee-ehm-poh, oh bah ee bee-ehn-eh?)
What caused the pain?	¿Qué causó el dolor? (Keh kah-oo-soh ehl doh-lohr)
What did you do that caused the pain?	¿Qué hacía cuando apareció el dolor? (Keh ah-see-ah koo-ahn-doh ah-pah-reh-see-oh ehl doh-lohr)
What makes the pain better?	¿Qué hace mejorar el dolor? (Keh ah-seh meh-hoh-rahr ehl doh-lohr)
What is wrong?	¿Qué pasa? (Keh pah-sah)
Is there any pain?	¿Tiene algún dolor? (Tee-eh-neh ahl-goon doh-lohr)
What is hurting you?	¿Qué le duele? (Keh leh doo-eh-leh)
How are you?	¿Cómo está? (Koh-moh ehs-tah)
Do you have vision problems?	¿Tienes problemas con la visión? (Tee-eh-nehs proh-bleh-mahs kohn lah bee-see-ohn)
Do you wear glasses?	¿Usas anteojos/lentes? (Oo-sahs ahn-teh-ohhohs/lehn-tehs)
Do you have problems with your teeth?	¿Tienes promblemas con los dientes? (Tee-eh-nehs prog-bleh-mahs kohn lohs dee-ehn-tehs)
At what time do you go to sleep?	¿A qué hora te acuestas a dormir? (Ah keh oh-rah teh ah-koo-ehs-tahs ah dohr-meer)
How many hours do you sleep?	¿Cuantás horas duermes? (Koo-ahn-tahs oh-rahs doo-ehr-mehs)
Do you wake up at night?	¿Te despiertas en la noche? (Teh dehs-pee-ehr-tahs ehn lah noh-che)
Have you had headaches?	¿Ha tenido dolor de cabeza? (Ah teh-nee-doh doh-lohr deh kah-beh-sah)
Do you have dizzy spells?	¿Tiene mareos? (Tee-eh-neh mah-reh-ohs)
Swelling of the ankles?	¿Hinchazón en los tobillos? (Een-chah-sohn ehn lohs toh-bee-yohs)
nausea	náusea (nah-oo-seh-ah)
normal	normal (nohr-mahl)
Are you nauseated?	¿Está nauseado?/¿Tiene náuseas? (Ehs-tah nah-oo-seh-ah-doh/ Tee-eh-neh nah-oo-seh-ahs)
Are you okay?	¿Está bien?/¿Se siente bien? (Ehs-tah bee-ehn/ Seh see-ehn-teh bee-ehn)

Do you feel
  nauseated?
¿Se siente nauseado?
(Seh see-ehn-teh nah-oo-
  seh-ah-doh)

Do you feel weak?
¿Se siente débril?
(Seh see-ehn-teh deh-beel)

Do you have pain?
¿Tiene dolor?
(Tee-eh-neh doh-lohr)

Is there any pain?
¿Tiene algún dolor?
(Tee-eh-neh ahl-goon doh-lohr)

Is there anything
  that worries you?
¿Hay algo que le preocupa?
(Ah-ee ahl-goh keh leh preh-oh-
  koo-pah)

Is there anything
  else bothering
  you?
¿Hay otra cosa que le moleste?
(Ah-ee oh-trah koh-sah keh-leh
  moh-lehs-teh)

Is there numbness/a
  tingling sensation/
  burning in your
  leg/arm/foot/
  hand?
¿Está entumecido/adormecido/
  tiene ardor en su pierna/
  brazo/pie/mano?
(Ehs-tah ehn-too-meh-see-doh/
  ah-dohr-meh-see-do/
  tee-eh-neh ahr-dohr ehn soo
  pee-ehr-nah/brah-soh/
  pee-eh/mah-noh)

Tell me if there is
  pain.
Dime si duele.
(Dee-meh see doo-eh-leh)

Tell me if it hurts.
Dime si esto te duele.
(Dee-meh see ehs-toh teh doo-
  eh-leh)

The pain is in one
  place?
¿El dolor es fijo?
(Ehl doh-lohr ehs fee-hoh)

The pain is local-
  ized, sharp.
El dolor está fijo, agudo.
(Ehl doh-lohr ehs-tah ehn ehl
  lah-dohl kohs-tah-doh)

The pain is on the
  side.
El dolor está en el lado/costado.
(Ehl doh-lohr ehs-tah ehn ehl
  lah-dohl kohs-tah-doh)

The pain is sharp?
¿El dolor es agudo?
(Ehl doh-lohr ehs ah-goo-doh)

What brought you
  to the hospital?
¿Qué lo trajo al hospital?
(Keh loh trah-hoh ahl
  ohs-pee-tahl)

What is the matter?
¿Qué le pasa/sucede?
(Keh leh pah-sah/soo-seh-deh)

What is the pain
  like?
¿Qué tipo de dolor tiene?
(Keh tee-oh deh doh-lohr tee-
  eh-neh)

What other discom-
  fort do you have?
¿Qué otra molestia tiene?
(Keh oh-trah moh-lehs-tee-ah
  tee-eh-neh)

What symptoms do
  you have?
¿Qué síntomas tiene?
(Keh seen-toh-mahs tee-eh-neh)

When you have
  pain, do you get
  nauseated?
Cuando tiene dolor, ¿le dan
  náuseas?
(Koo-ahn-doh tee-eh-neh doh-
  lohr, leh dahn nah-oo-seh-ahs)

CHAPTER 7: UNDERSTANDING THE PERSON

Let me know how
  you feel.
Dígame cómo se siente.
(Dee-gah-meh koh-moh seh
  see-ehn-teh)

My name is . . .
Mi nombre es . . . /Me llamo . . .
(Mee nohm-breh ehs/
  Meh yah-moh)s

Good-bye!
¡Hasta luego!
(Ahs-tah loo-eh-goh)

Hi!
!Hola!
(Oh-lah)

Good morning.
Buenos días.
(Boo-eh-nohs dee-ahs)

Good afternoon.
Buenas tardes.
(Boo-eh-nahs tahr-dehs)

Good evening.
Buenas noches.
(Boo-eh-nahs noh-chehs)

Do you speak
  English?
¿Habla inglés?
(Ah-blah een-glehs)

Thank you!
¡Gracias!
(Grah-see-ahs)

Thank you very
  much!
¡Muchas gracias!
(Moo-chahs grah-see-ahs)

You are welcome.
De nada.
(Deh nah-dah)

respect
respeto
(rehs-peh-toh)

the family
la familia
(lah fah-mee-lee-ah)

father
padre
(pah-dreh)

dad
papá
(pah-pah)

mother
madre
(mah-dreh)

mom
mamá
(mah-mah)

husband
esposo
(ehs-poh-soh)

wife
esposa
(ehs-poh-sah)

sister
hermana
(ehr-mah-nah)

brother
hermano
(ehr-mah-noh)

son
hijo
(ee-hoh)

daughter
hija
(ee-hah)

niece
sobrina
(soh-bree-nah)

nephew
sobrino
(soh-bree-noh)

grandmother
abuela
(ah-boo-eh-lah)

grandfather	abuelo
	(ah-boo-eh-loh)
grandparents	abuelos
	(ah-boo-eh-lohs)
aunt	tía
	(tee-ah)
uncle	tío
	(tee-oh)
stepfather	padrastro
	(pah-drahs-troh)
stepmother	madrastra
	(mah-drahs-trah)
stepson	hijastro
	(ee-hahs-troh)
stepdaughter	hijastra
	(ee-hahs-trah)
children	hijos
	(eeh-hohs)
great-grandparents	bisabuelos
	(bee-sah-boo-eh-lohs)
mother-in-law	suegra
	(soo-eh-grah)
father-in-law	suegro
	(soo-eh-grah)
sister-in-law	cuñada
	(koo-nyah-dah)
brother-in-law	cuñado
	(koo-nyah-doh)
cousins	primos
	(pree-mohs)
cousin (female)	prima
	(pree-mah)
cousin (male)	primo
	(pree-moh)
grandchildren	nietos
	(nee-eh-tohs)
godparents	padrinos
	(pah-dree-nohs)
godfather	padrino
	(pah-dree-noh)
godmother	madrina
	(mah-dree-nah)
Do you understand?	¿Comprende?/¿Entiende?
	(Kohm-prehn-deh/
	Ehn-tee-ehn-deh)
Are you cold?	¿Tiene frío?
	(Tee-eh-neh free-oh)
Are you hot?	¿Tiene calor?
	(tee-eh-neh kah-lohr)
Are you hungry?	¿Tiene hambre?
	(Tee-eh-neh ahm-breh)
Are you sleepy?	¿Tiene sueño?
	(Tee-eh-neh soo-eh-nyoh)
Are you thirsty?	¿Tiene sed?
	(Tee-eh-neh sehd)

Is that enough?	¿Es suficiente?
	(Ehs soo-fee-see-ehn-teh)
Is that a lot?	¿Es mucho?
	(Ehs moo-choh)
Is that too much?	¿Es demasiado?
	(Ehs deh-mah-see-ah-doh)
Are you comfortable?	¿Está cómoda?
	(Ehs tah koh-moh-dah)
A nurse will see you.	Una enfermera la atenderá.
	(Ooh-nah ehn-fehr-meh-rah lah ah-tehn-deh-rah)
Good!	¡Bueno!
	(Boo-eh-noh)
Good afternoon, Miss González.	Buenas tardes, señorita González.
	(Boo-eh-nahs tahr-dehs, seh-nyoh-ree-tah Gohn-sah-lehs)
Good luck!	¡Buena suerte!
	(Boo-eh-nah soo-ehr-teh)
Have a good day!	¡Pase un buen día!
	(Pah-seh oon boo-ehn dee-ah)
Hello.	Hola
	(Oh-lah)
I am through.	Ya terminé.
	(Yah tehr-mee-neh)
I will see you tomorrow.	Le veré mañana.
	(Lah beh-reh mah-nyah-nah)
I will return shortly.	Regresaré en seguida.
	(Reh-greh-sah-reh ehn seh-ghee-dah)
If you don't understand, please let me know.	Si no entiende, dígame por favor.
	(See noh ehn-tee-ehn-deh, dee-gah-meh pohr fah-bohr)
Visiting hours are from nine in the morning to nine at night.	Las horas de visita son de las nueve de la ma–ana a las nueve de la noche.
	(Lahs oh-rahs deh bee-see-tah shon deh lahs noo-eh-beh deh lah mah-nyah-nah ah lahs noo-eh-beh deh lah noh-cheh)
Visiting hours are from two to eight P.M.	Las horas de visita son de las dos a las ocho de la noche.
	(Lahs oh-rahs deh bee-see-tah sohn deh lahs dohs ah loahs oh-choh deh lah noh-cheh)

CHAPTER 8: BODY STRUCTURE AND FUNCTION

ligament	ligamento
	(lee-gah-mehn-toh)
organ	órgano
	(ohr-gah-noh)
pancreas	páncreas
	(pahn-kreh-ahs)
saliva	saliva
	(sah-lee-bah)

CHAPTER 9: GROWTH AND DEVELOPMENT

infancy | infancia
(een-fahn-see-ah)

CHAPTER 11: SAFETY

What can I help you with? | ¿En qué puedo ayudarlo?
(Ehn keh poo-eh-doh ah-yoo-dahr-loh)

This is the call bell. | Este es el timbre.
(Ehs-teh ehs ehl teem-breh)

coma | coma
(koh-mah)

comatose | comatoso
(koh-mah-toh-soh)

Call if you need help. | Llame si necesita ayuda.
(Yah-meh see neh-seh-see-tah ah-yoo-dah)

No smoking. | No se permite fumar.
(Noh seh pehr-mee-teh foo-mahr)

Wear this bracelet all the time. | Use esta pulsera todo el tiempo.
(Oo-seh ehs-tah pool-seh-rah toh-doh ehl tee-ehm-poh)

You cannot smoke here. | No puede fumar aquí.
(Noh poo-eh-deh foo-mahr ah-kee)

You cannot smoke in your room. | No puede fumar en el cuatro.
(Noh poo-eh-deh foo-mahr ehn ehl koo-ahr-toh)

CHAPTER 14: PREVENTING INFECTION

Wash well all fruits and vegetables. | Lave bien frutas y verduras.
(Lah-beh bee-ehn froo-tahs ee behr-doo-rahs)

Wash hands before eating. | Lave las manos antes de comer.
(Lah-beh lahs mah-nohs ahn-tehs deh koh-mehr)

bacteria | bacteria
(bahk-teh-ree-ah)

inflammation | inflamación
(een-flah-mah-see-ohn)

pathogen | patogénico
(pah-toh-heh-nee-koh)

CHAPTER 15: BODY MECHANICS

spinal | espinal
(ehs-pee-nahl)

CHAPTER 16: SAFELY HANDLING, MOVING, AND TRANSFERRING THE PERSON

I will put you on the stretcher. | Voy a ponerlo en la camilla.
(Boy ah poh-nher-loh ehn lah kah-mee-yah)

Sit in the chair. | Siéntese en la silla.
(See-ehn-teh-seh ehn lah see-yah)

Do you need the headboard up? | ¿Necesita levantar más la cabecera?
(Neh-seh-see-tah leh-bahn-tahr mahs lah kah-beh-seh-rah)

I am going to help you lie down. | Voy a ayudarlo a acostarse.
(Boy ah ah-yoo-dahr-loh ah ah-kohs-tahr-seh)

I am going to help you lie on the stretcher. | Voy a ayudarlo a acostarse en la camilla.
(Boy ah ah-yoo-dahr-loh ah ah-kohs-tahr-seh ehn lah kah-mee-yah)

I will help you sit. | Le ayudaré a sentarse.
(Leh ah-yoo-dah-reh ah sehn-tahr-seh)

Turn on your side. | Voltéese de lado.
(Bhol-teh-eh-seh deh lah-doh)

Turn to your side. | Voltéate de lado.
(Bhol-teh-ah-teh deh lah-doh)

CHAPTER 17: THE PERSON'S UNIT

These buttons move the bed up/down. | Estos botones mueven la cama arriba/abajo.
(Ehs-tohs boh-tah-nehs moo-eh-behn lah kay-mah ah-ree-bah/ah-bah-hoh)

You can raise the head. | Puede levantar la cabeza.
(Poo-eh-deh leh-bahn-tahr lah kah-beh-sah)

You can raise the feet. | Puede levantar los pies.
(Poo-eh-deh leh-bahn-tahr lohs pee-ehs)

The rails lower down. | El barandal se baja.
(Ehl bah-rahn-dahl seh bah-hah)

Your towels are in the bathroom. | Sus toallas están en el baño.
(Soos too-ahyahs ehs-tahn ehn ehl bah-nyoh)

There is an emergency light. | Hay una luz para emergencias.
(Ah-ee oo-nah loos pah-rah eh-mehr-hehn-see-ahs)

Pull the cord in the bathroom. | Jale el cordón en el baño.
(Hah-leh ehl kohr-dohn ehn ehl bah-nyoh)

The bell will sound. | La campana sonará.
(Lah kahm-pah-nah soh-nah-rah)

This button lowers (raises) the headboard.
Este botón baha (sube) la cabecera de la cama.
(Ehs-teh boh-tohn bah-hah (soo-beh) lah kah-beh-seh-rah deh lah kah-mah)

The chair turns into a bed.
Esta silla se hace cama.
(Ehs-tah see-yah seh ah-seh kah-mah)

This is the radio.
Este es el radio.
(Ehs-teh ehs ehl rah-dee-oh)

This is the call bell/buzzer.
Este es la campana/el timbre.
(Ehs-teh ehs lah kahm-pah-nah/ehl teem-breh)

You have a private bathroom.
Tiene un baño/inodoro privado.
(Tee-eh-neh oon bah-nyoh/ee-noh-doh-roh pree-bah-doh)

CHAPTER 18: BEDMAKING

linen
lino
(lee-noh)

Do you need more pillows?
¿Necesita más almohadas?
(Neh-seh-see-tah mahs ahl-moh-ah-dahs)

CHAPTER 19: PERSONAL HYGIENE

I am going to clean your teeth.
Voy a limpairle los dientes.
(Boy ah leem-pee-ahr-leh lohs dee-ehn-tehs)

Rinse your mouth.
Enjuague su boca.
(Ehn-hoo ah-geh soo boh-kah)

Here is a glass of water to rinse with.
Aquí está un vaso de agua para que se enjuague.
(Ah-kee-ehs-tah oon bah-soh deh ah-goo-ah pah-rah keh seh ehn-hoo-ah-geh)

Open your mouth, please.
Abra la boca, por favor.
(Ah-brah lah boh-kah, pohr fah-bohr)

There is a shower.
Hay una ducha/regadera.
(Ah-ee oo-nah doo-chah/reh-gah-deh-rah)

There is also a bathtub/tub.
También hay una bañera/tina.
(Tahm-bee-ehn ah-ee oo-nah bah-nyeh-rah/tee-nah)

Use dental floss.
Use hilo dental.
(Oo-seh ee-loh dehn-tahl)

CHAPTER 20: PERSONAL CARE AND GROOMING

Mrs. . . . , I need to help you change clothes.
Señora . . . , necesito ayudarle a cambiar su ropa.
(Se–ora . . . , neh-seh-see-toh ah-yoo-dahr-leh ah kahm-bee-ahr soo roh-pah)

CHAPTER 21: URINARY ELIMINATION

When was the last time you used the toilet?
¿Cuándo fue la última vez gue hizo del baño/que obró?
(Koo-ahn doh foo-eh lah ool-tee-mah behs keh ee-soh dehl bah-nyoh/keh oh-broh)

How often do you urinate?
¿Cuántas veces ornia?
(Koo-ahn-tahs beh-sehs oh-ree-nah)

Do you want the bedpan?
¿Quiere el pato/el bacín?
(Kee-eh-reh ehl pah-toh/ehl bah-seen)

Do you have problems with starting to urinate?
¿Tiene dificultad para empezar a orinar?
(Tee-eh-neh dee-fee-kool-tahd pah-rah ehm-peh-sahr ah oh-ree-nahr)

Do you want to pass urine?
¿Quiere orinar?
(Kee-eh-reh oh-ree-nahr)

Everytime you go to the bathroom to void, you must place the urine in the container.
Cada vez que vaya al baño a orinar, debe poner la orina en el recipiente.
(Kah-dah behs keh bah-yah ahl bah-nyoh ah oh-ree-nahr, deh-beh poh-nehr lah oh-ree-nah ehn ehl reh-see-pee-ehn-teh)

I will ask you to void.
Le diré que orine.
(Leh dee-reh keh oh-ree-neh)

CHAPTER 22: BOWEL ELIMINATION

Are you constipated?
¿Está esterñido?
(Ehs-tah ehs-treh-nyee-doh)

Do you have diarrhea?
¿Tiene diarrea?
(Tee-eh-neh dee-ah-reh-ah)

Do you wish to have a bowel movement?
¿Quiere evacuar/hacer del baño?
(Kee-eh-reh eh-bah-koo-ahr/ah-sehr dehl bah-nyoh)

A bowel movement.
Hacer del baño.
(Ah-sehr dehl bah-nyoh)

Do you want to have a bowel movement?
¿Quiere evacuar? ¿Quiere obrar?
(Kee-eh-reh eh-bah-koo-ahr/Kee-eh-reh oh-brahr)

I will collect a sample of feces.
Voy a recoger una muestra de excremento.
(Boy ah reh-koh-hehr oo-nah moo-ehs-trah deh ehx-kreh-mehn-toh)

CHAPTER 23: NUTRITION AND FLUIDS

Have you eaten?
¿Ha comido?
(Ah koh-mee-doh)

What did you eat?
¿Qué comido?
(Keh koh-mee-doh)

Do you take a special diet?
¿Toma dieta especial?
(Toh-mah dee-eh-tah ehs-peh-see-ah-lehs)

What foods do you like?	¿Qué alimentos le gustan? (Keh ah-lee-mehn-tohs leh goos-tahn)
What foods do you dislike?	¿Qué alimentos le disgustan? (Keh ah-lee-mehn-tohs leh dees-goos-tahn)
How many times do you eat per day?	¿Cuántas veces come por día? (Koo-ahn-tahs beh-sehs koh-meh pohr dee-ah)
What did you eat for breakfast?	¿Qué comió en el desayuno? (Keh koh-mee-oh ehn ehl deh-sah-yoo-noh)
I am going to give you a list.	Voy a darle una lista. (Boy ah dahr-leh oo-nah lees-tah)
For breakfast:	Para el desayuno: (Pah-rah ehl deh-sah-yoo-noh)
eggs	huevos (oo-eh-bohs)
toast	pan tostado (pahn tohs-tah-doh)
coffee	café (kah-feh)
milk	leche (leh-cheh)
juice	jugo (joo-goh)
fruit	fruta (froo-tah)
How do you like your coffee?	¿Comó le gusta el café? (Koh-moh leh goos-tah ehl kah-feh)
black	negro (neh-groh)
with cream	con crema (kohn kreh-mah)
with sugar	con azúcar (kohn ah-soo-kahr)
What kind of coffee?	¿Qué clase de café? (Keh klah-seh deh kah-feh)
regular	regular (reh-goo-lahr)
decaffeinated	descafeinado (dehs-kah-feh-ee-nah-doh)
instant	instantáneo (eens-tahn-tah-neh-oh)
What kind of juices?	¿Qué clase de jugos? (Keh klah-seh deh joo-gohs)
orange	naranja (nah-rah-hah)
grape	uva (oo-bah)
apple	manzana (mahn-sah-nah)
grapefruit	toronja (toh-rohn-hah)
prune	ciruela (see-roo-eh-lah)
tomato	tomate (toh-mah-teh)
How do you like the eggs fixed?	¿Cómo le gustan los huevos? (Koh-moh leh goos-tahn lohs oo-eh-bohs)
scrambled	revueltos (reh-boo-ehl-tohs)
over-easy	volteados (bohl-teh-ah-dohs)
fried	fritos (free-tohs)
hard-boiled	duros (doo-rohs)
with ham	con jamón (kohn hah-mahn)
We have cereals.	Tenemos cereales. (Teh-neh-mohs seh-reh-ah-lehs)
oatmeal	avena (ah-beh-nah)
cream of wheat	crema de trigo (kreh-mah deh tree-goh)
corn flakes	hojitas de maíz/corn flakes (oh-hee-tahs de mah-ees/hohrn fleh-ee-ks)
Do you like them hot/cold?	¿Le gustan calientes/fríos? (Leh goos-tahn kah-lee-ehn-tehs/free-ohs)
We have meats:	Tenemos carnes: (Teh-nehmohs kahr-nehs)
beef	res (rehs)
hamburger	hamburguesa (ahm-boor-geh-sah)
steak	bistec (bees-tehk)
roast	rostizado (rohs-tee-sah-doh)
pork	puerco (poo-ehr-koh)
chops	chuletas (choo-leh-tahs)
ribs	costillas (kohs-tee-yahs)
chicken	pollo (poh-yoh)
fried chicken	pollo frito (poh-yoh free-toh)
baked chicken	pollo asado (poh-yoh ah-sah-doh)
breast	pechuga (peh-choo-gah)
leg	pierna (pee-ehr-nah)
wings	alas (ah-lahs)
fish	pescado (pehs-kah-doh)

breaded	empanizado (ehm-pah-nee-sah-doh)	Do you want water?	¿Quere agua? (Kee-eh-reh ah-goo-ah)
broiled fish	pescado al horno (pehs-kah-doh ahl ohr-noh)	Do you need ice?	¿Necesita hielo? (Neh-seh-see-tah ee-eh-loh)
Among the vegetables that we serve are:	Entre los vegetales que servimos hay: (Ehn-treh lohs beh-heh-tah-lehs keh sehr-bee-mohs ah-ee)	The fork, spoon, and knife are wrapped in the napkin.	El tenedor, cuchara y cuchillo están envueltos en la servilleta. (Ehl teh-neh-dohr, koo-chah-rah ee koo-chee-yoh ehs-tahn ehn-boo-ehl-tohs ehn lah sehr-bee-yeh-tah)
potatoes	papas (pah-pahs)	There is a straw.	Hay un popote. (Ah-ee oon poh-poh-teh)
baked potatoes	papas asadas (pah-pahs ah-sah-dahs)	The salt and pepper are in these packets.	La sal y pimienta están en estos paquetes. (Lah sahl ee pee-mee-ehn-tah ehs-tahn ehn ehs-tohn pah-keh-tehs)
french fries	papas fritas (pah-pahs free-tahs)		
mashed potatoes	puré de papas (poo-reh deh pah-pahs)	The cover is hot.	La cubeirta está caliente. (Lah koo-bee-ehr-tah ehs-tah kah-lee-ehn-teh)
green beans	ejotes/habichuelas eh-hoh-tehs/ah-bee-choo-eh-lahs)	It keeps the food warm.	Guarda la comida tibia. (Goo-ahr-dah lah koh-mee-dah tee-bee-ah)
peas	chícharos (chee-chah-rohs)	Select your foods from the menu after breakfast.	Seleccione las comidas del menú después del desayuno. (Seh-lehk-see-oh-neh lahs koh-mee-dahs dehl meh-noo dehs-poo-ehs dehl deh-sah-yoo-noh)
corn	maíz/elote (mah-ees/eh-loh-teh)		
beans	frijoles/habas (free-hoh-lehs/ah-bahs)		
pinto beans	frijol pinto (free-hohl peen-toh)	dehydration	deshidratación (deh-see-drah-tah-see-ohn)
refried	refritos (reh-free-tohs)	nutrition	nutrición (noo-tree-see-ohn)
salad	ensalada (ehn-sah-lah-dah)	salt	sal (sahl)
lettuce	lechuga (leh-choo-gah)	Do you want:	¿Quiere: (Kee-eh-reh)
We also have desserts:	También tenemos postres: (Tahm-bee-ehn teh-neh-mohs pohs-trehs)	a glass of water?	un vaso de agua? (oon bah-soh deh ah-goo-ah)
ice cream	nieve/helado (nee-eh-beh/eh-lah-doh)	a glass of juice?	un vaso de jugo? (oon bah-soh deh hoo-goh)
vanilla	vainilla (bah-ee-nee-yah)	Do you want:	¿Quiere: (Kee-eh-reh)
chocolate	chocolate (choh-koh-lah-teh)	something to eat?	algo de comer? (ahl-goh deh koh-mehr)
strawberry	fresa (freh-sah)	something to drink?	algo de tomar/beber? (ahl-goh deh toh-mahr/beh-behr)
pies	pasteles (pahs-teh-lehs)	something to read?	algo de leer? (ahl-goh deh leh-ehr)
pecan	nuez (noo-ehs)	After meals.	Después de las comidas. (Dehs-poo-ehs deh lahs koh-mee-dahs)
apple	manzana (mahn-sah-nah)		
cookies	galletas (gah-yeh-tahs)	Are you hungry?	¿Tiene hambre? (Tee-eh-neh ahm-breh)
candy	dulces (dool-sehs)	Difficulty in swallowing . . .	Diffcultad al tragar . . . (Dee-fee-kool-tahd ahl-trah-gahr)
The water is in the glass/ pitcher.	El aqua están en el vaso/la jarra. (Ehl ah-goo-ah ehs-tah ehn ehl bah-soh/lah hah-rah)	Do you want a cup of coffee?	¿Quiere una taza de café? (Kee-eh-reh oo-nah tah-sah deh-kah-feh)

Do you want a glass of juice?	¿Quiere un vaso con jugo? (Kee-eh-reh oon bah-soh kohn hoo-goh)
Do you want a glass of water?	¿Quiere un vaso con agua? (Kee-eh-reh oon bah-soh kohn ah-goo-ah)
Do you want something to drink?	¿Quiere algo de tomar/beber? (Kee-eh-reh ahl-goh deh toh-mahr/beh-behr)
How do you like your eggs fixed?	¿Comó le gustan los huevos? (Koh-moh leh goos-tahn lohs oo-eh-bohs)
How do you like your coffee?	¿Cómo le gusta el café? (Koh-moh leh goos-tah ehl kah-feh)
How many glasses of water do you drink?	¿Cuántos vasos de agua toma? (Koo-ahn-tohs bah-sohs de ah-goo-ah toh-mah)
The meals are served at. . . .	Los alimentos se sirven a. . . (Lohs ah-lee-mehn-tohs seh seer-behn ah)
When was the last time you ate?	¿Cuándo fue la última vez que comió? (Koo-ahn-doh foo-eh lah ool-tee-mah behs keh koh-mee-oh)
You have to choose three meals a day.	Tiene que escoger tres comidas diarias. (Tee-eh-neh keh ehs-koh-hehr trehs koh-mee-dahs dee-ah-ree-ahs)

CHAPTER 25: MEASURING VITAL SIGNS

I will start by taking vital signs.	Voy a empezar por tomar los signos vitales. (Boy ah ehm-peh-sahr pohr toh-mahr lohs seeg-nohs bee-tah-lehs)
Take the temperature rectally.	Tome la temperatura por el recto. (Toh-meh lah tehm-peh-rah-too-rah pohr ehl rehk-toh)
bradycardia	bradicardia (brah-dee-kahr-dee-ah)
fever	fatal (fah-tahl)
pulse	pulso (pool-soh)
rectal	rectal (rehk-tahl)
stethoscope	estetoscopio (ehs-teh-tohs-koh-pee-oh)
systole	sístole (sees-toh-leh)
thermometer	termómetro (tehr-moh-meh-troh)

| I will take the radial pulse. | Voy a tomar su pulso radial. (Boy ah toh-mahr soo pool-soh rah-dee-ahl) |
| I will take your blood pressure. | Voy a tomar tu presión de sangre. (Boy ah toh-mahr too preh-see-ohn deh sahn-greh) |

CHAPTER 26: EXERCISE AND ACTIVITY

Please stay/ remain in bed.	Por favor, quédeses en la cama. (Pohr fah-bohr, keh-deh-seh ehn lah kan-mah)
Lift your arm.	Levanta tu brazo. (leh-bahn-tah too brah-soh)
Extend it.	Extiéndelo. (Ehx-tee-ehn-deh-loh)
Flex it.	Dóblalo. (Doh-blah-loh)
Rotate it.	Gíralo./Dale vuelta. (Hee-rah-loh/Dah-leh boo-ehl-tah)
Bend your elbow.	Dobla el codo. (doh-blah ehl koh-doh)
Turn your forearm.	Voltea el antebrazo. (Bohl-teh-ah ehl ahn-teh brah-soh)
Open your hand.	Abre tu mano. (Ah-breh too mah-noh)
Close it.	Ciérrala. (See-eh-rah-lah)
Open the fingers wide.	Separa bien los dedos. (Seh-pah-rah bee-ehn lohs deh-dohs)
Bend the wrist.	Dobla la muñeca. (Doh-blah lah moo-nyeh-kah)
Extend your wrist.	Extiende tu muñeca. (Ehx-tee-ehn-deh too moo-nyeh-kay)
Lift your leg.	Levanta la pierna. (Leh-bahn-tah lah pee-ehr-nah)
Bend it.	Dóblala. (Doh-blah-lah)
Bend your hip.	Dobla tu Cadera. (Doh-blah too kah-deh-rah)
Straighten your knee.	Endereza la rodilla. (Ehn-deh-reh-sah lah roh-dee-yah)
Move your leg.	Mueve tu pierna. (Moo-eh-beh too pee-ehr-nah)
Forward.	Adelante. (Ah-deh-lahn-teh)
Backward.	Atrás. (Ah-trahs)
Turn it to the left.	Voltéalo hacia la izquierda. (Bohl-teh-ah-loh ah-see-ah lah ees-kee-ehr-dah)
Turn it to the right.	Voltéalo hacia la derecha. (Bohl-teh-ah-loh ah-see-ah lah deh-reh-chah)
Lift your foot.	Levanta tu pie. (Leh-bahn-tah too pee-eh)

Bend your toes.	Dobla tus dedos (del pie). (Doh-blah toos deh-dohs (dehl pee-eh)	How long?	¿Cuánto tiempo? (Koo-ahn-toh tee-ehm-poh)
Lower your foot.	Baja el pie. (Bah-hah ehl pee-eh)	Rest now.	Descanse ahora. (Dehs-kahn-seh ah-oh-rah)
Flex the foot upward.	Dobla el pie hacia arriba. (Doh-blah ehl pee-eh ah-see-ah ah-ree-bah)	At what time do you go to sleep?	¿A qué hora se acuesta a dormir? (Ah keh oh-rah seh ah-koo-ehs-tah ah dohr-meer)
Straighten your leg.	Endereza tu pierna. (Ehn-deh-reh-sah too pee-ehr-nah)	Do you wake up at night?	¿Se despierta en la noche? (Seh dehs-pee-ehr-tah ehn lah noh-chen)
Please walk.	Camina, por favor. (Kah-mee-nah, pohr fah-bohr)	Are you cold?	¿Tiene frío? (Tee-eh-neh free-oh)
exercise	ejercicio (eh-hehr-see-see-oh)	Are you comfortable?	¿Está cómoda? (Ehs-tah koh-moh-dah)
syncope	síncope (seen-koh-peh)	Are you hurting?	¿Tiene dolor? (Tee-eh-neh doh-lohr)
Activities are part of the plan.	Las actividades son parte del plan. (Lahs ahk-tee-bee-dah-dehs sohn pahr-teh dehl plahn)	Are you sleepy?	¿Tiene sueño? (Tee-eh-neh soo-eh-nyoh)
Are you dizzy?	¿Tiene mareos? (Tee-eh-neh mah-reh-ohs)	Do you have chest pain?	¿Tiene dolor en el pecho? (Tee-eh-neh doh-lohr ehn ehl peh-choh)
Do you feel dizzy?	¿Se siente mareado? (Seh see-ehn-teh mah-reh-ah-doh)	Does it still hurt?	¿Todavía le duele? (Toh-dah-bee-ah leh doo-eh-leh)
Extend your arm.	Extiende tu brazo. (Ehx-tee-ehn-deh too brah-soh)	Does the pain move from one place to another?	¿El dolor se mueve de un lugar a otro? (Ehl doh-lohr seh moo-eh-beh deh oon loo-gahr ah oh-troh)
Extend your leg and foot.	Extiende tu pierna y pie. (Ehx-tee-ehn-deh too pee-ehr-nah ee pee-eh)	Has the pain gotten worse or gotten better?	¿Se ha puesto el dolor peor o mejor? (Seh ah poo-ehs-toh ehl doh-lohr peh-ohr oh meh-hohr)
Flex your foot upward.	Dobla el pie para arriba. (Doh-blah ehl pee-eh pah-rah ah-ree-bah)	How often do you have the pain?	¿Qué tan seguido tiene el dolor? (Keh tahn seh-gee-doh tee-eh-neh ehl doh-lohr)
Flex your arm.	Dobla tu brazo. (Doh-blah too brah-soh)	I am going to let you rest.	Voy a dejarlo descansar. (Boy ah deh-hahr-loh dehs-kahn-sahr)
Now raise the left arm.	Ahora levante el brazo izquierdo. (Ah-oh-rah leh-bahn-teh ehl brah-soh ees-kee-ehr-doh)	If it hurts, tell me.	Si duele, avísame. (See doo-eh-leh, ah-bee-sah-meh)
Turn the forearm.	Voltea el antebrazo. (Bhol-teh-ah ehl ahn-teh-brah-soh)	On a scale from 1 [insignificant] to 10 [unbearable]. . .	En una escala del 1 [insignificante] al 10 [intolerable]. . . (Ehn oo-nah ehs-kah-lah dehl oo-noh [een-seeg-nee-gee-kahn-teh] ahl dee-ehs [een-toh-leh-rah-bleh])

CHAPTER 27: COMFORT, REST, AND SLEEP

At what time do you get up?	¿A qué hora se levanta? (Ah keh oh-rah seh leh-bahn-tah)	Pain?	¿Dolor? (Doh-lohr)
At what time do you go to bed?	¿A qué hora se acuesta? (Ah keh oh-rah seh ah-koo-ehs-tah)	Point when it hurts.	Señale cuando duela. (Seh-nyah-leh koo-ahn-doh doo-eh-lah)
How many hours do you sleep?	¿Cuántas horas duerme? (Koo-ahn-tahs oh Drahs doo-ehr-meh)	Rest.	Descanse (Des-kahn-seh)
Do you sleep during the day?	¿Duerme durante el día? (Doo-ehr-meh doo-rahn-teh ehl dee-ah)		

CHAPTER 28: ADMISSIONS, TRANSFERS, AND DISCHARGES

I am going to ask many questions!
¡Voy a hacerle muchas preguntas!
(Boy ah ah-sehr-leh moo-chahs preh-goon-tahs)

The meals are served
Los alimentos se sirven
(Lohs ah-lee-mehn-tohs seh seer-behn)

at seven A.M.
a las siete de la ma–ana.
(ah lahs see-eh-teh deh lah mah-nyah-nah)

at eleven thirty.
a las once y media.
(ah lahs ohn-seh ee meh-dee-ah)

at five P.M.
a las cinco de la tarde.
(ah lahs seen-koh deh lah tahr-deh)

Phone for local calls.
Teléfono para llamadas locales.
(Teh-leh-foh-noh pah-rah yah-mah-dahs loh-kah-lehs)

This is the radio.
Este es el radio.
(Ehs-teh ehs ehl rah-dee-oh)

The television has four channels.
El televisor tiene cuatro canales.
(Ehl teh-leh-bee-sohr tee-eh-neh koo-ah-troh kay-nah-lehs)

Change into the gown.
Póngase esta bata.
(Phn-gah-seh ehs-tah bah-tah)

I need to ask you some questions.
Necesito hacerle unas preguntas.
(Neh-seh-see-toh ah-sehr-leh oo-nahs preh-goon-tahs)

I am going to give you a tour of the floor.
Voy a darle un recorrido por el piso.
(Boy ah dahr-leh oon reh-koh-ree-doh pohr ehl pee-soh)

This is the lobby.
Esta es la sala de espera.
(Ehs-tah ehs lah sah-lah deh ehs-peh-rah)

The elevators work twenty-four hours.
Los elevadores funcionan las veinticuatro horas.
(Lohs eh-leh-bah-dohrehs foon-see-oh-nahn lahs beh-een-tee-koo-ah-troh oh-rahs)

In case of fire, take the stairs.
En caso de fuego, use la escalera.
(Ehn kah-soh deh foo-eh-goh, oo-seh lah ehs-kah-leh-rah)

There are bathrooms for guests in the corner.
Hay baños para las visitas en la esquina.
(Hay bah-nyohs pah-rah lahs bee-see-tahs ehn lah ehs-kee-nah)

This is your room.
Este es su cuarto.
(Ehs-teh ehs soo koo-ahr-toh)

You can tape pictures to the wall.
Puede pegar retratos en la pared.
(Poo-eh-deh peh-gahr reh-trah-tohs ehn lah pah-rehd)

You can put cards on the shelf.
Puede poner trajetas en el estante.
(Poo-eh-deh poh-nehr tahr-hehtahs ehn ehl ehs- tahn-teh)

You can have flowers.
Puede tener flores.
(Poo-eh-deh teh-nehr floh-rehs)

This is the call bell/buzzer.
Esta es la campana/el timbre.
(Ehs-tah ehs lah kahm-pah-nah/ehl teem-breh)

This button lowers (raises) the headboard.
Este botón baja (sube) la cabecera de la cama.
(Ehs-teh boh-tohn bah-hah (soo-beh) lah kah-behseh-rah deh lah kah-mah)

Do you need more pillows?
¿Necesita más almohadas?
(Neh-seh–see-tah mahs ahl-moh-ah-dahs)

You have a private bathroom.
Tiene un baño/inodoro privado.
(Tee-eh-neh oon bah-nyoh/ee-noh-doh-roh pree-bah-doh)

There is a shower.
Hay una ducha/regadera.
(Ahee oo-nah doo-chah/reh-gah-deh-rah)

There is also a bathtub/tub.
También hay una ba–era/tina.
(Tahm-bee-ehn ah-ee oo-nah bah-nyeh-rah/tee-nah)

Your clothes go in the closet.
Su ropa va en el closet/ropero.
(Soo roh-pah bah ehn ehl kloh-seht/roh-peh-roh)

You can make local phone calls.
Puede hacer llamadas locales.
(Poo-eh-deh ah sehr-yah-mah-dahs loh-kah-lehs)

Dial 9, wait for the tone, then dial the number you want to call.
Marque el nueve, espere el tono, luego marque el número que quiera llamar.
(mahr-keh ehl noo-eh-beh, ehs-peh-reh ehl toh-noh, loo-eh-doh mahr-key ehl noo-meh roh keh kee-eh-rah yah-mahr)

You can call collect.
Puede llamar por cobrar.
(poo-eh-deh yah-mahr pohr koh-brahr)

You cannot smoke in your room.
No puede fumar en el cuarto.
(Noh poo-eh-deh foo-mahr ehn ehl koo-ahr-toh)

Did you bring a hearing aid?
¿Trajo un aparato para oír?
(Trah-hoh oon ah-pah-rah-toh pah-rah oo-eer)

Did you bring an artificial eye?
¿Trajo un ojo artificial?
(Trah-hoh oon prohs-teh tee-koh)

Did you bring an artificial limb?
¿Trajo un prostético?
(Trah-hoh oon oh-hoh ahr-tee-fee-see-ahl)

Did you bring contact lenses?
¿Trajo lentes de contacto?
(Trah-hoh lehn-tehs deh kohn-tahk-toh)

Did you bring dentures?
¿Trajo una dentadura postiza?
(Trah-hoh oon-ah dehn-tah-doo-rah pohs-tee-sah)

Did you bring glasses?	¿Trajo anteojos/lentes? (Trah-hoh ahn-teh-oh-hohs/ lehn-tehs)
Did you bring jewelry?/cash?	¿Trajo joyas?/diner? (Trah-hoh hoh-yahs/dee-neh-roh
I will show you your room.	Le mostraré su cuarto. (Leh mohs-trah-reh soo koo-ahr-tah)

CHAPTER 30: COLLECTING AND TESTING SPECIMENS

I am going to explain how to collect the urine.	Le voy a explicar cómo juntar la orina. (Leh boy ah ehx-plee-kahr koh- moh hoon-tahr lah oh-ree-nah)
Every time you urinate, put it in the container.	Cada vez que orine, póngala en el frasco. (Kah-dah behs keh oh-ree-neh, pohn-gah-lah ehn ehl frahs-koh)
The container will be kept in the bucket with ice.	El frasco se mantendrá en una tina con hielo. (Ehl frahs-koh seh mahn-tehn-drah ehn oo-nah tee-nah kohn ee-eh-loh)
Remember that you will do this for 24 hours.	Recuerde que hará esto por vein- ticuatro horas. (Reh-koo-ehr-deh keh ah-rah ehs- toh pohr beh-een-tee-koo-ah- troh oh-rahs)
If there is no ice in the bucket, call me.	Si no hay hielo en la tina, llámeme. (See noh ah-ee ee-eh-loh ehn lah tee-nah, yah-meh-meh)
I also need a urine sample.	También necesito una mues-tra de orina. (Tahm-bee-ehn neh-seh-see-toh oo-nah moo-ehs-trah deh oh-ree-nah)
I am going to ex- plain the col- lection of the urine.	Le voy a explicar la colección de orina. (Leh boy ah ehx-plee-kahr lah koh- lehk-see-ohn de oh-ree-nah)

CHAPTER 31: THE PERSON HAVING SURGERY

anesthesia	anestesia (ah-nehs-teh-see-ah)
embolism	embolismo (ehm-boh-lees-moh)

CHAPTER 32: WOUND CARE

hematoma	hematoma (eh-mah-toh-mah)
ulcer	úlcera (ool-seh-rah)

CHAPTER 34: OXYGEN NEEDS

Breathe in.	Respire. (Rehs-pee-reh)
Breathe out.	Saque el aire. (Sah-keh ehl ah-ee-reh)
Now, take a deep breath.	Ahora, respira hondo. (Ah-oh-rah, rehs-pee-rah ohn-doh)
Cough!	¡Tose! (Toh-seh)
Cough harder!	¡Tose más fuerte! (Toh-seh mahs foo-ehr-teh)
Let it out.	Exhala. (Ehx-ah-lah)
oxygen	oxígen (ohx-ee-heh-noh)
Are you having problems breathing?	¿Tiene problemas al respirar? (Tee-eh-neh proh-bleh-mahs ahl rehs-pee-rahr)
Cough deeply.	Tosa más fuerte. (Toh-sah mahs foo-ehr-teh)
Does it hurt to breathe?	¿Te duele al respirar? (Teh doo-eh-leh ahl toh-sehr)
Does it hurt to cough?	¿Te duele al toser? (Teh doo-eh-leh ahl toh-sehr)

CHAPTER 36: REHABILITATION AND RESTORATIVE CARE

independence	independencia (een-deh-pehn-dehn-see-ah)

CHAPTER 37: HEARING, SPEECH, AND VISION PROBLEMS

glaucoma	glaucoma (glah-oo-koh-mah)
vertigo	vértigo (behr-tee-goh)
vision	visión (bee-see-ohn)

CHAPTER 38: CANCER, IMMUNE SYSTEM, AND SKIN DISORDERS

cancer	cáncer (kahn-sehr)
chemotherapy	quimioterapia (kee-mee-oh-teh-rah-pee-ah)
What causes AIDS?	¿Qué causa el SIDA? (Keh kah-oo-sah ehl see-dah)
A virus known as HIV . . .	El virus causal del SIDA se conoce como VIH . . . (Ehl bee-roos kah-oo-sahl dehl see- dah seh koh-noh- seh koh-moh beh-ee-ah- cheh[VIH])
Who is at risk of getting AIDS?	¿Quién está en riesgo de contraer el SIDA? (Kee-ehn ehs-tah ehn ree-ehs-goh deh kohn-trah-ehr ehl see-dah)

sexually active homosexual and bisexual males or females

homosexuales activos y hombres o mujeres bisexuales
(oh-moh-sehx-oo-ah-lehs ahk-tee-bohs ee ohm-brehs oh moo-heh-rehs bee-sehx-oo-ah-lehs)

intravenous drug abusers

los que abusan de las drogas intravenosas
(lohs keh ah-boo-sah deh lahs droh-gahs een-trah-beh-noh-sahs)

hemophiliacs and recipients of blood/blood components

hemofílicos, donadores de sangre o transfusión con sangre contaminada
(eh-moh-fee-lee-kohs, doh-nah-doh-rehs deh sahn-greh oh trahns-foo-see-ohn kohn sahn-greh kohn-tah-mee-nah-dah)

fetus of infected mothers

fetos de madres contamnadas
(feh-tohs deh mah-drehs kohn-tah-mee-nah-dahs)

Infected persons can transmit the virus.

Las personas infectadas pueden transmitir el virus
(Lahs pehr-soh-nahs een fehk-tah-dahs poo-ehdehn-trahns-mee-teer ehl bee-roos)

Can casual contact cause AIDS?

¿Los contactos eventaules puden causar SIDA?
(Lohs kohn-tahk-tohs eh-behn-too-ah-lehs poo-eh-dehn kah-oo-sahr see-dah)

HIV is not transmissible by casual contact, nor . . .

El VIH no es transmitido en forma casual, ni por . . .
(Ehl VIH noh ehs trahns-mee-tee-doh ehn fohr-mah kah-soo-ahl, nee pohr:)

living in the same house as infected persons

vivir en la misma casa con personas infectadas
(bee-beer ehn lah mees-mah kah-sah kohn pehr-soh-nahs een-fehk-tah-dahs)

eating food handled by persons with AIDS

comer comida preparada por personas infectadas con SIDA
(koh-mehr koh-mee-dah preh-pah-rah-dah pohr pehr-soh-nahs een-fehk-tah-dahs kohn see-dah)

coughing, sneezing, kissing, or swimming with infected persons

tos, estornudo, besar, o nadar con personas infectadas
(tohs, ehs-tohr-noo-doh, beh-sahr oh nah-dahr kohn pehr-soh-nahs een-fehk-tah-dahs)

How serious is AIDS?

¿Qué tan serio es el SIDA?
(Keh tahn seh-ree-oh ehs-ehl see-dah)

AIDS has a high fatality rate approaching 100%.

El SIDA tiene una tasa cercana al 100 por ciento de mortalidad.
(Ehl see-dah tee-eh-neh oo-nah tah-sah sehr-kah-nah ahl see-ehn pohr see-ehn-toh deh mohr-tah-lee-dahd)

Is there a danger from donated blood?

¿Qué peligro hay por sangre donada?
(Keh peh-lee-groh ah-ee pohr sahn-greh doh-nah-dah)

The risk of contracting HIV is not high. Blood banks and other centers use sterile equipment and disposable needles.

El riesgo de contraer VIH no es alto. Los bancos de sangre y otros centros usan equipos estériles y agujas desechables.
(Ehl ree-ehs-goh deh kohn-trah-ehr VIH noh ehs ahl-toh. Lohns bahn-kohs deh sahn-greh ee oh-trohs sehn-trohs oo-sahn eh-kee-pohs ehs-teh-ree-lehs ee ah-goo-hahs deh-seh-chah-blehs)

The U.S. Public Health Service recommends:

El Departamento de Salud Pública de los Estados Unidos recomienda:
(Ehl Deh-pahr-tah-mehn-toh deh Sah-lood Poo-blee-kah deh lohs Ehs-tah-dohs Oo- nee-dohs reh-koh-mee-ehn-dah)

1. Know sexual background/ habits of partners.

1. Conozca los hábitos sexuales de su pareja.
(Koh-nohs-kah lohs ah-bee-tohs sex-oo-ah-lehs deh soo pah-reh-hah)

2. Use a condom or prophylactic.

2. Use un condón o profiláctico.
(Oo-seh oon kohn-dohn oh proh-fee-lahk-tee-koh)

3. If your partner is in a high risk group, cease sexual relations.

3. Si su compañera está en el grupo de alto riesgo, suspenda las relaciones sexuales.
(See soo kohm-pah-nyeh-rah ehs-tah ehn ehl groo-pah deh ahl-toh ree-ehs-goh, soos-pehn-dah lahs reh-lah-see-ohn-ehs sehx-oo-ahl-ehs)

4. Eliminate multiple sexual partners.

4. Elimine múltiples compa–eros sexuales.
(Eh-lee-mee-neh mool-tee-plehs kohm-pha-nyeh-rohs sehx-oo-ah-lehs)

5. Don't use intravenous drugs with contaminated needles; don't share needles or syringes.

5. No use drogas intravenosas con agujas contaminadas; no comparta agujas o jeringas.
(Noh oos-eh droh-gahs een-trah-veh-noh-sahs kohn ah-goo-hahs kohn-tah-mee-nah-dahs; noh kohm-pahr-tah ah-goo-hahs oh hehr-een-gahs)

CHAPTER 40: CARDIOVASCULAR AND RESPIRATORY DISORDERS

asthma   asma
          (ahs-mah)
cardiac   cardíaco
          (kahr-dee-ah-koh)

CHAPTER 41: DIGESTIVE AND ENDOCRINE DISORDERS

insulin   insulina
          (een-soo-lee-nah)
vomit   vómito
          (boh-mee-toh)

CHAPTER 42:URINARY AND REPRODUCTIVE DISORDERS

venereal venéreo
          (beh-neh-reh-oh)

CHAPTER 43: MENTAL HEALTH PROBLEMS

claustrophobia claustrofobia
                (klah-oos-troh-foh-bee-ah)
obsession   obsesión
                (ohb-seh-see-ohn)
panic   pánico
                (pah-nee-koh)

CHAPTER 44: CONFUSION AND DEMENTIA

delirious   delirio
            (deh-lee-ree-oh)

CHAPTER 45: DEVELOPMENTAL DISABILITIES

epilepsy   epilepsia
            (eh-peel-ehp-see-ah)

CHAPTER 46: SEXUALITY

sex   sexo
          (sehx-oh)
sexual   sexual
          (sehx-oo-ahl)

CHAPTER 47: CARING FOR MOTHERS AND NEWBORNS

Is he/she . . .   ¿Está . . .
                     (Ehs-tah . . .)
breast-feeding?   tomando pecho?
                     (toh-mahn-doh peh-choh)
taking formula?   tomando fórmula?
                     (toh-mahn-doh fohr-moo-lah)
What formula   ¿Qué fórmula toma?
   does he take?   (Keh fohr-moo-lah toh-mah)

How many ounces   ¿Cuántas onzas toma?
   does he take?   (Koo-ahn-tahs ohn sahs-toh-mah)
How often do you   ¿Qué tan a menudo alimenta al
   feed the baby?   bebé?
                     (keh tahn ah meh-noo-doh ah-lee-
                        mehn-tah ahl beh-beh)
Does he/she have: ¿Tiene: fiebre/diarrea/cólico?
   fever/diarrhea/   (Tee-eh-neh: fee-eh-breh/dee-ah-
   colic?   rreh-ah/ koh-lee-koh)
Does the baby   ¿Dureme el bebé toda la noche?
   sleep all night? (Doo-ehr-meh ehl beh-beh toh-dah
                        lah noh-cheh)
How many times   ¿Cuántas veces se despierta?
   does he wake   (Koo-ahn-tahs beh-sehs seh
   up?   dehs-pee-ehr-tah)
Does he cry a lot?   ?Llora mucho?
                     (Yoh-rah moo-choh)
When was the   ¿Cuándo fue la última vez que
   last time he   evacuó/hizo del baño?
   had a bowel   (Koo-ahn-doh foo-eh lah ool-tee-
   movement?   mah behs keh eh-bah-koo-oh/
                        ee-soh dehl bah-nyoh)
Is he urinating   ¿Orina bien?
   well?   (Oh-ree-nah bee-ehn)
Have you seen   ¿Ha visto sangre en la orina?
   blood in the   (Ah bees-toh sahn-greh ehn lah oh-
   urine?   ree-nah)
How many dia-   ¿Cuántos pañales le ha cambiado
   pers have you   desde ayer?
   changed since   (Koo-ahn-tohs pah-nyah-lehs leh
   yesterday?   ah kahm-bee-ah-doh dehs-deh
                        ah-yehr)
When did you   ¿Cuándo se díco cuenta de la piel
   notice the skin   rosada?
   rash?   (Koo-ahn-doh seh dee-oh koo-ehn-
                        tah deh lah pee-ehl roh-sah-dah)
How many times   ¿Cuántas veces ha vomitado?
   has he vomited?   (Koo-ahn-tahs beh-sehs ah boh-
                        mee-tah-doh)
Is it a lot?   ¿Es mucho?
                     (Ehs moo-choh)
Does the vomit   ¿Tiene sangre el vómito?
   have blood?   (Tee-eh-neh sahn-greh ehl
                        boh-mee-toh)
What color?   ¿De qué color?
                     (Deh keh koh-lohr)
Does it have un-   ¿Tiene restos de comida?
   digested food?   (Tee-eh-neh rehs-tohs deh
                        koh-mee-dah)
Does it smell   ¿Huele mal?
   bad?   (Oo-eh-leh mahl)
Is he coughing?   ¿Está tosiendo?
                     (Ehs-tah toh-see-ehn-doh)
Do not put on   No le ponga clzones de plástico!
   plastic pants!   (Noh leh pohn-gah kahl-sohn-ehs
                        deh plahs-tee-koh)

Sterilize the bottles.

Esterilice las botellas/ los biberones.
(Ehs-teh-ree-lee-seh lahs boh- teh-yahs/lohs bee-beh-roh-nehs)

Help him to burp.

Póngalo a repetir/eructar.
(Pohn-gah-loh ah reh-peh-teer/eh-rook-tahr)

Pat his back gently.

Dé palmaditas en la espalda.
(Deh pahl-mah-dee-tahs ehn lah ehs-pahl-dah)

sanitary

sanitario
(sah-nee-tah-ree-oh)

CHAPTER 48: ASSISTED LIVING

Take the medicine with juice.

Tome la medicina con jugo.
(Toh-meh lah meh-dee-see-nah kohn joo-goh)

Take it with a full glass of water.

Tómela con un vaso lleno de agua.
(Toh-meh-lah kohn oon bah-soh yeh-noh deh ah-goo-a)

Do not drink alcohol with this medicine.

No tome alcohol con esta medicina.
(Noh toh-meh ahl-kohl kohn ehs-tah meh-dee-see-nah)

It can cause drowsiness.

Le puede causar sueño.
(Leh poo-eh-deh kah-oo-sahr soo-eh-nyoh)

Do not drive!

¡No maneje/conduzca!
(Noh mah-neh-heh/ kohn-doos-kah)

Do not operate machinery!

¡No maneje/opere una máquina/ maquinaria!
(Noh mah-neh-heh/oh-peh- reh oo-nah mah-kee-nah/ah-kee-nah-ree-ah)

Take on an empty stomach.

Tómela con el estómago vacío.
(Toh-meh-lah kohn ehl ehs-toh-mah-goh bah-see-oh)

Take one hour before eating.

Tómela una hora antes de comer.
(Toh-meh-lah oo-nah oh-rah ahn-tehs de koh-mehr)

Take the medicine with food.

Tome la medicina con comida.
(Toh-meh lah mehdee-see-nah kohn koh-mee-dah)

medication

medicamento
(meh-dee-kah-mehn-toh)

medicine

medicina
(meh-dee-see-nah)

CHAPTER 49: BASIC EMERGENCY CARE

We are going to the hospital.

Vamos al hospital.
(Bah-mohs ahl ohs-pee-tahl)

We are going in the ambulance.

Vamos en la ambulancia.
(Bah-mohs ehn lah ahm-boo-lahn-see-ah)

D

MyPyramid Food Intake Pattern Calorie Levels

MyPyramid assigns Individuals to a calorie level based on their sex, age, and activity level.

The chart below identifies the calorie levels for males and females by age and activity level. Calorie levels are provided for each year of childhood, from 2-18 years, and for adults in 5-year increments.

	MALES				FEMALES		
Activity level	Sedentary*	Mod. active*	Active*	Activity level	Sedentary*	Mod. active*	Active*
AGE				AGE			
2	1000	1000	1000	2	1000	1000	1000
3	1000	1400	1400	3	1000	1200	1400
4	1200	1400	1600	4	1200	1400	1400
5	1200	1400	1600	5	1200	1400	1600
6	1400	1600	1800	6	1200	1400	1600
7	1400	1600	1800	7	1200	1600	1800
8	1400	1600	2000	8	1400	1600	1800
9	1600	1800	2000	9	1400	1600	1800
10	1600	1800	2200	10	1400	1800	2000
11	1800	2000	2200	11	1600	1800	2000
12	1800	2200	2400	12	1600	2000	2200
13	2000	2200	2600	13	1600	2000	2200
14	2000	2400	2800	14	1800	2000	2400
15	2200	2600	3000	15	1800	2000	2400
16	2400	2800	3200	16	1800	2000	2400
17	2400	2800	3200	17	1800	2000	2400
18	2400	2800	3200	18	1800	2000	2400
19-20	2600	2800	3000	19-20	2000	2200	2400
21-25	2400	2800	3000	21-25	2000	2200	2400
26-30	2400	2600	3000	26-30	1800	2000	2400
31-35	2400	2600	3000	31-35	1800	2000	2200
36-40	2400	2600	2800	36-40	1800	2000	2200
41-45	2200	2600	2800	41-45	1800	2000	2200
46-50	2200	2400	2800	46-50	1800	2000	2200
51-55	2200	2400	2800	51-55	1600	1800	2200
56-60	2200	2400	2600	56-60	1600	1800	2200
61-65	2000	2400	2600	61-65	1600	1800	2000
66-70	2000	2200	2600	66-70	1600	1800	2000
71-75	2000	2200	2600	71-75	1600	1800	2000
76 and up	2000	2200	2400	76 and up	1600	1800	2000

*Calorie levels are based on the Estimated Energy Requirements (EER) and activity levels from the Institute of Medicine Dietary Reference Intakes Macronutrients Report, 2002.
SEDENTARY = less than 30 minutes a day of moderate physical activity in addition to daily activities.
MOD. ACTIVE = at least 30 minutes up to 60 minutes a day of moderate physical activity in addition to daily activities.
ACTIVE = 60 or more minutes a day of moderate physical activity in addition to daily activities.

United StatesDepartment of Agriculture
Center for Nutrition Policy and Promotion
April 2005
CNPP-XX

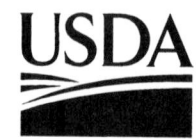

Glossary

abbreviation A shortened form of a word or phrase

abduction Moving a body part away from the midline of the body

abrasion A partial-thickness wound caused by the scraping away or rubbing of the skin

abuse The intentional mistreatment or harm of another person

accountable Being responsible for one's actions and the actions of others who performed delegated tasks; answering questions about and explaining one's actions and the actions of others

acetone A substance that appears in urine from the rapid breakdown of fat for energy; ketone body or ketone

activities of daily living (ADL) The activities usually done during a normal day in a person's life

acute illness A sudden illness from which a person is expected to recover

acute pain Pain that is felt suddenly from injury, disease, trauma, or surgery

adduction Moving a body part toward the midline of the body

admission Official entry of a person into an agency

adolescence The time between puberty and adulthood; a time of rapid growth and physical, sexual, emotional and social changes

advance directive A document stating a person's wishes about health care when that person cannot make his or her own decisions

affect Feelings and emotions

allergy A sensitivity to a substance that causes the body to react with signs and symptoms

alopecia Hair loss

ambulation The act of walking

AM care Early morning care

amputation The removal of all or part of an extremity

anaphylaxis A life-threatening sensitivity to an antigen

anesthesia The loss of feeling or sensation produced by a drug

anorexia The loss of appetite

anterior At or toward the front of the body or body part; ventral

antibiotic A drug that kills microbes that cause infections

anxiety A vague, uneasy feeling in response to stress

aphasia The total or partial loss *(a)* of the ability to use or understand language *(phasia)*; a language disorder resulting from damage to parts of the brain responsible for language

apical-radial pulse Taking the apical and radial pulses at the same time

apnea The lack or absence *(a)* of breathing *(pnea)*

arterial ulcer An open wound on the lower legs or feet caused by poor arterial blood flow

artery A blood vessel that carries blood away from the heart

arthritis Joint *(arthr)* inflammation *(itis)*

arthroplasty The surgical replacement *(plasty)* of a joint *(arthr)*

asepsis Being free of disease-producing microbes

aspiration Breathing fluid, food, vomitus, or an object into the lungs

assault Intentionally attempting or threatening to touch a person's body without the person's consent

assessment Collecting information about the person; a step in the nursing process

assisted living residence Provides housing, personal care, support services, health care, and social activities in a home-like setting

atrophy The decrease in size or the wasting away of tissue

autopsy The examination of the body after death

B

base of support The area on which an object rests

battery Touching a person's body without his or her consent

bed rail A device that serves as a guard or barrier along the side of the bed; side rail

benign tumor A tumor that does not spread to other body parts; it can grow to a large size

biohazardous waste Items contaminated with blood, body fluids, secretions, or excretions; *bio* means life, and *hazardous* means dangerous or harmful

Biot's respirations Rapid and deep respirations followed by 10 to 30 seconds of apnea

bisexual A person who is attracted to both sexes

blind The absence of sight

blood pressure The amount of force exerted against the walls of an artery by the blood

body alignment The way the head, trunk, arms, and legs are aligned with one another; posture

body language Messages sent through facial expressions, gestures, posture, hand and body movements, gait, eye contact, and appearance

body mechanics Using the body in an efficient and careful way

body temperature The amount of heat in the body that is a balance between the amount of heat produced and the amount lost by the body

boundary crossing A brief act or behavior outside of the helpful zone

boundary sign An act, behavior, or thought that warns of a boundary crossing or violation

boundary violation An act or behavior that meets your needs, not the person's needs

bradycardia A slow *(brady)* heart rate *(cardia)*; less than 60 beats per minute

bradypnea Slow *(brady)* breathing *(pnea)*; respirations are fewer than 12 per minute

braille A touch reading and writing system that uses raised dots for each letter of the alphabet; the first 10 letters also represent the numbers 0 through 9

breast-feeding Feeding a baby milk from the mother's breasts; nursing

Broca's aphasia Expressive aphasia; motor aphasia

C

calorie The amount of energy produced when the body burns food

cancer Malignant tumor

capillary A tiny blood vessel; food, oxygen, and other substances pass from the capillaries to the cells

cardiac arrest See "sudden cardiac arrest"

carrier A human or animal that is a reservoir for microbes but does not have the signs and symptoms of infection

case management A nursing care pattern; a case manager (an RN) coordinates a person's care from admission through discharge and into the home setting

catheter A tube used to drain or inject fluid through a body opening

catheterization The process of inserting a catheter

cell The basic unit of body structure

cerumen Earwax

chart The medical record; clinical record

Cheyne-Stokes respirations Respirations gradually increase in rate and depth and then become shallow and slow; breathing may stop (apnea) for 10 to 20 seconds

chronic illness An ongoing illness, slow or gradual in onset; it has no known cure; the illness can be controlled and complications prevented with proper treatment

chronic pain Pain lasting longer than 6 months; it is constant or occurs off and on

chronic wound A wound that does not heal easily

circumcision The surgical removal of foreskin from the penis

civil law Laws concerned with relationships between people

circadian rhythm Daily rhythm based on a 24-hour cycle; the day-night cycle or body rhythm

circulatory ulcer An open sore on the lower legs or feet caused by decreased blood flow through the arteries or veins; vascular ulcer

clean-contaminated wound Occurs from the surgical entry of the reproductive, urinary, respiratory, or gastrointestinal system

clean technique Medical asepsis

clean wound A wound that is not infected; microbes have not entered the wound

closed fracture The bone is broken but the skin is intact; simple fracture

closed wound Tissues are injured but the skin is not broken

cognitive function Involves memory, thinking, reasoning, ability to understand, judgment, and behavior

colostomy A surgically created opening (stomy) between the colon (colo) and abdominal wall

coma A state of being unaware of one's surroundings and being unable to react or respond to people, places, or things

comatose Being unable to respond to verbal stimuli

comfort A state of well-being; the person has no physical or emotional pain and is calm and at peace

communicable disease A disease caused by pathogens that spread easily; a contagious disease

communication The exchange of information—a message sent is received and correctly interpreted by the intended person

compress A soft pad applied over a body area

compound fracture An open fracture

compulsion Repeating an act over and over again

conscious Awareness of the environment and experiences; the person knows what is happening and can control thoughts and behaviors

confidentiality Trusting others with personal and private information

conflict A clash between opposing interests or ideas

congenital To be born with (congenitus)

constipation The passage of a hard, dry stool

constrict To narrow

contagious disease Communicable disease

contamination The process of becoming unclean

contaminated wound A wound with a high risk of infection

contracture The lack of joint mobility caused by abnormal shortening of a muscle

contusion A closed wound caused by a blow to the body; a bruise

convulsion See "seizure"

cotton drawsheet A drawsheet made of cotton; it helps keep the mattress and bottom linens clean

courtesy A polite, considerate, or helpful comment or act

crime An act that violates a criminal law

criminal law Laws concerned with offenses against the public and society in general

culture The characteristics of a group of people—language, values, beliefs, habits, likes, dislikes, customs—passed from one generation to the next

cyanosis Bluish color

D

Daily Value (DV) How a serving fits into the daily diet; expressed in a percent (%) based on a daily diet of 2000 calories

dandruff Excessive amounts of dry, white flakes from the scalp

deafness Hearing loss in which it is impossible for the person to understand speech through hearing alone

deconditioning The loss of muscle strength from inactivity

defamation Injuring a person's name and reputation by making false statements to a third person

defecation The process of excreting feces from the rectum through the anus; a bowel movement

defense mechanism An unconscious reaction that blocks unpleasant or threatening feelings

dehiscence The separation of wound layers

dehydration The excessive loss of water from tissues; a decrease in the amount of water in body tissues

delegate To authorize another person to perform a nursing task in a certain situation

delirium A state of temporary but acute mental confusion

delusion A false belief

delusion of grandeur An exaggerated belief about one's importance, wealth, power, or talents

delusion of persecution A false belief that one is being mistreated, abused, or harassed

dementia The loss of cognitive function that interferes with routine personal, social, and occupational activities

denture An artificial tooth or a set of artificial teeth

development Changes in mental, emotional, and social function

developmental disability (DD) A disability occurring before 22 years of age

developmental task A skill that must be completed during a stage of development

diabetic foot ulcer An open wound on the foot caused by complications from diabetes

diarrhea The frequent passage of liquid stools

diastole The period of heart muscle relaxation; the period when the heart is at rest

diastolic pressure The pressure in the arteries when the heart is at rest

digestion The process of physically and chemically breaking down food so that it can be absorbed for use by the cells

dilate To expand or open wider

diplegia Similar body parts are affected on both sides of the body

dirty wound An infected wound

disability Any lost, absent, or impaired physical or mental function

disaster A sudden catastrophic event in which people are injured and killed and property is destroyed

discharge Official departure of a person from an agency

discomfort Pain

disinfection The process of destroying pathogens

distal The part farthest from the center or from the point of attachment

distraction To change the person's center of attention

diuresis The process *(esis)* of passing *(di)* urine *(ur)*; large amounts of urine are produced—1000 to 5000 mL a day

dorsal Posterior

dorsal recumbent position The back-lying or supine position; the supine position with the legs together; horizontal recumbent position

dorsiflexion Bending the toes and foot up at the ankle

drawsheet A small sheet placed over the middle of the bottom sheet

dysphagia Difficulty *(dys)* swallowing *(phagia)*

dyspnea Difficult, labored, or painful *(dys)* breathing *(pnea)*

dysuria Painful or difficult *(dys)* urination *(uria)*

E

early morning care Care given before breakfast; AM care

edema The swelling of body tissues with water; swelling caused by fluid collecting in tissues

ego The part of the personality dealing with reality; deals with thoughts, feelings, reasoning, good sense, and problem solving

ejaculation The release of semen

elective surgery Surgery done by choice to improve the person's life or well-being

electrical shock When electrical current passes through the body

embolus A blood clot that travels through the vascular system until it lodges in a blood vessel

emergency surgery Surgery done at once to save life or function

emesis Vomitus

emotional illness Mental disorder, mental illness, psychiatric disorder

enema The introduction of fluid into the rectum and lower colon

enteral nutrition Giving nutrients into the gastrointestinal (GI) tract *(enteral)* through a feeding tube

enuresis Urinary incontinence in bed at night

epidermal stripping Removing the epidermis (outer skin layer) as tape is removed from the skin

episiotomy Incision *(otomy)* into the perineum

erectile dysfunction (DD) Impotence

ergonomics The science of designing a job to fit the worker

esteem The worth, value, or opinion one has of a person

ethics Knowledge of what is right conduct and wrong conduct

evaluation To measure if goals in the planning step were met; a step in the nursing process

evening care Care given at bedtime; PM care

evisceration The separation of the wound along with the protrusion of abdominal organs

expressive aphasia Difficulty expressing or sending out thoughts; motor aphasia, Broca's aphasia

expressive-receptive aphasia Difficulty expressing or sending out thoughts and difficulty understanding language; global aphasia, mixed aphasia

extension Straightening a body part

external rotation Turning the joint outward

F

fainting The sudden loss of consciousness from an inadequate blood supply to the brain

false imprisonment Unlawful restraint or restriction of a person's freedom of movement

fecal impaction The prolonged retention and buildup of feces in the rectum

fecal incontinence The inability to control the passage of feces and gas through the anus

feces The semi-solid mass of waste products in the colon that is expelled through the anus

fever Elevated body temperature

first aid Emergency care given to an ill or injured person before medical help arrives

flashback Reliving the trauma in thoughts during the day and in nightmares during sleep

flatulence The excessive formation of gas or air in the stomach and intestines

flatus Gas or air passed through the anus

flexion Bending a body part

flow rate The number of drops per minute *(gtt/min)*

Foley catheter An indwelling or retention catheter

footdrop The foot falls down at the ankle; permanent plantar flexion

Fowler's position A semi-sitting position; the head of the bed is raised between 45 and 60 degrees

fracture A broken bone

fraud Saying or doing something to trick, fool, or deceive a person

freedom of movement Any change in place or position for the body, or any part of the body, that the person is physically able to control

friction The rubbing of one surface against another

full-thickness wound The dermis, epidermis, and subcutaneous tissue are penetrated; muscle and bone may be involved

full visual privacy Having the means to be completely free from public view while in bed

functional incontinence The person has bladder control but cannot use the toilet in time

functional nursing A nursing care pattern focusing on tasks and jobs; each nursing team member has certain tasks and jobs to do

G

gait belt Transfer belt

gangrene A condition in which there is death of tissue

gastrostomy tube A tube inserted through a surgically created opening *(stomy)* in the stomach *(gastro)*; stomach tube

gavage The process of giving a tube feeding

general anesthesia The loss of consciousness and all feeling or sensation

geriatrics The branch of medicine concerned with the problems and diseases of old age and older persons; care of aging people

germicide A disinfectant applied to the skin, tissues, or non-living objects

gerontology The study of the aging process

global aphasia Expressive-receptive aphasia; mixed aphasia

glucosuria Sugar (glucos) in the urine (uria); glycosuria

glycosuria Sugar (glycos) in the urine (uria); glucosuria

goal That which is desired in or by the person as a result of nursing care

gossip To spread rumors or talk about the private matters of others

graduate A measuring container for fluid

ground That which carries leaking electricity to the earth and away from an electrical item

growth The physical changes that are measured and that occur in a steady, orderly manner

guided imagery Creating and focusing on an image

H

hallucination Seeing, hearing, smelling, or feeling something that is not real

harassment To trouble, torment, offend, or worry a person by one's behavior or comments

hazardous substance Any chemical in the workplace that can cause harm

healthcare-associated infection (HAI) An infection that develops in a person cared for in any setting where health care is given; the infection is related to receiving health care

health team The many health care workers whose skills and knowledge focus on the person's total care; interdisciplinary health care team

hearing loss Not being able to hear the normal range of sounds associated with normal hearing

hemiplegia Paralysis on one side of the body

hematoma A swelling (oma) that contains blood (hemat)

hematuria Blood (hemat) in the urine (uria)

hemiplegia Paralysis on one side of the body

hemoglobin The substance in red blood cells that carries oxygen and gives blood its color

hemoptysis Bloody (hemo) sputum (ptysis means to spit)

hemorrhage The excessive loss of blood in a short time

hemothorax Blood (hemo) in the pleural space (thorax)

hemorrhage The excessive loss of blood in a short time

heterosexual A person who is attracted to members of the other sex

high-Fowler's position A semi-sitting position, the head of the bed is raised 60 to 90 degrees

hirsutism Excessive body hair

holism A concept that considers the whole person; the whole person has physical, social, psychological, and spiritual parts that are woven together and cannot be separated

homosexual A person who is attracted to members of the same sex

hormone A chemical substance secreted by the endocrine glands into the bloodstream

horizontal recumbent position The dorsal recumbent position

hospice A health care agency or program for persons who are dying

hyperextension Excessive straightening of a body part

hyperglycemia High (hyper) sugar (glyc) in the blood (emia)

hypertension Blood pressure measurements that remain above (hyper) a systolic pressure of 140 mm Hg or a diastolic pressure of 90 mm Hg; high blood pressure

hyperthermia A body temperature (thermia) that is much higher (hyper) than the person's normal range

hyperventilation Respirations (ventilation) are rapid (hyper) and deeper than normal

hypoglycemia Low (hypo) sugar (glyc) in the blood (emia)

hypotension When the systolic blood pressure is below (hypo) 90 mm Hg and the diastolic pressure is below 60 mm Hg

hypothermia A very low (hypo) body temperature (thermia)

hypoventilation Respirations (ventilation) are slow (hypo), shallow, and sometimes irregular

hypoxemia A reduced amount (hypo) of oxygen (ox) in the blood (emia)

hypoxia Cells do not have enough (hypo) oxygen (oxia)

I

id The part of the personality at the unconscious level; concerned with pleasure

ileostomy A surgically created opening (stomy) between the ileum (small intestine [ileo]) and the abdominal wall

immunity Protection against a certain disease; protection against a disease or condition; the person will not get or be affected by the disease

implementation To perform or carry out nursing measures in the care plan; a step in the nursing process

impotence The inability to have an erection; erectile dysfunction

incident Any event that has harmed or could harm a patient, resident, visitor, or staff member

incision An open wound with clean, straight edges; usually intentional from a sharp instrument

indwelling catheter A catheter left in the bladder so urine drains constantly into a drainage bag; retention or Foley catheter

infancy The first year of life

infected wound A wound containing large amounts of microbes that shows signs of infection; a dirty wound

infection A disease state resulting from the invasion and growth of microbes in the body

infection control Practices and procedures that prevent the spread of infection

insomnia A chronic condition in which the person cannot sleep or stay asleep all night

intake The amount of fluid taken in

intentional wound A wound created for therapy

internal rotation Turning the joint inward

intravenous (IV) therapy Giving fluids through a needle or catheter inserted into a vein; IV and IV infusion

intubation Inserting an artificial airway

invasion of privacy Violating a person's right not to have his or her name, photo, or private affairs exposed or made public without giving consent

involuntary seclusion Separating a person from others against his or her will; keeping the person confined to a certain area or away from his or her room without consent

J

jaundice Yellowish color of the skin or whites of the eyes

jejunostomy tube A feeding tube inserted into a surgically created opening (stomy) in the jejunum of the small intestine

job description A document that describes what the agency expects you to do

K

Kardex A type of card file that summarizes information found in the medical record—drugs, treatments, diagnoses, routine care measures, equipment, and special needs

ketone Acetone, ketone body

ketone body Acetone; ketone

knee-chest position The person kneels and rests the body on the knees and chest; the head is turned to one side, the arms are above the head or flexed at the elbows, the back is straight, and the body is flexed about 90 degrees at the hips

Kussmaul respirations Very deep and rapid respirations

L

laceration An open wound with torn tissues and jagged edges

laryngeal mirror An instrument used to examine the mouth, teeth, and throat

lateral Away from the midline; at the side of the body or body part

lateral position The person lies on one side or the other; side-lying position

law A rule of conduct made by a government body

lice Pediculosis

libel Making false statements in print, writing, or through pictures or drawings

licensed practical nurse (LPN) A nurse who has completed a 1-year nursing program and has passed a licensing test; called *licensed vocational nurse (LVN)* in some states

licensed vocational nurse (LVN) Licensed practical nurse

lithotomy position The woman lies on her back with her hips at the edge of the exam table, her knees are flexed, her hips are externally rotated, and her feet are in stirrups

local anesthesia The loss of feeling or sensation in a small area

lochia The vaginal discharge that occurs after childbirth

logrolling Turning the person as a unit, in alignment, with one motion

low vision Eyesight that cannot be corrected with eyeglasses, contact lenses, drugs, or surgery

M

malignant tumor A tumor that invades and destroys nearby tissue and can spread to other body parts; cancer

malpractice Negligence by a professional person

mechanical ventilation Using a machine to move air into and out of the lungs

meconium A dark green to black, tarry bowel movement

medial At or near the middle or midline of the body or body part

medical asepsis Practices used to remove or destroy pathogens and to prevent their spread from one person or place to another person or place; clean technique

medical diagnosis The identification of a disease or condition by a doctor

medical record A written account of a person's condition and response to treatment and care; chart or clinical record

medical symptom An indication or characteristic of a physical or psychological condition

medication reminder Reminding the person to take drugs, observing them being taken as prescribed, and charting that they were taken

melena A black, tarry stool

menarche The first menstruation and the start of menstrual cycles

menopause The time when menstruation stops and menstrual cycles end

menstruation The process in which the lining of the uterus breaks up and is discharged from the body through the vagina

mental Relating to the mind; something that exists in the mind or is done by the mind

mental disorder Emotional illness, mental illness, psychiatric disorder

mental health The person copes with and adjusts to everyday stresses in ways accepted by society

mental illness A disturbance in the ability to cope with or adjust to stress; behavior and function are impaired; emotional illness, mental disorder, psychiatric disorder

metabolism The burning of food for heat and energy by the cells

metastasis The spread of cancer to other body parts

microbe A microorganism

microorganism A small (*micro*) living plant or animal (*organism*) seen only with a microscope; a microbe

micturition Urination or voiding

mite A very small spider-like organism

mixed aphasia Expressive-receptive aphasia; global aphasia

mixed incontinence Having more than one type of incontinence

morning care Care given after breakfast; hygiene measures are more thorough at this time

motor aphasia Expressive aphasia; Broca's aphasia

N

nasal speculum An instrument used to examine the inside of the nose

nasogastric (NG) tube A feeding tube inserted through the nose (*naso*) into the stomach (*gastro*)

nasoduodenal tube A feeding tube inserted through the nose (*naso*) into the *duodenum* of the small intestine

nasointestinal tube A feeding tube inserted through the nose (*naso*) into the small intestine (*intestinal*)

nasojejunal tube A feeding tube inserted through the nose (*naso*) into the *jejunum* of the small intestine

need Something necessary or desired for maintaining life and mental well-being

neglect Failure to provide the person with the goods or services needed to avoid physical harm, mental anguish, or mental illness

negligence An unintentional wrong in which a person did not act in a reasonable and careful manner and a person or the person's property was harmed

nocturia Frequent urination (*uria*) at night (*noct*)

non-pathogen A microbe that does not usually cause an infection

nonverbal communication Communication that does not use words

normal flora Microbes that live and grow in a certain area

NREM sleep The phase of sleep when there is *no rapid eye movement*; non-REM sleep

nursing Breast-feeding

nursing assistant A person who has passed a nursing assistant training and competency evaluation program; performs delegated nursing tasks under the supervision of a licensed nurse

nursing care plan A written guide about the person's care; care plan

nursing diagnosis Describes a health problem that can be treated by nursing measures; a step in the nursing process

nursing intervention An action or measure taken by the nursing team to help the person reach a goal

nursing process The method nurses use to plan and deliver nursing care; its five steps are assessment, nursing diagnosis, planning, implementation, and evaluation

nursing task Nursing care or a nursing function, procedure, activity, or work that can be delegated to nursing assistants when it does not require an RN's professional knowledge or judgement

nursing team Those who provide nursing care—RNs, LPNs/LVNs, and nursing assistants

nutrient A substance that is ingested, digested, absorbed, and used by the body

nutrition The processes involved in the ingestion, digestion, absorption, and use of foods and fluids by the body

O

objective data Information that is seen, heard, felt, or smelled; signs

observation Using the senses of sight, hearing, touch, and smell to collect information

obsession A recurrent, unwanted thought, idea, or image

obstetrics The branch of medicine concerned with the care of women during pregnancy, labor, and childbirth and for the 6 to 8 weeks after birth

old Persons between 75 and 84 years of age

old-old Persons 85 years of age and older

oliguria Scant amount (olig) of urine (uria); less than 500 mL in 24 hours

ombudsman Someone who supports or promotes the needs and interests of another person

open fracture The broken bone has come through the skin; compound fracture

open wound The skin or mucous membrane is broken

ophthalmoscope A lighted instrument used to examine the internal structures of the eye

optimal level of function A person's highest potential for mental and physical performance

oral hygiene Mouth care

organ Groups of tissues with the same function

orthopnea Breathing (pnea) deeply and comfortably only when sitting (ortho)

orthopneic position Sitting up (ortho) and leaning over a table to breathe (pneic)

orthostatic hypotension Abnormally low (hypo) blood pressure when the person suddenly stands up (ortho and static); postural hypotension

ostomy A surgically created opening

otoscope A lighted instrument used to examine the external ear and the eardrum (tympanic membrane)

output The amount of fluid lost

overflow incontinence Small amounts of urine leak from a bladder that is always full

oxygen concentration The amount (percent) of hemoglobin containing oxygen

P

pack A treatment that involves wrapping a body part with a wet or dry application

pain To ache, hurt, or be sore; discomfort

panic An intense and sudden feeling of fear, anxiety, terror, or dread

paralysis Loss of muscle function, loss of sensation, or loss of both muscle function and sensation

paranoia A disorder (para) of the mind (noia); false beliefs (delusions) and suspicion about a person or situation

paraphrasing Restating the person's message in your own words

paraplegia Paralysis in the legs and lower trunk

partial-thickness wound The dermis and epidermis of the skin are broken

parenteral nutrition Giving nutrients through a catheter inserted into a vein; para means beyond; enteral relates to the bowel

pathogen A microbe that is harmful and can cause an infection

patient-focused care A nursing care pattern; services are moved from departments to the bedside

pediatrics The branch of medicine concerned with the growth, development, and care of children: they range in age from newborns to teenagers

pediculosis Infestation with wingless insects; lice

pediculosis capitis Infestation of the scalp (capitis) with lice

pediculosis corporsis Infestation of the body (corporsis) with lice

pediculosis pubis Infestation of the pubic (pubis) hair with lice

peer Persons of the same age-group and background

penetrating wound An open wound in which the skin and underlying tissues are pierced

percussion hammer An instrument used to tap body parts to test reflexes; reflex hammer

percutaneous endoscopic gastrostomy (PEG) tube A feeding tube inserted into the stomach (gastro) through a small incision (stomy) made through (per) the skin (cutaneous); a lighted instrument (scope) used to see inside a body cavity or organ (endo)

pericare Perineal care

perineal care Cleaning the genital and anal areas; pericare

peristalsis Involuntary muscle contractions in the digestive system that move food down the esophagus through the alimentary canal; the alternating contraction and relaxation of intestinal muscles

personality The set of attitudes, values, behaviors, and traits of a person

phantom pain Pain felt in a body part that is no longer there

phlebitis Inflammation (itis) of a vein (phleb)

phobia An intense fear

planning Setting priorities and goals; a step in the nursing process

plantar flexion The foot (plantar) is bent (flexion); bending the foot down at the ankle

plaque A thin film that sticks to the teeth; it contains saliva, microbes, and other substances

plastic drawsheet A waterproof drawsheet made of plastic placed between the bottom sheet and the cotton drawsheet to protect the mattress and bottom linens from dampness and soiling; waterproof drawsheet

pleural effusion The escape and collection of fluid (effusion) in the pleural space

PM care Evening care

pneumothorax Air (pneumo) in the pleural space (thorax)

pollutant A harmful chemical or substance in the air or water

polyuria Abnormally large amounts (*poly*) of urine (*uria*)

posterior At or toward the back of the body or body part; dorsal

postmortem care Care of the body after (*post*) death (*mortem*)

post-operative After surgery

postpartum After (*post*) childbirth (*partum*)

postural hypotension Orthostatic hypotension

posture Body alignment

preceptor A staff member who guides another staff member

prefix A word element placed before a root; it changes the meaning of the word

pre-hypertension When the systolic pressure is between 120 and 139 mm Hg or the diastolic pressure is between 80 and 89 mm Hg

pre-operative Before surgery

pressure ulcer A localized injury to the skin and/or underlying tissue usually over a bony prominence; the result of pressure or pressure in combination with shear and/or friction

primary caregiver The person mainly responsible for providing or assisting with the child's basic needs

professional boundary That which separates helpful behaviors from behaviors that are not helpful

professionalism Following laws, being ethical, having good work ethics, and having the skills to do your work

professional sexual misconduct An act, behavior, or comment that is sexual in nature

primary nursing A nursing care pattern; an RN is responsible for the person's total care

pronation Turning the joint downward

prone position Lying on the abdomen with the head turned to one side

prosthesis An artificial replacement for a missing body part

protected health information Identifying information and information about the person's health care that is maintained or sent in any form (paper, electronic, oral)

proximal The part nearest to the center or to the point of origin

pseudodementia False (*pseudo*) dementia

psychiatric disorder Emotional illness, mental disorder, mental illness

psychiatry The branch of medicine concerned with mental health problems

psychosis A state of severe mental impairment

puberty The period when reproductive organs begin to function and secondary sex characteristics appear

pulse The beat of the heart felt at an artery as a wave of blood passes through the artery

pulse deficit The difference between the apical and radial pulse rates

pulse rate The number of heartbeats or pulses felt in 1 minute

puncture wound An open wound made by a sharp object; entry of the skin and underlying tissues may be intentional or unintentional

purulent drainage Thick green, yellow, or brown drainage

pyuria Pus (*py*) in the urine (*uria*)

Q

quadriplegia Paralysis in the arms, legs, and trunk; tetraplegia

R

radiating pain Pain felt at the site of tissue damage and in nearby areas

range of motion (ROM) The movement of a joint to the extent possible without causing pain

receptive aphasia Difficulty understanding language; Wernicke's aphasia

recording The written account of care and observations; charting

regional anesthesia The loss of feeling or sensation in a large area of the body

registered nurse (RN) A nurse who has completed a 2-, 3-, or 4-year nursing program and has passed a licensing test

regurgitation The backward flow of stomach contents into the mouth

reflex An involuntary movement

reflex incontinence The loss of urine at predictable intervals when the bladder is full

rehabilitation The process of restoring the person to his or her highest possible level of physical, psychological, social, and economic function

reincarnation The belief that the spirit or soul is reborn in another human body or in another form of life

relaxation To be free from mental and physical stress

religion Spiritual beliefs, needs, and practices

REM sleep The phase of sleep when there is *rapid eye movement*

remove easily The manual method device, material, or equipment used to restrain the person that can be removed intentionally by the person in the same manner it was applied by the staff

reporting The oral account of care and observations

reservoir The environment in which a microbe lives and grows; host

respiration Breathing air into (*inhalation*) and out of (*exhalation*) the lungs; the process of supplying the cells with oxygen and removing carbon dioxide from them

respiratory arrest When breathing stops; breathing stops but heart action continues for several minutes

respiratory depression Slow, weak respirations at a rate of fewer than 12 per minute

responsibility The duty or obligation to perform some act or function

rest To be calm, at ease, and relaxed; no anxiety or stress

restorative aide A nursing assistant with special training in restorative nursing and rehabilitation skills

restorative nursing care Care that helps persons regain health, strength, and independence

restraint Any manual method or physical or mechanical device, material, or equipment attached to or near the person's body that he or she cannot remove easily and which restricts freedom of movement or normal access to one's body; a drug that is used as a restriction to manage a person's behavior or restrict the person's freedom of movement and is not a standard treatment or dosage for the person's condition

retention catheter A Foley or indwelling catheter

reverse Trendelenburg's position The head of the bed is raised and the foot of the bed is lowered

rigor mortis The stiffness or rigidity (*rigor*) of skeletal muscles that occurs after death (*mortis*)

root A word element containing the basic meaning of the word

rotation Turning the joint

S

sanguineous drainage Bloody *(sanguis)* drainage

seclusion The involuntary confinement of a person alone in a room or area from which the person is physically prevented from leaving

seizure Violent and sudden contractions or tremors of muscle groups; convulsion

self-actualization Experiencing one's potential

self-esteem Thinking well of oneself and seeing oneself as useful and having value

self-neglect A person's behaviors that puts him or her at high risk for harm; health and safety are threatened

semi-Fowler's position The head of the bed is raised 30 degrees; or the head of the bed is raised 30 degrees and the knee portion is raised 15 degrees

semi-prone side position Sims' position

serosanguineous drainage Thin, watery drainage *(sero)* that is blood-tinged *(sanguineous)*

serous drainage Clear, watery fluid *(serum)*

service plan A written plan listing the services needed by the person and who provides them

sex Physical activities involving the reproductive organs; done for pleasure or to have children

sexuality The physical, emotional, social, cultural, and spiritual factors that affect a person's feelings and attitudes about his or her sex

sexual orientation Sexual arousal or romantic attraction to persons of the other gender (heterosexual), the same gender (homosexual), or both genders (bisexual)

shearing When skin sticks to a surface while muscles slide in the direction the body is moving

shock Results when organs and tissues do not get enough blood

side-lying position The lateral position

signs Objective data

simple fracture Closed fracture

Sims' position A left side-lying position in which the upper leg is sharply flexed so it is not on the lower leg and the lower arm is behind the person; semi-prone side position

skin tear A break or rip in the skin; the epidermis (top skin layer) separates from the underlying tissues

slander Making false statements orally

sleep A state of unconsciousness, reduced voluntary muscle activity, and lowered metabolism

spastic Uncontrolled contractions of skeletal muscles

sphygmomanometer A cuff and measuring device used to measure blood pressure

spore A bacterium protected by a hard shell

sputum Mucus from the respiratory system that is expectorated *(expelled)* through the mouth

standard of care The skills, care, and judgment required by a health team member under similar conditions

stasis ulcer Venous ulcer

sterile The absence of *all* microbes

sterile field A work area free of *all* pathogens and non-pathogens (including spores)

sterile technique Surgical asepsis

sterilization The process of destroying *all* microbes

stethoscope An instrument used to listen to sounds produced by the heart, lungs, and other body organs

stool Excreted feces

stoma An opening

stomatitis Inflammation *(itis)* of the mouth *(stomat)*

straight catheter A catheter that drains the bladder and then is removed

stress The response or change in the body caused by any emotional, physical, social, or economic factor

stress incontinence When urine leaks during exercise and certain movements that cause pressure on the bladder

stressor The event or factor that causes stress

subconscious Memory, past experiences, and thoughts of which the person is not aware; they are easily recalled

subjective data Things a person tells you about that you cannot observe through your senses; symptoms

suction The process of withdrawing or sucking up fluid *(secretions)*

sudden cardiac arrest (SCA) The heart and breathing stop suddenly and without warning; cardiac arrest

suffix A word element placed after a root; it changes the meaning of the word

suffocation When breathing stops from the lack of oxygen

suicide To kill oneself

suicide contagion Exposure to suicide or suicidal behaviors within one's family, one's peer group, or media reports of suicide

sundowning Signs, symptoms, and behaviors of AD increase during hours of darkness

superego The part of the personality concerned with right and wrong

supination Turning the joint upward

supine position The back-lying or dorsal recumbent position

suppository A cone-shaped, solid drug that is inserted into a body opening; it melts at body temperature

surgical asepsis The practices that keep items free of *all* microbes; sterile technique

symptoms Subjective data

syncope A brief loss of consciousness; fainting

system Organs that work together to perform special functions

systole The period of heart muscle contraction; the period when the heart is pumping blood

systolic pressure The amount of force needed to pump blood out of the heart into the arterial circulation

T

tachycardia A rapid *(tachy)* heart rate *(cardia)*; more than 100 beats per minute

tachypnea Rapid *(tachy)* breathing *(pnea)*; respirations are more than 20 per minute

tartar Hardened plaque

team nursing A nursing care pattern; a team of nursing staff is led by an RN who decides the amount and kind of care each person needs

terminal illness An illness or injury for which there is no reasonable expectation of recovery

tetraplegia Quadriplegia

thrombus A blood clot

tinnitus A ringing, roaring, hissing, or buzzing sound in the ears or head

tissue A group of cells with similar functions

tort A wrong committed against a person or the person's property

tracheostomy A surgically created opening *(stomy)* into the trachea *(tracheo)*

transfer Moving the person from one place to another; moving a person from one room or nursing unit to another

transfer belt A device used to support a person who is unsteady or disabled; gait belt

transgender A broad term used to describe people who express their sexuality or gender in other than the expected way; persons who are undergoing hormone therapy or surgery for sexual reassignment (female to male; male to female)

transsexual A person who believes that he or she is a member of the other sex

transvestite A person who dresses and behaves like the other sex for emotional and sexual relief; cross-dresser

trauma An accident or violent act that injures the skin, mucous membranes, bones, and organs

Trendelenburg's position The head of the bed is lowered and the foot of the bed is raised

tumor A new growth of abnormal cells; tumors are benign or malignant

tuning fork An instrument vibrated to test hearing

U

ulcer A shallow or deep crater-like sore of the skin or a mucous membrane

umbilical cord The structure that connects the mother and fetus; it carries blood, oxygen, and nutrients from the mother to the fetus

unconscious Experiences and feelings that cannot be recalled

unintentional wound A wound resulting from trauma

urge incontinence The loss of urine in response to a sudden, urgent need to void; the person cannot get to a toilet in time

urgent surgery Surgery needed for the person's health; it is done soon to prevent further damage or disease

urinary diversion A new pathway for urine to exit the body

urinary frequency Voiding at frequent intervals

urinary incontinence The loss of bladder control

urinary urgency The need to void at once

urination The process of emptying urine from the bladder; micturition or voiding

urostomy A surgically created opening (stomy) between the ureter (uro) and the abdomen

V

vaccination Giving a vaccine to produce immunity against an infectious disease

vaccine A preparation containing dead or weakened microbes

vaginal speculum An instrument used to open the vagina so it and the cervix can be examined

vascular ulcer A circulatory ulcer

vein A blood vessel that returns blood back to the heart

venous ulcer An open sore on the lower legs or feet caused by poor blood flow through the veins; stasis ulcer

ventral Anterior

verbal communication Communication that uses written or spoken words

vertigo Dizziness

vital signs Temperature, pulse, respirations, and blood pressure

voiding Urination or micturition

vomitus Food and fluids expelled from the stomach through the mouth; emesis

vulnerable adult A person 18 years old or older who has a disability or condition that makes him or her at risk to be wounded, attacked, or damaged

W

Wernicke's aphasia Receptive aphasia

will A legal document of how a person wants property distributed after death

withdrawal syndrome The person's physical and mental response after stopping or severely reducing the use of a substance that was used regularly

word element A part of a word

work ethics Behavior in the workplace

workplace violence Violent acts (including assault and threat of assault) directed toward persons at work or while on duty

wound A break in the skin or mucous membrane

Y

young-old Persons between 65 and 74 years of age

Key Abbreviations

A

A Axillary
AAMR American Association on Mental Retardation
AARP American Association of Retired Persons
ABC Airway, breathing, circulation
ABCD Airway, breathing, circulation, defibrillation
ABGs Arterial blood gases
ACS Acute coronary syndrome
ACTH Adrenocorticotropic hormone
AD Alzheimer's disease
ADA Americans With Disabilities Act of 1990
ADEAR Alzheimer's Disease Education and Referral Center
ADH Antidiuretic hormone
ADL Activities of daily living
AE Antiembolism, anti-embolic
AED Automated external defibrillator
AFB American Foundation for the Blind
AFO Ankle-foot orthosis
AHA American Hospital Association; American Heart Association
AIDS Acquired immunodeficiency syndrome
AIIR Airborne infection isolation room
ALF Assisted living facility
ALR Assisted living residence
ALS Amyotrophic lateral sclerosis
AMD Age-related macular degeneration
AMI Acute myocardial infarction
ANA American Nurses Association
Ap Apical

B

BLS Basic Life Support
BP Blood pressure
BPD Borderline personality disorder
BPH Benign prostatic hyperplasia
BRP Bathroom privileges

C

C Centigrade; Celsius
CAD Coronary artery disease
CBC Complete blood count
CCRC Continuing care retirement community
CDC Centers for Disease Control and Prevention
CEU Continuing education unit
CHF Congestive heart failure
cm Centimeter
CMG Case mix groups
CMS Centers for Medicare & Medicaid Services

CNA Certified nursing assistant, certified nurse aide
CNS Central nervous system
CO$_2$ Carbon dioxide
COPD Chronic obstructive pulmonary disease
CP Cerebral palsy
CPR Cardiopulmonary resuscitation
C-section Cesarean section
CVA Cerebrovascular accident
CXR Chest x-ray

D

DASH Dietary Approaches to Stop Hypertension
DD Developmental disability
DNR Do not resuscitate
DON Director of nursing
DRG Diagnosis-related groups
DS Down syndrome
DV Daily Value

E

ECG Electrocardiogram
ECHO Elder Cottage Housing Opportunity
ED Erectile dysfunction
EKG Electrocardiogram
EMS Emergency Medical Services
EMT Emergency medical technician
EPA Environmental Protection Agency
EPHI, ePHI Electronic protected health information
ET Endotracheal

F

F Fahrenheit
FBAO Foreign-body airway obstruction
FDA Food and Drug Administration

G

GED General equivalency diploma
GERD Gastroesophageal reflux disease
GH Growth hormone
GI Gastrointestinal
gtt Drops
gtt/min Drops per minute

H

HAI Healthcare-associated infection
HBV Hepatitis B virus
Hg Mercury
HHRG Home health resource groups
HIPAA Health Insurance Portability and Accountability Act of 1996
HIV Human immunodeficiency virus
HMO Health maintenance organization

I

I&O Intake and output
ICU Intensive care unit
ID Identification
IDCP Interdisciplinary care planning
IQ Intelligence quotient
IV Intravenous, intravenous infusion

J

JC Joint Commission
JRA Juvenile rheumatoid arthritis

L

L/min Liters per minute
LNA Licensed nursing assistant
LPN Licensed practical nurse
LVN Licensed vocational nurse

M

MCI mild cognitive impairment
MDRO Multidrug-resistant organism
MDS Minimum data set
MI Myocardial infarction
MID Multi-infarct dementia
mL Milliliter
MLT Medical laboratory technician
mm Millimeter
mm Hg Millimeters of mercury
MRSA Methicillin-resistant *Staphylococcus aureas*
MS Multiple sclerosis
MSDS Material safety data sheet

N

NAD National Association of the Deaf
NANDA North American Nursing Diagnosis Association
NATCEP Nursing assistant training and competency evaluation program
NCSBN National Council of State Boards of Nursing
NFLPN National Federation of Licensed Practical Nurses
NG Nasogastric
NIAAA National Institute on Alcohol Abuse and Alcoholism
NIDCD National Institute on Deafness and Other Communication Disorders
NIMH National Institute of Mental Health
NPO Non per os; nothing by mouth
NREM No rapid eye movement

O

O$_2$ Oxygen
OASIS Outcome and Assessment Information Set
OBRA Omnibus Budget Reconciliation Act of 1987
OCD Obsessive-compulsive disorder

OPIM Other potentially infectious materials
OR Operating room
OSHA Occupational Safety and Health Administration
oz Ounce

P

PACU Post anesthesia care unit
PASS Pull the safety pin, aim low, squeeze the lever, sweep back and forth
PDA Personal digital assistant
PEG Percutaneous endoscopic gastrostomy
PHI Protected health information
PICC Peripherally inserted central catheter
PPE Personal protective equipment
PPO Preferred provider organization
PTSD Post-traumatic stress disorder
PVS Persistent vegetative state

R

R Rectal
RA Rheumatoid arthritis
RACE Rescue, alarm, confine, extinguish

RAPs Resident assessment protocols
RBC Red blood cell
REM Rapid eye movement
RN Registered nurse
RNA Registered nurse aide
ROM Range of motion
RRT Rapid Response Team
RUG Resource utilization groups

S

SARS Severe acute respiratory syndrome
SCA Sudden cardiac arrest
SCD Sequential compression device
SIDS Sudden infant death syndrome
SMI Sustained maximal inspiration
SNF Skilled nursing facility
SpO₂ Oxygen saturation
SSE Soapsuds enema
STD Sexually transmitted disease

T

TB Tuberculosis
TBI Traumatic brain injury
TED Thrombo-embolic disease
TH Thyroid hormone; thyroxine
TIA Transient ischemic attack

TPN Total parenteral nutrition
TPR Temperature, pulse, and respirations
TRS Telecommunications Relay Services
TSH Thyroid-stimulating hormone
TTD Telecommunications Devices for the Deaf
TTY Teletypewriter
TURP Transurethral resection of the prostate

U

USDA United States Department of Agriculture
UTI Urinary tract infection

V

VF Ventricular fibrillation
V-Fib Ventricular fibrillation
VR Vancomycin-resistant *Enterococcus*

W

WBC White blood cell
WMSD Work-related musculoskeletal disorder

Index

Page reference followed by *b* indicates box, *f* indicates figure or illustration, and *t* indicates table.

824